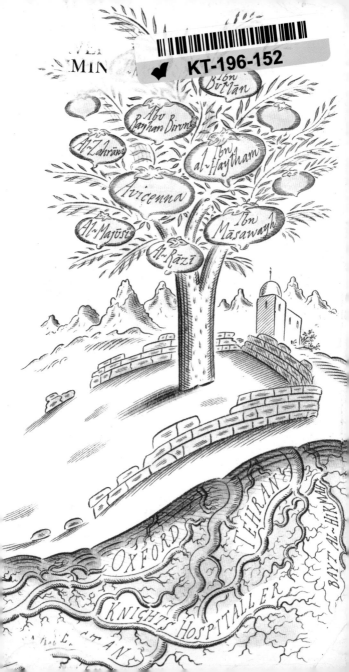

BU 2608431 7

THE UNIVERSITY OF BIRMINGHAM
LIBRARY SERVICES

Barnes Library

Collier, J. A. B.
Oxford handbook of clinical specialties / Judith Colli ...
2013
9th ed.

Classmark

RC 55

O

Control Number M0632708BU   Barcode 26084317

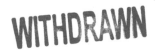
WITHDRAWN

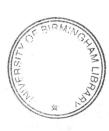

OXFORD
HANDBOOK
OF CLINICAL
SPECIALTIES

NINTH EDITION

JUDITH COLLIER
MURRAY LONGMORE
KEITH AMARAKONE

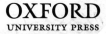
OXFORD
UNIVERSITY PRESS

OXFORD
UNIVERSITY PRESS Great Clarendon Street, Oxford OX2 6DP

Oxford University Press is a department of the University of Oxford. It furthers the University's objective of excellence in research, scholarship, and education by publishing worldwide. Oxford is a registered trade mark of Oxford University Press in the UK and certain other countries.

Published in the United States by Oxford University Press Inc., New York

© Oxford University Press, 2013

The moral rights of the authors have been asserted

First published 1987	Fifth edition 1999	**Translations:**	Greek
Second edition 1989	Sixth edition 2003	Spanish	Romanian
Third edition 1991	Seventh edition 2006	German	Russian Polish
Fourth edition 1995	Eighth edition 2008	Hungarian	Portuguese

All rights reserved. No part of this publication may be reproduced, stored in a retrieval system, or transmitted, in any form or by any means, without the prior permission in writing of Oxford University Press, or as expressly permitted by law, by licence or under terms agreed with the appropriate reprographics rights organization. Enquiries concerning reproduction outside the scope of the above should be sent to the Rights Department, Oxford University Press, at the address above.

You must not circulate this book in any other form and you must impose the same condition on any acquirer.

British Library Cataloguing in Publication Data

Data available

Library of Congress Cataloging in Publication Data
Data available

Typeset by GreenGate Publishing Services, Tonbridge, UK; printed in China on acid-free paper through C&C Offset Printing Co., Ltd

ISBN 978-0-19-959118-3

BIRMINGHAM UNIVERSITY LIBRARY

Drugs

Except where otherwise stated, recommendations are for the **non-pregnant adult** who is **not breastfeeding**. To avoid excessive doses in obese patients it may be best to calculate doses on the basis of ideal body weight (IBW): see p621.

We have made every effort to check this text, but it is still possible that drug or other errors have been missed. OUP makes no representation, express or implied, that doses are correct. Readers are urged to check with the most up-to-date product information, codes of conduct, and safety regulations. The authors and the publishers do not accept responsibility or legal liability for any errors in the text, or for the misuse or misapplication of material in this work.

►For updates/corrections, see oup.co.uk/academic/medicine/handbooks/updates.

26084317

Contents

Front cover
Back cover

The content of each chapter is detailed on each chapter's first page.

Preface

This is the first medical textbook to take the health of its readers seriously on the grounds that the health of one person (a patient) must not be bought at the expense of another (their doctor). It is an unsettling paradox that when we study medicine our own health goes out of the window (fig 1), with long hours of coal-face working often without joy or sustenance as our health is shattered by the weight of an over-full curriculum (no doubt because there are too many organs and we know far too much about them).

What can a book do about this defenestration (fig 1)? First of all the ideal book can (must!) be brief with a clear distinction between work and play. Secondly, such a book must furnish the mind: as we drill down into the minute structure of disease, there must be a corresponding search for the macroscopic, the human, and the universal. This book intends to make plain the idea that for every such spiral of down-drilling, there is a corresponding upward spiral (the swarf, fig 2) towards the

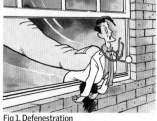
Fig 1. Defenestration

infinite—and we aim the help the reader find the jumping-off point where these spirals intersect, so that the movement down (reductionism) is complemented by a movement up (integrative medicine). Can this influence the heath of our readers? The answer lies in a single word: *enlightenment*.

The spiral illuminations at the beginning of each chapter (and scattered throughout the book) remind us to follow the movement up as well as the movement down. Follow the swarf! We should do this in our consultations, as well as in our reading. Never pass over an opportunity to widen the horizons of your patients, or to have your own horizons widened by your patient: what better way is there of reducing the size of their (and our) insoluble problems? Here, it is enough to point out that the well-furnished mind confers resilience to the body. We all know

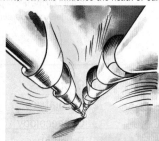
Fig 2. Swarf
"The way up is the way down... Whether on the shores of Asia, or in the Edgware Road."
The dry salvages TS Eliot; 1941

that stress brings on physical disease—and from this premise it is a short step to accept that a resilient mind is central to maintaining heath. We aim to find magnetic correspondences in the jumping-off points between the downward-drilling helix and the upward-spinning swarf-spirals using philosophy, literature, humour, and tinctures of hope. Ultimately we would like readers to develop their own methods, thereby converting passive acceptance of an overfull curriculum into wealth, life, and beauty.

JABC, KM & JML—*Preface to the 9th edition*—Cape Clear

Preface to the 1st Edition

When someone says that he is 'doing obstetrics'—or whatever, this should not hide the fact that much more is being done besides, not just a little of each of medicine, psychiatry, gynaecology and paediatrics, but also a good deal of work to elicit and act upon the patient's unspoken hopes and fears. At the operating table he must concentrate minutely on the problem in hand; but later he must operate on other planes too, in social and psychological dimensions so as to understand how the patient came to need to be on the operating table, and how this might have been prevented. All the best specialists practise a holistic art, and our aim is to show how specialism and holism may be successfully interwoven, if not into a fully watertight garment, then at least into one which keeps out much of the criticism rained upon us by the proponents of alternative medicine.

We hope that by compiling this little volume we may make the arduous task of learning medicine a little less exhausting, so allowing more energy to be spent at the bedside, and on the wards. For a medical student coming fresh to a specialty the great tomes which mark the road to knowledge can numb the mind after a while, and what started out fresh is in danger of becoming exhausted by its own too much. It is not that we are against the great tomes themselves—we are simply against reading them too much and too soon. One starts off strong on 'care' and weak on knowledge, and the danger is that this state of affairs becomes reversed. It is easier to learn from books than from patients, yet what our patients teach us may be of more abiding significance: the value of sympathy, the uses of compassion and the limits of our human world. It is at the bedside that we learn how to be of practical help to people who are numbed by the mysterious disasters of womb or tomb, for which they are totally unprepared. If this small book enables those starting to explore the major specialties to learn all they can from their patients, it will have served its purpose—and can then be discarded.

Because of the page-a-subject format, the balance of topics in the following pages may at first strike the reader as being odd in places. However, it has been our intention to provide a maximally useful text rather than one which is perfectly balanced in apportioning space according to how common a particular topic is—just as the great *Terrestrial Globes* made by George Phillips in the 1960s may seem at first to provide an odd balance of place names, with Alice Springs appearing more prominently than Amsterdam. To chart a whole continent, and omit to name a single central location out of respect for 'balance' is to miss a good opportunity to be useful. George Phillips did not miss this opportunity, and neither we hope, have we. It is inevitable that some readers will be disappointed that we have left out their favoured subjects (the Phillips' Globe does not even mention Oxford!). To these readers we offer over 300 blank pages by way of apology.

JABC & JML—*Preface to the 1st edition*—Ferring, 1987

Conflicts of interest: none declared

Because of numerous and well-publicized occasions where writers of guidelines recommending certain drugs turn out to have undisclosed financial contacts with the pharmaceutical industries concerned,[1] we wish to place on record that we have no contacts with any pharmaceutical company, and no pharmaceutical company employs us in any capacity, and neither have we received any financial input bearing upon our research for this publication. We have a policy of not seeing representatives from the pharmaceutical industry, or receiving their gifts or hospitality. We assert that the drugs recommended in this book have been selected on the basis of the best available evidence.

DRS LONGMORE, COLLIER, and AMARAKONE, 2012

Understanding our patients

Most of the time we treat our patients quite well, without ever really understanding them. The idea that we should strive to understand and empathize with *all* our patients is unreasonable. Out-patient clinics and surgeries would grind to a halt, and urgent visits would never get done. It is also possible that to do so would be counter-productive from the patient's point of view. For two human beings to understand each other's inner life is a rare event, and if we offered this understanding to all our patients they might become addicted to us, and be unable to get on with the rest of their lives. Nevertheless, it is good practice to try to understand *some* patients. Doing so may entail swallowing an alien world and digesting it rather slowly. Paradoxically, to achieve this, we very often need to keep our mouths shut, particularly with those in whom we have reached a therapeutic impasse—for example if the illness is untreatable, or the patient has rejected our treatment, or if the patient seems to be asking or appealing for something more. Eye contact is important here. One of the authors (JML) recalls forever his very first patient—found on a surgical ward recovering from the repair of a perforated duodenal ulcer: a nice simple surgical patient, ideal for beginners. I asked all the questions in the book, and knew all his answers and his physical features, even the colour of his eyes. Luckily, the house officer who was really looking after him did not ask so many questions, and knew how to interpret the appeal for help behind those eyes, and in his busy day found space to receive the vital clue beyond my grasp—that my patient was a drug addict and under great stress as he could no longer finance his activity.

So, the first step in trying to understand a patient is to sit back and listen. Next, if possible, it is very helpful to see your patient often, to establish rapport and mutual respect. If the relationship is all one way, with the doctor finding out all about the patient, but revealing nothing of him or herself, this mutual respect can take a very long time to grow. But beware of sharing too much of your own inner life with your patients: you may overburden them, or put them off. Different patients respond to different approaches. Understanding patients inevitably takes time, and it may be hard in a series of short appointments. A visit to the patient's home may be very revealing, but for many doctors trapped in hospital wards or clinics, this is impossible. But it is usually possible to have a longish private interview, and take whatever opportunity arises. We once worked with a consultant who infuriated his junior staff on busy ward rounds by repeatedly selecting what seemed to us the most boring and commonplace medical 'cases' (such as someone with a stroke) and proceeding to draw the curtain around the patient's bed to exclude us, and engage in what seemed like a long chat with the patient, all in very hushed voices, so that we never knew what he said—until Sister told us that he never said anything much, and simply received anything that was on the patient's mind. For the most part, he was swallowing their world in silence. We came to realize that there was nothing that these patients, robbed as they were of health and wholeness, appreciated more in their entire hospital stay.

What happens when two ward rounds collide?

We once worked with a splendid consultant, Dr B—, who, among other eccentric but lovable traits, believed that data such as an ECG should be interpreted according to the mood of the day and in the light of bedside nuances. He would not let us label old ECGs with the diagnosis accorded at the time of their recording, in case this conflicted with later nuances. So during ward rounds old ECGs would be unearthed and reinterpreted by the great man, as if he were a conductor wringing new meaning from a well-known score. Ward rounds tended to be rather slow and it so happened that faster, newer consultants would start overtaking us on ward rounds. But we noticed that some of their entourage would take this moment of impact to hive off from the fast ward round, and attach themselves to ours. The faster ward round moved on to some trite destination leaving us to tussle with the great questions of medicine.

Let us consider further this moment of instability and choice when the two ward rounds collide. As Paul Verlaine wrote, "There is nothing more precious than a song which is cloudy from the joining of the indistinct with the precise". We tend to over-value the precise and undervalue the indistinct. Like Dr B—, we need to re-interpret patients' exact words as if they were a musical score. All too often, though, we rely on summaries of our patients' stories, massacred by eloquent, but treacherous, medical jargon. Paul Verlaine knew what to do: "Take eloquence, and wring its neck" is his advice, if it's truth we are after. In its place he recommends systematic ambiguity and giving nuance free rein....

C ar nous voulons la Nuance encor,	For we want nuance,
Pas la couleur, rien que la Nuance!	Not colour, nothing but nuance!
Oh! la nuance seule fiance	Only nuance joins
Le rêve au rêve et la flûte au cor!	Dream to dream and flutes to horns!
	Paul Verlaine, *Art poétique*

So what *are* the facts? Give me hard facts and I will give you a diagnosis. That was the alluring but dangerous message from the fast ward round. And we all have to make our choice of when to hive off from this ward round and join Dr B—. If we can accord some ambiguity to the facts we may start to be of real use to our patients. After all, they have to live with the facts, so we may as well let the facts breathe and have a complicated life of their own. **_There is something undefined in every fact_**. Find what it is, and use the undefined as a vehicle to explore your patient's subtleties and contradictions.

So, in memory of Dr B—, we propose a new section in the Medical Notes called *Nuances*, to be placed before the *Functional Enquiry* and after the *History of the Presenting Complaint*. "The patient pointed to his ear when he said this" or "He was obviously frightened reliving this moment..." or "The patient ran out of language at this point..."

Running out of language is a sure sign that you are getting somewhere with our patient. Too much eloquence is fatal: this is Paul Verlaine's worthless jewel ("*ce bijou d'un sou*") that sounds hollow and fake when put to the test. We have to accept that language is not very good at dealing with pain—or any internal state.

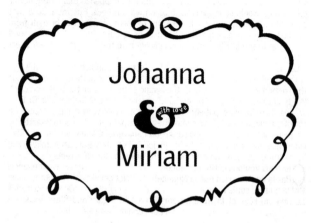

Johanna & with love Miriam

Acknowledgements

We thank those who have contributed their time and wisdom to previous editions: Dr Steven Emmet for detailed help in reading proofs; Professor Tor Chiu for his help with the *ENT* chapter; Natalie Langdown for help with autism; Professor Mark Lowenthal for his indefatigable help with *Paediatrics* and other chapters. We thank all the authors who have joined us for previous editions: Judith Harvey, Tim Hodgetts, Duncan Brown, Peter Scally, Mark Brinsden, Ahmad R. Mafi, and Tom Turmezei.

Specialist Readers We are hugely indebted to our Specialist Readers for their advice, encouragement, and constructive criticism. Each chapter in this book has benefitted from their trustworthy oversight. They are thanked individually at the beginning of each chapter.

Junior Readers It was our great pleasure to welcome a new team of Readers to the ninth edition of this book. Our Junior Readers showed commitment, intelligence, and ingenuity in their contributions to the referencing and cross-referencing of this edition. We have a better book for it. Thank you to Mathuranayagham Niroshan, Shahzad Arain, Rashmi Singh, Josh Hurn, Konstantinos Kritikos, Mark Cassar, William Hunt, David Lee, Aaron Lai, Winnie Chen, Yong De Jun, Pooja Sarkar, Xuebin Dong, Roland Bensted, and Fandy Wang.

Reader participation We have been very fortunate to receive so many well-considered suggestions and corrections to the book from readers . Their contributions have enhanced the book and we are grateful. Over the years the list has grown too large to accommodate in the book, so we now have a dedicated webpage for the purpose: **www.oup.com/uk/ohcs9acknowledgements.**

If you would like to give us feedback, correct a mistake, or make a suggestion, you can do so by filling in the comment card enclosed in this volume and posting it to us, or by going to our website: **www.oup.com/uk/ohcs9efeedback**.

How to use this book

This book has some useful features to help you get the most out of the information inside.

Quick chapter look-ups Index on the back cover refers to and aligns with the coloured tabs on the sides of the pages.

References ([1]) Every reference has an individual identification indicated by a pink superscript number. The full details of every reference are held online at **www.oup.com/ohcs9refs.**

Cross references There are cross references to other chapters within the book, to the *Oxford Handbook of Clinical Medicine (OHCM)*, and to other titles in the Oxford Medical Handbooks series.

Reference intervals Included inside the back cover. Conversion factors to and from SI units are given on the bookmark.

Right-hand vertical comments At the side of some tables and topics, an alternative opinion of the content inside.

Symbols and abbreviations See opposite.

Corrections and suggestions Found a mistake? Have a suggestion for the next edition? Let us know at **www.oup.com/uk/ohcs9efeedback.** Major changes are announced online at **www.oup.co.uk/academic/series/oxhmed/updates.**

A note on the use of pronouns

For brevity, the pronoun *'he'* or *'she'* has been used in places where *'he or she'* would have been appropriate. Such circumlocutions do not aid the reader in forming a vivid visual impression, which is one of the leading aims of good authorship. Therefore, for balance and fairness, and where sense allows, we have tried alternating *he* with *she.*

Symbols and abbreviations

▶▶	don't dawdle! Prompt action saves lives
▶	this phrase is important
👭 (👫)	more (or less) vital topic; a rough guide for 1st-time readers
🌀	an opportunity for holistic/non-reductionist thinking
🔥	conflict (controversial topic)
1,2,3	references at oup.co.uk/ohcs9refs
1,2,3	drug dose not in *BNF*, see oup.co.uk/ohcs9refs
#	fracture
ΔΔ	differential diagnosis
♂:♀	male to female ratio
↓	decreased
↔	normal (eg plasma level)
↑	increased
~	about
≈	approximately equal
–ve	negative
+ve	positive
∵	on account of/because of
∴	therefore
A&E	emergency department
A2A	angiotensin 2 receptor (blockers)
ABC	air, breathing, circulation
A(P)LS	advanced (paediatric) life support manuals
ABR	audiological brainstem responses
AC	*ante cibum* (before food)
ACE(i)	angiotensin-converting enzyme (inhibitor)
ACLS	advanced cardiac life support
ACTH	adrenocorticotrophic hormone
ADD	attention deficit disorder
ADH	antidiuretic hormone
AFP	α-fetoprotein (α=alpha)
AIDS	acquired immunodeficiency syn.
Alk	alkaline (phos=phosphatase)
ALL	acute lymphoblastic leukaemia
ALT	alanine aminotransferase
ANA	antinuclear antibody
ANF	antinuclear factor
ANS	autonomic nervous system
AP	anteroposterior
APH	antepartum haemorrhage
APLS	advanced paediatric life support
APM	auto-premotor syndrome
ARF	acute renal failure
ARM	artificial rupture of membranes
ASD	atrioseptal defect
ASO	antistreptolysin O (titre)
ASW	approved social worker
ATLS	Advanced Trauma Life Support manual; see www.trauma.org
ATN	acute tubular necrosis
AV	atrioventricular
AVM	arteriovenous malformation
βHCG	β-human chorionic gonadotrophin
BJGP	*British Journal of General Practice*
BMJ	*British Medical Journal*
BNA	borderline nuclear abnormality
BNF	*British National Formulary*
*BNF*c	children's *BNF*
BP	blood pressure
©	courtesy of the copyright holder

C3	complement
Ca	carcinoma
CBRN	chemical, biological, radiological, nuclear
CBT	cognitive-behaviour therapy
CCDC	consultant in communicable disease control
CCF	combined (right & left sided) cardiac failure
CHC	combined hormonal contraception
ChVS	chorionic villus sampling
CI	contraindications
CIN	cervical intra-epithelial neoplasia
CMV	cytomegalovirus; controlled mandatory ventilation
CNS	central nervous system
CoC	combined oral contraceptive
COM	chronic otitis media
CPA	care programme approach
CPAP	continuous +ve airways pressure
CPR	cardiopulmonary resuscitation
CRP	c-reactive protein
CRPS	complex regional pain syndrome
CSF	cerebrospinal fluid
CT	computer tomography
CVP	central venous pressure
CVS	cardiovascular system
CXR	chest x-ray
D	dimension (or dioptre)
D&C	dilatation (cervix) & curettage
D&V	diarrhoea and vomiting
dB	decibel
DHS	dynamic hip screw
DIC	disseminated intravascular coagulation
DIP	distal interphalangeal
DKA	diabetic ketoacidosis
dL	decilitre
DM	diabetes mellitus
DMSA	dimercaptosuccinic acid
DNA	deoxyribonucleic acid
DOH	Department of Health (NHS)
DPL	diagnostic peritoneal lavage
DRG	dorsal root ganglion
DSM-IV	*Diagnostic & Statistical Manual*, 4e
DUB	dysfunctional uterine bleeding
DVT	deep venous thrombosis
E-BM	evidence-based medicine
EBV	Epstein–Barr virus
ECG	electrocardiogram
ECT	electroconvulsive therapy
EEG	electroencephalogram
EIA	enzyme immunoassay
ENT	ear, nose and throat
ERPC	evacuation of retained products of conception
ESR	erythrocyte sedimentation rate
ET	endotracheal
FB	foreign body
FBC	full blood count
FCR	flexor carpi radialis
FDP	flexor digitorum profundus
FDS	flexor digitorum sublimis
FH	family history
FNA	fine needle aspiration

FNT	fetal nuchal translucency	LHRH	luteinizing hormone-releasing hormone
FSH	follicle-stimulating hormone		
G	gauge	LMP	day 1 of last menstrual period
g	gram	LMWH	low molecular weight heparin
G(γ)GT	gamma(γ)glutamyl trans-peptidase	LP	lumbar puncture
		LVH	left ventricular hypertrophy
G6PD	glucose-6-phosphate dehydrogenase	μ(g)	micro(gram)
		MAOI	monoamine oxidase inhibitor
GA	general anaesthesia	MCP	metacarpophalangeal
GCS	Glasgow coma scale	MCV	mean cell volume
GFR	glomerular filtration rate	MEA	microwave endometrial ablation
GH	growth hormone	MET	meta-analysis
GI	gastrointestinal	mg	milligrams (μg=microgram=mcg)
GP	general practitioner	MHA	Mental Health Act
h	hour	MI	myocardial infarction
Hb	haemoglobin	ML	millilitre
HBsAg	hepatitis B surface antigen	mmHg	millimetres of mercury
HBV	hepatitis B virus	MRI	magnetic resonance imaging
HCG	human chorionic gonadotrophin	MSU	midstream urine culture
HDL	high-density lipoprotein	MTP	metatarsophalangeal
HFOV	high-frequency oscillatory ventilation	mU	milliunit(s)
		MVA	motor vehicle accident
HIV	human immunodeficiency virus	N=20*	reference to a randomized trial of 20 patients (* or what ever number follows N)
HLA	human leucocyte alleles		
HPA	Health Protection Agency		
HPO	hypothalamic–pituitary–ovarian	n=63*	reference to a non-randomized trial of 63 patients (* or what ever number follows n)
HPV	human papilloma virus		
HRT	hormone replacement therapy		
HVS	high vaginal swab	N₂O	nitrous oxide
ibid	*ibidem* (Latin, in the same place)	NaCl	sodium chloride
IBW	ideal body weight	NAI	non-accidental injury
ICP	intracranial pressure	NBM	nil by mouth (no solids or fluids)
IE	infective endocarditis	NEJM	*New England Journal of Medicine*
Ig	immunoglobulin	NEPE	non-epileptic paroxysmal events
IHD	ischaemic heart disease	NGT	nasogastric tube
IM	intramuscular	NHS	National Health Service
INR	international normalized ratio of prothrombin time	NICE	National Institute for Health and Clinical Excellence
IOP	intraocular pressure	NICU	neonatal intensive care unit
IP	interphalangeal	NMJ	neuromuscular junction
IPPV	intermittent positive pressure ventilation	NOF	neck of femur
		NSAID	non-steroidal anti-inflammatory drug(s)
IPT	interpersonal therapy		
IQ	intelligence quotient	OAE	otoacoustic emissions
ISQ	*in status quo* (Latin, no change)	OED	*Oxford English Dictionary*, OUP
ISS	injury severity score	OHCM	*Oxford Handbook of Clinical Medicine* 8ᵉ, OUP
ITP	idiopathic thrombocytopenic purpura		
		OM	otitis media
ITU	intensive therapy unit	OME	otitis media with effusion
IU/iu	international unit	OMV	open mouth view
IUCD	intrauterine contraceptive device	ON	*omni nocte* (take at night)
IUI	intrauterine insemination	ORh−ve	blood group O, Rh negative
IV	intravenous	ORIF	open reduction and internal fixation
IVF	*in vitro* fertilization	OT	occupational therapist
IVI	intravenous infusion	PA	posteroanterior
IVU	intravenous urography	PₐCO₂	partial pressure of CO₂ in arterial blood
JVP	jugular venous pressure		
K⁺	potassium	PAN	polyarteritis nodosa
kg	kilogram	pANCA	perinuclear antineutrophil cytoplasmic antibody
kpa	kilopascal		
L	litre	PₐO₂	partial pressure of oxygen in arterial blood
LA	local anaesthesia		
LBC	liquid-based cytology	PC	*post cibum* (after food)
LCR	ligase chain reaction	PCA	patient-controlled anaesthesia
LDH	lactate dehydrogenase	PCOS	polycystic ovarian syndrome
LFT	liver function test	PCR	polymerase chain reaction
LH	luteinizing hormone	PCV	packed cell volume

PDA	patent ductus arteriosus	SGA	small-for-gestational age
PE	pulmonary embolus	SLE	systemic lupus erythematosus
PET	pre-eclamptic toxaemia	SNHL	sensorineural hearing loss
PG	pemphigoid gestations	SpO₂	pulse oximetry estimated S_aO_2; no allowance for carboxyhaemoglobin
PGD	preimplantation genetic diagnosis		
PICU	paediatric intensive care unit	SSRI	selective serotonin reuptake inhibitor(s)
PID	pelvic inflammatory disease		
PIP	proximal interphalangeal	stat	*statim* (Latin for once); single dose
PKU	phenylketonuria	STD	sexually transmitted disease
PMB	postmenopausal bleeding	STI	sexually transmitted infection
PMS	premenstrual syndrome	SUFE	slipped upper femoral epiphysis
PO	*per os* (Latin for by mouth)	SVC	superior vena cava
PoP	progesterone-only pill	SVP	saturation vapour pressure
POP	plaster of Paris	syn	syndrome
PPH	postpartum haemorrhage	T°	temperature, degrees Centigrade
PR	*per rectum*	t½	half life
PTR	prothrombin ratio	T3	triiodothyronine
PUO	pyrexia of unknown origin	T4	thyroxine
PUVA	psoralen-ultraviolet A	TB	tuberculosis
PV	*per vaginam* (via the vagina)	TBW	tension band wiring
QOF	quality & outcomes framework	TCRE	transcervical resection of endometrium
℞	treatment (prescribing drugs)		
RA	rheumatoid arthritis; regional anaesthesia	TED	transverse elastic graduated
		TENS	transcutaneous electrical nerve stimulation
RBC	red blood cell		
RCGP	Royal College of General Practitioners	TFT	thyroid function tests
		TIA	transient ischaemic attack
RCOG	Royal College of Obstetricians and Gynaecologists	ToP	termination of pregnancy
		TPH	transplacental haemorrhage
RCT	randomized controlled trial	TPR	temperature, pulse, and respirations
REM	rapid eye movement		
RMO	registered medical officer	TRTS	triage revised trauma score
RSD	reflex sympathetic dystrophy	TSH	thyroid-stimulating hormone
RSI	repetitive strain injury; rapid sequence induction	TSOH	transient synovitis of the hip
		U	unit(s)
RTA	road traffic accident(s)	U&E	urea and electrolytes
RTS	revised trauma score	UK	United Kingdom
RUQ	right upper quadrant	URTI	upper respiratory tract infection
RVH	right ventricular hypertrophy	US(s)	ultrasound (scan)
S₁S₂	1ˢᵗ and 2ⁿᵈ heart sounds	UTI	urinary tract infection
SAD	seasonal affective disorder	UV	ultraviolet
SALT	speech and language therapist	VLBW	very low birthweight infant
SAO₂	arterial blood O₂ saturation, ≈SpO₂ (allows for carboxyhaemoglobin)	VSD	ventriculoseptal defect
		VTE	venous thromboembolism
SBE	subacute bacterial endocarditis	VUR	vesico-ureteric reflux
SC	subcutaneous	WCC	white blood cell count
SCBU	special care baby unit	wt	weight
SE	side-effects	WR	Wasserman reaction
sec	second(s)	yrs, y	years
SFH	symphysis fundal height	ZN	Ziehl–Neelsen (stain for TB)
SERM	selective oestrogen receptor modulator		

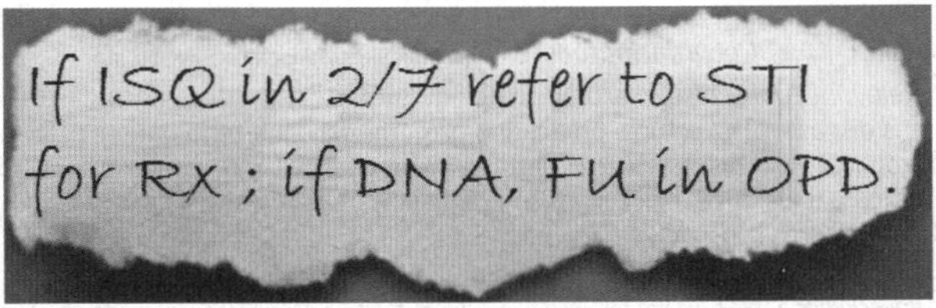

> If ISQ in 2/7 refer to STI
> for Rx ; if DNA, FU in OPD.

Fig 1. This plan is rendered almost unintelligible by over-use of abbreviations. It might mean: If *in status quo* (ISQ=no change in state) in 2 days' time (/7 in this context means days; /52 would mean weeks), refer to the Sexually Transmitted Infections clinic for treatment (℞)— if it turns out he does not arrive (DNA), follow-up at the out-patient department.[2]

1 Obstetrics

Sources RCOG *Green Top* guidelines; *Saving Mothers' Lives* (Confidential Enquiry). [1 Mat. mort 2011] *Cochrane database* (www.liv.ac.uk/lstm/ehcap/pc/nwc-pcl.html).

Relevant topics elsewhere: Neonatology, p107–22; breastfeeding, p124–6; rhesus disease, p116; ectopic pregnancy, p262; miscarriage/termination, p258–60; trophoblastic disease, p264; fibroids in pregnancy, p277; preterm/light-for-dates babies, p128; chickenpox in pregnancy, p144; parvovirus B19, p142; postnatal depression, p408.

1 The term *pregnancy-induced hypertension with proteinuria* is tending to replace the term *pre-eclampsia*. We have not followed this trend as to do so obscures the vital fact about pre-eclampsia: it may lead on to eclampsia. We favour *pre-eclampsia* because it is short and sends a shadow of a shiver down our spines, being a reminder of how dangerous it can be.

We thank Ms Alison Peattie, our Specialist Reader, and Mathuranayagham ...shan, our Junior Reader, for their contribution to this chapter.

The essence of reproductive health

Pregnancy is a risky affair for babies and mothers. The textbook causes of maternal mortality in the UK are pulmonary embolism, eclampsia, haemorrhage, infection, and cardiac diseases, with all the other causes being rare. But if an obstetrician could be granted one wish, it would not be to abolish these; rather it would be to make every pregnancy *planned* and *desired by the mother*. Worldwide, a woman dies every minute from the effects of pregnancy, and most of these women never wanted to be pregnant in the first place—but either had no means of contraception, or were without the skills, authority, and self-confidence to negotiate with their partners. So the real killers are poverty, ignorance, and the unwieldy desires of men, and the real solutions entail literacy, economic growth, and an equality of dialogue between the sexes. Any obstetric or governmental initiatives in reproductive health which do not recognize these facts are doomed.[2]

School-based sex education This *can* be effective, if linked to easy access to contraceptive services. This is the conclusion of a meta-analysis, taking into account cohort studies (if meta-analyses confine themselves to the 15 or so randomized studies, no benefit is shown).[3] It may be necessary to foster a knowledge-sharing, skill-promoting environment that is part of a continuing process, and not a 'one-off' affair—for educational programmes to work. *Adolescent pregnancy rates:* USA: 116/1000; UK: 57/1000; Canada: 50/1000. In 2007 in England & Wales 160 pregnancy were terminated in those <14 years old (out of ~200,000 terminations and ~650,000 live births).[4]

Definitions

Gravidity refers to the number of pregnancies that a woman has had (to any stage). *Parity* refers to pregnancies that resulted in delivery beyond 28 weeks' gestation. An example of the shorthand way of expressing pregnancies before and after 28 weeks is: para 2+1. This means that she has had 2 pregnancies beyond 28 completed weeks' gestation, and 1 which terminated prior to 28 weeks. If she is not pregnant at the time of describing her she is gravida 3, but if she is pregnant now she is gravida 4. Twins present a problem as there is controversy as to whether they count as 1 for both parity and gravidity or should count as 2 for parity.

It is unclear whether the cut-off point in these definitions should now be 24 weeks, to harmonize with the new definition of stillbirth (p82). In general, aim to use proper English rather than the shorthand described above, which is open to ambiguity. For example, when presenting a patient try something like: 'Mrs Cottard is a 32-year-old lady who is 15 weeks into her 4th pregnancy; the 3rd ended in a miscarriage at 17 weeks, and the others came to term with normal deliveries of children who are now 2 & 8.' The bald statement 'Para 2+1' is ambiguous, incomprehensible to the patient, and misses the point that the patient is now approaching the time when she lost her last baby.

Length of pregnancy: Normal pregnancy is 40 weeks from the LMP. Naegele's rule: expected delivery date (EDD) ≈ 1yr and 7 days after LMP minus 3 months (not if last period was a withdrawal bleed; for cycles shorter than 28 days, subtract the difference from 28; if longer, add the difference). A revised rule suggests the addition of 10 days rather than 7 is more accurate.

Obstetrics

The aim is to help prospective parents embark upon pregnancy under conditions most likely to ensure optimal fetal and maternal wellbeing. Babies conceived 18–23 months after a live birth have lowest rate of perinatal problems.[NICE] Reduce weight if obese (for risks of obesity see p7). Ensure the woman is rubella (±chickenpox, p144) immune prior to pregnancy; assess need for thromboprophylaxis in pregnancy (p16). Other areas include:

• Optimal control of chronic disease (eg diabetes) before conception. This is also important for hypothyroidism as the fetus cannot make thyroxine until 12 weeks and under-replacement may affect neurodevelopment. Strict diet is essential peri-conceptually for women with phenylketonuria (PKU).

• Stop teratogens or seek expert advice prior to conception (p29, p31). Paroxetine is associated with fetal heart defects in 1st trimester use, as is lithium (rate ↑ 8:1000 to 60:1000) with Ebstein's anomaly ↑ from 1 to 10 per 20 000.[RCOL] HIV drugs didanosine and efavirenz have teratogenic potential and avoidance may be possible[7] in first trimester (seek expert advice).

• Medication to protect the fetus from abnormality (eg folate supplements for neural tube defects, see p140 and below).

• Provide expert information for those at ↑ risk of abnormality so pregnancy or its avoidance is an informed choice, and any tests needed (eg chorionic villus sampling, p10) are planned. Regional genetic services give detailed pre-pregnancy counselling. See p154. In relevant ethnic populations, take blood for thalassaemia and sickle-cell tests (p22). If 'cut' (p247) offer defibulation.

• Avoidance of infection: eg sperm washing advised if HIV+ve male partner and HIV-ve woman

• If past/family history of thromboembolism, screen for thrombophilia.

Diet To prevent neural tube defects (NTD) and cleft lip, all should have folate-rich foods + **folic acid** 0.4mg daily >1 month pre-conception till 13wks (5mg/day if past NTD, on antiepileptics, p29, obese (BMI ≥30), HIV+ve on co-trimoxazole prophylaxis,[8] diabetic[RCOL] or sickle cell disease p19). Foods with >0.1mg of folic acid/serving: brussels sprouts, asparagus, spinach, blackeye beans, fortified cereals. Avoid liver & vit. A (vit. A embryopathy) & caffeine.

Smoking decreases ovulations, causes abnormal sperm production (± less penetrating capacity), ↑ rates of miscarriage (×2), and is associated with preterm labour and lighter-for-dates babies (mean is 3376g in non-smoker; smoker: 3200g), placenta praevia and abruption.[RCOL] Reduced reading ability in smokers' children up to 11yrs old shows that long-term effects are important. ~17% of smoking mothers stop before or in pregnancy.

Alcohol consumption High levels of consumption are known to cause the fetal alcohol syndrome (p138). Mild drinking eg 1–2u/wk has not been shown to adversely affect the fetus but alcohol does cross the placenta and may affect the fetal brain. Miscarriage rates are higher among drinkers of alcohol. NICE recommends <1u/24h. Binge drink (>5u/session) is especially harmful.[11] To cut consumption: see p513.

Spontaneous miscarriage (SM) Risk of miscarriage is 8.9% in women aged 20–40yrs, rising to 74.7% for women ≥45yrs. After 3 miscarriages, risk of next pregnancy failure is 44.6% for nullips aged 25–29yrs, and 35.4% for parous women.[12]

Recurrent spontaneous miscarriage See p261.

Search for those who need counselling most
• Diabetes mellitus
• Tropical travellers
• Frequent miscarriage
• Hypothyroidism
• Epilepsy
• Rubella-susceptible
• Pet-owners (toxoplasmosis risk is ↑)
• Phenylketonuria
• BP ↑
• SLE
• Genetic history, eg: •spina bifida etc. •thalassemia •Duchenne's •cystic fibrosis *et al*

For optimal care, when there are many features that need to be addressed an individualized care plan can help. The example below is of a care plan for diabetic women. The care plan is a chance for dialogue between the mother and her carers: all must sign-up to it. Placed in her notes it should be consulted throughout pregnancy when the woman is seen. In the case of a diabetic pregnancy the woman should be seen in a joint clinic where a multidisciplinary team is available comprising obstetrician, diabetes physician, diabetic specialist nurse, diabetes midwife, and dietician.

The care plan should cover the antenatal period and up to 6 weeks post-partum. It can be individualized, and generally includes advice about:
• Aspirin 75mg/24h PO until delivery to reduce pre-eclampsia risk.[13]
• Targets for glycaemic control (p24 for levels; pregnant mother to liaise every 2 weeks with diabetic team concerning blood readings).
• Retinal digital screening with mydriasis schedule (as soon as possible after pregnancy confirmed if not screened in previous 12 months; after 1st antenatal appointment and again at 16–20 weeks if retinopathy seen on initial screen in pregnancy and at 28 weeks if none seen at initial screening).[14] Up to 20% develop proliferative retinopathy.
• Renal screening schedule (for microalbuminuria as well as dipstix protein, at 1st appointment if not screened in previous 12 months). Refer to nephrologist if creatinine ≥120μmol/L or protein excretion >2g/day. Give thromboprophylaxis if protein excretion >5g/day.
• Fetal surveillance (eg 4 chamber and outflow tract echo at 20 weeks; ultrasounds at 28, 32, and 36 weeks for fetal growth and amniotic fluid depth and cardiotocogram eg twice weekly from 38 weeks if she chooses to await spontaneous labour rather than accepting induction/caesarean section when offered at 38 weeks) earlier if growth restriction seen.
• Plan for delivery. If co-morbidity such as neuropathy or obesity arrange anaesthetic assessment at 36 weeks.
• Diabetes care after delivery.

If macrosomia is found on ultrasound the consultant obstetrician should then write a clear plan to determine follow-up scans, fetal surveillance, and mode and time of delivery.

For postnatal care the care plan should include, as a minimum:
• Plan for managing glycaemic control (eg return to pre-pregnancy regimen).
• Neonatal care: feed as soon as possible then 2–3hrly to prevent hypoglycaemia. Check glucose level at 2–4h after birth, and if signs of hypoglycaemia. Give IV glucose to baby if symptomatically hypoglycaemic. Tube feed or give IV glucose if 2 consecutive readings <2mmol/L despite maximal feeding or if unable to feed. Do not discharge to community until >24h old, feeding well and able to maintain glucose levels.
• Contraception (currently mothers with the worst obstetric outcomes are the least likely to receive contraceptive advice).
• Follow-up care after discharge from hospital (eg glucose tolerance test 6 weeks postpartum and annually to see if still diabetic in gestational diabetes).
• How to access pre-pregnancy review prior to subsequent pregnancies.

The advantage of care plans is that by documenting the plan, it enables members of the team (including the mother and father, for they are frequently the most reliable at making sure things happen if they know what is expected) to check that pregnancy is monitored as planned.

Obstetrics

Most women in the UK have 'shared obstetric care'—ie most of their antenatal care is from the community midwife (±GP), with limited (or no) visits (usually 2) to the hospital to see the consultant under whose care they are delivered, returning home (eg after 6–72h) for postnatal care. A minority receive their complete care from hospitals and the usual reasons for this are that the complications envisaged make full consultant care desirable. Some women are cared for by community midwives and their GP, but increasingly, low-risk women are receiving all their care from midwives, with doctors involved only if complications arise. Delivery may be in hospital in consultant- or midwife-led units, or, more rarely, at home. ▶There is quite good evidence that consultant input into antenatal care of normal pregnancies achieves no added benefits (p8)—but risk factors making specialist visits and booking desirable are generally agreed (see MINIBOX).

Is it safe for low-risk mothers to deliver in high-technology hospitals? Here interventions with their complications are more common. In the UK this question is usually academic (unless a midwife-led delivery unit is available) as most GPs are reluctant to conduct births—and 6 months' training in obstetrics gives scant skill. The rising birth rate and service pressures are putting these big hospitals under great strain. In places (eg New Zealand, Holland) where delivery outside of big hospitals is the norm, there is fairly clear (but not uncontested●❋) evidence that on all measures, and in all but the highest risk groups, big hospitals come out less favourably. The few trials seeming to favour high-technology are now recognized to be seriously flawed.

Home delivery (Rare in England: 2.8% of births in 2007 at home, 2% in freestanding midwifery units, 3% in alongside midwifery units.) Data comparing morbidity and mortality in home vs hospital delivery is sparse but a 2008–10 (N=65,438) study showed increased morbidity and high rate of transfer in labour for nullips.[15] But an important observation is that rapid intervention is necessary to save life (maternal or fetal) in ~5% of low-risk pregnancies. This pinpoints the need for any domiciliary service to have good equipment available for home delivery and good emergency back-up (eg by emergency obstetric ambulance units—ie specially trained ambulance personnel who, it is hoped, will liaise directly with senior medical obstetric staff in hospital).

Birth centres offer homely birth in congenial surroundings (eg with purpose-designed *birthing pools*). Formerly, labour ward facilities were nearby,

Risk factor—*vis à vis:*
The mother
• >40yrs old
• Nullip <20 or >34yrs
• History of infertility
• ≥5 past pregnancies
• Multip <154cm tall
• Primip <158cm tall
• Obese with BMI ≥35
• Social deprivation
• HBsAg or HIV+ve p34
Past deliveries
• Preterm or small (<37 weeks, <2.5kg)
• Deformity, still-birth, or neonatal death
• Caesarean section
• Hysterotomy
• Retained placenta/PPH
• Placental abruption
• Had pelvic floor repair
• Instrumental deliveries
• Poor fetal growth or wellbeing
• Diabetes, ↑ BP, anaemia
• Malpresentations after 34 weeks
• Serum α-fetoprotein ↑
This pregnancy
• Cardiac/thyroid disease
• Renal/liver disease
• Multiple pregnancy
• Rh antibodies (p116)
• Autoimmune disorders
• Asthma/epilepsy

if needed, and the mother was attended by her GP and community midwife. A randomized trial showed that mothers' satisfaction is great, and nearly all requested this type of delivery for future births.[16] Such centres may offer a compromise to adherents of home delivery, and go a long way towards celebrating rather than medicalizing birth. But we note that new UK birth centres may be entirely run by midwives, so if an obstetrician is needed (or an epidural) a lengthy and possibly risky journey is needed.[17] www.birthchoiceuk.com.

Issues surrounding home delivery[1]

▶*Remember that normal delivery is a retrospective diagnosis.*

- In the UK, because of past hospital experience of many abnormal labours, GPs are often *very* wary of home birth.
- Medico-legal aspects tend to dominate thoughts about worst-case scenarios—so that few GPs willingly take on intrapartum care.
- It's not clear who is to do the doctor's ordinary work when absent on a home delivery, if a mother particularly wants their GP present. Some small surgeries have had to close during delivery as no locum was available—an unacceptable consequence of offering mothers extra choice. NB: in the UK, midwives, but not GPs, have a statutory duty to help at home deliveries.
- It is not clear if there are enough doctors or midwives with the necessary experience in suturing and neonatal resuscitation. Where there is a good team, there is no doubt that home delivery can be a safe and rewarding experience.
- Decisions about the place of labour are dynamic, and need revising (eg in 29%) as events in pregnancy unfold.
- Necessary equipment is not readily available, eg Entonox.®
- The key factor in increasing choice about home delivery is a good working relationship between the parents, the GP, and the midwife. Where this exists, ~70% of home delivery requests tend to come to fruition; where the GP is rated as being unsupportive, in a UK context, this figure drops to 54%.
- Everyone needs to know that transfer in labour is common in labours starting off as planned home deliveries (9–14% if multip, 36–45% if primip)—and there is excess morbidity for primips, though levels are still low.[18]
- It is salutary to note that <20% of pregnancies in England and Wales are considered 'normal' and without antenatal or postnatal complications.[19] If normal delivery is defined as delivery without use of general anaesthetic, induction, epidural, instrumentation or surgical intervention, the normal delivery rate in England in 2003 was 51%.[20] In the 2008–2010 study it was 58% for planned obstetric unit birth, 76% alongside midwifery unit, 83% freestanding midwifery unit and 88% for home birth.[18] However, over-medicalization is a real problem too, eg in ≥20% of labours (p58).
- Intrapartum perinatal mortality rate for intended home delivery (1994–2003) was 0.48:1000 births for intended home delivery, 1.42:1000 for unintended home delivery, and 6.05:1000 births for women transferred to another place for delivery.[21] Average intrapartum mortality for England and Wales for all births for this period was 0.79:1000 births.

Indications for intrapartum transfer

- Malpresentation or breech in labour
- Significant meconium-stained liquor
- Fetal heart monitoring indication including heart rate abnormalities (p44)
- Delay in 1st or 2nd stage labour
- Epidural pain relief requested
- Maternal T° >38, or twice T° >37.5, 2h apart
- Retained placenta (p86)
- Maternal BP raised +140/ and/or +/90
- Uncertainty if fetal heart heard
- Emergency: (ante/post-partum haemorrhage, cord presentation/prolapse, maternal collapse or need for advanced neonatal resuscitation)
- 3rd or 4th degree vaginal tear or other complicated perineal repair needed.

When considering transfer bear in mind imminence of birth.

Hormonal changes Progesterone, synthesized by the corpus luteum until 35 post-conception days and by the placenta mainly thereafter, decreases smooth muscle excitability (uterus, gut, ureters) and raises body temperature. *Oestrogens* (90% oestriol) increase breast and nipple growth, water retention, and protein synthesis. The maternal thyroid often enlarges due to increased colloid production. Thyroxine levels, see p25. Pituitary secretion of *prolactin* rises throughout pregnancy. Maternal *cortisol* output is increased but unbound levels remain constant.

Genital changes The 100g non-pregnant uterus weighs 1100g by term. Muscle hypertrophy occurs up to 20 weeks, with stretching after that. The cervix may develop ectropion ('erosions'). Late in pregnancy cervical collagen reduces. Vaginal discharge increases due to cervical ectopy, cell desquamation, and ↑ mucus production from a vasocongested vagina.

Haemodynamic changes *Blood:* From 10 weeks the plasma volume rises until 32 weeks when it is 3.8 litres (50% >non-pregnant). Red cell volume rises from 1.4 litres when non-pregnant to 1.64 litres at term if iron supplements not taken (↑18%), or 1.8 litres at term (↑30%) if supplements are taken—hence Hb falls due to dilution (physiological 'anaemia'). wcc (mean 10.5×10^9/L), platelets, ESR (up 4-fold), cholesterol, β-globulin, and fibrinogen are raised. Albumin and gamma-globulin fall. Urea and creatinine fall.

Cardiovascular: Cardiac output rises from 5 litres/min to 6.5–7 litres/min in the first 10 weeks by increasing stroke volume (10%) and pulse rate (by ~15 beats/min). Peripheral resistance falls (due to hormonal changes). BP, particularly diastolic, falls during the second trimester by 10–20mmHg, then rises to non-pregnant levels by term. With increased venous distensibility, and raised venous pressure (as occurs with any pelvic mass), varicose veins may form. Vasodilatation and hypotension stimulate renin and angiotensin release—an important feature of BP regulation in pregnancy.

Aorto-caval compression From 20 weeks the gravid uterus compresses the inferior vena cava (and to a lesser extent the aorta) in supine women reducing venous return. This reduces cardiac output by 30–40% (so-called supine hypotension). ►Placing the woman in left lateral position or wedging her tilting 15° to the left relieves the pressure and restores cardiac output.

Other changes Ventilation increases 40% (tidal volume rises from 500 to 700mL), the increased depth of breath being a progesterone effect. O_2 consumption increases only 20%. Breathlessness is common as maternal P_aCO_2 is set lower to allow the fetus to offload CO_2. Gut motility is reduced, resulting in constipation, delayed gastric emptying, and, with a lax cardiac sphincter, heartburn. Renal size increases by ~1cm in length during pregnancy.

Frequency of micturition emerges early (glomerular filtration rate ↑ by 60%), later from bladder pressure by the fetal head. The bladder muscle is lax but residual urine after micturition is not normally present. Skin pigmentation (eg in linea nigra, nipples, or as chloasma—brown patches of pigmentation seen especially on the face), palmar erythema, spider naevi, and striae are common. Hair shedding from the head is reduced in pregnancy but the extra hairs are shed in the puerperium.

Pregnancy tests Positive eg from 9 days post-conception (or from day 23 of a 28-day cycle) until ~20 weeks of pregnancy; they remain positive for ~5 days after miscarriage or fetal death. Otherwise, the false +ve rate is low. They detect the β-subunit of human chorionic gonadotrophin in early morning urine, so are positive in trophoblastic disease (p264).

♋Pregnancy and obesity[22] (BMI >30 at booking, p530)

Maternal obesity affects the fetus adversely, casting a long fat shadow over the baby's adult life (with risk of heart disease, diabetes, the metabolic syndrome and some cancers, eg breast, lung).[23] Epigenetic mechanisms (p653) mean that the over- (and under)nutrition may influence not just this baby, but subsequent generations down the centuries.[24] There is also risk of macrosomia, meconium aspiration.[25] Incidence is rising in the UK and women with a BMI >35 constitute 15% of mothers dying, and almost 50% of those dying from thromboembolism are obese.

For mothers, obesity increases prevalence of:
• Miscarriage
• Pre-eclampsia
• Gestational diabetes
• Thromboembolism
• Cardiac disease
• Induced labour
• Caesarean section
• Infection (eg post-op)
• PPH
• Maternal mortality
• Feeding by bottle

►As mothers may be more motivated to accept lifestyle modifications, pregnancy is a period during which obesity can be more effectively managed. Control of body weight during this period is vital. Aim to encourage weight loss well before embarking on planned pregnancy. NB: dieting during pregnancy may not be wise as low weight gain during pregnancy correlates with lighter babies more prone to postnatal problems.[26] Good evidence is lacking. Lowest neonatal mortality is for birth weights of 3500–4500g and maternal weight gain depending on BMI:[27]♋

BMI	<19.8	recommended weight total gain (not twins):	12.5–18kg
	19.8–26		11.5–16kg
	26.1–29.0		7–11.5kg
	>29		2*–6kg

*Assuming *personal coaching* and using a *food diary* ("I didn't eat the cake as I knew I'd have to write it down, so I chose fruit instead..."). Some may need no weight gain.♋ medicinenet.com/script/main/art.asp?articlekey=100897

2010 CMACE/RCOG guidelines recommend giving 5mg folic acid from 1 month before conception and for the first trimester if BMI ≥30 to prevent increased risk of neural tube defects. Obese women are more prone to vitamin D deficiency so ensure they are taking 10μg vitamin D supplementation while pregnant and breastfeeding. If BMI ≥30, screen for diabetes, eg oral glucose tolerance test at 24–28 weeks and consider heparin thromboprophylaxis for 7 days postnatally if one additional thrombotic risk factor (p16), with addition of TED stockings if 2 risk factors. Mobilize all obese women early. If women with BMI ≥30 require caesarean section, give IV prophylactic antibiotics and, if subcutaneous fat is >2cm thick, suture that separately, to prevent infection.

Women with BMI ≥40 should always receive 7-day postnatal heparin prophylaxis and TED stockings whatever the mode of delivery. They should have an antenatal consultation with an obstetric anaesthetist with an anaesthetic plan made for labour and delivery, and need 3rd trimester assessment to plan manual handling requirements and provision of appropriate TED stockings. When in labour inform anaesthetist. They should have continuous midwifery care and should have an IV sited early in labour. If operative delivery is required the attending anaesthetic should be a consultant (or signed off obese-competent) obstetric anaesthetist.

Obstetrics

"Eating for 2 is the only nice thing about being pregnant"

Obstetrics

The aims of antenatal care are to: • Detect any disease in the mother • Ameliorate the discomforts of pregnancy • Monitor and promote fetal well-being • Prepare mothers for birth • Monitor trends to prevent or detect any early complications of pregnancy: BP is the most important variable (eclampsia, p48). • Is thromboprophylaxis (p16) or aspirin (p3 and p31) needed?

Who should give antenatal care? Midwives may manage care, calling in doctors if risks (p4) *or specific needs arise*. Book by 12 weeks: see within 2 weeks if already ≥12 weeks pregnant. Women with BMI ≥35 need consultant care.

The 1st antenatal visit is very comprehensive. ►Find a language interpreter if she needs one. Avoid using relatives (confidentiality issues). *History:*
• Usual cycle length; LMP (a normal period?); see Naegele's rule (p1).
• Contraception; drugs; past history, eg surgery to abdomen or pelvis.
• Any fertility problems; outcome and complications of past pregnancies.
• Is there family history of diabetes, BP↑, fetal abnormality, or twins?
• Does she have concurrent illness (p20–35)? Has she been 'cut' (p247)? If past or family history of DVT or embolism, screen for thrombophilia.
• Is gestational diabetes (GDM) a risk? Screen (75g glucose tolerance test) at 18±28wks) if previous (GDM); at 24wks if BMI >30, previous baby >4.5kg, 1st degree relative diabetic, family origin (FO) from area of high risk of diabetes.
• Past mental illness? If serious (schizophrenia, bipolar disorder) or past post-natal problems, get antenatal assessment; put management plan in notes.
• Is she *poor* (eg gas/electricity supply cut off)? *Unmarried? Unsupported? Subject to domestic violence?* (p514) *A substance abuser?* (p362). 'Healthy Start Vitamins for Women'—folic acid + vitamins C & D (10µg/d) are free to some during pregnancy and for 1 year after birth (Healthy Start Scheme [UK]).
• Avoid pâtés & blue/soft cheese (eg Brie, Camembert, to avoid listeria, p35); Toxoplasmosis advice: p34. Avoid liver (p2). Advise UK mothers to have vitamin D (above) if family of origin is African, or as listed below,[1] or housebound, covered when outdoors, have BMI >30, or are diet vit. D depleted[2]

Examination: Check heart, lungs, BP, weight (record BMI), and abdomen. Is a cervical smear needed? Varicose veins? Sensitively ask if genitally 'cut' (p246).

Tests: Blood: Hb, group (antibodies if Rh–ve, p116), syphilis & rubella (±chicken-pox) serology, HBsAg (p36 & p26) HIV test; sickle test if black, Hb electrophoresis (p22) and 25-hydroxyvitamin D if relevant.[28] Take an MSU (protein; bacteria). Arrange tests to exclude Down's (p12). If she is foreign, a TB contact, or a hospital worker, consider *CXR* after 14 weeks.

Offer *early ultrasound* to establish dates, exclude multiple pregnancy and aid with Down's tests and an 18–20-week anomaly scan.

Suggest: Parentcraft/relaxation classes; dental visit. Enquire about problems and anxieties. Consider need for *iron and folate* (p85 and p22).

Advise on: Smoking, alcohol, diet, correct use of seat belts (above or below the bump, not over it) and adequate rest. Ensure knowledge of social security benefits. Usual exercise and travel are OK (avoid malarious areas) up to 36 weeks (singleton):[29] check with airline. Intercourse OK if no vaginal bleeding.

Later visits Check urine for albumin, BP, fundal height. Check lie and presentation at 36 weeks. Do Hb and Rh antibodies at 28 & 34 weeks and give anti-D then if needed (p9). Visits are at <12 weeks then at 16, 25, 28, 31, 34, 36, 38, 40, and 41 weeks (primip). Weigh only if clinically indicated.

The head is usually engaged (p40) by 37 weeks in Caucasian primips (if not, consider: large (or malpositioned) head, small pelvis or obstruction, placenta praevia, or wrong estimation of dates).

---

1 FO=family of origin from India, Pakistan, Bangladesh, Saudi Arabia, United Arab Emirates, Iraq, Jordan, Syria, Oman, Qatar, Kuwait, Egypt, or if black Caribbean.
2 Vitamin D containing foods include oily fish, meat, eggs, fortified margarine, and breakfast cereal.

Using anti-D immunoglobulin

Dose: 250u for gestations <20 weeks, 500u if >20 weeks, (1500u if no Kleihauer). Give in deltoid (buttock absorption too slow); IV$_{RCOL}^{30}$ or SC if bleeding disorder; as soon as possible after incident, by 72h (some protection if by 10d). From 20^{+0} weeks do Kleihauer test (FBC bottle of maternal blood; fetal RBCs therein are less susceptible to lysis, so can be counted to measure the bleed's volume). Don't give anti-D if already sensitized ie antibodies to anti-D are present.

Postnatal use: 500u is the normal dose after 20^{+0} weeks' gestation. 37% of Rh–ve women give birth to Rh–ve babies and these women do not need anti-D.

- Anti-D should be given to all Rh–ve women where the baby's group cannot be determined (eg macerated stillbirths), or if the baby's group is unknown 72h post delivery.
- Do a Kleihauer test on all eligible for anti-D. 500u anti-D can suppress immunization by up to 4mL of fetal red cells (8mL of fetal blood), but 1% of women have transplacental haemorrhage (TPH) of >4mL, especially after manual removal of placenta, and with caesarean section. A Kleihauer test is especially important in stillbirth, as massive spontaneous transplacental haemorrhage can be the cause of fetal death. Where >4mL TPH is suggested by the Kleihauer screen, a formal estimation of the TPH volume is required and 500u anti-D given for every 4mL fetal cells transfused (maximum 5000u anti-D at 2 IM sites/24h). Note: Kleihauer tests can be negative where there is ABO incompatibility as fetal cells are rapidly cleared from the maternal circulation. Liaise with the transfusion service. Check maternal blood every 48h to determine clearance of cells and need for continuing anti-D.
- Any mother receiving anti-D prenatally (see below), should also receive it postnatally unless she delivers an Rh-negative baby.

Use of anti-D in miscarriage in Rh–ve mothers

1 Anti-D should be given to all having surgical or medical terminations of pregnancy or evacuation of hydatidiform mole (p264), unless they are already known to have anti-D antibodies. Give 250u if <20 weeks; 500u (and Kleihauer) if >20^{+0} weeks' gestation.
2 Anti-D should always be given where spontaneous miscarriage is followed by medical or surgical evacuation.
3 Anti-D should be given where spontaneous complete miscarriage occurs after 12^{+0} weeks' gestation.
4 Threatened miscarriage ≥12^{+0} weeks give anti-D; if bleeding continues intermittently give anti-D 6-weekly until delivery.
5 Routine anti-D is not recommended with threatened miscarriage before 12 weeks' gestation (but consider if viable fetus, heavy or repeated bleeding, and abdominal pain).

Use of anti-D in pregnancy in Rh–ve mothers

1 Give anti-D 500u at 28 and 34 weeks to rhesus negative women (primip antenatal sensitization falls from 0.95% to 0.35%). Anti-D may still be detectable in maternal blood at delivery. Still give postnatal anti-D, if indicated (as above). Take 28-week blood sample for antibodies before 28-week anti-D.
2 When significant TPH may occur: with chorionic villus sampling; external cephalic version; APH; uterine procedures (eg amniocentesis, fetal blood sampling); abdominal trauma; intrauterine death. Use 250u before 20 weeks' gestation, 500u (and do Kleihauer) after 20 weeks.
3 Anti-D should be given in cases of ectopic pregnancy.
4 For threatened miscarriage, see above.

Obstetrics

'The first half of pregnancy can become a time of constant "exams" to see if the baby can be allowed to graduate to the second half of pregnancy'. Those at high and, increasingly, those at low risk of having an abnormal baby are offered prenatal diagnosis to allow better treatment of the expected defect, or (more often) if they would wish to terminate any abnormal fetus. Cell-free fetal DNA circulating in maternal blood may be useful in the future.

High-risk pregnancies • Maternal age >35 (chromosome defects).
• Previous abnormal baby or family history of inherited condition.

Problems ▶*Anxiety while false +ve results are sorted out is a big problem.*
• Terminating normal fetuses, eg ♂ fetus of carriers of x-linked conditions.
• Most abnormalities are in low-risk groups (∴ missable by selective screening).
• Services available, their quality, and populations made eligible vary widely.
• Termination of female fetuses in cultures valuing males more highly.
• Devaluation of positive view of handicapped or 'special needs' children.

Ultrasound at 11^{+0}–13^{+6} weeks dates pregnancy, screens for nuchal translucency (see BOX) and chorionicity (p68). Further anomaly scan is at ~18 weeks. Skilled operators detect many structural anomalies. See BOX opposite and p46. Ultrasound best detects externally impinging structural abnormality, eg anencephaly/spina bifida. Internal structural abnormality detection rate, eg for heart disease and diaphragmatic hernia, remains <50%. Fetuses with false +ve suggestion of abnormality are mostly associated with 'soft signs' on ultrasound, eg nuchal thickening (eg trisomy 21), choroid plexus cysts (trisomies 18 and 21), and echogenic bowel (trisomy 21 and cystic fibrosis). Use of 'soft signs' may increase false +ves 12-fold.

α-Fetoprotein (AFP) AFP is a glycoprotein synthesized by the fetal liver and GI tract. Fetal levels fall after 13 weeks, but maternal (transplacental) serum AFP continues to rise to 30 weeks. Maternal AFP is measured at 17 weeks. In 10% with a high AFP there is a fetal malformation, eg an open neural tube defect (but closed defects are missed), exomphalos, posterior urethral valves, nephrosis, GI obstruction, teratomas, Turner's syndrome (or normal twins). In ~30% of those with no malformation, there is an adverse outcome, eg placental abruption and third trimester deaths. ▶Monitor closely. 1 in 40 with a low AFP have a chromosomal abnormality (eg Down's). AFP is lower in diabetic mothers. NB: as this test is non-specific on its own, it is of use for preliminary screening; those with abnormal values may be offered further tests (see below, and p12 for the 'quadruple test').

Amniocentesis Use continuous ultrasound. Fetal loss rate is ~1% at ~16 weeks' gestation, but ~5% for early amniocentesis at 10–13 weeks (not recommended as ↑ talipes and respiratory problems). Amniotic fluid AFP is measured (a more accurate screen for neural tube defects than maternal serum), and cells in the fluid are cultured for karyotyping (+enzyme and gene probe analysis). Cell culture takes 3wks, so an abnormal pregnancy must be terminated at a late stage. Is anti-D needed (p9)?

Chorionic villus biopsy At 10+ weeks, placenta is sampled by transcervical or transabdominal approach under continuous ultrasound control. Karyotyping takes 2 days, enzyme and gene probe analysis 3 weeks, so termination for abnormality is earlier, safer, and less distressing than after amniocentesis. Fetal loss rate is ~4%. Use up to 20 weeks (cordocentesis preferable thereafter). It does not detect neural tube defects, may cause fetal malformation, and is not recommended in dichorionic multiple pregnancy.[31] Is anti-D needed (p9)?

Fetoscopy is carried out at ~18wks with ultrasound guidance to find external malformations, do fetal blood samples, or biopsy. Fetal loss rate is ~4%.

- Early scans (at 11–14 weeks) may detect 59% of those with structural abnormality and 78% of those with chromosome abnormality. It is best at detecting CNS defects, neck abnormalities, GI, and renal defects: less good for spina bifida, heart and limb defects. With a combination of early and later scans up to 81% of malformations may be diagnosed.[32]
- Fluid accumulation in the neck at 10–14 weeks' gestation (increased fetal nuchal translucency, FNT) may reflect fetal heart failure,[33] and be seen in serious anomaly of the heart and great arteries.[34] Meta-analysis shows that taking the 99th percentile as a cut off for cardiac screening enables 33% of heart abnormalities to be detected antenatally.[35] Referring 99th percentile fetuses for echocardiography may show 106 cardiac abnormalities per 1000 fetuses examined.[36]
- There is a strong association between chromosomal abnormality and FNT. In one study, 84% of karyotypically proven trisomy 21 fetuses had a nuchal translucency >3mm at 10–13 weeks' gestation (as did 4.5% of chromosomally normal fetuses).
- The greater the extent of FNT, the greater the risk of abnormality.
- Nuchal translucency screening may be used to see who may benefit from more invasive chorionic villus sampling (or amniocentesis p10, which may delineate the precise chromosomal abnormality, eg trisomies). Note: positive predictive value of screening is 4% so 96% of women with a 'positive' test undergo an 'unnecessary' invasive procedure (chorionic villus sampling in the first trimester or amniocentesis in the second trimester). If nuchal screening was used as the *only* screening test 2 or 3 normal pregnancies would be lost after chorionic villus sampling, and 1 after amniocentesis, for every 4 pregnancies correctly detected with trisomy 21.
- It is useful for screening twins as early detection is best, for if selective fetocide is to be used risk of miscarriage is 3-fold higher if done after 16 weeks. Monochorionic twins have a higher false +ve rate for nuchal translucency thickness than dichorionic twins or singletons. In the 25% of monochorionic twins with FNT discordance of >20 %, more than 30% had early fetal death or severe twin–twin transfusion syndrome (10% if less discordance).[37]
- Note that the degree of neck flexion during the ultrasound examination may influence nuchal measurements.
- Other 'soft markers' for Down's syndrome are fetal nasal bone appearance, the Doppler velocity wave form in the ductus venosus and tricuspid regurgitation.[38]
- Systematic review shows that of all chromosomally normal fetuses (euploid) with significant nuchal thickening, 70–90% have normal outcome, 2.2–10.6% miscarry, 0.5–12.7% have neurodevelopmental problems, and 2.1–7.6% of malformations were undiagnosed before birth.[39]

Obstetrics

The 1st antenatal diagnosis of Down's syndrome was in 1968. Initially there was amniocentesis for older mothers (Penrose noted an association with maternal age in 1933; see table). Then screening by blood test was introduced, then nuchal screening (p11).

Maternal age & Down's[1]		
Age of mother (yrs)[40]	Fetuses with Down's at 16 weeks[1]	Live births with Down's
15–19	—	1:1250
20–24	—	1:1400
25–29	—	1:1100
30–31	—	1:900
32	—	1:750
33	1:420	1:625
34	1:325	1:500
35[1]	1:250	1:350
36	1:200	1:275
34	1:150	1:225
38	1:120	1:175
39	1:100	1:140
40	1:75	1:100
41	1:60	1:85
42	1:45	1:65
43	1:35	1:50
44	1:30	1:40
≥45	1:20	1:25

From 2007, the UK NHS has aimed for screening tests giving detection rates of 75% with a false +ve rate of <3%. Tests estimate risk of Down's taking into account results from nuchal scanning, blood tests, and the woman's age. Where risk of Down's is >1:250 (~5% of pregnancies) she will be offered tests such as chorionic villus sampling (p10) and amniocentesis (p10). Early ultrasound is vital for dating pregnancies for these tests.

The combined test combines nuchal translucency (NT) + free β-human chorionic gonadotrophin (βHCG) + pregnancy associated plasma protein (PrAP-A or PAPP-A) + the woman's age. Used between 10 weeks 3 days and 13 weeks 6 days. It achieves detection rates of 95% of all aneuploidies, 86% trisomy-21, and 100% of trisomy-18 and trisomy-13. PrAP-A levels are ~19.6% lower in smokers.[41] In multiple pregnancy risk is calculated per pregnancy if monochorionic; per fetus when dichorionic or trichorionic.[42]

The integrated test This is better than the combined test if there are good facilities for NT measurements available and the woman is prepared to wait for 2nd trimester results. It involves NT + PrAP-A in the 1st trimester + the quadruple test in the 2nd trimester. Do not use 2nd trimester tests for triplets.[AFCE]

The quadruple test combines maternal α-fetoprotein (AFP) + unconjugated estriol + free βHCG or total βHCG + inhibin-A + the woman's age in the 2nd trimester. Use between 15 weeks + 0 days and 20 weeks + 0 days so useful for women presenting in the 2nd trimester.

The emotional cost to the mother is impossible to calculate:[43] 56 out of every 57 women under 37yrs old who had a +ve test proved, after amniocentesis, not to have an affected fetus. Amniocentesis causes fetal loss (~0.86%[44]), and these losses will sometimes be of normal babies. New screening regimens in the 1st trimester go some way to mitigating distress and anxiety.

We have no idea of the best way of counselling parents before the test. If we just hand out a leaflet, few will read it, and then when it comes to amniocentesis and termination, many will refuse—and the screening test wastes money, as well as laying health authorities open to litigation: "I never understood that I might lose a normal baby..." The alternative is to provide full details at the time of the initial blood test. The irony is that gaining informed consent is then the most expensive part of the test, and one which itself could cause much distress. ☺Imagine an overjoyed expectant mother arriving in the clinic serenely happy in fulfilling her reproductive potential: the quintessence of health. She leaves only after being handed ethical conundrums of quite staggering proportions, involving death, disease, and human sacrifices, and a timetable for their resolution that would leave even the most fast-moving philosopher breathless and disorientated, and which may leave her forever bereft of one of Nature's most generous gifts: the fundamental belief in one's own wholeness.

1 Sources vary: if we look just at births to mothers aged 35, the proportion with Down's in 4 studies was 1:265; 1:270; 1:350[40,45] and 1:400 (ACOG 1999)[46] Why the difference between 16wks and time of birth? Because of spontaneous miscarriages of fetuses with Down's syndrome between 16wks and birth.

Preimplantation genetic diagnosis (PGD) is an early form of prenatal diagnosis in which embryos created *in vitro* are analysed for well-defined genetic defects. Defect-free embryos are then used for implantation.

It is used in those with high risk of genetic disease, eg carriers of monogenic disease or chromosome structural abnormalities (eg translocations) who have repeatedly terminated pregnancies due to prenatal tests showing abnormality, who have concurrent infertility, who have had recurrent miscarriage (as occurs with translocation carriers), and for those with moral or religious objections to termination.

It has also been used to screen for aneuploidy (PGD-AS) in those undergoing *in vitro* fertilization hoping to enhance chance of ongoing pregnancy (eg in the case for women >37–40 years old—but see below).

Pioneered in the early 1990s, PGD has resulted in >1200 pregnancies (pregnancy rate 24%), of which 5% of babies had some kind of abnormality. PGD selection of embryos by HLA type so that a child born after using this technology can be used as a stem cell donor to save a sibling from certain conditions (eg with Fanconi anaemia, β thalassaemia, or leukaemia) is controversial, but possible. Some clinics select sex of implanted embryo eg for 'family balancing'.

Genetic analysis at the single cell level occurs using 1st polar body of an egg, or 2nd polar body (extruded after fertilization and completion of second meiotic division), or using blastomeres from cleavage-stage embryos. The blastocyst is the latest stage from which cells can be used but is little used as it leaves little time for analysis as embryos must be transferred before day 5 or 6. Biopsied surplus embryos can be cryopreserved but implantation rate for these is only 12%.

Fluorescence *in situ* hybridization (FISH) is used for analysis of chromosomes and polymerase chain reaction (PCR) for analysis of genes in monogenic diseases. PGD can currently be applied for detecting 33 monogenic diseases. Gene analysis for x-linked conditions has the advantage that healthy male embryos and non-carrier female embryos can be transferred. Sexing embryos for x-linked conditions remains useful for conditions where the single gene is not known (eg non-fragile-x x-linked mental retardation), has been judged too difficult a search, and for women eg over 37 who do not wish to wait for specific tests to be developed.

Pregnancy rates are 17% after testing for structural chromosome abnormality (including translocations), 16% after sexing, 21% after testing for monogenic diseases. This is lower than the expected rate of 20–25% expected for regular IVF. For PGD-AS 25% pregnancy rates are achieved overall for women of previously poor prognosis due to advanced maternal age (a lower proportion than those where preimplantation genetic screening is not used),[47] repeated IVF failure (but only 8% do get pregnant), and recurrent miscarriage (28% pregnancy rate achieved).

Obstetrics

The placenta is the organ of respiration, nutrition, and excretion for the fetus. It produces hormones for maternal wellbeing. It immunologically protects the fetus from rejection and allows the passage of maternal IgG antibodies.

Development At term the placenta weighs 1/7th the weight of the baby. It has a blood flow of 600mL/min. The placenta changes throughout pregnancy as calcium is deposited in the villi and fibrin on them. Excess fibrin may be deposited in diabetes and rhesus disease, so ↓ fetal nutrition.

Placental types *Velamentous* insertion (1%): umbilical vessels go within the membranes before placental insertion. *Placenta succenturia:* (5%) There is a separate (succenturiate) lobe away from the main placenta which may fail to separate normally and cause a PPH or puerperal sepsis. *Vasa praevia:* Fetal vessels from velamentous insertion or between lobes (succenturia, or bilobe placenta) risk damage at membrane rupture causing fetal haemorrhage. Caesarean delivery is needed (urgent if fetal compromise at membrane rupture, elective if detected antenatally by ultrasound). *Placenta membranacea* (1/3000) a thin placenta surrounds the baby. Some is in the lower segment so predisposes to APH. It may fail to separate in the 3rd stage. *Placenta accreta:* There is abnormal (morbid) adherence of all or part of the placenta to the uterus, termed *placenta increta* myometrium inflitrated, *placenta percreta* if penetration reaches the serosa. These 3 types predispose to PPH and need hysterectomy. Incidence ↑ with the number of previous caesarean sections. Diagnose prenatally (colour doppler US/MRI p78).

Placenta praevia The placenta lies in the lower uterine segment. It is found in ~0.5% of pregnancies. Risks are of significant haemorrhage by mother and fetus. Avoid PV examinations, advise against penetrative intercourse.[10] *Associations:* Caesarean section; sharp curette TOP; multiparity; multiple pregnancy; mother >40 years; assisted conception; deficient endometrium-manual removal of placenta, D&C, fibroids, endometritis . Ultrasound (US) at <24 weeks' gestation shows a low-lying placenta in 28% but with lower segment development only 3% lie low at term. Transvaginal ultrasound is superior to transabdominal for localizing placentas accurately, and, if combined with 3D power Doppler/MRI, diagnoses vasa praevia and placenta accreta. It has not been shown to increase bleeding. Repeat US at 32wks if major praevia, 36wks if minor.

Major placenta praevia (placenta covers the internal os) requires caesarean section for delivery. Minor placenta praevia (placenta in lower segment but does not cross the internal os): aim for normal delivery unless the placenta encroaches within 2cm of the internal os (especially if posterior or thick). Presentation may be as APH (separation of the placenta as the lower segment stretches causes bleeding) or as failure for the head to engage ie a high presenting part. Problems are with bleeding and with mode of delivery as the placenta obstructs the os and may shear off during labour, or may be accreta (5%), especially after a previous caesar (>24%). Poor lower segment contractility predisposes to postpartum haemorrhage. Caesarean section should be consultant-performed or supervised with consultant anaesthetic attendance at 38wks, (36–7wks with steroid cover, crossmatched blood + haematologist available,[48] if accreta suspected), at a hospital with blood bank and level 2 critical care beds.[49] Admitting those with major placenta praevia at ≤35 weeks' gestation so that immediate help is available, is controversial, and not practiced by many UK units but admit at 34wks if major praevia and there has been bleeding.

After delivery Examine the placenta for abnormalities (clots, infarcts, amnion nodosum, vasa praevia, single umbilical artery). Weigh the placenta (weight >25% of the baby suggests congenital nephrotic syndrome). Blood may be taken from the cord for Hb, Coombs' test, LFTs, and blood group (eg for ...is disease), or for infection screens, if needed.

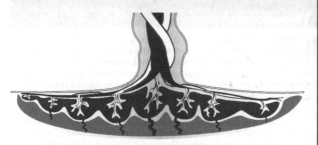

Fig 1. Seven spiral arteries are here seen to have been successfully invaded by trophoblast and they are now flooding the vast intervillous spaces with hot maternal blood—producing the slow whooshing crescendos heard by the ultrasound probe as the backdrop to the faster fetal heart beat. To get to the fetus proper, nutrients have a 6-part journey: maternal blood space → syncytiotrophoblast → trophoblast basement membrane → capillary basement membrane → capillary endothelium → fetal blood.[50]

In pre-eclampsia, trophoblast invasion is too shallow: there is no progress beyond the superficial portions of the uterine spiral arterioles. So these spiral arterioles retain their endothelial linings and remain narrow-bore, high-resistance vessels, resulting in poor maternal blood flow. The mother may raise her blood pressure to compensate for this—but the price may be eclampsia (p49).[51]

Plasma chemistry in pregnancy

	Non-pregnant		Trimester 1		Trimester 2		Trimester 3	
Centile	2.5	97.5	2.5	97.5	2.5	97.5	2.5	97.5
Na⁺ mmol/L	138	146	135	141	132	140	133	141
Ca²⁺ mmol/L	2	2.6	2.3	2.5	2.2	2.2	2.2	2.5
*corrected	2.3	2.6	2.25	2.57	2.3	2.5	2.3	2.59
Albumin g/L	44	50	39	49	36	44	33	41
AST IU/L	7	40	10	28	11	29	11	30
ALT IU/L	0	40	6	32	6	32	6	32
TSH	0	4	0	1.6	1	1.8	7	7.3

*Calcium corrected for plasma albumin (*OHCM* p670)

Other plasma reference intervals (not analysed by trimester)

	Non-pregnant	Pregnant
Alk phos IU/L	3–300	≤450 (can be ↑↑ in normal pregnancies)
Bicarbonate mmol/L	24–30	20–25
Creatine μmol/L	70–150	24–68
Urea mmol/L	2.5–6.7	2–4.2
Urate μmol/L	150–390	116–276 (24wks), 110–322 (32wks), 120–344 (36wks)

- C-reactive protein does not change much in pregnancy.
- Platelets ≥150 ×10⁹/L (beware if 120×10⁹/L see p48).
- TSH may be low <20 weeks in normal pregnancy (suppressed by HCG); see above & p25.
- Protein S falls in pregnancy, so protein S deficiency is difficult to diagnose.
- Activated protein C (APC) resistance is found in 40% of pregnancies so special tests are needed when looking for this. Genotyping for factor V Leiden and prothrombin G20210 are unaffected by pregnancy.

♱ ▶Pregnancy is a hypercoagulable state: consider need for thromboprophylaxis pre-pregnancy, at booking, if admitted to hospital, throughout the antenatal period, at start of labour and once delivered. If needed refer to Trust-nominated expert in thrombosis in pregnancy. Screen women with non-oestrogen provoked thromboembolism for thrombophilia before the next pregnancy.

▶In all pregnant women avoid immobility and dehydration.

▶For women with 3 or more persisting risk factors (MINIBOX), consider antenatal and postnatal low molecular weight heparin (LMWH) prophylaxis, starting as early in pregnancy as possible as risk is throughout (risk↓ by ≤60–70%). Continue normal dose prophylaxis when admitted in labour. Treat for 6 weeks postpartum, and supply graduated compression stockings postpartum.

▶If BMI >40, or caesarean in labour, give LMWH for 7 days postpartum.

Thromboprophylaxis after vaginal delivery:

Risk factors: (Thrombophilia/past thromboembolism considered separately.) If BMI >40 offer treatment. Offer to all women with two of the risk factors opposite (see MINIBOX).

Treatment: Treat with low molecular weight heparin (LMWH) eg enoxaparin starting as soon as possible after delivery (as long as no postpartum haemorrhage and ≥4h after epidural catheter siting or removal—6h if that was traumatic). Continue for 7 days including at home. Dose of **enoxaparin**: if the early pregnancy weight (EPW) is 50–90kg, give 40mg/24h SC; if EPW <50kg, give 20mg/24h SC; if EPW 91–130kg give 60mg/24h SC, if EPW 131–170kg give 80mg/24h SC, if EPW >170kg give 0.6mg/kg/24h SC. If heparin is contraindicated, use TED compression stockings (TED= transverse elastic graduated). If 3 or more risk factors give stockings and LMWH.

Women with past venous thromboembolism (VTE) ± thrombophilia: Action depends on risk: VH = very high; HR = high risk; IR = intermediate risk.

• (VH) If recurrent VTE (+antiphospholipid syndrome or antithrombin deficiency) or already on long-term warfarin, use high-dose prophylactic LMWH, eg enoxaparin 40mg/12h SC if 50–90kg EPW (or 75% of weight adjusted therapeutic dose (WATD)). WATD=1mg/kg/12h (kg is the EPW), prenatally and 1.5mg/kg/24h postnatally. This is given prenatally. Withhold at onset of labour (halve to /24h the day before and the day of induction). Give for 6wks postpartum or revert to warfarin day 5–7 postnatally.

• (HR) Previous VTE unprovoked/idiopathic or oestrogen (or pregnancy)-related; or VTE + (1st degree relative with VTE or thrombophilia); or VTE + documented thrombophilia: give LMWH antenatally and 6 weeks postpartum.

• (IR) If a single previous VTE provoked by major risk factor no longer present and no other risk factors give LMWH for 6wks postpartum (PP).

Women with asymptomatic thrombophilia: See p33.

Risk factors
• Age >35 years old
• Early pregnancy BMI >30
• Smoker
• Parity ≥3
• Multiple pregnancy
• Assisted reproduction
• Gross varicose veins
• Paraplegia
• Sickle cell disease/SLE
• Nephrotic syndrome
• Some cardiac causes
• Past thromboembolism[1]
• Thrombophilia
• Myeloproliferative dis.
• Inflammatory bowel dis.
• Hyperemesis/dehydration
• Pre-eclampsia
• Immobility for ≥3 days eg symphysis pubis dysfunction
• Ovarian hyperstimulation
• Major infection (eg pyelonephritis, wound infection) so hospital admission
• Labour lasting >24h
• Mid-cavity forceps
• Elective caesarean
• Blood loss >1L/transfused
• Surgery in puerperium eg evacuation of retained products of conception
• Postpartum sterilization
• Long travel time (≥4h)

Obstetrics

ˉˢtrogen related provoked thromboembolism eg previous major surgery is not a risk factor.

University of Birmingham
Barnes Library

Title: Core clinical cases in psychiatry : a problem-solving approach /
ID: 5526170531
Due: 05/07/2019 23:59:00 BST

Total items: 1
28/06/2019 12:41

Check your library account at
www.findit.bham.ac.uk

Contact us at
www.intranet.birmingham.ac.uk/justask

►Before prescribing any drug, think—Is it necessary? Is it safe? Consult *Data-sheets* ± a national teratology information service (tel 0191 232 1525[uk]).

Symptoms and signs in the first 10 weeks: Early symptoms are amenorrhoea, nausea, vomiting, and bladder irritability. Breasts engorge, nipples enlarge (darken at 12 weeks), Montgomery's tubercles (sebaceous glands on nipples) become prominent. Vulval vascularity increases and the cervix softens and looks bluish (4 weeks). At 6–10 weeks the uterine body is more globular. Temperature rises (<37.8°C).

Headaches, palpitations, and fainting are all commoner in pregnancy. Dilated peripheral circulation ↑sweating and feeling hot. Management: Increase fluid intake: take showers. If feels faint from postural hypotension, stand slowly.

Urinary frequency is due to pressure of the fetal head on the bladder in later pregnancy. Exclude UTI.

Abdominal pain: See p38.

Breathlessness is common. See p6.

Constipation tends to occur as gut motility decreases. Adequate oral fluids and a high-fibre diet help combat it. Avoid stimulant laxatives—they increase uterine activity in some women. Increased venous distensibility and pelvic congestion predispose to *haemorrhoids* (if they prolapse, rest the mother head down, apply ice packs and replace them) and *varicose veins*. Resting with feet up and properly worn elastic stockings help.

Reflux oesophagitis and heartburn occur as pyloric sphincter relaxation allows irritant bile to reflux into the stomach. Cigarettes and spices should be avoided, small meals taken, and antacids may be used. Use more pillows, and a semi-recumbent position.

Third trimester backache: Due to pelvic ligament and muscle relaxation, pain tends to be worse at night. A firm mattress, flat shoes, standing with back straight, and pelvic support from physiotherapy all help.

Carpal tunnel syndrome (p714) in pregnancy is due to fluid retention. Advise wrist splints until delivery cures the problem.

Itch/itchy rashes are common (up to 25%) and may be due to the usual causes (*OHCM* p64, check LFT—see p26) or to pruritic eruption of pregnancy (PEP = *prurigo of pregnancy*)—an intensely itchy papular/plaque rash on the abdomen and limbs. PEP is most common in first pregnancies beyond 35 weeks' gestation. Emollients and weak topical steroids ease it. Delivery cures it. If vesicles are present, think of *pemphigoid gestationis* (PG): a rare (1 : 50,000) condition which may cause fatal heat loss and cardiac failure; the baby may be briefly affected; refer early (prednisolone may be needed). PG may recur in later pregnancies.

Ankle oedema: This is a very common, almost normal, manifestation of pregnancy. Measure BP and check urine for protein (pre-eclampsia, p48). Check legs for DVT. It often responds to rest and leg elevation. Reassure that it is harmless (unless pre-eclampsia).

Leg cramps 33% get cramp, the latter half of pregnancy, severe in 5%, often worse at night. Raising the foot of the bed by 20cm will help.

Chloasma: This is a patch of darker pigmentation, eg on the face: p586.

Nausea affects ~80%. *Vomiting* occurs in ~50%. It may start by 4 weeks and decline over the following weeks. At 20 weeks 20% may still vomit. Most respond to frequent small meals, reassurance, and a stress-free environment. It is associated with good outcome (fewer fetal losses). Hyperemesis: p18.

This is defined as persisting vomiting in pregnancy which causes weight loss (>5% of pre-pregnancy weight) and ketosis. It affects 1% of pregnant women. Risk is increased in youth, non-smokers, primips, working outside home, pre-existing diabetes, hyperthyroidism, psychiatric illness, family history, those with previous eating disorders and multiple or molar pregnancy (hence the idea that excessively high HCG levels may be the cause—whereas steeply rising oestrogens may cause the very common feature of morning sickness). Rarely, hyperemesis has been fatal. Recurrence rate 15% (10% if changed paternity).[53]

Presentation Inability to keep food or fluids down; weight ↓ (2–5kg) ± nutritional deficiency, dehydration, hypovolaemia, tachycardia, postural hypotension, electrolyte disturbance with hypokalaemia and hyponatraemic shock, polyneuritis (B vitamins ↓), behaviour disorders, liver and renal failure. There may be ptyalism (inability to swallow saliva) and spitting.

Tests Do PCV and U&E to help guide IV fluid regimen. 50% have abnormal LFTs (usually raised aminotransferase and bilirubin). TFTs are abnormal in 60% of those with hyperemesis. This is biochemical hyperthyroidism with raised free thyroxine and suppressed TSH. In women with hyperemesis thyroxine is converted to reverse tri-iodothyronine in the tissues which is physiologically inactive so stimulating metabolic rate less and conserving energy stores. The severity of hyperemesis correlates with the degree of biochemical hyperthyroidism, and those with abnormal TFTs require longer hospitalization to prevent readmission. The biochemical hyperthyroidism settles as vomiting settles so does not require treatment in its own right. Chart losses, weigh, record pulse and standing and lying blood pressure. Exclude UTI. Do ultrasound scan to exclude twins or hydatidiform mole.

Treatment Admit to hospital. Give thromboprophylaxis (eg enoxaparin 40mg/24h SC) and anti-embolic stockings. Spend time optimizing psychological wellbeing. Is she worried about how her other children are being cared for?

Most settle with due *care and attention*. If not too severe it may settle with rest, ginger, pyridoxine, dry bland food, and carbonated drinks. Routine thiamine supplementation is wise for all women admitted (eg thiamine 25–50mg/8h PO) or if IV required 100mg diluted in 100mL normal saline given over 60min, repeated at weekly intervals. This is to prevent development of Wernicke's encephalopathy (see *OHCM* p707)—which is then associated with 40% fetal loss. Correct dehydration with IV infusion (eg with normal saline infusion with potassium added to each bag as guided by U&E). Beware rapid reversal of hyponatraemia which can cause fatal central pontine myelinosis.[54] If condition does not improve after rehydration anti-emetics may be needed eg cyclizine 50mg/8h PO/IM or IV. Other recognized anti-emetics used: metoclopramide, prochlorperazine, chlorpromazine, domperidone, ondansetron.[55] Phenothiazines can cause drowsiness, extrapyramidal side effects, and oculogyric crisis. Those resistant to conventional treatments may respond to steroid treatment, eg hydrocortisone 100mg twice daily followed by 40mg prednisolone/24h tapering down. Prednisolone can then usually be reduced to 2.5–10mg/24h by 20 weeks' gestation. If it is needed long-term screen for UTI and gestational diabetes. Prednisolone is metabolized by the placenta, fetal blood levels are low and adverse fetal effects have not been reported.

Parenteral nutrition may, very rarely, be needed—*OHCM* p574. If nutritional support is required both nasojejunal tube feeding and percutaneous endoscopic gastrostomy have been successfully used.[56] Parenteral nutrition has been found to be associated with serious complications (eg line sepsis). ►Get a dietician's help.

Sickle-cell disease (SCD) is caused by a group of haemoglobin disorders (single gene recessive) which predispose to 'sickling' of red cells in low oxygen conditions causing vaso-occlusion in small vessels, and cells prone to increased haemolytic breakdown. Disease complications include painful crises, stroke, pulmonary hypertension, renal dysfunction, leg ulcers, retinal disease, avascular necrosis (eg of hip). Pregnancy complications include maternal painful crises, prematurity and fetal growth restriction. Some studies suggest increased maternal infection, thromboembolic events and pre-eclampsia. Most prevalent in those of African descent it is also prevalent in the Caribbean, Middle East, Mediterranean, parts of India, South and Central America. There are 100–200 pregnancies in women with SCD in the UK annually.

Preconception Women with SCD should be under annual clinic review to monitor disease. Arrange sickle specialist preconception review. Advice should cover factors affecting sickling crises (cold, hypoxia, dehydration-hence nausea and vomiting of pregnancy, over-exertion, stress). Pregnancy worsens anaemia, so ↑ risk of crises and acute chest syndrome (ACS)-chest pain, cough, tachypnoea and new infiltrates on CXR: treat as for pneumonia+blood transfusion. Screen for red cell antibodies (if present ↑risk of haemolytic disease of newborn). Pregnancy ↑ risks of infection (especially UTI). Address ↑ risk of fetal growth restriction (hence ↑ induction, ↑caesarean section rates). Address chance of fetus being affected (partner's blood to check carrier/haemoglobinopathy status: genetic counselling if needed). Assess current disease: echocardiography if not done in last year to exclude pulmonary hypertension (tricuspid regurgitant jet velocity >2.5m/s high risk, p20); BP & urinalysis, U&E, LFT; retinal screening (proliferative retinopathy common); screen for iron overload if multiply transfused (if significantly overloaded, preconception chelation therapy is advised). SCD is a hyposplenic state; advise daily penicillin or erythromycin and update vaccines: hepatitis B, single dose haemophilus influenza B & meningococcal C, 5-yearly pneumococcal, and annual H1N1 with seasonal influenza. Stop ACE/A2A drugs & hydroxycarbamide ≥3 months, preconceptually. Give 5mg folic acid daily (p2) preconceptually (requirement ↑ as haemolysis).

Antenatal care Ensure preconception measures addressed. Manage by specialist multidisciplinary team if possible; if not, by 'high-risk' team using protocols. If fetus has haemoglobinopathy risk, offer prenatal testing by 8–10 weeks. From 12 weeks give 75mg aspirin daily to reduce risk of developing pre-eclampsia. Suggest graduated compression stockings in pregnancy. If hospitalized, give heparin thromboprophylaxis. Check BP at all antenatal visits and an MSU monthly. Offer viability scan at 7–9 weeks, dating scan at 11–14, anomaly scan at 20, and growth scan 4-weekly from 24 weeks. Only supplement iron if proven deficiency. Blood transfusion is not routine; if needed for sickling complication use fully compatible rhesus C,D,E and Kell typed CMV-negative blood (if so, transfusion regimen may be needed for rest of pregnancy). Top up transfusions may be needed if Hb falls to 6 or by 2g/dL from booking. *Crises* affect 27–50%. Admit if fever, severe or atypical pain, chest pain, or breathless. If pain needs IV opiates use morphine/diamorphine (not pethidine, it risks fits); give nasal O₂ if oxygen sats <95% (take to ITU if O₂ sats not maintained), and adequate fluid intake 60mL/kg/h PO/IV unless pre-eclampsia (then specialist advice). Exchange transfusion is needed for acute chest syndrome or if stroke.

Intrapartum care Aim for delivery at 38 weeks at hospitals able to manage SCD and high-risk pregnancy. Keep warm and hydrated in labour/post-partum. Monitor fetus, and maternal O₂ sats. Avoid pethidine (above). Give 7d heparin thromboprophylaxis post vaginal delivery, 6 weeks if caesarean. Progestogenic contraception is that of choice.

In pregnancy cardiac output (co) increases to a maximum of 30–40% > non-pregnant levels by ↑ heart rate and stroke volume. Twins ↑ co 30% more.

Heart disease affects <1% of pregnant women. Examine the heart carefully early in all pregnancies. Ask the opinion of a cardiologist if there is doubt: •Past history (eg congenital heart disease, rheumatic fever). •Previous Kawasaki disease (now a more common cause of acquired heart disease than rheumatic fever). •Murmurs (other than 5–7 in the list below).

60% of maternal cardiac deaths occur after delivery. Cardiac failure can occur at any stage in pregnancy (risk ↑ in later pregnancy, and highest in the early puerperium). Eisenmenger's syndrome risks maternal mortality (MM) of 30%; pulmonary hypertension (MM= 30–50%); coarctation of the aorta (surges of BP↑ in the proximal segment), severe aortic or mitral stenosis, and inoperable cyanotic heart disease are associated with ↑MM, so advise against pregnancy—or arrange meticulous specialist care. Seek pre-pregnancy advice for those with Marfan's or Ehlers–Danlos. Termination may be medically advised.

Prosthetic valve anticoagulation: Get expert help. Warfarin risks fetal harm (p640); heparin risks valve thrombosis.[58] Some use IV **heparin** infusion weeks 6–12 and 37–term+7d; warfarin with target level of INR of 3 at other times.

Antenatal management Regular visits to cardiologist/obstetric combined clinic. Prevent anaemia, obesity, and smoking. Ensure sufficient rest. Treat hypertension. Treat infections early. Examine carefully to exclude pulmonary oedema and arrhythmias at all visits. Heart failure requires admission.

Labour Outcome is worst for mothers unable to ↑ their cardiac output (rare). Have O_2 and drugs to treat cardiac failure to hand. Avoid lithotomy position (dangerous ↑ venous return after labour—the best position is semi-sitting). Aim for vaginal delivery at term with a short 2nd stage (lift-out forceps or ventouse). Pain relief should be good. Epidurals are safe if hypotension is avoided. Beware large volumes of IV fluids. Avoid ergometrine (use **oxytocin**, if necessary). Caesarean section should not be done (except during eclampsia) if in heart failure. Heart failure is most likely within the first 24h after delivery, so ensure careful observations at this time.

Cardiac failure If symptoms or signs found, admit for bed rest, and treatment with diuretics ± digoxin. If acute failure develops, give 100% oxygen, nurse semi-recumbent, and give **furosemide** 40mg IV slowly (<4mg/min), **morphine** 10mg IV. Are vasodilators (nitrates or hydralazine) needed? Seek advice on ACE inhibitors. If there is no improvement, consider ventilation.

Arrhythmias *Atrial fibrillation:* Is there mitral stenosis?—admit. ℞ is as for the non-pregnant and may include digitalization or cardioversion. *Narrow complex tachycardia:* may precipitate cardiac failure. If Valsalva manoeuvre and carotid massage fail, anaesthetize and cardiovert.

These signs may be normal in pregnancy
1 Oedema and an increased pulse volume.
2 Vigorously pulsating neck veins (but JVP should not be ↑).
3 The apex beat is forceful (but <2cm lateral to midclavicular line).
4 The first heart sound is loud and a third heart sound can be heard in 84%.
5 An ejection systolic murmur is heard in 96% of women.
6 Systolic or continuous murmurs over either 2nd intercostal spaces 2cm from sternal edge, modified by pressure may be from mammary vessels.
7 Venous hums may be heard in the neck (modified by posture).
8 cxr may show slight cardiomegaly, ↑ pulmonary vascular markings, distension of pulmonary veins due to ↑ cardiac output.

For puerperal depression, see p408.

Try to avoid drugs in pregnancy (eg in depression, cognitive-behaviour therapy is a favoured alternative) but sometimes psychotropics are essential, eg if the mother is neglecting herself or her pregnancy. If used, psychotropic drugs must be combined with well-planned psychosocial support from a trusted confidant of the patient. In those with history of major depression, relapse is higher if prophylactic drugs are discontinued.[59] If used, aim for monotherapy.

Depression in pregnancy—*Unipolar:* For diagnosis, see p336. Try to wait until the 2nd trimester before prescribing. Most experience is with tricyclics such as amitriptyline, and these have lowest known risk in pregnancy,[60]—and are therefore the 1st choice when drugs are essential. They are more dangerous than SSRIs in overdose. It is wise to discuss decisions with another doctor, or your local drug information service. Problems are unlikely, but the exact risk of teratogenesis is unknown. Withdrawal effects have been seen in neonates, eg agitation ± respiratory depression with amitriptyline, and colic, spasms, and hyper- or hypotension with imipramine, convulsions with clomipramine. Get a second opinion if ECT may be indicated. SSRIs should only be used with caution: fluoxetine has lowest known risk in pregnancy. They may cause persistent pulmonary hypertension if used after 20 weeks' gestation. ▶Avoid paroxetine (teratogenic—see p2: neonatal convulsions can be a withdrawal reaction[61] and 1st trimester use may be associated with cardiac malformations).[62] In general, breastfeeding is contraindicated, as metabolites pass to the baby (imipramine, nortriptyline, and sertraline have lowest levels; highest with citalopram and fluoxetine).

Bipolar: Lithium (Li+, p354) *is* linked with teratogenicity (heart defects, including Ebstein's anomaly, p2). Offer specialist fetal echocardiography at 16 weeks in those women electing to stay on Li+. Used outside the 1st trimester, lithium can still cause problems with the fetal renal and thyroid function. Monitor drug levels frequently (exactly 12h post-dose 4-weekly to 36wks, then weekly, and keep the dose as low as possible, and, in general, aim for a level of <0.4mmol/L). Do not change brands, as bioavailability varies. Do extra monitoring during intercurrent illness, D&V, and when poor compliance or toxicity is suspected (tremor, drowsiness, visual disturbance). Deliver in hospital. Monitor fluid balance and avoid dehydration in labour. If lithium is stopped for a pregnancy or labour, restart it within a few days of birth. High doses are excreted in breast milk, so breastfeeding is contraindicated.

Phenothiazines for schizophrenia in pregnancy There is conflicting data on safety—but there is agreement that most pregnancies will be unaffected. Pre-birth exposure may result in a syndrome of hyperreflexia, hypertonia, and tremor, which may persist for the first months of life. NB: rates of fetal abnormality are increased in schizophrenia, even in those taking no drugs. NICE warn of possible raised prolactin levels (hence reduced fertility) with amisulpride, sulpiride, and risperidone; gestational diabetes from weight gain with olanzapine; fetal agranulocytosis if breastfeeding mother on clozapine; and extrapyramidal symptoms in neonate if mother on depot antipsychotics. Low-dose typical antipsychotics eg chlorpromazine are favoured by NICE.

Anxiety in pregnancy Benzodiazepines may be linked to fetal malformation and should be avoided. Avoid diazepam around the time of delivery, as withdrawal may occur in the baby (floppy baby syndrome). Avoid β-blockers, as these retard fetal growth. Relaxation techniques (p344) and supportive psychotherapy (p380) are far more appropriate.

⚕ ►Even a small PPH may become life threatening if the mother is anaemic. Anaemia predisposes to infection, makes heart failure worse, and is the main cause of perinatal problems associated with malaria. Above all, anaemia is a leading mechanism by which poverty exacts its morbid toll in pregnancy.

WHO definition of anaemia of pregnancy Hb <11g/dL. By this standard 50% of women not on haematinics become anaemic. The fall in Hb is steepest around 20 weeks' gestation, and is physiological (p6).

Who is prone to anaemia? Those who start pregnancy anaemic, eg from menorrhagia, hookworm, malaria, with haemoglobinopathies; those with frequent pregnancies, twin pregnancy, or a poor diet.

Antenatal screening includes Hb estimation at booking, at 28 and 36 weeks. In black patients do sickle-cell tests; in others of overseas descent consider Hb electrophoresis for other haemoglobinopathies. From malarious areas consider malaria, and thick films. See p27.

Treatment Pregnancy increases iron needs by 700–1400mg (per pregnancy), provided for by a pregnancy-induced 9-fold increase in iron absorption. Iron and folate supplements (and prevention against hookworm and malaria) are recommended in many developing countries.[63]

Offer *oral iron* (eg ferrous sulfate 200mg/24h PO; twice-weekly may be sufficient if unable to tolerate this)[64] if likely to be iron deficient (see above) or would refuse transfusion if haemorrhaging (p85). *Parenteral iron* may be given (to those with iron deficiency anaemia not tolerating oral iron) as **iron dextran** or **iron sucrose**. Beware anaphylaxis. Use only if cardiopulmonary resuscitation facilities to hand. Hb rises over 6 weeks, so late severe anaemia (Hb <9g/dL) may need blood transfusion. One unit of blood increases the Hb by ~0.7g/dL.

Thalassaemias (*OHCM* p336) These globin chain production disorders are found in Mediterranean, Indian, and South-east Asian populations. Although anaemic, never give parenteral iron as iron levels are usually high. Seek expert advice as to use of oral iron and folate. β-thalassaemia does not affect the fetus but in homozygotes regular transfusions sustain life only until young adulthood. There are α chains in fetal HbF, so in α-thalassaemias the fetus may be anaemic or, if severe, stillborn. Mothers carrying lethally affected hydropic fetuses risk severe pre-eclampsia, and delivery complications due to a large fetus and bulky placenta. Prenatal diagnosis is possible by chorionic villus sampling (p10) for thalassaemias anticipated by parental blood studies.

Sickling disorders can affect people of African origin, Saudi Arabians, Indians, Mediterranean, South and Central American populations. *Sickle-cell trait* is not usually a problem. *Sickle-cell disease* see page 19. *Sickle-cell haemoglobin c disease* is a milder variant of sickle-cell disease. Hb levels are usually near normal so women may be unaware they are affected. They are still susceptible to sickling crises in pregnancy and the puerperium, so antenatal diagnosis is essential. Prenatal sickle-cell diagnosis is possible by chorionic villus sampling.

►Aim for diagnosis at birth (cord blood) at the latest so that penicillin pneumococcal prophylaxis may be started (*OHCM* p334).

Obstetrics

Without interventions ~15% babies acquire HIV if the mother is +ve (↑ risk in Africa; but HIV-2 transmitted less). ►Vertical transmission occurs during vaginal delivery (1st twins are twice as often infected as 2nd). Membrane rupture for >4h doubles risk then ↑ by 2%/h for 24h. Breast feeding doubles risk. Maternal anti-retroviral use, elective caesarean delivery, and bottle feeding attains ≤2% risk.

Offer HIV tests at booking, if declined, again at 28wks. If HIV status unknown in labour rapid (20min) tests are available and are recommended. If positive in labour; use drugs to reduce maternal–fetal transmission (below; seek expert advice). If HIV+ve arrange multidisciplinary care with HIV physician to monitor viral loads, drug regimens and toxicity monitoring. Check for hepatitis B & C, varicella zoster, measles & toxoplasmosis antibodies. Offer hepatitis B, pneumococcal and influenza vaccines (safe in pregnancy). Screen for genital infections at booking and at 28wks. Treat infections, even if asymptomatic (to reduce risk of pre-term birth). Women needing highly active antiretroviral treatment (HAART) for their own health (symptomatic HIV/falling or low CD4 lymphocyte count <350×10⁶/L) should continue treatment throughout pregnancy and postpartum. If on HAART at booking; screen for gestational diabetes and warn of ↑risk of premature labour. If on co-trimoxazole for pneumocystis ji*roveci* prophylaxis (CD4 <200×10⁶/L) add pre-pregnancy/1st trimester 5mg folic acid/day. Women not needing antiretrovirals for their own health should start HAART 20–28wks, taking until delivered. (If good CD4 levels, viral load <10,000 copies/mL, and elective caesarean delivery planned zidovudine monotherapy orally from 20–28wks, IV in labour is an alternative.) Plan mode of delivery by 36wks.

Premature labour If membranes rupture >34wks expedite delivery, whatever the maternal viral load. If membranes rupture <34wks give steroids (p51), give erythromycin (p50), ensure mother takes usual HAART regimen, seek HIV specialist advice on how to optimize her regimen to reduce fetal transmission eg maternal nevirapine crosses placenta with long fetal plasma concentration, plus zidovudine infusion. Determine delivery balancing risks of prematurity, and infection. Manage preterm labour without membrane rupture as if HIV-ve.

Delivery *Vaginal delivery:* Offer to women with viral loads <50 copies/mL, (<400 copies/mL if on HAART).[48,NICE] Continue HAART in labour. Avoid fetal blood sampling/scalp electrodes. Avoid amniotomy unless delivery imminent. Oxytocin can be used for augmentation. Low cavity forceps are preferred over ventouse (less fetal trauma). Avoid mid-cavity or rotational forceps.

Caesarean section: Offer elective caesarean section at 38 weeks' gestation to women if on zidovudine monotherapy (above), if on HAART with viral loads > those above, or if co-infected with hepatitis c. If viral load is <50 copies/mL, and elective section needed, plan for 39+ weeks (this viral load level is acceptable for vaginal delivery so membrane rupture is not of consequence).

Postpartum Avoid breastfeeding in resource-rich countries (breastfeeding doubles HIV transmission risk). Cabergoline 1mg PO within 24h of birth is recommended to suppress lactation. Newborns are treated within 4h of birth eg zidovudine twice daily for 4 weeks; HAART if high risk eg untreated mothers; mother with viral loads >50copies/mL despite being on HAART. Co-trimoxazole (PCP) prophylaxis is given to babies at high risk of transmission. Babies are tested at day 1, 6wks and 12wks for HIV with confirmatory test at 18 months. Affected women should have annual smears. Condoms, intrauterine systems (eg Mirena®) and depot progesterone injections are all suitable for women on HAART. Some antiretrovirals are enzyme inducers so may effect efficiency of progesterone only, and combined (so use high dose) pills. Check if maternal MMR vaccine (if CD4 count >200/mL, contraindicated if lower), and varicella zoster vaccine (only if CD4 count >400/mL) required.

Obstetrics

▶Meticulous control around conception decreases malformation rates.

Preconception Avoid unplanned pregnancy. Adjust insulin to optimize control preconception (values as antenatally, below). Aim for HbA1c of ≤6.1% (avoid pregnancy if HbA1c >10%). Give 5mg folic acid daily preconception (p2). Arrange dietetic review. Stop oral hypoglycaemics (except metformin), statins, ACE and A2A inhibitors (use other antihypertensive p31, if needed). Treat retinopathy pre-pregnancy. Retinopathy screen; ≤20% develop proliferative retinopathy. Nephropathy may worsen; if severe, avoid pregnancy. DM may develop in pregnancy (GDM, p8). Glycosuria unrelated to DM is common (GFR ↑ and tubular glucose reabsorption ↓). Non-diabetic blood glucose levels in pregnancy are constant (3.5–4.5mmol/L) except after meals. Fetal glycaemia follows maternal. Compensatory fetal hyperinsulinaemia promotes fetal growth.

Complications *Maternal:* Hypoglycaemia unawareness (esp 1st trimester) so warn about it. Hydramnios (?fetal polyuria), preterm labour, stillbirth. *Fetal:* Malformation rates ↑ ×3 (sacral agenesis, almost exclusive to diabetic offspring, is rare; CNS & CVS malformations much commoner). Babies may be macrosomic (too large) or growth restricted. *Neonatal risks:* Hypoglycaemia, Ca²⁺↓, Mg²⁺↓, and RDS (p118), polycythaemia—so more neonatal jaundice.

Antenatal care Use care plan & review in joint clinic (p3). Confirm gestation with early ultrasound. Detailed abnormality scan at 19–20 weeks. Fetal echo at 18–20 weeks. Educate about benefits of normoglycaemia. Aim for home monitored glucose 1h after every meal (postprandial) and before bed. Insulin needs increase by 50–100% as pregnancy progresses so review regularly. Aim for fasting level 3.5–5.9mmol/L; 1h post-prandial level <7.8mmol/L. Give Glucogel® and glucagon kit (ensure partner knows how to use). Exclude ketoacidosis if unwell. Assess renal function; refer to nephrologist if creatinine >120μmol/L, protein excretion >2g/24h (use thromboprophylaxis if >5g/24h). Admit if adequate control unachievable at home. Metformin can be used in pregnancy.

Monitor fetal growth & wellbeing by ultrasound and cardiotocography (p3).

Delivery Deliver the baby where there are good neonatal facilities. NICE recommends elective delivery at 38 weeks.⁶⁶ₙᵢcₑ *In labour:* Avoid acidosis and monitor the fetus (p44). Avoid maternal hyperglycaemia (causes fetal hypoglycaemia). Monitor glucose; prevent hyperglycaemia with extra insulin (may need 5u/h) if glucocorticoids are used in preterm labour. Aim for vaginal delivery with labour of <12h. Beware shoulder dystocia with macrosomic babies. With elective delivery, give normal insulin the evening before induction. During labour give 1L of 5–10% **glucose**/8h IVI with 1–2u **insulin**/h via a pump. Aim for a blood glucose of 4.5–5.5mmol/L (check hourly). Insulin needs fall as labour progresses and immediately postpartum. Stop infusions at delivery. Return to pre-pregnancy regimen. Do a caesarean section if labour is prolonged. Clamp cord early (polycythaemia risk).

Postnatal •Encourage breastfeeding (metformin and glibenclamide are compatible with breastfeeding). •Encourage pre-pregnancy counselling *before* next pregnancy (p2) to transfer to insulin if needed. •If preproliferative retinopathy review ophthalmologically for 6 months. •Discuss contraception.

Gestational diabetes (OGTT glucose ≥7.8mmol/L, OHCM p198) *Incidence:* 3%.⁶⁷ For screening and who to screen see p8. Monitor glucose if diagnosed. If levels not controlled by diet and exercise over 1–2 weeks consider oral hypoglycaemics (metformin, glibenclamide–note NICE and product characteristic sheets conflicting advice) or insulin. 50% get full DM, so give lifelong dietary advice and follow-up.⁶⁸ Check fasting glucose 6 weeks postpartum.

▶Exercise, a good diet, and no smoking all help lower this risk.

*See diabetic care plan p3.

▶Whenever a mother isn't quite right postpartum, check her TSH & free T_4—but note that any apparent hypothyroidism may be transitory.

Biochemical changes in normal pregnancy NB: normal pregnancy mimics hyperthyroidism (pulse ↑, warm moist skin, slight goitre, anxiety).
• Thyroid binding globulin & T_4 output rise to maintain free T_4 levels, p15.
• High levels of HCG mimic thyroid stimulating hormone (TSH).
• There is reduced availability of iodine (in iodine-limited localities).
• TSH may fall below normal in the first trimester (suppressed by HCG).
• The best thyroid tests in pregnancy are free T_4, free T_3, and TSH.

Pre-pregnancy hyperthyroidism Treatment options include antithyroid drugs (but 60% relapse on stopping treatment), radioactive iodine (contraindicated in pregnancy or breastfeeding: avoid pregnancy for 4 months after use), or surgery. Fertility is reduced by hyperthyroidism.

Hyperthyroidism in pregnancy (Usually Graves' disease.) There is ↑ risk of prematurity, fetal loss, and, maybe, malformation. Severity of hyperthyroidism often falls in pregnancy. Transient exacerbations may occur (1st trimester & postpartum). Propylthiouracil is the best treatment.[69] Keep dose as low as possible. Monitor ≥monthly. Some advocate stopping antithyroid drugs in the last month of pregnancy. Propylthiouracil is preferred postpartum (less concentrated in breast milk). If hyperthyroidism cannot be controlled by drugs, partial thyroidectomy can be done in the 2nd trimester. TRAb (TSH-receptor stimulating antibodies): ↑levels can cause fetal hyperthyroidism after 24wks causing premature delivery; craniosynostosis so intellectual impairment; goitre so polyhydramnios; extended neck in labour. Note labour, delivery, surgery, and anaesthesia can precipitate thyroid storm (fever, tachycardia, changed mental state—agitation, psychosis, coma) requiring urgent treatment.

Hypothyroidism Associated with relative infertility, untreated hypothyroidism risks ↑ rates of miscarriage, stillbirth, premature labour, and abnormality. Optimize T_4 preconception (p2). Increase levothyroxine by 30% as soon as knows pregnant.[70] Monitor replacement by T_4 and TSH measurement 6-weekly. Aim for TSH ≤2.5mu/L. Use pre-pregnancy levothyroxine doses postpartum.

Postpartum thyroiditis Prevalence: 5%. Hyperthyroidism is followed by hypothyroidism (~4 months postpartum). The hyperthyroid phase does not usually need treatment as it is self-limiting. If treatment is required β-blockers are usually sufficient. Antithyroid drugs are ineffective as thyrotoxicosis is from thyroid destruction releasing thyroxine, rather than increased synthesis. Monitor the hypothyroid phase for >6 months, and treat if symptomatic. Withdraw treatment after 6–12 months for 4 weeks to see if long-term therapy is required. 90% have thyroid antiperoxidase antibodies; 5% of antibody positive women become permanently hypothyroid each year so monitor annually. Hypothyroidism may be associated with postpartum depression, so check thyroid status of women with postpartum depression.

Neonatal thyrotoxicosis Seen in 1% of babies of women with past Graves' disease, as TRAb crosses the placenta. Signs: fetal tachycardia (>160/min) in late pregnancy ± intrauterine growth restriction. If mother has been on antithyroid drugs signs may not be manifest until the baby has metabolized the drug (7–10 days postpartum). Test thyroid function in affected babies frequently. Antithyroid drugs may be needed. It resolves spontaneously at 2–3 months, but perceptual motor difficulties, and hyperactivity can occur later in childhood.

Thyroid antibodies Presence of these increase rates of miscarriage and preterm delivery; randomized studies suggest thyroxine treatment may reduce miscarriage in euthyroid women with antibodies.[71]

▶Get expert help *promptly*. Jaundice in pregnancy may be lethal. Know exactly what drugs were taken and when (*prescribed* or *over-the-counter*). Where has she travelled to? What lifestyle or occupational risks are there?

Jaundice occurs in 1 in 1500 pregnancies. Viral hepatitis and gallstones may cause jaundice in pregnancy and investigation is similar to the non-pregnant. Those with Gilbert's and Dubin–Johnson syndrome (*OHCM* p714) do well in pregnancy (jaundice may be exacerbated with the latter).

Tests Do all the usual tests (*OHCM* p250), eg urine tests for bile, serology, LFTs, and ultrasound.

Intrahepatic cholestasis of pregnancy[72,NICE] Incidence: 0.1–1.5% pregnancies in Europe. There is pruritus, especially of palms and soles in the second half of pregnancy. Liver transaminases are mildly ↑ (<300u/L) in 60%, ↑ bilirubin in 25%. Exclude viral hepatitis. There is risk of preterm labour, fetal distress, and stillbirth, so monitor fetal wellbeing. Give **vitamin K** 10mg PO/24h to the mother, and 1mg IM to the baby at birth. **Ursodeoxycholic** acid reduces pruritus and abnormal LFTs. Symptoms resolve within days of delivery. It is a contraindication to oestrogen-containing contraceptive pills. It recurs in 40% pregnancies.

Acute fatty liver of pregnancy Incidence: 1 : 6600–13,000 deliveries—so it is rare but grave. The mother develops abdominal pain, jaundice, headache, vomiting, ± thrombocytopenia and pancreatitis. There is associated pre-eclampsia in 30–60% (±postpartum). It usually occurs after 30 weeks. There is hepatic steatosis with micro-droplets of fat in liver cells. Deep jaundice, uraemia, severe hypoglycaemia, and clotting disorder may develop causing coma and death. Monitor BP. Give supportive treatment for liver and renal failure and treat hypoglycaemia vigorously (CVP line). Correct clotting disorders. Enlist haematologist's help. Expedite delivery. Epidural and regional anaesthesia are CI. Monitor postpartum. Beware PPH and neonatal hypoglycaemia. Mortality can be as low as 18% maternal and 23% fetal.

Some other causes of jaundice in pregnancy
• Viral hepatitis; ALT ↑, eg >200u/L; maternal mortality ↑ (~20%) in E virus,[48,NICE] treatment is supportive. Hepatitis C is thought to affect <1% of women in the UK at present. Vertical transmission affects about 5% of babies. Elective caesarean delivery is only recommended for those with coexistent HIV.[48,NICE] Passive antibodies transferred from the mother wane by 18 months. Check baby for HCV RNA at 2–3 months (& 12 months, and anti HCV antibody at 12–18 months), refer baby to paediatric hepatologist if HCV RNA positive.[73] Currently screening is not planned. Refer infected women for specialist treatment to clear the viral infection after birth (*OHCM* p470).
• The jaundice of severe pre-eclampsia (hepatic rupture and infarction can occur); ALT <500u/L; bilirubin <86μmol/L.
• Rarely, complicating hyperemesis gravidarum (can be fatal); ALT <200u/L.
• Hepatitis may occur if halothane is used for anaesthesia (so avoid it).
• HELLP syndrome (haemolysis, elevated liver enzymes, and low platelet count). Incidence in pregnancy: 0.1–0.6%; in pre-eclampsia: 4–12%. It causes upper abdo pain, malaise, vomiting, headache, jaundice, microangiopathic haemolytic anaemia, DIC, LDH ↑, ALT ↑ <500u/L, bilirubin <86μmol/L. It recurs in 20%. Treatment: get expert help. Admit; deliver if severe.

Hepatitis B Check HBsAG in all women with jaundice and look for IgM anti-HBc to detect acute infection. Avoid contact with blood during delivery and be careful with disposal of 'sharps'. Babies need immunoglobulin and vaccination at birth (p151). Transplacental infection may be reduced by maternal lamivudine[74] (seek expert advice). Offer vaccination to all the family.

Malaria in pregnancy

In any woman who presents with odd behaviour, fever, jaundice, sweating, DIC, fetal distress, premature labour, seizures, or loss of consciousness, always ask yourself: ►*Could this be malaria?* If so, do thick and thin films. Confirm (or exclude) pregnancy. Seek expert help, eg from Liverpool, below.

Falciparum malaria is dangerous (and complicated) in pregnancy, particularly in those with no malaria immunity. Cerebral malaria has a 50% mortality in pregnancy. 3rd-stage placental autotransfusion may lead to fatal pulmonary oedema. Hypoglycaemia may be a feature (both of malaria itself and secondary to quinine). There is increased susceptibility to sepsis. Women with coexistent HIV have less good pregnancy outcomes (fetal and maternal).

Other associations between *falciparum* malaria and pregnancy are anaemia, miscarriage, stillbirth, low birth weight, and prematurity. PPH is also more common. Hyperreactive malaria splenomegaly (occurs typically where malaria is holoendemic) may contribute to anaemia via increased haemolysis.

Vivax malaria is less dangerous, but can cause anaemia and ↓ birth weight.

Treating malaria ►*OHCM* p396; ►►cerebral malaria, *OHCM* p397. In severe *falciparum* artesunate 2.4mg/kg IV at 0, 12, & 24h then daily until can take oral artesunate+clindamycin is 1st line, if available (tel 08451 555000 tropical medical registrar for advice/supply), or load with quinine 20mg/kg IVI over 4h in 5% glucose (max 1.4g) (do not load if on quinine/mefloquine). Then 10mg/kg IVI over 4h in 5% glucose every 8h with 450mg clindamycin/8h IV. Beware hypoglycaemia with quinine. Switch to artesunate regimen as soon as it is available.[75] When severe treat on ITU. If haematocrit <20% give slow transfusion of packed cells, with 20mg furosemide. Include the volume of packed cells in fluid balance calculations. Consider exchange transfusion. Beware hyperpyrexia (fan, give paracetamol); renal failure; pulmonary oedema; and sepsis (if shock do blood cultures give IV ceftriaxone). Get expert help. Uncomplicated *falciparum* and resistant *vivax* are treated for 7 days with quinine 600mg with clindamycin 450mg/8h PO. Non-resistant *vivax, ovale* and *malariae* are treated with chloroquine orally over 3 days with weekly dose to prevent relapse during pregnancy. 3 months after delivery (and G6PD testing) primaquine is then given for *ovale* and *vivax* prevention of relapse.

If infection peripartum, anticipate fetal distress, fluid-balance problems, and hypoglycaemia in labour. Monitor appropriately. After any infection send placenta for histology and placental, cord, and baby blood (weekly×4) for blood films to check if baby infected (0.3–4% are), and treat baby if infected.

Prevention in UK women Advise against visiting malarious areas. If it is unavoidable, give prophylaxis (*OHCM* p396). Emphasize importance of preventive measures such as mosquito nets and insect repellents. Normal dose chloroquine and proguanil if *P. falciparum* strains are sensitive. With proguanil, give concurrent folic acid 5mg/day. If chloroquine resistance mefloquine is best.

Mefloquine is recommended for 2nd and 3rd trimester use.[76] Heed strict contraindications (eg epilepsy, neuropsychiatric disorder). If unsuitable, Malarone® (atovaquone-proguanil, with folic acid) is an alternative in 2nd and 3rd trimester for chloroquine or mefloquine resistant areas. 1st trimester prophylaxis is a problem. Seek expert advice (eg tel 0845 602 6712).

Mothers living in endemic areas Chemoprophylaxis improves birthweight (by ~250g, with fewer very low birthweight babies). Red cell mass also rises. WHO advises intermittent preventive treatment (IPT) eg with 2 or 3 doses of sulfadoxine-pyrimethamine (SP) during pregnancy, but monthly doses are better if HIV +ve.[78] But SP causes Stevens–Johnson syndrome in 1 in 7000, and resistance to SP has spread fast, so new IPT regimens need urgent evaluation in pregnancy.[79] Dihydroartemisinin-piperaquine (Artekin®) is a good candidate.[80]

►If in doubt, phone an expert, eg, in the UK, at Liverpool (tel. 0151 705 3100).

Obstetrics

Note: Values considered normal when not pregnant may reflect decreased renal function in pregnancy. Creatinine >75µmol/L and urea >4.5mmol/L merit further investigation. See p15. Glycosuria in pregnancy may reflect altered renal physiology and not necessarily imply hyperglycaemia.

▶Treat asymptomatic bacteriuria in pregnancy. Check that infection and bacteriuria clear with treatment.

Asymptomatic bacteriuria Found in 2% of sexually active women it is commoner (up to 7%) during pregnancy—especially in diabetics and in those with renal transplants. With the dilatation of the calyces and ureters that occurs in pregnancy, 25% will go on to develop pyelonephritis, which can cause fetal growth restriction, fetal death, and premature labour. This is the argument for screening all women for bacteriuria at booking. If present on 2 MSUs treatment is given (eg **amoxicillin** 250mg/8h PO with a high fluid intake). Test for cure after 1 and 2 weeks. If the organism is not sensitive to amoxicillin, consider nitrofurantoin 50mg/6h PO with food. It recurs in 30% (so keep screening).[81]

Pyelonephritis This may present as malaise with urinary frequency or as a more florid picture with raised temperature, tachycardia, vomiting, and loin pain. It is common at around 20 weeks and in the puerperium. Urinary infections should always be carefully excluded in those with hyperemesis gravidarum and those admitted with premature labour. Treatment is with bed rest and plenty of fluids. After blood and urine culture give IV antibiotics (eg **ampicillin** 500mg/6h IV, according to sensitivities) if oral drugs cannot be used (eg if vomiting). Treat for 2–3 weeks. MSUs should be checked every fortnight for the rest of the pregnancy. 20% of women having pyelonephritis in pregnancy have underlying renal tract abnormalities and an IVU or ultrasound at 16 weeks' postpartum should be considered. In those who suffer repeated infection, **nitrofurantoin** (100mg/24h PO with food) may prevent recurrences. Avoid if the glomerular filtration rate is <50mL/min. SE: vomiting, peripheral neuropathy, pulmonary infiltration, and liver damage.

Chronic renal disease With mild renal impairment (pre-pregnancy creatinine <125mmol/L) without hypertension there is little evidence that pregnancy accelerates renal disorders. Patients with marked anaemia, hypertension, retinopathy, or heavy proteinuria should avoid pregnancy as further deterioration in renal function may be expected. Close collaboration between physicians and obstetricians during pregnancy in those with renal disease is the aim. Induction of labour may become advisable in those with hypertension and proteinuria, or if fetal growth is retarded.

Pregnancy for those on dialysis is fraught with problems (fluid overload, hypertension, pre-eclampsia, polyhydramnios). A 50% increase in dialysis is needed. Live birth outcome is 50–70%. Outcome is better for those with renal transplants, but up to 10% of mothers die within 7 years from birth.

Obstetric causes of acute tubular necrosis Acute tubular necrosis may be a complication of any of the following situations:
• Septicaemia (eg from miscarriage with infection, or pyelonephritis).
• Haemolysis (eg sickling crisis, malaria).
• Hypovolaemia, eg in pre-eclampsia; haemorrhage (APH, eg abruption, PPH, or intrapartum); DIC; miscarriage—or adrenal failure in those on steroids not receiving booster doses to cover labour.

Whenever these situations occur, monitor urine output carefully (catheterize the bladder). Aim for >30mL/h output. Monitor renal function (U&E, creatinine). Dialysis may be needed (*OHCM* p304).

Obstetrics

►The key to successful pregnancy is access to good preconception counselling (p2). Anti-epileptic drugs are normally specialist initiated; ask for a review if pregnancy may be considered.

►If seizures occur in pregnancy, think *could this be eclampsia?*

Epilepsy *de novo* is rare in pregnancy. Epilepsy affects ~0.5% of women of childbearing age so a unit with 3000 deliveries per year has ~15 pregnant epileptic women at any one time. Seizure rates worsen in most women having >1 seizure/month. Sleep deprivation in the last month of pregnancy may contribute to seizures. It is unusual for seizures to recur in pregnancy when preceded by a long seizure-free period.

Complications—*Maternal:* ↑ Risk of 3rd trimester vaginal bleeding. 1% convulse in labour. *Fetal:* • Haemorrhagic disease of newborn can occur with enzyme inducers (below). • Congenital malformation (UK register suggests 6.2% affected with sodium valproate, 2.2% with carbamazepine, 3.2% with lamotrigine).[82] Malformation is commoner if ≥2 anticonvulsants are used and with higher doses. *Fetal valproate syndrome:* Signs: major organ system anomalies ± autism ± small ears, small broad nose, a long upper lip, shallow philtrum & micro/retrognathia.[1] *Cleft lip:* Associated with maternal epilepsy only, the relative risk for a fetus having clefts compared to the non-epileptic population is 1.0 if the mother develops epilepsy after the pregnancy; 2.4 if she develops it after conception (but has no drugs); 4.7 if fetus is exposed to anticonvulsants. Phenytoin and phenobarbital cause clefts and congenital heart disease. *Neural tube defects* are commoner with valproate (& carbamazepine) so screen for these (p10). Reduced cognitive function is seen with valproate (at age 3);[83] seen as lower intelligence quotient (also seen in the offspring of those having frequent tonic clonic seizures in pregnancy).[84]

Management ►Get expert help (refer to epilepsy specialist to optimize and monitor medication: only make antiepileptic changes on expert advice). Carbamazepine may be drug of choice in pregnancy.[85] Lamotrigine dose usually needs to be increased in pregnancy to maintain seizure control. Where anticonvulsants are needed keep the dose of the chosen drug as low as possible. Aim for 1 drug only. Give **folic acid** supplements, eg 5mg/24h PO from prior to conception. Give **vitamin K** 20mg/24h PO to the mother from 36 weeks if she is taking enzyme inducers, ie carbamazepine, ethosuximide, phenytoin, primidone, phenobarbital (oxcarbazine and topiramate are subjects of debate). Screen for neural tube defects and heart disease if relevant (above). Treat status epilepticus as in the non-pregnant but monitor the fetus. It is associated with significant fetal and maternal mortality. Deliver in hospital with resuscitation facilities (1–2% epileptic women convulse in labour and the subsequent 48 hours) and avoid early discharge. Give baby **vitamin K** 1mg IM at birth. If seizures are likely, to avoid dropping the baby during a seizure, advise changing the baby on mat on floor, and feeding sitting on floor supported by cushions; only bath the baby with supervision. Mothers showering, not bathing reduces risk of drowning. Mothers may breastfeed (phenobarbital can cause drowsiness in the baby). Ask for review of epilepsy drugs postnatally eg at 12 weeks.

Encourage mother to register pregnancy at www.epilepsyandpregnancy.co.uk. or tel 0800 389 1245.

---

[1] Of those affected 62% had musculoskeletal abnormalities, 26% had cardiovascular abnormalities, 22% had genital abnormalities, and 16% had pulmonary abnormalities.[86]

Rheumatoid arthritis is usually alleviated by pregnancy (but exacerbations may occur in the puerperium). Methotrexate use is contraindicated (teratogenic); sulfasalazine may be used (give extra folate). Azathioprine use may cause intrauterine growth restriction and penicillamine may weaken fetal collagen. Non-steroidal anti-inflammatories can be used in the first and second trimesters but are not recommended in the third as they can cause premature closure of the ductus arteriosus and late in pregnancy have been associated with renal impairment in the newborn. Anti-tumour necrosis factor TNF-alpha therapies have not shown problems; but experience is limited.[87] Congenital heart block is a rare fetal feature. Deliver babies with heart block as below.

Systemic lupus erythematosus SLE exacerbations are commoner in pregnancy and the puerperium. Most are mild to moderate involving skin, but those with renal involvement and hypertension may deteriorate and are prone to pre-eclampsia. Of those with SLE glomerulonephritis and a creatinine >130μmol prior to conception only 50% achieve a live birth. Pre-eclampsia, oligohydramnios, and intrauterine growth restriction may occur. Both hydralazine and methyldopa can be used in pre-eclampsia.

Planned pregnancy should be embarked on after 6 months' stable disease without requiring cytotoxic suppression. Disease suppression may be maintained with azathioprine and hydroxychloroquine. Aspirin 75mg daily should be started prior to conception and continued throughout pregnancy, and the fetus should be carefully monitored.

Rarely, the fetus is affected by maternal antibodies that cause a self-limiting sunlight sensitive rash (usually face and scalp) for which no treatment is required; or anti-Ro or anti-La antibodies irreversibly damage the fetal heart conduction system causing congenital heart block (~65% require a pacemaker). Deliver by caesarean or monitor fetal blood gases in labour.

Mothers requiring ≥ 7.5mg daily prednisolone in the 2 weeks before delivery should receive **hydrocortisone 100mg/6h** IV in labour.

Antiphospholipid syndrome Those affected have antiphospholipid antibodies (lupus anticoagulant and/or anticardiolipin antibodies on 2 tests taken >8 weeks apart) ± past arterial thrombosis, venous thrombosis, or recurrent pregnancy loss. It may be primary, or follow other connective tissue disorder (usually SLE in which it occurs in 10%). Outcome: Untreated, <20% of pregnancies proceed to a live birth due to 1st trimester loss or placental thrombosis (causes placental insufficiency, leading to intrauterine growth restriction and fetal death).

Careful regular fetal assessment (Doppler flow studies and ultrasound for growth) is required from 20 weeks as appropriate obstetric intervention can substantially increase the number of live-born babies.

Management: Affected women are treated from conception with aspirin 75mg daily and heparin eg enoxaparin 40mg SC/24h from when fetal heart identified (~6 weeks) until 34 weeks. Those who have suffered prior thromboses receive heparin throughout pregnancy. See p33.

Postpartum use either heparin or warfarin (breastfeeding contraindicated with neither) as risk of thrombosis is high.

Pregnancies in those with SLE (especially with renal disease) and antiphospholipid syndrome require specialist management.

Hypertension in pregnancy

Chronic hypertension is hypertension predating pregnancy or developing before 20 weeks' gestation. *Gestational hypertension* is that, without proteinuria, which develops after 20 weeks' gestation. Hypertension with proteinuria is *pre-clampsia* see p48–49.

Chronic hypertension *Preconception:* ACE inhibitors, A2A blockers and chlorothiazide risk congenital abnormality so change these pre-conception to more suitable preparation and encourage low sodium intake or use of salt substitute. Atenolol, labetalol, metoprolol and methyldopa are licensed for use throughout pregnancy. *Antenatal:* Ensure suitable antihypertensive is being used (above). Aim for BP <150/90 (140/90 if end organ damage), but with diastolic ≥80. If hypertension is secondary to another disorder involve a specialist in hypertensive disorders. Give aspirin 75mg/24h/PO from 12 weeks until the baby is born. At 28–30 and 32–34 weeks arrange ultrasound to assess fetal growth, amniotic fluid volume and umbilical artery velocity: if normal at 34 weeks do not repeat. If fetal activity is abnormal arrange cardiotocography (CTG). During labour, monitor BP hourly if BP <159/109, continuously if ≥160/100. If severe hypertension does not respond to treatment advise operative delivery. Give oxytocin alone at 3rd stage of labour. Postnatally check BP on days 1, 2, and once on days 3–5 and at 2 weeks. Change methyldopa to another antihypertensive post delivery as risk of postnatal depression. Avoid diuretics if breastfeeding (labetalol, atenolol, metoprolol, captopril, and enalapril are safe).

Gestational hypertension needs assessment in secondary care, with urine testing for proteinuria with automated reagent strip readings or urine protein/creatinine ratio testing. Check urine and BP weekly if mild (BP 140/90–149/99) but start treatment eg with labetalol PO if >150/100 and check BP and urine twice weekly. If BP ≥160/110 admit to hospital, measure BP 4 times daily and check urine daily and check FBC, U&E, AST/ALT and bilirubin at presentation and weekly. If BP is mild do ultrasound/CTG as above but do ultrasound fortnightly if BP severe. Repeat CTG if there is a PV bleed, abdominal pain, reduced fetal movements or maternal deterioration. Aim for delivery after 37 weeks unless pre-eclampsia (p49) supervenes. During labour continue antihypertensives, monitor BP hourly (continuously if >160/110). If BP is outside target range (>160/110) advise operative delivery. Continue antenatal hypotensives postnatally (as above), reducing treatment if BP <130/80. Review at 2 and 6 weeks. If treatment is still needed at 6 weeks arrange review with specialist in hypertensive disorders.

Obstetrics

▶*Investigate any unexplained calf or chest symptoms today.* Thromboembolism is a chief UK cause of maternal death. VTE risk rises 6-fold in pregnancy (~0.1–0.2% of pregnancies: 20–50% occur antenatally—in *any* trimester. For those at special risk see p16. 50% of those with 1st VTE have *thrombophilia* (p33), so check for this. Where clinical suspicion is strong but tests negative, start treatment; stop only after repeat negative tests 1 week later.[88] Before starting heparin take blood for: FBC, U&E, LFTs, coagulation screen.

Pulmonary embolism Small emboli may cause unexplained pyrexia, syncope, cough, chest pain, and breathlessness. Pleurisy should be considered due to embolism unless there is high fever or much purulent sputum. Large emboli present as collapse with chest pain, breathlessness, and cyanosis. There will be a raised JVP, third heart sound, and parasternal heave.

Tests: Do CXR (normal in 50%). Scan legs for venous thrombi (if thrombi seen V/Q and CTPA (below) not needed as treatment indicated). Blood gases may be helpful (P_aO_2↓; P_aCO_2↓). If PE still suspected do V/Q scan, spiral CT, or CT pulmonary angiography (CTPA). Maternal breast radiation is higher with CTPA increasing lifetime breast cancer risk by 13% but V/Q increases risk of childhood cancer more, as fetal radiation is higher. Exclude neonatal hypothyroidism after CTPA as iodinated contrast medium is used.

Treatment: Massive emboli may require prolonged cardiac massage, thrombolysis, percutaneous catheter thrombus fragmentation or pulmonary embolectomy. Give unfractionated heparin eg 80u/kg IV stat then 18u/kg/h IVI in 0.9% saline by syringe pump. Omit the stat dose if thrombolysis has been used. Monitor APTT at 6h from stat dose and after dose changes, and /24h. (Target value APTT 1.5–2.5.) Adjust dose as needed[89] (usual 1000–2000u/h). After 3–7 days IV heparin maintain on longterm heparin (eg 10,000u/12h sc) with careful monitoring. Problems: maternal osteopenia (reversible on stopping); thrombocytopenia; allergic skin rashes; alopecia. Monitor platelets every 2–3 days from day 4.

For less massive emboli, low molecular weight heparin (LMWH) eg enoxaparin (see below) is good treatment. (Warfarin is teratogenic in pregnancy —Conradi–Hünermann syndrome, p640 and is used antenatally up to 36 weeks only in those with artificial heart valves.) SC heparin is continued throughout pregnancy (see below). Treat for at least 6 weeks postpartum and 3 months from embolus. Some choose **warfarin** instead after 3 days postpartum.

Deep vein thrombosis (DVT) Suspect if leg pain/discomfort (especially left); swelling; oedema; ↑T°; ↑WCC; lower abdominal pain. *Tests:* Compression duplex ultrasound. If iliac vein thrombosis suspected (back pain/entire limb swollen) do MRI or contrast venography. If iliac thrombosis consider use of inferior vena caval filter perinatally.[89][RCOL] *Treatment:* Use class 2 compression stockings. Initially elevate the leg; then mobilize wearing stockings. Give heparin throughout pregnancy eg enoxaparin 1mg/kg/12h sc (based on early pregnancy weight). Check platelets every 2–4 days (2–14 days if on LMWH). Stop injections at onset of labour, 24h before planned delivery. Do not use regional anaesthesia until >24h since last dose LMWH. If caesarean section, use drains and wound clips or interrupted sutures in case of wound haematoma. Restart heparin 3h post-op (or >4h from epidural; do not remove epidural catheter within 12h of LMWH use).

Postpartum enoxaparin can be reduced to 1.5mg/kg/24h. If warfarin chosen (after 3rd day) postpartum, monitor INR meticulously. Treat for at least 6 weeks postpartum and 3 months from thrombosis. Compression stockings should be worn for 2 years (reduces post-thrombotic syndrome incidence from 23% to 11%).[89][RCOL] Both heparin and warfarin are fine if breastfeeding.

Prophylaxis See p16.

Thrombophilia is a tendency to increased clotting and many underlying causes are now known to contribute. Collectively, the conditions below affect at least 15% of Western populations, but are found in 50% of those with episodes of venous thromboembolism. Conditions include:

- Factor V Leiden mutation* decreases factor V breakdown by protein C (activated protein C (APC) resistance). This affects ~4% of the population and increases thrombotic risk 5–8.3 times (heterozygotes). Homozygous individuals have 10–34 times the risk of venous thromboembolism.
- Protein C deficiency* (affects 0.3% of population; increasing thrombotic risk 2–4.8 times).
- Protein S deficiency* (affects 2% of population; ↑ thrombotic risk 3.2 times).
- Antithrombin III deficiency* (affects 0.02% of population; thrombotic risk is increased 4.7–10 times).
- Acquired thrombophilia. This is lupus anticoagulant ± cardiolipin antibody*. Women with lupus anticoagulant risk arterial and venous thrombosis; in atypical veins, eg portal or arm.
- G20210A mutation of the prothrombin gene (1% of the population). Thrombotic risk is increased 3–10 times for heterozygotes, 26.4 times in homozygotes
- Homozygosity for the thermolabile variant of methylene tetrahydrofolate reductase (C677T MTHFR), which leads to homocysteinaemia (10% of the population). No association was found between venous thromboembolism and homozygosity for C677T MTHFR mutation, perhaps because plasma homocysteine reduces in pregnancy and folic acid supplements ameliorate hyperhomocysteinaemia.
- Dysfibrinogenaemia is rare, and the thrombotic risk variable.

Pregnancy is an acquired risk factor for venous thromboembolism; the postnatal period being especially risky. The difficulty is to know who has thrombophilia, and what risk this poses to a pregnant woman. Past thrombosis increases risk, as does family history so thromboprophylaxis is recommended for those with history of thromboembolism and known thrombophilia or family history of thromboembolism (p16) both antenatally and postnatally. Treatment is stratified according to risk. For risks see p16.

Women with asymptomatic thrombophilia: Women without past thromboembolic history but with the higher risk thrombophilias ie antithrombin deficiency, more than one thrombophilic defect (including homozygous factor V Leiden, homozygous G20210A mutation, and compound heterozygotes of factor V Leiden and G20210A mutations); and women with other thrombophilias but additional risk factors need expert advice as to whether antenatal thromboprophylaxis is required in addition to postnatal use on an individual basis. Women with lower risk thrombophilias but no additional risk factors can have careful surveillance antenatally and 7 days of postnatal low molecular weight heparin.

It is not felt that all women should be screened for thrombophilia; although screening is recommended for those with a family history of thromboembolism and those with past history of idiopathic, or unprovoked thromboembolism (ie not oestrogen or pregnancy related). Screening is also recommended in those with second-trimester pregnancy loss, severe or recurrent eclampsia, and intrauterine growth restriction.

Low molecular weight heparin is recommended for those with thrombophilia and past history of thromboembolism (see p16). The thrombophilias marked * above, and acquired protein c resistance are risk factors for developing pre-eclampsia so aspirin 75mg/24h PO is recommended from 12 weeks until delivery.[90]

Obstetrics

Investigating rash in pregnancy[91] Investigate maculopapular rashes for rubella and parvovirus B19 (p142) (both these can infect the fetus) and measles. If maternal measles within 6 days before or after birth, the neonate needs human normal immune globulin 0.6mL/kg to max 5mL to prevent infection. Maternal chickenpox (p144) in 1st 24h of rash, from 20 weeks' gestation merits oral aciclovir. Hospitalize her for IV aciclovir if immunosuppressed, very dense or haemorrhagic lesions, neurological or respiratory symptoms. Mothers in contact with rashes (15min, same household or room, face to face contact); test for parvovirus B19 (asymptomatic infections affect fetus as often as symptomatic), and rubella (unless vaccinated ×2 or antibody level ≥10IU/mL ×2, or 1 of each). If she has chickenpox contact and is susceptible (confirmed by urgent blood test), varicella zoster immune globulin (VZIG) can be given within 10 days of exposure but still manage her as if infectious 8–24 days post VZIG; and advise her to see GP if she develops a rash as protection not always effective.

Rubella Childhood vaccination prevents rubella susceptibility. ►Asymptomatic reinfection can occur making serology essential in all pregnant rubella contacts. Routine antenatal screening finds those needing puerperal vaccination (avoid pregnancy for 1 month: vaccine is live). Symptoms (p142) are absent in 50%. The fetus is most at risk in the 1st 16 weeks' gestation. 50–60% of fetuses are affected if maternal primary infection is in the 1st month of gestation: <5% are affected if infection is at 16 weeks. Risk of fetal damage is much lower (<5%) with reinfection. Cataract is associated with infection at 8–9 weeks, deafness at 5–7 weeks (can occur with 2nd-trimester infection), cardiac lesions at 5–10 weeks. Other features: purpura, jaundice, hepatosplenomegaly, thrombocytopenia, cerebral palsy, microcephaly, IQ ↓, cerebral calcification, microphthalmia, retinitis, growth disorder. Miscarriage or stillbirth may occur. If suspected in the mother seek expert help. Take antibody levels 10 days apart and look for IgM antibody 4–5 weeks from incubation period or date of contact.

Cytomegalovirus (CMV) In the UK, CMV causes more congenital retardation than rubella. Maternal infection is mild (or ↑T°, lymphadenopathy, rash & sore throat). Up to 5:1000 live births are infected; 5% develop early multiple handicaps, and have cytomegalic inclusion disease with nonspecific signs like rubella syndrome + microcephaly, hydrops, & choroidoretinitis. Another 5% later develop cerebral calcification (IQ ↓); sensorineural deafness and psychomotor retardation. Δ: (tricky; ask lab). Paired sera. Are IgM and IgG antibodies found? Amniocentesis at >20wks + shell viral culture can detect fetal transmission. Also do throat swab, urine culture, and baby's serum after birth. Reducing exposure to toddlers' urine (the source of much infection) in pregnancy limits spread. NB: reactivation of old CMV may occur in pregnancy; it rarely affects the baby. One way to know that +ve serology does not reflect old infection is to do serology (or freeze a sample) pre-pregnancy. R: Hyperimmune globulin may have a role.

Toxoplasmosis 40% of fetuses are affected if the mother has the illness (2–7:1000 pregnancies); the earlier in pregnancy the more the damage. Symptoms are like glandular fever. Fever, rash, and eosinophilia also occur. If symptomatic, the CNS prognosis is poor. Diagnose by reference laboratory IgG and IgM tests. *Maternal, R (Royal College Regimen):* Start spiramycin promptly in infected mothers, eg 1.5g/12h PO. In symptomatic non-immune women test every 10 weeks through pregnancy. If infected consider amniocentesis to see if the fetus is infected. If the fetus is infected, give the mother pyrimethamine 50mg/12h as loading doses on day 1, then 1mg/kg/day + sulfadiazine 50mg/kg/12h + calcium folinate 15mg twice weekly all until delivery. *Affected babies:* (diagnose by serology—>90% asymptomatic). Intracranial calcification, hydrocephalus, choroidoretinitis if severely affected. Encephalitis, epilepsy, mental and physical retardation, jaundice, hepatosplenomegaly, thrombocytopenia, and skin rashes occur. Treat with 4-weekly courses of pyrimethamine, sulfadiazine and calcium folinate × 6, separated by 4 weeks of **spiramycin**. Prednisolone is given until signs of CNS inflammation or choroidoretinitis abate. *Prevention:* Avoid eating raw meat, wash hands if raw meat touched, wear gloves if gardening or dealing with cat litter, and avoid sheep during lambing time.

HIV See p23. It is a sad fact that for many women in some resource-poor countries access to retrovirals in pregnancy is still not an option (only 45% in 2008),[92] and the mainstays of prelabour caesarean section and avoidance of breastfeeding, so successful in reducing transmission, are also not an option. It is estimated 430,000 infants and children are infected with HIV each year.

Intrauterine syphilis Maternal screening occurs (UK screen 55,700 to prevent 1 case. In some parts of London 2:1000 women are infected); if infection found treat the mother with procaine **penicillin 600mg/24h IM** daily for 10 days. ~⅓ are stillborn. Neonatal signs: rhinitis, snuffles, rash, hepatosplenomegaly, lymphadenopathy, anaemia, jaundice, ascites, hydrops, nephrosis, meningitis, ±keratitis, and nerve deafness. Nasal discharge exam: spirochetes; x-rays: perichondritis; *CSF:* ↑Monocytes and protein with +ve serology. *Treatment:* Give **procaine penicillin 37mg/kg/24h IM** for 3 weeks.

Listeria Affects 6–15:100,000 pregnancies. Maternal symptoms: fever, shivering, myalgia, headache, sore throat, cough, vomiting, diarrhoea, vaginitis. Miscarriage (can be recurrent), premature labour, and stillbirth may occur. Infection is usually via infected food (eg milk, soft cheeses, pâté). ▶Do blood cultures in any pregnant patient with unexplained fever for ≥48h. Serology, vaginal and rectal swabs do not help (can be commensal). See *OHCM* p409.

Perinatal infection usually occurs in 2nd or 3rd trimester. 20% of affected fetuses are stillborn. An early postnatal feature is respiratory distress from pneumonia. There may be convulsions, hepato-splenomegaly, pustular or petechial rashes, conjunctivitis, fever, leucopenia. Meningitis is commoner after perinatal infection. Diagnose by culture of blood, CSF, meconium, and placenta. Infant mortality: 30%. Isolate baby (nosocomial spread can occur). Treat with **ampicillin 50mg/kg/6h IV** and **gentamicin 3mg/kg/12h IV** until 1 week after fever subsides. Monitor levels.

Sheep-borne conditions Listeriosis, toxoplasmosis, and ovine chlamydia (*Chlamydophila abortus*) can be contracted from sheep. Ovine chlamydial infection is rare; can cause DIC, septicaemia, and renal failure in pregnant women and miscarriage of the fetus. Diagnose by serology; treat with erythromycin or tetracycline. ▶Pregnant women should not handle sheep or lambs.[1]

---

1 'TORCH' infections: **T**oxoplasmosis, **O**ther (eg syphilis, cocksackie, leptospira, Q fever, Lyme disease, malaria), **R**ubella, **C**MV, **H**erpes (and hepatitis). 1st 4 are acquired antenatally (herpes & hepatitis usually perinatally). Other agents: chickenpox p144; HIV, p144–5. See also erythrovirus (=parvovirus B19, p142). Zoster reactivation in pregnancy is not a risk for the baby.

✚ **Hepatitis B virus (HBV)** All mothers should be screened for HBsAg. Carriers have persistent HBsAg for >6 months. High infectivity is associated with HBeAg so anti-HBe antibodies are negative. Without immunization 95% of babies born to these mothers might develop hepatitis B, and 93% of the babies would be chronic carriers at 6 months. If the mother develops acute infection in the mid- or third trimester there is high risk of perinatal infection. Her risk of death is 0.5–3%. Most neonatal infections occur at birth but some (especially in the East) are transplacental; hence the seeming failure of vaccination in up to 15% of neonates adequately vaccinated. Most infected neonates will develop chronic infection and in infected males lifetime risk of developing hepatocellular cancer is 50%; 20% for ♀. Most will develop cirrhosis, so immunization is really important. ▶Give immunoglobulin (200u IM) and vaccinate babies of carriers and infected mothers at birth. See p151. In uncomplicated hepatitis HBV DNA is cleared, anti-core antibodies develop, followed by anti-HBe antibodies with the decline and disappearance of HBeAg and HBsAg at 3 months. Do serology of vaccinated baby at 12–15 months old. If HBsAg–ve and anti-HBs is present, the child is protected.

Hepatitis C See p26.

Hepatitis E Risk of maternal mortality is ↑ (25% if in 3rd trimester); death is usually postpartum, preceded by fulminant hepatic failure, coma, and massive PPH. 33–50% of babies become infected. A vaccine is being developed.

Herpes simplex (HSV) Neonatal infection can cause blindness, IQ↓, epilepsy, jaundice, respiratory distress, DIC, and death (in 30%, even if treated).

Prevalence of past (2°) HSV infection is ~25% and recurrence in pregnancy is not usually a problem thanks to maternal antibodies. If a mother develops primary (1st-ever) genital herpes in pregnancy, refer to a genitourinary clinic to screen her (and her partners) for other infections and confirm it is primary. If in last trimester give her oral *aciclovir* or *valaciclovir* ± elective caesarean if 1° infection within 6 weeks of her due date. Type-specific HSV diagnosis: PCR.

If active primary infection lesions at time of delivery do a caesar, even if membranes have ruptured up to 4h previously. If a mother with primary lesions does deliver vaginally risk of infection to the baby is 41%, so give mother (by IVI in labour) and newborn high-dose *aciclovir* (p200; do PCR at birth). Try to avoid fetal blood sampling, scalp electrodes, and instrumental delivery. Neonatal infection usually appears at 5–21 days with grouped vesicles/pustules on a red base, eg at the presenting part or sites of trauma (eg scalp electrode) ± periocular and conjunctival lesions. Non-vesicular rashes also occur.

Varicella zoster If mothers develop chickenpox in last 7 days of pregnancy aim for delivery after 7 days, give babies varicella immune immunoglobulin (VZIG) at birth and monitor for 28 days; and treat with aciclovir if neonate develops chickenpox. Babies of non-immune mothers also need VZIG if contacts in 1st 7 days of life. Earlier in pregnancy, if women with no personal history of chickenpox have had significant (eg 15 min) chickenpox contact; check blood for varicella antibodies; if none, give VZIG, and manage as still potentially infectious 8–28 days later and notify doctor if develops rash. Women developing chickenpox in pregnancy should avoid contact with pregnant women, and have oral *aciclovir* 800mg 5×daily PO for 7 days if >20wks if presenting within 24h of rash. Hospitalize if chest, CNS symptoms, dense/haemorrhagic rash or immunocompromized. Fetal varicella syndrome (FVS) complicates ~1% fetuses of mothers infected at 3–28 weeks of pregnancy by reactivation in utero. FVS features: skin scarring, eye defects (microphthalmia, chorioretinitis, cataracts), neurological abnormalities (microcephaly, cortical atrophy, IQ↓, bowel and bladder sphincter disturbances). Refer to fetal medicine specialist for detailed ultrasound at 16–20wks, or 5wks post-infection.[93]

Chlamydia trachomatis Associations: low birthweight, premature membrane rupture, fetal death. ~30% of infected mothers have affected babies. Conjunctivitis develops 5–14 days after birth and may show minimal inflammation or purulent discharge. The cornea is not usually involved. *Complications:* Chlamydia pneumonitis, pharyngitis, or otitis media. *Tests: Special swabs are available but may be unreliable.* See p285. *Treatment:* Local cleansing of eye + erythromycin 12.5mg/kg/6h PO for ~3 weeks eliminates lung organisms. Give parents/partners erythromycin[94] or azithromycin 1g PO single dose.

Gonococcal conjunctivitis Occurs within ~4 days of birth, with purulent discharge and lid swelling, ± corneal hazing, corneal rupture, and panophthalmitis. Note, 50% will also have concurrent chlamydial infection. *Treatment:* Infants born to those with known gonorrhoea should have cefotaxime 100mg/kg IM stat, and chloramphenicol 0.5% eye-drops within 1h of birth. For active gonococcal infection give benzylpenicillin 50mg/kg/12h IM and 3-hourly 0.5% chloramphenicol drops for 7 days. Isolate the baby.

Ophthalmia neonatorum This is purulent discharge from the eye of a neonate <21 days old. There are many causes: chlamydiae, herpes virus, staphylococci, streptococci, pneumococci, *E. coli*. *Tests:* Swab for bacterial and viral culture, microscopy (look for intracellular gonococci), and chlamydia (eg immunofluorescence). Treat gonococcus and chlamydia as above; other infections with neomycin drops or ointment (allows chlamydia detection—not so with chloramphenicol).

Clostridium perfringens: Suspect this in any complication of criminal abortion and when intracellular encapsulated Gram +ve rods are seen on genital swabs. It may infect *in utero* deaths or any other anaerobic site (eg haematomas). *Signs:* Endometritis→septicaemia/gangrene→myoglobinuria→renal failure→death. *Treatment:* • Surgically debride all devitalized tissue. • Hyperbaric O_2. • High-dose IV benzylpenicillin (erythromycin if serious penicillin allergy). The use of gas gangrene antitoxin is controversial. Seek expert help.

Preventing neonatal group B strep (GBS) sepsis Give all women IV antibiotics at labour's start or on membrane rupture if: • +ve GBS screening swab (vaginal or perineal; do at 35–37wks • Any baby previously infected with GBS • Any documented GBS bacteriuria (regardless of level of colony-forming units/mL) in this pregnancy • Recent swab result unknown and gestation <37wks unless –ve swab in last 5wks• • Any intrapartum fever • If a woman is GBS+ve (swab or bacteriuria), with prelabour rupture of membranes at term, treat with GBS antibiotic prophylaxis and induce labour • If culture result unknown and membranes are ruptured at term for >18h: GBS prophylaxis (eg penicillin).g[15361281]

TB All babies born into households with TB, to immigrant mothers from areas with a high TB prevalence, or who will travel to such areas should have BCG (Bacillus Calmette-Guérin) vaccination after birth 0.05mL intradermally at deltoid's insertion: 0.03mL if using a multiple puncture gun. Babies not vaccinated in hospital are unlikely to be vaccinated in the community.[95] Give other vaccinations as usual, avoiding the BCG vaccinated arm for 3 months. Separate babies from mothers with active or open TB until she has had 2 weeks of R and is sputum -ve. BCG vaccinate the baby and treat with isoniazid until he or she has a +ve skin reaction. Consider CXR in pregnant women with cough, fever, or weight loss (esp. if recent immigrant). Encourage breastfeeding.

✠ ►With any pain in pregnancy think, is this onset of labour? If pain is in the second half of pregnancy think is this pre-eclampsia? (check BP and urine protein).

►Women with chest, back or epigastric pain severe enough for opiates need full investigation including cardiac causes (ECG, CXR, troponin, echocardiography, CT angiography + CT/MRI chest scan).

Abdominal pain may be from ligament stretching or from symphysis pubis strain. In early pregnancy remember miscarriage (p260) and ectopics (p262).

Abruption The triad of abdominal pain, uterine rigidity, and vaginal bleeding suggests this. It occurs in between 1 in 80 and 1 in 200 pregnancies. Fetal loss is high if >50% of placenta affected. A tender uterus is highly suggestive. Ultrasound may be diagnostic (but not necessarily so). A live viable fetus merits rapid delivery as demise can be sudden. Prepare for DIC, which complicates 33–50% of severe cases, and beware PPH, which is also common. See p56.

Uterine rupture See p80.

Uterine fibroids For torsion and red degeneration, see p277.

Uterine torsion The uterus rotates axially 30°–40° to the right in 80% of normal pregnancies. Rarely, it rotates >90° causing acute uterine torsion in mid or late pregnancy with abdominal pain, shock, a tense uterus, and urinary retention (catheterization may reveal a displaced urethra in twisted vagina). Fibroids, adnexal masses, or congenital asymmetrical uterine anomalies are present in 90%. Diagnosis is usually at laparotomy. Delivery is by caesarean section.

Ovarian tumours Torsion, rupture, see p282. **Pyelonephritis** See p28.

Appendicitis Incidence: ~1 : 1000 pregnancies. It is not commoner in pregnancy but mortality is higher (esp. from 20wks). Perforation is commoner (15–20%). Fetal mortality is ~1.5% for simple appendicitis; ~30% if perforation. The appendix migrates upwards, outwards and posteriorly as pregnancy progresses, so pain is less well localized (often para-umbilical or subcostal—but right lower quadrant still commonest)[96] and tenderness, rebound, and guarding less obvious. Peritonitis can make the uterus tense and woody-hard. Don't delay surgery!—laparotomy over site of maximal tenderness with patient tilted 30° to the left by an experienced obstetric surgeon (laparoscopy appears to be safe)[97]

Cholecystitis Incidence 1–6 per 10,000 pregnancies. Pregnancy encourages gallstone formation due to biliary stasis and increased cholesterol in bile. Symptoms are similar to the non-pregnant with subcostal pain, nausea, and vomiting. Jaundice is uncommon (5%). Ultrasound confirms the presence of stones. The main differential diagnosis is appendicitis, and laparotomy or laparoscopy is mandatory if this cannot be excluded. Surgery should be reserved for complicated non-resolving biliary tract disease during pregnancy as in >90% the acute process resolves with conservative management. For patients requiring surgery, laparoscopic cholecystectomy can be a safe and effective method of treatment, but uterine perforation or injury is a risk.

Rectus sheath haematoma Very rarely, bleeding into the rectus sheath and haematoma formation can occur with coughing (or spontaneously) in late pregnancy causing swelling and tenderness. Ultrasound is helpful. *ΔΔ*: Abruption. *Management:* Laparotomy (or perhaps laparoscopy—but not in late pregnancy) is indicated if the diagnosis is in doubt or if there is shock.[98,99]

Pre-eclampsia Abdominal pain may complicate pre-eclampsia by liver congestion. Rarely, in severe pre-eclampsia the liver ruptures.

Pancreatitis in pregnancy is rare, but mortality is high (37% maternal; 5.6% fetal). Diagnose by urinary diastase in 1st trimester when amylase may be low.[100]

Obstetrics

The uterus occupies the pelvis and cannot be felt *per abdomen* until ~12 weeks' gestation. By 16 weeks, its fundus lies half way between the symphysis pubis and the umbilicus. By 20–24 weeks it reaches the umbilicus. In a primip, the fundus is under the ribs by 36 weeks. At term the uterus lies a bit lower than at 36 weeks, as the head descends into the pelvis. Some midwives prefer to measure the symphysis fundal height (**SFH**) in cm from the symphysis pubis (after voiding urine). From 16 weeks the SFH increases ~1cm/week.

The symphysis fundal height during pregnancy		
As a rule of thumb: at	16–26 weeks	the SFH (cm) ≈ dates (in weeks)
	26–36 weeks	the SFH (cm) ± 2cm ≈ dates
	36 weeks to term	the SFH (cm) ± 3cm ≈ dates

SFH is used as a rough guide to find babies small for gestational age (p52). Suspect this if the measurement lies >1–2cm outside these ranges given above. NB: more false positives will occur with the simpler rule of *weeks of gestation = cm from pubic symphysis to fundus.*[101,102]

Other reasons for discrepancy between fundal height and dates: • Inaccurate menstrual history • Multiple gestation • Fibroids • Polyhydramnios • Adnexal mass • Maternal size • Hydatidiform mole.

On inspecting the abdomen note any scars from previous operations. Caesarean section scars are usually Pfannenstiel ('bikini-line'). Laparoscopy scars are just below and parallel to the umbilicus or in the left upper quadrant (Palmer's point). It is common to see a line of pigmentation, the linea nigra, extending in the midline from pubic hair to umbilicus. This darkens during the first trimester (the first 13 weeks).

Palpating the abdomen Measure the SFH and listen to the *fetal heart*. After 32 weeks palpate laterally to assess the lie, then bimanually palpate over the lower uterine pole for presentation and degree of engagement. Pawlik's grip (examining the lower pole of the uterus between the thumb and index fingers of the right hand) can also be used for assessing the degree of engagement. Watch the patient's face during palpation and stop if it causes pain. Obesity, polyhydramnios, and tense muscles make it difficult to feel the fetus. Midwives are skilled at palpation, so ask them if you need help.

It is important to determine the *number of fetuses* (p68), the *lie* (longitudinal, oblique, or transverse), the *presentation* (cephalic or breech, fig **2**), and the *engagement*. Ultrasound is useful here. Note the amount of liquor, the apparent size of the fetus, and any contractions or fetal movements seen or felt.

Auscultation The fetal heart may be heard by Doppler ultrasound from ~12 weeks and with a Pinard stethoscope from ~24 weeks.

Fetal movements[103] 1st noted by mothers at 18–20wks, movements ↑ until 32wks then plateau at average 31/h. Fetuses sleep for 20–40-min cycles day and night (rarely >90mins). Maternal posture affects detection (lying> sitting>standing). If mothers feel movements reduced at 28+wks, advise lying semi-recumbent for 2h; if <10 movements arrange same day CTG (p44), and next available ultrasound if reduction persists or IUGR (p52)/stillbirth risk.

Engagement The level of the head is assessed in 2 ways: engagement, or fifths palpable abdominally. Engagement entails passage of the biggest diameter of the presenting part through the pelvic inlet. Fifths palpable abdominally states what you can feel, and makes no degree of judgment on degree of engagement of the head. In primigravida the head usually enters the pelvis by 37 weeks, otherwise causes must be excluded (eg placenta praevia or fetal abnormality). In multips the head may not enter the pelvis until onset of labour.

Position–ie which way is the fetus facing? (figs 1 & 2)		
Occipitoanterior	**Occipitolateral**	**Occipitoposterior**
Back easily felt	Back can be felt	Back not felt
Limbs not easily felt	Limbs lateral	Limbs anterior
Shoulder lies 2cm from midline on opposite side from back	Midline shoulder	Shoulder 6–8cm lateral, same side as back
Back from midline=2–3cm	6–8cm	>10cm

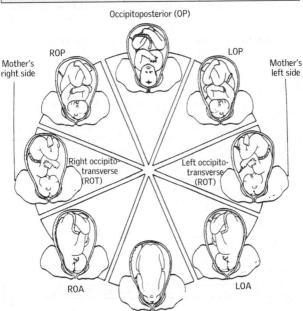

Occipitoposterior (OP)

ROP — LOP

Mother's right side — Mother's left side

Right occipito-transverse (ROT) — Left occipito-transverse (ROT)

ROA — LOA

Occipitoanterior (OA) Front

Fig 1. Fetal positions.

©OUP

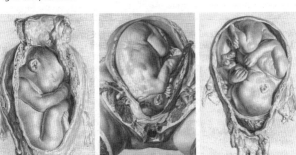

Fig 2. Use figure 1 to help determine the lie, the presentation, and the position from these dissections by William Hunter (1718–83).

William Hunter (1718–1783). *Anatomia uteri humani gravidi tabulis illustrata* (The anatomy of the human gravid uterus exhibited in figures).

The ideal pelvis This has a rounded brim, a shallow cavity, non-prominent ischial spines, a curved sacrum with large sciatic notches and sacrospinous ligaments >3.5cm long. The angle of the brim is 55° to the horizontal, the AP diameter at least 12cm and transverse diameter at least 13.5cm. The subpubic arch should be rounded and the intertuberous distance at least 10cm. A *clinically favourable* pelvis is one where the sacral promontory cannot be felt, the ischial spines are not prominent, the subpubic arch and base of supraspinous ligaments both accept 2 fingers, and the intertuberous diameter accepts 4 knuckles when the woman is examined.

The true pelvis Anteriorly there is the symphysis pubis (3.5cm long) and posteriorly the sacrum (12cm long).

Zone of inlet: Boundaries: Anteriorly lies the upper border of the pubis, posteriorly the sacral promontory, laterally the ileopectineal line. Transverse diameter 13.5cm; AP diameter 11.5cm.

Zone of cavity: This is the most roomy zone. It is almost round. Transverse diameter 13.5cm; AP diameter 12.5cm.

Zone of mid-pelvis: Boundaries: Anteriorly, the apex of the pubic arch; posteriorly the tip of the sacrum, laterally the ischial spines (the desirable distance between the spines is >10.5cm). Ovoid in shape, it is the narrowest part.

Zone of outlet: The pubic arch is the anterior border (desirable angle >85°). Laterally lie the sacrotuberous ligaments and ischial tuberosities, posteriorly the coccyx.

Head terms The *bregma* is the anterior fontanelle. The *brow* lies between the bregma and the root of the nose. The *face* lies below the root of the nose and supraorbital ridges. The *occiput* lies behind the posterior fontanelle. The *vertex* is the area between the fontanelles and the parietal eminences.

Moulding The frontal bones can slip under the parietal bones which can slip under the occipital bone so reducing biparietal diameter. The degree of overlap may be assessed vaginally.

Presentation	Relevant diameter presenting	
Flexed vertex	Suboccipitobregmatic	9.5cm
Partially deflexed vertex	Suboccipitofrontal	10.5cm
Deflexed vertex	Occipitofrontal	11.5cm
Brow	Mentovertical	13cm
Face	Submentobregmatic	9.5cm

Movement of the head in labour (normal vertex presentation)

1 Descent with increased flexion as the head enters the cavity. The sagittal suture lies in the transverse diameter of the brim.
2 Internal rotation occurs at the ischial spine level due to the grooved gutter of the levator muscles. Head flexion increases. (The head rotates 90° if occipitolateral position, 45° if occipitoanterior, 135° if occipitoposterior.)
3 Disengagement by extension as the head comes out of the vulva.
4 Restitution: as the shoulders are rotated by the levators until the bisacromial diameter is anteroposterior, the head externally rotates the same amount as before but in opposite direction.
5 Delivery of anterior shoulder by lateral flexion of trunk posteriorly.
6 Delivery of posterior shoulder by lateral flexion of trunk anteriorly.
7 Delivery of buttocks and legs.

Obstetrics

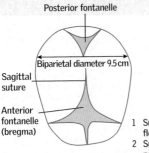

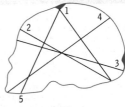

Posterior fontanelle

Biparietal diameter 9.5 cm

Sagittal suture

Anterior fontanelle (bregma)

1 Suboccipitobregmatic 9.5 cm
  flexed vertex presentation
2 Suboccipitofrontal 10.5 cm
  partially deflexed vertex
3 Occipitofrontal 11.5 cm deflexed vertex
4 Mentovertical 13 cm brow
5 Submentobregmatic 9.5 cm face

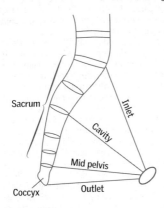

Sacrum

Inlet

Cavity

Mid pelvis

Coccyx

Outlet

Fig 1. Pelvic diameters *vs* fetal head.

'Life forced her through this gate of suffering' DH Lawrence, *Sons and Lovers.*

In high-risk pregnancy, antepartum cardiotocography and biophysical profiles by ultrasound (p46) are used to monitor fetal activity and responsiveness. The aim is to detect intrauterine hypoxia prenatally.

Cardiotocography (CTG): Doppler ultrasound detects fetal heart beats and a tocodynamometer over the uterine fundus records any contractions. A continuous trace is printed over ~30min (eg a paper speed of 1cm/min) with the mother lying semi-recumbent, or in the left lateral position or half-sitting position. A normal trace in an afebrile mother at term who is not having drugs has a base rate of 110–160 beats/min, with a variability of >5 beats/min, and at least 2 accelerations (a common response to movement or noise) of an amplitude ≥15 beats/min over a 20-min period. (Fetal heart rate falls by ~1 beat/min/week from 28 weeks.) CTG needs to be done every 24h antenatally to identify the changing fetal heart rate pattern associated with hypoxia (loss of baseline variability with decelerations).

Intrapartum monitoring Death and disability due to complications of labour occur in <1 : 300 labours. Intrapartum fetal heart rate monitoring aims to detect patterns known to be associated with fetal distress—a diagnosis supported by fetal hypoxia (acidosis) on blood sampling.

Intermittent auscultation (IA) at the end of contractions (to listen for decelerations) with Doppler or Pinard stethoscope is used for low-risk labours. Use every 15min in 1st stage, 5min throughout 2nd stage. If abnormality noted (below) or intrapartum problems occur, start *continuous fetal heart rate (FHR) monitoring.* This has poor predictive value, overdiagnosing fetal distress even if used with fetal blood sampling. Its value is uncertain even in high-risk labours, for which it is used throughout labour, ideally with a scalp electrode, but it is associated with reduced neonatal seizures.[104] Where scalp electrode is used it is also possible to monitor the *fetal electrocardiogram:* ST waveform analysis is associated with fewer babies with severe metabolic acidosis, less fetal blood sampling, less neonatal encephalopathy, and fewer operative vaginal deliveries (but not caesarean sections).[105] *Indications:* High-risk pregnancy; use of oxytocin; abnormality on intermittent auscultation (decelerations noted after a contraction, or rate <110 or >160 beats/min); fresh meconium passed, p72, (consider too if just meconium stained liquor); maternal pyrexia (T° >37.5 2h apart, or once T° >38); fresh bleeding in labour; maternal request.[106 NICE] *Disadvantages:* Limited maternal mobility and effort.

Management of a poor trace:
• Lie the mother on her left side and give O₂. Stop **oxytocin**. If there is uterine hypercontractility give tocolysis with 0.25mg **terbutaline** SC.
• Take fetal blood sample. If you do not have this facility, consider rapid delivery if the trace does not improve.

Fetal blood sampling: Use to check for hypoxia in presence of pathological FHR trace, but not if acute compromise (eg deceleration lasting >3 min). Take with mother in left lateral position. Fetal acidosis reflects hypoxia. Scalp blood pH of >7.25 is normal, repeat in <1h if FHR remains pathological. If 7.21–7.24 it is borderline, repeat within 30min if FHR remains pathological, sooner if other abnormality. If <7.2 call consultant obstetrician.[106 NICE] Levels <7.2 require immediate delivery unless in second stage when a level as low as 7.15 may be acceptable. CI maternal infection (HIV, hepatitis viruses, and herpes), fetal suspected clotting disorder, <34 weeks' gestation.

Fetal pulse oximetry Knowledge of fetal oxygen saturation is not associated with reduction in rate of caesarean section or with improved condition of the newborn.[107]

Fetal heart rate patterns and their clinical significance (Figs 1 & 2)

The normal pattern is described opposite. Accelerations suggest intact sympathetic activity and are rarely associated with hypoxia.

Loss of baseline variability Baseline variability of >5 beats/min shows response to vagal tone, sympathetic stimuli, and catecholamines in a well-oxygenated fetal brainstem. Loss of baseline variability may reflect a preterm fetus who is asleep, drug effects (eg diazepam, morphine, phenothiazine), or hypoxia.

Baseline tachycardia Heart rate >170 beats/min is associated with maternal fever, or β-sympathomimetic drug use, chorioamnionitis (loss of variation too), and acute/subacute hypoxia. Persistent rates >200 are associated with fetal cardiac arrhythmia.

Baseline bradycardia A heart rate <110 beats/min is rarely associated with fetal hypoxia (except in placental abruption). It may reflect ↑ fetal vagal tone, fetal heart block, or, if spasmodic, cord compression.

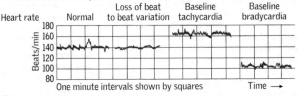

Fig 1. Rate patterns.

Early decelerations coinciding with uterine contractions reflect increased vagal tone as fetal intracranial pressure rises with the contraction. **Late decelerations**, when the nadir of the deceleration develops some 30sec after the peak of the uterine contraction, reflect fetal hypoxia, the degree and duration reflecting its severity. **Variable decelerations**, both in degree and in relation to uterine contractions, may represent umbilical cord compression around the limbs or presenting part.

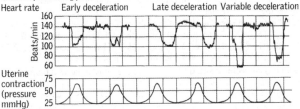

Fig 2. Fetal heart deceleration patterns.

Pathological CTG pattern [106 NICE] This has 2 or more non-reassuring features (baseline rate 100–109 or 161–180 beats/minute; variability < 5 beats/minute for ≥40 but <90 minutes; typical variable decelerations with >50% contractions, occurring over 90 minutes; or a prolonged deceleration of <3 minutes) or 1 abnormal feature (rate <100 or >180 beats/minute; variability <5 beats/minute for ≥90 minutes; atypical variable decelerations with > 50% contractions, or late decelerations, both over 90 minutes: or a single prolonged deceleration of >3 minutes).

♯ In each ultrasound examination, examine placental site and structure, assess liquor volume and fetal structure, and wellbeing (see below).

Early in pregnancy If there is bleeding and pain, ultrasound can confirm ectopic or viable intrauterine pregnancy—at 4 weeks + 3 days for regular 28–day cycle with transvaginal scan. Where there is discrepancy between uterine size and dates, gestation can be estimated, a viable fetus ascertained (not missed miscarriage, p260), or twins (and if monochorionic or dichorionic see p68) diagnosed—especially important after the use of fertility drugs or in the presence of hyperemesis gravidarum (also to exclude hydatidiform mole).

Estimating gestation Crown–rump length is measured at 6–12 weeks (~10mm at 7 weeks; ~55mm at 12). From 12 weeks the biparietal diameter can be measured (and femur length from 14 weeks so there are 2 independent estimations with each scan). Biparietal diameter measurements to estimate age are most accurate up to 20 weeks (unreliable from 34 weeks). Knowing-gestational age is vital in managing rhesus disease and in diabetic pregnancy (p24). It also helps if the date of the LMP is unknown, or cycles are irregular.

Fetal abnormality See *fetal nuchal translucency*, p11; MINIBOX. Many units offer routine scans to find abnormality at 18–20 weeks. With the best machines and sonographers, an increasing range of markers of fetal abnormality are discernible, eg nuchal thickness in Down's syndrome, but the sign is also +ve in ~6% of normal pregnancies. The more such markers, the greater the chance of abnormality (see p10 for 'soft signs'). It is hard to know how to counsel women before these discerning scans: full informed consent is time-consuming, and itself causes psychopathology (p12). Another problem is that many fetuses with chromosomal abnormalities suggested by early scans will spontaneously miscarry in subsequent weeks, and one will have overburdened the mother needlessly.

Indications for scanning for abnormality
• Family history of neural tube defect
• Maternal diabetes
• Maternal epilepsy
• Oligohydrammios
• Multiple pregnancy

Fetal echocardiography Offered to high-risk groups (personal or 1st degree relative history of heart disease; associated with ↑ nuchal thickness) it is traditionally offered at specialist centres at 22–24 weeks. Scanning at 12–15 weeks at these centres may exclude most major abnormalities.[108]

Biophysical profile scoring Ultrasound of the fetus in the womb over a period of up to 30min aims to assess if the fetus is being affected by acute or chronic asphyxia. With acute asphyxia the fetus loses active biophysical variables regulated by central nervous system outflow (fetal breathing, gross body movement, fetal flexor tone, and heart rate accelerations with fetal body movement). Reduction in amniotic fluid demonstrated by pockets of fluid of less than 1cm depth measured in 2 perpendicular planes is taken to indicate chronic asphyxia. By use of specific criteria for these 5 variables, a 'wellbeing' score can be reached. Management protocols according to score then help guide the obstetrician as to when intervention should take place.

Ultrasound is used as an adjunct to the diagnostic procedures of amniocentesis, fetoscopy, cordocentesis, and chorionic villus biopsy.

In pregnancies where fetal growth is of concern (p52) growth can be monitored by regular scans; the abdominal to skull circumference ratio is of interest. Fetal weight can be estimated when planning vaginal delivery of breech presentation (but less accurate for larger fetuses).

In later pregnancy, lie and presentation fetus can be determined. If there is APH, placenta praevia can be excluded and the placenta examined for abruption. With secondary PPH, retained products of conception may be visualized.

Side-effects

Ultrasound is one of the safest tests ever invented; nevertheless, over the years, fears have been expressed about inducing childhood cancers. There is now good evidence that this does not occur. There is one randomized trial indicating that *repeated* ultrasound with Doppler is associated with an increased risk (1.65) of birthweights below the third centile.

Doppler ultrasound and fetal wellbeing

Doppler ultrasound is a technique that can be used to assess circulation on both sides of the placenta. It has not been shown to be of use as a screening tool in routine antenatal care but it has been shown to be of use in high-risk pregnancies. Waveform outlines (velocimetry) have been seen to be abnormal in small babies who ultimately died or were severely ill perinatally, and babies known to be small from real-time ultrasound have been shown not to be at risk if umbilical artery waveforms were normal, but if end-diastolic signals are absent the baby is likely to be hypoxic and acidotic. In management of growth-retarded babies uncomplicated by other obstetric problems surveillance using Doppler velocimetry is more cost-effective than use of cardiotocography, and may be sufficient as the sole extra means of surveillance (in addition to ultrasound examination of biophysical parameters). Doppler is useful in determining severity of twin–twin transfusion (p68) in monochorionic twins.[109] ►Consider caesarean section if umbilical artery Doppler velocimetry shows absent or reversed end-diastolic velocities in pregnancies complicated by intrauterine growth restriction and hypertension—to prevent postnatal problems such as cerebral haemorrhage, anaemia, and hypoglycaemia. These changes correlate with placental intervillous space ischaemia and spasm or occlusion of tertiary stem arterioles on the fetal side of the circulation. Placental intervillous ischaemia leads to centralization of fetal circulation so that blood returning from the placenta is shunted to fetal brain, coronary arteries, and adrenals. Intervention studies based on knowledge of abnormal umbilical waveform patterns have resulted in babies small-for-gestational age (SGA) with abnormal waveform patterns being ~500g larger than expected when the mothers were given low-dose aspirin rather than placebo from the time of diagnosis. It is also the case that low-dose aspirin delays the onset of hypertension and reduces its severity in primiparous mothers whose babies had abnormal umbilical waveforms. However, aspirin has not been shown to be of benefit in low-risk pregnancies.

Obstetrics

Pre-eclampsia Terminology: see footnote on p0. This is pregnancy-induced hypertension (PIH) with proteinuria ± oedema. A multisystem disorder originating in the placenta, the primary defect is failure of trophoblastic invasion of spiral arteries (fig 1, p15) leaving them vasoactive—properly invaded they cannot clamp down in response to vasoconstrictors and this protects placental flow. Increasing BP partially compensates for this. Pre-eclampsia also affects hepatic, renal, and coagulation systems. It develops after 20 weeks and usually resolves within 10 days of delivery. Eclampsia (1 in 2000 maternities) is a major cause of maternal death and fetal morbidity/mortality. Pre-eclampsia may be asymptomatic, so frequent screening is vital. It may recur in a subsequent pregnancy.

Risk factors: High risk: • Chronic hypertension • Hypertension in previous pregnancy • Chronic kidney disease • Diabetes mellitus • Autoimmune disease (SLE, antiphospholipid, thrombophilia). Moderate risk: • 1st pregnancy • ≥40y • Pregnancy interval >10y BMI ≥35kg/m² • FH pre-eclampsia • Multiple pregnancy. If 1 high-risk or 2 moderate-risk factors take aspirin 75mg/24h PO from 12th week of pregnancy until delivery to prevent eclampsia.

Fetal: Hydatidiform mole (↑BP at 20 weeks); multiple pregnancy; placental hydrops (eg rhesus disease). Fetal causes all have increased placental bulk.

Effects of pre-eclampsia: Plasma volume ↓; peripheral resistance ↑; placental ischaemia. If the BP is >180/140mmHg microaneurysms develop in arteries. DIC may develop. Oedema may develop suddenly (eg weight ↑ by 1kg suddenly). Proteinuria is a late sign, meaning renal involvement, which may be detected earlier by doing urate levels (>0.29mmol/L at 28 weeks, >0.34mmol/L at 32 weeks, and >0.39mmol/L at 36 weeks suggest pre-eclampsia). Initially glomerular filtration is normal and only serum urate is ↑; later urea *and* creatinine increase. The liver may be involved (contributing to DIC)—and HELLP syndrome (p26) may be present with placental infarcts. Fetal asphyxia, abruption, and small babies (p52 & p47) may also occur. *Late effects (mother):* Hypertension and renal failure (sometimes); she should be encouraged to accept screening for hypertension.[110]

Preventing eclampsia Antenatal BP checks/urinalysis; use of $MgSO_4$: see below. Uterine artery Doppler scans can identify high-risk women in whom low-dose aspirin use results in a significant reduction in pre-eclampsia.

Symptomatic pre-eclampsia may mimic flu, with *headache, chest* or *epigastric pain, vomiting,* and *pulse* ↑—but also *visual disturbance, shaking, hyperreflexia,* and *irritability.* The mother is now in danger of *generalized seizures* (eclampsia) and treatment must occur. Death may be imminent from *stroke* (commonest), *hepatic, renal,* or *cardiac failure.* ▶Prophylactic magnesium sulfate halves risk of eclampsia, and may ↓maternal deaths. (Doses of >50g magnesium sulfate may be toxic to preterm fetal brains.)[111]

Management *Early phase:* Admit if BP rises by >30/20mmHg over booking BP, if BP ≥160/100, if ≥140/90 + proteinuria (1+), or there is growth restriction. In hospital, measure BP 2–4-hourly, (thigh cuff if arm circumference ≥41cm),[112] weigh daily, test all urine for protein; regularly monitor fluid balance, check U&E, LFT, and platelets (beware falls to <110 × 10⁹/L). Do cardiotocography (p44) on admission: repeat if PV bleed, abdo pain, ↓fetal movements or deteriorating maternal condition; and US scan to check growth, amniotic fluid volume and umbilical artery velicometry. In asymptomatic pre-eclampsia, treat if systolic BP ≥160, eg methyldopa 250mg to 1g/8h under supervision in hospital, in order to buy time for fetal maturation, and if all other variables are satisfactory. If signs worsen deliver the baby (liaise with paediatricians). Delivery is the only cure. Give all pre-eclamptic women H_2-blockers at onset of labour. Beware BP rise if anaesthetic induction needed.

Managing severe pre-eclampsia

This applies to those with BP >160/110 with proteinuria *or* BP ≥140/90 with proteinuria plus one or more of:

- Seizures
- Headache or epigastric pain
- Platelets <100 × 10⁹/L
- Visual disturbance
- Papilloedema
- ALT >70u/L
- Clonus (>3 beats)
- Liver tenderness or HELLP (p26)

▸▸ Continuously monitor maternal oxygen saturation, and BP.

▸▸ Use prophylactic magnesium sulfate: 4g (8mL of 50% solution) IVI over 15min in 100mL 0.9% saline; then maintenance as below.

▸▸ Catheterize: measure urine output (eg use urometer) & T° hourly; FBC, U&E, LFTs, creatinine every 12–24h. If platelets <100 × 10⁹/L do clotting studies.

▸▸ Monitor fetal heart rate; assess liquor volume and fetal growth by scan; umbilical cord Doppler if possible. Use monitoring in labour.

▸▸ *Delivery is the only cure for these women.* When a decision is made to deliver, contact on-call consultant, anaesthetist, and senior labour ward midwife. Deliver appropriately (eg <34 weeks usually by caesar). Give **steroids** if <34–36 wks, (p51). At 3ʳᵈ stage of labour give 5u **oxytocin** IM/IV slowly.

Treatment of hypertension: Beware: automated BP devices underestimate BP.

▸▸ If BP >160/110mmHg or mean arterial pressure >125mmHg, use **labetalol** 20mg IV increasing after 10min intervals to 40mg then 80mg until 200mg total is given. Aim for BP 150/80–100mmHg. Alternative is **hydralazine** 5mg slowly/20min til 20mg given (unless pulse>120bpm) after 500mL colloid IV.

▸▸ Give prophylactic H₂ blockers until normal postnatal care starts.

▸▸ Restrict fluids to 80mL/h. Hourly urine output. Renal failure is rare. Maintain fluid restriction until postpartum diuresis. Fluid restriction is inappropriate if there is haemorrhage.

Treatment of seizures (eclampsia):

▸▸ Treat a first seizure with 4g **magnesium sulfate** in 100mL 0.9% saline IVI over 5min + maintenance IVI of 1g/h for 24h. Beware ↓ respiration.

▸▸ If recurrent seizure give 2g IVI magnesium sulfate over 5 min.

▸▸ Check tendon reflexes and respiratory rate every 15min.

▸▸ Stop magnesium sulfate IVI if respiratory rate <14/min or tendon reflex loss, or urine output <20mL/h. Have IV **calcium gluconate** ready in case of MgSO₄ toxicity: 1g (10mL) over 10 min if respiratory depression.

▸▸ Use diazepam once if fits continue (eg 5–10mg slowly IV). If seizures continue, ventilate and consider other causes (consider CT scan).

Pitfalls in the management of eclampsia and pre-eclampsia

- Belief that the disease behaves predictably, and that BP is a good marker.
- Ignoring mild proteinuria; even if 1+, the patient may be dead within 24h.
- Believing antihypertensives stop pre-eclampsia (they may stop stroke). They don't. Only delivery cures. Diuretics deplete plasma volume, and are especially contraindicated (except in the rare left ventricular failure or laryngeal oedema complicating pre-eclampsia). Continue antihypertensives postpartum; wean off slowly. Avoid methyldopa (depression).
- Believing that delivery removes risk. In the UK, 44% of eclamptic fits are postpartum: half of these are >48h postpartum. Continue vigilance until clinically and biochemically normal. Avoid discharge <5 postnatal days.
- Ergometrine should not be used for the 3ʳᵈ stage (it ↑ BP and risks stroke).
- Not replacing significant blood loss *meticulously*. Risks are hypovolaemia or fatal fluid overload ± acute respiratory distress syndrome. Have one person (the most experienced) in charge of all the IVIs.
- Failure to inform anaesthetists early and use intensive care facilities.
- Not asking GP to check for proteinuria at 6 weeks (13% have renal disease or underlying hypertension). Refer to physician if proteinuria still present.

Obstetrics

▶This is a leading cause of perinatal mortality and morbidity.

Premature infants are those born before 37^{+6} weeks' gestation. Prevalence: ~6% of singletons, 46% of twin, 79% of triplet or higher-order deliveries. About 1.4% are before 32^{+0} weeks—when neonatal problems are greatest. In 25%, delivery is elective (p62). 10% are due to multiple pregnancy; 25% are due to APH, cervical incompetence, amnionitis, uterine abnormalities, diabetes, polyhydramnios, pyelonephritis, or other infections. In 40% the cause is unknown, but abnormal genital tract colonization (bacterial vaginosis) with ureaplasma and *Mycoplasma hominis* is implicated, as either a risk factor or risk marker. If treating 2nd trimester vaginosis is necessary, use macrolide or **clindamycin**, (not metronidazole which is associated with ↑ premature birth rates).[113]

Prophylactic antibiotics in spontaneous preterm labour with intact membranes increase risk of cerebral palsy,[1] and are not recommended.[114]

Managing preterm rupture of membranes (PROM) Admit; do T° MSU, and HVS—using a sterile bivalve speculum. Assess for causes/associations: eg abruption, twins, and polyhydramnios. If liquor is not obvious its presence is suggested if nitrazine sticks (pH-sensitive) turn black (false +ve with infected vaginal discharge, semen, blood, and urine). Give corticosteroids[115] (see opposite page). In 80%, membrane rupture initiates labour. The problem with the 20% who do not go into labour is balancing advantages of remaining *in utero* (maturity and surfactant ↑) against the threat of infection (causes 20% of neonatal deaths after PROM). Intrauterine infection supervenes after membranes have ruptured in 10% by 48h, 26% by 72h, 40% by >72h. Prophylactic erythromycin 250mg/6h PO for 10 days or until delivery reduces births within 42 hours. If infection develops, do blood culture and give IV antibiotics (eg **ampicillin** 500mg/6h IV + **gentamicin** 3–5mg/kg/8h over ≥3mins IV) and expedite labour (p62). Antibiotics for ~24h pre-labour, ↓ rates of intraventricular haemorrhage and periventricular malacia (below) in the baby. If labour supervenes, allow it to progress. If liquor stops draining for >48h (rare) slowly mobilize the mother.

Management of preterm labour In 50% contractions cease spontaneously. Treating the cause (eg pyelonephritis) may make it cease. Give corticosteroids (p51). Attempts to suppress contractions (tocolysis) are unlikely to succeed if membranes are ruptured or the cervix >4cm dilated. The rationale for tocolytic drug use was that delay of preterm labour would improve fetal outcome without causing harm to mother or fetus. Trials have shown them to be of almost no clinical benefit, and only nifedipine is associated with improvement of fetal outcome. It is quite reasonable not to use tocolytic drugs; though they may be considered desirable in certain circumstances eg to give time for corticosteroids to work, or for *in utero* transfer. Use only between 24–33 weeks. Consider transfer to hospital with NICU facilities. Call paediatrician to attend to the baby at birth. See cord-cutting recommendations opposite.

Tocolytics Absolute CI: chorioamnionitis, fetal death or lethal abnormality, condition (fetal or maternal) needing immediate delivery. Relative CI: fetal growth restriction or distress, pre-eclampsia, placenta praevia, abruption, cervix >4cm. β-sympathomimetics, associated with maternal fluid overload and pulmonary oedema are not recommended. Atosiban (licensed in Europe) has fewer maternal effects, has not been shown to benefit the fetus. Nifedipine is as effective, and associated with less newborn respiratory distress and admission to intensive care. Regimen: **nifedipine** 20mg PO then 10–20mg/6–8h according to uterine activity (unlicensed use). Use up to 48h. SE: ↓ BP; headache; flushing; pulse ↑ (transient); myocardial infarction (very rare); CI: heart disease (caution diabetes, multiple pregnancy as pulmonary oedema risk).[116]

---

1 Co-amoxiclav or erythromycin in threatened preterm labour with intact membranes ↑ risk cerebral palsy: the number needed to harm with erythromycin is 64 and with co-amoxiclav 79.[117,118]

Glucocorticoids *Dose:* Betamethasone 12mg IM with a 2nd dose 12–24h later (or dexamethasone 6mg/12/h ×4 doses).

These help fetal surfactant production, lowering mortality (by 31%) and complications of RDS (p118) by 44%. They also help close patent ductuses and protect against periventricular malacia, a cause of cerebral palsy.

• Use in all women (but note cautions, below) at risk of iatrogenic or spontaneous preterm birth between ~24+0 and ~34+6 weeks.[119 RCOL]
• If growth restriction too, use up to 35+6 weeks.
• If risk at 23+0–23+6 weeks use only on senior advice.
• Use before all elective Caesarean sections up to 38+6 weeks.
• Consider use at 35–6 weeks if delivery expedited for pre-eclampsia (NICE).[120]
• Use with caution if maternal systemic infection eg TB, maternal sepsis: if overt chorioamnionitis seek senior opinion before use. If diabetic, monitor glucose.

Benefit occurs within 24h (and lasts for 7 days). Repeat doses (eg every 2wks until 33wks' gestation or delivery) did more harm than good in the MACS study (babies weighed less, had smaller heads).[121] A further 'rescue' dose is only recommended if the first course was given before 26 weeks and a new obstetric indication arises.[119]

Magnesium sulphate Studies show a neuroprotective effect if given antenatally for babies<34 weeks' gestation. It is estimated that 63 women will need treatment to prevent one case of cerebral palsy. Australian draft national clinical guidelines recommend a maternal loading dose of 4g IV over 20–30 minutes followed by 1g/h maintenance infusion for up to 24h (or birth, if earlier), and use if fetus <30 weeks' gestation.[122]

Delivery Babies delivered at <28 weeks' gestation should be delivered in a room with temperature of 26°c, wrapped in food grade plastic wrap or bag without drying after birth and be placed under heat whilst stabilizing (keep wrapped until temperature checked in NICU).[123] Older babies are wrapped in dry towels. A 3-min delay in cutting the cord, (if premature babies are vigorous and not needing active resuscitation), and holding the baby 20cm below the introitus, results in higher haematocrit levels, and reduces transfusion and oxygen supplement requirements in premature babies, and reduces rates of intraventricular haemorrhage, but increases need for phototherapy.[123]

Prematurity, survival, and disability—the figures
• Cerebral palsy is present in 20% of surviving babies born at 24–26 weeks' gestation (compared with 4% at 32 weeks) in a large French study.[124]

Viability thresholds for very premature babies have reduced by 1 week per decade for the last 40 years. Survival before 22 weeks is very rare. In 1995, 1% of babies born at 22–23 weeks survived to leave hospital; 11% at 23–24; 26% at 24–25; 44% at 25–26. Of surviving babies born between 23–24 weeks two-thirds had moderate or severe disability; by 25 to 26 weeks two-thirds had no or only mild disability. These figures have lead to guidelines for consideration of treatment at different gestations, eg not resuscitating babies of less than 22 weeks' completed gestation unless specifically requested by parents after discussion with senior paediatrician; but normally admitting babies of >23 weeks' completed gestation to neonatal intensive care.[125] The figures for England, Wales and Northern Ireland were that 58% of babies born at 24 weeks' gestation survived the neonatal period, increasing to 77% at 25 weeks; (85% at 26 weeks; 92% at 27 and 28 weeks; 96% at 29 weeks; 97% at 33 weeks).[126]

Obstetrics

BIRMINGHAM UNIVERSITY LIBRARY

▶When talking to parents, avoid the term *growth retardation* as this may imply to them the inevitability of mental handicap—which is not the case. Distinguish premature babies from those who are small-for-gestational age (SGA): they are at risk from different problems after birth.

Causes of growth restriction (IUGR) Growth restricted neonates are those weighing < the 10th centile for their gestational age (*Tables*, p129).

Maternal factors: Multiple pregnancy, malformation, infection, smoking, diabetes, BP ↑, Hb ↓, pre-eclampsia, heart or renal disease, asthma.

~10% are to mothers who only ever produce small babies.

Asymmetric growth restriction: Where placental insufficiency was the cause, head circumference is relatively spared (the baby has been starved).

Antenatal diagnosis 50% are undetected before birth, and many babies suspected of IUGR do not have it. Measuring fundal height progress from the symphysis pubis is recommended by NICE to measure growth, (ideally use with centile charts). Oligohydramnios and poor fetal movements are other indications of placental insufficiency. If growth restriction is suspected, monitor growth *in utero* by serial ultrasounds of head circumference and abdominal circumference. If umbilical cord Doppler blood flows are normal the outcome of growth restricted pregnancies is better (fewer premature births and stillbirths). Those with abnormal Dopplers may benefit from maternal low-dose aspirin (p47), eg 75mg/24h PO. Biophysical profile monitoring (p46) and antenatal cardiotocography (p44) are used to try to detect those babies who are becoming hypoxic *in utero* and who would benefit from delivery to prevent stillbirth. Advise the mother to stop smoking, and to take plenty of rest.

Labour and aftercare Growth restricted fetuses are more susceptible to hypoxia, so monitor in labour (p44). If steroids needed, note later gestation (p51). After birth, temperature regulation may be a problem, so ensure a warm welcome; nurse those <2kg in an incubator. After being relatively hypoxic *in utero* the Hb at birth is high, so jaundice is more common. They have little stored glycogen so are prone to hypoglycaemia. Feed within 2h of birth and measure blood glucose before each 3-hourly feed. If hypoglycaemic despite regular feeds, transfer to a special care unit. They are more susceptible to infection. Routine induction at 36 weeks does not show benefit over induction if needed.[127]

Distinguishing growth restriction from prematurity Before 34 weeks' gestation there is no breast bud tissue; from then it develops at 1mm diameter/week. Ear cartilage develops between 35 and 39 weeks so premature babies' ears do not spring back when folded. Testes lie in the inguinal canal at 35 weeks, in the scrotum from 37. Labia minora are exposed in premature girls. Skin creases on the anterior ⅓ of the foot appear by 35 weeks (on anterior ⅔ by 39, and all over from 39). 'Prems' have red, hairy skin. Vernix is made from 28 weeks and is maximal at 36 weeks. Prems do not lie with legs flexed until 32 weeks. All limbs are flexed from 36 weeks.

Effects of IUGR in adult life By age 23yrs, milder cognitive problems have often been overcome[128]—but new problems begin to be manifest:
• Hypertension
• Type 2 diabetes mellitus
• Coronary artery disease
• Autoimmune thyroid disease.

So fetal malnutrition casts a long shadow. Specific early deficiencies are important too (eg iodine, iron).

Large for gestational age

These are babies above the 90th centile in weight for gestation.

Causes: Constitutionally large (usually familial—the largest 10% of the population); maternal diabetes (p24); hyperinsulinism; Beckwith–Wiedemann syndrome (p638).

Labour and aftercare: Large babies risk birth injury (see *impacted shoulder*, p72). Large babies are prone to immaturity of suckling and swallowing and may need temporary tube feeding. They are prone to hypoglycaemia and hypocalcaemia. Polycythaemia may result in jaundice. They are also prone to left colon syndrome: a self-limiting condition clinically mimicking Hirschsprung's disease (p130) whereby temporary bowel obstruction (possibly also with meconium plug) occurs. Rarely, there is renal vein thrombosis.

Definition Prolonged pregnancy is defined as that exceeding 42 completed weeks of pregnancy (gestation having been assessed by ultrasound at <16 weeks' gestation).

Incidence 5–10% of pregnancies.

Problems
- Possible placental insufficiency
- Larger fetuses (25% >4000g)
- Fetal skull more ossified so less mouldable
- Increased meconium passage in labour (25-40%)
- Increased fetal distress in labour
- Increased caesarean rates for labours after 41 completed weeks.

Management At 38-week visit discuss what is recommended if spontaneous labour does not occur by 41 completed weeks, including membrane sweep and induction. Arrange for visit at 41 weeks if not delivered.

1 Membrane sweep. On vaginal examination as much membrane is swept from the lower segment as possible by a finger inserted through the cervix. It is thought to induce natural prostaglandins. This may cause discomfort and a little bleeding but may induce labour 'naturally'. 8 women are membrane swept for 1 formal induction avoided. Offer at 40- and 41-week visit in nullips, at 41 weeks in multips.

2 A policy of induction after 41 completed weeks' pregnancy does reduce fetal death rate.[129] NICE says to offer induction between 41[+0] and 42[+0] weeks.[130] Induction is with vaginal prostaglandin followed by oxytocin (p62). After induction, monitor the fetus in labour (p44). It is estimated that 500 inductions are needed to prevent 1 perinatal death.

3 If the woman declines induction then arrange twice weekly cardiotocography (p44), and ultrasound estimation of amniotic fluid depth to try to detect fetuses who may be becoming hypoxic. Doppler studies of cord blood flow may be used to look for absent end-diastolic flow as a predictor of fetal compromise.

Interestingly, if one looks at the perinatal mortality figures for England, Wales, and Northern Ireland in 2005, the stillbirth rate was 1:1000 total births, and neonatal death rate 0.6:1000 live births for gestations of 42+ weeks; compared with stillbirth rates of 2:1000 and neonatal deaths of 1:1000 for gestations of 37–41 weeks.[131] NICE warns that their advice may not hold equal weight for all ethnic groups in the UK as Asians have excess fetal mortality, but especially after 37 weeks gestation.[130]

Signs of postmaturity in the baby: Dry, cracked, peeling, loose skin; decreased subcutaneous tissue; meconium staining of nails and cord.

▶▶Fetal distress

Fetal distress signifies hypoxia. Prolonged or repeated hypoxia causes fetal acidosis. An early sign may be the passage of meconium in labour (p72). Other signs that the fetus may be hypoxic are a fetal tachycardia persisting above 160 beats/min (tachycardia may also occur if the mother has a high temperature or is dehydrated). Hypoxia may also be reflected by loss of variability of the baseline in the fetal heart rate trace and slowing and irregularity of the heart rate (especially late decelerations p45). ▶▶If the heart rate falls below 100 beats/min urgent assessment is required. Hypoxia may be confirmed by the use of fetal blood sampling (p44). When significant hypoxia appears to be present (eg pH <7.24), deliver promptly (by the quickest route available, eg caesarean section or vaginal extraction). In complete anoxia the pH falls by 0.1 unit/min.

▶▶Obstetric shock

Most obstetric shock is associated with severe haemorrhage (see MINIBOX). It should be remembered that with placental abruption, actual bleeding may be far in excess of that revealed *per vaginam* (p56).

Causes
• Severe haemorrhage
• Ruptured uterus (p80)
• Inverted uterus (p86)
• Amniotic fluid embolus (p89)
• Pulmonary embolism
• Septicaemia
• Adrenal haemorrhage

Vomiting, diarrhoea, and abdominal pain may be signs of genital sepsis. There may be rash (generalized streptococcal maculopapular). Fever may be absent. Persistent tachycardia, peripheral vascular shutdown, increased respiratory rate, oliguria, metabolic acidosis, and reduced oxygen saturation indicate critical illness needing urgent management. DIC may develop; so may uterine atony with subsequent massive haemorrhage. There may be hypothermia and hypotension. Check blood gases to detect metabolic acidosis. Unfortunately young women can maintain blood pressure, appearing deceptively well and talking until sudden cardiovascular decompensation occurs. Septicaemia may lack classical signs (eg pyrexia) and must be considered where profound persisting shock is present, be appropriately investigated (eg blood cultures), and treated immediately suspected, eg **cefuroxime** 1.5g/8h IV + **metronidazole** 500mg/8h IVI + **gentamicin** 1.5mg/kg/8h IV given over >3min; (do levels, but levels not needed acutely, see *OHCM* p371), without waiting for microbiology results. Liaise with microbiologists. Nurse on critical care unit with critical care anaesthetic help.

Prompt resuscitation is required (see individual pages for management). Renal function and urine output should always be measured after shock has occurred (p28). A late complication can be Sheehan's syndrome (also called Simmonds' disease) whereby pituitary necrosis leads to lack of thyroid-stimulating hormone, adrenocorticotrophic hormone, and the gonadotrophic hormones, hence leading to hypothyroidism, Addisonian symptoms, and genital atrophy.

Obstetrics

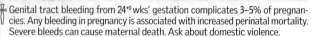

Genital tract bleeding from 24^{+0} wks' gestation complicates 3–5% of pregnancies. Any bleeding in pregnancy is associated with increased perinatal mortality. Severe bleeds can cause maternal death. Ask about domestic violence.

▶ Avoid vaginal examination: placenta praevias may bleed catastrophically.

Dangerous causes Abruption, placenta praevia, vasa praevia (here the baby may bleed to death).

Other uterine sources: Circumvallate placenta, placental sinuses.

Lower genital tract sources: Cervical polyps, erosions and carcinoma, cervicitis, vaginitis, vulval varicosities.

Placental abruption ('accidental haemorrhage') Part of the placenta becomes detached from the uterus. The outcome depends on the amount of blood loss and degree of separation. It may recur in subsequent pregnancies (4%: 19–24% if twice). *Associations* pre-eclampsia, smoking, IUGR (p52), PROM (p50), multiple pregnancy, polyhydramnios, ↑ maternal age, thrombophilia, abdo trauma, assisted reproduction, cocaine/amphetamine use, infection, non vertex presentation. Bleeding may be well localized to one placental area and there may be delay before bleeding is revealed.

Consequences: Placental insufficiency may cause fetal anoxia or death. Compression of uterine muscles by blood causes tenderness, and may prevent good contraction at all stages of labour, so beware a PPH (which occurs in ~25%). Posterior abruptions may present with backache. There may be uterine hypercontractility (>7 contractions per 15min). Thromboplastin release may cause DIC (10%). Concealed loss may cause maternal shock after which beware renal failure and Sheehan's syndrome (p55).

Placenta praevia (For terminology and complications, see p14.) The placenta lies in the lower uterine segment. Bleeding is always revealed.

Distinguishing... *Abruption*	From *Placenta praevia*
Shock out of keeping with visible loss	Shock in proportion to visible loss
Pain constant	No pain
Tender, tense uterus	Uterus not tender
Normal lie and presentation	Both may be abnormal
Fetal heart: absent/distressed	Fetal heart usually normal
Coagulation problems	Coagulation problems rare
Beware pre-eclampsia, DIC, anuria	Small bleeds before large

Note: the risk of PPH is increased in both conditions. The lower segment may not contract well after a placenta praevia.

Management of APH *Always admit.* ▶▶If bleeding is severe call emergency ambulance, put up IVI, take bloods, and raise legs. Give O$_2$ at 15L/min via mask with reservoir. On admission, if shocked give fresh ABO Rh compatible or 0 Rh−ve blood (eg 6u, 2 IVIs) fast until systolic BP >100mmHg. Send blood for clotting screen. Catheterize bladder; keep urine output >30mL/h. Call anaesthetist to monitor fluids (CVP lines help). *Summon expert help urgently.* If bleeding is severe, *deliver*—caesarean section for placenta praevia (sometimes for abruption, or induction). Beware PPH (manage 3rd stage with Syntometrine®).

For milder bleeding, set up IVI, do Hb, crossmatch, coagulation studies, and U&E. Check pulse, BP, and loss regularly. Establish diagnosis (ultrasound of placenta, speculum examination). If placenta praevia is the diagnosis, keep in hospital until delivery (usually by caesarean section at 37–38 weeks). If pain and bleeding from a small abruption settles and the fetus is not compromised the woman may go home (after anti-D, if indicated; 6-weekly if recurrent bleeds), but then treat as 'high-risk' pregnancy (serial scans). Arrange follow-up.

Obstetrics

'Labour is one of the shortest yet most hazardous journeys humans make in their lifetime.' From the 1ˢᵗ trimester, the uterus has Braxton Hicks contractions (ie non-painful 'practice' contractions, eg to ≤15mmHg pressure; in labour pressure is ~60mmHg). They are commonest after 36 weeks.

Normal labour (fig 1) ~60% of births are normal and need no intervention (we over-medicalize ≥20% of labours, intervening unnecessarily).[132]

Normal labour occurs after 37wks' gestation and results in spontaneous vaginal delivery of the baby within 24h of the onset of regular spontaneous contractions. It is often heralded by a 'show', ie a plug of cervical mucus and a little blood as the membranes strip from the os (membranes may then rupture).

The first stage of labour *Latent phase* (not necessarily continuous): there are painful contractions, the cervix initially *effaces* (becomes shorter and softer) then dilates to 4cm. *Established phase:* contractions with dilatation from 4cm. A satisfactory rate of dilatation from 4cm is 0.5cm/h. The 1ˢᵗ stage generally takes 8–18h in a primip, and 5–12h in a multip. During the first stage check maternal ʙᴘ, and ᴛ° 4-hourly, pulse hourly; assess the contractions every 30min, their strength (you should not be able to indent the uterus with the fingers during a contraction) and their frequency (ideally 3–4 per 10min, lasting up to 1min). Note frequency of bladder emptying. Offer vaginal examination eg every 4h to assess the degree of cervical dilatation, the position and the station of the head (measured in cm above the ischial spines) and note the degree of moulding (p42). Note the state of the liquor (p73). Auscultate fetal heart rate (if not continuously monitored), by Pinard or Doppler every 15min, listening for 1min after a contraction. When to use continuous monitoring? See p44.

The second stage *Passive stage* is complete cervical dilatation (but no desire to push. In *active stage,* the baby can be seen, there is full dilatation with expulsive contractions and maternal effort (using abdominal muscles and the Valsalva manoeuvre until the baby is born (see *Movement of head in labour,* p42). Discourage supine maternal position in 2ⁿᵈ stage. Encourage mother to adopt a comfortable position. Check ʙᴘ and pulse hourly, ᴛ° 4-hourly , assess contractions half-hourly, auscultate for 1min after a contraction every 5min, offer vaginal examination hourly, and record urination during 2ⁿᵈ stage. If contractions wane, oxytocin augmentation may be needed.

As the head descends, the perineum stretches and the anus gapes. Expect birth within 3h from active 2ⁿᵈ stage in primips (refer to obstetrician if not imminent at 2h); expect birth within 2h in a multip (refer if birth not imminent at 1h). Prevent a precipitate delivery (and so intracranial bleeding) by pressure over the perineum. 1-min delay in clamping the cord is recommended in vigorous term babies.[123] 3-min delay benefits premature babies (↓ anaemia).[133]

The third stage is delivery of the placenta. As the uterus contracts to a <24-week size after the baby is born, the placenta separates from the uterus through the spongy layer of the decidua basalis. It then buckles and a small amount of retroplacental haemorrhage aids its removal.

Signs of separation: Cord lengthening → rush of blood (retroplacental haemorrhage) *per vaginam* → uterus rises → uterus contracts in the abdomen (felt with hand as a globular mass). Physiological (natural) 3ʳᵈ stage takes ≤1h.

Use of Syntometrine® (**ergometrine maleate 500µg ɪᴍ + oxytocin 5ᴜ ɪᴍ**) as the anterior shoulder is born decreases third stage time (to ~5min), and decreases the incidence of ᴘᴘʜ, but may cause problems for undiagnosed twins. It can precipitate myocardial infarction and is contraindicated in those with pre-eclampsia, severe hypertension, severe liver or renal impairment, severe heart disease and familial hypercholesterolaemia. If ʙᴘ not measured in labour give just **oxytocin**.[134] Examine the placenta to check it is complete.

▶ Is thromboprophylaxis needed? (p16)

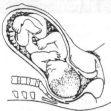

(1)
1st stage of labour. The cervix dilates. After full dilatation the head flexes further and descends further into the pelvis.

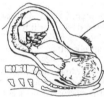

(2)
During the early second stage the head rotates at the levels of the ischial spine so the occiput lies in the anterior part of pelvis. In late second stage the head broaches the vulval ring (crowning) and the perineum stretches over the head.

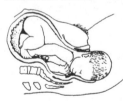

(3)
The head is born. The shoulders still lie transversely in the midpelvis.

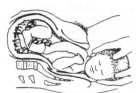

(4)
Birth of the anterior shoulder. The shoulders rotate to lie in the anteroposterior diameter of the pelvic outlet. The head rotates externally, 'restitutes', to its direction at onset of labour. Downward and backward traction of the head by the birth attendant aids delivery of the anterior shoulder.

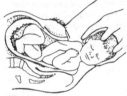

(5)
Birth of the posterior shoulder is aided by lifting the head upwards whilst maintaining traction.

Fig 1. Normal labour

Obstetrics

This is rupture of the membranes prior to the onset of labour in women at or over 37 completed weeks gestation. It occurs in 8–10% of pregnancies. Infection of the lower genital tract or amnion is a known aetiological factor.

When there is prelabour rupture of membranes risk of serious infection is increased (1% versus 0.5% for women with intact membranes). 60% of women will go into spontaneous labour within 24 hours.

If a woman has prelabour membrane rupture she should be offered a choice of induction or expectant management. If spontaneous labour has not commenced by 24h then NICE states that it is appropriate to induce labour.$_{NICE}^{139}$ Vaginal prostaglandin is the preferred method of trying to induce labour. (NICE notes that special product characteristics say use vaginal prostaglandins with caution, or that they should not be used in those with ruptured membranes but there is over 20 years UK experience with these. So obtain and document informed consent with their use.)

Until labour is commenced or if expectant management is chosen to continue beyond 24h ask the woman to take her temperature 4-hourly in waking hours and report to hospital immediately if she develops fever or if there is change in colour or smell of vaginal loss. Bathing and showering do not increase, but sexual intercourse may increase risk of infection. If there are signs of infection give a full course if IV antibiotics (p50).

Monitor fetal heart rate at 1st contact and every 24h after membrane rupture whilst the woman is not in labour. Ask her to report if there are reduced fetal movements. Those giving birth after 24h of ruptured membranes should deliver where there are neonatal care facilities, and advise to stay in hospital for 12h after birth.

Babies are most susceptible to infection within 12h of birth. Observe at 1h, 2h and then 2-hourly for further 10h. Observations should include, general wellbeing, chest movement and nasal flare, capillary refill, feeding, muscle tone, temperature, respirations and heart rate. If there is any suggestion of sepsis in the baby call a neonatal care specialist. Mothers should also be advised to report any health concerns with the baby in the 1st 5 days of life.

~20% of UK labours are induced artificially, usually because it has been decided that to remain *in utero* is relatively more risky for the fetus than to be born, but in some it is because of risk to the mother. 75% of inductions are for hypertension, pre-eclampsia, prolonged pregnancy, or rhesus disease. Other indications are diabetes, previous stillbirth, abruption, fetal death *in utero*, and placental insufficiency.

▶Inducing mothers at 41+ weeks aims to reduce stillbirth rates.

Contraindications Cephalopelvic disproportion which is absolute, malpresentations other than breech or face presentation, fetal distress, placenta praevia, cord presentation, vasa praevia, pelvic tumour, previous repair to cervix. Cone biopsy requires caution.

Cervical ripeness When an induction is being planned the state of the cervix will be assessed. In 95% of women at term the cervix is ripe. If primips are induced with an unripe cervix (Bishop's score ≤3, see below) the rates of prolonged labour, fetal distress, and caesarean section are increased. This is less marked in multips.

Modified Bishop score	0	1	2
Cervical dilation (cm)	0	1–2	3–4
Length of cervix (cm)	>2	1–2	<1
Station of head (cm above ischial spines)	−3	−2	−1
Cervical consistency	Firm	Medium	Soft
Position of cervix	Posterior	Middle	Anterior

A score of >5 is 'ripe'. An unripe cervix may be ripened using prostaglandin (PGE2) vaginal gel (1mg) the evening before or the morning of induction (use 2mg for unfavourable primip cervix). If antenatal fetal heart rate monitoring is indicated, this should commence before prostaglandin insertion. If there is failure to ripen (occurs in 12%) PGE2 may be repeated 6–8h later. If the cervix still remains unripe consider caesarean section. PGE2 may stimulate uterine contractions or precipitate labour.

Once the cervix is ripe, rupture the membranes (amniotomy) and start intrapartum fetal heart rate monitoring using a scalp clip or pulse oximetry (less invasive, see *OHCM* p148). Oxytocin is given IV in 5% dextrose using a pump system (eg Ivac®). Infusions start at 1–4 milliunits (MU) per min, increasing every 30min until 3–4 contractions occur every 10min (usually at a rate of 4–10MU/min: occasionally 20MU/min may be needed); max dose 5U/day. Monitor the fetal heart and stop if distress or uterine hyperstimulation. Beware using large volumes of IV fluid (if >4 litres, there is risk of water intoxication—ie confusion, convulsions, and coma). Use standard strength solutions as per *BNF*. When the cervix is 5cm dilated the uterus is more sensitive to oxytocin and 8MU/min may be sufficient to maintain contractions. Note: the Dublin regimen (p64) results in most women going into spontaneous labour.

Misoprostol (a prostaglandin E1 analogue) PO or PV is as effective at cervical ripening and inducing labour as PGE2 and oxytocin. Oral route (eg 50µg 4-hourly) has fewer problems with uterine hyperstimulation.[135] NICE says use only use for labour induction after intrauterine death.

Problems of induction •Failed induction (15%) •Uterine hyperstimulation (1–5%) •Iatrogenic prematurity •Infection •Bleeding (vasa praevia) •Cord prolapse (eg with a high head at amniotomy) •Caesarean section (22%) and instrumental delivery rates (15%) are higher •Uterine rupture (rare).

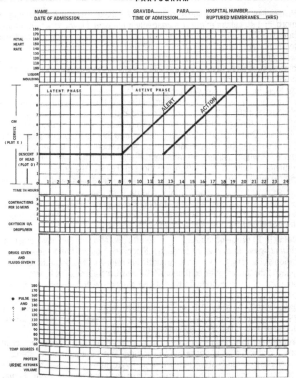

Fig 1. Example of a partogram. It has a steep x/y gradient of ratio 1:1. Less steep ratios (eg 2:1) may predispose to premature intervention, as does inclusion of the 'latent' phase on the partogram.

Reproduced with permission from the Oxford Handbook of Obstetrics and Gynaecology, 2nd edition.

Historically, this emanated from Dublin, a centre of excellence for labouring mothers with coherent labour management plans, and low caesarean section rates (eg 5% *vs* 24% for other centres): forceps rates were ~10%. The cardinal features were to have only women in active 1st stage of labour (p58) on labour ward; to assess regularly (eg hourly for 1st 3h, subsequently every 2h) to check that cervical dilatation was progressing well—and to take action if not. Membranes would be ruptured if no progress after 1h, and labour augmented with oxytocin in primiparous women with single, cephalic presentation babies, if unsatisfactory cervical dilatation within the next hour (or in subsequent time periods). Satisfactory dilatation was considered 1cm/h. Mothers had a personal midwife throughout labour. Women were kept informed of their progress, given an estimated time of delivery and assured that delivery should be within 12h of entering the labour ward. Caesarean section would be performed on those for whom delivery not imminent at 12h. The system was very efficient, with unit delivery costs ⅓ of those in the UK at the time.

The problem with active management is that it is very medicalized, with amniotomy, frequent examinations, and IVI lines needed. Over time this has been felt to be unacceptable and although amniotomy and augmentation have a role in delay in labour; current recommended time scales are slower. Below are the recommendations of *NICE*.[109] For normal labour see page 58.

Delay in 1st stage of labour This is <2cm/h dilatation in 4h in any woman; or slowing in progress in 2nd or subsequent labours. Consider the descent and rotation of the fetal head and the strength and frequency of contractions. When delay is diagnosed offer continuous fetal heart monitoring (p44). If delay diagnosed, offer amniotomy (advise it will <labour by 1h and may ↑ pain and contraction strength). Re-examine 2h later; if <1cm progress and amniotomy at 1st declined, offer again; if has had; consider oxytocin augmentation; explaining that augmentation increases pain and strength of contractions. Ensure adequate pain relief. Offer epidural before oxytocin started.

Augmentation This recognizes that a primiparous uterus is an inefficient organ of birth that is *not* prone to rupture—but the multiparous uterus is an efficient organ that *is* rupture-prone. Oxytocin may be used to enhance efficiency in the primiparous uterus without maternal danger. Oxytocin may be dangerous to multips as delay is likely to be from obstructed labour, so a decision to use it must only be made by a senior obstetrician. Continuous fetal heart monitoring should commence when oxytocin used. See p62, p44. Advise examination 4h later: if >2cm dilatation, continue oxytocin, examining 4hrly; if <2cm dilatation get obstetric review; caesarean section may be needed.

Delay in 2nd stage of labour If delivery not imminent within 1 hour after onset of active 2nd stage (p58) in multips; or after 2h in primips call obstetrician experienced in operative delivery. Offer amniotomy if membranes not ruptured. Ensure adequate anaesthesia/analgesia. Ensure obstetric review every 15–30mins. If 2nd stage prolonged or fetal compromise consider instrumental delivery (p76) with adequate analgesia/anaesthesia. Caesarean section (p78) should be advised if vaginal birth is not possible.

Meconium in liquor At amniotomy this suggests placental insufficiency. Meconium other than light staining in good liquor volume prompts fetal blood sampling and scalp clip electronic monitoring—or prompt caesarean section (fetal blood pH low, or very thick meconium).

▶Pain relief in labour is our greatest gift to womankind; however, in the UK NHS 25% of mothers said they didn't get the relief they needed.[132]

Not everyone wants natural birth: don't make people feel guilty about requesting pain relief. The ideal analgesia must be harmless to mother and baby, must allow good maternal cooperation, and must not affect uterine contractility.

Education That given by the National Childbirth Trust meets all these criteria. Education about labour reduces fear; breathing exercises and relaxation techniques teach the mother ways to combat pain herself.

Waterbirth Labouring in water has been shown to reduce need for regional anaesthesia.[136] It is recommended by NICE with the advice that water temperature be checked hourly and kept <37.5° to prevent maternal pyrexia.[109]NICE

In the first stage, **narcotic injections** are often tried, eg pethidine 50–150mg IM (not if birth expected in <2–3h as neonatal respiratory depression may occur, reversible with naloxone 0.1–0.2mg as a single dose IM). Expect analgesia by 20min and to last 3h. NB: doses frequently produce vomiting, but no relief of pain. Other SE: disorientation, ↓gastric emptying (nausea, vomiting), neonatal respiratory depression and drowsiness. CI: mother on MAOIs (p368). Give with antiemetic. Women should not enter water within 2h of injection.[109]NICE

Nitrous oxide (50% in O_2 = Entonox®) can be inhaled throughout labour and is self-administered using a demand valve. CI: pneumothorax. It can make the woman feel nauseated and light-headed.

Pudendal block (sacral nerve roots 2, 3, and 4) uses 8–10mL of 1% lidocaine (= lignocaine) injected 1cm beyond a point just below and medial to the ischial spine on each side. It is used with perineal infiltration for instrumental delivery, but analgesia is insufficient for rotational forceps.

Spinal block See p634; used for rotational delivery or caesarean section.

Epidural anaesthesia See p67. Pain relief is by anaesthetizing pain fibres carried by T11–S5. Epidurals may be started during latent 1st phase of labour,[109]NICE and continued until placenta delivered, and any perineal repair completed. Set up IVI. Give IV ephedrine and volume preload.[52]RCOL Check BP, every 5min for 15min, and electronically monitor fetal heart for 30 mins after the epidural is set up, and after top ups. Top-ups are required ~2-hourly. Recall anaesthetist if inadequate pain relief within 30mins. Assess level of sensory block hourly. Epidurals may be helpful for the following: OP position (p71), breech, multiple pregnancy, preterm delivery, pre-eclampsia, forceps delivery, incoordinate uterine contractions. *Problems:* For those due to technique, see p635. There may be postural hypotension (IV fluids, nurse 15° to left side), urinary retention (catheterize regularly), paralysis (pelvic floor muscle paralysis reduces rotation and voluntary effort in 2nd stage, perhaps increasing need for forceps). Aim for delivery within 4h of full dilatation. Oxytocin for 2nd stage in primips and delaying pushing until 1–2h post full dilatation, or strong desire to push, reduces forceps rates.

After delivery: urinary retention and headache (esp. after dural puncture).

Epidural anaesthesia for those having heparin thromboprophylaxis: When low molecular weight heparin (LMWH) is used, wait 12h after heparin dose before inserting block or removing catheter (24h if on therapeutic rather than prophylactic dose of heparin).[52]RCOL Wait at least 4h after block siting before next dose of LMWH. Aim to give LMWH at 18.00h each day. Beware use of other anticoagulants or non-steroidal anti-inflammatory drugs. Inductions may need to be timed around heparin doses. Heparin use can preclude use of regional anaesthesia (eg in spontaneous labour). All patients must be extremely vigilantly monitored to detect new numbness; weakness; bowel or bladder dysfunction. Any neurological problem must be investigated as an emergency.

Combined spinal epidural (CSE) anaesthesia gives quicker pain relief, with little or no motor blockade in most mothers, allowing standing, walking, sitting, and voiding urine. A large-bore needle is put into the epidural space, and a fine-bore needle put through that to puncture the subdural space. (Cerebrospinal fluid can be aspirated via the spinal needle to confirm placement.) A small dose of opiate (eg fentanyl) and anaesthetic is used intrathecally to give pain relief during the 1st stage. An epidural catheter threaded into the epidural space allows top up with anaesthetic to give more profound analgesia for 2nd stage. The patient can control the dose, and this leads to a dose reduction of 35%, and reduces motor blockade. Women should inform their midwife if they notice light-headedness, nausea, or weak legs. Spontaneous delivery rates are not better than with traditional epidural. Systematic review (n=2658) found that apart from quicker onset of action there was no difference when compared to *low-dose* epidural in terms of mobilization in labour, modes of birth, maternal satisfaction, post dural puncture headache, blood patch, or maternal hypotension.[137] ►Skilled anaesthetic help is vital.

Incidence[uk] Twins: 3:200 pregnancies; triplets: 1:10,000.

Predisposing factors Previous twins; FH of twins (dizygotic only); ↑ maternal age (<20yrs 6.4:1000; >25yrs 16.8:1000); induced ovulation and IVF (1% of all UK pregnancies of which 25% are ≥twins); race origin (1:150 pregnancies for Japanese, 1:23 in Nigerian Yoruba women). The worldwide rate for monozygotic (of which 75% monochorionic ie shared placenta) twins is constant at ~4:1000.

Features Early pregnancy: uterus large for dates; hyperemesis. Later there may be polyhydramnios. The signs are: >2 poles felt; a multiplicity of fetal parts felt; 2 fetal heart rates heard (reliable if rates differ by >10 beats/min). Ultrasound confirms diagnosis (at 11^{+0}–13^{+6} weeks distinguishes monochorionic from dichorionic twins by placental masses, lambda or T sign, membrane thickness).

Complications during pregnancy • Polyhydramnios • Pre-eclampsia (10% in singleton pregnancies; 30% in twins) • Anaemia commoner (iron and folate requirements increased) • APH incidence rises (6% for twins *vs* 4.7% for singletons) from both abruption and placenta praevia (large placenta).

Fetal complications Perinatal mortality ↑ (8:1000 singletons; 36.7:1000 for twins; 73:1000 for triplets; 204:1000 for higher multiples). The main problem is prematurity. Mean gestation for twins is 37 weeks, for triplets 33 weeks. Growth restriction (p52) is commoner (growth rate=singletons until 24 weeks, may slow thereafter). Malformation rates ↑ ×2–4, especially if monozygotic. Severe disability rate 1.5% for singletons, 3.4% for twins. Ultrasound is the main diagnostic test. Selective feticide (eg with intracardiac potassium chloride)[1] is best used before 20 weeks in the rare instances where it is indicated. With monochorionic pregnancies, placental vascular anastomoses may result in disparate twin size and one being born plethoric (so jaundiced later), the other anaemic ie twin-twin (feto–fetal) transfusion (FFT). Placental anastomosis laser coagulation can treat. Rarely, a fetus dying *in utero* shrinks and mummifies (fetus papyraceous) which may be aborted later or delivered prematurely.

Complications of labour PPH (4–6% in singletons, 10% in twins). Malpresentation is common (cephalic (Ce)/Ce 40%, Ce/breech (Br) 40%, Br/Br 10%, Ce/transverse (Tr) 5%, Br/Tr 4%, Tr/Tr 1%). Vasa praevia rupture; cord prolapse (0.6% singleton, 2.3% twins); premature placental separation and cord entanglement (especially monoamniotic). Undiagnosed twins with syntometrine use.

Management
• Ultrasound at 11^{+0}–13^{+6} weeks for viability, chorionicity, nuchal translucency, malformation: monthly from 20wks (2-weekly if monochorionic: membrane folding suggests FFT).[138] Check fetal growth using 2 biometric variables. Name twins eg left, right. Discordant growth of ≥25% indicates growth restriction and tertiary centre referral. Refer also if FFT; fetal anomaly; monochorionic (MC) +monoamniotic; or MC+diamniotic (triplets); discordant death.
• Check FBC at 20–24 weeks. Give aspirin >12wks if risks indicate (p48).
• More antenatal visits, eg weekly from 30 weeks (risk of eclampsia ↑).
• Tell the mother how to identify preterm labour, and what to do.
• Offer elective birth at 37^{+0} wks for uncomplicated dichorionic twins; at 36^{+0} wks (+steroids p51), for uncomplicated monochorionic twins; at 35^{+0} weeks (+steroids) for uncomplicated triplets.[NICE] Use IV access in labour and anaesthetist availability at delivery. Have paediatricians (one per baby) present at delivery in case resuscitation needed (2nd twins have a higher risk of asphyxia). Most women spontaneously deliver before these dates.

Terminology: Monochorionic twins or triplets share the placenta. If *Monoamniotic* they share one amniotic sac; if di-amniotic there are 2 sacs, triamniotic, there are 3. One placenta risks fetofetal transfusion, 1 sac risks entanglements.

1 In monochorionic twins, total cord coagulation is required to avoid haemorrhage from the co-twin into the dying fetus. Potassium is CI (could pass to other twin).[138] Ethical and legal considerations are complex.

With >4 million IVF babies born worldwide[141] since 1978 it is apparent that there are increased problems for pregnancy and offspring, not merely those of multiple pregnancy. These are:

- Multiple birth: affects 1 in 4 IVF pregnancies. Monozygotic twins are also commoner. The rate of triplets was 5× pre-IVF rates by 1998 but are now only twice, as only 2 eggs are implanted into women <40 years old. Meta-analysis shows that 1 fresh embryo transfer with a frozen embryo months later if unsuccessful gives as good results as 2 embryos transfer.[142]
- Older mother effects: so more pre-eclampsia, pregnancy induced hypertension, caesarean section delivery, and diabetes in the mothers (all of which have implications for offspring).
- Donor egg problems: pregnancy-induced hypertension is 7.1 times more common if nulliparous women receive donated eggs than for standard IVF.
- Genetic defects: Beckwith–Wiedemann syndrome is 6 times commoner in IVF babies and there is concern that intracytoplasmic sperm injection (ICSI) techniques could encourage chromosomal abnormalities or cystic fibrosis in offspring of men with azoospermia or oligospermia, so screening of these men for cystic fibrosis carrier status and chromosomal abnormalities before performing ICSI is recommended.
- Low birthweight is 1.75 times commoner for singleton IVF babies compared to naturally conceived babies (and very low birthweight 2.7–3 times commoner). Part of this is due to prematurity, part to growth restriction. Interestingly low birthweight is particularly correlated to the number of gestation sacs at earliest scan, even if a baby ends up as a singleton. IVF twins are less commonly low birthweight compared to naturally conceived twins.
- Vasa praevia (p14) rates increased, possibly up to 1 : 300.[143]
- Prematurity is twice as common in IVF singleton babies compared to those naturally conceived, 3 times more common for prematurity <32 weeks. Again it is commoner if there was originally >1 gestation sac. There is less difference between IVF and naturally conceived twins.
- Perinatal mortality is ↑ 60% in IVF conceived singletons (but natural conception after delay ↑ mortality ×3 compared to quick conception).
- Abnormality rates are slightly increased (in singletons too).

Bringing up one child is difficult: twins are often very very difficult—but triplets is more than very very very difficult—and are frequently a source of significant psychopathology. Even 4 years after their birth, all mothers in one triplets study[144] suffered from exhaustion and emotional distress. The relationship with the children was often difficult (aggression and conflicts). One-third of mothers had sufficient depression to require psychotropic medication, and one-third spontaneously expressed regrets about having triplets. If triplets are reduced to twins *in utero*, subsequently one-third of mothers will suffer emotional problems (persistent sadness and guilt) up to 1 year. However, adjustment had occurred in ~90% by 2 years after birth.[145]

Legislation in most developed countries is trying to limit the numbers of embryos that may be implanted at *in vitro* fertilization in order to reduce higher-order pregnancies (already there has been a reduction by 25% since 1998). The UK current practice is to implant only 2 embryos in mothers <40yrs; though 3 may be implanted if she is >40 yrs.[146]

Breech presentation The commonest malpresentation: 40% of babies are breech at 20 weeks, 20% at 28 weeks, but only 3% at term. In pregnancy it is normal for the buttocks to come to lie in the fundus. *Conditions predisposing to breech presentation:* •Contracted pelvis •Bicornuate uterus •Fibroid uterus •Placenta praevia •Oligohydramnios •Spina bifida •Hydrocephalic fetus. Ultrasound may show the cause and influence the management.

Extended breech presentation is commonest—ie flexed at the hips but extended at the knees. **Flexed breeches** sit with hips and knees both flexed so that the presenting part is a mixture of buttocks, external genitalia, and feet. **Footling breeches** are the least common. The feet are the presenting part and this type has the greatest risk (5–20%) of cord prolapse.

Diagnosis of breech presentation Diagnose antenatally. The mother may complain of pain under the ribs. On palpation the lie is longitudinal, no head is felt in the pelvis, and in the fundus there is a smooth round mass (the head) which can be ballotted, a sensation akin to quickly sinking an apple in water.

External cephalic version (ECV)[147][RCOG]—turning the breech by manoeuvring it through a (usually forward), somersault. Turn the baby only if vaginal delivery planned. Version at 36 weeks is recommended for primips, 37 weeks for multips. Success rate 40% primips (67% if spinal block used),[148] 60% multips. Tocolysis can ↑success rates. *Version contraindications:* •Placenta praevia •Multiple pregnancy (except delivery of 2nd twin) •APH in last 7 days •Ruptured membranes •Growth restricted babies •Abnormal cardiotocography •Mothers with uterine scars, uterine abnormality •Pre-eclampsia, pre-eclampsia, or hypertension (risk of abruption is increased) •Unstable lie. Monitor CTG (p44). Give anti-D (500u) to rhesus -ve patients. Emergency caesarean rate after ECV is 0.43%.[149]

Mode of delivery Planned caesarean section may provide better outcome for the fetus *vs* vaginal delivery. A large multicentre trial (*n* = 2088) published in 2000 suggested it is.[151] Re-analysis and later data questions that conclusion.[152] Others suggest that with careful selection vaginal delivery remains a safe option.[153] Evidence is less clear for pre-term singletons and twins. (RCOG recommends caesarean if 1st twin breech; vaginal delivery if 2nd twin breech.) If vaginal delivery occurs, attendants experienced at breech delivery should be present. These are becoming harder to find.

CI to vaginal route [150][RCOL]
• Inadequate pelvis
• Footling breech
• Kneeling breech
• Baby >3800 or <2000g
• Previous caesarean
• Hyperextended neck
• Lack of clinician experienced in breech delivery
• Concomitant condition. CI vaginal delivery

Assisted breech delivery The breech engages in the pelvis with the bitrochanteric diameter (9.5cm) transverse. With further descent through the pelvis, rotation occurs so the bitrochanteric diameter lies anteroposteriorly as it emerges from the birth canal, being born by lateral flexion of the trunk. External rotation then occurs so that this diameter is again transverse. The shoulders enter the pelvis with the bisacromial diameter transverse and rotate through 90° emerging in the AP diameter. The head enters the pelvis with the sagittal suture transverse and rotates 90°. When the body is completely born it is allowed to hang for about 1–2 mins until the nape of the neck is well seen. The body is then lifted above the vulva by an assistant, the head being delivered with forceps.

▶Check baby for hip dislocation (↑incidence): also, if vaginal delivery, for Klumpke's paralysis (p764) and signs of CNS injury.

Occipitoposterior presentation (OP) In 50% of patients the mothers have a long 'anthropoid' pelvis. Diagnosis may be made antenatally by palpation (p40). On vaginal examination the posterior fontanelle will be found to lie in the posterior quadrant of the pelvis. Labour tends to be prolonged because of the degree of rotation needed, so adequate hydration and analgesia (consider epidural) are important. During labour 65% rotate 130° so that the head is occipitoanterior at the time of birth, 20% rotate to the transverse and then arrest ('deep transverse arrest'), 15% rotate so that the occiput lies truly posterior and birth is by flexion of the head from the perineum. Although in 73% delivery will be a spontaneous vaginal delivery, 22% will require forceps and 5% a caesarean section.

Face presentation Incidence 1:994. 15% are due to congenital abnormality such as anencephaly, tumour of or shortened fetal neck muscles. Most occur by chance as the head extends rather than flexes as it engages. Antenatal diagnosis: the fetal spine feels S-shaped, the uterus is ovoid without fullness in the flanks and there is a deep groove between the occiput and the back. On early vaginal examination, the nose and eyes may be felt but later this will not be possible because of oedema. Most engage in the transverse (mentobregmatic diameter ≈9.5cm). 90% rotate so that the chin lies behind the symphysis (mentoanterior) and the head can be born by flexion. If the chin rotates to the sacrum (mentoposterior), caesarean section is indicated.

Brow presentation This occurs in 1:755 deliveries and is often associated with a contracted pelvis or a very large fetus. Antenatal diagnosis: the head does not engage (mentovertical diameter ≈13cm) and a sulcus may be felt between the occiput and the back. On vaginal examination the anterior fontanelle and supraorbital ridges may be felt. Deliver by caesarean section.

Transverse lie (compound shoulder presentation) This occurs in 1 in 400 deliveries and is usually in multiparous women (see MINIBOX). Antenatal diagnosis: ovoid uterus wider at the sides, the lower pole is empty, the head lies in one flank, the fetal heart is heard in variable positions. On vaginal examination with membranes intact no distinguishing features may be felt, but if ruptured and the cervix dilated, ribs, shoulder, or a prolapsed hand may be felt. The risk of cord prolapse

Typical causes
• Multiparity
• Multiple pregnancy
• Polyhydramnios
• Placenta praevia
• Arcuate/septate uterus
• Contracted pelvis ...

is high. External cephalic version (p70) may be attempted from 32 weeks. If malpresentation persists or recurs caesarean section will be necessary. Those with persistent instability of lie need hospital admission from 37 weeks (to prevent cord prolapse at home when the membranes rupture) and decision as to elective caesarean section.

Obstetrics

This is descent of the cord through the cervix, either alongside (*occulta*) or in front of the next presenting part (*overt*) in the presence of ruptured membranes. It is an emergency because cord compression causes fetal asphyxia. Cord prolapse is the wildcard that makes every home delivery a gamble with death.[154] But with speedy intervention, neonatal deaths may be kept to <10%.[155]

Incidence 0.1–0.6%; ↑ if: 2ⁿᵈ twin, footling breech, shoulder presentation, polyhydramnios, unengaged head, transverse or unstable lie, male. If cord presentation is noted prior to membrane rupture, carry out caesarean section. Whenever you rupture membranes, remember that cord prolapse is possible, eg if the presenting part is poorly applied. External cephalic version is also a risk.

Presentation The problem is obvious if the cord is at the introitus. But the only sign may be fetal bradycardia or variable fetal heart decelerations: always do a vaginal exam in this context to exclude prolapsed cord.

Action Get help. Activate alarms. Tell labour ward. Keep cord in vagina (minimal handling prevents spasm). Stop the presenting part from occluding the cord:
▶▶Displace the presenting part by putting a hand in the vagina; push it back up (towards mother's head) during contractions. NB: there is little evidence that replacing the cord above the presenting part helps (*not* recommended).[156] ʀᴄᴏɢ
▶▶Use gravity, either place the woman head down (left-lateral position) or get her into knee–elbow position (kneeling so rump higher than head).
▶▶Infuse 500mL saline into bladder via an IVI giving set taped to a catheter(16G). Remember to empty the bladder before any attempt at delivery/extraction.
▶▶Tocolysis (**terbutaline** 0.25mg SC) reduces contractions and helps bradycardia.

In general, if the fetus is alive, immediate caesarean is best. If cervix fully dilated and the presenting part is low in pelvis, delivery by forceps (if cephalic) or by breech extraction (by an experienced obstetrician) is best if it leads to birth in <15min. The paediatrician will take paired cord blood samples for pH and base excess (if normal, intrapartum hypoxic brain injury is 'excluded').

▶▶Impacted shoulders (shoulder dystocia) [157] ʀᴄᴏɢ

This is inability to deliver the shoulders after the head has been delivered. RCOG definition: a delivery requiring additional obstetric manoeuvres to release the shoulders after gentle downward traction has failed. The incidence is 0.6% deliveries (UK and USA). There can be high rate of fetal mortality and morbidity. Postpartum haemorrhage occurs in 11% of mothers and 3.8% get 4ᵗʰ degree perineal tears whether or not manoeuvres are used. Brachial plexus injuries occur in 4–16% (1 : 2300 live births UK) of which 10% are left with permanent disability. A common cause of litigation: note which shoulder is anterior as posterior shoulder injuries are not considered due to accoucheur (maternal propulsive forces may contribute to injuries).

Associations: •Large/postmature fetus (but most babies >4800g do not develop it and 48% that do weigh <4000g), eg maternal BMI >30kg/m² •Induced or oxytocin augmented labours •Prolonged 1ˢᵗ or 2ⁿᵈ stage or secondary arrest •Assisted vaginal delivery •Previous shoulder dystocia (1–16%). Most occur in women with no risk factors. •Suggest caesarean birth to diabetic mothers with macrosomic fetuses; discuss it if previous shoulder dystocia.

Management The danger is death from asphyxia. ▶▶Speed is vital as the cord is usually squashed at the pelvic inlet.
• Use the McRoberts (hyperflexed lithotomy) position. It is successful in 90%. Abduct, rotate outwards, and flex maternal femora so each thigh touches the abdomen (1 assistant to hold each leg). This straightens the sacrum relative to the lumbar spine and rotates the symphysis superiorly helping the impacted shoulder to enter the pelvis without manipulating the fetus.

Obstetrics

- Apply suprapubic pressure for 30sec: with flat of hand laterally in the direction baby is facing, and towards mother's sacrum. Apply steady traction to the fetal head towards the floor. This aims to displace the anterior shoulder allowing it to enter the pelvis.
- If this fails, check anterior shoulder is under the symphysis (here the diameter of the outlet is widest); if not rotate it to be so and repeat traction.
- If this fails, rotation by 180° so posterior shoulder now lies anteriorly may work, as may delivery of the posterior arm. Episiotomy helps rotations/arm delivery.
- If these have failed, alternatives now include getting the mother into 'all fours position'; maternal symphisiotomy; or replacement of the fetal head by firm pressure of the hand to reverse the movements of labour and return the head to the flexed occipito-anterior position and caesarean delivery. The baby is likely to be severely acidotic at this stage.
- If the baby dies prior to delivery, cutting through both clavicles (cleidotomy) with strong scissors assists delivery.
- Check the baby for damage, eg Erb's palsy (fig 1, p77) or fractured clavicle.
- Beware PPH or 4th degree vaginal tears in the mother.

In the notes, record time of delivery of head; direction head faced after restitution; manoeuvres (timing & sequence); time of delivery of body; who and when present; Apgar of baby at birth; umbilical cord blood acid–base measurement.

Meconium-stained liquor

In late pregnancy, it is normal for some babies to pass meconium (bowel contents), which stains the amniotic fluid a dull green. This is not significant. During labour, fresh meconium, which is dark green, sticky, and lumpy, may be passed. This may be a response to the stress of a normal labour, or a sign of distress, so transfer to a consultant unit and commence continuous fetal heart rate monitoring (p44). Aspiration of fresh meconium can cause severe pneumonitis. Routine suction of nasopharynx and oropharynx prior to birth is not recommended. Only suction airway if there is thick/tenacious meconium in oropharynx. Have a healthcare professional trained in advanced neonatal support in attendance (p107) to suck out pharynx and trachea under direct vision using a laryngoscope if the baby has depressed vital signs. Observe babies after light staining present for 2 hours; if more significant staining, for 12 hours.[NICE]

Meconium aspiration in some countries has been reducing. This is, in part, thought due to a reduction in births of babies >41 weeks' gestation.[158] Surfactant may reduce the need for extracorporeal oxygenation.[159]

Team-work, obstetric emergencies, and debriefing

There is no finer example of interdisciplinary working than when midwife, obstetrician, and paediatrician (with porters, lab staff, and others) unite to achieve optimal outcomes in difficult obstetric practice. But outcomes are frequently not optimal, and the reason is usually poor team-work—not always because of overwork: 25% of obstetricians and 58% of midwives freely admit goals are not shared between professions.[160]

One way forward is regular meetings, agreement on spheres of leadership, auditable standards, simulations, and debriefing after emergencies, emphasizing that we cannot control the ever-present threat of disasters, and that when these occur it is structures not individuals that need interrogating.[161]

We should also debrief patients after disasters and near-misses. This can help avoid post-traumatic stress disorder and fear of future births.[156]

Dystocia is difficulty in labour, implying problems with one or more of the '3 P's:

1 *Passages*—there may be soft tissue (eg fibroid or cervical dystocia after cervical biopsy or genital mutilation, p247) or bony obstruction.

2 *Passenger*—owing to a large baby; see also impacted shoulders/shoulder dystocia (p72) or an abnormal presentation.

3 *Propulsion*—thanks to the uterine powers.

Cephalopelvic disproportion is the appropriate label if diameters are unfavourable (p42) and/or the head is big; but see the box for a critique of this idea.

The pelvis The ideal pelvis has a round (*gynaecoid*) brim, but 15% of women have a long oval (*anthropoid*) brim. A very flat brim (*platypelloid* fig 1) is less favourable; it occurs in 5% of women over 152cm (5ft), but in 30% of women <152cm.

Kyphosis, scoliosis, sacralization of the L5 vertebra, spondylolisthesis and pelvic fractures all affect pelvic anatomy. Rickets and polio were important causes of pelvic problems. Suspect pelvic contraction if the head is not engaged by 37 weeks in a Caucasian primip (do ultrasound to exclude placenta praevia).

Presentation & lie Cephalic presentations are less favourable the less flexed the head is. Transverse lie and brow presentations always need caesarean section: face and OP (p71) presentations may deliver vaginally but are more likely to fail to progress. Breech presentation is most unfavourable if the fetus >3.5kg.

The uterine powers Contractions start in the fundus and propagate downwards. The intensity and duration of contractions are greatest at the fundus, but the contraction reaches its peak in all parts of the uterus simultaneously. Normal contractions occur at a rate of 3 per 10min, they should last up to 75sec. The contraction peak usually measures 30–60mmHg, and the resting uterine tone between them should be 10–15mmHg. Uterine muscle has the property of retraction: this shortening of the muscle fibres encourages cervical dilatation.

Uterine dysfunction/functional dystocia is easily diagnosed in labour by lack of cervical dilatation over 2h associated with weak contractions.[161] (If contractions are good, failure to progress is usually due to cephalo-pelvic disproportion.) Contractions may be hypotonic (↓resting tone, low contraction peaks) or they may be normotonic but too infrequent, or they may be coupled (2 contractions coupled too close together are inefficient).[162]

If membranes are intact, amniotomy may be tried. If cervical dilatation <1cm/h, oxytocin may help (p64). Whenever oxytocin is used, discuss with a senior obstetrician and limit geometric dose increase to nullips (multips may be very sensitive to oxytocin). 40min may be needed for assessing dose changes (don't expect progress to be as fast as with normal labour: median rate =1.4cm/h for nullips and 1.8cm/hour for multips).[163] Despite oxytocin, 'failure to progress' is *the* major problem for many women in the 1st stage of labour.

Pain and fear cause release of catecholamines which can inhibit uterine activity. So adequate analgesia is needed (p66) and may speed labour's progress.

Consequences of prolonged labour Neonatal mortality rises as does maternal morbidity (especially from infection).

NB! ►Modern management of labour entails careful monitoring of progress (p64) to diagnose and treat delay promptly.
►When there is dystocia, ask "is safe vaginal delivery possible?"

Most women have an abnormal pelvis!

The ideal pelvis, just like the ideal woman, is a male construct that does not exist. Reducing the pelvis to a few dimensions belies its complexity, and this reductionism is one reason why pelvimetry (bedside, ultrasound, or MRI) is disappointing and leads to unnecessary caesarean sections. ►*The only valid test of labour is labour itself*. Another reason is that pelvimetry perpetuates the myth that bones are static. There is a dialogue between the baby and the pelvis: the baby's skull moulds to its shape (p90) and the pelvis responds to pregnancy-associated hormones (eg relaxin). These induce resorption of the symphyseal margins (symphyseolysis) and change the fibrocartilaginous disc, increasing symphyseal width (eg by ~100%) and mobility.[164–166]

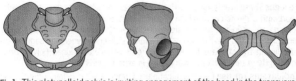

Fig 1. This platypelloid pelvis is inviting engagement of the head in the transverse position. Because the pelvis is so flat, deep transverse arrest is a particular risk.

Redrawn from López-Zeno, J, Glob. libr. women's med with permission from Sapiens Global Library, Ltd.

Obstetrics

Operative delivery 10–13% of births UK. A companion in labour; an upright or lateral position for delivery; avoidance of epidural or delay in pushing with epidural, reduce the need for operative deliveries.

Conditions of use The head must be engaged, the membranes ruptured, the position of the head known and the presentation suitable, ie vertex or face (mentoanterior); cephalo–pelvic disproportion must be absent (moulding not excessive); the cervix must be fully dilated; the uterus contracting; and analgesia adequate (epidural or perineal infiltration if episiotomy); pudendal blocks may be sufficient for mid-cavity forceps and ventouse deliveries but not for Kielland's. The bladder must be empty. A neonatal resuscitator should attend.

Forceps These are designed with a cephalic curve, which fits around the fetal head, and a pelvic curve which fits the pelvis. Short-shanked (eg Wrigley's) forceps are used for 'lift out' deliveries, when the head is on the perineum; long-shanked (eg Neville Barnes) for higher deliveries, when the sagittal suture lies in the AP diameter. Kielland's forceps have a reduced pelvic curve, making them suitable for rotation (only in experienced hands).

Indications for use Forceps may be used where there is delay in the second stage: this is frequently due to failure of maternal effort (uterine inertia or just tiredness), epidural analgesia, or malpositions of the fetal head. They may be used when there is fetal distress or a prolapsed cord, or eclampsia—all occurring only in the second stage. They are also used to prevent undue maternal effort, eg in cardiac disease, respiratory disease, pre-eclampsia. They are used for the after-coming head in breech deliveries. See BOX, OPPOSITE.

Technique Learn from demonstration. The following is an *aide-mémoire* for non-rotational forceps. Place the mother in lithotomy position with her bottom just over the edge of the delivery bed. Use sterilizing fluid to clean the vulva and perineum; catheterize; check the position of the head. Insert pudendal block, infiltrate episiotomy site (not necessary if she has an epidural). Assemble the blades to check they fit, with the pelvic curve pointing upwards. The handle which lies in the left hand is the left blade and is inserted first (to the mother's left side) and then the right: the handles should lock easily. Traction must not be excessive (the end of bed is not for leverage!). Synchronize traction with contractions, guiding the head downwards initially. Episiotomy may be needed when the head is at the vulva. Change the direction of traction to up and out as the occiput clears the symphysis pubis. If baby needs resuscitation, give to resuscitator.

Forceps complications: Maternal: Trauma (commoner than with ventouse). Fetal: facial bruising, VII paralysis (usually resolves); brachial plexus injury.

Ventouse The ventouse, (vacuum extractor), causes less maternal trauma than forceps (but still affects ~11%). It is preferred worldwide (but not in the UK). It may be used in preference to rotational forceps. As traction is applied, with the cup over the posterior fontanelle, rotation during delivery occurs. It should not be used if the head is above the ischial spines. It is contraindicated for face presentations and for babies <34+0 wks; caution if 34+1–36+0 wks. A cup is applied with a suction force of 0.8kg/cm². The baby's scalp is sucked up to form a 'chignon', which resolves in 2 days. There is increased rate of fetal cephalhaematoma (p90), failed delivery, fetal retinal haemorrhages compared to forceps.

After delivery Give vitamin K (p120). Give regular analgesia. Document time and volume of 1st void urine (catheterize for 12h if epidural). Pass catheter if residual suspected. Is thromboprophylaxis needed (p16)? Arrange physiotherapy to reduce incontinence. Discuss future delivery; >80% will be vaginal but individual plan if 3rd or 4th degree tear with this delivery.

Indications for operative delivery

Relative indications (caesarean an alternative)
• Delay or maternal exhaustion in second stage.
• Dense epidural block with diminished urge to push.
• Rotational instrumental delivery needed for malposition of head.
• Suspected fetal distress.

Specific indications for forceps (forceps delivery is usually superior to ventouse or caesarean in these circumstances)
• Assisted breech delivery, forceps to deliver head.
• Assisted delivery of preterm infant <34 weeks' gestation.
• Controlled delivery of head at caesarean section.
• Assisted delivery with face presentation.
• Assisted delivery with suspected coagulopathy or thrombocytopenia in fetus (but note coagulopathy is a relative CI to forceps).
• Instrumental delivery where maternal condition precludes pushing (eg cardiac disease, respiratory disease).
• Cord prolapse in second stage of labour.
• Instrumental delivery under GA.

Operative delivery likely to fail (Consider delivery in theatre)
• Maternal BMI >30
• Big baby (estimated weight >4kg)
• OP presentation (p71)
• Midcavity if >¹/₅ head palpable per abdomen

► Abandon operative vaginal delivery if no progression with each pull and delivery not imminent with 3 pulls by experienced operator.

Obstetric brachial plexus injury (OBPI)

OBPI complicates <0.5% of live births.

Risk factors: Large birthweight; shoulder dystocia with prolonged 2ⁿᵈ stage of labour; forceps delivery; vacuum extraction; diabetes mellitus; breech presentation. Formerly, the cause of OBPI was excessive lateral traction applied to the fetal head at delivery, in association with anterior shoulder dystocia.

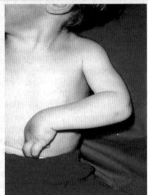

Instrumental-associated OBPI may arise because of nerve stretch injuries after rotations of >90° or from direct compression of the forceps blade in the fetal neck.[168] Not all cases of brachial plexus palsy are attributable to traction. Intrauterine factors may play some role.[169]

Fig 1. Brachial plexus injury.

Management: 10–20% need surgical intervention for optimal results.[170]

Some injuries will be permanent.[171] See p764 for orthopaedic insights.

▶If previous section, localize placenta by ultrasound to see if praevia. If colour flow Doppler suggests accreta/percreta (p14), offer MRI to clarify invasion.[37, 2]

Incidence WHO says to aim for <15%. It is ≥24% of UK labours (30% in the USA) 9–16% are pre-labour.[172] *Maternal mortality:* ~1 per 100,000. Morbidity is higher—eg infection, ileus, and thromboembolism. For 1st operations 25% are due to failure to progress, 28% for fetal distress, 14% for breech; of 2nd caesareans 44% have had previous section. Use of support in labour, induction at 41 weeks, consultant involvement in decision to section, fetal blood sampling when fetal monitoring is used, and use of a 4 hour partogram with action line all help reduce incidence of caesarean sections. 9:1000 will require ITU care.

Lower uterine segment incision Joel Cohen incision (straight incision 3cm above symphysis pubis) with blunt dissection thereafter is recommended (reduces blood loss). Fetal laceration rate is 2%.

Classical caesarean section (vertical incision) Rarely used. Indications:
• Very premature fetus, lower segment poorly formed • Fetus lies transverse, with ruptured membranes and liquor draining • Structural abnormality makes lower segment use impossible • Constriction ring present • Fibroids (some)
• Some anterior placenta praevia when lower segment abnormally vascular
• Mother dead and rapid birth desired.

Before an emergency section ▶Explain to the mother what is to happen.
• Activate the anaesthetist, theatre staff, porters, and paediatrician.
• Have the mother breathe 100% O_2 if there is fetal distress.
• Neutralize gastric contents with 20mL of 0.3 molar sodium citrate, and promote gastric emptying with metoclopramide 10mg IV. (NB: there is no time for H_2 agonists to work; ranitidine is kept for elective sections, eg 150mg PO 2h before surgery.) Consider pre-operative emptying of stomach (eg if prolonged labour or opiate given). The stomach should be routinely emptied prior to extubation to minimize risk of post-operative aspiration. See Mendelson's syndrome, p80.
• Take to theatre (awake); set up IVI. Take blood for crossmatch, eg 2u; if for abruption (6u and 2 IVIs if previous section and anterior placenta praevia—see below).
• Catheterize the bladder. Tilt 15° to her left side on operating table.
• Use pulse oximetry peri/post-operatively if dark skinned.
• Tell the paediatrician if the mother has had opiates in the last 4h.
• Offer prophylactic antibiotics given before skin incision.[48, NICE]
• Remember thromboprophylaxis (see OPPOSITE).

Avoid halothane for obstetric procedures because uterine muscle relaxation increases bleeding. Other anaesthetic problems include vomiting on induction (use rapid sequence induction, p626), and light anaesthesia (out of consideration for the baby) causing paralysed awareness. ▶In reducing maternal mortality, the importance of having an experienced anaesthetist is vital. When appropriate, offer regional anaesthesia. Document indication for and urgency of operation. Note: in 2002–3 only 8% of caesarean sections were under GA.

Indications for elective caesarean section • Known cephalo–pelvic disproportion • Placenta praevia • Morbid adherent placenta (accreta/percreta p14) • Breech presentation (offer version at 37 weeks) • Twins where 1st twin not cephalic • Some malpresentations (p71) • After vaginal surgery (suburethral repair; vesico–vaginal fistula repair) • Some maternal infections, eg herpes (p36), hepatitis C+HIV (p26), some with HIV (p23) • Maternal request (NICE).[48, NICE]

10% go into labour before expected date of operation at 39 weeks, so plan for this. Plan elective caesarean section after 39 completed weeks gestation (to reduce incidence of neonatal respiratory problems).[173] Give antenatal corticosteroids (p51) for all elective caesareans up to 38^{+6} weeks.[119, RCOG]

Emergency section may be needed because of antenatal complications, eg severe pre-eclampsia, abruptio placentae (baby still alive). In others, the need becomes apparent during labour: fetal distress; prolapsed cord (if fetus alive); after failed induction; or failure to progress.

Trial of scar in labour: See p80. Beware oxytocin. *Antibiotic prophylaxis* is recommended. Infection (wound, endometritis, and UTI) is reduced by IV antibiotics (eg 2g cefradine at induction, 1g at 6h and 12h post-op) for both emergency and elective sections. Longer courses do not appear to be superior, nor do more expensive second-generation cephalosporins. *Abdominally placed cervical cerclage* if cerclage in place and delivery by caesarean the suture can be left for future pregnancy.[174]

Management of women already on thromboprophylaxis[52] If on high dose or 75% of weight adjusted therapeutic dose prophylaxis (see p16) halve to same dose/24h as was previously being given/12h, on the day before planned caesarean. For all on prophylaxis omit dose on morning of caesarean and give 3h post-op unless epidural used: see p66. 2% of women will get a wound haematoma.

At caesarean section Remove placenta by controlled cord traction (less endometritis than manual removal). In Rh−ve mothers, remove all excess blood from peritoneal cavity. Use a Kleihauer test (p9) to determine dose of anti-D.

After caesarean section [175] Give one-to-one support in recovery unit. Aim for baby/mother skin to skin contact (beware chilling baby). Check pulse, respiration rate (RR), BP, and sedation levels at least half hourly for 1st 2h, then hourly for 24h and until 2h after epidural or patient-controlled opiate analgesia discontinued). Use MEOWS (modified early obstetric warning score chart). After epidural, remove urinary catheters when mobile or 12h after last top-up dose (whichever is later). After GA, give extra midwife support to help establish breastfeeding. Mobilize early. Remove wound dressing at 24h. Give analgesia (ibuprofen + co-codamol if pain severe, co-codamol if moderate, paracetamol if mild). Average hospital stay is 3–4 days but mothers can be discharged after 24h if they wish and are well. Discuss reason for caesarean section and birth options in future.

Prophylaxis against thromboembolism
- Women with no risk factors undergoing elective caesarean section in an uncomplicated pregnancy require only early mobilization and good hydration.
- All women having elective caesarean who have 1 or more risk factors for thromboembolism (MINIBOX p16) should be considered for low molecular weight heparin for 7 days postnatally.
- All women having an emergency caesarean section should be considered for low molecular weight heparin for 7 days postnatally.
- Women who have had a thromboembolism in pregnancy should receive thromboprophylaxis for 6 weeks postpartum.
- All women having thromboprophylaxis antenatally should have it for 6 weeks postpartum. See p16.

Ruptured uterus is rare in the UK (0.5–2:10 000 deliveries in an unscarred uterus but 1:100 deliveries in parts of Africa). Associated maternal mortality is 5%, and the fetal mortality 30%. ~70% of UK ruptures are due to dehiscence of caesarean section scars. Lower-segment scars are far less likely to rupture (<0.74%) than the classical scars (2–9%)—see p78. Other risk factors: •Obstructed labour in the multiparous, especially if oxytocin is used •Previous cervical surgery •High forceps delivery •Internal version •Breech extraction. Rupture is usually during the third trimester or in labour.

Vaginal birth after caesarean (trial of scar): Vaginal birth will be successful in 72–76%. Endometritis, need for blood transfusion, uterine rupture and perinatal death (↑ by 2–3:10,000 births—mainly due to increased stillbirth at around 39 weeks: this increases mortality to that of a firstborn) are commoner than with elective repeat caesarean.[176] Neonatal respiratory problems are, however, reduced. 24–28% undergo repeat emergency section. Of 9 ruptures in 4021 women undergoing trial of scar; there were no maternal or fetal deaths.[177] Use fetal monitoring.[48,NICE]

Signs and symptoms Rupture is usually in labour. In a few (usually a caesarean scar dehiscence) rupture precedes labour. Pain is variable, some only having slight pain and tenderness over the uterus. In others pain is severe. Vaginal bleeding is variable and may be slight (bleeding is intraperitoneal). Unexplained maternal tachycardia, sudden maternal shock, cessation of contractions, disappearance of the presenting part from the pelvis, and fetal distress are other presentations. Postpartum indicators of rupture: continuous PPH with a well-contracted uterus; if bleeding continues postpartum after cervical repair; and whenever shock is present.

Management If suspected in labour, perform laparotomy, deliver the baby by caesarean section, and explore the uterus. ▸▸ •Give O₂ at 15L/min via a tight-fitting mask with reservoir •Set up IVI •Crossmatch 6u of blood and correct shock by fast transfusion. •Arrange laparotomy. The type of operation performed should be decided by a senior obstetrician; if the rupture is small, repair may be carried out (possibly with tubal ligation); if the cervix or vagina are involved in the tear, hysterectomy may be necessary. Care is needed to identify the ureters and exclude them from sutures. Give post-operative antibiotic cover, eg ampicillin 500mg/6h IV and gentamicin 3–5mg/kg/8h IV over 3min (unless there is renal impairment). 85% of spontaneous ruptures require hysterectomy, but >66% of ruptured scars are repairable.

▸▸Mendelson's syndrome

This is the name given to the cyanosis, bronchospasm, pulmonary oedema, and tachycardia that develop due to inhalation of gastric acid during general anaesthesia. Clinically it may be difficult to distinguish from cardiac failure or amniotic fluid embolism. Pre-operative H₂ antagonists, sodium citrate, gastric emptying, cricoid pressure (p626), the use of cuffed endotracheal tubes during anaesthesia, and pre-extubation emptying of stomach aim to prevent it (p78).

Management ▸▸Tilt the patient head down. Turn her to one side and aspirate the pharynx. Give 100% oxygen. Give aminophylline 5mg/kg by slow IVI and hydrocortisone 200mg IV stat.[178] The bronchial tree should be sucked out using a bronchoscope under general anaesthesia. Antibiotics, eg ampicillin and gentamicin (as above), should be given to prevent secondary pneumonia. Ventilation conducted on intensive care may be needed. Physiotherapy should be given during convalescence.

Stillbirths are those babies born dead after (but that were alive at—see BOX) 24 weeks' completed gestation. Rate: 1:200 total births. Death *in utero* can occur at any stage of pregnancy or labour. Delivery is an emotional strain for mother and attendant staff: labour may seem futile, mothers may feel guilty—or punished.

Some hours after a fetus has died *in utero* the skin begins to peel. At delivery such fetuses are described as *macerated*, as opposed to *fresh* stillbirths. If left, spontaneous labour usually occurs (80% within 2 weeks, 90% within 3 weeks). Coagulopathy (p88) occurs in 10% within 4 weeks of late IUFD: 30% thereafter.

Causes of stillbirth *Antepartum:* Malformation (6% have chromosomal anomalies); congenital infection (TORCH p35), pre-eclampsia; APH (p56); maternal disease (hypertension, renal, diabetes); hyperpyrexia (T° >39.4°C); post-maturity. *Intrapartum:* Abruption; maternal and fetal infection; cord prolapse/ knots; uterine rupture. In 50% no cause is found. Multiple pregnancy ↑ risk (16.6:1000).Increasing maternal age, smoking and obesity increase incidence.

Diagnosis The mother usually reports absent fetal movements. No heart sounds (unreliable). Diagnose by absent fetal movement (eg heart beat) on ultrasound. It may help the mother to see lack of heart beat. Mothers sometimes feel passive movements after death. Repeat ultrasound, if mother requests. If mother alone at diagnosis; offer to call a companion.

Management ▶If mother Rh -ve give anti-D (p9). Do Kleihauer on *all* women to diagnose fetomaternal haemorrhage (FMH)—a cause of stillbirth; and to determine anti-D dose. If large FMH diagnosed; repeat Kleihauer at 48h to check fetal cells cleared. Check maternal T°, BP, urine for protein, and blood clotting screen if fetus not thought recently demised. Advise delivery if pre-eclampsia, abruption, sepsis, coagulopathy or membrane rupture. If safe, the mother may want to go home after diagnosis to reflect, collect things, and make arrangements. If not induced in 48h check for coagulopathy twice weekly. Labour is induced using mifepristone orally, adding prostaglandin (or misoprostol) vaginally. Amniotomy is traditionally contraindicated as it risks ascending infection. Oxytocin augmentation may be needed later. If vaginal scar seek consultant advice re induction/ augmentation. Deliver away from sounds of babies, if possible.

Ensure good pain relief in labour (if epidural, check clotting tests all normal and no sepsis). Do not leave the mother unattended. When the baby is born wrap it (as with any other baby) and offer to the mother to see and to hold—if she wishes. A photograph may be taken for her to take home, a lock of the baby's hair and palm-print given (keep in notes for later if not wanted then). Unseen babies can be difficult to grieve for. Naming the baby and holding a funeral service may help with grief. Remember thromboprophylaxis if needed (p16). Discuss lactation suppression and contraception.

Labour ward procedure (to try to establish cause) *Maternal tests:* Kleihauer (above); FBC, CRP, LFT, TFT, HbA1c, glucose, blood culture, viral screen (TORCH^Etc* screen p35), thrombophilia screen, antibodies (anti-red cell, anti-Ro, anti-La, alloimmune antiplatelet, if indicated[179]), MSU, urine for cocaine (if indicated and permission given), cervical swabs, parental chromosomes, if indicated.[179] *Fetal tests* Fetal and placental swabs. Cord blood in lithium heparin tube for infection. Thorough examination of the stillbirth. Take time to talk to parents about how helpful a post-mortem may be to them, in understanding what happened, and planning further pregnancies. If post-mortem is refused, MRI (may miss significant pathology and is not routinely available), cytogenetics (use fetal skin, cartilage and placenta, this can also be used for sexing babies which may be difficult in macerated and very premature stillbirths) ± small volumes of tissue for metabolic studies, and placental histology may be acceptable but are less informative and still need written parental consent.

---

* '**TORCH**' infections: **T**oxoplasmosis, **O**ther (eg syphilis), **R**ubella, **C**MV, **H**erpes (and hepatitis)^et al

- Give parents a follow-up appointment to discuss causes found by the above tests. Consider a domiciliary visit if parents prefer. Refer for genetic counselling if appropriate.

- In England, a *Certificate of Stillbirth* is required (issued by obstetrician or midwife attending birth), that the mother (or father, if married at time of birth) is required to take to the Registrar of Births and Deaths within 42 days (21 days in Scotland, 5 days in Northern Ireland) of birth for fetuses born after 24 weeks' completed gestation. If there is developmental or ultrasound evidence that the fetus was not alive at 24 completed weeks' gestation (eg in cases of fetus papyraceous, or after selective fetal reduction before 24 weeks), then such a certificate is not issued,[180] but evidence for the fact why the fetus is not believed to have been alive at 24 completed weeks should be written in the woman's notes. The father's name only appears in the register if the parents are married, or if both parents make the registration, or the father signs a Form of Declaration (available from Registrar). Registration can be delegated to a health care professional or hospital bereavement officer.

- The Registrar then issues a Certificate of Burial or Cremation which the parents then give to the undertaker (if they have chosen a private funeral—in which case they bear the cost of the funeral), or to the hospital administrators if they have chosen a hospital funeral—for which the hospital bears the cost. Parents are issued with a Certificate of Registration to keep which has the name of the stillborn baby (if named), the name of the informant who made the registration, and the date of stillbirth.

- UK hospitals are directed by the Department of Social Security to offer 'hospital' funerals for stillborn babies (arranged through an undertaker). If the parents offer to pay for this, the hospital may accept. The hospital should notify the parents of the time of the funeral so that they may attend, if they wish. With hospital funerals a coffin is provided and burial is often in a multiple-occupancy grave in a part of the graveyard set aside for babies. The hospital should inform parents of the site of the grave. Graves are unmarked, so should the parents not attend the funeral and wish to visit later it is recommended that they contact the graveyard attendants for the grave to be temporarily marked. Parents may buy a single occupancy grave, if they wish, on which they can later erect a headstone. Hospitals can arrange cremations, but the parents pay for this. Tell parents that there may not be any ashes after cremation.

- Arrange a follow-up appointment with the obstetrician to discuss implications for future pregnancy, and the cause (if known) of the stillbirth. Give parents the address of a local branch of an organization for bereavement counselling, eg SANDS.[181] Grief may take a long time to resolve (p498) and parents may find it difficult to contact ordinary medical staff without the 'excuse' provided by asking about the baby's ailments.

Each maternity unit should have a bereavement counsellor to support the mother and father, and help guide them through the formalities.

In the UK statutory maternity pay and the maternity allowance and social fund maternity payments are payable after stillbirth.

After stillbirth Be vigilant to possible depression. In next pregnancy after unexplained stillbirth recommend obstetrician antenatal care and delivery, and screen for diabetes. If there was evidence of growth restriction assess growth by serial ultrasound biometry in subsequent pregnancies.[179]

Primary PPH is the loss of greater than 500mL (definitions vary) in the first 24h after delivery. This occurs after ~6% of deliveries; major PPH (>1 litre) in 1.3%. Causes: uterine atony (90%), genital tract trauma (7%), clotting disorders—p88 (3%). Death rate: 2/yr in the UK; 125,000/yr worldwide.

Risk factors for PPH: *Antenatal* • Previous PPH or retained placenta • BMI>35kg/m² • Maternal Hb<8.5g/dl at onset of labour • Antepartum haemorrhage • Multiparity 4+ • Maternal age 35y+ • Uterine malformation or fibroids • A large placental site (twins, severe rhesus disease, large baby) • Low placenta, • Overdistended uterus (polyhydramnios, twins) • Extravasated blood in the myometrium (abruption). *In labour* • Prolonged labour (1ˢᵗ, 2ⁿᵈ or 3ʳᵈ stage) • Induction or oxytocin use • Precipitant labour • Operative birth or caesarean section. ▸Book mothers with risk factors for obstetric unit delivery.

Management • Give oxytocin 5u slowly IV. • Call emergency ambulance unit (p4)—if not in hospital. Give high-flow O_2 as soon as available. • Set up IVI (2 large-bore cannulae). • Call anaesthetist (a CVP line may help guide fluid replacement, but not if it causes delay). • If shocked give Gelofusine® or fresh blood of the patient's ABO and Rh group (uncrossmatched group O Rh –ve in emergency) fast until systolic BP >100mmHg and urine flows at >30mL/h (catheterize the bladder). • Is the placenta delivered? If it is, is it complete? If not, explore the uterus. • If the placenta is complete, put the patient in the lithotomy position with adequate analgesia and good lighting. Check for and repair trauma. • If the placenta has not been delivered but has separated, attempt to deliver it by controlled cord traction after rubbing up a uterine contraction. If this fails, ask an experienced obstetrician to remove it under general anaesthesia. Beware renal shut down.

   If bleeding continues despite all the above, give 10 units of **oxytocin** in 500mL dextrose saline, eg at a rate of 15 drops/min. Bimanual pressure on the uterus may decrease immediate loss. Inform consultant. Check that blood is clotting (5mL should clot in a plain round-bottomed glass tube in <6min); formal tests: platelets, prothrombin ratio, kaolin–cephalin clotting time, fibrin degradation products. Involve consultant haematologist if coagulopathy. Intravenous tranexamic acid eg 1g may also reduce bleeding. Explore the uterus for possible rupture. If uterine atony is the cause, and the circulation is still compromised, give **carboprost** 250μg (15-methyl prostaglandin F2α) eg as Hemabate® 1mL deep IM. If no response to 2 doses, >15min apart consider other method eg hysterectomy. SE: nausea, vomiting, diarrhoea, T° ↑; (less commonly—asthma, BP ↑, pulmonary oedema). It controls bleeding in ~88%. If atony persists despite drugs a B-Lynch brace uterine suture[182] may well stop bleeding (can be used in conjunction with vessel ligations). Rarely, uterine packing, internal iliac artery or uterine vessel ligation or embolization, or hysterectomy is needed to stop bleeding. Ask a haematologist's advice on clotting factor replacement (fresh frozen plasma contains all of them; the cryoprecipitate has more fibrinogen, but lacks antithrombin III).

Secondary PPH This is excessive blood loss from the genital tract after 24h from delivery. It usually occurs between 5 and 12 days and is due to retained placental tissue or clot. Secondary infection is common. Uterine involution may be incomplete. If bleeding is slight and there is no sign of infection it may be managed conservatively—but heavier loss, the suggestion of retained products on ultrasound, or a tender uterus with an open os requires exploration. Crossmatch 2 units of blood pre-operatively. Give antibiotics (eg ampicillin 500mg/6h IV, metronidazole 1g/12h PR) if there are signs of infection. Carefully curette the uterus (it is easily perforated at this stage). Send curettings for histology (excludes choriocarcinoma).

- Know maternal attitude to transfusion at booking.
- Give oral iron and folate to mother to maximize haemoglobin stores (parenteral iron if does not respond—p22 (not if thalassaemia)).
- Book for delivery where there are good facilities to deal with haemorrhage promptly (including facilities for hysterectomy, balloon angioplasty to stabilize loss, and interventional radiology techniques such as uterine artery embolization), and with critical care facilities and cell salvage if the mother is high risk, eg if placenta praevia.
- Ensure consultant obstetrician and anaesthetist assess antenatally to make plans for labour.
- Arrange ultrasound to know placental site.
- Inform consultant when admitted in labour. Ensure experienced staff conduct labour. Give oxytocin as soon as the baby is delivered. Do not leave the mother alone for first hour post-delivery.
- Consultant obstetrician and anaesthetist should perform caesarean section if required.
- Cell savers which wash the woman's own blood so that it may be returned may be acceptable to some women (suitable for intra-abdominal blood not contaminated by amniotic fluid).[172]
- Haemorrhage should be dealt with promptly, and clotting disorders excluded early. Involve a consultant obstetrician early (to decide if intervention may be needed eg embolization of uterine arteries, B-Lynch suture, internal iliac ligation or hysterectomy), and a consultant anaesthetist (for help with fluid replacement and for use of intensive care facilities). Liaise with a consultant haematologist. Avoid dextran (adversely affects haemostasis), but Gelofusine® is useful. Erythropoietin is not an effective alternative to transfusion as it takes 10–14 days to work.
- Ensure the woman does not want to change her mind and receive a transfusion.
- Should the woman die of exsanguination both bereaved relatives and distressed staff should be offered support.

Obstetrics

Third stage of labour (p58) is considered delayed if not complete by 30 minutes with active management, by 60 minutes with physiological 3rd stage. A placenta not delivered by then will probably not be expelled spontaneously. The danger with retained placenta is haemorrhage. Associations: • Previous RP or uterine surgery • Preterm delivery • Maternal age >35y • Placental weight <600g • Parity >5 • Induced labour • Pethidine used in labour.

Management If the placenta does not separate readily, avoid excessive cord traction—the cord may snap or the uterus invert. Check that the placenta is not in the vagina. Palpate the abdomen. If the uterus is well contracted, the placenta is probably separated but trapped by the cervix. Wait for the cervix to relax and release it. If the uterus is bulky, the placenta may have failed to separate. Rub up a contraction, put the baby to the breast (stimulates oxytocin production). Give 20IU oxytocin in 20mL saline into umbilical vein and proximally clamp cord. Empty the bladder (a full bladder causes atony). If the placenta still does not deliver within further 30mins, offer examination to see if manual removal is needed (delay may precipitate a PPH). Examination needs analgesia or anaesthesia. Stop if examination is painful.[106][NICE]

Manual removal Set up IVI and crossmatch blood (eg 2u). Call the anaesthetist to arrange anaesthesia. The procedure can be done under epidural if *in situ*. Obtain consent. With the mother in lithotomy position, using aseptic technique, place one hand on the abdomen to stabilize the uterus. Insert the other hand through the cervix into the uterus. Following the cord assists finding the placenta. Gently work round the placenta, separating it from the uterus using the ulnar border of the hand. When separated it should be possible to remove it by cord traction. Check that it is complete. Give oxytocic drugs and start antibiotics, eg **doxycycline** 200mg stat, 100mg/24h and **metronidazole** 500mg/8h IV.

Rarely, the placenta will not separate (placenta accreta) and hysterectomy may be necessary—by a senior obstetrician.

▸▸Uterine inversion

Inversion of the uterus is rare. It may be due to mismanagement of the third stage, eg with cord traction on an atonic uterus (between contractions) and a fundal insertion of the placenta. It may be completely revealed, or partial when the uterus remains within the vagina. Even without haemorrhage the mother may become profoundly shocked.

Management The ease with which the uterus is replaced depends on the amount of time elapsed since inversion, as a tight ring forms at the neck of the inversion. With an inversion noted early before shock sets in, replacement by hand may be possible. If shock has ensued, set up a fast IVI and infuse colloid or blood. Summon expert help. Under halothane anaesthesia to relax the uterus, hold the uterus in the vagina with one hand. Run two litres of warm 0.9% saline fast into the vagina through cystoscopy tubing (or with a funnel and tube) with an assistant holding the labia encircled tightly around the operator's arm to prevent the fluid running away. Running the fluid through a silastic ventouse cap held in the vagina improves the 'vaginal seal'. The hydrostatic pressure of the water should reduce the uterus. Once the inversion has been corrected, give ergometrine to contract the uterus and prevent recurrence. Prophylactic antibiotics are advisable.

Obstetrics

✠ **DIC** in pregnancy is always secondary to stimulation of coagulation by pro-coagulant substance release in the maternal circulation. Known triggers are: retention of a dead fetus (of greater than 20 weeks' gestation which has been dead for >3 weeks); pre-eclampsia; placental abruption; endotoxic shock; amniotic fluid embolism; placenta accreta; hydatidiform mole; prolonged shock from any cause; acute fatty liver of pregnancy (p26). *Pathogenesis:* Thromboplastins are released into the circulation, fibrin and platelets are consumed as intravascular clotting occurs. *Tests:* Kaolin–cephalin clotting time ↑ (↓ factors II, V, VII), fibrinogen ↓, fibrin degradation products ↑. In situations where DIC is a possibility send blood for crossmatch, platelets, partial thromboplastin time or accelerated whole blood clotting time, prothrombin time, fibrinogen estimation, and fibrin degradation products. Preliminary results should be available in 30min. *Management:* Presentation may be as heavy bleeding and shock, and the first measures must be the correction of shock. ▶▶Give O₂ at 15 L/min via a tight fitting mask with reservoir. Set up at least 1, preferably 2, wide-gauge IVIs, take bloods as above, and give blood fast (group-compatible blood—available in 5–10min or o Rh–ve blood if desperate). Stored blood is deficient in clotting factors. Give fresh frozen plasma to normalize the kaolin–cephalin clotting time and the prothrombin time. Platelets are indicated with prolonged bleeding and low platelet count. Calcium is sometimes needed to counteract citrate in stored blood (eg 10mL of 10% **calcium gluconate** IVI, eg after 6u of blood). Seek expert help from a haematologist. The condition is usually self-limiting if the stimulus can be removed. In the case of intrauterine death and abruption (p56) removal of the uterine contents is the way to correct the stimulus, and this should be done as promptly as possible. *Mortality:* <1% if placental abruption; 50–80% if infection/shock.

Autoimmune thrombocytopenic purpura (AiTP) Incidence 1–2:10,000 pregnancies. IgG antibodies cause thrombocytopenia (associated with increased bone marrow megakaryocytes) in the mother and, being able to cross the placenta, they cause thrombocytopenia in ~10% of fetuses. Exclude systemic lupus erythematosus in the mother (thrombocytopenia may be an early presentation; do DNA binding, *OHCM* p540). Consider maternal HIV. If maternal platelets fall below 20 × 10⁹/L or 50 × 10⁹/L near delivery, give steroids. Rarely, splenectomy is necessary during pregnancy (ideally in the second trimester). Immunoglobulin IgG 0.4g/kg IV for 5 days is sometimes used near expected date of delivery, inducing maternal and fetal remission for up to 3 weeks, but it is extremely expensive. Aim for non-traumatic delivery for both mother and baby. Neonatal platelet count may fall further in the first days of life, then gradually rise to normal over 4–16 weeks. Treatment is not needed unless surgery is contemplated. Maternal mortality due to AiTP is now negligible, but fetal mortality remains (due to intracranial bleeding). Take cord blood at delivery. If platelets <20 × 10⁹/L give baby IgG 1g/kg IVI at birth. If platelets low at birth observe baby for 2–5 days as further falls likely.

Causes of thrombocytopenia in pregnancy

1 Spurious (try citrated bottle).
2 Pregnancy-associated thrombocytopenia (benign gestational thrombocytopenia)—mild and self-limiting (platelets stay above 100 × 10⁹/L).
3 Autoimmune thrombocytopenia.
4 Pre-eclampsia (platelets may fall early, preceding clotting abnormality).
5 DIC (above) and haemolytic uraemic syndrome (p176)/thrombotic thrombocytopenic purpura (2 ends of a microangiopathic spectrum, *OHCM* p332).
6 Folate deficiency.
7 Congenital (May–Heggin anomaly, hereditary macrothrombocytopenia).
8 Marrow disease; hypersplenism.

Amniotic fluid embolism

This condition, with a mortality of up to 61% (20% in 2006–8) with sudden dyspnoea and hypotension heralded in 20%, by seiz... develop DIC, and of those who survive the initial collapse 70% go... pulmonary oedema (acute respiratory distress syndrome, ARDS, ... There may be premonitory symptoms such as breathlessness, chest pa... ing cold, light-headedness, restlessness, distress, panic, paraesthesiae in fin-gers, nausea and vomiting.[183] These may be from immediately before until up to 4h before collapse. An anaphylactic type of response occurs to (possibly abnormal) amniotic fluid in the maternal circulation. *Presentation* is often at the end of the first stage of labour or shortly after delivery but can complicate amniocentesis, or termination of pregnancy, abruption, trauma, caesarean section, and has even occurred up to 48h postpartum. Medical induction does appear to double risk, although absolute excess risk is low.[184]

Management
▸▸ The first priority is to prevent death from respiratory failure. Give mask oxygen and call an anaesthetist urgently. Endotracheal intubation and ventilation may be necessary. Set up IVI in case DIC should supervene. Cardiovascular collapse is due to left ventricular failure. DIC and haemorrhage then usually follow. Treatment is essentially supportive—important steps are detailed below. Diagnosis may be difficult: exclude other causes of obstetric shock (p55).
▸▸ Cardiopulmonary resuscitation if indicated.
▸▸ Give highest available O_2 concentration. If unconscious, ventilate and use 100% inspired O_2.
▸▸ Monitor for fetal distress.
▸▸ If hypotensive, give fluids rapidly IVI to increase preload. If still hypotensive consider inotropes: **dobutamine** (a better inotrope than dopamine), eg in a dose range of 2.5–10µg/kg/min IVI may help.
▸▸ Pulmonary artery catheterization (Swan–Ganz catheter if available) helps guide haemodynamic management.
▸▸ After initial hypotension is corrected, give only maintenance requirements of fluid to avoid pulmonary oedema from acute respiratory distress syndrome. Transfer to intensive care unit as soon as possible.
▸▸ Treat DIC with fresh whole blood or packed cells and fresh frozen plasma. Use of heparin is controversial; there are insufficient data to warrant routine heparinization.
▸▸ If the mother dies it is recommended to deliver the baby abdominally. Perimortem caesarean within 5 minutes can aid resuscitation of the mother.

Most mortality occurs in the first hour. Mortality rates reported: 26.4–61%. (In 2006–8 there were and 13 deaths in England and Wales.) Report suspected cases to National Amniotic Fluid Embolism Register (at UKOSS).[1] Should the woman die, perform autopsy as soon as possible. Specifically request that the lungs be examined for the presence of amniotic squames or lanugo hair (histology and immunochemistry to confirm the diagnosis). In future complement measurement or serological or lung tissue tests for fetal antigen sialyl Tn may be the tests of choice.

1 UKOSS The National Perinatal Unit, Old Road Campus, Old Road, Headington, Oxford, OX37LF, e-mail www.npeu.ox.ac.uk

Give all babies with signs of trauma **vitamin K** 1mg IM at birth (unless already given as part of routine measures).

To the baby—*Moulding:* This is a natural phenomenon, not an injury. The skull bones can override each other (p42) to reduce the diameter of the head. Moulding is assessed by degree of overlap of the overriding at the sutures. If moulding is absent, skull bones are felt separately. With slight moulding, the bones just touch, then they override but can be reduced; finally they override so much that they cannot be reduced. Excessive moulding during labour indicates cephalo–pelvic disproportion, and can result in intracranial damage.

Cephalhaematoma: This is a subperiostial swelling on the fetal head, and its boundaries are therefore limited by the individual bone margins (commonest over parietal bones). It is fluctuant. Spontaneous absorption occurs but may take weeks and may cause or contribute to jaundice.

Caput succedaneum: This is an oedematous swelling of the scalp, superficial to the cranial periosteum (which does not, therefore, limit its extent) and is the result of venous congestion and exuded serum caused by pressure against the cervix and lower segment during labour. The presenting part of the head therefore has the swelling over it. It gradually disappears in the first days after birth. When ventouse extraction is used in labour a particularly large caput (called a chignon) is formed under the ventouse cup.

Erb's palsy: See fig 1, p77. This may result from a difficult assisted delivery, eg shoulder dystocia (so ↑ × 10 in UK diabetic pregnancies).[RCOG] The baby's arm is flaccid and the hand is in the 'porter's tip' posture (p764). Exclude a fractured clavicle and arrange physiotherapy. If it has not resolved by 6 months, the outlook is poor.

Subaponeurotic haematoma: Blood lies between the aponeurosis and the periosteum. As haematoma is not confined to the boundaries of one bone, collections of blood may be large enough to result in anaemia or jaundice. They are associated with vacuum extractions.

Skull fractures: These are associated with difficult forceps extractions. They are commonest over parietal or frontal bones. If depressed fractures are associated with CNS signs, ask a neurosurgeon if the bone should be elevated.

Intracranial injuries: Intracranial haemorrhage is especially associated with difficult or fast labour, instrumental labour, and breech delivery. Premature babies are especially vulnerable. Normally a degree of motility of intracranial contents is buffered by cerebrospinal fluid. Excessive moulding and sudden changes in pressure reduce this effect and are associated with trauma. In all cases of intracranial haemorrhage check babies' platelets. If low, check mother's blood for platelet alloantibodies (PLA1 system). Subsequent babies are at equal risk. IV maternal immunoglobulin treatment is being evaluated.

Anoxia may cause intraventricular haemorrhage (p108). Asphyxia causes intracerebral haemorrhage (often petechial) and may result in cerebral palsy. Extradural, subdural, and subarachnoid haemorrhages can all occur. Babies affected may have convulsions, apnoea, cyanosis, abnormal pallor, low heart rate, alterations in muscle tone, restlessness, somnolence, or abnormal movements. Treatment is supportive and expectant. See p108 & p110.

Obstetric anal sphincter injury (OASI) is common, and is not totally preventable by episiotomy (p93). Of the 1% who suffer anal sphincter injury with vaginal delivery ~30% have problems with flatus incontinence, 8% problems with liquid stool incontinence, and 4% with solid stool (though usually less than once a week). Faecal incontinence is a source of misery, and requires expert attention.

Risk of mechanical injury is greatest after the first vaginal delivery. Traumatic stretching of the pudendal nerves occurs in >30% of primips, but is mostly asymptomatic, or mildly/transiently so. These patients are at ↑ risk in subsequent deliveries (cumulative pudendal nerve injury is well recognized). Other risk factors: • Baby >4kg • Persistent occipito-posterior position • Induced labour • Epidural • 2nd stage >1h • Midline episiotomy • Forceps.

If rectal incontinence occurs, and especially if there is a recto–vaginal fistula, get expert surgical help.[186] If symptomatic or abnormal anorectal manometry or abnormality on endoanal ultrasound after previous repair, consider elective caesarean for subsequent delivery, as 17–24% develop worsening faecal symptoms after subsequent vaginal delivery.[187] Elective caesarean may not protect against symptoms caused by pudendal nerve neuropathy.[188]

Vesicovaginal fistula

This abnormal opening between bladder and vagina leading to urinary incontinence, a common sequel to obstructed labour is thought to affect 3 million women worldwide,[189] now almost exclusively in developing countries.

Obstructed labour is particularly a problem for malnourished girls who become pregnant before full pelvic maturation. In obstructed labour the pelvic head progressively compresses the soft tissues of vagina, bladder, and rectum against the pelvis causing ischaemic damage to these tissues and fetal asphyxiation. 2 days after the fetus dies it becomes macerated, softens, and can be vaginally expelled. A few days later the mother passes sloughed ischaemic tissue leaving a fistula between bladder, urethra, and vagina or rectum and vagina (or both). Damaged tissues adjacent to the sloughed tissue heal poorly, often with fibrosis. Vagina and rectum may later stenose; chronic pyelonephritis and renal failure can ensue. Incontinent women are often shunned by family, divorced by their husbands, and stigmatized (especially in cultures where the affliction is believed to be punishment by God).

Treatment is with continuous urinary drainage for 3 months if presenting with vesicovaginal fistula early (<3 months postpartum) or surgery if later. Operation is most successful for 1st operation and small defects (<2cm) with successful closure rates of up to 85% (but 16–32% of these women remain incontinent).

Good obstetric management of obstructed labour prevents fistulas. Early treatment can allow healing without recourse to surgery. Sadly it is those parts of the world where there is poor access to obstetric facilities where women develop fistulas and where the chance of having subsequent repair is also limited. Read.[1]

1 Living with obstetric fistula (A patient's Journey) F Aliyu 2011 BMJ 342 1360

Obstetrics

▶Examine gently. Unless marked bleeding, allow the mother some bonding time with baby before examination and repair.[106]NICE

Perineal tears These are classified by the degree of damage caused. Risk factors for development are discussed on p91.

Labial tears Common; these heal quickly and suturing is rarely helpful.

First degree tears These tears are superficial and do not damage muscle. Suture unless skin edges well apposed to aid healing.[106]NICE

Second degree tears These lacerations involve perineal muscle. Repair is similar to that of episiotomy (see below).

Third degree tears Damage involves the anal sphincter muscle. Classification:
3a External anal sphincter (circular fibres) thickness <50% torn;
3b External anal sphincter thickness >50% torn;
3c Both external and internal anal sphincters (longitudinal fibres) torn.

If rectal mucosa also involved it is a **fourth degree tear**. See p91. Repair by an experienced surgeon, under epidural or GA in theatre with intra-operative antibiotic cover. Rectal mucosa is repaired first using absorbable suture from above the tear's apex to the mucocutaneous junction. Muscle is interposed. Vaginal mucosa is then sutured. Internal anal sphincter is repaired with interrupted sutures. Overlap and repair severed ends of the external anal sphincter. Finally repair skin. Give antibiotic prophylaxis with 3rd and 4th degree tears. Give high-fibre diet and lactulose for 10 days to avoid constipation. Arrange pelvic floor exercise physiotherapy for 6–12 weeks. Arrange consultant obstetrician follow-up at 6–12 weeks; if pain or incontinence refer to specialist gynaecologist or colorectal surgeon for endoanal ultrasound or manometry.[187]NICOL

Episiotomy This is performed to enlarge the outlet, eg to hasten birth of a distressed baby, for instrumental or breech delivery, to protect a premature head, and to try to prevent 3° tears (but anal tears are not reduced by more episiotomies in normal deliveries). Rates: 8% Holland, 12% England, 50% USA.◀

The tissues which are incised are vaginal epithelium, perineal skin, bulbocavernous muscle, superficial, and deep transverse perineal muscles. With large episiotomies, the external anal sphincter or levator ani may be partially cut, and ischiorectal fat exposed.

Technique: Hold the perineal skin away from the presenting part of the fetus (2 fingers =in vagina). Infiltrate area to be cut with local anaesthetic, eg 1% lidocaine (=lignocaine). Still keeping the fingers in the introitus, cut mediolaterally towards the ischial tuberosity, starting midline (6 o'clock), so avoiding the Bartholin's glands.

Repair: (See fig 1) NB: use resorbable suture—eg polyglactin 910. In lithotomy, and using good illumination, repair the vaginal mucosa first. Start above the apex using continuous non-locked stitches 1cm apart, 1cm from wound edges. Tie off at mucocutaneous junction of fourchette. Then repair muscles with continuous non-locked technique[106]NICE to obliterate any dead spaces. Finally close the skin with subcuticular stitch. Perform rectal examination afterwards to check sutures have not penetrated the rectal mucosa.

Problems with episiotomy: Bleeding (so may increase chance of spread of HIV from mother to baby); infection and breakdown; haematoma formation. For comfort some suggest ice packs, salt baths, hair dryer to dry perineum. 60% of women suffer perineal damage (episiotomy or tear) with spontaneous vaginal delivery; rectal diclofenac can provide effective analgesia. Superficial dyspareunia: see p310. If labia minora are involved in the skin bridge, the introitus is left too small. If the deep layers are inadequately sutured, the introitus becomes rather rounded exposing the bladder to coital thrusts.

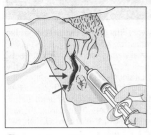

1. Swab the vulva towards the perineum. Infiltrate with 1% lidocaine (→arrows).

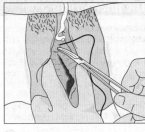

2. Place tampon with attached tape in upper vagina. Insert 1st suture above apex of vaginal cut (not too deep as underlying rectal mucosa nearby).

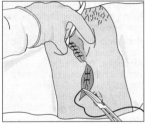

3. Bring together vaginal edges with continuous stitches placed 1cm apart. Knot at introitus under the skin. Appose divided levator ani muscles.

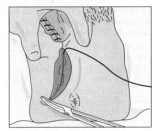

4. Close perineal skin (subcuticular continuous stitch is shown here).

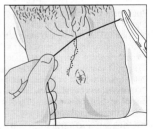

5. When stitching is finished, remove tampon and examine vagina (to check for retained swabs). Do a **PR** to check that apical sutures have not penetrated rectum.

Fig 1. Repairing an episiotomy.

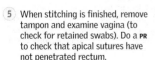
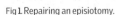

The puerperium is the 6 weeks after delivery. The uterus involutes, from 1kg weight at delivery to 100g. Felt at the umbilicus after delivery, it is a pelvic organ at 10 days. Afterpains are felt (especially while suckling) as it contracts. The cervix becomes firm over 3 days. The internal os closes by 3 days, the external os by 3 weeks. Lochia (endometrial slough, red cells, and white cells) is passed *per vaginam*. It is red (*lochia rubra*) for the 1st days, then becomes yellow (*lochia serosa*) then white over the next 10 days (*lochia alba*), until 6 weeks. The breasts produce milky discharge and colostrum during the last trimester. Milk replaces colostrum 3 days after birth. Breasts are swollen, red, and tender with physiological engorgement at 3 to 4 days.

The first days Is thromboprophylaxis needed? (p16) If Rh–ve, give anti-D, within 72h, p9. Check T°, BP, breasts, legs, lochia, fundal height if heavy PV loss. Teach pelvic floor exercises. Persistent *red lochia*, failure of *uterine involution*, or *PPH* (p84) suggest retained products. *Sustained hypertension* may need drugs (OHCM p134). ►Check rubella immunity. Vaccinate if non-immune (simultaneously but different limb from anti-D, or wait 3 months).[190] Check Hb on postnatal day 1 or ≥day 7: postpartum physiological haemodilution occurs from days 2–6. Discuss contraception (see BOX OPPOSITE).

Puerperal pyrexia is T° >38°C in the first 14 days after delivery or miscarriage. Examine fully (chest, breasts, legs, lochia, and bimanual vaginal examination). Culture MSU, high vaginal swabs, blood, and sputum. 90% of infections will be urinary or of the genital tract. Superficial perineal infections occur around the second day. *Endometritis* gives lower abdominal pain, offensive lochia, and a tender uterus (on bimanual vaginal exam). Endometritis needs urgent IV antibiotics (below) and uterine curettage. For breast infection give **flucloxacillin 250mg/6h PO** early for ≥10 days, to prevent abscesses. Suckling or breast expression should continue to prevent milk stagnation. Even if the cause of pyrexia is unknown, it is wise to treat with **amoxicillin 500mg/8h PO/IV + metronidazole 400mg/8h PO**. NB: puerperal infection can be prevented by cleansing the birth canal at every vaginal examination with 0.25% chlorhexidine.

Superficial thrombophlebitis This presents as a painful tender (usually varicose) vein. Give NSAID, eg **ibuprofen 400mg/8h PO** PO. Bandage and elevate the leg. Recovery is usual within 4 days. *Deep vein thrombosis:* See p32.

Puerperal psychosis (1:500 births): ►See p408. This is distinguished from the mild depression that often follows birth by a high suicidal drive, severe depression (p336), mania, and more rarely schizophrenic symptoms (p358) with delusions that the child is malformed. If an acute organic reaction (p350) is present, suspect puerperal infection. Presentation is by day 7 postpartum in 50%, by 3 months in 90%. Onset is usually sudden and deterioration rapid. Refer to heath trust's community psychiatric team for pregnancy. Admission to specialist mother and baby unit may be needed. See p408 for a fuller discussion of postnatal depression. 10% of mothers develop postnatal depression; in ⅓ -½ of these depression is severe.

The 6-week postnatal examination gives a chance to: • See how mother and baby relate. • Do BP & weight. • Do FBC if anaemic postnatally. • Arrange a cervical smear due. • Check contraceptive plans are enacted (see OPPOSITE). • Ask about depression, backache, incontinence. Ask: "Have you resumed intercourse?"(CEMACE recommends abstinence or 'gentle intercourse' for first 6 weeks postpartum to prevent fatal air embolism).[191] Sexual problems are common, and prolonged: ~50% report that intercourse is less satisfactory than pre-pregnancy, with major loss of libido, and dyspareunia the chief complaints. Vaginal examination to check healing is *not* usually needed.

Lactational amenorrhoea (LAM)[192] This is Nature's contraception. Breast-feeding delays return of ovulation (suckling disrupts frequency and amplitude of gonadotrophin surges so that although there is gonadotrophin rise in response to falling placental sex steroids after delivery, ovulation does not occur). Women who are fully breastfeeding day and night (ie breast milk is baby's sole nutrient), and are less than 6 months postpartum, and amenorrhoeic can expect this method to be 98% effective. Average 1st menstruation in a breastfeeding mother is at 28.4 weeks (range 15–48). Contraceptive efficacy of LAM is decreased after 6 months, if periods return, if breastfeeding frequency reduces, night feeding stops, there is separation from the baby (eg return to work), if the baby receives supplements, or if mother or baby become ill or stressed. In the UK although 69% of mothers initiate breastfeeding only 21% still feed at 6 months. Aim for additional contraception once decreased efficacy is anticipated.

Progesterone only Pill (PoP, p302) These may be started any time post-partum but if started after day 21 additional precautions are needed for 2 days. They do not affect breast milk production. Low doses (<1%) of hormone are secreted in the milk but have not been shown to affect babies.

Combined Pills Start at 3 weeks if not breastfeeding. They affect early milk production and are not recommended if breastfeeding until 6 months (but can be used from 6 weeks if other methods unacceptable). Levels of hormone in breast milk are similar to that of ovulatory cycles.

Emergency contraception Use of progesterone method (p299) is suitable for all. It is not needed before 21 days postpartum.

Depot injections These are not recommended until 6 weeks in those breast-feeding (theoretical risk of sex steroid to baby's immature nervous system and liver). **Medroxyprogesterone acetate** 150mg given deep IM 12-weekly can start 5 days postpartum if bottle feeding, or **norethisterone enanthate** 200mg into gluteus maximus 8-weekly (licensed for short-term use only, but can be given immediately postpartum when medroxyprogesterone use can cause heavy bleeding).

Progesterone implants Insertion is not recommended until 6 weeks in those who are breastfeeding. 0.2% of daily dose of etonogestrel is excreted in breast milk. Implant at 21–28 days in those bottle feeding.

Intrauterine contraceptive devices (IUCD) These should be inserted within the first 48h postpartum or delayed until 4 weeks. This is to minimize risk of uterine perforation at insertion. **Levonorgestrel**-releasing intrauterine devices are also inserted at 4 weeks.

Diaphragms and cervical caps The woman needs to be fitted at 6 weeks as different sizes may be required from previously. Alternative contraception is needed from day 21 until the new ones are confidently handled.

Sterilization Unless sterilization highly advisable at caesarean section (eg repeated sections, family complete), it is best to wait an appropriate interval as immediate postpartum tubal ligation has possible increased failure rate and is more likely to be regretted.

Obstetrics

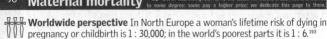

Ideas, beliefs, art, work: none are worth sacrificing life for; the one thing worth sacrificing life for is life itself. All mothers sacrifice themselves to some degree: some pay a higher price: we dedicate this page to them.

Obstetrics

Worldwide perspective In North Europe a woman's lifetime risk of dying in pregnancy or childbirth is 1 : 30,000; in the world's poorest parts it is 1 : 6.[193]

Maternal mortality is defined in the UK as the death of a mother while pregnant or within 42 days of the pregnancy ending, from any cause related to or aggravated by the pregnancy or its management, but not from accidental or incidental causes (called *coincidental* deaths). Deaths are subdivided into those from '*direct causes*'—those in which the cause of death is directly attributable to pregnancy (eg abortion, eclampsia, haemorrhage)—and *indirect* deaths—those resulting from previous existing disease or disease developed during pregnancy, and which were not due to direct obstetric causes but were aggravated by pregnancy (eg heart disease). *Late deaths* are those occurring between 42 days and 1 year after termination, miscarriage, or delivery that are due to direct or indirect maternal causes.

History Since 1952 there have been 3-yearly confidential enquiries into maternal deaths. Prior to 1979, many deaths were considered to have had 'avoidable factors' (denoting departures from acceptable standards of care by individuals, including patients) but since 1979 the wider term of 'substandard care' has been used to cover failures in clinical care and other factors, such as shortage of resources and back-up facilities. Reports allow analysis, reflection, and recommended actions so each death should improve future care.

Maternal mortality has reduced since reports started, (deaths per 100,000 *maternities* (live birth, or stillbirth ≥24wks' gestation) were 67.1 in 1955–7, 33.3 in 1964–6 & 11.39 in 2006–8 of which direct deaths were 4.67/100,000).[194 Mat. mort 2011]

Internationally, figures are given from death certification (rather than proactive case seeking as in the UK), and expressed per 100,000 *live births*. This would give a 2006–8 figure of 6.69. Rates rise with maternal age (especially ≥40yrs). Multiple pregnancy ↑ risk ×3.9. Risk of dying in pregnancy, childbirth, or from abortion is 1 : 65 in developing countries (1 : 9000 in the UK). Note: pregnancy is very protective as all-cause mortality in 15–45-yr-old women is 58.4 : 100,000/year (ie rates of death 4 × *lower* in pregnancy and 1 year after).

In 2006–8, 261 UK deaths were recorded excluding 33 late direct and 24 late indirect deaths. 107 were direct obstetric deaths; 154 were indirect and 50 were coincidental (in no way related to pregnancy, eg car accident). Death was increased in non-whites (×3.5 if black, ×1.5 if Asian), if partner unemployed (×6). 26% of those dying were poor attenders, or had not booked by 18 weeks' gestation (in 2010, 87% of pregnant women had booked by 13 weeks); 19% of those dying were obese or morbidly obese, and 16.6% were substance abusers.

In 2006–8 genital sepsis was the chief cause of direct death in the UK (24.2% of direct, excluding late deaths), and cardiac disease the commonest cause overall. Other direct (excluding late) causes: pre-eclampsia (17.7%); thromboembolism (16.8%); amniotic fluid embolism (12.1%); early pregnancy (10.2%, mainly ectopic pregnancy at 5.6%); haemorrhage (9.25%); anaesthetic (6.5%); fatty liver (2.8%). Deaths from suicide were as rare as from amniotic fluid embolism.

59% of women dying had undergone caesarean section (and 21 babies born at the 38 peri/postmortem caesareans were live born, 9 dying neonatally).

The maternal mortality rate was lower than in the previous triennium for direct deaths (4.67 vs 6.24 : 100,000), and again there were more indirect than direct deaths. Care was considered substandard in 70% of cases of direct and 55% cases of indirect death in 2006–8. 'Substandardness' includes pregnant women who refuse medical advice, lack of knowledge skills to recognize severity of illness, and lack of consultant support and of patient assessment.

This is the number of stillbirths and deaths in the 1st week of life (early neonatal deaths)/1000 births. Stillbirths only include those fetuses of >24 weeks' gestation; if a fetus of <24 weeks' gestation is born showing signs of life, and then dies, this is counted as a perinatal death in the UK (if dying within the 1st 7 days). Neonatal deaths are those infants dying up to and including the 28th day after birth. Other countries use different criteria—including stillbirths from 20 weeks and neonatal deaths up to 28 days after birth, so it is not always easy to compare statistics.

Perinatal mortality is affected by many factors. Rates are high for *small* (61% of deaths in babies <2500g) and *preterm* babies (70% of deaths occur in the 5% who are preterm). See p50 & p128. *Regional variation* in the UK is quite marked. There is a *social class variation* with rates being less for social classes 1 and 2 than for classes 4 and 5. *Teenage mothers* have higher rates than mothers aged 20–29. From 35yrs rates rise until they are 1.5-fold higher than the low-risk group (25–35yrs) by age >40. *Second babies* have the lowest mortality rates. Mortality rates are doubled for fourth and fifth children, trebled by sixth and seventh (this effect is not independent of social class as more lower social class women have many children). Rates are lower for *singleton births* than for multiple (↑×10 for triplets *vs* singletons).[195] Time to conception also has an influence with mortality rates being 3 times more if it has taken a long time to conceive compared with short time (in Denmark).[196] Perinatal mortality in UK* (*figures exclude Scotland) is twice as high in offspring of mothers of black ethnicity; 1.5 times commoner if of Asian ethnicity.[197]

Perinatal mortality rates in the UK have fallen over the years from 62.5:1000 in 1930–5 to 7.6:1000 in 2009 for UK*. Declining mortality reflects improvement in standards of living, improved maternal health, and declining parity, as well as improvements in medical care. The main causes of stillbirth were congenital abnormalities (9%), antepartum/intrapartum haemorrhage (11%), placental conditions (12%) in 2009. The cause in 28% of stillbirths was unexplained. The main causes of neonatal death were prematurity (48%) and malformation (22%).

Examples of how changed medical care may reduce mortality

- Worldwide, treatment of syphilis, antitetanus vaccination (of mother during pregnancy), and clean delivery (especially cord techniques) have the greatest influence in reducing perinatal mortality.
- Antenatal detection and termination of malformed fetuses.
- Reduction of mid-cavity procedures and vaginal breech delivery.
- Detection of placenta praevia antenatally.
- Prevention of rhesus incompatibility.
- Preventing progression of preterm labour.
- Better control of diabetes mellitus in affected mothers.
- Antenatal monitoring of 'at risk' pregnancies.

While we must try to reduce morbidity and mortality still further, this must not blind us to other problems that remain, such as the 'over-medicalization' of birth; the problem of reconciling maternal wishes to be in charge of her own delivery with the immediate needs of the baby; and the problem of explaining risks and benefits in terms that both parents understand, so that they can join in the decision-making process.

Obstetrics

98 **2 Paediatrics**

*who are you, little i
(5 or 6 years old)
peering from some high window
e e cummings*

Other relevant pages: Orthopaedics (Chapter 11); Infectious disease (OHCM
p372–447); perinatal infection p36; child psychiatry p389; play therapy p377;
squint p422; retinoblastoma p421; pain p718; syndromes: p638–55.

We thank Professor Robert Tasker, our Specialist Reader, and Dr Shahzad
Arain, our Junior Reader, for their contribution to this chapter.

Growing up can seem like joining the points on a growth chart, with the chief desiderata being that we should not cross the dotted centiles of our pre-determined course, set out *in utero*, and ending in adulthood or death (these states being synonymous in the mind of the average alienated 15-yr-old). Examples of points on our metaphysical growth chart might be realizing that we are individuals, next that we lead separate lives to our parents and carers. Next may come a view that there is a divinity shaping our lives; this may give way to a more subtle view that this divinity has ceased to care much about us, one way or another, and that we are alone with each other, those tantalizing other minds that, in order to survive, we must learn to read. At last, standing on our own two feet, supported and constrained by the dotted lines of our allowed variability, we realize that our hard-won independence may be an illusion (interdependence not independence is the human rule). Even our own unitary ego may come to look fragile compared with the system of interacting, conflicting processes which perpetually dissolve and reform in strange or familiar patterns of personal identity.

Where is the child in front of you on his or her own unique journey through this landscape? You'd better find out if you want to cure some difficult problems—or perhaps you had better ignore this question. After all, the ward-round has just moved on, and you don't want to be left behind with a perplexed child on the point of confounding you. Sometimes it is enough to look after the body, thereby allowing the soul to look after itself.

We cannot hope to enable children to realize their full potential—for, unsurprisingly, potential is only ever lost. The egg has more potential than the embryo (its sex, for example, is yet to be determined). The child has more potential than the medical student who is forever closing off lines of enquiry to concentrate on one thing. So if potential can only be lost we must aim for potential to be lost in the least harmful way.

The essence of paediatrics is aligning embryology, growth and development, family interactions, and preventive and therapeutic measures to achieve a person who is capable of making choices. Happy or free? Creative or reasonable? Self-destructive and isolated, or participatory and social? We cannot hand down the answers—we just peddle our wares down this one-way street. Ask children what childhood is for, and they will tell you "Preparation. Learning. A time to become yourself...".[1] This is why paediatrics must be holistic—otherwise it will not contribute to these aims. It is against this background of enabling children to become themselves that paediatricians practise their art and their science.

We note with great interest that most patients between the ages of 15 and 20 who have acute leukaemia treated by paediatricians are cured—up to 63%, whereas <50% of this group survive if treated in adult units.[2] This chapter aims to explain how this difference might arise—and to encourage the reader to extend the skills learned in paediatrics to *all* branches of medical practice.

There are 3 aims. **1** To establish a good relationship with the child and parents, so that if difficult treatment is required (or there is nothing wrong) the parents trust you and are able to accept this. **2** Reaching a diagnosis or differential diagnosis. **3** Placing the diagnosis in the context of the child and family. There is no one treatment for pneumonia, or diabetes, or anything else (same disease, but different contexts require different treatments). Try to avoid any hurry or distractions. Introduce yourself; explain your role in the ward or consulting room. Take a history from as many sources as possible—the child, mother, father, and any significant other—but beware allowing the child to feel marginalized, so address yourself to the child first, and last.

Presenting complaints Record the child's and parents' own words.

The present illness When and how did it start? Was he/she well before? How did it develop? What aggravates or alleviates it? Has there been contact with infections? Has the child been overseas recently?

Especially in infants, enquire about feeding, excretion, alertness, and weight gain. After ascertaining the presenting complaint, further questioning is to test the various hypotheses of differential diagnosis.

Past *In utero:* Any problems (eg PET, rubella, Rh disease); drug exposure?
At birth: Gestation, duration of labour, mode of delivery, birthweight, resuscitation required, birth injury, malformations.
As a neonate: Jaundice, fits, fevers, bleeding, feeding problems.

Ask about later illnesses, operations, accidents, screening tests, drugs, allergies, immunization, travel, and drug or solvent abuse.

Development (p220) Does the mother remember milestones reliably?

Drugs Prescribed, recreational, *in utero*, and over-the-counter. Drug intolerances, adverse drug reactions, and true allergies (ie rashes; anaphylaxis).

Family history Stillbirths, TB, diabetes mellitus, renal disease, seizures, jaundice, malformations, others. Are siblings and parents alive and well? Find out about late-onset diseases with a genetic component.[1] Consanguinity is common in some cultures and may be relevant to disease.

Social history It may be vital to know who the father is, but damaging to ask directly. Asking about the 'family unit', or drawing a family tree (*OHCM* p21) is a way forward. Allow information to surface slowly, eg after chats with friendly nurses. Ask about play, eating, sleeping (excessively wrapped or liable to cold?), schooling and pets. Who looks after the child if the parents work? What work do they do? Is paternity leave available? Is it taken?[2] Ask about their hopes, fears, and expectations about the child's illness and hospital stay.

⚙️**Child-centred care** Taking into account the preferences of the child can be difficult, but it is our duty to discover these preferences, and this process starts with taking the history. It will often be the case that the child does not appear to want the treatment on offer (eg an IVI for dehydration). Explanation sometimes leads to co-operation, but if this is not the case talk to colleagues to see what the alternatives are—and whether beneficence trumps ignoring autonomy. Beware overruling the child—but sometimes it is your duty to do so. *Privacy, dignity, and confidentiality* are easy to pay lip-service to, but hard to ensure in busy wards, where space is at a premium. During an average stay in hospital most patients and their relatives overhear confidential exchanges, and only a few recall being offered a screen to preserve privacy during examinations.[3] ▶If the family does not speak your language, find an interpreter.

---

1 For example, if a parent has had a myocardial infarction before 40yrs old, do serum lipids (>40% of these children will turn out to have hyperlipidaemia: the sooner it is treated, the better, p156). 💉
2 Emotional/behaviour problems are commoner at 3yrs old if no paternity leave was taken.[4] *n=19,000* In the UK, 81% of fathers in professions get paternity leave *vs* 46% of those in less skilled work.

	Neonate	Toddler	Older child
Cardio-respiratory	Tachypnoea, grunts wheeze, cyanosis, cold sweats (heart failure)	Cough, exertional dyspnoea	Cough, wheeze sputum, chest pain
Gut	Appetite, D&V, feeding problems, stool frequency Jaundice	Appetite, D&V, stool frequency	Appetite, D&V, abdominal pain, stool frequency
Genitourinary	Wet nappies (how often?)	Wet nappies (how often?)	Haematuria, dysuria, sexual development
Neuromuscular	Seizures; attacks; jitters	Seizures, drowsy hyperactive hearing↓ vision↓ gait	Headaches, fits, odd sensations, drowsy, schooling, vision hearing, co-ordination
ENT; teeth	Noisy breathing	Ear discharge	Earache, discharge, sore throat

Systems review—questions coming to the fore depend on age:

General weight, appetite, fevers, fatigue, lumps, everything else OK?

Paediatrics

"He went white, then red, then blue" If it's hard to ask the right questions, it can be harder still to interpret the answers. Each time a story is told (first to the grandmother, then to the GP, then to the junior doctor and consultant) a new layer of meaning, colour, or ambiguity is disclosed, like swirling spirals of colour on a collective gobstopper. Don't be impatient to get at the truth: suck it and see: the flavour may be as important as all the 'facts'. Often there are *no* unbiased facts, just 5 diverging stories. As Virginia Woolf once said, in cases such as these, *truth is only to be had by laying together many varieties of error.*[5]

Shakespeare's Sister
Girton & Newnham 1928

Wait on events; learn who you can trust, and accept that all 'conclusions' are, provisional—as is the case with any professional historian who juggles his tinted and tainted sources.

Paediatric encounters are among the best places to start the process of becoming an expert in this generic skill of balancing different sources. In adult medicine we typically pay 100% attention to what the patient says about his or her symptoms, and 0% to what anyone else says. With pre-verbal infants, the reverse is true—underlying the point that we should not assume that patients have the most privileged access to their symptoms.

If taking the history is not going well, stop taking it: just hang around and see what happens: learn to waste time.

A single routine will not work for all children. If the child is very ill, examination is limited (p103). Also, points in the examination assume varying importance depending on age (for neonates, see p114). But it is helpful to have some sort of standard: here we look at a boy of 3 years who is being seen because of vomiting. Not everything on even this slimmed-down page will need to be done. The more experienced you are, the better you will be able to judge when and how to take short cuts. Don't mistake taking short cuts for being lazy. Use the time saved to be available to answer questions, and to address the fears and hopes of the parents and child. NB: there is no correct order: be opportunistic, eg with younger children on a lap listen to heart when there are gaps in crying.

1 Wash and warm your hands. Encourage both parents to be present.

2 Regard the child (eg while feeding). Is he ill or well?[1] Restless, still, or playing? If crying, is it high pitched or normal? Is he behaving normally? Any jaundice, cyanosis, rashes, anaemia, or dehydration (p235)? Is he moving normally? Does anything hurt, eg neck, abdomen, limbs?

3 Talk to the child. Explain what you are doing. This helps you both relax, and enjoy the occasion (*not* a trivial point: a happy doctor is an engaged doctor; an engaged doctor is more open to subtle signs). If he seems anxious, examine his teddy in a playful way, to allow him to build up trust. Asking about pets or siblings often helps.

4 If quiet or asleep, now is the time to get any listening done, so examine his heart, lungs, and abdomen. Use a warm stethoscope. Undress in stages.

5 Examine finger nails, then the hands, radial pulse, BP, axillary and neck nodes, neck lumps. Is there neck stiffness? (a 'useless' sign in infants)

6 Size and shape of head (p224). Facial symmetry. In a baby, does the anterior fontanelle (between the parietal and frontal bones) feel tense (intracranial pressure ↑) or sunken (dehydration)?

7 Is there mucus in the nose? Leave ears and throat alone at this stage.

8 Count the respirations. Is there intercostal recession (inspiratory indrawing of the lower costal area, signifying ↑work of breathing)?

9 Percuss the chest if >2yrs old (not very reliable even then), and palpate the abdomen. Is it distended, eg by spleen, liver, fluid, flatus, faeces?

10 Undo the nappy, if worn. Have an MSU pot to hand. If urine is passed, make a clean catch (p174). Inspect the nappy's contents. Examine the genitalia/anus. Find the testes. Rectal examination is very rarely needed.

11 Note large inguinal nodes. Feel femoral pulses.

Neurological examination After completing the above, much will have been learned about the nervous system; if in doubt, check: *Tone:* Passively flex and extend the limbs (provided this will not hurt). *Power and co-ordination:* Watch him walk, run, and pick up a small toy and play with it, with each hand in turn. *Reflexes:* Look for symmetry. *Sensation:* Light touch and pain testing are rarely rewarding. Fundi.

Ears/throat Leave to the end, as there may be a struggle. Mother holds the child on her lap laterally, one hand on the forehead, holding his head against her chest, and the other round his arms. Examine ear drums (p536) first (less invasive). Then, hold the child facing outwards, one arm around his arms, one on his forehead. You can then introduce a spatula and get one good look at mouth and tonsils. Inspect the teeth.

Growth Chart height, weight, and head circumference (p224).

TPR charts Pulse and respiratory rate; T° (rectal T°: normally <37.8°C).

Finally ask child and parents if there is anything else you should look at.

1 In the mood of *la belle époque*, get the *whole* picture as a gestalt flash, and mirror that genius of photography, Jaques Lartigue: "I open my eyes, then I close them, then open them again, wide, and hey presto! I capture the image with everything...and what I hold onto is something living, that moves and feels".

Paediatrics

Is this child seriously ill? [APLS]

(NICE 2007)

Recognizing the need of prompt help is a central skill of paediatrics. It can be uncanny to watch the moment of transformation that this recognition brings to a normally laid-back, easy-going doctor who is now galvanized into an efficient, relentless device for delivering urgent care—*'omitting nothing necessary and adding nothing superfluous'*, a frame of mind recommended by Graham Greene for murder, but equally well suited to curing disease. If you are new to paediatrics, take every opportunity to observe such events, and, later, closely question the doctor about what made her act in the way she did, using this page to prepare your mind to receive and retain her answers.

Typical causes
- Sepsis, meningitis[et al]
- D&V/gastroenteritis
- Obstruction, eg volvulus
- Arrhythmias
- Hypoglycaemia
- U&E imbalance
- Metabolic errors
- Myocarditis
- Congenital heart dis.
- Cardiomyopathies
- Intussusception (p172)
- DIC (p120 & OHCM p346)
- Haemolytic uraemic syn.
- Reye's syndrome (p652)

Airway, breathing, circulation: then dynamic inverse 'traffic light' assessment

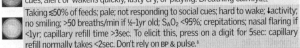

Taking most feeds OK; normal colour (lips, tongue, skin); responds to social cues, alert or wakens quickly, lusty cry, or playing. Breathing calmly.[67][NICE]

Taking ≤50% of feeds; pale; not responding to social cues; hard to wake; ↓activity; no smiling; >50 breaths/min if ½-1yr old; S_AO_2 <95%; crepitations; nasal flaring if <1yr; capillary refill time >3sec. To elicit this, press on a digit for 5sec: capillary refill normally takes <2sec. Don't rely on BP & pulse.[8]

Pale; mottled; ashen; blue. Doesn't stay awake when roused. [1] Consciousness↓ (not engaging; apathy; coma); skin turgor↓. Any **GRUNTING** signs?

→ Grunting; weak or continuous high-pitched cry; tachypnoea >60 breaths/min.
→ Rib recession; retraction of sternomastoid, use of alae nasae; wheeze; stridor.
→ Unequal or unresponding pupils; focal CNS signs; fits; marked hypotonia.[9]
→ Not using limbs/lying still; odd or rigid posture decorticate (flexed arms, extended legs); or decerebrate (arms + legs extended).
→ T° ≥38°C if <6 months or ≥39° especially if cold or shutdown peripheries.
→ I'm having a bad feeling about this baby. ►Learn to trust your judgment.[1]
→ Neck rigidity, non-blanching rash, meningism, bulging fontanelle, etc.
→ Green bile in vomit[10](≈GI obstruction,[11] eg atresia, volvulus, intussusception).[12]

When assessing response level, use the Glasgow coma scale (if <4yrs, p201) or AVPU. A=alert; V=responds to voice; P=responds to pain; U=unresponsive.

Age—Reference interval for:	Breathing rate	Pulse	Systolic BP
<1yr	30-40/min	110-160/min	70-90mmHg
2-5yr	20-30/min	95-140/min	80-100mmHg
5-12yr	15-20/min	80-120/min	90-110mmHg
>12yr	2-16/ min	60-100/min	100-120mmHg

Action—if very ill → 100% O_2 by tight-fitting mask with reservoir, then:
- Immediate IV access. Go intraosseous if access cannot be found (p236).
- Colloid: 20mL/kg bolus IV; repeat if no better. ≥40mL/kg; call PICU.
- Do blood glucose (lab and ward test); U&E (ask specifically for HCO_3^-, and, if vomiting, Cl^-); FBC; thick film if tropical travel possible or unknown.
- Crossmatch blood if trauma is possible, or patient looks anaemic.
- Consider the need for CXR, MSU, and lumbar puncture.
- Do swabs, blood culture (+suprapubic urine aspirate if <1yr, before starting blind treatment with IV antibiotics, eg ceftriaxone or cefotaxime, p202).
- If worsening, insert CVP. Get expert help; do blood gases ± clotting screen.
- Ventilation may be needed if very sick, to offload the heart.
- If perfusion↓ despite 60mL/kg colloid or CVP >10cmH₂O, consider inotropes, p203.

1 DOH[UK] free DVD *Spotting the Sick Child* (cat n° 40630): tel 08701 555455 dh@prolog.uk.com + NICE 2006
2 This is a reason to spend hours and hours on the wards: to gain the experience that validates 'bad feels'. We once asked an obstetrician how he had recognized placenta praevia during a vaginal exam in labour: "It was easy" he said; "I felt sick and started to sweat as soon as my finger entered the os".

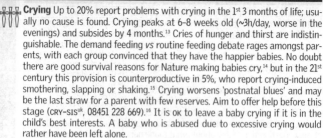

Crying Up to 20% report problems with crying in the 1st 3 months of life; usually no cause is found. Crying peaks at 6–8 weeks old (~3h/day, worse in the evenings) and subsides by 4 months.[13] Cries of hunger and thirst are indistinguishable. The demand feeding *vs* routine feeding debate rages amongst parents, with each group convinced that they have the happier babies. No doubt there are good survival reasons for Nature making babies cry,[14] but in the 21st century this provision is counterproductive in 5%, who report crying-induced smothering, slapping or shaking.[15] Crying worsens 'postnatal blues' and may be the last straw for a parent with few reserves. Aim to offer help before this stage (CRY-SIS^uk, 08451 228 669).[16] It is ok to leave a baby crying if it is in the child's best interests. A baby who is abused due to excessive crying would rather have been left alone.

- Don't make parents feel inadequate; foster a spirit of practical optimism with parents taking it in turns to sleep. Explain normal crying and sleeping.
- Baby-centred approach to help parents help the baby deal with discomfort.
- Help parents recognize when their baby is tired and hungry ('read-your-baby' lessons may be needed),[17] and to apply a consistent approach to care.
- Vocal (singing), vestibular (rocking, going for a drive) or tactile stimulation (hugs) may help.[18] Encourage help from friends/family. Simplify daily living.
- If not coping, admit to a parenting centre or hospital;[19] don't over-medicalize!

3-month colic (Paroxysmal crying with pulling up of the legs, for >3h on ≥3days/wk). Cows' milk protein allergy, transitory lactose intolerance,[20] and parental discord are implicated[1]. There is an association with feeding difficulties.[21] Also, blunted rhythm in cortisol production is reported, suggesting delay in establishing circadian activity of the hypothalamic–pituitary–adrenocortical axis and associated sleep-wake cycles.[22] **R:** Movement (carry-cot on wheels) is often tried and may help.[23] Let the baby **finish the first breast first**^Fisher's rule (hindmilk is easier to digest).[24] Pre-incubation of feeds with **lactase** (eg 2 drops of **Colief Infant Drops®** per formula feed, left in the fridge for 4–12h[25] before heating) helps.[26] If breastfeeding: express ~15mL of milk into a sterilized container; add 4 drops of Colief®; feed to the baby on a sterilized plastic spoon, then start breastfeeding at once. Alternative: **dimeticone** (simeticone) drops (40mg/mL; 2.5mL po with feeds). Few other drugs are licensed at this age. Consider 1mL of 30% **glucose** po[27] or **fennel** seed oil emulsion.[28] There is some evidence probiotics (*Lactobacillus reuteri*) may be beneficial.[29] If breastfeeding, a 'low-allergen' diet may help.[30] Soya milk used to be tried, but is not recommended (∵ high levels of oestrogens). **Reassure strongly; reduce stress;**[31] encourage **grandparent** involvement. Remember: a crying baby may be a sign of major relationship problems.

Nappy rash/diaper dermatitis 4 types (may co-exist).[32]
1 The common 'ammonia dermatitis'—red desquamating rash, sparing skin folds, due to moisture retention, not ammonia.[33] It responds to frequent nappy changes (cloth nappies retain more moisture than disposables), or nappy-free periods, careful drying, and emollient creams. Best treatment: leave nappy off. Use barrier cream: eg Sudocrem® (zinc oxide cream).
2 Candida/thrush is isolatable from ~½ of all nappy rashes. Its hallmark is satellite spots beyond the main rash. Mycology: see p598. Treatment: as above, + **clotrimazole** (± 1% **hydrocortisone** cream, no stronger, eg as Canesten HC®). One trial favours thrice-daily **mupirocin** ointment.[N=20] Avoid oral antifungals (hepatotoxic) and gentian violet (staining is disliked).
3 Seborrhoeic dermatitis: a diffuse, red, shiny rash extends into skin folds, often occurs with other seborrhoeic areas, eg occiput (cradle cap). **R:** as for 1.[35]
4 Isolated, psoriasis-like scaly plaques (p594), which can be hard to treat.

---

1 Consider this: are stressed parents simply more likely to report colic?

Vomiting

Effortless regurgitation of milk is common during feeds ('posseting'). Vomiting between feeds is also common. Ask about carpets: significant vomiting in a baby will have caused lots of damage to the parent's carpets. No damage: unlikely to be pathological. Causes: gastro-oesophageal reflux, over-feeding (150mL/kg/day is normal), pyloric stenosis (projectile, at ∼8 weeks old), or UTI. Rarer causes: pharyngeal pouch, metabolic conditions, almost any other illness. Gastroenteritis is uncommon in babies as their feed is usually sterile. Observing feeding is helpful in deciding if vomiting is projectile (eg over the end of the cot), suggesting pyloric stenosis. *Bilious (green) vomiting:* Get urgent help, p130; consider duodenal obstruction or volvulus.

☼Chronic childhood illness, and family support

Diseases such as severe asthma, CNS disease, and neoplasia may cause disintegration of even the most apparently secure families: ►*consequent strife and marital breakdown may be more severe and have more far-reaching consequences than the illness itself.*

Remember that illness makes families poor, and movement down the social scale leads to unpredictable consequences in housing and (un)employment. Families experiencing housing instability and food insecurity (without homelessness or hunger) are known to miss out on health care.[37] n=12,746

Marital disharmony may seem to be beyond the scope of paediatrics, but any holistic view of child health *must* put the family at the centre of *all* attempts to foster child health and wellbeing.

We see many families coping well with severe, prolonged illness in a child. But don't presume that because things are OK in clinic today, you can afford to neglect the fostering of family life. Given a certain amount of stress almost *all* families will show psychopathology, in time. Your job is to prevent this if possible. Counselling skills are frequently needed (p380)—but do they work? Various tools are helpful in answering this:[38]

- Communication is vital in any family, and this can be measured by scales such as the Communication Skills Test (CST).[1]
- The Dyadic Adjustment Scale (DAS) looks at the emotional interaction within a marriage or any other pairing.[39]
- The Miller Social Intimacy Scale (MSIS) looks at intimacy in relationships, and intimacy is, beyond doubt, a source of strength within a family experiencing illness in a child.
- Specific therapies validated in randomized trials in families coping with severe chronic illness in a child include Emotionally Focused Marital Therapy (EMT), with these benefits:[40]
  - Higher overall levels of marital adjustment (on the DAS scale). None of the couples receiving the active therapy deteriorated by >7 points, whereas one-third of couples in the control group had such a deterioration (which shows the stress these families were under, and supports the notion that family psychopathology in the face of chronic childhood illness is an evolving phenomenon—*the stress is reversible if you take certain steps*).
  - Better levels of intimacy as measured on MSIS scale, with effects persisting for at least 5 months.
  - Lower rates of negative communication (on the CST score).
  - NNT=2 (2 couples need treating for one to improve).

"I lost everything when my son got sick... I lost my job and then my home...then I read my husband's suicide note."

---

1 Full instruments available in: K Corcoran *Measures for clinical practice: A sourcebook*. New York.

Temperature Rectal is most reliable.[41-43] In the axilla: use an electronic or chemical dot thermometer. In the ear: use an infra-red tympanic thermometer.[2007][NICE]

3 questions to ask: *How severe are the symptoms?* and *How appropriate is the child's response to the illness?* The symptom may be severe (eg "terrible diarrhoea all over the cot") without being biologically serious (if the baby is alert, drinking, wetting many nappies, and behaving as usual), but ANY apparently mild symptom should set your internal alarm bell ringing if:[44,45]
• Less than half the usual amount of feed has been taken in the last day.
• There is breathing difficulty, or high-pitched continuous moans or cries.
• There is a history of being pale, mottled, cyanosed, and hot.
• Dull expression; apathetic; uninterested in you; drowsy; dehydrated.
• A significant reduction in the number of wet nappies in the last 24h.
• Blood in diarrhoea, or seizures, or tachycardia not explained by pain or fever.
The 3rd question is: *Is neutropenia possible* (eg on chemotherapy)?

Assess the **'traffic light' way,** p103, paying especial attention to red signs (pale, mottled, ashen blue, not staying awake when roused, etc). Always listen to your sixth sense: act if you have a bad feeling about this. Then observe the limbs: pain causes *pseudoparalysis,* eg with legs in a frog position (hips & knees semiflexed, feet rotated outward), eg in osteomyelitis, or septic arthritis.[46-48] The above signs carry extra weight if immunocompromised (eg neonates; post measles; AIDS; cystic fibrosis; leukaemia; chemotherapy/malignancy; absent spleen; B/T cell dysfunction); congenital anomaly or foreign body, eg an indwelling IVI line (bacteria may be unusual and of low virulence).[49]

Fever (meningitis, p202; pneumonia, p160; UTI, p174.) Fever is the major acute presentation in paediatrics, eg from viruses, otitis media, or pharyngitis (p564), and prognosis is good. Here, fever *may* help (aids neutrophil migration; ↑bioactivity of cytokines, ↑interferon and ↑ T-cell proliferation).[49] The challenge is to treat serious bacterial infections promptly, without medicalizing normal childhood ills. *Do MSU within 24h of fever onset. Is LP needed?* see above & p206.

Bacteraemia occurs in ~4% of febrile children and, in most, a source of infection is found by a good history and examination, blood & urine cultures, FBC/ film, CXR ± LP (see above), etc. Rapid virology is becoming available—eg PCR and direct fluorescent assay (for adenoviruses).[50] ESR >30mm/h and ↑C-reactive protein also indicate bacterial infection—eg *Strep pneumoniae, N. meningitidis.* Sometimes the child (esp. between 3 and 24 months of age) has T° ⩾39°C and WCC >15×10⁹/L, but despite being feverish, he does not look ill, and no obvious focus of infection can be found. This can be due to **occult bacteraemia,** which is usually transient and self-limiting (although a small but significant number of these children may develop a serious bacterial infection). *Management:* Management of the febrile child is very resistant to written guidelines. NICE guidance (2007) gives a framework for the under 5s, but a large amount of clinical acumen is still needed. If in doubt, ask for senior help. If they look toxic, do bloods and a blood culture. If you have not identified a source for the infection, then do a full septic screen. With a sick patient, however, there should be no delay: give **cefotaxime 50mg/kg/6h** or **ceftriaxone[1] 50mg/kg/24h** (for weights <50kg). Most patients <3 months with a fever should be admitted, those under 1 month will invariably need at least 48h of IV antibiotics. There is some leeway if aged 1-3 months: those that look unwell, or have a WCC >15 or <5 will need an LP and antibiotics, but if investigations are normal and they look well some infants may be suitable for observation only/ outpatient management—this will depend on the experience of the practitioner, observational skills of the parent and ease of follow-up.[51,52]

1 Concomitant R with calcium contraindicates ceftriaxone use in neonates (?older children too): it causes precipitation in the lungs. Other CI: neonatal jaundice, albumin↓, acidosis, ↓bilirubin binding.

90% of neonates are perfectly healthy: the best plan is to return these babies to the mother with no interference, to augment bonding.[55] Mother-and-baby skin-to-skin contact is ideal, rather than swaddling or nursery cots, and is the best way to maintain temperature.[56] A paediatrician or nurse trained in advanced neonatal resuscitation should attend the following births: emergency caesars, breeches, twins, forceps for fetal distress, intrapartum bleeding, prematurity, hydrops fetalis, eclampsia and thickly stained meconium liquor.

Before birth Check the equipment. Get a warm blanket. Heat the crib.

At birth If pulse <100, poor colour or respiratory effort, set a clock in motion, and see OPPOSITE. Be alert to:

- Hypothermia (use heat lamp).
- Hypoglycaemia: glucose 10%, 2.5mL/kg IV.
- Pethidine toxicity: naloxone 200μg (60μg/kg stat) IM or 10μg/kg repeated every few min; contraindicated in maternal opioid abuse.
- Anaemia (heavy fetal blood loss?)—give 10mL/kg of 0.9% NaCl over 10-20 seconds.
- Is there lung disease or congenital cyanotic heart disease (p136)? Transfer to NICU/SCBU for monitoring.
- Suck out oropharynx (*before* stimulating breathing!) only if meconium aspiration likely and the baby is flat.
- 21% O₂ (air) is better than 100% O₂.[54,57]

Endotracheal intubation is a key skill: use 3.5mm uncuffed, unshouldered tubes on term infants; 3mm if 1.25–245kg (2.5mm if smaller). Learn from experts. Have many sizes to hand. Practise on models.

Prognosis Mortality for *prems* is 315/1000 if 5min Apgar score 0–3, *vs* 5/1000 if score is ≥7. Corresponding figures *at term* are 244/1000 & 0.2/1000. If a term infant with Apgar score ≤3 has a low arterial pH (≤7), risk of neonatal death increases 8-fold.[58] Survival in those needing CPR (cardiac resus) is 63% for infants of 0.5–1.5kg, compared with 88% in these weight groups if CPR is not needed. Severe intraventricular haemorrhage is seen in 15% of those needing CPR *vs* 5% in those who don't.

Dry the baby (unless <28 wks); place under radiant heat.
↓
Set a clock in motion; assess *colour, tone, breathing & pulse.*
If not breathing after ∼60sec:
↓
Control the airway
(head in the neutral position)
↓
Support breathing: 5 inflation breaths; aim for inflation pressure of 20cm H₂O (max 40cm H₂O). Confirm response: visible chest movements or ↑heart rate.
↓
If no response, check *head position* and try a *jaw thrust*; then 5 inflation breaths. Confirm response: visible chest movements or ↑ heart rate.
↓
If still no response, get 2ⁿᵈ person to help with airway control and inflation breaths. Any sucking out of the pharynx should be under direct vision.[59]
- Repeat 5 inflation breaths
- Insert oropharyngeal airway
- Repeat inflation breaths
Consider intubation. Confirm response: visible chest movements or increased heart rate.
↓
When chest is moving, continue with ventilation breaths if no spontaneous breathing.
↓
Check heart rate; if absent or <60 *start chest compressions.* Do 3 chest compressions to 1 breath, for 30sec
↓
Reassess pulse: if improving, stop chest compressions. If not breathing, go on ventilating. If heart rate still↓ continue ventilation & chest compressions.
↓
Consider *IV or umbilical access* & *drugs,* eg adrenaline (epinephrine): 10μg/kg (0.1mL 1:10,000/kg) IV.

At all stages ask *Do I need help?*

Paediatrics

Apgar	Pulse	Respirations	Muscle tone	Colour	On suction
2	>100	Strong cry	Active	Pink	Coughs well
1	<100	Slow, irregular	Limb flexion	Blue limbs	Depressed cough
0	0	Nil	Absent	All blue or white	No response

Neonatal intensive care is a technological development of the basic creed of first aid— ABC; airway, breathing, and circulation. There is also an E. Epithelial cells determine whether low birthweight babies survive outside the uterus. They manage all interactions with the *ex utero* world: •Lung mechanics/gas exchange •Renal tubular balance of fluid and electrolytes •Barrier functions of the gut and skin for keeping bacteria out and water in, plus enabling digestion •Intact neuroepithelium lining of the ventricles of the brain and retina.[60]

Monitor $T°$, pulse, BP (intra-arterial if critical), respirations, blood gases (S_AO_2 ± intra-arterial electrode), U&E, bilirubin, FBC, weight, weekly head circumference.

The patient is usually a premature baby. His mortal enemies are: cold, hypoxia, hypoglycaemia (p112), respiratory distress syndrome (p118), infection (p112); intraventricular haemorrhage; apnoea; necrotizing enterocolitis (p120).[1] *You* may become the problem: overzealous investigation/handling is damaging,[61] as is under-intervention.[62] Getting the balance right is vital.

Cold With their small volume and relatively large surface area, this is a big problem for small babies. Incubators allow temperature (as well as humidity and F_iO_2) to be controlled, and also afford some protection against infection. F_iO_2 is the fraction of O_2 in inspired air, ie 0.6=60% O_2.

Apnoeic attacks *Prevalence:* 25% of neonates <2.5kg; 90% if <1kg. *Causes:* Respiratory centre immaturity; aspiration; heart failure; infection; $P_aO_2\downarrow$; glucose↓; $Ca^{2+}\downarrow$; seizures; patent ductus (PDA); $T°\uparrow$ or ↓; exhaustion; airway obstruction. If stimulating the baby doesn't restore breathing, suck out the pharynx and use bag-and-mask ventilation. Avoid wild P_aO_2 fluctuations to prevent ROP (below). *Tests:* CXR; U&E; infection screen; glucose; Ca^{2+}; Mg^{2+}. R_x: If aspiration is the problem, give small frequent feeds, or continuous tube feeds. Monitor S_AO_2 continuously; if hypoxic despite an ambient O_2 of 40%, consider CPAP or IPPV. Caffeine citrate 20mg/kg PO/IVI stat, then 5mg/kg once daily starting 24h after stat dose—some neonates may need 10mg/kg; neonates >44 weeks postmenstrual age may need 10mg/kg/12h (fewer SE than theophyllines).[63]

Nasal CPAP ± doxapram *may* prevent hypoventilation. If apnoea is seizure-related, see p112. *Stopping ventilation:* Try 4–5 days after apnoea has stopped. *Prevention:* Betamethasone intrauterine maturation (p51).[64]

RoP (retinopathy of prematurity) A disorder of the developing retina. Major risk factors are low birth weight and prematurity. Exposure to supplemental oxygen is a cause, in particular large fluctuations in P_aO_2, so careful titration of O_2 levels has led to a decrease in the incidence of ROP. Abnormal fibrovascular proliferation or retinal vessels may lead to retinal detachment and visual loss. *Prevalence (lower limits):* <1000g: 53%; ≤1250g: 43%; ≤1500g: 35%.[65] *Classification:* There are 5 stages, depending on site involved, the degree of retinal detachment, and extent (measured as clock hours in each eye). *Treatment:* Diode laser therapy causes less myopia than cryotherapy. Screening: see BOX.

IVH (intraventricular haemorrhage)[2] occurs in 25% if birthweight ≤1500g.[66] Preterm infants are at risk of IVH due to unsupported blood vessels in the subependymal germinal matrix and the instability of blood pressure associated with birth trauma and respiratory distress. Delayed cord clamping in prems may ↓risk.[67] Suspect in neonates who deteriorate rapidly (esp. in week 1). *Signs:* Seizures; bulging fontanelle and cerebral irritability but many will have no clinical symptoms.[68] *Tests:* Ultrasound; CT. *Complications:* IQ↓, cerebral palsy, hydrocephalus (see DRIFT[3]). Many survive unscathed. R_x: Meticulous nursing; head elevation; circulatory support, seizure control (p112).

---

1 UK *perinatal death trends:* deaths from congenital defects and hypoxia are 50% of 1980s rates, but death rates for infection are similar. Rates of multiple births and their problems are rising.[69]
2 *Other types of bleeding:* subdural; subarachnoid; parenchymal. MRI shows that 26% of 'normal' babies have small bleeds, probably from skull pressure at delivery. Bleeds were not found in caesarean births.[70]
3 DRIFT aims to treat IVH-associated hydrocephalus.

With our first breath pulmonary vascular resistance falls, and there is a rush of blood to our lungs.[71] This is partly mediated by endogenous nitric oxide (NO). This breath initiates changes from fetal to adult circulation—a process which may be interrupted in various conditions, eg meconium aspiration, pneumonia, respiratory distress syndrome, diaphragmatic hernia, group B strep infection, and pulmonary hypoplasia.[72]

Pulmonary hypertension arises as a consequence of these adverse events. It may also be due to hypertrophy of the muscular layer in the pulmonary arteries (primary pulmonary hypertension).

The chief diagnostic features are a background (eg meconium aspiration) and persisting desaturation despite intensive O_2 use. When it is suspected, arrange immediate echocardiography, and get help. Echo will show right-to-left shunting via the ductus arteriosus in the absence of structural heart disease.

Inhaled nitric oxide (iNO)[1] helps promote adult circulation and improves pulmonary outcomes for prems (eg 1000-1250g) who are at risk from BPD (p119).[73,74] It also ↓need for extracorporeal membrane oxygenation (below). It may also ↓risk of brain injury. iNO relaxes smooth muscle by ↑production cyclic guanosine monophosphate. (NB: sildenafil inhibits its degradation—and may also have a role).[75,76] iNO may be associated with ↑risk of intraventricular haemorrhage.[77] Alternatives: adenosine, tolazoline, and epoprostenol (prostacyclin).[78] Ventilate (p110) gently, and correct reversible contributory factors (hypothermia, polycythaemia, hypocalcaemia, hypoglycaemia). Give surfactant as indicated (p118).

Persistent pulmonary hypertension occurs in ~0.2% of live births.[79] Mortality is 10-20% despite high-frequency ventilation, surfactant, inhaled nitric oxide, and extracorporeal membrane oxygenation—but is much higher when these therapies are not available.[80]

Extracorporeal membrane oxygenation (ECMO) ECMO is a complex procedure (done in specialized units) providing lifesupport for respiratory failure, which obviates the need for lung gas exchange.

One trial showed that ECMO done after referral to one of 5 UK ECMO centres ↓deaths from respiratory failure (oxygenation index ≥40).[2] The trial was stopped early because the scrutineers found the results so strongly favoured ECMO over traditional measures: 32% died in the ECMO group, compared with 59% in the control group. The advantage was upheld irrespective of the primary diagnosis, or the type of referring centre. The number of infants suffering severe disability at follow-up at 1yr was 1 in each group.[81] N=185

Criteria which may make ECMO cost-effective: weight >2kg; no major congenital malformations or CNS abnormality on ultrasound; gestation >34 weeks; oxygen index (OI) >40 (unresponsive to NO inhalation).

NB: more premature babies *may* benefit, eg when problems with circuitry and heparinization are solved. Need for ECMO may be ~1 : 4000 live births. It is thought to be economically worthwhile.[82,83]

Screening for retinopathy of prematurity[84]

Screening is recommended if <1500g or <32 weeks' gestation.
If ≤27 weeks, screen at 30-31 weeks postmenstrual age.
If born at 27-32 weeks then screen at 4-5 weeks post natal age.
Screening ought to be repeated 1-2 weekly depending on severity of disease.
It must be done by an experienced ophthalmologist.

---

1 In one good trial a 24-day course of iNO started at 20 parts per million (for 48-96h, reducing at weekly intervals to 10, 5, and 2 ppm).[85] *NB*: iNO is new, expensive, and uncertain; await more data before using.
2 **What is the oxygen index (OI)?** In the equation, MAP is the mean airway pressure in cmH_2O.[86] F_iO_2 is the partial pressure of inspired O_2. $OI = (F_iO_2 \times MAP) \div P_aO_2$

This is a skill to be learned at the cot side. Nurses and specialist respiratory therapists will help you. Needs of apparently similar babies vary, so what follows is only a guide to prepare your mind before teaching. Continuous refinement in the light of transcutaneous and blood gas analysis is needed. The aims are to improve gas exchange, decrease work of breathing, and enable ventilation for those with respiratory depression or apnoea.

Non-invasive ventilation

HFNC (high-flow nasal cannula) A high flow nasal cannula delivers a distending positive pressure to the airways similar to CPAP. Humidifying the gas delivered decreased side effects of mucosal dryness. Use of HFNC may reduce the number of ventilated days compared to CPAP, but it is not yet considered to be standard practice.[87]

CPAP (continuous positive airways pressure) Pressure is raised throughout the respiratory cycle, so assisting spontaneous inspiration. With skill, this method has few complications, and is useful as a first stage in ventilating a baby before it is known whether he or she will need IMV.

NIPPV (nasal intermittent positive pressure ventilation) This combines nasal CPAP with superimposed ventilator breathing at a set pressure—it can be used as a bridge between invasive ventilation and nasal CPAP.

Invasive ventilation

Invasive ventilation is broadly composed of *conventional mechanical ventilation* (CMV) (a.k.a. intermittent mandatory ventilation (IMV)) and *high frequency ventilation* (HFV).

TCPL (time-cycled pressure limited ventilation) Continuous flows of heated and humidified gas pass via an endotracheal tube. The breath delivered is set by peak inspiratory pressure (PIP) and either the absolute inspiratory time (T_1), or the inspiratory:expiratory ratio (I:E ratio). The delivered tidal volume is dependent on lung compliance and resistance. Nasotracheal siting is best (fewer tube displacements).[88] TCPL allows the infant to make respiratory efforts between ventilator breaths which can lead to dysynchrony between the ventilator and the baby. *Initial settings:* Choose to give good chest inflation and air entry on auscultation and adequate transcutaneous O_2 readings. Typical settings might be T_1 0.32sec, 40 cycles/min, inspiratory pressure 14–18cmH$_2$O, and PEEP 5cmH$_2$O. Adjust in the light of blood gas analysis.

PTV (patient-triggered ventilation), including SIMV and SIPPV. PTV combines TCPL ventilation with a sensor which detects spontaneous breaths. The ventilator then delivers a breath which is synchronized with the infant's own inspiratory effort. In PTV, inspiratory and end-expiratory pressure is set by the operator, but the rate (within limits) set by the baby. PTV is associated with a shorter duration of ventilation.[89,90] Hiccups cause problems if abdominal movement is used to detect inspiration.

HFV (high-frequency ventilation) delivers small volumes of gas at very rapid rates. Its aim is to reduce ventilator-associated lung injuries. There are several different types—high-frequency positive pressure ventilation (HFPPV), jet ventilation, flow interrupted and oscillatory ventilation (HFOV). HFPPV may reduce incidence of air leak compared to CMV (see BOX 4).[91]

Paralysis Pancuronium (eg 30μg/kg IV; then 10μg/kg every 1.5–4h to maintain paralysis) prevents pneumothorax ± IVH (p108) in asynchronous respiratory efforts (eg needing unexpectedly high P_1).[92]

Factors associated with a good outcome from ventilation

▶*Don't base decisions on when to ventilate solely on degree of prematurity.* Factors associated with a better outcome: antenatal corticosteroids, singleton pregnancy, ♀ sex, and higher birthweight (in 100g increments). Each of these equates with 1 extra week of gestation in determining prognosis.[93] In this study of infants born at 22 to 25 weeks' gestation, 49% died, 61% died or had profound impairment (eg neurosensory disability, IQ↓, or cerebral palsy), and 73% died or had some impairment.

Some complications of mechanical ventilation of neonates

Because of the positive pressure it produces, positive pressure ventilation will cause some haemodynamic compromise (hypotension, ↓cardiac output).

Lung Pneumothorax; pulmonary haemorrhage; bronchopulmonary dysplasia (p119); interstitial pulmonary emphysema; pneumonia. Multidrug-resistant organisms are often the cause of late-onset ventilator-associated pneumonia (cefepime has a role here).[94] Post extubation atelectasis may be more frequent after nasal intubation (esp. in very-low-birthweight infants).[95]

Airways Upper airway obstruction (worse in inspiration and may cause stridor). Consider bronchoscopy (may show supraglottic lesions). Laryngomalacia gastro-oesophageal reflux also occur, but more rarely.[96]

Others Patent ductus arteriosus; ↑intracranial pressure ± intraventricular haemorrhage (p108); retinopathy of prematurity (p108); subcutaneous emphysema; pneumomediastinum; pneumopericardium; pneumoperitoneum (transdiaphragmatic); air embolus.

Weaning from the ventilator

Decrease the rate of IMV and lower P_I by 2cmH$_2$O at a time; try extubating if blood gas OK with ~4cmH$_2$O PEEP and a PIP of 12-14 with spontaneous breaths over a backup rate of 5.

Racemic adrenaline doesn't stop intubation-associated ↑upper airways resistance.[97]

Nasal intermittent positive pressure ventilation (NIPPV) delivers ventilator breaths via nasal prongs. If each breath is synchronized with the baby's own inspiratory efforts, this may prevent the need for re-intubation.[98]

Other factors

Pain relief/sedation: Consider 5% **glucose** IVI with **morphine** 25-100µg/kg over ≥5min, then 5-40µg/kg/h. This is thought safe, and lowers catecholamine concentrations (an objective correlate of pain and stress which helps form pain assessment tools[99]) —only quasi-valid![100]

Air leak: Air ruptures alveoli tracking along vessels and bronchioles (pulmonary interstitial emphysema), and may extend intrapleurally (pneumothorax + lung collapse), or into the mediastinum or peritoneum. Associated with high PIP, it is less common with HFOV. *Signs:* Tachypnoea, cyanosis, chest asymmetry. The lateral decubitus CXR is often diagnostic if you have time. ▶▶Prompt 'blind' needle aspiration of a pneumothorax may be needed. Aspirate through the second intercostal space in the midclavicular line with a 25G 'butterfly' needle and a 50mL syringe on a 3-way tap. If the leak is continuous, use underwater seal drainage.

Paediatrics

Sepsis Common (1-10/1000 births), and commonly overwhelming (mortality 15-50%). Here, signs may be minimal, or as opposite (BOX). *Action:* ABC (p108). Clear the airway; intubate and ventilate if necessary. This should correct acidosis, so bicarbonate is rarely needed. Set up a colloid IVI (20mL/kg initially). Exclude hypoglycaemia; do blood gases. *Infection screen:* •Blood culture, virology, FBC, platelets, glucose, CXR. •Lumbar puncture: CSF (p202) for urgent Gram stain, cell count, protein & glucose level, culture, and virology. •Stool: for virology. •Urine: microscopy, culture, and virology. •ENT swabs: for culture. *Antibiotics:*[101] In **early onset infection** (ie neonates <48h old), group B streps and *E. coli* (+ any organism prevalent in your NICU) are common. Treat with benzylpenicillin and gentamicin for 10-14 days. An alternative is amoxicillin and cefotaxime, but this may be less effective.[102] *Doses:* Benzylpenicillin: 50mg/kg/12h (increase to 8-hrly once >1wk old); gentamicin 4mg/kg/24h IV (36-hrly in prems <32 weeks' gestation). *Note on dilutions* Dilute 600mg of benzylpenicillin in 1.6mL of water; 600mg of the powder displaces 0.4mL, so final concentration is 300mg/mL. In **late-onset infection** (ie neonates over 48h old), coagulase -ve staphs and listeria are possible, so regimens include flucloxacillin + gentamicin, amoxicillin + cefotaxime or amoxicillin + gentamicin. **Vancomycin** or **teicoplanin** (p195) may be used. If the CSF suggests meningitis, see p202.

Neonatal seizures (~4/1000 births) *Causes:* Hypoxic-ischaemic encephalopathy (due to birth asphyxia/respiratory distress etc); infection (meningitis/encephalitis); intracranial haemorrhage/infarction; structural CNS lesions (focal cortical dysplasia/tuberous sclerosis); metabolic disturbance (hypoglycaemia; $\downarrow Ca^{2+}$; $\uparrow\downarrow Na^+$; $\downarrow Mg^{2+}$); metabolic disorders (urea cycle disorders/amino acid metabolism). *Diagnosis:* Can be difficult as there may only be subtle clinical signs of seizures (see BOX 2). EEG can confirm seizure activity.

Treatment: ABC. Turn on the side. Ask an experienced nurse to help.
• Rule out or treat reversible causes such as hypoglycaemia and electrolyte disorders.
• Start on empirical antibiotics if possible sepsis.
• Investigate to find cause of seizures.
• If prolonged or repeated seizures consider anticonvulsants. *First line* **Phenobarbital** Loading dose: 20mg/kg IV as slow injection. *Second line:* Phenytoin 18mg/kg IVI *Other agents:* clonazepam; midazolam; paraldehyde. If fits continue: **pyridoxine** 50-100mg IV + 50-100mg/day PO (?for *all* <2yrs old with undiagnosed seizures: in case of pyridoxine deficiency).Autosomal recessive[103]
Hypocalcaemia: Use low PO_4^{3-} milk + calcium gluconate 10%, 4.4mL/kg/day PO (IV: 0.5mL/kg diluted in 4.8mL/kg of saline over 5-10min). Monitor ECG. NB: American experts use higher IV emergency doses: 2mL/kg of a 10% solution.
Hypomagnesaemia: Give 100mg/kg of **MgSO₄** 10% (=100mg/mL),[3] IV over >10min.[104]

Shock *Causes:* Blood loss (placental haemorrhage, twin-twin transfusion; intraventricular haemorrhage; lung haemorrhage); capillary plasma leaks (sepsis, hypoxia, acidosis, necrotizing enterocolitis); fluid loss (D&V; ↑insensible loss; inappropriate diuresis); cardiac causes (hypoxia, hypoglycaemia, L to R shunts, valve disease, coarctation). *Signs:* Pulse ↑; BP ↓; urine output ↓; coma. *Management:* ABC. Ventilate as needed. Treat causes. Aim for a CVP of 5-8cm-H₂O. Give colloid 10-20mL/kg IV as needed. Inotropes may be used, eg **dopamine** 3-20µg/kg per min[4] ± **dobutamine** 5-20µg/kg/min as needed[105] (*may* act synergistically; detailed dosing: p203). There is scant experimental evidence for this regimen, and there may be side effects (blunting of respiratory drive; endocrine/immunological impairment; GI function↓).[106] Milrinone: see BNFc If the pH is <7.2, **sodium bicarbonate**, eg 1-2mmol/kg IV as a 4.2% solution, may be indicated (if adequate ventilation; don't mix with inotropes).

Problems with neonatal sepsis

Diagnosis is often hard, as signs may be non-specific, and cultures take time—and time is never on your side. ►Sepsis is always in the differential diagnosis of any unwell neonate.

Non-specific and probably unreliable tests: C-reactive protein, FBC and film: looking at the ratio of immature to total neutrophils *may* help.

NB: it's possible that looking for soluble immunological mediators may help: ideal ones may be interleukin-1 receptor antagonist (IL-1ra), and interleukin-6 (IL-6). Specificity: 92% and 83%, respectively. Circulating intercellular adhesion molecule-1 (cICAM-1) is less reliable.[107]

Definitive cultures of blood*et al* take ~48-72h.

12 predictive signs for severe illness if <1 week old:
• Seizures[15]
• Stiff limbs[15]
• Cyanosis[13]
• Capillary refill ≥3sec[10]
• Difficulty feeding[10]
• Severe chest indrawing[9]
• T° ≤35.5°[9]
• Movement only when stimulated[7]
• Respiratory rate ≥60[3]
• Lethargy[3]
• Grunting[3]
• T° ≥37.5°[3]
A rule requiring any one sign has high sensitivity (87%) and specificity (74%). The number in blue refers to the odds ratio.[108]

Normal values are often hard to define, eg a CSF WCC of up to 10/mm³ with 60% polymorphs may be normal in neonates.

Changing patterns of antibiotic resistance Ampicillin/amoxicillin and gentamicin is a safe combination for most neonates. This duo may reduce over-use of **vancomycin**.[109–112]

Drug pharmacokinetic problems These are only partly obviated by doing plasma levels. Creatinine, sex, and birthweight influence what is an acceptable level in complex ways. With aminoglycosides, adjust dose as indicated in the *Data sheet* if renal function is poor. If doing levels is problematic, **cefotaxime** is a good alternative (p202).[113] **Gentamicin:** see p175.

Subtle manifestations of neonatal seizures

Unless you have a high index of suspicion, you may miss seizures referable to the brainstem, eg nystagmus, conjugate eye movements, posturing, sucking movements, lip smacking, etc. Grand mal is rare. EEGs are helpful in diagnosing when unsure. Always look for metabolic abnormalities (these are treated with metabolic approaches; don't rely on conventional anticonvulsants).[114]

Paediatrics

The aim is to screen for abnormality, and to see if the mother has any questions or difficulties. The following is a recommended routine before the baby leaves hospital—or during the 1st week of life for home deliveries. Before the examination find out if the birthweight was normal. Was the birth and pregnancy normal? Is mother Rh-ve? Find a quiet, warm, well-lit room. Enlist the mother's help. Explain your aims. Does she look angry or depressed? Listen if she talks. Examine systematically, eg head-to-toe. Wash your hands meticulously. Note observations (eg τ°; rectal is more reliable than tympanic).[115,166]

Head Circumference (50th centile=35cm, p224), shape (odd shapes from a difficult labour soon resolve), fontanelles (tense if crying or intracranial pressure↑; sunken if dehydrated). *Eyes:* Red reflex (absent in cataract & retinoblastoma); corneal opacities; conjunctivitis. *Ears:* Shape; position. Are they low set (ie below eyes)? The tip of the nose, when pressed, shows jaundice in white babies. Breathing out of the nose (shut the mouth) tests for choanal atresia. Ensure oto-acoustic screening is done (p548). Are follow-up brainstem evoked responses needed?[117] *Complexion:* Cyanosed, pale, jaundiced, or ruddy (polycythaemia)? *Mouth:* Look inside; insert a finger: is the palate intact? Is suck good? Does the baby's face look normal? Dysmorphism can be difficult to detect soon after birth as the baby may have some puffiness in the face.

Arms & hands Single palmar creases (normal or Down's). Waiter's (porter's) tip sign of Erb's palsy of C5 & 6 trunks (p77; p766). Number of fingers. Clinodactyly (5th finger is curved towards the ring finger, eg in Down's).

Thorax Watch respirations; note grunting and intercostal recession (respiratory distress). Palpate the precordium and apex beat. Listen to the heart and lungs. Inspect the vertebral column for neural tube defects.

Abdomen Expect to feel the liver. Any other masses? Inspect the umbilicus. Is it healthy? Flare suggests sepsis. Next, lift the skin to assess skin turgor. Inspect genitalia and anus. Are the orifices patent? Ensure in the 1st 24 hours the baby passes urine (consider posterior urethral valves in boys if not) and stool (consider Hirschprung's, cystic fibrosis, hypothyroidism). Is the urinary meatus misplaced (hypospadias), and are both testes descended? The neonatal clitoris often looks rather large, but if very large, consider CAH, p134. Bleeding PV may be a normal variant following maternal oestrogen withdrawal.

Legs Test for congenital dislocation of the hip (p684). Avoid repeated tests as it hurts, and may induce dislocation. Can you feel femoral pulses (to 'exclude' coarctation)? Note talipes (p684). Toes: too many, too few, or too blue?

Buttocks/sacrum Is there an anus? Are there 'mongolian spots'? (blue—and harmless). Tufts of hair ± dimples suggest bifida occulta? Any pilonidal sinus?

CNS Assess posture and handle the baby. Intuition can be most helpful in deciding if the baby is ill or well. Is he jittery (hypoxia/ischaemia, encephalopathy, hypoglycaemia, infection, hypocalcaemia)? There should be some control of the head. Do limbs move normally. Is the tone floppy[2] or spastic? Are responses absent on one side (hemiplegia)? The Moro reflex rarely adds important information (and is uncomfortable for the baby). It is done by sitting the baby at 45°, supporting the head. On momentarily removing the support the arms will abduct, the hands open and then the arms adduct. Stroke the palm to elicit a grasp reflex. Is the baby post-mature, light-for-dates, or premature (p128)?

▶Discuss any abnormality with the parents *after liaising with a senior doctor.*

---

1 The neonatal period is the 1st 28 days of life; if prem, 44 completed weeks of the infant's conceptional age (=the chronological age plus gestational age at birth).[118]
2 Causes of floppiness: Sepsis; hypoglycaemia; dehydration; hypothermia; trauma/abuse; myopathy; poor nutrition; botulism (may look like near sudden infant death syndrome)[119]; maternal drugs (lorazepam; clozapine); alcohol withdrawal; rickets; Down's, Ehlers-Danlos, or Prader-Willi syndromes; cerebral palsy; CNS syndromes—eg muscular dystrophy, myasthenia, Zellweger leukodystrophy, Guillain-Barré—or myotonic dystrophy (shake hands with the mother: she may have delayed release of grip).[120]

Neonatal jaundice is common, occurring in 60% of neonates.[121] Most do not need any treatment. Jaundice is caused by raised bilirubin levels. When severe, or not properly managed, kernicterus, a permanent form of brain damage, may occur. Transcutaneous bilirubin levels measured by midwives in homes may prevent kernicterus in babies discharged early by allowing early detection of jaundice. In non-Caucasians, the device needs recalibration: don't rely on tests such as pressing the nose.[122] Management of severe neonatal jaundice typically involves phototherapy, and exchange transfusion if very severe. The threshold levels for these treatments varies with gestational age, and postnatal age. (see NICE GUIDELINES at www.nice.org.uk/cg98)

Hyperbilirubinaemia (<200µmol/L) after 24h is usually 'physiological':
1 Increased bilirubin production in neonates due to shorter RBC lifespan.
2 Decreased bilirubin conjugation due to hepatic immaturity.
3 Absence of gut flora impedes elimination of bile pigment.
   Exclusive breastfeeding (esp. if there are feeding difficulties→↓intake→dehydration→↓bilirubin elimination + ↑enterohepatic circulation of bilirubin—not *usually* a reason to stop[123]).

Visible jaundice within 24h of birth is always abnormal. *Causes:* ►Sepsis or:
• *Rhesus haemolytic disease:* +ve direct Coombs test (DCT, p117).
• *ABO incompatibility:* (mother O; baby A or B, or mother A and baby B, or vice versa) DCT +ve in 4%; indirect Coombs +ve in 8%. Maternal IgG anti-A or anti-B haemolysin is 'always' present.[124]
• *Red cell anomalies:* congenital spherocytosis (fragility tests/EMA binding, p196); glucose-6-phosphate dehydrogenase deficiency (do enzyme test).[125]

Tests: FBC; film; blood groups (eg rare group incompatibility.); Coombs test; urine for reducing agents; syphilis/TORCH[et al] screen, p34.[126]

Prolonged jaundice (not fading after 14 days) *Causes:* breastfeeding; sepsis (UTI & TORCH, p34); hypothyroidism; cystic fibrosis; biliary atresia if conjugated and pale stools. *Galactosaemia:* urine tests for reducing agents (eg Clinitest®) are +ve, but specific tests (Clinistix®) for glycosuria are –ve (an insensitive test; galactose-1-phosphate uradyl transferase levels diagnostic).

Kernicterus refers to the clinical features of acute bilirubin encephalopathy (ABE): lethargy/poor feeding/hypertonicity/opisthotonus/shrill cry—and chronic bilirubin encephalopathy, as well as the yellow staining in the brain associated with ABE. Risk is increased with extremely high bilirubin levels (360µmol/L (lower in prems)). Long-term sequelae include athetoid movements, deafness, and ↓IQ. It is prevented by phototherapy (below) ± exchange transfusion.[127]

Phototherapy uses light energy to convert bilirubin to soluble products (lumirubin and other isomers) that can be excreted without conjugation. This occurs most efficiently when blue light with a wavelength of ~460nm is used.[128] Efficacy depends on irradiance (measured in µW/cm²)—so exposing baby will lead to more rapid reduction in serum bilirubin, as will using light from above and below. SE: T°↑↓; eye damage (baby will need eye protection); diarrhoea; separation from mother; fluid loss. *Intense phototherapy* is an adjunct to exchange transfusion.[129,130] To decide when to start phototherapy/exchange transfusion use NICE guidelines(www.nice.org.uk/cg98), or your unit's protocol.

Exchange transfusion Uses warmed blood (37°C), 160ml/kg (double volume), given ideally via umbilical vein IVI, with removal via umbilical artery. Monitor ECG, U&E, Ca²⁺, bilirubin, clotting, FBC, and glucose. Consider more exchanges if bilirubin goes on rising. *Stop* if the pulse rate fluctuates by >20 beats/min. ►*Ensure the volumes exchanged always balance.* If anaemic, consider a simple fresh blood transfusion (20mL/kg). *Complications* (may be fatal): Pulse↓, apnoea, platelets↓, glucose↓, Na⁺↓,[131] O₂ Hb saturation↓ (as fetal Hb↓).[132]

Physiology When a RhD−ve mother delivers a RhD+ve baby a leak of fetal red cells into her circulation may stimulate her to produce anti-D IgG antibodies (isoimmunization). In later pregnancies these can cross the placenta, causing worsening rhesus haemolytic disease (*erythroblastosis fetalis*) with each successive Rh+ve pregnancy. First pregnancies may be affected due to leaks, eg: • Threatened miscarriage • APH • Mild trauma • Amniocentesis • Chorionic villous sampling • External cephalic version.

An affected oedematous fetus (with stiff, oedematous lungs) is called a *hydrops fetalis*. Anaemia-associated CCF causes oedema, as does hypoalbuminaemia (the liver is preoccupied by producing new RBCs). ΔΔ: Thalassaemia; infection (eg toxoplasmosis, CMV, p34); maternal diabetes.

Clinical Rh disease ▸ *Test for D antibodies in all Rh-ve mothers, at booking, 28 & 34 weeks' gestation.* Anti-D titres <4u/mL (<1:16) are very unlikely to cause serious disease; it is wise to check maternal blood every 2 weeks. If >10u/mL, get the advice of a referral centre: fetal blood sampling ± intraperitoneal (or, with fetoscopy, intravascular via the cord) transfusion may be needed.

Signs
• Jaundice—eg on day 1
• Yellow vernix
• CCF (oedema, ascites)
• Hepatosplenomegaly
• Progressive anaemia
• Bleeding
• CNS signs
• Kernicterus (p115)

Expect fetal Hb to be <7g/dL in 10% of those with titres of 10–100u/mL (75% if titres >100u/mL).

Do regular ultrasound (+amniocentesis if anti-D titre >4u/mL). Timing is vital. Do it 10 weeks before a Rh-related event in the last pregnancy (eg if last baby needed delivery at 36 weeks, expect to do amniocentesis at 26 weeks). Fetuses tolerating high bilirubins may be saved risky transfusions (fatality 2–30%) if monitored by serial measurements of fetal Hb (by fetoscopy or non-invasive middle cerebral artery peak velocity) and daily ultrasound to detect oedema, cardiomegaly, pericardial effusion, hepatosplenomegaly, or ascites.[133]

Anti-D is the chief antibody. Others: Rh C, E, c, e, Kell, Kidd, Duffy (all are IgG). Low concentrations sometimes produce severe disease.

Prognosis is improving. Mortality is <20% even for hydropic babies. Note that maternal antibodies persist for some months, and continue to cause haemolysis during early life.[134]

Exchange transfusion *Indications/technique:* If Hb <7g/dL, give 1st volume of the exchange transfusion (80mL/kg) as packed cells, and subsequent exact exchanges according to response. ▸ *Keep the baby warm.*

Ultraviolet photodegradation of bilirubin (with phototherapy lamp) may be all that is needed in less than severe disease. Give extra water (30mL/kg/24h PO). Avoid heat loss. Protect the eyes. Keep the baby naked.

Giving Rh-ve mothers anti-D immunoglobulin (p9) This strategy has markedly reduced need for exchange transfusion (cost per QALY ≈£11,000–52,000, see *OHCM* p12).[135,136]

ABO incompatibility 1 in 45 of group A or B babies born to group O mothers will have haemolysis from maternal antibodies. Exchange transfusion may be needed, even in first-borns.

Paediatrics

Hydrops fetalis: management

- Get expert help.
- At birth, take cord blood for Hb, PCV, bilirubin (conjugated and unconjugated), blood group, Coombs test,[1] serum protein, LFT, and infection screen (p112) to find the cause—eg isoimmunization; thalassaemia; infection (eg toxoplasmosis, syphilis, parvoviruses, CMV p34); maternal diabetes; twin-twin transfusion; hypoproteinaemia.
- Expect to need to ventilate with high inspiratory peak pressure and positive end pressure. HFOV may have a role, p110.◆✷
- Monitor plasma glucose 2–4-hourly, treating any hypoglycaemia.
- Drain ascites and pleural effusions if severe.
- Correct anaemia.
- Vitamin K 1mg IM, to reduce risk of haemorrhage.
- If CCF is present, **furosemide** may be needed, eg 1–2mg/kg/12h IV.
- Limit IV fluids to 60mL/kg/24h (crystalloid); if exchange transfusing, aim for a deficit of 10–20mL/kg. Monitor urine output.
- Prognosis: 90% of those with non-immune hydrops die *in utero*; 50% die postnatally. Babies with non-immune hydrops not secondary to infection have a good neurological outcome.[137]

Biliary atresia

Incidence 1:17,000. This is rare but serious. Apparently healthy term babies have jaundice, yellow urine and pale stools due to biliary tree occlusion by angiopathy at around week 3 of life. The spleen becomes palpable after the 3rd or 4th week—the liver may become hard and enlarged. Early surgery (Kasai procedure = hepatoportoenterostomy—the extrahepatic biliary tree is identified, a cholangiogram performed to check diagnosis, and an intestinal limb (Roux-en-Y) is attached to drain bile from the porta hepatis) has a good chance of restoring flow of bile to bowel eg in 60%, but if presenting for operation late (eg at 100 days) Kasai procedure is unlikely to be successful due to advanced liver damage and cirrhosis; and the baby will likely need liver transplant in 1st year of life. It can occur in premature babies. 20% have associated cardiac malformations: polysplenia and situs inversus. Babies may be excessively hungry. Refer all term babies jaundiced at 1 week (preterm at 3) for conjugated/unconjugated bilirubia. Breast milk jaundice has ↑ unconjugated bilirubin. Conjugated bilirubin >25 may reflect serious liver disease (<20 µmol is normal). Ultrasound may help with diagnosis. Percutaneous liver biopsy may show bile duct proliferation and bile plugs. Babies suspected of biliary atresia should be assessed in a liver unit.

Paediatrics

---

1 The direct Coombs test (DCT) identifies red cells coated with antibody or complement and a positive result usually indicates an immune cause of haemolysis (OHCM p330).

RDS is due to a deficiency of alveolar surfactant, which is mainly confined to premature babies. Insufficient surfactant leads to alveolar collapse; re-inflation with each breath exhausts the baby, and respiratory failure follows. Hypoxia leads to ↓cardiac output, hypotension, acidosis and renal failure. It is the major cause of death from prematurity. *Infants at risk:* 91% if 23–25 weeks; 52% if 30–31 weeks.[132] Also: maternal diabetes, males, 2nd twin, caesareans.

Signs Respiratory distress shortly after birth (1st 4h)—tachypnoea (>60/min), grunting, nasal flaring, intercostal recession and cyanosis. CXR: diffuse granular patterns (ground glass appearance) ± air bronchograms.

Differential diagnosis *Transient tachypnoea of the newborn (TTN)* is due to excess lung fluid. It usually resolves after 24h. *Meconium aspiration* (p120); congenital pneumonia (group B strep); tracheo-oesophageal fistula (suspect if respiratory problems after feeds); congenital lung abnormality; sepsis.

Prevention Betamethasone or dexamethasone should be offered to all women at risk of preterm delivery from 23–35 weeks (p51); mothers at high risk should be transferred to perinatal centres with experience in managing RDS.

Treatment[132] Learn at the cot side. Delay clamping of cord by 3 min (p51) to promote placento–fetal transfusion. Give oxygen via an oxygen–air blender, using lowest concentration of O_2 possible provided there is an adequate heart rate response. If spontaneously breathing stabilize with CPAP (5–6cm H_2O). Babies at high risk of RDS should get natural surfactant (reduces mortality and air leaks). If gestation ≤26wks, intubate and give prophylactic surfactant via ET tube ± 2 further doses if ongoing O_2 demand/ventilation requirement. Rock gently to aid spread in the bronchial tree. Monitor O_2, as needs may suddenly↓.[139] Aim for sats between 85–93% to reduce risk of retinopathy of prematurity and bronchopulmonary dysplasia.[132] Some centres give a dose of surfactant then extubate pending developments; others keep the baby intubated and extubate as tolerated.

• Wrap up warmly and take to NICU/SCBU incubator.
• If blood gases worsen, intubate and support ventilation (p110), *before* fatigue sets in. ↑P_aCO_2 suggests that the minute volume is too low.
• *Traditional ventilator settings:* (p110) On connecting the endotracheal tube, check chest movement is adequate and symmetrical. Listen for breath sounds. P_aO_2 is increased by ↑mean pressure (not too high). P_aCO_2 is decreased by ↑minute volume (↑ breath frequency) by lessening expiratory time. One option is *high-frequency oscillatory ventilation (HFOV)*. Ask a senior colleague for advice.[140,141]
• ▶If any deterioration, consider: blocked or dislodged tube (a common occurrence), infection, faulty ventilator, or pneumothorax.
Fluids: Give 10% glucose IVI (p123). *Nutrition:* Get help. Inositol is an essential nutrient promoting surfactant maturation and plays a vital role in neonatal life. Supplementing nutrition of prems with inositol reduces complications (IVH, p108; bronchopulmonary dysplasia, p119).[142] Full parenteral nutrition can be started on day 1. *Minimal* enteral feeding can also be started on day 1.[132]

Signs of a poor prognosis Persistent pulmonary hypertension, large right to left shunt via the ductus; ↑dead-space fraction in lungs.[143]

☼If, despite everything, hypoxia worsens, the baby is dying. Confer with your senior. Explain what is happening to the parents, and that the baby will feel no pain. Encourage christening, or what is congruent with parents' beliefs. Relieve pain (p172); keep the baby comfortable. In the light of dialogue with parents and nurses it may be appropriate to disconnect the tubes, so allowing the parents to hold the baby, and, in so doing, to aid their grief. NB: contact your Trust's head and defence organization if legal issues beckon.[144]

Communicating with parents

Take time to explain to parents exactly what is happening to their baby—not just for the respiratory distress syndrome, but for *any* serious diseases. Structured, tested interviews yield these guidelines:[145]

• Ask both parents to be present (plus a nurse whom they trust).
• Hand your bleep to a colleague. Allow time. Call the parents by name.
• Look at the parents (mutual gaze promotes trust).
• Name the illness concerned with its complications. Write it down.
• Give support group details: www.cafamily.org.uk tel: 020 7240 0671 for a list.
• Elicit what the parents now know. Clarify or repeat as needed.
• Answer any questions. Arrange follow-up (<50% may be remembered).

Doctors' decisions are increasingly being questioned by parents. If you and your team are sure your actions are in the child's best interests, and the parents take a different view, take any steps you can to resolve the issue in a non-confrontational way. Violent fights between doctors and parents endanger other children (some UK units have had to be evacuated while police are called). You should know emergency procedures for contacting the High Court to settle the issue (go through the on-call manager: your Trust can make applications day or night). Failure to get Court approval will leave you open to criticism from the European Court of Human Rights, which is likely to take the view that 'do not resuscitate' notices fail to guarantee respect for the child's 'physical and moral integrity'—guaranteed by Article 8 of the Convention on Human rights—see Glass *vs* United Kingdom, 2004 (61827/00).[146]

Bronchopulmonary dysplasia (BPD)

This complicates ventilation for RDS in 40% of babies of <1kg birthweight.[147] There is persistent hypoxia ± difficult ventilator weaning—eg still requiring ventilation at 36 weeks postmenstrual age (eg S_aO_2 ≤88% in air). Classically, BPD is mainly from barotrauma and oxygen toxicity, whereas surfactant-related BPD is multifactorial with airway infections triggering inflammatory cascades. (Without surfactant, many would not survive to get BPD.)[148] Oxidative processes may also play a key role, but antioxidants are unproven.[149]

Tests: CXR: hyperinflation, rounded, radiolucent areas, alternating with thin denser lines. *Histology:* necrotizing bronchiolitis with alveolar fibrosis.

Mortality: Variable, ∴ complex interaction with surfactant use.[150]

Early sequelae: ↓IQ; cerebral palsy; feeding problems. O_2 desaturation during feeds is not uncommon. Visuospatial abilities at age 5½yrs are only reduced in those with the severest forms of chronic lung disease.[151]

Late sequelae: By adolescence/early adulthood the main changes remaining are airways obstruction, airways hyper-reactivity, and hyperinflation.

Prevention: Steroids (antenatal & postnatal); surfactant and 'suitably high' calorie feeding.[152]

Pulmonary hypoplasia

Suspect this in all infants with persisting neonatal tachypnoea ± feeding difficulties, particularly if prenatal oligohydramnios. Hypoplasia may be a consequence of oligohydramnios, eg in Potter's syndrome or premature rupture of the membranes. In diaphragmatic hernia it is a consequence of the 'space-occupying lesion'. Cystic adenomatoid malformations are another cause. CXR is likely to be misleadingly reported as normal. The condition need not be fatal: postnatal catch-up growth occurs.

Differential: RDS, meconium aspiration, sepsis, or primary pulmonary hypertension.[153] Some degree of pulmonary hypoplasia is the price of adopting an expectant plan for early spontaneous rupture of the membranes, but despite this, expectant management leads to fewer deaths.[154]

Necrotizing enterocolitis (NEC) is an inflammatory bowel necrosis. Pre-maturity is the chief risk factor: if weight <1500g, 5–10% develop NEC. Other risk factors: enteral feeds, bacterial colonization, mucosal injury, rapid weight gain.[155] *Signs:* If mild, just some abdominal distension. A little blood/mucus may be passed PR. If severe, there is sudden abdominal distension, tenderness (± perforation), shock, DIC & mucosal sloughing. Pneumatosis intestinalis (gas in the gut wall seen on x-ray) is pathognomonic for NEC. *R:* Stop oral feeding[156] (except oral probiotics, eg *Bifidobacteria infantis*, which can help);[157] barrier nurse; culture faeces; crossmatch (may get anaemic); give antibiotics: eg ce-fotaxime + vancomycin.[158] Liaise with surgeon; repeated imaging and girth measurement. Platelets mirror disease activity; <100×10⁹/L is 'severe'.[159]
Laparotomy indications: Progressive distension, perforation (up to 50% die).
Prophylaxis: Expressed breast milk; probiotics;[160] oral antibiotics.[16] NNT≈10.

Meconium aspiration syndrome (MAS) occurs in the term/near term in-fant when meconium, the faecal material that accumulates in the fetal colon during gestation, is passed *in utero*, leading to meconium stained amniotic fluid (MSAF). MSAF occurs in ~8–25% of births, usually due to fetal distress or advance fetal age. MAS occurs in only 5% of these infants;[162] it is defined as respiratory distress in the infant born through MSAF which cannot otherwise be explained. Aspiration of meconium mostly occurs pre-birth.[163] It may lead to airway obstruction, surfactant dysfunction, pulmonary vasoconstriction, infection and chemical pneumonitis. Intrapartum suctioning of the oro/naso-pharynx is not recommended.[164] Endotracheal suctioning is only needed for those infants who aren't vigorous at birth.[164] Cricoid and/or chest compression at birth to prevent aspiration have not been shown to be useful.[165] Surfactant, ventilation, inhaled nitric oxide and antibiotics are all used.[166]

Vitamin K deficiency bleeding (VKDB=haemorrhagic disease of the newborn) occurs from days 2–7 postpartum. *Cause:* No enteric bacteria to make vit K. The baby is usually well, apart from bruising/bleeding. Prothrombin & partial throm-boplastin times (PT & PTT)↑; platelets ↔. *Prevention:* (Many regimens) vit K 1mg (0.4mg/kg if prem) IM (if at ↑risk¹)—or 2 doses of oral colloidal (mixed micelle) phytomenadione 2mg at birth, repeated in ≤7d; if breastfed, give a 3ʳᵈ dose at 1 month old; not needed if bottle-fed (already fortified). NB: a weak correlation[167] with cancers caused a scare, but there is no hard evidence. *R:* Plasma, 10mL/kg IV & vit K (≤1mg slow IV) for active bleeding (monitor coagulation).[168]

Disseminated intravascular coagulation (DIC) *Signs:* Septic signs (ill); pete-chiae; venepuncture oozings; GI bleeding. *Tests:* Platelets↓; schistocytes (frag-mented RBCs); INR↑; fibrinogen↓; partial thromboplastin time↑; D-dimer↑ (hard to interpret if birthweight low).[169,170] *Treatment:* Get help; treat cause (eg NEC, sepsis *etc*); give vit. K ≤1mg slow IV± platelet transfusion (aim for >30×10⁹/L).
• Fresh plasma±cryoprecipitate,[1] 10mL/kg IV↑ ± heparin IV ± protein C.[171,172]
• If bleeding still continues, consider exchange transfusion.

Autoimmune thrombocytopenia (ITP) <10% of babies of women with ITP are thrombocytopenic (p88). *Alloimmune thrombocytopenia* (1:2000 births; via fetomaternal incompatibility of platelet antigens). It develops *in utero*. 50% are 1ˢᵗ born (it recurs in ~80% of later pregnancies with same or ↑severity). If affected *in utero* 25% have CNS problems. Platelets fall for 48h post-delivery. Treat severe thrombocytopenia with *compatible platelets* or *irradiated mater-nal platelets*. IV Ig 400mg/kg/day[6] for 48h and steroids may help. *Platelet transfusion via cordocentesis* from 24wks may be needed in later pregnan-cies. Diagnose by detecting *maternal platelet allo-antibody* against father's platelets. Do *neuroimaging* on all patients.[173]

---

1 Asphyxia, bleeding problems, cholestasis—or mother with liver disease or on carbamazepine, pheno-barbital, phenytoin, rifampicin, or warfarin.

Minor neonatal problems

Most neonates have a few minor lesions; the more you examine neonates the better you will become at reassuring mothers.[174]

Strawberry naevus: Typically disappear by age 2.

Milia: 1–2mm pearly white/cream papules caused by retention of keratin in dermis. Found on forehead, nose, cheeks. Will resolve spontaneously.

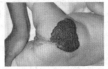

Fig 1. Strawberry naevus.

Erythema toxicum (neonatal urticaria): These are harmless red blotches, often with a central white pustule which come and go in crops. Described as 'flea bitten' in appearance. They last ~24h, in contrast to septic spots which are smaller and not mobile. *Miliaria crystallina* (a prickly-heat like-rash) develops due to transient sweat-pore disruption[175] or immaturity[176]—hence its characteristic 1–2mm retention vesicle.[177] Prevalence: ≤8%.[178] In *miliaria rubra* there is a surrounding flush.

Stork mark: These are areas of capillary dilatation on the eyelids, central forehead and back of the neck—where the baby is deemed to have been held in the stork's beak. They blanch on pressure and fade with time.

Harlequin colour change: Transient, episodic, demarcated erythema on left or right, with simultaneous contralateral blanching—occasionally related to use of systemic prostaglandin E1 (no need to stop: the condition is self-limiting).[179]

Peeling skin/desquamation: Common in postmature babies, it does not denote future skin problems. Olive oil prevents skin folds from cracking.

Petechial haemorrhages, facial cyanosis, subconjunctival haemorrhages: These temporary features generally reflect suffusion of the face during delivery (sometimes inaccurately referred to as 'traumatic asphyxia').

Swollen breasts: These occur in both sexes and occasionally lactate (witch's milk). They are due to maternal hormones and gradually subside if left alone, but if infected need antibiotics. Milk may persist until 2 months old.[180]

The umbilicus: It dries and separates through a moist base at about day 7. Signs of infection: odour, pus, periumbilical red flare, malaise. Isolate the baby, take swabs and blood cultures, give antibiotics. Granuloma: exclude a patent urachus and cauterize with a silver nitrate stick.

Sticky eye: (commonly from an unopened tear duct, p418.) Swab to exclude *ophthalmia neonatorum* (p36)/chlamydia (special swab). When vertically transmitted sexual infections occur, liaise with your microbiologist and local genitourinary medicine (GUM) clinic.[181]

Feeding anxieties: Healthy term babies require little milk for the first few days and early poor feeding is not an indication for investigation or bottle top-ups. The exceptions are babies of diabetic mothers, and light-for-dates babies, because of their risk of hypoglycaemia.

New babies may have difficulty co-ordinating feeding and breathing, and briefly choke, gag, or turn blue. Exclude disease, check feeding technique (too much? too fast?) and reassure.

Regurgitation is often due to overfilling a tiny stomach with milk and air. Check feeding technique; if bottle fed, is the teat too big for the mouth or the hole too small or the amount too great?

Winding during feeds may help but is not essential to health.

Red-stained nappy: This is usually due to urinary urates but may be blood from the cord or baby's vagina (oestrogen withdrawal bleed).

Neonatal sneezing clears nasal amniotic fluid.[182] If jittery ± T°t/ muscle hypertonia, suspect fluoxetine or opiate withdrawal.[182,183] RSV (p160) is another cause.

Paediatrics

Breastfeeding (± expressed breast milk, p124–6) is the ideal way to feed term babies; if <2kg, powder sachets of breast milk fortifiers (eg Cow & Gate) have a role. In prems, extrauterine growth restriction and neurodevelopmental delay from under-feeding is only partly preventable by oral/tube feeding—owing to fear of necrotizing enterocolitis.[1] Parenteral nutrition can meet many of their nutritional needs, but has significant side effects—intestinal atrophy, sepsis, increased susceptibility to inflammatory stimuli, and systemic inflammatory responses.[184]

Nasogastric tube feeding *Indications:* Any sick infant who is too ill or too young to feed normally (eg respiratory distress syndrome). Expressed breast milk or formula milk is fed via a naso- or orogastric tube either as a bolus or as a continuous infusion. If gastro-oesophageal reflux or aspiration is a problem, then a silastic naso-jejunal tube can be used. After entering the stomach, the tube enters the jejunum by peristalsis: confirm its position on x-ray. When the baby improves, start giving some feeds by mouth (PO), eg by increasing the ratio of oral to nasogastric feeds, either in whole feeds, or by fractions of each feed. If during oral feeds, cyanosis, bradycardia, or vomiting supervene, you may be trying too soon.

Trophic feeding *Synonyms:* Minimal enteral or hypocaloric feeding; gut priming.

Rationale: If prems go for weeks with no oral nutrition, normal GI structure and function are lost despite an anabolic body state. Villi shorten, mucosal DNA is lost, and enzyme activity is less. Early initiation of subnutritional enteral feeding may help by promoting gut motility and bile secretion, inducing lactase activity, and by reducing sepsis and cholestatic jaundice.[185]

Technique: Typically, milk volumes of ~1mL/kg/h are given by tube starting on day 2–3. Use expressed breast milk (or a preterm formula, eg Nutriprem®).

Effects: Studies show that weight gain and head growth is better, and that there are fewer episodes of neonatal sepsis, fewer days of parenteral nutrition are needed, and time to full oral feeding is less. If too much is given, NEC (p120) may ensue.[186]

Eligibility: Experience shows that almost all prems with non-surgical illness tolerate at least some milk as trophic feeds.[187]

Parenteral nutrition (PN, via a central vein). Indications: post-op; trauma; burns; if oral nutrition is poor (eg in ill, low-birthweight babies) and necrotizing enterocolitis (when the gut must be 'rested'). *Day-by-day guide:* see BOX. ▶*Sterility is vital*; prepare using laminar flow units. Monitoring must be meticulous.[2]

Daily checks: Weight; fluid balance; U&E; blood glucose; Ca²⁺. Test for glycosuria. Change IVI sets/filters; culture filters, Vamin®, and Intralipid® samples.

Weekly: Length; head circumference; skinfold thickness. LFT; Mg²⁺; PO₄³⁻; alk phos; ammonia; triglycerides; FBC; ESR/CRP (helps determine if there is sepsis).

Complications: Infection; acidosis; metabolic imbalances; thrombophlebitis; hepatobiliary stenosis; cholelithiasis; osteopenia.[188] If plasma PO₄³⁻↓, consider giving PO₄³⁻ (1mmol/kg/day for neonates, 0.7mg/kg/day if 1–24 months old) as the potassium salt. Mix with glucose, but not Vamin® or trace element mixtures. PN is complex: get expert help. In addition, some precipitation errors are preventable by using computer-based decision support.[189]

Stopping IV nutrition Do in stages to prevent hypoglycaemia.

---

1 *What is it about NEC which makes oral feeding problematic?* Relevant factors: •Ischaemia •Introduction of novel metabolic substrate into the gut •Gut maturation •Inflammation—proinflammatory cytokines (tumour necrosis factor-α, interleukin IL-6, IL-18, and platelet-activating factor) •Paucity of protective Gram +ve organisms. ▶The best way of providing protective bacteria with feeds is unknown.[190]
2 See British Association for Parenteral and Enteral Nutrition *Guidelines*, ISBN 1-899467-408

Fig 1. 'Gavage' (from an old French word meaning 'to gorge') denotes a controversial farming and gastronomic method entailing insertion of a long funnel into a goose's throat. Down this funnel is pumped a slurry of ground corn and water, to produce obesity—and, to some palates, a delicious (if unnaturally fatty) pâté—*pâté de foie gras*. On the neonatal unit, gavage feeding should not be quite so enthusiastic. But French farmers were right about one thing: *bolus* gavage feeding is better than *continuous* tube feeds, at least with regard to trophic feeding.[191]

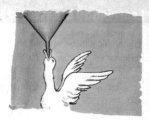

Type of baby	Day of PN	Age days	PROTEIN Vaminolact®; mL	CARBOHYDRATE Glucose 10%; mL	FAT Intralipidy® 20%; mL	Na	K	Ca	PO₄	FLUID PN vol. mL¹
Neonates & low-birth-weight babies	1	3	~14	97.5	2.5	3	3	1	0.4-1	120
	2	4	~20	115	5	3	3	1	0.4-1	150
	3	5	~26	115	10	3	3	1	0.4-1	165
	M	>5	≤35	100	15	3	3	1	0.4-1	165
Infants >1 month¹ & <10kg	1		~12	95-125	5	2.5	2.5	0.6	0.4	120-150*
	2		~18	80-110	10	2.5	2.5	0.6	0.4	120-150*
	M		~24	65-125	15	2.5	2.5	0.6	0.4	120-150*
10-30kg	1&2		~8	23.5-78.5	7.5	2	2	0.2	0.1	45-100*
	M		16-18	7-57	10-15	2	2	0.2	0.1	45-100*
>30kg	1&2		14-10	26-56	5	1.5-2	1.5-2	0.2	0.1	45-75*
	M		14.5	14-51.5	10-12.5	1.5-2	1.5-2	0.2	0.1	45-75*

Parenteral nutrition: day-by-day guide. ▶All values are per kg/day

The IONS (mmol) columns above are Na, K, Ca, PO₄.

Note: M=maintenance. *See p234 for 24h fluid requirement. ▶See datasheets/SPC data

Trace elements: Peditrace® eg 1mL/kg (max 10mL) if renal function OK—caution if prolonged treatment, eg >1 month, or if ↓biliary excretion (stop if cholestasis); checking Mn⁺ may be needed. *Vitamins:* Solivito N®: add 1mL/kg/day (max 10mL) to Vaminolact® (protect from light). Cater for A, D, & K with Vitalip N® 1-4mL/kg/day (max 10mL/kg/day) to Intralipid®. ▶These values are a guide only. *Individual needs vary greatly.* Supplementing very preterm infants with selenium is controversial. It may help reduce sepsis; data are dominated by one large trial from areas with low selenium levels and may not be readily translated elsewhere.[192] Get expert help.

1 This is the total volume of fluid required (60 & 90mL/kg for days 1 & 2).

It is better to be apprenticed antenatally to a breastfeeding mother than to rely on simple encouragement and leaflets.[193]

Reflexes Rooting (searching, with wide-open mouth)→suckling (jaw goes up and down while the tongue compresses the areola against the palate)→swallowing reflex (as milk hits the oropharynx, the soft palate rises and shuts off the nasopharynx; the larynx rises, and the epiglottis falls, closing the trachea).

Skill Don't assume this comes naturally; commonly, learning to breastfeed is as hard as learning to drive—and as anxiety-provoking. The best way to learn is from an experienced person in comfortable surroundings—eg sitting in an upright chair, rather than inadequately propped up in bed. Reassure that a few problematic feeds do not mean that the baby will starve, and that bottle feeding is needed. *Most term babies have plenty of fuel reserves* (earthquake infant-victims may survive for >1 week)—and perseverance will almost always be rewarded. Furthermore, 'top-up' bottle feeds may undermine confidence, and, by altering the GI milieu, diminish the benefits of breastfeeding.

A good time to start breastfeeding is just after birth (good bonding; PPH risk↓), but labour procedures may make this hard, eg intrapartum pethidine ± instrumental delivery, T° and BP measurements, washing, weighing, going to a postnatal ward. ▶*It is never too late to put to the breast, provided lactation has been maintained.*

Beware of intervening too quickly without observing the mother's efforts. Rather than saying "that's completely wrong: do it like this..." try "good: you and your baby are going to get on fine. One extra tip might be..."

From the baby's viewpoint, breastfeeding entails taking a large mouthful of breast-with-nipple, which he or she gets to work on with tongue and jaw. Ensure the baby is close to the mother with the shoulders as well as the head facing the breast—which, if large, may need supporting (mother's fingers placed flat on the chest wall at the base of the breast: avoid the 'scissors' grip which stops the baby from drawing the lactiferous sinuses into his mouth).

• Avoid forcing the nipple into the mouth; so do not place a hand over his occiput and press forwards. Cradle the head in the crook of the arm.
• Explain the signs of correct attachment:
   •Mouth wide open, and chin touching the breast (nose hardly touching).
   •The baby should be seen to be drawing in breast, not just nipple.
   •Lower lip curled back, maximally gobbling the areola (so angle between lips >100°). (Don't worry about how much areola can be seen above the top lip: this gives little indication of where the tongue and lower jaw are.)
   •Slow, rhythmic, and deep jaw movements, as well as sucking movements. The 1st few sucks may be fast, shallow, and non-nutritive: here the baby is inducing the 'let-down' reflex, which promotes flow.
• When helping with placing, it is quite appropriate to 'tease' the baby by brushing his lip over the nipple, and then away. This may induce a nice big gape. With one movement bring to the breast, aiming his tongue and lower jaw as far as possible from the base of the nipple—so his tongue can scoop in the nipple and a good mouthful of breast.
• Keeping on the postnatal ward for a few days, and having the mother learn with an experienced, friendly midwife is very helpful, but this is rare in the UK, as cost and other pressures make admissions shorter.

Paediatrics

It is good for every breastfeeding mother to learn this skill (access to teaching is *required* before the accolade of 'baby-friendly' can be granted to UK hospitals). There are at least 4 times when expressing is valuable:

• To relieve (sometimes very) painful breast engorgement between feeds.
• To keep milk production going when it is necessary to give nipples a rest owing to soreness—which is quite a common problem.
• To aid nutrition if sucking is reduced for any reason (eg prematurity or cleft lip).
• If the mother is going to be separated from her baby for a few feeds, eg going out to work.

The best way to learn is from a midwife, and by watching a mother who is already successfully expressing milk. Pumps are available from any chemist. If not, wash hands, and dry on a clean towel. Then, try to start flow by:

• Briefly rolling the nipple: this may induce a let-down reflex, especially if the baby is nearby.
• Stroke the breast gently towards the nipple.
• With circular movements, massage the breast gently with the 3 middle fingers.

Applying warm flannels, or expressing in the bath may aid flow, eg while the mother is learning, and only a few drops are being expressed.

Teach the mother to find the 15 or so ampullae beneath the areola: they feel knotty once the milk comes in. Now with the thumb above the areola and the index finger below, and whole hand pressing the breast back on the chest wall, exert gentle pressure on the ampullae. With rhythmic pressure and release, milk should flow. Use a sterile container.

Take care that the fingers do not slip down on to the nipple, and damage the narrowing ducts. Fingers tire easily: practice is the key. Concentration is also needed to be sure to catch oddly angled jets.

If kept in a fridge, the milk lasts 24–48h. Frozen milk should be used within 3 months. It is thawed by standing it in a jug of warm water. Any unused milk should be discarded after 24 hours, not refrozen. NB: it is known that the antioxidant level of stored breast milk falls, but it is not known if this matters. Refrigeration is better than freezing and thawing.[194]

Paediatrics

Factors which make starting breastfeeding harder • Family pressures, including partner's hostility (10% breastfeed vs ~70% if he approves).
• If mother and baby are separated at night in hospital.
• Urbanization/unfriendly working environments.
• Cultural reframing of breasts as sex objects; no non-sexual role models.
• The commitment a breastfeeding mother makes is huge and sustained—24/7 for many months (WHO advises exclusive breastfeeding for 6 months).[1] ❧❀

☼Breastfeeding advantages ► Mutual gaze ↑emotional input from mother.
• Sucking promotes uterine contractions, so avoiding some PPHs.
• Breastfeeding-induced oxytocin surges promote trust and diminish fear.[195,196]
• Less insulin resistance, BP↑ & obesity (growth is less rapid, p181)[197] due to ↑breast milk Long-Chain Polyunsaturated Fatty Acids.[198] ►LCPUFAs may also ↑IQ.[199]
• Breast milk is cheap and clean, and gives babies an attractive smell.
• Colostrum has endorphins: good for birth-associated stress?[200]
• IgA, macrophages, lymphocytes (with interferon) and lysozyme protect from infection. Acids in breast milk promote growth of friendly lactobacilli in the baby's bowel. Gastroenteritis may be less severe if the mother makes and transfers antibodies (an 'immune dialogue'). NB: one meta-analysis casts doubt vis à vis prems and infection.[201]
• Infant mortality, otitis media, pneumonia & diarrhoea are less if breastfed.[202]
• Breast milk contains less Na⁺, K⁺ and Cl⁻ than other milk, so aiding homeostasis. If dehydration occurs, risk of fatal hypernatraemia is low.
• Exclusive breastfeeding may ↓risk of: type 1 DM, rheumatoid arthritis, inflammatory bowel disease, food allergy/atopy (if family history +ve).[203–205] To reduce allergies, the USA Pediatric Academy[207] says to delay weaning till 6 months old,[208] and cows' milk to 1yr, egg to 2yrs, and peanuts, tree nuts & fish to 3yrs old. This may be valuable in prems;[209] evidence is conflicting in term babies.[210]
• Breastfeeding helps mothers lose weight, and is contraceptive (unreliable!).
• Some protection in premenopausal years against maternal breast cancer.

Why is feeding on demand to be encouraged?
• It keeps the baby happy, and enhances milk production.
• Fewer breast problems (engorgement, abscesses).

NB: feeding by routine is possible with a structured plan (see the *New contented little baby book*),[211] which may help to promote a diurnal sleep cycle.

NB: although co-sleeping (a baby sleeping in the parental bed) can aid parental sleep, there is a risk of inadvertent smothering (p148).

Contraindications to breastfeeding • An HIV +ve mother in developed countries • Amiodarone • Antimetabolites • Antithyroid drugs • Opiates. See *BNF*.

Problems Treat *breast engorgement* by better breast technique and better latching-on; aim to keep breasts empty, eg by hourly feeds or milk expression. If a *breast abscess* forms, discard the milk if it is pus-like. Give the mother flucloxacillin 250mg/6h PO (it is safe for her baby). Surgery may be needed. Treat *sore nipples* by ensuring optimal attachment (p124), and moist wound healing (paraffin gauze dressing or glycerin gel)[212] *not* by resting, except in emergency.

Prematurity Preterm breast milk is the best food for prems. Give unheated, via a tube (p122). Add vitamins D 1000u/day and κ (p122). Phosphate supplements may be needed. Even term babies may (rarely) develop rickets ± hypocalcaemia (eg fits, recurrent 'colds', lethargy, or stridor) if exclusively breastfed, unless vitamin supplements are used (p150).

---

1 However, evidence is insufficient to say confidently "Breastfeed exclusively for 6 months" in developed countries, as breast milk may not meet full energy needs of some infants at 4-6 months old—and there may be risk of specific nutritional deficiencies. Further evidence is awaited.[113]

Bottle feeding

There are few contraindications to breastfeeding but many pressures not to (p126). In many communities >50% mothers are breastfeeding at 2 weeks but this reduces to ≤40% at 6 weeks. Most change to bottle because of lack of knowledge or no encouragement. Advertising also has a role. The WHO/UNICEF *International Code of Marketing of Breastmilk Substitutes* bans promotion of bottle feeding and sets out requirements for labelling and information on feeding.[214] The advantage of bottle feeding is that fathers and others can help; Knowing how much milk the baby is taking can be reassuring to mothers.

Teats Babies fed with a cross-cut teat (lets the baby determine rate) cry less and spend more time awake and content than babies fed with standard teats.

Standard infant formulas (Cows' milk 'humanized' by reducing the solute load and modifying fat, protein, and vitamin content.) As with breast milk, the protein component is whey-based. Many brands are available, eg SMA Gold Cap®. Brands are similar so shopping around for a brand which 'suits better' is unlikely to be an answer to feeding problems.

Follow-on formula milks are like standard formulas, but the protein component is casein-based (∴ delays stomach emptying and allows less frequent feeds). These are marketed to satisfy hungrier babies before they start weaning. Typical age of use: 6–24 months. SMA White® is an example.

Soya milks These are no longer recommended. They contain high levels of phyto-oestrogens which have oestrogen-like properties. This could affect immunity and thyroid function, as well as the more obvious hormonal disruption, especially in boys. Soya milks are still on sale in the supermarket: try to discourage parents from their use. Soya milk is *not* indicated in re-establishing feeding (regrading) after gastroenteritis.

Hydrolized formula is a cows' milk formula where protein is hydrolized into short peptides (eg Nutramigen®). Indications: *cows' milk allergy* (seen in 1% of babies, eg with bloody diarrhoea ± perioral rash) or *soya allergy*; prevention of atopy (eg in babies with a strong family history). Cows' milk can be reintroduced eg at 1 year (can be risky: so do so in hospital).

Specialist milks Many types exist (eg for gastro-oesophageal reflux, malabsorption, metabolic diseases, etc). Get help from a paediatric dietician.

Preparing feeds Hands must be clean, equipment sterilized, and boiled water used—infective gastroenteritis causes many deaths in poor countries and considerable morbidity in the UK. Powder must be accurately measured. Understrength feeds lead to poor growth and overstrength feeds have caused dangerous hypernatraemia, constipation, and obesity.

Feeding After the first few days, babies need ~150mL/kg/24h (30mL=1oz) over 4-6 feeds depending on age and temperament. If small-for-dates up to 200mL/kg/day is needed; if large-for-dates, <100mL/kg. Feeds are often warmed; there is no evidence that cold milk is bad. Flow should almost form a stream; check before each feed as teats silt up. The hole can be enlarged with a hot needle. Bottles are best angled so that air is not sucked in with milk.

Weaning Introduce solids at 4–6 months by offering cereal or puréed food on a spoon. Don't add cereals to bottles. After ~6 months follow-on formula may be tried; lumpy food is started so that the baby can learn to chew. Normal supermarket cows' milk *may* be used from when the baby is ~1 year old, but it may still be too rich in protein, Na^+, K^+, phosphorus—and is poor in iron, trace elements, linoleic and alpha-linolenic acids[1] and vitamins C & B complex. Infants must be able to cope with its higher solute load.[215]

---

1 Docosahexaenoic acid (DHA) is the main lipid in our brain—derived endogenously via α-linolenic acid (ALA). Several studies have tried to improve blood DHA concentrations of formula-fed infants by ↑ ALA in feeds and measuring changes in growth & development. Results are far from clear.[216]

Some definitions *Preterm:*[1] A neonate whose calculated gestational age from the last menstrual period is <37 completed weeks—ie premature.

Low birth weight (LBW): Birth weight of <2500g regardless of gestational age. Thus a LBW baby may not be small for gestational age (see below) if they are born preterm. 6% of UK infants are <2500g at birth, and 50% of these are preterm. 10% of pregnancies end in spontaneous preterm delivery, and 70% of all perinatal deaths occur in preterm infants.

Very low birth weight (VLBW): Birth weight of <1500g regardless of age.

Extremely low birth weight (ELBW): Birth weight <1000g regardless of age.

Small for gestational age (SGA): Typically SGA refers to a birth weight below the 10th percentile (SGA^W). However, SGA may also refer to reduced length (SGA^L) or a combination of both (SGA^{W+L}). SGA^L children have normal body proportions except for head circumference (HC), which is *relatively* larger in many of these children. SGA^{L+W} babies still have a smaller HC at the age of ~6 years compared with SGA^L children. *Chief causes:* ▶Poverty/poor social support may account for 30% of variance in birthweights.[217] Constitutional/familial factors are also important. *Other causes:* Malformation; twins; placental insufficiency (maternal heart disease, BP↑, smoking, diabetes, sickle-cell disease, pre-eclampsia).[218] Gestational age (based on LMP and ultrasound) is more important for predicting survival than the birthweight alone.

Intrauterine growth restriction (IUGR) refers to a small subgroup of babies with proven intrauterine growth restriction (eg due to placental restriction, toxic effects or fetal infections). Infants with SGA need not have suffered IUGR, and those with brief IUGR may be born at a normal weight so are not SGA.

Are SGA effects permanent? 90% of SGA catch up growth in the first 2 yrs, however as adults they are on average 1 standard deviation shorter than the mean adult height.[219] There may be an association between SGA and adult risk of coronary heart disease and obesity.[219]

Causes of prematurity are mostly unknown; smoking tobacco, poverty, and malnutrition play a part. Others: past history of prematurity; genitourinary infection/chorioamnionitis (eg *ureaplasma*[220])[2]; pre-eclampsia; polyhydramnios; closely separated pregnancies; twins; uterine malformation; placenta praevia; abruption; premature rupture of the membranes. Labour may be induced early on purpose or accidentally (p62).

Estimating the gestational age Use the Dubowitz score (p228).

Management If 32 weeks or less, transfer *in utero* to a special centre, if possible.◆※ Once born, ensure airway/breathing is optimal; protect from cold. Take to NICU/SCBU. Plan supplemental breast milk or low-birth-weight formula if <2kg. Measure blood glucose before each 3-hourly feed. Tube feed if oral feeds are not tolerated. If oral feeding is contraindicated (eg respiratory distress) IV feeding is needed (p122).

Survival if very premature 40% of infants born before 23 weeks die on labour ward (↑ by 8% since 1995). Of those surviving labour ward, 75% died on the neonatal unit. 47% survive at 24 weeks and 67% at 25 weeks.^{EPICure2}

Mortality is associated with intracranial abnormalities seen ultrasonically.

Disability *As a percentage of live births:* if 23 weeks' gestation: 5% had no or minor subsequent disability (24 weeks ≈ 12%; 25 weeks ≈ 23%). Morbidity relates to cerebral palsy, squint, and retinopathy (p108).[221][▷150]

Disability may be subtle but specific: one pattern is ↓numeracy if gestation is <30/40, from ↓grey matter in the left parietal lobe.[222] ADD risk↑ (p212).

---

1 Premature is now used as a synonym for preterm; beware older books, as premature once meant birthweight <5lbs (2.5kg), before the difference between light-for-dates and preterm was recognized.
2 Ureaplasma also causes neonatal sepsis, resp. distress & intraventricular haemorrhage. Screening mothers in pregnancy can ↓rates of prem birth (3% *vs* 5.3% in the control group).[223]

Is this baby small for gestational age?

Use centile charts which take into account that first-borns are lighter than subsequent births: the table below gives sample data.

Weeks gestation	Tenth centile weight (grams)				
	First born: Boy	Girl	Subsequent births:	Boy	Girl
32	1220	1260		1470	1340
33	1540	1540		1750	1620
34	1830	1790		2000	1880
35	2080	2020		2230	2100
36	2310	2210		2430	2310
37	2500	2380		2600	2480
38	2660	2530		2740	2620
39	2780	2640		2860	2730
40	2870	2730		2950	2810

Very low birthweight: 1-1.5kg; *extremely low birthweight:* 500-999g.

Paediatrics

Preventing neonatal deaths—worldwide[224]

Each year, of the 130 million babies who are born, ~4 million die in the 1st 4 weeks of life (the neonatal period)—most from preventable causes. Two-thirds occur in India, China, Pakistan, Nigeria, Bangladesh, Ethiopia, the Democratic Republic of the Congo, Indonesia, Afghanistan, and Tanzania. Most of the deaths are caused by pre-term births, infections, respiratory problems, and tetanus. (Malaria and some diarrhoeal diseases are less important in the neonatal period except in those areas of the highest neonatal mortality.) Prevention depends on:

• Tetanus vaccination, access to antibiotics and breastfeeding advice.
• Sanitary delivery rooms with basic emergency services (caesarean sections and blood transfusion; obstructed labour is a major problem).
• Preventing and managing low birthweight. Low birthweight affects 14% of births worldwide, but accounts for ~70% of neonatal deaths. Managing low birthweight babies need not require expensive technology. Much could be achieved by application of known primary care principles of warmth, feeding, and the prevention and early treatment of infection.
• Preventing maternal mortality (0.5 million maternal deaths/yr) is a prerequisite for preventing many neonatal deaths. In one small but harrowing study from Gambia *all* the children born to mothers who died from pregnancy-related causes were themselves dead at one year.[225]

MDG-4 *Millennium Development Goals* are internationally 'agreed' commitments to reduce poverty and ill-health. The 4th goal aims to reduce mortality in under-5s by ⅔ before 2015. The developing world spends $2 billion annually on this. It is estimated that another $4 billion is needed to do the job.

Non-pharmacological methods to reduce pain in neonates

Pain relief through non-nutritive sucking (NNS), rocking, massage, 20% sucrose (12mg may be enough),[226] distilled water and expressed breast milk (EBM) have been studied in a randomized way—in the context of a heel-prick. Duration of cry and Douleur Aiguë du Nouveauné score were used as objective measures of pain. Pain scores and duration of crying were lowest in the NNS and rocking groups compared with sucrose, distilled water, expressed breast milk and massage.[227] Other trials show that for venepuncture, breastfeeding or glucose plus use of a pacifier provides good analgesia.[228,229] Other alternatives: kangaroo care; morphine; fentanyl. Whenever you hear **siren cry** (sequence of almost identical cries with a period of 1sec) think: "How can I help this baby? What is going wrong?"[230]

Less pain=less stress=better babies

▶Bilious (green) vomiting in neonates always needs urgent help (paediatric surgeon + neonatology team) for prompt investigation and management.[231]

Hirschsprung's disease Occurs in 1 in 5000 births.[232] Congenital absence of ganglia in a segment of colon (or in the rare 'long-segment' disease, can be all the way up to the stomach) leading to functional GI obstruction, constipation and megacolon. Faeces may be felt *per abdomen*, and PR exam may reveal tight anal sphincter and explosive discharge of stool and gas. ♂:♀ ≈ 3:1. *Complications:* GI perforation, bleeding, ulcers, enterocolitis (may be life-threatening). Short-gut syndrome after surgery. *Tests:* Diagnosis through rectal suction biopsy of the aganglionic section, staining for acetylcholinesterase-positive nerve excess, is most accurate.[233] Excision of the aganglionic segment is needed ± colostomy.

Oesophageal atresia (OA) + Tracheo-oesophageal fistula (TOF) A spectrum of abnormalities with OA plus a distal TOF being the most common (86%). Isolated OA (7%) and TOF without OA (4%) can also occur.[234] *Prenatal signs:* Polyhydramnios; small stomach. *Postnatal:* Cough, airway obstruction, ↑secretions, blowing bubbles, distended abdomen, cyanosis, aspiration. *Δ:* Inability to pass a catheter into the stomach; x-rays show it coiled in the oesophagus. Avoid contrast imaging. *℞:* Stop feeding, suck out oesophageal pouch. Primary surgical repair is possible in the majority of cases.[235] 50% have other anomalies.

Congenital diaphragmatic hernia (CDH) A developmental defect in the diaphragm allowing herniation of abdominal contents into the chest. Leads to impaired lung development (pulmonary hypoplasia and pulmonary hypertension). *Incidence:* 1:3700.[236] *Diagnosis:* Prenatal: ultrasound; postnatal: CXR. *Signs:* Difficult resuscitation at birth; respiratory distress; bowel sounds in one hemithorax (usually left so heart is best heard on the right). pH <7.3 and cyanosis augur badly (∴ lung hypoplasia).[237] *Associations:* other malformations (neural tube in 50%); trisomy 18; chromosome deletions eg at 15q2, Pierre Robin (p138).[238] *Treatment:* •*Prenatal:* Fetal surgery is not usually practical or available (tracheal obstruction may be tried: it encourages lung growth, so pushing out other viscera)—but premature birth may be caused.[239] •*Postnatal:* Insert a large-bore nasogastric tube when diagnosis suspected: at birth if prenatal diagnosis. The aim is to keep all air out of the gut. Facemask ventilation is contraindicated (so immediately intubate, ventilate, and paralyse, with minimal pressures). Get surgery in an appropriate centre.

Inguinal hernias These are due to a patent processus vaginalis (the passage which ushers the descending testicle into the scrotum). They present as a bulge lateral to the pubic tubercle, eg during crying. In one series (n=6361), ♂:♀×5:1; there were 59% right, 29% left, and 12% bilateral hernias (almost all indirect), with a hydrocele in 19%.[240] Incarceration occurred in 12%. Most surgeons aim to repair these promptly (laparoscopic repair is possible)[241] to avoid incarceration. Hydroceles are hard to distinguish from incarceration—explore if in doubt.

Hydroceles in infancy A processus vaginalis patent at birth, and allowing *only fluid* from the peritoneal cavity to pass down it, generally closes during the first year of life—so no action is usually needed. If it persists until the age of 2 it may need surgical exploration.[242] If the fluid-filled sac is adjacent to the spermatic cord, it is called an encysted hydrocele or a spermatic cord cyst. If the proximal opening of the processus vaginalis is wide, a true inguinal hernia is formed, and action is always required.[243]

Imperforate anus Covers a variety of anorectal abnormalities. Babies may have an associated fistula starting in the rectum. Most girls have a posterior fourchette fistula; boys have a posterior urethral fistula (may pass meconium in urine). Absence of perineal fistula in boys indicates communication with the urethra (so colostomy may be required). Do GU imaging to show commonly associated GU abnormalities. Posterior sagittal anorectoplasty is possible.[244] Babies with Trisomy 21 commonly have imperforate anus without fistula.

Mid-gut malrotations ▶Bilious neonatal vomiting merits immediate surgical referral (pass NGT).[245] Absent attachment of the small intestine mesentery can cause mid-gut volvulus or obstruction of the third part of the duodenum by fibrotic bands. Presentation may be late; passage of blood per rectum heralds mid-gut necrosis—and is an indication for emergency surgical decompression.

Acute gastric volvulus causes non-bilious vomiting, epigastric distention and signs of pain, and is often associated with abnormalities of adjacent organs. There may also be feeding difficulty. Anterior fixation of the stomach to the anterior abdominal wall may be needed after upper GI imaging.

Anterior abdominal wall defects

Gastroschisis (Fig 1): A paraumbilical defect with evisceration (extrusion of viscera) of abdominal contents. *Incidence:* ~1.6:10,000; rising (especially in babies of young mothers[246] or fathers[247]—or, in multips, if there has been a new father for this pregnancy (hence the idea that maternal immune factors play a role)).[248] Another hypothesis is that it is caused by a vascular

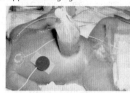
Fig 1. Gastroschisis.

event related to cocaine use. Corrective surgery has a good outcome in 90% (so deliver where there are good paediatric surgical facilities, if diagnosed pre-natally—aim to diagnose at ultrasound).[249,250] Manage as per diaphragmatic hernia: aim to have no air in the gut, so intubate and paralyse at birth if in respiratory distress.

Exomphalos (omphalocele) (Fig 2): Ventral defects of the umbilical ring with herniation of abdominal viscera (which are covered in peritoneum) are common and often associated with malformations such as chromosomal, cardiac, or genitourinary abnormalities. A small exomphalos may contain only a Meckel's diverticulum while a large defect may contain the stomach, liver and bladder. The growth of viscera outside the abdominal cavity may lead it to be proportionally small making reduction of visera more difficult. *Antenatal:* Most are identified by routine fetal anomaly scans (AFP↑ too).[252] *Postnatal management:* • Protect herniated viscera • Maintain fluids and electrolytes. • Prevent hypothermia, gastric decompression, prevention of sepsis, and maintenance of cardiorespiratory stability. • Primary or staged closure may be used to repair the defect. With big defects, closure can cause respiratory insufficiency, haemodynamic compromise, dehiscence, and inability to close the abdomen and subsequent death.[252] After pulmonary and other comorbidities have stabilized, the omphalocele may gradually be reduced with a loose elastic bandage, with **delayed closure** at 6 to 12 months old.[252,253]

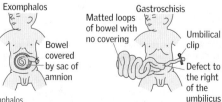

Exomphalos — Bowel covered by sac of amnion

Gastroschisis — Matted loops of bowel with no covering — Umbilical clip — Defect to the right of the umbilicus

Fig 2. Exomphalos.

Paediatrics

Pre-auricular tags are markers of GU problems; consider GU ultrasound.[254]

Undescended testis—cryptorchidism (2–3% of neonates, 15–30% of prems; bilateral in 25% of these). On cold days retractile testes may hide in the inguinal pouch, eluding all but the most careful examination (eg while squatting, or with legs crossed, or in a warm bath they may be 'milked' down into position). These retractile testes need no surgery. If truly undescended it will lie along the path of descent from the abdominal cavity. Early (eg at 1 year) fixing within the scrotum (orchidopexy) may prevent infertility and reduces later neoplasia (untreated, risk is ↑ >5-fold). Intranasal gonadotrophin-releasing hormone is unreliable. NB: biopsy may cause later malignancy.[255]

Posterior urethral valves present with oligohydramnios or absent or feeble voiding (± uraemia and a palpable bladder). *Micturating cystogram:* posterior urethral dilatation. Laser resection is possible. *Antenatal diagnosis:* ultrasound scan (USS) shows GU dilatation.

Hypospadias (narrow meatus on ventral penis) Avoid circumcision: use foreskin for preschool repair; attend to aesthetic considerations.[256]

Epispadias (meatus on dorsum of penis) May occur with bladder extrophy.

Some congenital/genetic disorders

Horseshoe kidney (crossed-fused kidney): Symptoms: Silent or obstructive uropathy ± renal infections. USS diagnosis: kidneys 'too medial'; lower pole 'too long'; anterior-rotated pelvis; poorly defined inferior border; isthmus often invisible.[257]

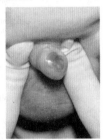

Fig 1. Epispadias.

Autosomal recessive polycystic kidney disease and congenital hepatic fibrosis (ARPKD-CHF) is characterized by cystic dilations of the collecting ducts associated with biliary dysgenesis and perioportal fibrosis. PKHD1 is the responsible gene (on short arm of chromosome 6). Typically diagnosed by prenatal ultrasound (hyperechogenic, large kidneys ± oligohydramnios). Affects 1 in 40,000. Severe cases lead to pulmonary hypoplasia. 80% of those infants that survive the 1st month of live will live to 15. Affected children tend to develop hyponatraemia, hypertension and renal failure. The histology of the liver is always abnormal. Survivors risk UTIs and portal hypertension with haematemesis.[258]

Ectopic kidney: May be seen on US scan (eg pelvic mass) or renal scintigraphy. Associations: anorectal abnormalities, UTIs; calculi.[259]

Renal agenesis causes oligohydramnios, Potter's facies + death if bilateral. VACTERL association (vertebral, anal, cardiac, tracheoesophageal, renal and limb anomalies). *Diagnosis:* prenatal US scan.[260]

Patent urachus: Urine leaks from the umbilicus. *Image:* excretory urogram.

Bladder extrophy: Pubic separation with bladder exposure.[261]

Double ureter: Associations: ureterocele, UTI, pyelonephritis; may be symptomless.

Renal tubular defects: (eg renal glycosuria, cystinuria, or diabetes insipidus). In *renal tubular acidosis* conservation of fixed base is impaired, causing metabolic acidosis + alkaline urine. *Symptoms:* Failure to thrive; polyuria; polydipsia.[262]

Wilms' nephroblastoma This is the commonest renal tumour of childhood (6–7% of all malignancies).[263] It is an undifferentiated mesodermal tumour of the intermediate cell mass. It may be sporadic, or familial (2%), or associated with Beckwith–Wiedemann syndrome (BWS, p638), aniridia, GU malformations (eg cryptorchidism), and retardation (WAGR).[1] One of the Wilms' tumour genes (WT1 on chromosome 11) encodes a protein which is a transcriptional repressor downregulating IGF-II, an insulin-like growth factor.[264]

Median age at presentation: 3.5yrs. 95% are unilateral. Staging:

    I Tumour confined to the kidney
   II Extrarenal spread, but resectable
  III Extensive abdominal disease
  IV Distant metastases
   V Bilateral disease

The patient: Features include fever, flank pain, an abdominal mass. Haematuria is not common. Ultrasound: renal pelvis distortion; hydronephrosis. *CT/MRI* provide the detailed anatomical information needed for surgical planning.[265]

Management: Avoid biopsy; nephrectomy + **vincristine** and **actinomycin** for 4 weeks pre-op can cure. A 2-drug regimen is recommended for early Wilms' (without radiotherapy); more advanced stages need a 3-drug regimen + radiotherapy.[266] Genetic and biological factors guide risk categorization and help individualize care.[267,268] N=382 *Prognosis:* ~90% long-term survival.[269]

Paediatrics

---

1 Retardation is not always a feature: see *Clin Dysmorphol* 2007 16 69.[270]

This is rare, but devastating for the parents. It can be an endocrinological emergency: *refer promptly.* ▶Distinguish genetic, gonadal, phenotypic (affected by sex hormone secretion etc), psychological, and social-role sexualities. Male sex differentiation depends on SRY genes (on Y chromosomes) transforming an indifferent gonad into a testis; its products (testosterone & Mullerian inhibiting substance) control fetal sex differentiation.[1 271]

Ask about Exposure to progesterone, testosterone, phenytoin, aminoglutethamide? Past neonatal deaths (adrenogenital syndrome recessive). Note phallic size and urethral position. Are the labia fused? Have the gonads descended? Undescended impalpable testes are more likely to signify intersexuality than palpable maldescended testes—likewise with severity of hypospadias.[272]

Tests Buccal smear (Barr body suggests ♀); WBC mustard stains make Y chromosomes fluoresce; these take <24h *vs* 5 days for chromosome analysis. If there is a phallus and buccal smear is '♀', diagnose adrenogenital syndrome or maternal androgens (drugs, tumours) or true hermaphroditism, ie ovary and testis coexist (1 on each side) 46,XY, 46,XX, 45,XO/46,XY or 45,X/47,XYY mosaic.[273] If a phallus and the buccal smear is ♂, tell mother the baby is a boy.

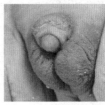

Fig 1. Ambiguous genitalia.

Don't rely on appearances whenever there is: bilateral cryptorchidism (at term), even if a phallus is present; unilateral cryptorchidism with hypospadias; penoscrotal or perineoscrotal hypospadias. Arrange examination by a paediatric endocrinologist to exclude androgen resistance (eg testicular feminization).[1] Genetic tests are also vital: eg terminal deletion of 10q deletes genes essential for normal male genital development.[274]

NB: if the stretched phallus is <25mm long, normal procreation is unlikely. If there is uncertainty due to a short penis, a paediatric endocrinologist may try 3 days' treatment with human chorionic gonadotrophin. If the baby is a boy, the penis will grow (possibly even to normal length) after 5 days.[275]

Aromatase deficiency CYP19 genes are needed for normal oestrogenization: recessive mutations cause ambiguous genitalia in 46,XX individuals; at puberty there is hypergonadotropic hypogonadism, with no secondary sexual characteristics, except for progressive virilization. Boys have normal male sexual differentiation but are tall with brittle bones. Oestrogen receptor gene mutations are similar.[276] Note that sexual differentiation of the brain is mostly dependent on prenatal exposure to testosterone, and congenital aromatase deficiency is thought not to disturb the maleness of brain development in men. But it is not known if this is true for sexually dimorphic brain areas possibly related to sexual orientation and gender identity,[277,278] eg the bed nucleus of the stria terminalis (BSTC is bigger in men but not in some male transsexuals).[279]

Congenital adrenal hyperplasia (From ↑secretion of androgenic hormones ∴ deficiency of 21-hydroxylase, 11-hydroxylase, or 3-β-hydroxysteroid dehydrogenase). Cortisol is inadequately produced, and the consequent rise in adrenocorticotrophic hormone leads to adrenal hyperplasia and overproduction of androgenic cortisol precursors. CAH is a leading cause of male pseudohermaphroditism. *Incidence:* 1:14000.[280] *Signs:* Vomiting, dehydration, and ambiguous genitalia. Girls may be masculinized. Boys may seem normal at birth, but have precocious puberty, or ambiguous genitalia (↓androgens in 17-hydroxylase deficiency), or incomplete masculinization (hypospadias with cryptorchidism from ↓3β-hydroxysteroid dehydrogenase). Hyponatraemia (with paradoxically ↑urine Na⁺) and hyperkalaemia are common. ↑Plasma 17-hydroxyprogesterone in 90%; urinary 17-ketosteroids↑ (not in 17-hydroxylase deficit).

▶▶Emergency treatment of adrenocortical crisis

Babies may present with an adrenocortical crisis (circulatory collapse) in early life. Other presentations include hyponatraemic seizures in infancy (often misdiagnosed as a febrile convulsion). ▶▶Urgent treatment is needed with 0.9% saline IVI (3–5g Na⁺/day), glucose, **fludrocortisone** 0.1mg/day PO and **hydrocortisone**—neonate: 10mg slow IV stat, then 100mg/m² daily by IVI; child 1 month–12yrs: 2–4mg/kg/6h; if >12yrs: 100mg/6–8h slow IV.

Assigning sex and gender

▶There are two pieces of information every new parent is asked: the weight and the sex. It is traumatic for them not to be able to tell. However, don't shy away from telling patients that you do not know whether their baby is a boy or girl, and that tests must be done (it may be wise to await results before naming the child). This is unsatisfactory, but much better than having to re-assign gender. This is why a neonate with ambiguous genitalia is a sexual emergency. Choice of gender must take into account chromosomal and gonadal sex, the hormonal milieu during fetal life, surgical aspects, internal anatomy, fertility, psychosexual development, and adult sexual function. NB: ♀ karyotype does not guarantee absence of intra-abdominal testes—so future risks of malignancy have to be assessed too.[281]

Your job may be to assemble an optimum team: ie a paediatric endocrinologist with psychological expertise, and a laparoscopic surgeon skilled in neonatal cystoscopy and genitography as well as in reconstruction.

Prenatal preparation entails comparing prenatal karyotype with US genital scans to formulate an intersex differential diagnosis—but US scans are unreliable in >50% of ♀ pseudohermaphroditism.[282,283] NB: it is common to assign ♀ gender when in doubt,[284] but while some favour a gender compatible with the chromosomal sex, if possible, others point out that this is a simplification as we don't fully understand determinants of gender role (social sex).[285,286] It is important not to think simply in terms of what promotes the greatest efficiency in the act of sexual intercourse.[287]

Advise against registering the birth until a definite treatment plan is in place. Once registered, legal sex cannot be changed in most countries.

Screening for congenital adrenal hyperplasia

The common cause of adrenal hyperplasia is one of ~10 gene defects (6p21.3; the gene is called *CYP21*) that cause deficiency of 21-hydroxylase (which mediates the penultimate step in cortisol biosynthesis). Corticotrophin-induced accumulation of 17OH-progesterone leads to ↑levels of testosterone (via hepatic conversion). Most affected infants are also salt losers, as 21-hydroxylase is needed for aldosterone biosynthesis, and in boys this is usually the sole early manifestation (excess virilization may be early or in adulthood). Biochemical screening is rarely universal, but some centres use it in boys, aiming for diagnosis before life-threatening adrenal hyperplasia. (Girls are detected by finding virilization at neonatal examination providing the baby is not misdiagnosed as a boy—also prenatal diagnosis is possible, and treatable by giving the mother dexamethasone from early in pregnancy.)

One difficulty is the diversity in time of onset and clinical presentation despite identical cyp21 mutations, making adrenal hyperplasia a continuum of disorders. Treatment is medical and surgical (clitoral reduction and vaginoplasty). Growth and fertility are also impaired.[288]

---

1 Androgens cause maleness in 46, XY individuals, provided no mutations in the X-linked androgen receptor occur. Mutations cause more or less complete androgen insensitivity and female phenotype, with normal levels of testosterone and dihydrotestosterone (DHT). If there is partial insensitivity, topical (periscrotal) DHT (Andractim®) has been used to augment maleness, but if *in vitro* functional assays show this is impossible, babies are usually brought up as girls.[289]

Paediatrics

Incidence 8:1000 births (the most common type of birth defect).[290] 2 questions: *Has the defect lead to decompensation?* Poor feeding, dyspnoea, hepatomegaly, engorged neck veins, pulse↑ (or ↓, premorbidly) •↓Systemic perfusion: weak pulse ± acidosis. •Pulmonary venous congestion: *Is there cyanosis?* All defects can cause decompensation. Only right to left shunts cause cyanosis: some babies will seem well, but blue.

Acyanotic causes (left to right shunt; NB: if pulmonary hypertension develops watch for shunt reversal + cyanosis, Eisenmenger, p642). Atrio-septal defects (ASD), VSD, aortopulmonary window, patent ductus (PDA). Coarctation of the aorta. Any mild isolated valve lesion (eg pulmonary stenosis; prevalence 1:1000).[291]

Cyanotic causes (R to L shunt) Fallot's (p642, *OHCM* p151), transposition of great arteries; tricuspid or pulmonary atresia, total anomalous pulmonary venous return (TAPVR). Hypoplastic left heart syndrome. Truncus arteriosus.

Tests FBC, CXR, P_aO_2 (in air & 100% O_2), ECG, 3D echo, cardiac catheter. *VSD:* (25% of cases) Symptoms: usually mild. Signs: harsh, loud, pansystolic 'blowing' murmur ± thrill. ECG: normal at birth. Later left (or combined) ventricular hypertrophy. CXR: pulmonary engorgement. Course: 20% close spontaneously by 9 months (*maladie de Roger*). Large defects may need surgery. *ASD:* (7% of cases) Symptoms: usually none. Signs: widely split, fixed S_2 + systolic murmur due to a pulmonary flow murmur (upper left sternal edge).[292] The ASD itself does not cause a murmur. CXR: cardiomegaly, globular heart (primum defect). ECG: RVH ± incomplete R bundle branch block. *Patent ductus:* Signs: failure to thrive, pneumonias, CCF, SBE, collapsing pulse, thrill, S_2↑, systolic pulmonary area murmur, or continuous machinery hum. CXR: vascular markings↑, big aorta. ECG: LVH. **Dexamethasone** in preterm labour helps close PDAS, as does **ibuprofen** 10mg/kg slow IV, then 5mg/kg after 24 & 48h is similar to **indometacin** 0.1mg/kg/24h (3 doses IV over 30min if 2–7 days old; see *BNF*c).[293] Meta-analyses favour indometacin.[294] Beware: oliguria; renal failure; ↓platelets.[295] *Coarctation:* Aortic constriction makes feeling femoral pulses hard; BP↑ in the arms (±epistaxis) and ↓ in legs, absent foot pulses, ± systolic murmur at the left sternal edge and back, heart failure. Think of this whenever there is shock, eg on days 3–10, when the ductus closes. CXR: rib notching (very late). ECG: LVH. *Transposition of great arteries (TGA):* Cyanosis, CCF, ± systolic murmur. CXR: egg-shaped heart. ECG: RVH. Balloon atrial septostomy allows oxygenated blood to reach the aorta via ASD. Correction is possible.[296] *Pulmonary stenosis:* Pulmonary thrill and systolic murmur. See *OHCM* p142.

Treatment •Treat heart failure in babies with nasogastric feeds, sitting upright, O_2, furosemide ~1mg/kg/24h slow IV ± spironolactone; digoxin (see *BNF*c) is rarely used. •You may be advised to keep the ductus open in duct-dependent cyanotic conditions with alprostadil (10 nanograms/kg/min by IVI initially); intubate and ventilate if needed before transfer to specialists; during transfer be alert to: T°↓; Ca²⁺↓; glucose↓; hypovolaemia, apnoea. Open-heart surgery using hypothermia and circulatory arrest is possible at any age, eg for: Fallot's, VSD, TGA, total anomalous pulmonary venous drainage (in which pulmonary veins drain, eg into the portal system, causing CCF). Balloon valvuloplasty decreases need for open surgery in pulmonary stenosis (there is more of a problem with restenosis and residual incompetence with aortic valvuloplasty). It is also employed in coarctation. Systemic to pulmonary shunts to enlarge an underdeveloped pulmonary arterial tree, before inserting a valve-bearing conduit is an example of palliative surgery.

Prenatal screening echocardiography Sensitivity: 88%; specificity and +ve predictive value: 100%. Intrauterine cardiac intervention is possible.[297]

We hear benign flow murmurs (eg parasternal low-frequency 'twangs' in early systole) in ~80% of children, at some time (eg with fever, anxiety, exercise). *Still's murmur* is an example, and may be abolished by hyperextension of the back, and neck. Lack of other features distinguishes these from malformations: *no* clubbing; *no* cyanosis; *no* thrills; *no* rib recession; *no* clicks; *no* arrhythmias; normal pulses & apex; *no* failure to thrive. When in doubt, get a skilled echocardiogram. CXR & ECG often mislead.[298] Another (validated) option is to use an electronic stethoscope and e-mail the sounds to a cardiologist.[299]

Questions to ask yourself while listening to the 2nd heart sound (S_2)
• Is it a double sound in inspiration, and single in expiration? (Normal)
• Is S_2 split all the time? (ASD—atrial septal defects)
• Is S_2 never split, ie single? Fallot's; pulmonary atresia; severe pulmonary stenosis; common arterial trunk; transposition of the great arteries (the anterior aorta masks sounds from the posterior pulmonary trunk).
• Is the pulmonary component (2nd part) too loud? (Pulmonary hypertension)
NB: the 2nd heart sound is more useful diagnostically than the first.

Points to note on hearing murmurs If you have an ear for detail! *Timing:*
• *Ejection systolic* (innocent, or semilunar valve or peripheral arterial stenosis).
• *Pansystolic* with no crescendo-decrescendo (VSD, mitral incompetence).
• *Late systolic*, no crescendo-decrescendo (mitral prolapse, *OHCM* p138).
• *Early diastolic* decrescendo (aortic or pulmonary incompetence).
• *Mid-diastolic* crescendo-decrescendo (↑atrio-ventricular valve flow, eg VSD, ASD; or tricuspid or mitral valve stenosis). An opening snap (*OHCM* p138) and presystolic accentuation suggest the latter.
• *Continuous murmurs* (PDA, venous hum, or arterio-venous fistula).

Loudness: The 6 grades for systolic murmurs: (Thrills mean pathology.)
1 Just audible with a quiet child in a quiet room. *2* Quiet, but easily audible.
3 Loud, but no thrill. *4* Loud with thrill.
5 Audible even if the stethoscope only makes partial contact with skin.
6 Audible without a stethoscope.

Place:

AS = aortic stenosis; PS = pulmonary stenosis

AS Sternum PS
ASD Still's
VSD Mitral incompetence

Accentuating/diminishing manoeuvres *Inspiration:* Augments systemic venous return ('negative' pressure draws blood from abdomen into the thorax), and therefore the murmurs of pulmonary stenosis and tricuspid regurgitation. *Expiration:* Augments pulmonary venous return and decreases systemic return, and therefore VSD, mitral incompetence, and aortic stenosis too. In (mild) pulmonary stenosis, the ejection click is augmented by expiration. *Valsalva manoeuvre:* ↓Systemic venous return and benign flow murmurs, but ↑ murmurs from mitral incompetence and sub-aortic obstruction. *Sitting or standing* (vs lying): ↓Innocent flow murmurs, but ↑ murmurs from subaortic obstruction or from a venous hum (places to listen: right base; below left clavicle; neck—it is abolished by gently pressing the ipsilateral jugular; PDA murmurs are similar, but no change with posture).

Catheter findings	
Pulmonary stenosis	RV pressure↑; pulmonary artery pressure↓. If peak systolic gradient ≤25mmHg at ~6 months old, it's likely to be benign[291]
+ foramen ovale	As above with right atrial pressure↑ and P_aO_2↓
VSD	RV pressure↑; RV O_2 >R atrial O_2
ASD	Right atrial pressure & oxygenation↑ compared with IVC
Patent ductus	RV pressure↑; pulmonary artery O_2 >RV O_2
Fallot's tetrad	See p642 *OHCM* p151; LV O_2↓, RV O_2↓[292] & P_aO_2↓

Paediatrics

This is the chief facial malformation. It results from failure of fusion of maxillary and premaxillary processes (during week 5). The defect runs from lip to nostril. It may be bilateral, when there is often a cleft in the palate as well, with the premaxillary process displaced anteriorly. Palate clefts may be large or small (eg of uvula alone). *Incidence:* ~2:1000. ♂:♀ > 1:1 *Causes:* Genes, benzodiazepines, antiepileptics, rubella. Other malformations are common, eg trisomy 18, 13–15, or Pierre Robin short mandible (causing cyanotic attacks). *Prevention:* Quit smoking pre-pregnancy.[293] Folic acid ≥6mg/day periconception ± multivitamins.[294,295] Avoidance of anti-epileptics. *Interdisciplinary treatment:* Orthodontist, plastic surgeon, oral surgeon, GP, paediatrician, speech therapist. Feeding with special teats may be needed before plastic surgery (usually, lip repair at 3 months, and palate at 1yr; some surgeons do lip at 1 week old). Repair of unilateral complete or incomplete lesions often gives good cosmesis. If bilateral, there is always some residual deformity. Surgery may involve iliac bone grafts + insertion of Gore-Tex® membranes.[296] *Complications:* Otitis media, aspiration, post-op palatal fistulae, poor speech (speech therapy helps). Social adjustment↓.[297] Avoid taking to NICU—may ↓bonding—a big problem (also the dopaminergic 'high' a normal baby's smile induces in the mother's putamen may be subverted by the defect).[298]

Other head & neck malformations Spina bifida: p140

Eyes Anophthalmos: there are no eyes; rare; part of trisomy 13–15.
Ectopia lentis: Presents as glaucoma with poor vision. The lens margin is visible; seen in Marfan's (OHCM p720), Ehlers–Danlos (p642), homocystinuria; incidence: <1:5000; autosomal-dominant (a-Dom) or recessive (a-R). *Cataract:* Rubella, Down's, others: recessive or sex-linked. *Coloboma:* Notched iris with a displaced pupil; incidence: 2:10,000; (a-R). *Microphthalmos:* Small eyes; 1:1000; due to rubella—or genetic (a-Dom).
Ears Accessory auricles: seen in front of the ear; incidence: 15:1000.
Deformed ears: Treacher–Collins' syndrome (p655).
Low-set ears: associations—Down's syndrome; congenital heart disease.
Nose/throat *Choanal atresia:* Signs: postnatal cyanotic attacks; nasal catheter doesn't go into the pharynx because of nasal malformation. *Incidence:* ≤1:5000. *Surgery:* consider a micro-endoscopic nasal approach.[299] *Congenital laryngeal stridor:* (∵ laryngeal webs or laryngomalacia: the larynx is unable to stay open. *Signs:* shrill inspirations; dyspnoea. *Surgery:* endoscopic.
Laryngeal atresia: Breaths don't expand the lungs, which are hypoplastic. Look for coexisting anomalies.[300] *Branchial fistula:* These open at the front of sternomastoid (a remnant of the 2nd or 3rd branchial pouch). *Incidence:* <1:5000. Branchial and thyroglossal cysts: p576.
Skull & spine *Brachycephaly:* Short, broad skull from early closure (craniostenosis) of the coronal suture; incidence: <1:1000; Down's-associated or a-Dom. *Cleidocranial dysostosis:* No clavicles (so shoulders meet). Slow skull ossification, no sinuses, high-arched palate; incidence <1:5000; a-Dom.
Craniofacial dysostosis: Tower skull, beaked nose, exophthalmos. Δ: spiral CT. Klippel-Feil syndrome (p648): fused cervical vertebra (so the neck is short).
CNS Hydrocephalus: incidence 0.3-2:1000. Ante- or neo-neonatal injury, infection, or genes (sex-linked) may cause aqueduct stenosis. Dandy–Walker syndrome (p640); Arnold–Chiari malformation (OHCM p708). *Microcephaly:* *Causes:* genetic,[301] intrauterine viruses (eg rubella), hypoxia, x-rays, maternal alcohol. *Incidence:* 1:1000. Recurrence risk: 1:50.
Fetal alcohol syndrome Severity depends on how much alcohol the mother has had in pregnancy. Features: microcephaly, short palpebral fissure, hypoplastic upper lip, absent philtrum, small eyes, IQ↓, cardiac malformations.

Head and neck words

To outsiders, it seems as if paediatricians are obsessed with measuring head circumference and head shape, and translating the latter into Latin—as if defining the *outside* could explain what what is going on *inside*. To insiders, though, ►*it is to diagnose and treat craniostenois that we we measure heads.* So... always know where your patient is on his or her centile charts.

Craniostenosis=craniosynostosis=premature closure of one or more of the skull's fibrous sutures by ossification. It affects ~1:2000 of whom 2–11% have a family history. 15–40% have one of 180 recognised syndromes (with a family history it's 50%). Normal time for sutures to close is 3–9 months for the metopic (frontal) suture, 29–39yrs for other sutures (saggital, coronal, lamboid). The skull compensates for closure by growing in the direction parallel to the closed suture. If the compensatory growth allows insufficient space for the growing brain there will be ↑ICP ± visual loss, sleep impairment (obstructive sleep apnoea), eating problems and ↓IQ. Babies with insufficient head growth (centile charts p222-4) or skull deformity need assessment by a craniofacial surgeon. 4–20% of children with single suture closure have raised intracranial pressure, up to 60% if more than one suture involved. Look for papilloedema. Skull x-ray: single closed suture. CT: structural brain abnormalities and suture fusion and will diagnose deformational plagiocephaly (due to absent suture) and pansynostosis secondary to micephaly. Subarachnoid spaces are larger in microcephaly. Surgery at 6-12 months aims to normalise the cranial vault and to allow for brain growth.

Cyclopia: A single eye in the area normally occupied by the root of the nose, which is missing, or present in the form of a proboscis (a tubular appendage) located above the eye. In some, it can be viewed as an extreme form of hypotelorism. It may be part of trisomy 13 (Patau's syndrome).

Dolicephalic: The head is elongated, eg as in Marfan's, or El Greco portraits.

Dystopia canthorum: Intercanthal distance is increased, but not the interpupillary or (bony) interorbital distances.

Holoprosencephaly: (a whole, ie single-sphered, brain) Hypotelorism with cleft palate ± premaxillary agenesis ± cyclopia ± cebocephaly (see above)—follows failure of the lateral ventricles to separate (defective cleavage of the prosencephalon), eg with fusion of the basal ganglia.

Lissencephaly: Smooth cortex with no convolutions (agyria).

Metopic suture: This is the same as the frontal suture.

Micrognathia: The mandible is too small.

Neurocranium: That part of the skull holding the brain.

Oxycephalic (=turricephaly=acro-cephaly) The top of the head is pointed.

Plagiocephaly: If fully expressed, synostosis affects coronal (rarely lambdoidal) sutures (±palpable bony ridge) with a flat forehead and elevation of the orbit on one side. Minor (unfused) plagiocephalic asymmetry is common in infants sleeping on their backs, improves with time, and is of no significance. Associations: scoliosis and pelvic obliquity (fig 1).

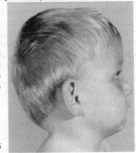

Rachischisis: Spinal column fissure.

Sinciput: Anterior, upper part of head.

Viscerocranium: Facial skeleton.

Wormian bones: Supernumerary bones in the sutures of the skull.

Fig 1. Plagiocephaly.

Neural tube defects result from failure of the neural tube to close between the 3rd and 4th week of *in utero* development.

Myelodysplasia: Any neuroectoderm defect, eg of the cord, either multiple anterior horns, several central canals, failure of cord fusion so that there is a flat neural plaque, not a fused tube (*myelocele*), or a double neural tube (*diplomyelia*), or herniation through a bony defect as a *meningocele* (contains dura & arachnoid) or meningomyelocele (the cord is involved too, fig 1). *Spina bifida* implies an incomplete vertebral arch (*spina bifida occulta* if covered by skin). *Anencephaly* implies absent skull vault and cerebral cortex. *Encephalocele* means that part of the brain protrudes through the skull.

Incidence in Europe ~4000 preventable NTDs/yr.[311] *Risk* increases with young primips, lower social class, and homozygosity for a point mutation (c677→T; prevalence ≈10%, interfering with folate metabolism). *Recurrence risk* rises 10-fold if one pregnancy is affected, 20-fold if 2, 40-fold if 3 pregnancies affected; and 30-fold if a parent is affected. See below for risk reduction.

Neurological deficit is variable, depending on level of the lesion and the degree to which the lower cord functions independently from the upper cord. The defect may progress after birth; hydrocephalus gradually worsens mental performance. A child who learns to walk during his 2nd year may subsequently outgrow his ability to support (weight increases as the cube of surface area, power only as its square). Those with lumbosacral myelomeningoceles usually learn to walk with callipers by the age of 3, but ≤20% with higher lesions ever walk. When there is paralysis below L3, as unopposed hip flexors and adductors are likely to dislocate the hips; only 5–13% retain their ability to walk.[312]

Postnatal surgery Firm guidelines on whom to treat often prove simplistic in individual infants. The final outcome of early closure of the defect depends on the state of the kidneys after multiple UTIs, and the extent of delayed hydrocephalus (requiring ventriculoperitoneal CSF shunts). Early post-operative mortality may account for ~25% of deaths. Many operations may be needed for spinal deformity (often severe and very hard to treat).

Intrauterine diagnosis A maternal serum α-fetoprotein >90u/mL at 18 weeks detects ~80% of open spina bifidas and 90% of anencephalics, but also 3% of normal singleton fetuses, twins, and some with exomphalos, congenital nephrosis, urethral valves, Turner's syndrome, trisomy 13, and oligohydramnios. Amniocentesis and skilled ultrasound ↑pick-up rates further.

Intrauterine surgery (*eg at 23 weeks' gestation*) This is very controversial.

Hurdles for the developing child

• Urinary and faecal incontinence. Penile appliances, urinary diversions, or intermittent self-catheterization save laundry and bed sores. Regular evaluation of bladder function is essential (surgery may or may not help).[1]
• The mother who 'does it all' can prevent maturity developing.
• Immobility. Mobility allowances are small and of little help.
• Social and sexual isolation, if a special school is needed.[313]

Prevention In mothers who have already had an affected baby, there is good evidence that folic acid (eg 5mg/day—or if diabetic, obese, on anti-epileptics, p2) given from before conception (as the neural tube is formed by 28 days, before pregnancy may even be recognized) reduces the risk of recurrence of neural tube defects by 72%. If no previous neural tube defects, 0.4mg of folic acid is recommended in the months before conception and for 13 weeks after; see p2.[314] Many mothers don't take folate pre-conception, hence the call for folate-fortification of bread etc. This is adopted in the USA, but is not ideal, as presentation of low B12 states may be delayed (see BOX 1).[315–317]

1 Untethering the spinal cord may be indicated: seek expert advice. See *J Urol* 2007 331.[318]

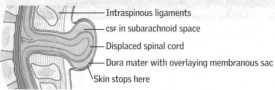

— Intraspinous ligaments
— CSF in subarachnoid space
— Displaced spinal cord
— Dura mater with overlaying membranous sac
— Skin stops here

Fig 1. Meningomyelocele.

Should we fortify staple foods with folic acid?

This is done in many places but not in Europe, from inertia as much as from regard to civil liberties/freedom of choice, but this inertia is being overtaken by research showing that the hoped-for decline in neural tube defects is not occurring—as most people are ignorant of (or do not act on) advice to take folic acid before conception.[319] Inertia is reasonable, perhaps, as some unforeseen harm may occur from fortification. If fortification is favoured, fortification of flour is one attractive option.[320] 40 countries have tried this; success in preventing NTDs ranges from 19% to 78%.[321]

So what harm could there be from folic acid? It can correct anaemia due to a low B_{12}—and hence might mask the underlying disease, and allow development or progression of B_{12}-related neuropathy and subacute combined degeneration of the spinal cord, if diagnosis depended on the presence of anaemic symptoms. This possibility may be partly overcome by educating ourselves, so that we do not believe that macrocytic anaemia is a necessary sign of B_{12}-related neurological disorders.[322] Another argument in favour of universal fortification is that significant neuropsychiatric morbidity is also preventable by folic acid supplementation.[323] the FACIT trial 2007

Who wants a nanny state stuffing chemicals down our throats?

Involuntary euthanasia for some neonates with spina bifida?

Deliberate termination of life of newborns with meningomyelocele is practiced openly only in the Netherlands. '**Unbearable and hopeless suffering**' is the single most cited criterion for this termination, together with the statement that '**there are no other proper medical means to alleviate this suffering**'.[324] Covert termination may or may not be more widespread. There are many sides to this question and many assumptions behind the phrases in blue which need examining. How to decide? We cannot decide here: only bear in mind one question "How can rational compassionate people reach diametrically opposed positions?"

   Part of the answer is to realize that we ourselves change over time and then to go on to ask how this change comes about. What changes? As a thought experiment, catalogue what changes when you change your mind. The facts? Fashion? The context? Experience? Other people's expectations of what your role is? A paralysing ability to see both sides of every question, like mirrors reflecting each other *ad infinitum*? Changing our mind is a process well worth studying. It is as if we are relieved when the seesaw swings from one stable-and-smug state of knowing-with-certainty to another. We hastily brush away the inelegant internal manoeuvrings which precede change. But hold on...it is these inelegant manoeuvres which validate us as human beings. So...let's try getting more comfortable with being uncomfortable. And perhaps this leads us to a yardstick to help answer the question: which position augments our humanity most?

Must suffering always be alleviated?

MeaslesND, rubellaND, mumpsND, and erythroviruses

Measles (RNA paramyxovirus) *Spread:* Droplets. *Incubation:* 7-12 days; infective from prodrome (cough, conjunctivitis, T°↑) until 5d after rash starts. *Koplik spots* (fig 1) are pathognomonic. They are often fading as the rash appears (eg behind ears, on day 3-5, spreading down the body, becoming confluent). Δ: IgM & IgG +ve;[325] PCR for typing. *Complications:* More common if <5yrs or >20yrs. Otitis media is most common complication. Croup, tracheitis and bronchiolitis occur in infants. Pneumonia is the most common cause of death in measles. Older patients may develop encephalitis—of these 15% die; 25% develop fits, deafness, or ↓cognition. *Subacute sclerosing parencephalitis* is a chronic complication of measles which develops 7-13yrs after primary infection with progressive changes in behaviour, myoclonus, choreoatheotosis, dystonia, dementia, coma and death. ℞: Isolate—in hospital, if the patient is ill or immunocompromised or malnourished, or has pneumonitis, CNS signs, or dehydration; then:

Fig 1. Koplik spots.
Courtesy of CDC.

- Ensure adequate nutrition (catabolism is very high). Continue breastfeeding, even during diarrhoea. Pass a nasogastric feeding tube if intake is poor.
- In the developing world, need for vitamin A arises; consider 2 doses, + 1 more at 6 weeks later (p450). CI: pregnancy; known not to be deficient.
- Treat secondary bacterial infection; antibiotics such as amoxicillin for otitis media and pneumonia. Prophylactic antibiotics have no clear role.[326]

Immunization: p151. Only 80% effective.[327] *Prognosis:* Good in rich countries; in poor areas death rate is ~10%.[328] (0.9 million/yr, mostly in Africa).[329]

Rubella (RNA virus). *Incubation:* 2-3wks. *Infectivity:* 5 days before to 5 days after start of rash. *Signs:* Macular rash; suboccipital lymphadenopathy. *Immunization:* Live virus, p151.[330] *Complications:* Small joint arthritis. Malformations *in utero* (p34). Infection during the 1st 4 weeks: eye anomaly (70%); wks 4-8: cardiac abnormalities (40%); wks 8-12: deafness (30%).

Mumps (RNA paramyxovirus) *Spread:* Droplets/saliva. *Incubation:* 14-21d. *Immunity:* Lifelong, once infected. *Infectivity:* 7 days before and 9 days after parotid swelling starts. *Signs:* Prodromal malaise; T°↑; painful parotid swelling, becoming bilateral in 70% (ΔΔ: Sjögren's; leukaemia; dengue; herpes-virus; EBV; HIV; sarcoid; pneumococci; haemophilus; staphs; anaphylaxis; blowing glass or trumpets; drugs; fig 2). *Complications:* Usually none; orchitis (± infertility), arthritis, meningitis, pancreatitis, myocarditis, deafness, myelitis. ℞: Rest. *Vaccine:* p151, for *any* non-immune adult or child (SE: rare parotitis/pancreatitis).

Erythrovirus ('fifth disease', erythema infectiosum; parvovirus B19; fig 3). *Signs:* Usually a mild, acute infection, with malar erythema ('slapped cheek') and a rash mainly on the limbs (**gloves and socks syndrome**, in adults).[331] By the time this appears, infectivity has waned. Constitutional upset is mild. Arthralgia is commoner in adults—who may present as 'glandular fever' (false +ve Paul-Bunnell).[332] Spread by droplet[331] is rapid in closed communities. It can also cause the marrow to stop making RBCs (aplastic crisis)—serious if RBC lifespan is already short (eg sickle-cell disease, thalassaemia, spherocytosis, HIV). Δ: IgM (PCR if immunocompromized). ℞: Transfusions and immunoglobulins are rarely needed.[331] *Pregnancy:* Risk of fetal death is ~10% (esp. midtrimester)[333]—eg from hydrops fetalis ∴ inhibition of multiplication and lysis of erythroid progenitor cells (monitor AFP for several weeks; if it rises abnormally, do ultrasound). *Fetal/neonatal problems:* **hydrops** (in ~3%; treat by intrauterine transfusion if severe); growth retardation, meconium peritonitis, myocarditis, glomerulonephritis, placentomegaly, hepatomegaly, oedema, pancytopenia. Respiratory insufficiency/death is rare. 10% of those affected before 20 weeks miscarry; in the rest, risk of congenital abnormality is ~1%.[334]

Hand, foot & mouth disease The child is mildly unwell; develops vesicles on palms, soles, and mouth. They may cause discomfort until they heal, without crusting. *Incubation:* 5–7 days. *Treatment* is symptomatic. *Cause:* Coxsackie-virus A16 or enterovirus 71 (suspect in outbreaks with herpangina, meningitis, flaccid paralysis ± pulmonary oedema). Herpangina entails fever + sore throat + vesicles or macerated ulcers (on palate or uvula, which heal over 2 days) ± abdominal pain and nausea. This has nothing to do with the bovine form.

Herpes infections See *OHCM* p400–1. Varicella zoster/chickenpox: p144.

Roseola infantum This is a common, mild, self-limiting illness in infants, causing $T^\circ\uparrow$, then a maculopapular rash on subsidence of fever at the end of the 4th febrile day. Uvulo-palatoglossal junctional ulcers may be a useful early sign.[335] *Cause:* Herpes virus 6 (HHV6; double-stranded DNA). It is related to other herpes viruses (HSV 1 & 2, varicella zoster, EBV & CMV). Interaction between host immunities and other viruses may lead to cellular immunodeficiency and fatal illness. *Synonyms:* exanthem subitum, fourth disease, 3-day fever. It is neurotropic (a rare cause of encephalitis/focal gliosis on MRI, maybe accounting for why the not uncommon roseola 'febrile fits' tend to occur *after* the fever).[336]

Other causes of rashes in children See also skin diseases section (p582).
• A transient maculopapular rash is a feature of many trivial viral illnesses (but a few macules may be a sign of early meningococcaemia).
• Purpuric rashes: meningococcaemia (p202); Henoch–Schönlein purpura (p197); idiopathic thrombocytopenic purpura (check FBC and film).
• Drug rashes (maculopapular) from eg penicillins or phenytoin are common.
• Scabies (p608); insect bites.
• Eczema (p596); urticaria (p584); psoriasis—guttate psoriasis may follow a respiratory tract infection in children (p594); pityriasis rosea (p602).
• Still's disease: transient maculopapular rash, fever, and polyarthritis.

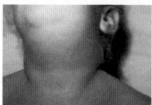
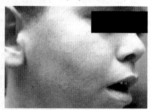

Fig 2. Mumps: generalized salivary swelling.   **Fig 3.** Slapped cheeks (parvovirus B19).
Both images courtesy of *CDC*.

Paediatrics

Managing distressing fever in viral illnesses

▶Unwrap ▶rehydrate ▶antipyretics ± *tepid* sponge (a partly validated alternative/additional method;[337] NB: cold water may vasoconstrict). Antipyretics aren't always needed[338] (↑mortality if used in severe sepsis,[339] and paracetamol is implicated in asthma/eczema).[340, n=205,487] Keep records of quantity used. Ibuprofen at 10mg/kg/8h (~100mg/8h if 1–4yrs old; twice this if 7–10yrs) is better than paracetamol at 15mg/kg/6h, so try it first. Giving both alternately is a bit better than giving one alone, if sustained effects are needed.[341, N=165]

Oral paracetamol doses *1–3 months old:* 30–60mg/8h. Children over 3 months use maximum of 4 doses/24h then doses are: *3–6 months* 60mg/4–6h; *6 months–2yrs* 120mg/4–6h; *2–4 years* 180mg/4–6h; *4–6 years* 240mg/4–6h; *6–8 years* 240–250mg/4–6h; *8–10 years* 360–375mg/4–6h; *10–12 years* 480–500mg/4–6h; *12–16 years* 480–750mg/4–6h; *16+ years* 500mg–1g/4–6h. Maximum of 4 doses in 24h.

Paracetamol suppositories are available (60, 125, or 250mg).

Chickenpox is a primary infection with varicella-zoster virus. Shingles (*OHCM* p400) is a reactivation of dormant virus in posterior root ganglia.

Chickenpox *Signs:* Crops of skin vesicles of different ages, often starting on face, scalp or trunk. The rash is more concentrated on the torso than the extremities. *Incubation:* 11-21 days. *Infectivity:* 4 days before the rash, until all lesions have scabbed (~1wk). *Spread:* Droplets. It can be caught from someone with shingles. It is one of the most infectious diseases known. 95% of adults have been infected; immunity is lifelong. *Tests:* Fluorescent antibody tests and Tzanck smears are rarely needed. *ΔΔ:* Hand, foot, and mouth disease; insect bites; scabies; rickettsia. *Course:* T°↑; rash starts 2 days later, often starting on the back: macule→papule→vesicle with a red-surround→ulcers (eg oral, vaginal)→crusting. 2-4 crops of lesions occur during the illness. Lesions cluster round areas of pressure or hyperaemia. *Complications:* If spots are blackish (*purpura fulminans*) or coalescing and bluish (necrotizing fasciitis), get urgent help on ITU; avoid ibuprofen. Be alert to pneumonia, meningitis, myelitis, CNS thrombi, DIC, LFT↑, Guillain-Barré, Henoch-Schönlein, nephritis, pancreatitis, myositis, myocarditis, orchitis, cerebellar ataxia. If susceptible, *live attenuated vaccine* pre-cytotoxics/steroids may be wise. *Immunization:* occurs in the US/Japan/Australia and other countries, but is not routine in the UK. Reasons not to vaccinate include paradoxically increasing shingles/chickenpox in adults[342] and lack of cost-effectiveness.[343] *Dangerous contexts:* Immunosuppression; cystic fibrosis; severe eczema; neonates. *R:* Keeping cool may reduce lesion numbers. **Calamine lotion** soothes. Trim nails to lessen damage from scratching. Consider daily antiseptic for spots (chlorhexidine). **Flucloxacillin** 125-250mg/6h PO if bacterial superinfection—treat for septicaemia if worsening. **Antivaricella-zoster immunoglobulin** (if ≤10 days post-exposure) + **aciclovir** if immuno-suppressed or on steroids (it's licensed as a 7-day course in chickenpox); begin within 24h of the rash. In renal failure, ↓ dose. There is *no* clear evidence on aciclovir ↓complications if immunocompetent, but it may help severe symptoms, eg in adolescents, or 2nd or 3rd family contacts. If used, use at the 1st sign of infection, or as a 7-day *attenuating dose* of 10mg/kg/6h starting 1wk post-exposure. **Famciclovir** is less well-studied.[344]

Shingles *Treatment:* Oral analgesia. Ophthalmic shingles: p420. Aciclovir may reduce progression of zoster in the immunocompromised (may be rampant, with pneumonitis, hepatitis, and meningoencephalitis). Aciclovir IVI dose: 10mg/kg/8h (over 1h), with concentration <5mg/mL, over >1h.

Varicella in pregnancy Pneumonitis and encephalitis are no commoner in pregnancy, despite pregnancy being an immunocompromised state (1 in 400 and 1 in 1000, respectively). Infection in the 1st 20 weeks (esp. 13-20 weeks) may cause varicella zoster virus (vzv) fetopathy in 2%.[345] *Signs of vzv fetopathy* are variable, eg cerebral cortical atrophy and cerebellar hypoplasia, manifested by microcephaly, convulsions and IQ↓; limb hypoplasia; rudimentary digits ± pigmented scars. Maternal shingles is *not* a cause. If the mother is affected from 1 week before to 4 weeks after birth, babies may suffer severe chickenpox. Give the baby zoster immunoglobulin 250mg IM at birth; if affected, isolate from other babies, and give aciclovir.

Infection is preventable by pre-pregnancy vaccination with live varicella vaccine,[346] but testing for antibodies pre-conceptually is expensive, and cost-effectiveness depends on local rates of seronegativity. ~80% of those who cannot recall any previous chickenpox are, in fact, immune.[347]

Varicella zoster globulin prevents infection in 50% of susceptible contacts, eg 1000mg IM (adults). Infection in pregnancy merits **aciclovir** (it's probably OK for the fetus). Chickenpox at birth is a problem. Barrier nursing mothers causes distress and is of unproven value. Infant mortality: up to 20%.[348]

In many sub-Saharan countries, ~40% of all under-5 mortality is a result of AIDS. If an HIV +ve mother breastfeeds, this ↑risk of vertical transmission by ~50%. Mothers with HIV should bottle feed in the UK, but in countries without reliable clean water, breastfeeding is less risky than bottle feeding.[349,350] Infection can occur from the 1st trimester; ~50% of infections occur at the time of delivery, and are more likely if mothers have symptomatic HIV infection or a high viral load[1]. Transmission rates with full intervention (ie antiretrovirals around birth, caesarean section, no breastfeeding) are <5%. In a cohort of 330 HIV +ve mothers, those with the p24 antigen had a 3-fold risk of transmission compared with those who were p24 -ve. For caesarean section and zidovudine in preventing vertical transmission, see p34. PCP (below). CMV may be fatal in infants whose mother's HIV status wasn't recognized in pregnancy.[351] **Diagnosing vertically acquired HIV-1** *Don't use standard tests* (placentally transferred IgG lasts for ≤18 months). Virus culture and PCR are reliable, and more sensitive than finding p23 antigen in blood. HIV-specific IgA doesn't cross the placenta, but only occurs in 50% of infected infants <6 months old. Discuss with lab. ▶Aim to diagnose 95% of infected infants before the age of 1 month. Monitoring CD4 counts (OHCM p413) helps in staging HIV. The all clear can only be given if all tests are negative at 18 months.

Consider HIV in children with: PUO; lymphadenopathy; hepatosplenomegaly; persistent diarrhoea; parotid enlargement; shingles; extensive molluscum; platelets↓; recurrent slow-to-clear infections; failure to thrive; clubbing; unexplained organ disease;[352] TB; pneumocystosis; toxoplasmosis; cryptococcosis; histoplasmosis; CMV; LIP (below). *Suspect non-vertical HIV seroconversion illness if:* T°↑, fatigue, rash, pharyngitis, lymphadenopathy, oral ulcers, D&V, headache, myalgia, arthralgia, meningism, peripheral neuropathy, thrush, weight↓, night sweats, genital ulcers, WCC↓; platelets↓; transaminases↑.[353]

HIV & the lung: TB; lymphocytic interstitial pneumonia (LIP), immune reconstitution inflammatory syndrome, malignancy, bronchiectasis.[354] *LIP:* tachypnoea; hypoxia; clubbing; diffuse reticulonodular infiltrates on CXR; bilateral hilar lymphadenopathy. It is not AIDS-defining. It is less serious than pneumocystosis.

Prognosis By 3yrs old, up to half with early-onset opportunistic infection have died *vs* 3% of those with no such infection. Children with slow progression of HIV have persistent neutralizing antibodies. Transplacental passage of maternal neutralizing antibody may also have a role.

Guidelines for preventing pneumocystosis (PCP) with co-trimoxazole		
Age/HIV status	*PCP prophylaxis*	*Do CD4 cell counts at:*
0-5wks, HIV exposed	No	1 month
5wks-4 months, HIV exposed	No	3 months
4-12 months: -HIV infected	Yes	6, 9, and 12 months
-Status unknown	Yes	6, 9, and 12 months
-No HIV infection	No	No monitoring needed
1-5yrs, HIV infected	Yes, if CD4 <500/µL*	At least every 3-4 months
6-12yrs, HIV infected	Yes, if CD4 <200/µL*	At least every 3-4 months
	*or CD4 %age <15%	

Ensure full course of vaccines (+*Pneumococcus*; avoid live vaccines if very immunocompromised, and BCG if symptomatic and TB prevalence is low).[355,356]

Highly active antiretroviral therapy[HAART] Use PENTA regimen. [Pediatric Eurpean Network for the Treatment of AIDS][357] (OHCM p413). Those with AIDS-defining conditions or CD4 <15% (esp. if falling) should start HAART at once. If few symptoms and CD4 stable at >20% get advice.[358] *Obstacles:* Poor adherence (unpleasant tasting pills); SE (lipids↑, glucose↑, bone metabolism↓); lack of family routines.[359] Diarrhoea-related morbidity:[360] micronutrient (eg Zn) zinc supplementation helps.[361] ▶Teach HIV+ve children about safe sex and other HIV issues before puberty.

1 NB: it is perfectly possible for a woman who has vertical HIV to produce HIV -ve babies.

▶Involve social services *today* when issues of abuse arise. Read what follows with local child protection and NICE guidelines,[362] and relevant legislation in your country, eg in England, the *Children's Act* (states that *the child's welfare is always paramount*). Abuse may be physical, sexual, emotional, or by neglect. In *Munchausen's by proxy*, a parent fabricates alarming symptoms in their child to gain attention via dangerous interventions. *Risk factors:* Birthweight <2500g; mother <30yrs; unwanted pregnancy; stress; poverty.[363] *Prevalence:* 1% of A&E work.[364] ◆ *Suspect abuse if:* Disclosure by child, or:

• Odd story, incongruent with injuries; odd mode of injury; odd set of signs.
• Late visit to an unknown doctor, or taken by someone who is not a parent.
• History inconsistent with the child's development. Can the baby really walk?
• Efforts to avoid full examination, eg after an immersion burn.
• Psychological sequelae (stress; depression) from sexual or emotional abuse.[1]
• Unexplained fractures, eg forearm or rib (esp. posterior, from squeezing).[365]
• Buttock, perineum or face injury; intracranial bleeds;[366] torn lingual frenulum; vitreous/retinal bleeds, hyphaema (p452), lens dislocation, bulging fontanelle; head circumference↑ ± xanthochromia; ▶if in doubt, do CT. *Also:* Cigarette burns; whip marks (outline of belt/buckle, or double electric flex); bruised non-mobile baby; signs of suffocation; fingermark bruising; perforated pharynx.[367]

▶NB: site or type of fracture can never be *relied on* to distinguish abuse from an accident (extraordinary things, even spiral fractures, can happen in play).

ΔΔ: Osteogenesis imperfecta; osteoporosis, eg from propionic acidaemia.[368,369]

Dangerous questions Although non-medical, these need addressing because we are not simply technicians following protocols, and they influence what we do, how we react to child abuse, and how society perceives our role.

• Could *proving* of abuse be more destructive than the abuse itself?[1] Note that even if the answer is yes, society places a duty on us to report abuse.
• Is it better for him to be loved and battered than neither?
• Is help from the extended family more desirable than the law? Is it possible that the parents can grow through crisis, as abuse is discussed and help given?

Remember that the first aim is to prevent organ damage, murder, and other significant harm. If this is a real danger ▶contact the duty social worker to-day—eg for an emergency protection order. Offer help to the parents. Learn to listen, leaving blame and punishment to judges. Find out about local policies and referral routes. Remember that often our duty is not to diagnose child abuse, but to recognize *possible* abuse, and then to get help.

Sexual abuse This may be prevented by teaching about 'personal safety' and how to say 'No'. Know your local guidelines. Inform Social Services. If you do not, ask yourself with whom you are colluding. Forensic specimens (eg pubic hair, vaginal swabs) are to be taken by an expert who knows how to be gentle, and to avoid a 'second rape'. Prepubertal venereal disease means abuse until proven otherwise. Does abuse cause psychological harm? Yes, usually, but the position is complex. See p323.

Repertoire of actions in primary care ▶After informing Social Services, liaise with health visitor (may be a very helpful source of information) or NSPCC (National Society for the Prevention of Cruelty to Children).

• Admission to a place of safety (eg hospital or foster home).
• Continuing support for parents and protection for siblings.
• Prevention: encourage impulses to be shared, and not acted on.
• Attend a case conference (social worker, health visitor, paediatrician; police).[2]

---

1 K Hulme 1984 *Bone People*. This novel tests Samuel Johnson's aphorism that 'it is better that a man should be abused than be forgotten'. Read it before making quick judgments about families.

A possible sequence of events might be:

Unexplained signs (or disclosure, or allegations), eg odd bruising

↓

'Testing of professional hypotheses' ≈ weighing it up in your own mind

↓

'Clarification by discussion with an experienced colleague' ≈ tell your boss

↓

'Reach a critical threshold of professional concern' ≈ you're both worried

↓

'Weigh the pros and cons of breaking confidentiality' ≈ you must breach confidentiality if doing so prevents a serious crime against a child.

↓

'Sharing concerns with statutory agencies' ≈ phone Social Services/police

↓

'Act within a timeframe not detrimental to the child' ≈ aim to do it now

↓

'Contemporaneous records detailing all your sources'≈ write it down now

↓

'Preliminary consultation with all concerned': don't promise to keep secrets

↓

'Strategic multidisciplinary discussion' ≈ is an abuse investigation needed?

↓

If so, 'Instigation of child abuse investigation' ≈ plan case conference

↓

'Must parents/child be present?' ≈ bend the ear of the conference chairman

↓

Tell parents & child (if appropriate) what your report to conference will be

↓

Case conference timed to let doctors fulfil their major role ≈ ?get a locum

↓

Register your dissent (if any) to the conference conclusions in its minutes

↓

Child is placed on a Register indicating that questions of abuse are unresolved and that the child remains at risk

↓

'Establish networks for information exchange, discussion & advice' ≈ follow up by Social Services, or a national society protecting children from cruelty (NSPCC)

↓

Second (review) conference to weigh new evidence

↓

Death of a child

↓

Agencies must issue reports to the Area Child Protection Committee UK

↓

Judge issues life sentence (♂ breadwinner removed from family for 10yrs)

↓

No ♂ role model for siblings ≈ perpetuation of cycles of poverty and abuse

↓

Unexplained bruising in a member of the next generation

↓

Man hands on misery to man [*]

M an hands on misery to man.
It deepens like a coastal shelf.
Get out as early as you can,
And don't have any kids yourself   *Philip Larkin, *This Be The Verse*

Not all our efforts to protect children end thus. Successes are frequent. And of course this sequence oversimplifies...the sign ≈ is not meant flippantly: it is intended as shorthand, denoting the exercise of reflection, good judgment, action, and the following of agreed procedures.

Paediatrics

2 The UK Families at Risk Review (2008) specifies joined-up agencies that 'ensure' that there is 'no wrong door' that families knock on—all doors lead to getting the correct help. Also: •Confirm social services referrals in writing •Question other's opinions if you disagree. •Document all phone-calls •Record discussions if there is disagreement over risk of deliberate harm.

Definition Sudden unexplained infant death refers to unexpected death <12 months where a cause is not immediately obvious *prior* to investigation. It includes deaths due to infection, metabolic errors, accidental suffocation and SIDS. Sudden infant death syndrome (SIDS) is 'Sudden death under 12 months old, which is unexpected after a thorough case investigation, including a complete autopsy, examination of the death scene, and review of the clinical history.' ▶SIDS is the leading 'cause' of death in infants aged over 1 week old.

Putative causes:
Obstructive apnoea:
• Inhalation of milk
• Airways oedema
• Passive smoking
Central apnoea:
• Faulty CO_2 drive
• Prematurity
• Brainstem gliosis
Others:
• Long Q–T interval[1]
• Staph infection[2]
• Overheating
• ↑Vagal tone or Mg^{2+}↑
• Immature diaphragm
• Genetic & viral causes

Epidemiology Peak incidence: 1–4 months; risk↑ if: poor, parents are smokers, baby is male or premature, winter, previous sibling affected by SIDS; co-existing minor upper respiratory infection is common, co-sleeping. There are many causal theories (SEE MINIBOX).

Sleeping supine ('back to sleep', even for short naps),[370] preventing overheating, and cigarette smoke exposure are the chief preventive interventions: risk from passive smoking is dose-dependent, and often at least doubles risk.[371]

The face is an important platform for heat loss—and it is known that the incidence of SIDS is ~5–10-fold higher among infants usually sleeping prone (17-fold higher if sleeping in a room separated from parents): ▶so always recommend sleeping supine. Advise as follows:
• Do not overheat the baby's bedroom. Aim for a temperature of 16–20°C.
• Do not use too much bedding, and avoid duvets if less than 1 year of age.
• If ill or feverish, consult a GP—do not increase the amount of bedding.
• Have feet come down to the cot's end to avoid under-blankets migration.
• While sleeping, avoid heaters, hot water bottles, electric blankets, and hats. Do wrap up for trips out in winter, but unwrap once indoors, even if this means disturbing the baby. Never tuck in blankets higher than the armpit.[372]
• Babies >1 month do not need to be kept as warm as in hospital nurseries.
• Avoid co-sleeping if possible and never, even if very tired (new parents!), if parents are deep sleepers, or if they have had any alcohol or drugs.[373,374]

Autopsy is unrevealing; minor changes are common; petechial haemorrhages over pleura, pericardium, or thymus, and vomit in the trachea may be agonal events. *Causes to exclude:* sepsis, metabolic defects (eg MCAD deficiency; medium-chain acyl-CoA dehydrogenase↓, p183); heart defects; and always bear in mind the possibility of murder.

Action after failed resuscitation in the Emergency Department
• Document all interventions, venepuncture sites, and any marks on the baby. You don't have to keep all tubes *in situ*, but ensure that someone who did not intubate confirms endotracheal placement of the tube before extubation.
• Take samples of blood for culture, CSF for culture/PCR, urine, and stool.
• Keep all clothing and the nappy.
• Explain clearly to parents that despite your best efforts, the baby has died.
• Unless the cause is obvious, be non-committal about cause of death. Explain the baby *must* have a post mortem (this is a coroner's case).
• Contact the consultant on call, the police, child protection team, and the coroner at once; also GP, health visitor, and any other involved professions.

1 Risk↑ if Q–T corrected for rate (QT^c) ≥440msec. QT^c=(Q–T)/($\sqrt{R–R}$).[375,376] LQTS genes are important.[377]
2 Staphs in mattress foam are implicated (∴ do not reuse); Jenkins 2005[378,379]

How the GP can help the family on the first day
• A prompt visit to express sympathy emphasizing that no one is to blame.
• Explain about the legal requirement for an autopsy and coroner's inquest. The parents may be called upon to identify the body.
• Bedding may be needed to help find the cause of death.

Subsequent help
Don't *automatically* suppress lactation, but if this becomes necessary cabergoline (250μg/12h PO for 48h) is preferred to bromocriptine. NB: continued lactation may be an important way of grieving for some mothers.

Many parents will not want anxiolytics, but may want hypnotics.

Advise the parents of likely grief reactions (guilt, anger, loss of appetite, hearing the baby cry). Make sure that the coroner informs you of the autopsy result; take some trouble to explain these to the parents. They should already have a routine appointment with a consultant paediatrician. This can provide helpful reinforcement and encouragement to the parents and yourself. The parents may find an electronic apnoea alarm reassuring in caring for later infants. Ask if they would like to join a self-help group. Programmes exist to prevent a future SID—eg the CONI programme (care of next infant).

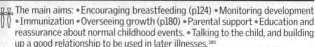

The main aims: • Encouraging breastfeeding (p124) • Monitoring development • Immunization • Overseeing growth (p180) • Parental support • Education and reassurance about normal childhood events. • Talking to the child, and building up a good relationship to be used in later illnesses.[380]

Monitoring The most cost-effective times to screen are unknown. A *best buy* might be checks after birth (p114), at 4–6 weeks; arrange vaccinations and DOH vitamin drops (A, D & C, unless sure that diet/sunlight is adequate[1]), then:

1–9 months:	Hips, testes descent, CVS examination.
18–24 months:	*Educate* on diet, dental care, accidents; walking (look for waddling), social and linguistic milestones; Hb if *iron deficiency* likely—it may well be. *Any parental depression?*
4 years:	Testes descent, CVS examination. Nutrition, dental care.

At each visit: • Encourage airing of queries • Ask about, and test for, squint, vision and deafness • Chart centiles. *Beware reading too much into a single test*. Remember to correct age for prematurity. Note the milestones below. There is much individual variation.

1 month:	Lifts head when prone; responds to bell; regards face.
2 months:	Holds head at 45° when prone; vocalizes; smiles.
4 months:	Uses arm support when prone; holds head steady when supported while sitting; reaches out; spontaneous smiling.
6 months:	Bears some weight on legs; on pulling to sitting, there is no head lag; reaching out; transfers things from hand to hand.
≥1 year:	Just stands; walks using a table's support; clashes cubes; pincer grip; can say 'Mummy' ± 'Daddy'. Plays 'pat a cake'.
18 months:	Can walk backwards; scribbles; 2-cube tower. 2–4 words. Recognizes/shows interest in TV images, eg of a dog. NB: drooling ± throwing items on the floor is abnormal by now.
2 years:	Kicks a ball; overarm 'bowling'; gets undressed.
3 years:	Jumps; can stand on one foot; copies; can build an 8-cube tower; knows his first and last name; dressing needs help.
4 years:	Stands on 1 foot for >4sec; picks the longer of 2 lines.

Health promotion in refugee children/asylum-seekers Unaccompanied children may request asylum explicitly or implicitly. Our job is to look after them, not to interpret laws. ☙ Tell immigration officers/police that children cannot be detained even if there is doubt about a child's age. UK immigration officers must abide by the UN convention on the Rights of the Child (1989). This stipulates that each State must ensure the rights of each child within its jurisdiction *without discrimination of any kind*. Any child who has been tortured has the right to physical and psychological recovery and social integration. (Prison is not a form of social integration.) Take any opportunity to promote children's health. If from areas of chronic conflict, don't assume the child has been vaccinated. Start from scratch. Test for TB (skin test) and give BCG, or refer to a chest clinic if needed. See Home Office[381] & Royal College Guidelines.[382] Paediatricians and GPs can promote refugee health by:

• Documenting development, ensuring nutrition, and treating physical illness.
• Easing access to antenatal and all other preventive care activities.
• Identifying depression/anxiety, and picking up clues that torture may have taken place: nightmares; hallucinations; panic attacks; sexual problems; phobias; difficulties with relationships. These may also be signs that the child has been recruited to fight other people's wars. Treating childhood depression is controversial (SSRI, p390) *but not treating it may be worse*.[383]
• Recognizing and treating TB and HIV (eg if vertically transmitted, look for persistent oral candida, caries, UTIs, widespread lymphadenopathy, hepatosplenomegaly; failure to thrive; developmental delay). See p145.
• Liaising with social services to ensure housing and schooling.

2 months	**Pediacel®**, ie 5-in-1 diphtheria + tetanus + acellular pertussis + inactivated polio + haemophilus B (HIB); if prem, still give at 2 months; can give if ≤10 yrs if missed vacs + **Prevenar 13®** (13-valent pneumococcal).
3 months	**Pediacel®** + **Neisvac C®** or **Meningitec®** (Meningitis C vaccine)
4 months	**Pediacel®** + **Prevenar 13®** + **Neisvac C®** or **Meningitec®**
12 months	**Menitorix®** (*H. influenzae* with meningitis C)
13 months	**MMR^L** or **Priorix®^L** (Measles, Mumps & Rubella) + **Prevenar 13®**
3¼-5yrs	**Repevax®** or **Infanrix-IPV®** (Diphtheria, tetanus, pertussis & polio) + **Priorix®^L** or **MMR^L**
13-18⁺yrs	**Revaxis®** (low-dose diphtheria, tetanus, inactivated polio; can also be used for primary vaccination if >10yrs). **Gardasil®** (against human papilloma virus) protects somewhat against cervical cancer: see p272.
70-80yrs	**Zostavax®** for herpes zoster (licensed but not marketed in UK)[385]
Any age	BCG^L (not universal in UK) If at ↑risk of TB, eg for all from high-prevalence country, ie >40:100,000/yr, or a visitor to such a country for >1 month. May start at 3 days old. **Hepatitis B:** p263; universal (WHO advice) or if at ↑risk. **Hepatitis B** may be given at any age if presents late. One-off **pneumococcal vaccine** with 23-valent Pneumovax II® (**Prevenar 13®**×2, as above, if <2yrs); yearly **'flu vaccine** if risk↑: see *OHCM* p390. Consider 2nd pneumococcal vaccine if at ↑risk after >5yrs.[386]
Pregnant	Pertussis (as **Repevax®**) and flu, as indicated.
Adults any	Tetanus and diphtheria boosters (**Revaxis®**, as above). Travellers: p367.

►An acute febrile illness is a contraindication to any vaccine. Note: Give live vaccines either together, or separated by ≥3 weeks.

Don't give live vaccines if primary immunodeficiency, or if on steroids (≥2mg/kg/day of prednisolone); but if HIV+ve, give all immunizations (including live) except for BCG, in areas where TB prevalence is low.

Hepatitis B (Engerix B®): see *OHCM* p262. Give at birth, 1 & 2 months, if mother is HBsAG +ve—0.5mL IM via anterolateral thigh. If birthweight ≤1500g give Hep B immunoglobulin as well as vaccine, regardless of mother's e-antigen status. If at term, give Hep B Ig unless mother is anti-HBe +ve.

HPV vaccination to prevent cervical cancer: see p272.

Chickenpox vaccination: In the USA this is routine and has greatly reduced incidence and hospitalizations/mortality.[387] Eradication is impossible.

Immunization in immunodeficiencies: See Royal College Guidelines.

Can the pain of the injection be reduced? Topical lidocaine–prilocaine 5% cream (EMLA®) and oral glucose at the time of vaccination does decrease the latency to 1st cry, and other objective markers of pain.[388]

MMR is not just for children: In the UK, in 2005, mumps rates rose 10-fold (to 5000/month), eg among students who were too old to have had full vaccination. Any non-immune adult is eligible for MMR (exclude pregnancy). If >18 months, the 2 doses of MMR should be separated by 3 months. MMR vaccine may also be offered to unimmunized, or measles-only immunized or seronegative post-partum women. *Does MMR vaccine cause autism?* No. Large-scale studies find no link and *The Lancet* has withdrawn the paper suggesting a link. Some parents prefer single M, M, & R injections, but the rationale is unclear.

What sort of needle? For IM vaccination, WHO advises that needles are 25mm long (blue in the UK).[389] Stretch the skin flat between thumb and forefinger to aid a deep injection—and make the angle (needle to skin) 90°. The subcutaneous route is OK for MMR; bunch the skin up, and inject at 45° into fat.

---

1 Adequate sunlight to prevent rickets is a big issue, especially north of Oxford (51°45') as UV-B is too scarce to make active vitamin D in winter.[390-392] Risk of rickets↑ if: skin pigmented; sunscreens or concealing clothing used; staying indoors to play video-games⬤⬤ (the old and institutionalized are at ↑risk too); obesity; malabsorption; renal and liver disease; using anticonvulsants. Good vit. D status in pregnancy (p8) helps neonatal bones, immune function, and lungs (asthma risk↓ by 40%⬤⬤).[393]

Paediatrics

▶It is as important to be able to love the handicapped and to respect their carers as it is to prevent the handicap; in doing the first we become more human. In the second, do we risk our own inappropriate deification?

Gene probes use recombinant DNA technology to identify specific mutations causing genetic diseases (eg Huntington's chorea; muscular dystrophy; polycystic kidneys; cystic fibrosis; thalassaemias) to DNA markers scattered throughout our genome. Using fetal DNA from amniotic fluid cells (amniocentesis) in the 2nd trimester, or from chorionic villus sampling in the 1st.

Enzyme defects Many of the inborn errors of metabolism can be diagnosed by incubation of fetal tissue with a specific substrate.

Chromosomal studies can be undertaken on cultured cells or on direct villus preparations. The most important abnormalities are aneuploidies (abnormalities in chromosome number)—eg trisomy 21, 18, and 13.

Screening for chromosomal abnormalities (eg the fragile X syndrome, p648) may be performed on at-risk mothers who may be carriers.

Non-disjunction After meiosis one gamete contains two chromosomes 21 (say)[11] and the other gamete has no chromosome 21. After union of the 1st gamete with a normal gamete, the conceptus has trisomy 21, and develops Down's syndrome (50% spontaneously abort). This is the cause in ≥88% of Down's babies, and relates to maternal age (p12).

Robertsonian translocations (fig 1) entail a fusion between the centromeres of 2 chromosomes with loss of the short arms forming a chromosome with two long arms, one derived from each chromosome. They involve any 2 of chromosomes 13, 14, 15, 21 & 22 (all acrocentric, ie the centromere is close to one end; the short arms contain few genes). This translocation trisomy 21 is the cause in 4% of Down's syndrome (unrelated to maternal age). If the father carries the translocation, risk of Down's is 10%; if it is the mother, the risk is 50%. 0.3% of mothers have this translocation.

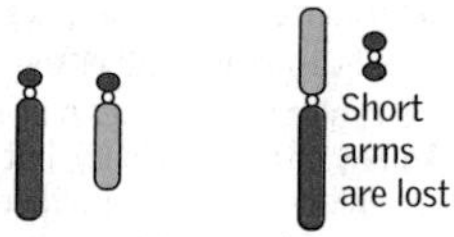

Short arms are lost

Two acrocentric chromosomes

A Robertsonian translocation

Fig 1. A chromosome with 2 long arms.

Balanced translocations entail no net gain or loss of chromosomal material, two chromosomes have been broken and rejoined in the wrong combination.

Mosaicism A trisomy may develop during early divisions of a normal conceptus (∴ somatic, not germline). If the proportion of trisomy 21 cells is low (eg 4%) CNS development may be 'normal'. It accounts for ≤8% of Down's babies.[394]

Other chromosomal abnormalities Edward's (p642), Klinefelter's (p646), Patau's (p650), and Turner's (p655) syndromes. In the *cri-du-chat* syndrome there is deletion of the short arm of chromosome 5, causing a high-pitched cry, CVS abnormalities, microcephaly, and widely spaced eyes, and a 'moon' face.

Down's syndrome *Causes:* See above. *Recognition at birth:* Flat facial profile, abundant neck skin, dysplastic ears, muscle hypotonia, and x-ray evidence of a dysplastic pelvis are the most constant features. Other features: see BOX. Widely spaced 1st & 2nd toes and a high-arched palate are more visible later. If uncertain, it is best to ask an expert's help, rather than baffle the mother by taking karyotype tests "just in case it's Down's".[2] *Associated problems:* Duodenal atresia; VSD; patent ductus; AVSD (foramen primum defects, p136); and, later, a low IQ and a small stature. Helping the mother accept her (often very lovable) child may be aided by introducing her to a friendly mother of a baby with Down's syndrome. *Prenatal diagnosis:* p10–12.

1 Chromosome 21 contains only 225 genes: most of its DNA is apparently meaningless.
2 Even in good hands, accuracy of suspicion is only 64%, so at some stage karyotyping is needed.[395]

Paediatrics

Ways of looking at genetic diseases such as Down's syndrome

The swot's approach: Learn the clinical manifestations—it might be asked in an exam. In the case of Down's syndrome, this person will focus on features such as a simian palmar crease, hypotonia, flat face/round head, protruding tongue, broad hands, upward slanted palpebral fissures and epicanthic folds, speckled irises (Brushfield spots); mental and growth retardation; pelvic dysplasia, cardiac malformations, short, broad hands, hypoplasia of middle phalanx of (incurving) 5th finger, intestinal atresia, and high arched palate. Associations learned about:[396][NICE]

- Lung problems (lung capacity is reduced in almost 100%)
- Hearing loss (60%)
- Congenital heart disease (40%)
- Digestive problems 6%
- Leukaemia
- 44% survive to age 60 yrs. 50% of adult survivors develop Alzheimer's.

The problem with this approach is that it does not make us good doctors because it is not much help to people and their families.

The dangerous young idealist: Down's syndrome is preventable. The focus should be on prenatal diagnosis and termination of affected fetuses. Down's cases are unfortunate. They are a burden to the State (he might argue). Their claims on scarce health resources are burdensome. Normal people should take priority.

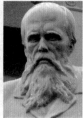

Fig 1. Dostoevsky.
Courtesy of Dr C Joyce.

The problem with this approach is that no-one is genetically normal. This man has engaged in too much abstract thought, and as Dostoevsky has said: 'too much abstract thought makes men cruel'. *Crime and Punishment*

The health needs approach: This approach starts by asking: How can I help? Health maintenance for Down's children is more important, not less, compared with the needs of other children—because their families are vulnerable, and many conditions are more likely in those with Down's. Examples are otitis media, thyroid disease, congenital cataracts, leukaemoid reactions, dental problems, and feeding difficulties.[397]

The patient-centred approach: Let's go down to the farm and milk the cow. *Let's see how muddy we can get...*

Different approaches are needed at different times: a key skill in becoming a good doctor is to be able to move seamlessly from one approach to another—and knowing when to adopt which approach.

Dostoevsky muddies the waters of abstract thought...so let's see just how muddy we can get.

The American College of Medical Genetics screens for:

Organic acid disorders:	*Fatty acid disorders:*	*Amino acid disorders:*
β-ketothiolase deficiency	Carnitine uptake defect	Arginosuccinic acidaemia
Glutaric acidaemia type 1	Long-chain hydroxyacyl-coa dehydrogenase lack	Citrullaemia
Hydroxymethylglutaric acidaemia	Medium-chain acyl-coa dehydrogenase deficiency	Homocystinuria
Isovaleric acidaemia		Maple syrup urine disease
3-methylcrotonyl-coa carboxylase deficiency	Trifunctional protein deficiency	Phenylketonuria
Methylmalonic acidaemia	Very-long-chain acyl-coa dehydrogenase deficit	Tyrosinaemia type 1
Multiple carboxylate deficiency	*Haemoglobin disorders:*	*Other congenital diseases:*
Propionic acidaemia	Hb S/β-thalassaemia	Biotinidase deficiency
	Hb S/C disease	Adrenal hyperplasia
	Sickle-cell anaemia	Hypothyroidism
		Cystic fibrosis
		Galactosaemia
		Hearing disorders

The great question is: Just because a disease can be screened for, should it be screened for? Answer: Only if the Wilson criteria are met: see p486.

Goal To provide accurate, up-to-date information on genetic conditions to enable families and patients to make informed decisions.

▶Genetic counselling is best done in regional centres to which you should refer families (nearest centre: UK tel.: 020 7794 0500). *Don't do blood tests on children lightly which might have long-term consequences, unless some form
of treatment is available. The child may never forgive you for labelling him
or her.*

In order to receive most benefit from referral:

• The affected person (proband) ideally comes with family (spouse, parents,
children, siblings); individuals can of course be seen alone as well.
• The family should be informed that a detailed pedigree (family tree) will be
made, and medical details of distant relatives may be asked for.
• Irrational emotions (guilt, blame, anger) are common. Deal with these sensitively, and do not ignore. *Remember:* you do not choose your ancestors, and
you cannot control what you pass on to your descendants.
• Warn patients that most tests give no absolute 'yes' or 'no' but merely 'likely'
or 'unlikely'. In gene tracking, where a molecular fragment near the gene is
followed through successive family members, the degree of certainty of the
answer will depend on the distance between the marker and the gene (as
crossing-over in meiosis may separate them).
• Accept that some people will not want testing, eg the offspring of a Huntington's chorea sufferer—or a mother of a boy who might have fragile X
syndrome, but who understandably does not want her offspring labelled
(employment, insurance, and social reasons). Offer a genetic referral to ensure that her decision is fully informed (but remember: 'being fully informed'
may itself be deleterious to health and wellbeing).

Naming chromosomes Autosomes are numbered 1 to 22 roughly in order of
size, 1 being the largest. The arms on each side of the centromere are named 'p'
(petite) for the short arm, and 'q' for the long arm (there's always a long Q for a
short P). Thus 'the long arm of chromosome 6' is written '6q'.

Chromosomal disorders include Down's (trisomy 21, p152), Turner's (45,X0,
p655) and Klinefelter's (47,XXY, p646) syndromes. Many genes are involved
when the defect is large enough to be seen microscopically.

Autosomal-dominants Adult polycystic kidney (16p), Huntington's chorea,
(4p). A single copy of a defective gene causes damage. Some people inheriting
the defective gene are phenotypically normal (=*reduced penetrance*).

Autosomal recessives Infantile polycystic kidney; cystic fibrosis (7q),
β-thalassaemia, sickle cell (11p), most metabolic conditions, and almost all
which are fatal in childhood. In general, both genes must be defective before
damage is seen, so carriers are common. Both parents must be carriers for
offspring to be affected, so consanguinity (marrying relatives) increases risk.

X-linked Duchenne muscular dystrophy, p642; haemophilia A & B; fragile X
(p648). In female (XX) carriers a normal gene on the 2nd X chromosome prevents bad effects manifesting. Males (XY) have no such protection.

NB: being pregnant and unwilling to consider termination does *not* exclude one
from undergoing useful genetic counselling.

'Couple screening' A big problem with counselling is the unnecessary alarm
caused by false +ve tests. In cystic fibrosis screening (analysis of cells in
mouthwash samples) this is reducible by 97% (0.08% *vs* 3.2%) by screening
mother and father together—who need only get alarmed if *both* turn out
to be screen-positive. The trouble with this is false reassurance. Many forget
that they will need future tests if they have a different partner, and those who
do not are left with some lingering anxieties.

Genetic counselling to try to influence pregnancy outcome?

Three contrasting principles:
1 The parents must decide: counselling must be non-directive.
2 Every newborn child has the right to be born healthy, if possible.
3 Every child has a right to be born.

Non-directive counselling is something of a mantra among counsellors, partly as a reaction to Nazi eugenic abuses, and partly because of an un-willingness to promulgate a single view of what is right in what can be a very complex area. Public health doctors are questioning this obedience to the non-directive ethic because, from their point of view, it makes attain-ment of their chief goal more difficult—namely to improve the health and wellbeing of all residents, including newborns. For example, we should tell pregnant women not to drink much alcohol, public health doctors assert, be-cause this is necessary to prevent the fetal alcohol syndrome. The same goes for other syndromes. When we know what to do we should state clearly and unequivocally what the mother should do. This is our duty to her and her unborn child.

Let us examine the public health doctor's standpoint more closely. He wants to improve health. To do this, it is necessary to define health. We have done this elsewhere (p470) and have argued that health entails more than just soundness of body and mind. It is not clear that an autocratic society in which patients were told what to do would be more healthy than a society of autonomous individuals each addressing the great questions of health and existence from his or her own viewpoint.

Another problem for the public health doctors is that, in the case above, it is not clear whether the directive 'don't drink if you are pregnant' would lead to fewer children with the fetal alcohol syndrome. It might lead to more orphans (a mother knows she is doing wrong, feels guilty, avoids health professionals, and dies of some unforeseen consequence of pregnancy, or from guilt-borne suicide).[398]

As ever, the way forward is not by abstract thought but by getting to know our patients better. There may be rare occasions when we know our patients well enough to risk "You are mad not to follow this advice...". But mostly we can-not be sure that this injunction will work, and it is wiser to explore the patient's world view and their expectations, and then use this knowledge to reframe the benefits of our proposed action in a way that makes sense to the individual concerned, taking into account his or her culture and system of beliefs.

In the UK, the Children's Act states that the welfare of the child is para-mount. What this means in the context of a family is open to interpretation.

Paediatrics

Childhood obesity is rising fast in the West.[1] Half the children born in the UK will soon be obese—by the time they are 10[399]💬—with inevitable consequences for heart disease and cancer. It is known for example that there is a higher prevalence of colorectal cancer in men who were overweight during adolescence. Similar effects are seen for cancers of the endometrium, kidney, gallbladder, and breast.[400] Consequences *vis à vis* insulin resistance: >30% of obese children have insulin resistance (detailed on p252),[2] and ~25% of all adolescents have 3 or more features of the metabolic syndrome x: obesity, hypertension, dyslipidaemia, and poor glycaemic control.[401] ▶Risk factors for adult heart disease and DM begin to cluster in 'normal' children.[402] Primary prevention must start in childhood.💬 Hence the need for recognizing small differences from normal in apparently health children. See BP table below, and p226 for centile BMI charts defining obesity by age. But do not focus exclusively on weight. Insulin resistance starts before the teenage years—and may occur in children of near-normal weight.[403] *UK incidence of type 2 DM in children: 0.2:100,000[404](↑×13 if Asian). When to start prevention?* It is never too early (obesity can start with bottle feeding)[405]—and it's often too late. Re-educate parents, teachers, and children; encourage exercise—and less: •Fast foods[406] •Soft drinks[407] •TV[408] •Sun-bathing (melanoma).[409] Cognitive therapy (p373) may be the best approach to re-orientate adolescents towards health.[410]

We assume that growth and development somewhere in the middle of our centile charts is optimal. But these charts are not goals—they are statements of heights and weights for particular historical populations. Now population weights are moving up, what appears normal to parents (and us) may in fact be detrimental. For example, in Plymouth, in the UK, mean weights of toddlers are now 460g heavier than the historic reference population.[411]

Age	Significant hypertension		Severe hypertension	
(Years)	Systolic mmHg	Diastolic mmHg	Systolic mmHg	Diastolic mmHg
Birth	≥96mmHg[3]		≥106mmHg[3]	
<2	≥112	≥74 [k4]	≥118	≥82 [k4]
3-5	≥116	≥76 [k4]	≥124	≥84 [k4]
6-9	≥122	≥78 [k4]	≥130	≥86 [k4]
10-12	≥126	≥82 [k4]	≥134	≥90 [k4]
13-15	≥136	≥86 [k5]	≥144	≥92 [k5]
16-18	≥142	≥92 [k5]	≥150	≥98 [k5]

Take ≥3 BPs (snugly fitted cuff of bladder-width >75% of upper arm length) >1 week apart (in general) before diagnosing hypertension. As the 5th Korotkoff sound (k5) is inaudible, use k4 for diastolic BPs, until adolescence.💬 Some BP standards break populations by age, sex, and height, but this doesn't greatly change hypertension prevalence.[412,413] Ambulatory BPs can show that white coat hypertension is about as common in children as in adults.[414,415] But beware automated devices: mercury sphygmomanometers are more accurate, and are of negligible risk to health.

---

1 Health Survey 2005; >25% are currently overweight/obese.[416]
2 Viner R 2005 *Arch Dis Child* **90** 10[417] *Correlates of 'normal children' in the top quintile of postprandial glucose (7.4–11.4mmol/L):*
•Lower vasodilatation to acetylcholine (Ach, P <0.005) and sodium nitroprusside (SNP, P <0.02) than those in the lower quintile (3.9–4.9mmol/L).
•↑Waist-to-hip ratio and ↑fasting insulin resistance.
•↑Fasting triglycerides & cholesterol (r–0.4, P <0.05).[418] **MODY**=maturity onset diabetes of the young.
3 Doppler may be needed. Often only systolic BPs are recordable. Values need adjusting if taller or shorter than expected for age (tables are available); compared with a 50th height-centile the reference interval is 1–4mmHg lower for a child on the 5th height-centile (1–4mmHg higher if on 95th centile).[419]

Causes of raised blood pressure in children

Neonates: Renal artery stenosis (or thrombosis), congenital renal malformations, coarctation of the aorta, bronchopulmonary dysplasia.

Infants: Renal parenchymal disease, coarctation, renal artery stenosis.

6–10yrs olds: Renal artery stenosis, renal diseases, primary hypertension.

Adolescence: Primary hypertension, renal diseases, syndrome x.

Stridor Acute stridor may be a terrifying experience for children; this fear may lead to hyperventilation, which worsens symptoms. Causes: p566. The leading causes to be distinguished are viral croup, bacterial tracheitis and epiglottitis (rare in the UK since haemophilus vaccination)—see BOX. Don't forget to consider inhaled foreign body if history doesn't seem quite right.

Investigations: This is a clinical diagnosis. Lateral neck x-ray (fig 1) may show an enlarged epiglottis, but this wastes time at a dangerous and critical time.

Croup (acute laryngotracheobronchitis) *Signs:* Stridor, barking cough, hoarseness from obstruction in the region of the larynx. *Age:* <6yrs. *Epidemics:* Autumn. *Causes:* Parainfluenza virus (1, 2, 3), respiratory syncytial virus, measles (rare). *Pathology:* Subglottic oedema, inflammation, and exudate. Croup is classified into mild/moderate and severe disease. *R:* Mild/moderate may be sent home if settles—eg with **dexamethasone**, 0.15mg/kg PO stat (some give more[420]) *or* prednisolone 1–2mg/kg stat. Anecdotal evidence says that warm, humid air helps, but mist tents have lost favour: they frighten, and subsequent hyperventilation worsens distress. *In hospital:* Aim for minimal interference and careful watching (TPR; S$_A$O$_2$) by experienced nurses. *Watch for severe signs:* Restlessness; cyanosis (give O$_2$); sternal retractions; rising pulse/respiratory rate; tiredness. If severe, use nebulized **adrenaline**[421] 1:1000 (5mL); if poor response, repeat, and take to ITU. Remember: volume of stridor is a factor of flow; in severe disease, stridor will be very soft. Failure to improve with steroids / nebulized adrenaline should prompt the consideration of **bacterial tracheitis**. This is defined by the presence of thick mucopurulent exudate and tracheal mucosal sloughing that is not cleared by coughing, and risks occluding the airway. There is often a history of a viral infection (such as croup) with an acute deterioration. Pronounced tracheal tenderness may be present.

▸▸*Managing suspected epiglottitis Stay calm! Avoid examining the throat.* This may precipitate obstruction. Do not bleed the patient or upset him. Summon the most experienced anaesthetist. Ask her to make the diagnosis by laryngoscopy. If epiglottitis (a cherry-red, swollen epiglottis), electively intubate *before* obstruction occurs. (A smaller diameter endotracheal tube than normal for that age may be needed). The cause is usually *Haemophilus influenzae* type b, treat with a 3rd generation cephalosporin (eg **cefotaxime**, 25–50mg/kg/8h IV). Bacterial tracheitis also benefits from early intubation, allowing pulmonary toilet and improved ventilation. Treat with cefotaxime + flucloxacillin. **Hydrocortisone** may be given in both, but isn't of proven value.

Diphtheria is caused by the toxin of *Corynebacterium diphtheriae*. It usually starts with tonsillitis ± a false membrane over the fauces. The toxin may cause polyneuritis, often starting with cranial nerves. Shock may occur from myocarditis, toxaemia, or cardiac conducting system involvement. Other signs: dysphagia; muffled voice; bronchopneumonia; airway obstruction preceded by a brassy cough (laryngotracheal diphtheria); nasal discharge with an excoriated upper lip (nasal diphtheria). If there is tachycardia out of proportion to fever, suspect toxin-induced myocarditis (do frequent ECGs). Motor palatal paralysis also occurs causing fluids to escape from the nose on swallowing.

Diagnosis: Swab culture of material below pseudomembrane; PCR.[422]

Treatment: ▸▸Diphtheria antitoxin: 10,000–30,000u IM[12](any age; more if severe, see *BNF*) and **erythromycin**; give contacts 7 days' **erythromycin** syrup: <2yrs old 125mg/6h PO (500mg per 6h if >8yrs) *before swab results are known.*

Risk ↑ if: Homeless/refugee; aged 3–6yrs old; in 'asocial' families. There is a now partly controlled[423] resurgence of diphtheria in north-west and central Russia[424] (relevant to travellers born before 1942, when vaccination started).

Prevention: Isolate until 3 –ve cultures separated by 48h. Vaccination: p151.

Paediatrics

Croup ... distinguished from ... bacterial tracheitis ... and ... Epiglottitis		
Common	Uncommon	Rare
6 months – 6 years	6 months – 14 years	2–7 years
Onset over a few days	Viral prodrome for 2-5 days, then rapid deterioration	▸▸Sudden onset
Stridor only when upset	Continuous stridor	▸▸Continuous stridor
Stridor sounds harsh	Stridor may be biphasic	▸▸Stridor softer, snoring
Swallows oral secretions	Swallows oral secretions	▸▸Drooling of secretions
Voice hoarse	Very hoarse	▸▸Voice muffled
Likely to be apyrexial	Moderate-high fever, appear toxic	▸▸Toxic and feverish (eg T° >39°C)
Barking cough	Barking cough	Cough not prominent

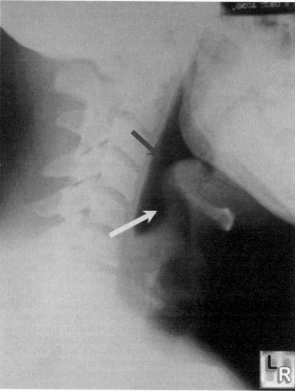

Fig 1. Lateral radiograph of the neck showing an enlarged epiglottis (red arrow) and thickening of the aryepiglottic folds (yellow arrow). There is reversal of the normal lordotic curve in the cervical spine and slight dilatation of the hypopharynx. learningradiology.com NB: the aryepiglottic folds are mucous membranes extending on each side between the lateral border of the epiglottis and the summit of the arytenoid cartilage. They form the lateral border to the top of the larynx.

Courtesy of Dr William Herring.

Paediatrics

▶If severely ill, think of staphs, streps, TB, and HIV (pneumocystosis, *OHCM* p154). *In chronic cough think of:* •Pertussis •TB •Foreign body •Asthma.

Acute bronchiolitis is *the* big lung infection in infants; coryza precedes cough, low fever, tachypnoea, wheeze, inspiratory crackles, apnoea, intercostal recession ± cyanosis. *Typical cause:* Winter respiratory syncytial virus (RSV); single-stranded RNA. *Others:* Mycoplasma, parainfluenza, adenoviruses. Those <6 months old are most at risk. *Signs prompting admission:* Poor feeding, >50 breaths/min, apnoea, dehydration, rib recession, patient or parental exhaustion. *Tests:* PCR/fluorescent antibody tests rarely contribute. If severe: CXR (hyperinflation); blood gases/SpO₂; FBC.[425] *R:* O₂ (stop when SpO₂ ≳92%);[426] nasogastric feeds. 5% need ventilating (mortality ≈1%; 33% if symptomatic congenital heart disease). Don't use bronchiodilators and steroids routinely.[427,428] Meta-analyses don't support ribavirin,[429] antibiotics (except possibly clarithromycin[430]), inhaled steroids,[431] physio,[432] or prevention with palivizumab (unless concurrent chest disease, chronic lung disease or history of prematurity).[427]

Pneumonia[433,434] *Signs:* T°↑, malaise, poor feeding, tachypnoea, cyanosis, grunting, rib recession;[435] older children may have typical lobar signs (pleural pain, crackles, bronchial breathing). *Admit:* if SpO₂ <90%; <6months; signs of respiratory distress; suspected MRSA; or concerns about observation at home.[434] *Tests:* Consider CXR/FBC/blood and sputum cultures. Detection of influenza / respiratory viruses decreases likelihood of needing antibiotics. Viral LRTI is more common than bacterial infection in children <2, so those with mild symptoms can typically be discharged without antibiotics (ensure follow up if symptoms persist). *Oral R:* Amoxicillin is 1ˢᵗ-line; alternatives: co-amoxiclav, cefaclor, erythromycin, azithromycin, clarithromycin.[433] *HIV+ve/multi-drug resistance:* Ask lab (cefepime may work).[436] *Causes:* Pneumococcus, Mycoplasma (hence erythromycin), Haemophilus, Staphs, TB, viral. *Monitor:* TPR; SpO₂.[437]

TB Suspect if: overseas contacts, HIV+ve; odd CXR *Signs:* Anorexia, low fever, failure to thrive, malaise. Cough is common (may be absent). *Diagnosis:* Tuberculin tests (*OHCM* p398); culture + Ziehl-Neelsen stain of sputa (×3) and gastric aspirate. CXR: consolidation, cavities. Miliary spread (fine white dots on CXR) is rare but grave. *R:* Get expert help. 6-month supervised plan:[438] isoniazid 15mg/kg PO 3 × a week + rifampicin 15mg/kg/PO ac 3 times a week + pyrazinamide (1ˢᵗ 2 months only) 50mg/kg PO 3 times a week. Monitor U&E & LFT before and during treatment. Stop rifampicin if bilirubin↑ (hepatitis). Isoniazid may cause neuropathy (give concurrent pyridoxine). ▶Explain the need for prolonged treatment. Multiple drug resistance: *OHCM* p409. *Prophylaxis:* If TB-with-HIV, co-trimoxazole prophylaxis is likely to be needed (pneumocystosis, p145).[438]

Whooping cough *(Bordetella pertussis) Signs:* Apnoea; bouts of coughing ending with vomiting (± cyanosis) worse at night or after feeds. Whoops (not always heard) are caused by inspiration against a closed glottis. Co-infection with RSV (above) is common. *Peak age:* Infants, with a 2ⁿᵈ peak in those >14.[439] In the UK, the illness is often mild, with 1% needing admission (eg with secondary pneumonia); but severe in the very young (may be fatal).[440] *Δ:* PCR; culture is unsatisfactory. Fluorescent antibody tests of nasopharyngeal aspirates is specific but insensitive. Absolute lymphocytosis is common (may be very high). *Incubation:* 10–14 days. *Complications:* Prolonged illness (the '100-day cough'). Coughing bouts may cause petechiae (eg on cheek), conjunctival, retinal & CNS bleeds, apnoea, inguinal hernias±lingual frenulum tears. Deaths may occur (esp. in infants), as may late bronchiectasis. *R:* Erythromycin is often used in those likely to expose infants to the disease (benefit unproven). Admit if <6 months old (risk of apnoea). May need ventilating and even ECMO (p109). *Vaccine:* p151, not always effective. 30% of severe infections are via a fully vaccinated sibling.

Many children with cough and wheeze do not fit into the categories opposite, and are too young for a diagnosis of asthma to be made with confidence. These infants often end up being treated with escalating bronchodilator therapy with frequent courses of antibiotics against uncultured organisms. While it is true that asthma can begin in infancy, most of these chesty infants do not have asthma—but we tend to prescribe 'just in case'. As the natural history of symptoms is to vary from hour to hour, sometimes we *appear* to be successful. NB: *viral wheeze/virally induced respiratory distress* or *virally induced lower airways disease (VILAD)* may be the appropriate label here: it is a non-atopic disorder; *respiratory syncytial virus* is more often the culprit rather than *Haemophilus*. An alternative diagnosis is *altered awareness of minor symptoms*, or *multi-trigger wheezing* to exercise, smoke, cold air, viruses and allergens.[441] When viruses are looked for (found in 80%), it turns out that together rhinoviruses, coronaviruses, human metapneumovirus, and human bocovirus account for 60% of viruses.[442] Although symptom scores and need for GP consultations are highest in infants with RSV, they are similar in infants infected with other viruses.[442]

The role of passive smoking is uncertain. 'Happy wheezers' (ie undistressed) probably need no treatment, but if chest symptoms start very early in life, a sweat test is needed to rule out cystic fibrosis. Between these ends of the spectrum of 'chestiness' lie those who clearly need some help. These may benefit from inhaled β_2-agonists (via a spacer) ± inhaled steroids, given for ~8 weeks in the lowest effective dose (not if this would mean almost continuous exposure). Assess benefit by ↓ in sleep disturbance. If ill enough to consider admission to ITU, 3 days' oral prednisolone 2mg/kg/day can ↓ duration of symptoms in children 6–35 months old with VILAD.[443] Other randomized trials disagree, so steroids may be best reserved for the aptopic.[444]

Aim to engage in a constructive dialogue with parents so that they understand that treatment is often unsuccessful, but that their child is unlikely to come to harm, while he or she is 'growing out of it'.

If cough is a chronic problem, exclude serious causes (eg TB; foreign body; asthma) and reassure. There is no good evidence that brand name cough medicines are better than placebo—but they may help the parents.

Alternative therapies: Prevention and treatment of winter chestiness/ upper respiratory infections (URTI) may be possible with herbal remedies ± vitamin C. Parents may ask about this. Chizukit®, for example, has 50mg of echinacea (*E. purpurea* + *E. angustifolia* roots) plus 50mg of propolis, and 10mg of vitamin C per mL. **Echinacea** is considered to be an immune stimulant (animal studies show effects on cytokines, macrophages, and natural killer cells). In the Coleman meta-analysis (children + adults), echinacea ↓ risk of URTI by 58% (by 86% in one trial when combined with vit C).[445] It can ↓duration of URTI by 1–3 days. **Propolis** is found in beehives and is said to be anti-infective. Vitamin C is possibly immunomodulatory. In one randomized study, reductions of >50% were seen in diagnoses of URTI, otitis media, pneumonia, and tonsillo-pharyngitis. Follow-up was poor because of its unpleasant taste.[446] (Do not assume that herbs and vitamins are harmless: apoptosis may be affected, and ↑risk of neoplasia in adults has been suggested)[444]—see also salicylate poisoning, p192.

This is one of the commonest autosomal recessive diseases (~1:2000; ~1:22 of Caucasians are carriers); it reflects mutations in the cystic fibrosis trans-membrane conductance regulator gene (CFTR) on chromosome 7, which codes for a cyclic AMP-regulated sodium/chloride channel. There is a broad range of severity of exocrine gland function, leading to meconium ileus in neonates (and its equivalent in children), lung disease akin to bronchiectasis, pancreatic exocrine insufficiency and a raised Na^+ sweat level—depending in part on the type of mutation (often ΔF_{508}; but other mutations, eg in intron 19 of CFTR, cause lung disease but no increased sweat Na^+).

Antenatal (p152) carrier-status testing is possible, as is preimplantation analysis after *in vitro* fertilization: at the 8 cell stage, 1 cell is removed from the embryo, and its DNA analysed; only embryos without the cystic fibrosis gene are reimplanted. This may be more acceptable than fetal terminations.

Diagnosis 10% present with meconium ileus as neonates. Most present later with recurrent pneumonia (±clubbing), steatorrhoea (if >7g/day/100g of undigested fat), or *slow growth. Sweat test*[1]: Sweat Cl⁻ <40mmol/L is normal (CF probability is low); >60mmol/L supports the diagnosis. Intermediate results are suggestive but not diagnostic of cystic fibrosis.[447] The test is capricious, so find an experienced worker (there are false positives and false negatives; see OPPO-SITE). Sweat is collected onto filter paper fixed to the forearm.[448] *Other tests:* IRT/DNA (below)[2]; CXR: shadowing suggestive of bronchiectasis (esp. upper lobes); malabsorption screen; glucose tolerance test; spirometry; sputum culture. Mycobacterial colonization affects up to 20%; consider if rapid deterioration.

Neonatal screening using immunoreactive trypsin (IRT): Dried blood samples at 3 days old, after consent (the French regimen). If IRT↑, DNA analysis is done on the same sample—looking for ≥30 mutations (gives 85% coverage).[449] This is routine on the newborn blood spot screening (Guthrie card).[450]

R ►*Genetic counselling* (p154). Long survival depends on antibiotics and good nutrition. *Respiratory problems (neutrophilic airway inflammation):* Start physiotherapy (×3/day) at diagnosis. Teach parents percussion + postural drainage. Older children learn forced expiration techniques. Organisms are usually *Staph aureus*, *H. influenzae* (rarer), and *Strep pneumoniae* in younger children. Eventually >90% are chronically infected with *Pseudomonas aeruginosa. Burkholderia cepacia* (*Ps cepacia*) is associated with rapid progression of lung disease (prompt diagnosis using PCR may be available: isolate the patient). Treat acute infection after sputum culture using higher doses, and for longer than normal. If very ill, **ticarcillin**, 80mg/kg (max 3.2g)/6–8h IV (if aged >1 month) + **gentamicin**, p175, or **ceftazidime** (50mg/kg/8h IV) alone may be needed 'blind'. Nebulizing ticarcillin and tobramycin at home *does* prevent admissions. **Colistin** and **meropenem** are reserved for panresistant *P. aeruginosa.*[451] In reversible airway obstruction, give inhaled salbutamol. Look for *Aspergillus* in sputum. Ensure full vaccination (+pneumococcal). Methicillin-resistant *Staph aureus* is unlikely to do great harm to the lungs.[451]

Gastrointestinal problems & nutrition: Energy needs rise by ~130% (∵ chronic lung inflammation). Most have steatorrhoea from pancreatic malabsorption and need enzymes: Pancrex v® powder mixed with tepid food for infants—and Pancrex v Forte® for older children, ≤10 tabs/meal—to give regular,

---

1 Explain the test and the reason for doing it. Give written information sheet. Other rules:
  • Sweat tests can be done at 2wks old in infants >3kg who are normally hydrated and without significant systemic illness. In term infants, sweat sodium and chloride can be high in the first 7 days.
  • Delay sweat tests if oedematous or if on systemic steroids. (Flucloxacillin is OK.)
  • For safety, do not do it on O_2 by an open delivery system (headbox & nasal prong O_2 are OK).
  • Stimulation, collection, storage, and analysis of sweat must be done according to written standards. Sweat should be collected for <30min and ≥20min.[452]

2 Having 2 mutations is associated with severe disease ($\Delta f508$, w1282x, g542x, n1303k, 1717-1g→a). Carrying one mutation may not be so bad (3849 + 10 kb → A T).[453]

formed, non-greasy bowel actions. Most older children have enzymes in microspheres (eg Creon®) so fewer tablets are needed. Omeprazole (or cimetidine, or ranitidine) helps absorption by ↑duodenal pH.[454] If all this controls steatorrhoea, a low-fat diet is not needed, but vitamins are still needed (A & D, eg as Abidec® 0.6mL/24h PO for infants or as multivitamin capsules 2/24h PO for older children). Diet should be high calorie/high protein.

Complications of CF
• Haemoptysis
• Pneumonia
• Pneumothorax
• Pulmonary osteo-arthropathy
• Diabetes mellitus
• Cirrhosis
• Cholesterol gallstones
• Fibrosing colonopathy
• Male infertility

Fine-bore nasogastric feeding is needed only if weight cannot otherwise be maintained.

GI obstruction if Creon® is omitted: admit urgently to a specialist centre for medical treatment (avoid laparotomy unless perforation imminent).

Impaired glucose tolerance: Risk rises with age and is higher if homozygous for ΔF508 mutations. Insulin may be needed; optimize diet, then optimize dose, not vice versa. Only try oral hypoglycaemics if nutrition is satisfactory.[455]

Psychological help: Parents and children need expert counselling—and transitional clinics with multidisciplinary teams when transferring from paediatric to adult services. The Cystic Fibrosis Research Trust can help here.

Meconium ileus Presents with failure to pass stool or vomiting in the 1st 2 days of life. Distended loops of bowel are seen through the abdominal wall. A plug of meconium may show as a firm mass in one such loop. In causes other than CF, lateral decubitus films show fluid levels. Tiny bubbles may be seen in the meconium ('inspissated'). *Options:* • Nasogastric tube drainage • Washout enemas • Excision of the gut containing most meconium.

Prognosis Death may be from pneumonia or cor pulmonale. Most survive to adulthood (median survival is >31yrs, and possibly >50yrs for those born after 2000).[456,457] 5-year survivorship models take account of forced expiratory volume in 1sec (% of expected), gender, weight-for-age z score, pancreatic function, plasma glucose, *Staph aureus* and *Burkholderia cepacia* infection, and number of acute lung exacerbations/yr.[458]

Newer options *Recombinant human deoxyribonuclease (rhDNase)* has been shown to improve lung function and reduce the number of pulmonary exacerbations—and, over the long term, the natural (untreated) increase in elastase activities and interleukin-8 concentrations can be curtailed.[459]

Lung transplantation (heart + lung, or double lung) is getting safer; consider in those who are deteriorating (FEV₁ <30% of expected) despite maximum therapy, provided nutrition is good, and there is no TB or aspergillus. Good results are limited by donor availability (avoid raising hopes).

Gene therapy aims to deliver normal copies of the cystic fibrosis gene into patients, so allowing them to make CFTR protein. Viral vectors and liposomes have been used to get the gene into cells.[460]

Pitfalls of the sweat test[461]

False-positive sweat test: May be seen in atopic eczema, adrenal insufficiency, ectodermal dysplasia, some types of glycogen storage diseases, hypothyroidism, dehydration, malnutrition. On the first day of life, up to 25% of normal newborns show a sweat sodium concentration >65mmol/L, but this rapidly declines on the second day after birth.

False-negative sweat test: Oedema is the most important cause. Poor technique can also give false negative results.

In the developed world, asthma is *the* leading chronic illness in children.[463] It implies reversible airway obstruction (peak flows vary by >20%) ± wheeze, dyspnoea, or cough. >20% wheeze at some time. *Prevalence* ↑ *if:* Birthweight↓; family history; bottle fed; atopy; ♂; pollution;[464] past lung disease; paracetamol use.[465] *Genetics:* Asthma susceptibility genes are described (eg ADAM33).*Triggers:* Pollen; dust; feathers; fur; exercise; viruses; chemicals; smoke; traffic. *ΔΔ:* Foreign body; pertussis; croup; pneumonia/TB (do CXR!);[466] hyperventilation; aspiration; cystic fibrosis (wet cough, starting at birth, failure to thrive).*Severe asthma:* (Not *always* distressed.) Too breathless to speak/feed; >40 breaths/min <5y >30 if 5–12y, ≥25 if >12y; pulse >140 beats/min <5y; >125 if 5–12y, ≥110 if >12y; pulse ≥120 (or >130 if <5yrs); peak flow ≤½ predicted 5–12yrs, 33–35% if >12yrs. *Life-threatening if:* Peak flow <⅓ of predicted •Cyanosis •Silent chest •Fatigue or exhaustion •Confused/agitation/↓consciousness/coma.

Treatment •Avoid triggers •Check inhaler technique: metered dose inhaler (MDI)[1] + Spacer[2] below the age of ~8. Then powders which need high inspiratory flow (≥60L/min) in the starting phase; or propellant systems (need constant flow, 40–90L/min) with long duration; ▶*teaching both at once doesn't work!*[467]
•Address fears •Have a self-management plan •Check compliance •Give a peak flow meter •Rescue **prednisolone** may be needed at any time, 1–2mg/kg/day PO for ≥48h. Step up when needed, and back down as symptoms allow, to avoid over-treatment.

1 Occasional β-agonists via pMDI.[1] If needed ≥3×/week, add step 2 (also if >5 yrs and many exacerbations, or asthma wakes from sleep >once/wk).
2 Add inhaled steroid,[2] eg **beclometasone**: specify brand[468] as potencies vary: Clenil Modulite® 50µg is a lower-potency CFC-free inhaler; Qvar® 50µg (CF free) is high-potency. Use up to 200µg of Clenil®/12h.[469]
3 Review diagnosis; check inhaler use/concordance; eliminate triggers; monitor height. *If <5yrs:* Add 1 evening dose of **montelukast** 4mg as a mouth-dissolving capsule. *If >5yrs:* Add inhaled **salmeterol** 50µg/12h (long-acting β-agonist); monitor closely; stop if of no help. If symptomatic ↑ inhaled steroid and try **montelukast** 5mg or **theophylline**, eg Slo-Phyllin® 125–250mg/12h PO if 6–12yrs. If problems remain, add in step 4.
4 Refer to specialist (± CXR).[470] ↑Inhaled steroid (Clenil® 400µg/12h).
5 Add **prednisolone** (if >5yrs) at lowest dose that works; check: growth.

Dose examples: β-*agonists:* **Salbutamol** 100µg via MDI as needed, with spacer. Admit if an attack is not controlled by 2–4 puffs/20–30min (max 10 puffs). *Antimuscarinics:* **Ipratropium** 20µg/8h by aerosol if ~6yrs old; 40µg/8h if older. *Treating severe asthma* Calmness helps. ★Give these treatments if the above life-threatening signs are present, or if not improving 15–30min after R starts.

1	Sit up; high-flow 100% O₂ if S_pO₂ <92% in air	6	Consider 1 IV dose of **magnesium sulfate**, 40mg/kg over 20min (≤2g); intracellular Mg²⁺ is↓[471]
2	**Salbutamol**: 5mg O₂-nebulized in 4mL saline (2.5mg if <5y) ±15µg/kg slow IV (monitor ECG)		
3	**Prednisolone** soluble tabs, 1–2mg/kg to max 40mg (60mg if already on steroids & <12yr), 50mg >12y	7	Peak flow before & after each nebulizer; normal values, see BOX
4	Oxygen nebulised ipratropium 250µg if <12y, 500µg if >12y	8	Nebulizers as needed, eg at 30 min, 1h, 2h, 3h & 4h with ipratropium 0.25mg mixed in if needed
5	★**Aminophylline** 5mg/kg IV over 20min (not if already on a xanthine); then IVI aminophylline (BOX)	9	Take to ITU if exhausted, confused, coma, or refractory to R and needing IVI salbutamol (2µg/kg/min)

Before discharge ensure: •Peak flow >75% of predicted •Good inhaler technique •Is stable on discharge regimen •Taking inhaled steroids+oral prednisolone •Written management plan •Follow-up: GP in 1 week; in clinic in ~4 weeks.

Prevention ↓Triggers.[472] A Mediterranean diet rich in fruit (esp. if eaten by the mother in pregnancy) may help.[473] Homeopathy[474] and flu vaccination don't help.

Paediatrics

Peak flow (litres/min) in normal boys and girls (5–18 years)

Height cm	Mean	3rd centile	Height cm	Mean	3rd centile
100	110		150	360	300
113	160	100	155	400	320
120	210	140	160	420	350
125	240	160	165	450	370
130	260	190	170	470	400
135	290	220	175	500	430
140	310	240	180	520	450
145	350	270	185	550	470
			190	570	500

Lung function measurements cannot reliably guide management in those <5yrs old.

Inhaler and nebulizer questions

- If <8yrs old, pressurized metered dose inhalers (pMDI)[1] with a spacer[2] are best for routine use in stable asthma for both steroids and bronchodilators.
- Nebulizers are not more efficacious than a well-used inhaler.
- Avoid using dry powder inhalers + pMDIs as techniques get muddled.
- *Is there a better alternative to nebulizers* (bulky and need servicing)? Evidence supports valved holding chambers (eg AeroChamber Plus®).[2475]
- Do combined inhalers offer added value? The SMART study Symbicort® maintenance & relief therapy shows real benefit from a fixed dose of long-acting β-agonist (**formoterol**) with budesonide (4.5/80µg/day + additional puffs for symptom relief). Doctor dependency was less, and there were fewer exacerbations.[476]

Continuous IVI of aminophylline

After loading dose[3] of 5mg/kg IV	Aminophylline mg/kg/h ▸Monitor ECG
1 month–12yrs	1.0
Children >12yrs	0.5–0.7

▸Confer with experts; target serum level: 10–20mg/L. SE: BP↓; arrhythmias; arrest if ≥25mg/L.

Pitfalls in managing asthma

- Reluctance to diagnose until a serious attack occurs.
- Faulty inhaler technique. Watch the patient operate the device.
- Inadequate perception of, and planning for, the severe attack.
- Unnoticed, marked diurnal variation in airways obstruction. Always ask about nocturnal waking; it is a sign of dangerous asthma.
- Being satisfied with less than total symptom control.
- Forgetting to start prophylaxis—and not using oral prednisolone early.
- Too much inhaled steroid (>400µg beclometasone or >800µg of budesonide)/day if ≤12yrs old:[477] [4] *consider adrenal insufficiency if ↓consciousness*; do blood glucose; IM hydrocortisone may be needed. Monitoring growth is *not* a good way to screen for adrenal suppression (cortisol ≤500nmol/L).[478]

---

1 pMDI=press-and-breathe pressurized meter dose inhaler—as recommended by NICE.
2 *Spacers*: (eg **AeroChamber®**—a responsive inspiratory valve allows opening on minimal effort to aid inhalation; it closes before exhalation disturbs retained aerosol) Static charge is a problem. Clean monthly. Wash in detergent. Dry in air. Wipe mouthpiece clean of detergent before use. Replace yearly.
3 If previous theophyllines used but level is subtherapeutic, a unique loading dose may be tried; to help calculate this, increasing a dose by 1mg/kg causes an increase in serum theophylline of ~2µg/mL. Get help. Erythromycin ↑aminophylline's half-life—also ciprofloxacin, propranolol, and the Pill. Drugs which ↓↑½: phenytoin, carbamazepine, barbiturates, and rifampicin. Do plasma concentrations.
4 Anti-IgE agents may ↓ need for steroids. **Omalizumab** is a recombinant humanized monoclonal antibody directed against IgE and can inhibit the immune system's response to allergen exposure. It prevents IgE from attaching to mast cells, reducing IgE mediated inflammation.[479]

Paediatrics

Signs Fever, splenomegaly, clubbing, splinter haemorrhages, anaemia, rash, heart failure, microscopic haematuria, new murmur (eg with known congenital heart lesion or IV line *in situ*). *Typical cause:* Streps; staphs.[480]

Tests Blood cultures (different times and different sites), echocardiograms.

Blind treatment After 3 blood cultures: benzylpenicillin 25mg/kg/4h IV + gentamicin (p175); get microbiological help.

Preventing endocarditis Prophylactic antibiotics are now generally not recommended. Advise on oral hygiene.[481]

Rheumatic fever

This is a systemic febrile illness caused by a cross-sensitivity reaction to Group A β-haemolytic streps, which, in the 2% of the population that is susceptible, may result in permanent damage to heart valves. It is common in developing countries, but is rare in the West, but pockets of resurgence sometimes occur in the USA in overcrowded areas (favours streptococcal spread). Some specific Group A streptococcal serotypes are known to be particularly rheumatogenic—eg type 5 of the M-protein serotypes. Other ubiquitous serotypes appear to be non-rheumatogenic (eg type 12).[482] Incidence: 500,000/yr (worldwide).[483]

Jones diagnostic criteria are said to be over-rigorous (will miss some cases)[484]—but here they are: elicit 2 major criteria or 1 major and 2 minor *plus* evidence of preceding strep infection: scarlet fever, a throat swab with β-haemolytic streptococci or a serum ASO titre >333U/L (reference intervals vary).[485]

Major criteria: (revised 2001)
- Carditis (1 of: changed murmur; CCF; cardiomegaly; friction rub; +ve echo)
- Polyarthritis (often migratory)
- Erythema marginatum, *OHCM* p564
- Subcutaneous nodules
- Sydenham's chorea (p654).

Minor criteria:
- Fever
- ESR >20mm or C-reactive protein↑
- Arthralgia, ie pain but no swelling
- ECG: PR interval >0.2sec
- Previous rheumatic fever or rheumatic heart disease.

Don't count arthralgia if polyarthritis is used as a major criterion; likewise for long P-R if carditis is used. *Joints:* Knees, ankles, elbows & wrists may be *very* tender, but no permanent sequelae. *Echo criteria:* Mitral regurgitant jet is: >1cm; holosystolic (throughout systole); visible in 2 planes; mosaic pattern (ie chaotic flow).

The *MacCallum plaque*[1] is at the base of the posterior mitral leaflet. Aortic, pulmonary and tricuspid valves are affected in descending order of frequency.

Treatment of rheumatic fever Rest/immobilization helps joints and heart. Aspirin (high-dose, p646; but get advice *re* Reye's, p652). If severe, get help. Prednisolone (below) *may* help.[486] Penicillin for pharyngitis (~125mg/6h PO) preceded by one dose of benzylpenicillin (25mg/kg IM or IV). *Sydenham's chorea:* unless mild, consider prednisolone (2mg/kg/day[5] for 4wks, then taper; halves time to remission to ≤8 weeks; emotional and learning difficulties can take far longer to resolve).[487] Consider haloperidol; valproic acid; carbamazepine.[488]

Prevention *Primary:* Where incidence is high, this might be worthwhile, but might entail giving IM penicillin for sore throats.[489] *Secondary:* Symptoms are often worse on recurrence of rheumatic fever—eg seen in 2.6%.[480] Prevent with phenoxymethylpenicillin 125mg/12h <6y; 250mg/12y >6y.[491]

---

1 MacCallum's plaque is due to subendocardial Aschoff bodies: these are a classic histological feature of rheumatic fever. They are perivascular with a necrotic core set in a layer of lymphocytes. Nodules are found in joints, tendons, heart, and blood vessels. They heal with extensive myocardial fibrosis.

PANDAS *(paediatric autoimmune neuropsychiatric disorders associated with strep infections).* Suspect this in those with tics (or Tourette's syndrome, *OHCM* p692) and obsessive–compulsive disorder. Anorexia nervosa *may* also be a feature. Antibiotics and **risperidone** have been tried.[492–494] See p654.

Diarrhoea may be an early sign of *any* septic illness. Faeces are sometimes so liquid they are mistaken for urine. NB: it is *normal* for breastfed babies to have liquid stools.

Gastroenteritis Rotavirus is the most common cause of gastroenteritis in infants and children. It causes ~600,000 childhood deaths/yr (a vaccine is available).[496] *Other enteric viruses:* Norovirus (most common cause in adults), astrovirus; adenovirus. *Treatment:*[497] ▶If dehydrated, see p234. Weigh, to monitor progress and quantify dehydration, if a recent previous weight is known. Start oral **rehydration therapy** (ORT), eg Dioralyte®, at 50mL/kg over 4h (≈1mL/kg every 5mins). Continue breastfeeding. If child refuses ORT, offer other fluids (eg bottle milk/water—not fruit juice) or consider ORT via a nasogastric tube. IV therapy is reserved for those who deteriorate or are in shock. Reintroduce milk after 4h of rehydration with ORT (even if <6 months), or sooner if he recovers and is hungry (starving harms).[498] Use of antiemetics (ondansetron 0.1–0.15mg/kg) has been shown to decrease vomiting[499] and reduce need for IV fluids, hospital admission[450] and overall costs,[451] but isn't officially recommended. *Complications:* Dehydration; malnutrition; temporary sugar intolerance after D&V with explosive watery acid stools. (Rare; manage with a lactose-free diet.) Post-enteritis enteropathy resolves spontaneously after ~7wks. *Tests:* Stool: look for bacteria, ova, cysts, parasites. *Prevention:* Hygiene, good water & food, education, fly control.

Classification diarrhoea by mechanism *Secretory* (↓absorption or ↑secretion) Stool is watery even if fasting, eg: cholera, *C. difficile, E. coli*, carcinoid. *Osmotic:* (↑osmotic load in gut lumen). Stool is watery, acidic, and +ve for reducing substances; to detect mix 5 drops of stool + 10 drops H₂O + 1 Clinitest® tablet, eg: galactose, glucose, sorbitol, or lactose intolerance, laxative abuse. *Motility disorders: Increased:* Thyrotoxicosis, irritable bowel syndrome dumping syndrome. Decreased: Pseudo-obstruction, intussusception (eg <4yrs old). *Inflammatory:* (eg bloody diarrhoea), salmonella, shigella, campylobacter, rotavirus, amoebiasis, NEC (p120), Crohn's/UC (look for weight↓; anaemia; WBC↑; platelets↑; ESR↑), coeliac disease, haemolytic uraemic syndrome (p176).

Malnutrition

Rising food prices + global warming + political corruption ≈ malnutrition + war

▶Being a major cause of death and misery, this is a global issue for us all. *Kwashiorkor* is due to ↓intake of protein & essential amino acids. *Signs:* Poor growth; diarrhoea; apathy; anorexia; oedema; skin/hair depigmentation; distended abdomen; glucose↓; K⁺↓; Mg²⁺↓; Hb↓; cholesterol↓; albumin↓. ℞: Re-educate child, family, and politicians. Offer a gradually increasing, high-protein diet + vitamins. *Marasmus* is lack of calories + discrepancy between height and weight. It is HIV-associated.[502] *Signs:* distended abdomen, diarrhoea, constipation, infection; albumin↓. Mid-arm circumference <9.9cm (any age) predicts severe malnutrition better than being <60% of median weight for age, or 85% of median height for age and 70% of median weight for height. Most can be treated at home with fortified ready-to-use foods if >6 months.[503] Parenteral feeding may be needed to restore hydration and renal function. Next offer a balanced diet with vitamins. Despite this, stature and head circumference may remain poor. Kwashiorkor and marasmus may coexist (*protein-energy malnutrition*).[504] *Prevention:* ▶Stop man-made activity contributing to climate instability. ▶Stop biofuels supplanting food crops. ▶Give to charity www.oxfam.org (to pay for fertilizers, high-yield seeds, and simple irrigation schemes). Medically, we often target the malnourished (z score -2, p227) at aged ½–5yrs, found by screening, but better results are got by giving *universal* help at ½–2yrs in at-risk places.[505]

Paediatrics

How does poverty impinge on childhood mortality & morbidity?

Worldwide, poor mothers are at ↑ risk of death: there is no worse start to life than the death of one's mother (100% fatal to her babies in some places).

Poverty-associated short stature, BMI <18.5 (p530) and iron deficiency in mothers accounts for 20% of maternal mortality.

Malnutrition causing stunting causes ~2.2 million deaths/yr and 21% of disability-adjusted life years (DALYs) in children <5yrs old.[506]

Deficiencies in vitamin A and zinc cause 1 million deaths/yr. Zinc supplementation[1] cannot always be relied on to ↓morbidity in children recovering from diarrhoea and respiratory illness in developing countries.[507] Prevention of the poverty which caused the diarrhoea is more important.

Not breastfeeding for the 1st 6 months of life (especially non-exclusive breastfeeding) causes 1.4 million deaths/yr in children <5yrs old.[508] NB: the position is further complicated by the fact that proteins, fat concentrations and caloric value in breast milk from undernourished mothers are lower than in breast milk from well-nourished mothers.

1–4 above account for 35% of child deaths and total global disease burden. In many other conditions (eg diarrhoeal diseases, HIV, asthma, obesity) poverty plays a leading role. But the main health issue is that it's harder to educate yourself if you live in a slum. ▶ No power≈no light≈no homework≈no learning≈an early death.

"I heard one person starve I heard many people laughing"

Paediatrics

Southern diarrhoea is only an excuse for northern amnesia

As you read this page two events unfold: in the northern hemisphere a child is born with a silver spoon in his mouth, his future assured thanks to incubators, ventilators, wealth, and family planning. Diametrically opposed to this birth another occurs in the southern hemisphere where the silver was mined for that lovely spoon. This child, according to our stereotype, must "Wait for his future like a horse that's gone lame *To lie in the gutter and die with no name*".[509] We assume that this death is from diarrhoeal diseases that we are all working, more or less efficiently, towards controlling—and we are pleased to blame non-human agencies for these deaths.

This model of our imperfect world does not stand up to scrutiny for two reasons: one is easy to understand (the diarrhoea was the mode of dying not the cause of death, which was poverty) and the other is impossible to understand—we didn't just let him die. We wanted him to die: in fact we killed him: in some cases, literally. Follow this well-documented thought sequence: There are too many homeless children living in my back yard→This threatens health and hygiene→How do we deal with this?→Other threats to health and hygiene are vermin→Street children are a sort of vermin→Vermin need eradicating→Let's shoot the vermin→Extrajudicial shooting of children—as occurred in Rio de Janeiro in 1994 and Sao Paulo in 2004.[510] In the former, most 'ordinary decent folk' approved of the killings when they phoned a local radio station, as the events unfolded... "*I killed you because you had no future.*"[511]

💭 The point of all this is to illustrate that if we want to do something for children it is no good just doing something about the big killers, such as diarrhoea, and it's no good simply attacking poverty, for there is something dark in our human heart which needs addressing before merely statistical or biological interventions have any chance of success. There is only one way of influencing human nature for the better, and that is through dialogue. So, in this sense, the treatment of diarrhoea is dialogue. Without such dialogue the rich wring their hands while poverty wrings necks.

Materialism is at war with altruism, and always what there is no progress and no silver lining.

---

1 Strategies for supplementing vit A (in neonates & late infancy), Zn & Fe for children and universal promotion of iodized salt can improve nutrition and prevent related diseases, and may reduce stunting at 36 months by 36% and mortality between birth and 36 months by about 25%.[512]

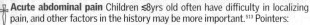

Acute abdominal pain Children ≤8yrs old often have difficulty in localizing pain, and other factors in the history may be more important.[513] Pointers:
• Hard faeces suggest that constipation is the cause (p210).
• In those of African or Mediterranean origin, suspect sickle-cell disease.
• Do tuberculin test (*OHCM* p398) if travel or other factors suggest TB risk.
• In children with pica (p210), do a blood lead level (and ferritin).
• Abdominal migraine is suggested by periodic abdominal pain with vomiting especially if there is a positive family history.
• If any past UTI, suspect GU disease (eg renal colic or hydronephrosis).

Common physical causes Gastroenteritis; UTI; viral illnesses (eg tonsillitis associated with mesenteric adenitis); and appendicitis.

Rarer causes Mumps pancreatitis; diabetes; volvulus; intussusception; Meckel's diverticulum; peptic ulcer; Crohn's/ulcerative colitis; Hirschsprung's disease; Henoch–Schönlein purpura and hydronephrosis. Consider menstruation or salpingitis in older girls. ►In boys always check for a torted testis.

Tests ►Always microscope and culture the urine. Others: consider plain abdominal x-ray; ultrasound; FBC; ESR; renal imaging, barium studies.

Appendicitis (*OHCM* p610) is rare if <5yrs, but perforation rates are high in this group (nearing 90%). Think: how can I tell this from other causes of abdominal pain? •Clues in the history: increasing pain in right lower quadrant, no previous episodes, anorexia, slight vomiting, absence of cough and polyuria. •Examination hint: fever and pulse↑ are likely; if the child appears well and can sit forward unsupported, and hop, appendicitis is unlikely. •Tests have very low positive and negative predictive values.

Gastro-oesophageal reflux/oesophagitis Presents with regurgitation, distress after feeds, apnoea, pneumonia, failure to thrive, and anaemia. *Tests:* Endoscopy + evaluation with an oesophageal pH probe is more reliable than barium studies. Ultrasound is not much help. *Treatment:* Reassurance; avoid over feeding (a common cause). Drugs may be needed, eg an antacid + sodium/magnesium alginate, eg for term infants, **Infant Gaviscon®** dual dose sachets, 1 dose mixed with 15mL boiled (cooled) water. This paste is given by spoon after each breast feed. If bottle fed, give each half of a dual sachet dose dissolved in 4oz of feeds. Carobel® thickens the feeds. If this fails, some experts use domperidone ± omeprazole (or similar). Most resolve by 6–9 months; if not, consider fundoplication, eg if there is failure to thrive, severe oesophagitis, apnoea, or bleeding.

Abdominal distension

Always remember acute GI obstruction as a cause; also consider:

Air:	Ascites:	Solid masses:	Cysts:
Faecal impaction	Nephrosis	Wilms' tumour	Polycystic kidney
Air swallowing	Hypoproteinaemia	Neuroblastoma	Hepatic; dermoid
Malabsorption	Cirrhosis; CCF	Adrenal tumour	Pancreatic

Hepatomegaly Infections: many, eg infectious mononucleosis, CMV.
Malignancy: leukaemia, lymphoma, neuroblastoma (see below).
Metabolic: Gaucher's and Hurler's diseases, cystinosis; galactosaemia.
Others: sickle-cell disease and other haemolytic anaemias, porphyria.

Splenomegaly All the above causes of hepatomegaly (not neuroblastoma).

Neuroblastoma This may be thought of as an embryonal neoplasm, derived from sympathetic neuroblasts. presenting with decreasing frequency from birth to 5yrs of age. Some forms regress, while others present after 18 months old (eg with metastases ± DVT) are highly malignant (outlook is poor and has not improved over the last 25yrs). *Prevalence:* 1:6000–1:10,000—the most common solid tumour in the under-5s. *Signs:* Abdominal swelling. *Metastatic*

Paediatrics

sites: Lymph nodes, scalp, bone (causing pancytopenia ± osteolytic lesions). In 92%, urinary excretion of catecholamines (vanillylmandelic & homovanillic acids) are raised. *Treatment:* Refer to special centre. Excision (if possible) and chemotherapy (eg cyclophosphamide + doxorubicin). *Prognosis:* Worse if certain genotypes (pseudodiploid karyotypes, chromosome 1p deletions, N-*myc* gene amplifications), less mature catecholamine synthesis, and if >12 months old. Those <1yr do best. *Prevention:* Pre-morbid screening by looking for excretion of catecholamines in the urine detects disease early, but may not to save lives.[514] Uncertainty is added by a 2008 study which appeared to record lower mortality in a screened group, (although it was a very large study, it is dubious, being retrospective).[515]

Recurrent abdominal pain ≥10% of children >5yrs suffer recurrent abdominal pains interfering with normal activity. Is there organic disease? No cause is found in most, but don't let this encourage complacency (you may delay diagnosis of *Crohn's* or *peptic ulcer*) or lead to zealous diagnosis of underlying psychological problems (now thought to be less important, but do consider it: who is present when the pain starts; what, or who, makes the pain better?). NB: long-term follow-up indicates a 4-fold ↑risk of psychological problems manifesting in adult life. Consider: gastro-oesophageal reflux, small bowel dysmotility, gastritis, duodenitis, carbohydrate malabsorption (eg lactose, sorbitol), abdominal migraine. *Who to investigate:* There are no rules. Do an MSU. Be suspicious if pain is unusual in terms of site, character, frequency, or severity. Whenever symptoms are present for more than a few months recheck for associated features, eg in inflammatory bowel disease (Crohn's) there may be no diarrhoea in 50%, according to one careful study,[516] but poor growth is often the clue that prompts further tests.

Coeliac disease: an example of malabsorption

Malabsorption typically presents with diarrhoea, failure to thrive ± anaemia (folate↓; ferritin↓), possibly with abdominal protrusion, everted umbilicus and wasted buttocks (if late-presenting). As subclinical/latent forms exist, investigate any unexplained anaemia, fatigue, 'irritable bowel' symptoms, diarrhoea, weight↓, arthralgia, eczema, and short stature. Patients may present at *any* age. Coeliac disease may cause short stature without overt gastrointestinal signs or symptoms. There may be a deceleration on the growth chart after introduction to gluten at weaning (4–6 months). See fig 1. *Cause:* Enteropathy induced by gluten (in wheat, barley, and rye). *Δ:* Serological tests show raised IgA anti-tissue transglutaminase (IgA-tTG), anti-gliadin (IgA-AGA), and endomysial antibodies (EMA). Also measure total IgA—if deficient measure IgG anti-gliadin antibodies.[517] Serology is less reliable if

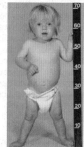

Fig 1. Coeliac disease

<18mths—IgA-AGA may be most useful in this age group.[518] Confirm by finding villous atrophy on small bowel biopsy (endoscopic under GA is better than Crosby capsule). Villi return to normal on the special diet; avoid a gluten challenge test unless diagnosis is in doubt.[519] *R: Gluten-free diet:* no wheat, barley, rye (no bread, cake, pasta, pizza, pies). Rice, maize, soya, potato, and jam are OK (also ≤25g/day of *pure* oats).[520] Canadian Celiac Assoc. 2007 Gluten-free biscuits, flour, bread, and pasta are prescribable. Minor dietary lapses may matter. *Other causes of malabsorption:* Cystic fibrosis; post-enteritis enteropathy; giardia; rotaviruses; bacterial overgrowth; milk sensitivity; worms; short bowel syndrome. *Coeliac associations:* Diabetes mellitus (type I).

Infantile hypertrophic pyloric stenosis Presents at 3-8 weeks (♂:♀≈4:1) with vomiting which occurs after feeds, and becomes projectile (eg vomiting over far end of cot). Pyloric stenosis is distinguished from other causes of vomiting by the following:

• The vomit does not contain bile, as the obstruction is so high.
• No diarrhoea: constipation is likely (occasionally 'starvation stools').
• Even though the patient is ill, he is rarely obtunded: he is alert, anxious, and always hungry—and possibly malnourished, dehydrated.
• The vomiting is extremely large volume and within minutes of a feed.

Observe left-to-right LUQ (left upper quadrant) peristalsis during a feed (seen in late-presenting babies). Try to palpate the olive-sized pyloric mass: stand on the baby's left side, palpating with the *left* hand at the lateral border of the right rectus in the RUQ, during a feed from a bottle or the left breast. There may be *severe* water & NaCl deficit, making urine output & plasma Cl⁻ (also K⁺ & pH) vital tests to guide resuscitation and determine when surgery is safe (Cl⁻ should be >90mmol/L). The picture is of hypochloraemic, hypokalaemic metabolic alkalosis. NB: don't rush to theatre.[521][n=84] *Imaging:* Ultrasound detects early, hard-to-feel pyloric tumours, but is only needed if examination is -ve.[522] Barium studies are 'never' needed. *Management:* Correct electrolyte disturbances. Before surgery (Ramstedt's pyloromyotomy/ endoscopic surgery) pass a wide-bore nasogastric tube.

Intussusception The most common cause of intestinal obstruction in children.The small bowel telescopes, as if it were swallowing itself by invagination. Patients may be any age (typically 5-12 months; ♂:♀≈3:1) presenting with *episodic* intermittent inconsolable crying, with drawing the legs up (colic) ± vomiting ± blood PR (like red-currant jam or merely flecks—a late sign). A sausage-shaped abdominal mass may be felt. He may be shocked and moribund. In between pains there may be no signs. *Tests/Management:* The least invasive approach is ultrasound with reduction by air enema (preferred to barium). CT may be problematic, and is less available. There may be a right lower quadrant opacity ± perforation on plain abdominal film. Doppler studies to show bowel viability have been used but are non-standard. If reduction by enema fails, reduction at laparoscopy or laparotomy is needed. Any necrotic bowel should be resected. *Pre-op care:* ►►Resuscitate, crossmatch blood, pass nasogastric tube. NB: children over 4 years old present differently: rectal bleeding is less common, and they have a long history (eg >3 weeks) ± contributing pathology (cystic fibrosis, Henoch–Schönlein or Peutz–Jeghers' syndromes; ascariasis, nephrosis or tumours such as lymphomas—in the latter obstructive symptoms caused by intussusception are the most frequent mode of presentation). Recurrence rate: ~5-15% in infants.[523]

Post-op pain relief Morphine IVI: child's loading dose: 100μg/kg in 30min, then ~20-30μg/kg/h (prem neonates 50μg/kg, then 5-20μg/kg/h) or diclofenac 0.3-1mg/kg/12h (max 75mg/12h for ≤2 days) if over 2yr (eg a 12.5mg suppository every 12h if ~1yr old). Ibuprofen dose: 7.5mg/kg/6h PO (syrup is 100mg/5mL). Pre-op (pre-emptive) tramadol also has a few advocates (~0.5-1mg/kg[61]).[524][n=45]

Phimosis The foreskin is too tight, eg due to circumferential scarring; retraction over the glans is impossible, eg with foreskin ballooning on voiding ± balanitis. *It is normal to have a simple non-retractile foreskin up to the age of 4yrs.* By 11yrs or older, prevalence is <8%.[525] Time or a wait-and-see policy will usually obviate the need for circumcision. *Forced* retraction may be causative, not therapeutic. 0.05% betamethasone cream also helps (esp. before 8yrs. Use twice-daily with stretching exercises for 15 days, then daily for 15 days.[526]

Other surgical problems: *appendicitis, hernias, volvulus, torsion of the testis, acute abdomen:* p170, p130, *OHCM* p654; *OHCM* p608.

Paediatrics

Presentation ▸Often the child may be *non-specifically* ill. Infants may present with collapse and septicaemia, and toddlers as vomiting, 'gastroenteritis', failure to thrive, colic, or PUO. Many with dysuria and frequency have *no* identifiable UTI, and often have vulvitis. The urinary tract is normal in most with UTI, but ~35% have vesico-ureteric reflux (VUR), ~14% have renal scars (most have reflux too), ~5% have stones, ~3% develop hypertension. Each year in the UK, 10–20 children enter endstage renal failure programmes because of reflux and chronic pyelonephritis complications. UTI is a common source of morbidity.[1]

Definitions *Bacteriuria:* Bacteria in urine uncontaminated by urethral flora. It may be *covert* ('no' symptoms), and can lead to renal scarring, BP↑, and, rarely, chronic renal failure. *UTI* denotes symptomatic bacteriuria that may involve different GU sites (∴ loin/suprapubic tenderness; fever; dysuria). *Chronic pyelonephritis* is a histological/radiological diagnosis. Juxtaposition of a cortex scar and a dilated calyx is the key feature. It is a big cause of hypertension and can result in renal failure, eg if the kidneys are congenitally dysplastic. During micturition, urine may *reflux* up ureters, seen on a micturicating cystogram (requires catheterization) or MAG3 scan (catheterization not needed)—grades: *I* Incomplete filling of upper urinary tract, without dilatation. *II* Complete filling ± slight dilatation. *III* Ballooned calyces. *IV* Megaureter. *V* Megaureter + hydronephrosis.

UTI incidence Boys: ≤0.23%/yr; girls: 0.31–1%; ratios are reversed in neonates. *Recurrence:* 35% if >2yrs old. *Prevalence of covert bacteriuria* in schoolgirls: ~3%. *Prevalence of associated GU anomalies:* 40% (½ have reflux; others: malpositions, duplications, megaureter, hydronephrosis). *Renal scars and age:* We used to concentrate on treating babies early, thinking new scars were rare after 4yrs old, but prospective ^{99m}Tc dimercaptosuccinate (DMSA) scintigraphy (the best test) shows new scars appearing on repeat scans in 43% of those <1yr old, 84% of those aged 1–5, and 80% of those >5yrs old.

Tests Dipstick all ward urines. If nitrites or WCC +ve, get a clean catch (or a suprapubic aspirate or catheter sample; bag urines have many false positives from vulvitis or balanitis). Wash the genitals gently with water, and tap repeatedly in cycles of 1min with 2 fingers just above the pubis, 1h after a feed, and wait for a *clean voided urine (CVU) sample*, avoiding the stream's 1st part. Do prompt microscopy[2] & culture. >10^8 organisms/L of a pure growth signifies UTI. For suprapubic aspiration, ward ultrasound helps identify a full bladder. Method: clean skin over the bladder; insert a 21G needle in the midline 1cm above symphysis pubis. Aspirate on advancing (any organisms found are significant). *Ultrasound (US):* US is cheap, non-invasive, getting more accurate, and is worthwhile in 1st UTIs (a good prenatal scan may suffice);[527] *sensitivity, specificity, positive predictive value, and negative predictive value* for detecting reflux are 18%, 88%, 23%, and 83%, respectively.[528] A right kidney longer than the left by ~10 mm is a good predictor of an abnormal DMSA scan.[529] Reserve renography for: infants *Recurrent* UTI and +ve family history of GU abnormality. If these are present and US is normal, proceed to ^{99}*Technetium renography*—static for scarring (^{99m}Tc DMSA scan, dynamic for obstructive uropathy) ± *isotope cystography. Micturicating cystourethrography (MCU)* is still the best way of excluding reflux—but it is said that if DMSA is negative, MCU 'never' shows significant reflux.[530] In general, it is *not* needed in over 1yr olds if initial tests are normal, pyelonephritis is unlikely, there is no family history of reflux, and there are no *recurrent* UTIs; it is invasive and unpleasant, but careful preparation with play therapy (p377) mitigates this. If it is done ill-advisedly on an uncomprehending and angry toddler, it may constitute assault. NB: operating on reflux is unlikely to improve renal function.[531]

---

1 Prevalence unknown as under-reported. See *Urol Clin North Am* 2008 35 47
2 Microscopy is more reliable than stix tests for nitrites & leucocytes: *Effective Health Care* 2004 8.6

Antibiotic treatment *Age <3 months:* IV amoxicillin + gentamicin (below) or IV cephalosporin alone (p106). *Child >3 months with uncomplicated lower UTI:* 3-day course of **trimethoprim**[1] 50mg/5mL, 4mg/kg/12h (max 200mg) PO ± prophylaxis (see below), nitrofurantoin, or amoxicillin/co-amoxiclav • Avoid constipation • ↑Oral fluids • Encourage full voiding • Repeat MSU. ►Resistance to trimethoprim and ampicillin renders monotherapy insufficient in some places.[532]

If the child or infant is ill (pyelonephritis + septicaemia) and blind parenteral therapy is needed, ►►gentamicin (5–7mg/kg/day) may be given in a once-a-day regimen (IM if IV access fails). In one study, children and infants were randomly assigned to once-daily gentamicin 5mg/kg/day[2] or 2.5mg/kg/8h slowly IV, where kg = lean body weight if obese.[2] There was no difference in efficacy, nephrotoxicity, ototoxicity, or renal scarring.[533] If neonate >35 weeks postmenstrual age, 2.5mg/kg/12h IV, slowly: consider a longer course if premature (gestation <34 weeks).[534] Do levels.[3] IV cefotaxime and co-amoxiclav are alternatives.

Treating ureteric reflux If prophylactic antibiotics fail, ureteric reimplantation can reduce reflux, but scarring remains. Keep on antibiotic prophylaxis.

Prevention Just one episode of reflux of infected urine may initiate renal scarring, so *screening* for bacteriuria is useless: damage is too quick. But once a UTI is suggested (eg by stix) treat it *at once*, before you know culture sensitivities, as renal damage may be about to happen. Obtain 2 high-quality urine samples for analysis. Consider prophylaxis if recurrent UTI, significant GU anomaly/renal damage. *Example:* **trimethoprim prophylaxis** (2mg/kg at night, max 100mg), eg while awaiting imaging—and sometimes indefinitely (optimum duration is unknown, but may be after 2 negative cystograms, if the indication is reflux). Consider screening siblings for reflux. Prophylaxis can be stopped after reflux has been ruled out if there is no scarring.

Surgical correction of moderate reflux is 'unlikely to be beneficial', and in minor reflux is 'likely to be harmful' (carefully made EBM phrases!)

---

1 Trimethoprim every 12h, eg if aged 6 weeks-6 months 25mg; 6 months–6yrs 50mg, 6–12yrs 100mg.
2 Assumes normal renal function; give lower dose if the patient is obese, based on **lean body weight** estimated by the 50th centile on weight-for-age charts. See *OHCM* p738.
3 Levels may not be needed if **gentamicin** is given for <72h (usually the case). One-hour post-dose (peak) serum gentamicin concentration should be 5–10mg/L (3–5mg/L for streptococcal or enterococcal endocarditis); pre-dose ('trough') concentration should be <2mg/L in neonates and <1mg/L in others on a once-daily regimen (<1mg/L for streptococcal or enterococcal endocarditis—*BNF* advice). In neonates phlebotomy is difficult and causes anaemia—so an example of monitoring advice from one NICU is: No levels before 48h of therapy unless proven infection requiring gentamicin and one of: •Perinatal asphyxia •Congenital renal defects •Renal insufficiency (creatinine >133μmol/L, ie >1.5mg/dL). www.cop.ufl.edu/wppd/research/sample7.pdf

Acute kidney injury AKI (Previously *acute renal failure*): Characterized by a rapid rise in creatinine or development of oliguria/anuria.[535] *Causes* in developed nations AKI occurs secondary to cardiac surgery, bone marrow transplantation, toxicity (NSAIDs, aminoglycosides, vancomycin, aciclovir and contrast nephropathy) and sepsis,[536] in the tropics causes include: diarrhoea/dehydration (50%);[537] glomerulonephritis (34%); drug-induced haemolysis in G6PD deficiency (5%); snake bite (4%); haemolytic uraemic syndrome (2%); myoglobinuria (*OHCM* p307). *Severity:* The paediatric RIFLE criteria stratifies severity of AKI based on changes in the creatinine, estimated creatinine clearance and urine output.[538] *ATN causes:* • Crush injury • Burns • Dehydration • Shock • Sepsis • Malaria.

Plasma chemistry: $K^+\uparrow$; creatinine↑; urea↑; $PO_4^{3-}\uparrow$ or $\leftrightarrow$; $Ca^{2+}\downarrow$; $Na^+\downarrow$; $Cl^-\downarrow$. MSU: Are there red cell casts (=GN)? If no RBCs seen but Labstix +ve for RBCs, consider haemo/myoglobinuria (*OHCM* p307). *Other tests:* ECG, serum and urine osmolality, creatinine, acid-base state, PCV, platelets, clotting studies (DIC), C_3, ASO titre, ANA (antinuclear antibody). *Radiology:* ►Arrange prompt abdominal ultrasound. Are the ureters dilated (eg stones: 90% radio-opaque)? If so, urgent surgery may be required. *Treatment:* Remove or reduce the cause promptly.

• Treat shock and dehydration (p234)—then:
• If urine/plasma (U/P) osmolality ratio is >5 the kidneys concentrate well; the oliguria should respond to rehydration. If the U/P ratio is low, try for a diuresis: **furosemide 2–5mg/kg/6h** IV slowly, (get help if more needed).
• Monitor BP. If BP↑↑: **nitroprusside** (p177).
• 24h fluid requirement: Avoid overhydration. Replace losses + insensible loss (12–15mL/kg). Aim for weight loss (0.5%/day).
• Give no K^+. Monitor ECG. Tall T-waves and QRS slurring prompt urgent lowering of K^+, with IV **salbutamol 4µg/kg or 5mg** nebulized (2.5mg if <25kg). A less easy to use alternative (if >1month old) is glucose with soluble insulin. Also consider **polystyrene sulfonate resins 0.5–1g/kg** max 60g PO and **calcium gluconate** (10%, 0.5mL/kg IV over 10min; monitor ECG: stop IVI if heart rate↓) to counteract electrophysiological effect of hyperkalaemia.
• High-energy, low volume infant renal formulas may prevent fluid excess.
• Consider renal replacement therapy as soon as fluid overload occurs. Many centres now prefer continuous haemofiltration to peritoneal dialysis.[536]
• ►Improvement is ushered in with a diuretic phase.

Haemolytic uraemic syndrome (HUS) *Essence:* Acute microangiopathic haemolytic anaemia (schistocytes, burr cells, *OHCM* fig 2 p327 & fig 3 p323), thrombocytopenia , renal failure + endothelial damage to glomerular capillaries. Typical HUS (95%) is associated with diarrhoea, atypical HUS (5%) is not (it is a disease of complement dysregulation).[539] *Typical HUS* is more frequent in the summer months, and typically occurs in children <3yrs. It is associated with Shiga toxin producing *E. coli* type 0157:H7.[540] *Other causes:* Shigella, HIV, SLE, drugs, tumour, scleroderma, BP↑. *Signs:* Colitis→haemoglobinuria→oliguria ± CNS signs→encephalopathy→coma. LDH↑. WCC↑. Coombs -ve. PCV↓. *Mortality:* 5–30%. ADAMTS13 helps with risk statification. *Treatment:* Supportive. Get help. Antibiotics, fibrinolytics, and anticoagulation are not used.[541] Treat renal failure (above). Relapses in TTP may be preventable by steroids, splenectomy, or vincristine.

Chronic renal failure *Causes:* Congenital dysplastic kidneys, pyelonephritis, glomerulonephritis, chronic infection, reflux nephropathy; AKI leading to cortical necrosis. ►Monitor growth, BP, U&E, Ca^{2+} (often ↓), PO_4^{3-} (often ↑).
The Child: Weakness, tiredness, vomiting, headache, restlessness, twitches, BP↑, hypertensive retinopathy, anaemia, failure to thrive, seizures, and coma.
Treatment: (See BOX). Talk with experts about haemodialysis & transplants.

Get a dietician's help. Calorie needs may not be met if vomiting is a problem. Eggs & milk may be appropriate (high biological protein value). Provide protein at a level of 2.5g/kg/24h. Vitamin drops may be needed. Nasogastric or gastrostomy tube feeding has a role. Growth hormone therapy combined with optimal dialysis improves growth: see *BNF*.

Acidosis is common, needing no treatment if serum bicarb is ≥20mmol/L.[1]

Renal osteodystrophy: A bone disease resulting from poor mineralization due to renal failure, causing poor growth, muscle weakness, slipped epiphyses, bone pain, and bone deformity (±cranial nerve lesions).[542] It is like rickets and low bone turnover osteomalacia (osteoblast and osteoclast activity ↓) osteomalacia. If glomerular filtration falls to ≤25% of normal, compensatory mechanisms to enhance phosphate excretion fail; resulting hyperphosphataemia promotes hypocalcaemia, so PTH rises, which enhances bone resorption to release Ca^{2+} in an attempt to correct hypocalcaemia. PTH↑ leads to marrow fibrosis (osteitis fibrosis cystica). Also, the failing kidneys cannot convert enough 25-hydroxycholecalciferol to active 1,25-dihydroxycholecalciferol, so GI calcium absorption falls, so worsening hypocalcaemia. ℞: Aim to normalize calcium and ↓associated hyperphosphataemia. Keep PTH within normal limits in predialysis children and 2-3 times over upper normal limit in those on dialysis. Avoid aggressive use of calcium-based phosphate binders and vit D derivates to prevent PTH oversuppression and development of adynamic bone disease. NB: there is little paediatric experience with calcimimetics, eg **cinacalcet**, that directly stimulate Ca^{2+}-sensing receptors and potently suppress PTH secretion without increasing Ca^{2+}.[543]

Hyperphosphataemia is treated with phosphate binders, eg **calcium carbonate** taken just before food. Dose: see *BNF*[c] section 9.5.2.2. This combines with dietary phosphate to form calcium phosphate, which is expelled in faeces. If there are episodes of Ca^{2+}↑, **sevelamer** may have a role (a synthetic calcium- and aluminium-free phosphate binder).[544]

If Ca^{2+} is low despite correcting serum phosphate, give 1,25-dihydroxycholecalciferol (**calcitriol**), eg 15 nanograms/kg/24h PO max 250 nanograms (increased in increments of 5ng/kg until Ca^{2+} and alk phos are normal, PTH level is reduced to 200–400pg/mL). X-ray evidence of healing rickets may also exist. Then reduce dose. SE: ↓renal function, hypercalcaemia, and hyperphosphataemia. Because normal bone requires adequate levels of PTH to promote bone modelling, oversuppression of PTH must be avoided to avoid adynamic osteodystrophy.

Anaemia is common, and is the result of ↓erythropoietin (± poor iron and folic acid intake). A typical Hb is 6–9g/dL. Do not transfuse, as this suppresses erythropoietin production. Erythropoietin may be indicated (sc in pre-dialysis and peritoneal dialysis patients, and IV if on haemodialysis).

▶▶Hypertensive emergencies

Get expert help. While awaiting this, use sodium nitroprusside 0.5μg/kg/min IVI, increased in 200 nanogram increments as needed, up to 8μg/kg/min IVI by pump (allows precise control). Protect from light. Monitor BP continuously; ↑dose slowly to the required level. CI: severe hepatic impairment. Withdraw over ≥20min to prevent rebound hypertension. If used for >1 day, cut dose to 4μg/kg/min IVI. Labetalol is an easy-to-use alternative, eg 0.25mg/kg/dose IV, doubled every 15min (as needed) up to 3mg/kg/h IV; CI: phaeochromocytoma.[545,546]

---

1 If pH ≤7.2, bicarbonate may be needed (by IVI if arrhythmias): get help as response is unpredictable, and dosing is difficult. Typical oral dose: 1-3mmol/kg/day in divided doses; bicarbonate 500mg capsules have ~6mmol of HCO_3^- (& Na^+).[198] Infant HCO_3^- deficit in mmol ≈ 0.3 × weight (kg) × base deficit (mmol/L) or 0.5 × weight (kg) × (20−serum HCO_3^-). In children it is 0.5 × weight (kg) × (24−serum HCO_3^-). Ask the expert what proportion of this deficit should be given IVI and over how long.[347]

Paediatrics

Acute nephritis *Essence:* Haematuria & oliguria (±BP↑, ± uraemia) produced by an immune glomerulonephritis (GN) in the kidney. *Peak age:* 7yrs.
Uncomplicated presentation:
Haematuria; oliguria; BP↑ (50%); periorbital oedema; fever; GI disturbance; loin pain.
Complicated presentations:
• *Hypertensive encephalopathy:* Restless; drowsy; bad headache; fits; vision↓; vomiting; coma.
• *Uraemia:* Acidosis, twitching, stupor, coma.

Causes of nephritis
• β-haemolytic strep via a preceding sore throat
• Henoch–Schönlein purpura
• Toxins or heavy metals
• Berger's dis. (*OHCM* p708)
• Malignancies
• Viruses
• Bacteria (IE/SBE; syphilis)
• Renal vein thrombosis

• *Cardiac:* Gallop rhythm, cardiac failure ± enlargement, pulmonary oedema.

Blood tests: Urea↑ in ⅔; ESR↑; acidosis. Complement (C_3) often ↓ 2–8 weeks after onset (not in Henoch–Schönlein purpura). Also ASO titre, antinuclear factor (ANA), anti-DNA antibodies (if SLE suspected), anti-neutrophil cytoplasmic (ANCA) antibodies (if vasculitis suspected), syphilis serology, blood cultures, virology. *MSU:* Count RBCs, WBCs, hyaline, granular casts; red cell casts mean glomerular bleeding. Skilled phase-contrast microscopy detects odd-shaped red cells, signifying glomerular bleeding. This change may not be present at first. 24h urine for protein and creatinine clearance. Check urine culture, and specific gravity (normal range: infants ~1.002–1.006; child/adult ~1.001–1.035).
Other tests: Renal ultrasound; renal biopsy, check platelets & clotting pre-op.

Poststreptococcal glomerulonephritis (PSGN) presents 7–21 days after a streptococcal infection (pharyngitis, impetigo) with gross haematuria (cola-coloured urine) and oedema + hypertension, malaise, anorexia, fever and abdominal pain. *Urine:* Proteinuria, RBC casts ± oliguria. *Blood:* ↑urea, ↑creatinine, ↓C_3. Recent streptococcal infection should be confirmed (serum ASO titre). Typically, renal biopsy is not needed. *R:* Na^+ restriction, diuretics, antihypertensives. Restrict protein in oliguric phase. Give **penicillin** orally for 7–10 days. Check BP often. If encephalopathy, give **nitroprusside** (p177). Oedema resolves in 5–10 days; however, hypertension, haematuria and proteinuria may last for several weeks. Prognosis is very good (95% full recovery).

Nephrotic syndrome (nephrosis) Oedema, proteinuria (>40mg/m^2/h), hypoproteinaemia ± hypercholesterolaemia. In 90% the cause is unknown, but any of the causes of nephritis (above) can cause nephrosis too. *Histology:* Usually minimal change GN (often associated with allergy and IgE production).[1] *Symptoms:* Anorexia, GI disturbance, infections, irritability; then oedema (periorbital, genital), ascites, oliguria. *Urine:* Frothy; albuminous ± casts; Na^+↓ (secondary hyperaldosteronism). *Blood:* Albumin↓ (so total Ca^{2+}↓); urea and creatinine usually normal. *Renal biopsy:* Reserve this for older children with any of: haematuria, BP↑, urea↑, if protein loss is unselective (ie large molecular weights as well as small), and treatment 'failures'. SE: haematuria; haematoma.[548][n=111] *Complications:* Pneumococcal peritonitis or other spontaneous infections. Consider pneumococcal vaccination if >2yrs. *Treatment:* Get help. Limit oedema with protein-controlled (3g/kg/24h) low-Na^+ diet (<50mmol/24h). Consider **furosemide** 0.5–1mg/kg/8h slow IV/PO + **spironolactone** (1–3mg/kg/24h PO, max 9mg/kg/24h if resistant—use lower doses in neonates). **Prednisolone** 60mg/m^2/day (max 80mg) for 6 weeks, then 40mg/m^2/48h for ≥6 weeks. 90% respond in 8 weeks. If steroid toxicity and relapsing NS, consider **cyclophosphamide**, eg 2mg/kg/day for ≥8 weeks (SE: haemorrhagic cystitis; WCC↓). If still relapsing, levamisole may help. Steroid-dependent NS may be treated with ciclosporin.[549] Ciclosporin is nephrotoxic.[550] ►Monitor BP. Control minimizes later renal failure.

---

1 Acharya B 2005 *Am J Nephrol* 1 30. Genetic variations in the IL-4 and IL-13 genes may be associated with predisposition to nephritic syndrome with minimal change glomerulonephritis.[551]

Steroids in nephrotic syndrome

In nephrotic syndrome, protein leaks from blood to urine through glomeruli, causing hypoproteinaemia and oedema. Before steroids (and antibiotics), many died from infections. Most children with nephrotic syndrome respond to corticosteroids, but many experience a relapsing course with recurrent oedema and proteinuria. Corticosteroids reduce mortality to ~3%, with infection remaining the most important cause of death. NB: steroids cause obesity, poor growth, BP↑, diabetes, osteoporosis, avascular necrosis (hip), and adrenal suppression.[552]

Steroid-resistant proteinuria and ACE-i

Enalapril is used in courses of >2yrs: dose example: 1 month–12yrs: initially 100µg/kg/day (monitor BP carefully for 1-2h; increase as needed to 0.5mg/kg/12h (maximum). In one study, urine protein electrophoresis showed a reduction of 80% and 70% in the total protein and albumin, respectively, after enalapril. Some patients become free of proteinuria. ACE-i are discontinued if renal failure occurs, eg during infections.[553,554]

Is growth normal? is a key question in determining the health of a child. Take any opportunity to weigh and measure a child. A series of plots on centile charts (p224) shows if growth is slow (growth curve crosses the centiles). NB: the growth rate in mid-childhood is 5-6cm/yr; this accelerates at puberty (peak height velocity) before epiphyses start to fuse.

Failure to thrive means poor weight gain in infancy (falling across centile lines). Head circumference is preserved relative to height, which is preserved relative to weight. In 95% this is due to not enough food being offered, or taken. Worldwide, poverty is *the* big cause; in the UK it is difficulty at home, neglect, unskilled feeding, or not enough breast milk (top-up bottles *may* be needed). *Idiosyncratic growth pattern* is one cause, or normal child of short stature (↓birthweight, short siblings or parents)—likely if he is a contented child.

Features to note:
• Signs of abuse (p146)
• Feeding patterns
• Behaviour
• Activity level
• Family finances
• Health and happiness
• Chart parental heights
• Any parental illnesses?
• Dysmorphic face

Be sceptical about reliability of data. Is the birthweight accurate? Was the child clothed during weighings? Length measurements are particularly error-prone: growth velocity is more useful than measurements done at a one time. *Issues to address:* Feeding and maternal interaction are most important. Is the child anorectic or ravenous—'hyperphagic short stature'?[555] Also:
• If breastfeeding, does he get a good mouthful of breast? (p124)
• If bottle feeding, does the teat's hole allow milk to flow through?
• Does weight gain return if the child is removed from the family?
• Is there evidence relevant to child protection proceedings?

Tests: Check feeding technique. It is a great skill to know *when* to investigate. It's better from the child's point of view to ask a trusted colleague's advice *before* painful tests. In one study only 39 of 4880 tests were helpful.[556]

Options are: MSU (expect false +ves if bags are used; but avoid routine suprapubic aspirations); U&E/glucose, LFT, Ca²⁺, proteins, immunoglobulins, CRP, TSH; FBC; sweat test; urinary amino ± organic acid chromatography; stools (MC&S ± sugar detection); CXR, renal or CNS ultrasound, skeletal survey for dwarfism and abuse; jejunal biopsy; ECG/echo. In *non-organic failure to thrive*, studies favour weekly visits from trained lay visitors.[557]

Short stature is a height <3ʳᵈ centile (p224). Use the method shown on the charts to correct for mid-parental height (short stature may represent 'regression towards the mean' of their heights). ►*Any chronic disease can cause short stature.* Hypopituitarism (an important cause of short stature) usually manifests after age 2yrs: look for relative obesity, without any other explanation for low growth velocity (ie <25ᵗʰ centile; measure for ≥1yr, see p226). Deficiency of growth hormone (GH) is shown by an impaired rise (peak GH <15MU/L) after a stimulus (eg sleep or hypoglycaemia, induced by IV insulin (*OHCM* p224), or an arginine stimulation test. Preschool screening for short stature is the aim. To be effective, start synthetic GH early. **Somatotropin** example: 23-39µg/kg/day SC; expect growth velocity to ↑ by ≥50% from baseline in year 1 of treatment. Other pituitary hormones may also be deficient (*OHCM* p224).

Typical causes:
• Constitutional (~80%)—if both parents short
• Psychological neglect
• Poverty; physical abuse
• Drugs: eg steroids
• Genetic: eg Turner's or cystic fibrosis
• Ineffective diet (coeliac)
• Inflammatory bowel dis.
• Hypothyroidism
• Infection (eg UTI; TB)
• GH↓ (as above)
• Rarities, eg Noonan, p650

Causes of height↑: Thyrotoxic; precocious puberty; Marfan's; homocystinuria. *Causes of weight↑:* Snacks^etc; not enough exercise; hypothyroidism; Cushings'; Prader-Willi, p652; Bardet-Biedl, p638; Cohen syndrome (hypotonia, obesity, prominent front teeth; seizures); polycystic ovary, p252.[558]

Paediatrics

It is clear that some populations are inherently shorter than others, and this poses problems when using UK90 growth charts (i.e charts for children >4); which are based on cohorts of UK children in the 1980s (see also p224). Consider these facts:

- The Dutch are the tallest *nation* on earth (mean ♂ height 1.84m): the tallest *population group* is the Masai people (eg in Tanzania and Kenya).
- African and Afro-Caribbean 5–11-yr-olds height is ~0.6 standard deviations scores (SDs) greater than white children living in England.
- Gujarati children and those from the Indian subcontinent (except those from Urdu- or Punjabi-speaking homes) have heights ~0.5 SDs less than white children living in England.
- Gujarati children's weight-for-height is ~0.9 SDs less than expected for Afro-Caribbeans, or white children in England—so Gujarati children's weight is ~1.5 SDs less than for white children living in England.
- Urdu and Punjabi weight is ~0.5 SDs < expected for white UK children.
- Published charts have centile lines 0.67 SDs apart; for height and weight shift the centile lines up by 1 centile line division for African-Caribbeans.
- Re-label Gujarati children's weight charts, so the 0.4th centile becomes the ~15th centile, and the 2nd weight centile becomes the ~30th centile.
- For most other Indian subcontinent groups, height & weight need shifting down, eg relabel the 0.4th & 2nd centile lines 1.5th & 6th respectively. NB: Sikh children are taller and heavier than Caucasians.[560]
- Body mass index centiles are said to be appropriate for African-Caribbeans, but recalculate as above for Indian subcontinent children, except for Gujarati-speaking children (0.4th & 2nd centiles→4th & 14th).

Trends towards tallness with each generation occur at varying rates in all groups, so 3rd generation immigrants are taller than expected using 2nd generation data. Intermarriage adds further uncertainty. NB: to print the *new CDC charts*, see www.cdc.gov/nchs/about/major/nhanes/growthcharts/clinical_charts.htm

NB: obesity (±diabetes) in school children is a big public health issue. See p156 for preventing 'adult' diseases by measures starting in childhood.

Paediatrics

Paediatrics

Hypothyroidism Thyroid hormone is necessary for growth and neurologic development. Dysfunction may occur in the neonate, infant or during childhood. *Congenital:* Thyroid scans divide these into 3 groups: athyreosis; thyroid dysgenesis; dyshormonogenesis. Also remember maternal antithyroid drugs (p25, eg propylthiouracil). *Acquired:* Prematurity; Hashimoto's thyroiditis; hypopituitarism; x-rays; Down's syndrome. *Signs:* May be none at birth—or prolonged neonatal jaundice, widely opened posterior fontanelle, poor feeding, hypotonia, and dry skin are common. Inactivity, sleepiness, slow feeding, little crying, and constipation may occur. Look for coarse dry hair, a flat nasal bridge, a protruding tongue, hypotonia, umbilical hernia, slowly relaxing reflexes, pulse↓, and poor growth and mental development if it has not been picked up. Other later signs: IQ↓, delayed puberty (occasionally precocious), short stature, delayed dentition.[561] *Universal neonatal screening:* Cord blood or filter paper spots (at ~7 days, from heel prick) allow early diagnosis (the 'Guthrie card'). They *do* prevent serious sequelae. Act on high *and* low TSHs (may indicate pituitary failure).[562] *Tests:* T₄↓, TSH↑ (but undetectable in secondary hypothyroidism), ^{131}I uptake↓, Hb↓. Bone age is less than chronological age. As it is unwise to x-ray the *whole* skeleton, the left wrist and hand are most commonly used. There are a large number of ossification centres. Each passes through a number of morphological stages, and using comparisons with key diagrams from 'normal' populations, a rough bone age can be determined. There is no hard-and-fast answer to the question of how much discrepancy (eg 2yrs) between skeletal and chronological years is significant.

Levothyroxine (LT4): Start neonates with ~15μg/kg/day; adjust by 5μg/kg every 2 weeks to a typical dose of 20–50μg/day. <2yrs start with 5μg/kg/day (max 50μg) adjust by 10–25μg every 2–4 weeks; >2yrs start with 50μg and adjust by 25μg every 2–4 weeks (eg to 25–75μg/day; adult doses are reached by 12yrs).[563,564] Adjust according to growth and clinical state. *Avoid high TSH levels.* Those with athyreosis need the highest doses of T₄ and the closest monitoring early on. Those with dysgenesis and dyshormonogenesis need more attention later.

Hyperthyroidism *Typical child:* Pubertal girl. *Signs/ lab features:* OHCM p210. Fine-needle cytology of goitres may show *juvenile autoimmune thyroiditis*. **Carbimazole** starting dose: ~250μg/kg/8h. Adjust according to response.[565] **Propylthiouracil:** 2.5mg/kg/8h (/12h in neonates) PO until euthyroid—then adjust dose; expect remission in ~67%.[566] Higher doses may be needed. Typical maintenance dose: ⅓–⅔ of remission-inducing dose.

Thyroid disease in pregnancy and neonates See p25.

The glycogen storage disorders (CSD) result from defects in enzymes required for the synthesis and degradation of glycogen. Abnormal stores are deposited in liver, muscle, heart, or kidney. In some types there are CNS effects. Most types (there are >12) are autosomal recessives. There is considerable variability in severity and prognosis. Early diagnosis and treatment are important for minimizing organ damage. Types include: von Gierke disease (type I, p655), Pompe's disease (type II, p652), Cori disease (type III—hypoglycaemia, hepatomegaly, with failure to thrive), Anderson disease (type IV), McArdle disease (type V), Hers disease (type VI) and Tauri disease (type VII—phosphofructokinase↓—like McArdle's, but with haemolysis and gout: diagnose by muscle enzyme assay). Treatment depends on type.

In McArdle's, (most common CSD in adolescents) the cause is myophosphorylase deficiency. Stiffness and myalgia follow exercise. Venous blood from exercised muscle shows ↓levels of lactate & pyruvate. ↓phosphorylase staining in muscle biopsy confirms diagnosis. There may be myoglobinuria. *Treatment:* No extreme exercise. Oral glucose and fructose may help.

These are often diagnosed by a urine metabolic screen (eg amino acids, organic acids, carbohydrates, mucopolysaccharides—in deciding which tests to do, get help; interest the lab in your problem). Typical signs: diarrhoea, lethargy, respiratory distress, metabolic acidosis (± odd body smells), jaundice, hypoglycaemia, U&E imbalance, fits, and coma. Features may be intermittent, and provoked by crises (eg infection; dehydration). In addition, look for:

Urine amino acids ↑ in:
• Alkaptonuria
• Canavan leucodystrophy
• Cystinosis
• Cystathioninuria
• Fructose intolerance
• Galactosaemia
• Hartnup disease
• Homocystinuria
• Hyperammonaemia

Physical sign:	Possible significance:
Hepatosplenomegaly	Eg amino acid and organic acid disorders, lysosomal storage diseases (Anderson–Fabry disease[1])
Coarse facies	Mucopolysaccharidoses, eg Hurler's syndrome, p646, gangliosidoses, mannosidoses
WCC↓, platelets↓	Organic acidurias
Hypoglycaemia	Many diseases, eg von Gierke's syndrome; MCADD[2]
Mental retardation	See p216
Failure to thrive	Aminoacidurias, organic aciduria, cystinuria, lactic acidosis, storage diseases

Paediatrics

PKU (phenylalanine ketonuria)—*Cause:* Mutation of phenylalanine hydroxylase (PAH) gene (chromosome 1—autosomal recessive) leading to absent or reduced activity of phenylalanine hydroxylase. Classic PKU leads to gradual mental impairment. The defect leads to ↓CNS dopamine, reduced protein synthesis, and demyelination.[567] Milder forms of hyperphenylalaninaemia can occur with different mutations to the same gene, or mutations in co-factor tetrahydrobiopetrin (BH₄). *Clinical features:* Fair hair, fits, eczema, musty urine. The chief manifestations is ↓IQ (eg dyscalculia ± poor spelling ± ↓cognition).[568] *Tests:* Hyperphenylalaninaemia (reference interval: 50–120µmol/L). Treatment instigated in infants with levels >360µmol/L—to avoid ↓IQ which may start with levels of >394µmol/L.[569] *Treatment:* Get expert help. *Diet:* protein substitute that lacks phenylalanine but is enriched in tyrosine. Aim to keep phenylalanine levels to <360µmol/L[570] by prescribing artificial food substitutes (amino acid drinks) to give <300mg–8g of natural protein/day (depending on age and severity of phenylalanine hydroxylase deficiency).[571] Hypomyelination may be proportional to degree of phenylketonaemia, but some studies fail to show stricter diets are associated with higher IQs. Despite treatment, children are more prone to depression, anxiety, phobic tendencies, isolation, and a less 'masculine' self-image.[572] Adherence to the diet may be poor (it's unpalatable).[573] Also, the diet may cause changes of questionable significance in levels of selenium, zinc, iron, retinol, and polyunsaturated fatty acids.[574]

Prevention of manifestations: Screen blood at 1 week (using a heel-prick and filter paper impregnation—the Guthrie test). *Maternal phenylketonuria* ▶Preconception counselling is vital. Effects on the baby: facial dysmorphism, microcephaly, growth retardation, IQ↓.

1 Anderson–Fabry disease may present with torturing, lancinating pains in the extremities (± abdomen) made worse by cold, heat, or exercise. It is a neuritis (vasculitis of the vasa nervorum). By adolescence, angiokeratomata appear (clusters of dark, non-blanching, petechiae) in the 'bathing trunk' area (esp. umbilicus & scrotum). Also: paraesthesiae, corneal opacities, hypohidrosis, proteinuria and renal failure. It may respond to enzyme Rₓ (α-galactosidase is ↓). Carbamazepine may help the pain.

2 MCAD deficiency is screened for in neonates on the same sample as for PKU & hypothyroidism. It's an autosomal recessive (mutation of the **m**edium-**c**hain **a**cyl-co**a** **d**ehydrogenase gene; ACADM; 1p31). Signs: hypoketotic hypoglycaemic coma; metabolic acidosis; LFT↑; medium chain dicarboxylic aciduria; 'SIDS'. ♀:♂≈1:1. Rₓ: avoid fasting; diet to give more calories from carbohydrates & proteins, while minimizing lipids. It is the chief inherited disorder of mitochondrial fatty acid oxidation in N. Europe. Carrier rate: 1:65.

Puberty may start as early as ~8yrs in girls and ~9yrs in boys. Refer to a pae-diatric endocrinologist if onset before this. ♀:♂ ≈10:1.[575] Causes may be central (gonadotrophin dependent, eg craniopharyngioma or pituitary tumour) or pe-ripheral (eg testis or adrenal problem, or HCG↑ from rare tumours 'anywhere').

Biology Think of each physical signs of puberty as a bioassay for a separate en-docrine event. Enlargement of the testes is the 1st sign of puberty in boys, and is due to pulses of pituitary gonadotrophin. Breast enlargement in girls and penis enlargement in boys is due to gonadal sex steroid secretion. Pubic hair is a mani-festation of adrenal androgen production. Growth in boys accelerates when testis volume reaches 10–12mL (if measured by comparison with orchidometer beads rather than ultrasound, expect overestimates by up to 60%).[576] Girls start to grow more quickly once their breasts have started to develop. Stage 4 breast development is a prerequisite for menarche (in most girls). The best sign that precosity is pathological is when this consonance of puberty goes awry: in Cush-ing's syndrome, pubic hair is 'too much' for the testicular volume; in hypothyroid-ism, the testes are large (FSH↑ as TSH↑↑) while growth velocity is low.[577]

Sexual signs may be obvious or subtle.[1] Gynae-comastia may worry boys.[2] One consequence is short stature caused by early fusion of epiphyses. Premature adrenal maturity (adrenarche) may presage insulin resistance. Ask about general hypothalamic dysfunction? Polyuria, polydipsia, obesity, sleep, and temperature regulation. There may also be signs of ICP↑ visual disturbance.

Rare causes
• Stress (eg adoption)
• CNS tumours/empty sella
• Craniopharyngioma
• Thyroid disorders
• Choriocarcinoma
• Meningoencephalitis
• McCune–Albright syn.
• 21-hydroxylase lack
• Rare genetic defects

If onset is before 2yrs, suspect a hypothalamic hamartoma. LH receptor gene mutations cause sporadic or familial male gonadotrophin-independent precocious puberty.

Tests Growth charts; puberty staging (Tanner charts); CNS CT/MRI; bone age (skeletal x-ray); urinary 17-ketosteroids; karyotype; adrenal, testis & pelvic♀ ultrasound, T4; TSH; LH; FSH; HCG; AFP; GH; pituitary tests (OHCM p224); oestro-gen/testosterone (if no adrenal source of ↑testosterone is found, left vs right spermatic vein sampling may suggest one testis has a tiny Leydig cell tumour or hyperplasia).[578] Virilizing 21-hydroxylase deficiency is confirmed by ↑17-hydroxyprogesterone on ACTH stimulation.[579]

Management: a physiological approach Initiation of puberty depends on release from inhibition of neurons in the medial basal hypothalamus that secrete gonadotrophin-releasing hormone (GnRH), and on decreasing hypo-thalamic-pituitary sensitivity to –ve feedback from gonadal steroids. These changes are accompanied by ↑frequency and magnitude of 'pulses' of LH. GnRH pulses are needed for normal gonadal function. Continuous high levels of GnRH paradoxically suppress secretion of pituitary gonadotrophins; this forms the basis for treating precocious puberty with synthetic GnRH analogues (nasal or SC). There is a reversal of gonadal maturation and all the clinical correlates of puberty (not for pubic hair, as there is no change in the secretion of androgens by the adrenal cortex). There is deceleration in skeletal maturation. Treatment is continued eg up to 11yrs. Families need reassurance that the child will de-velop normally. Endogenous oestrogen accelerates growth (♂ & ♀), as well as mediating ♀ sexual characteristics: testolactone can help by ↓its biosynthesis. Anti-androgens (eg flutamide) and spironolactone also have a role.[580]

---

1 Eg in boys: rapid growth of penis and testes; ↑frequency of erections; masturbation; appearance of pubic hair; body odour; acne—maybe a tendency to high IQ; tenergy expenditure ± tantrums/impulsive anger; early occurrence of capacity for frank sexual imagery in dreams and daydreams; early capacity for erotic and sexual arousal in relation to visual imagery, visual perception, and tactile sensation.
2 There is often transient oestrogen/testosterone imbalance early in ♂ puberty. Try to avoid tests (test-osterone, oestradiol; gonadotrophins; karyotype if testes <6mL). Reassure, and delay requests for mam-moplasty.

Type 1 DM is the third most common chronic disease in UK children (after asthma and cerebral palsy). *Don't medicalize the young person, but do personalize the medicine.* Paternalistic care almost never achieves good results. Good care of the child with diabetes requires involving the family unit *and* carers at school—over 50% of American children report being prevented from self-management of diabetes or using a bathroom at school.[581]

Typical presentation: Several weeks of polyuria, lethargy, polydipsia, and weight loss ±infection, poor growth; ketosis.[1] *Typical age:* 4–12yrs.[2] *Diagnostic criteria:* Based on WHO criteria:[582] signs of hyperglycaemia with ↑venous blood glucose, ie ≥11.1 mmol/L (random) or ≥7mmol/L (fasting), or raised venous blood glucose on 2 occasions without symptoms. Oral glucose tolerance tests are rarely required in children, but they are based on glucose levels at 0h and 2h post a 1.75g/kg glucose load, R: Should be delivered by a multidisciplinary paediatric diabetes care team—which provides 24h access to advice.[583] For diabetic ketoacidosis see p188. If non-ketotic, IV fluids are rarely needed. Inform children and parents that they may experience a partial remission phase ('honeymoon period') with the start of insulin. *Starting insulin:* Discuss with paediatric endocrinologist and use local protocols. One regimen would be to estimate total daily requirement of insulin (0.8–1 units/kg/24h for prepubertal children; 1.5units/kg/24h if pubertal)—this daily dose should be ⅓ rapid acting (eg Novorapid®) and ⅔ long-acting (eg protaphane). ⅔ of the daily dose should be given pre-breakfast, and ⅓ should be given pre dinner.[584] Tailor insulin regimen to your patient and their family. They may benefit from a continuous subcutaneous insulin infusion. *Diet:* Ask a paediatric dietician. Energy needs ≈1500kcal/m² or 1000kcal +100 to 200kcal for each year of age. Aiming for 30% of this with each major meal, and 10% as a bedtime snack suits some children. Giving ~20% of calories as protein, ~50% as unrefined carbohydrate, and ≤30% as fat is a rule of thumb. If the child is mildly to moderately symptomatic and clinically well, subcutaneous insulin and oral diet and fluids may be begun at diagnosis, avoiding hospital admission.[585]

Type 2 DM is rare in children (0.2:100,000;[586] ↑×13 if of Asian extraction); but insulin resistance/pre-syndrome x is burgeoning: ►see p156 for prevention.

Have a detailed written care plan What other things should a newly diagnosed child and his or her family know?

• Insulin: doses (eg during illness); practice self-injecting skills on oranges.
• Diet: What? When? Why important? What do you do if the child is hungry?
• Can blood glucose be monitored accurately? Watch the carer's technique.
• What does the carer do if the blood sugar is not well controlled?
• Does the parent or carer know what 'well controlled' means?
• Too much insulin? *Signs:* weakness→hunger→bolshy→faintness→sweating→ abdo pain→vomiting→fits→coma. Some units practise hypoglycaemia (glucose <2mmol/L) on the ward (ie no breakfast after morning insulin). Explain symptoms as they happen, and reversal with drinks (or Glucogel® oral gel).
• What should happen if the child misses a meal, or is sick afterwards?
• What happens to insulin requirements during 'flu and other illnesses?
• Who does mother or father contact in emergency? Give written advice.
• Is the GP told of discharge/follow-up plans? His role is vital in encouraging optimism, and in keeping in touch with those who skip appointments.[587]
• Encourage membership of a *Diabetic Association* (UK tel: 0207 323 1531).

---

1 Mean duration of symptoms pre-diagnosis is 30 days. Feeding with cows' milk, and infant exposure to enteroviruses, may ↑incidence. 10% have mild coeliac disease, so screening these patients is wise.

2 *Genes & environment:* DM was a disease of the over-5s, but in the UK, incidence is rising in infancy from ~1:10,000 in 1985–90 to >1.6:10,000. Islet cell antibodies are found in HLA-DR3/4 DQ8[588] (but not HLA-B15) children. ≥4 genes are important (6q partly determines islet sensitivity to damage), but most susceptibility is environmentally acquired. Most with type 1 DM have antibodies to cows' milk albumin which react with β-cell surface proteins. Also, mumps, rubella, coxsackie & CMV have the potential to injure β-cells (exact role unclear). If one child in a family has DM, risk to siblings is >5%.

MODY: maturity onset diabetes of the young[589]

MODY is a autosomal dominant kind of non-ketotic diabetes, in childhood or young adults. The defect is one of pancreatic beta cell dysfunction—leading to impaired insulin secretion.[590] ≥6 causal genes exist. MODY is caused by single gene defects, as opposed to type 1 & type 2 diabetes which are have polygenic and environmental causes. Classic MODY accounts for <5% of all childhood diabetes in Caucasians.[591]

MODY2 (GCK subtype) is caused by mutations in the glucokinase gene on chromosome 7. Glucokinase converts glucose to glucose-6-phosphate, which is needed to stimulate insulin secretion by the beta-cells. There is mild, asymptomatic, stable hyperglycaemia from birth. Microvascular disease is rare. Drugs are rarely needed.

MODY3 (HNF1A subtype) is the most common type. It is caused by a defect on chromosome 12 leading to a progressive decrease in insulin production. It features severe hyperglycaemia after puberty, which often leads to a diagnosis of type 1 DM. Despite progressive hyperglycaemia, sensitivity to sulfonylureas is retained for years. Diabetic retinopathy and nephropathy often occur in MODY3. Frequency of cardiovascular disease is not increased. Owing to the pleiotropic character of transcription factors, most MODY subtypes are diseases with multi-organ involvement in addition to diabetes.

MODY5 (HNF-1B) is more frequent than originally thought. It is associated with pancreatic atrophy, renal abnormalities, and genital tract malformations.

MODY 1, 4 & 6 These subtypes of MODY are all rare.

Molecular diagnosis matters because it has important consequences for prognosis, family screening, and management. Although MODY is dominantly inherited, expression varies, so a family history of DM is not always present.

Paediatrics

Hypoglycaemic coma

▸▸Get IV access. Get help. Intra-oral GlucoGel® has a role if IV access fails.
▸▸Give glucose 5mL/kg of 10% IVI, or by rectal tube if no IV access, with glucagon 0.5–1mg IM or slowly IV (0.5mg if <25kg). *Expect quick return to consciousness*. If not, recheck glucose; if low, give IV dexamethasone (p200); if normal, ask yourself *is this is a post-ictal state after a hypoglycaemic fit?* Here, giving more glucose worsens cerebral oedema.

'What are the aims of routine follow-up in the diabetes clinic?'

- To approach normoglycaemia via motivational education. Group learning is better than didactic doctor-sermons.
- To prevent complications (esp. renal & retinal). Check growth & fundi (dilate pupils; retinopathy takes ~10yrs to develop). Blood: glucose, Hb_{A1c}, microalbuminuria—present in 25% after 10yrs (50% after 20yrs): ▸reducible to 15% if glucose well-controlled; microalbuminuria may spontaneously reverse.
- If normoglycaemia is unachievable, choose the best compromise with the child's way of life and strict glucose control.
- Insulin-storing pen-shaped injectors allow flexibility in the timing and dose of insulin, delivering a variable dose (2u/push) without inconvenient drawing up of insulin (eg during a party).
- Introduce to a friendly diabetic nurse-teacher; ask "Is real-time *continuous* glucose monitoring indicated?". Feedback helps motivation and safety.

Just 100 years ago, DKA was universally fatal. The first patient to receive insulin (on January 11th 1922), was Leonard Thompson—a 14-yr-old boy, who went on to live a further 13 years. DKA results from a deficiency of insulin, often in combination with increased levels of counter-regulatory hormones (catecholamines, glucagon, cortisol and growth hormone—eg due to sepsis). The big concern with childhood DKA, (as opposed to adult DKA), is the increased frequency of cerebral oedema (see BOX), which occurs in ~1% of childhood DKA and has a mortality of 25%. Other fatal events in DKA include hypokalaemia and aspiration pneumonia (use NGT if semi-conscious and protect airway).

The patient Listlessness; confusion; vomiting; polyuria; polydipsia; weight loss; abdominal pain. *Look for:* Dehydration; deep and rapid (Kussmaul) respirations; ketotic (fruity-smelling) breath; shock; drowsiness; coma.

Diagnosis Requires the combination of *hyperglycaemia* (≥11mmol/L), *acidosis* (venous pH <7.3) and *ketones* in urine and blood. *Severity* is categorized by degree of acidosis: mild—pH <7.3; moderate—pH <7.2; or severe—pH <7.1

Management Do GCS (p720; p201 if <4yrs). True coma is rare (<10%) in DKA: exclude other causes of coma; remember DKA may be precipitated secondarily. Take the following action if shocked, consciousness↓, coma, or vomiting.[1]

• *Resuscitate: ABC:* Oropharyngeal airway 100% O_2 ± NGT. Consider intubation. Give 10mL/kg IV boluses of 0.9% saline only if shocked, to a max. of 30mL/kg: over-enthusiastic fluid resuscitation may cause cerebral oedema. Consider ITU if BP↓, or <2yrs, or ward staff busy (all children with DKA initially require high level of nursing care—usually 1:1).

• *Rapidly confirm diagnosis:* with history, finger-prick glucose + ketones; venous blood gas; urine dip for ketones/glucose.

• *Formal investigations:* Weigh; FBC; U&E; glucose; Ca^{2+}; PO_4^{3-}; blood gas; ECG monitoring (look for peaked T-waves of hyperkalaemia), lab urine.

• *Use clinical signs to assess dehydration* (BOX 2) Now calculate the volume of fluid to be replaced (fluid requirement): ie maintenance fluid *plus* the dehydration deficit *minus* any fluid already given as resuscitation fluid. It should be given at a constant steady rate over the 1st 48h. (see worked example).

• *Start IV fluids:* Start with 0.9% saline + 20mmol KCl/500mL. When blood glucose falls to 14mmol/L use 0.9% saline + 5% glucose + 20mmol KCl /500mL. After 12h, if plasma sodium is stable, change to 0.45% saline + 5% glucose + 20mmol KCl/500mL.

• *Start IV insulin only after 1h of IV fluids:* Cerebral oedema may be more likely if insulin is started early. There is no need for an initial bolus of insulin. Use a 1 unit/mL solution of fast acting insulin (eg Actrapid®). Run at 0.1 units/kg/h. Ensure there is glucose in the IV fluids when venous glucose is <14mmol/L. Do NOT stop insulin at this stage it is still required to switch off ketogenesis. Once pH >7.3 and glucose is <14mmol/L consider reducing insulin to 0.05units/kg/h.

• *Stop IV insulin:* When blood ketone levels are <1.0mmol/L, and patient is able to tolerate food, give a dose of subcutaneous insulin; feed the patient. Stop infusion 10–60mins after subcutaneous insulin injection

Avoid bicarbonate in DKA: it can increase the risk of cerebral oedema. If acidosis persists, consider ↑dose of insulin (more glucose may be needed in the IV fluids). Ask yourself: is this child septic?

Ongoing monitoring • Hourly blood glucose • CNS status ≥half-hourly. • Nurses must tell you of headache or behaviour change promptly as these may indicate cerebral oedema (BOX) • Hourly fluid balance • Blood gases 2h after starting IVI, then 4-hourly. Have a dedicated line for drawing blood. • If a central venous catheter (CVC) is used to aid monitoring, consider DVT prophylaxis.[2,592] • Weigh twice daily • Monitor ECG for T-wave changes • Infection screen.

Pitfalls in diabetic ketoacidosis

Cerebral oedema (MINIBOX) is a big threat, and is almost exclusively a condition of childhood. Pathophysiology is poorly understood: it usually occurs 4–12h from the start of treatment, but it may be present at onset of DKA or up to 24h afterwards, presenting as a sudden CNS deterioration after an initial improvement. It is the major cause of death in diabetic children, not the much-feared hypoglycaemia *Leukocytosis* (even a leukaemoid reaction) may occur without any infection. *Infection*: (there may be no fever). Do MSU, blood cultures, and CXR. Start broad-spectrum antibiotics (p202) if infection suspected. *Creatinine:* some assays for creatinine crossreact with ketone bodies, so plasma creatinine may not reflect true renal function. *Hyponatraemia* (from osmotic effects of glucose): if <120mmol/L, search for other causes, eg triglycerides↑↑. Hypernatraemia >150mmol/L may be treated with of 0.45% saline to start with (0.9% saline thereafter). *Ketonuria* does not equate with ketoacidosis. Normal individuals may have ketonuria after an overnight fast. Not all ketones are due to diabetes—consider alcohol, if glucose normal. Test plasma with Ketostix® or Acetest® to demonstrate ketonaemia. *Acidosis* without gross elevation of glucose may occur, but consider poisoning, eg with aspirin.

CNS deterioration
If warning signs: headache, ↓pulse, ↑BP, restlessness, irritability, focal neuorology (CN palsies), posturing, ↑ICP, or falling consciousness:
►►Call your senior
►►Exclude hypoglycaemia
►►Mannitol 0.25–1.5g/kg IVI or NaCl 2.7% 5mL/kg
►►Restrict IV maintenance fluids by ½ and replace deficit over 72h
►►Move to PICU and do CT
►►Treat sepsis vigorously

Serum amylase is often raised (up to 10-fold), and nonspecific abdominal pain is common even in the absence of pancreatitis.

Degree of dehydration[1]

• *Mild*—is hard to detect; it approximates to ~**3%** weight loss.
• *Moderate*—dry mucous membranes and ↓skin turgor: ~**5%**.
• *Severe*—sunken eyes and ↓capillary refill time: ~**8%**
Overestimation of dehydration is dangerous—►don't use an estimation of greater than 8%. NB: 8% dehydrated = water deficit of 80mL/kg

Calculating fluid requirement in DKA[1]

Hourly rate = (48h maintenance + deficit - fluid already given) ÷ 48

The BPSED[1] suggests the following maintenance requirements based on weight (different from standard APLS rates):

<12.9kg	80mL/kg/24h	35–59.9kg	45mL/kg/24h
13–19.9kg	65mL/kg/24h	>60kg	35mL/kg/24h
20–34.9kg	55mL/kg/24h		

A 20kg 6-year-old boy who is 8% dehydrated, and who has already had 20mL/kg of saline will require:

$$(48h \text{ maintenance} + \text{deficit} - \text{fluid already given}) \div 48$$
$$\approx 55mL \times 20kg \times 2 \text{ (as 48h)} + (80mL/kg \times 20kg) - (20mL \times 20kg) \div 48$$
$$\approx (2200mL + 1600mL - 400mL) \div 48$$
$$\approx 3400mL \div 48 = 71mL/h$$

---

1 Guidelines for the management of DKA in children, British Society for Paediatric Endocrinology and Diabetes (BPSED) 2009—available at: http://www.bsped.org.uk/clinical/docs/DKAGuideline.pdf. These have been endorsed by NICE.

2 Because thrombotic complications are rare, heparin isn't usually needed and is not recommended as part of standard therapy, but see brighton-healthcare.nhs.uk/diabetes/newpage17.htm[593] SE: thrombotic thrombocytopoenia.[594]

3 Note that pooling of KCl and insulin may cause uneven delivery in some IVI containers, so repeated mixing may be needed.[595]

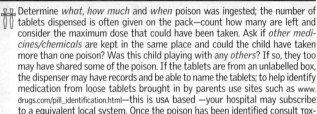

Determine *what, how much* and *when* poison was ingested; the number of tablets dispensed is often given on the pack—count how many are left and consider the maximum dose that could have been taken. Ask if *other medicines/chemicals* are kept in the same place and could the child have taken more than one poison? Was this child playing with any *others*? If so, they too may have shared some of the poison. If the tablets are from an unlabelled box, the dispenser may have records and be able to name the tablets; to help identify medication from loose tablets brought in by parents use sites such as www.drugs.com/pill_identification.html—this is USA based —your hospital may subscribe to a equivalent local system. Once the poison has been identified consult TOX-BASE (www.toxbase.org) or local equivalent.

►Contact a National Poisons Information Service (NPIS, eg 0844 892 0111 in UK). *Examination:* Look for signs of toxidromes. (see BOX). Ensure complete set of vital signs are obtained. Note GCS and pupils.

Principles of management

- As always: ABC is your priority. Also check blood glucose.
- Consider intubation if GCS <8, or respiratory failure; if GCS 8–14 consider oral/nasopharyngeal airway (caution if vomiting) and put in recovery position.
- Maintain BP; correct hypoglycaemia; monitor urine output.
- Baseline studies may include: FBC, U&E; glucose; ECG
- Do a blood gas: a metabolic acidosis with an increased anion gap can be due to drugs such as metformin; alcohol; ethylene; toluene; cyanide; isoniazid; iron; aspirin; paraldehyde or other causes (DKA; lactic acidosis)
- Certain drugs can be measured in serum—so test for paracetamol; ethanol; methanol; ethylene glycol; salicylates; iron; anti-convulsants; lithium; digoxin; theophylline; carboxyhaemaglobin if these are suspected.
- The mainstay of care is *supportive management.*
- Consider *gastric decontamination*—discuss with a toxicologist.
- *Ipecac syrup*, or any form of forced vomiting, is no longer recommended.[596] *Activated charcoal* is controversial as there is no evidence it improves clinical outcome.[597] It is most effective (in volunteer studies) if given within 1h of ingestion. Concerns exist about the risk of aspiration of charcoal if the patient vomits (increased in hydrocarbon poisonings) or becomes drowsy. Avoid with lithium, alcohol, cyanide, iron ingestions or rapid acting ingestions.[597] *Cathartics* and *Gastric lavage* are virtually never indicated.[598-600] *Whole bowel irrigation* should not be routinely used, but it may be of benefit in sustained released ingestions.[601] Only use after consulting NPIS or if specifically recommended in TOXBASE.[600]
- Determine if a *specific antidote* is available (see below and p192-3).

Specific antidotes

- *Beta-blockers:* cause hypotension, bradycardia, heart block and heart failure. Monitor ECG; atropine 40µg/kg IV for bradycardia, then glucagon (50–150µg/kg IV + infusion of 50µg/kg/h in 5% glucose). Consider adrenaline or dopamine infusions.
- *Carbon monoxide:* High flow oxygen and mannitol for cerebral oedeme. Severe cases may benefit from hyperbaric oxygen therapy.
- *Digoxin:* Atropine is used if bradycardic. Digoxin specific antibody (Digibind®) is used in those with severe dysrhythmias/hyperkalaemia. Historically use of calcium in digoxin-induced hyperkalaemia has been avoided due to fears about cardiac tetany: this has recently been considered less likely.[601]
- *Opioids:* use IV naloxone 10µg/kg; if no response try 100µg/kg (max 2mg). An infusion may be required.
- *Methanol/ethylene glycol:* Fomepizole.[602] Contact poisons unit promptly.
- *Sulfonylureas:* ?Try octreotide.[603] Other antidotes: OHCM p852.

- *Opioid*—eg morphine, codeine, methadone, oxycodone, heroin—bradycardia, hypotension, decreased respiratory rate, and pin-point pupils.
- *Cholinergic*—eg organophosphates; pilocarpine—*(DUMBELLS):* Diarrhoea; Urination; Miosis; Bradycardia; Emesis; Lacrimation; Lethary; Salivation.
- *Anticholinergic*—eg antihistamines, tricyclic antidepressants, deadly nightshade, atropine—these patients are *Hot as a hare, Red as a beet, Dry as a bone, Blind as a bat and, Mad as a hatter*—with hyperthermia, facial flushing, dry skin, dilated pupils, and delirium. They also have tachycardia and urinary retention.
- *Sympathomimetic*—eg cocaine, amphetamines, pseudoephedrine—patient is tachycardic, hypertensive, hyperthermic and has dilated pupils. Risk of seizures.

Iron poisoning

Iron is a common childhood poison. It is absorbed as Fe^{2+}, oxidized to Fe^{3+} and bound to transferrin. Toxicity occurs when transferrin binding capacity is reached.

Identify the exact preparation, as formulations contain different amounts of elemental iron. A 200mg $FeSO_4$ tablet contains ~65mg elemental iron. 125mg/mL $FeSO_4$ drops contain 25mg iron/mL. A 300mg ferrous fumarate tablet may contain 100mg of iron (depends on brand), whereas a 300mg ferrous gluconate tablet may only contain 35mg of iron. Expect mild toxicity at doses of >20mg/kg of elemental iron. Mod-severe toxicity occurs with doses of >60mg/kg.[604,605]

Presentation: Patients may have ingested tablets, liquid or multi-vitamins containing iron. He may present with nausea, vomiting, haematemesis, diarrhoea, altered mental status or hypotension. Between 6–12 hours there may be a phase of apparent improvement. Between 12–24 hours cardiovascular collapse and massive GI bleeding can occur. Severe metabolic acidosis may develop as each Fe^{3+} ion combines with water to produce $3H^+$ and $FeOH^3$. Renal and hepatic failure may ensue. Hepatotoxicity is a marker of severity and is a common cause of death. Survivors may develop pyloric strictures after 4–6 weeks secondary to scarring. *Tests:* Baseline blood gas, serum iron concentration, U&E, FBC, glucose. Iron levels at 4–6h help determine level of severity. Levels of <350µg/dL (~60µmol/L) are associated with minimal symptoms. Levels >500µg/dL (~90µmol/L) are associated with serious toxicity. An abdominal radiograph may show tablets within the gut and reveal a bezoar. ▶In servere toxicity do not wait for tests: start desferrioxamine.

Management:
- Obtain expert help as this is one of the few instances when gastric lavage/endoscopy to remove tablets in the stomach may be recommended.
- Activated charcoal is not given as it has no effect on iron absorption.
- Whole bowel irrigation may help (esp. in slow-release preparations).[606]
- Supportive care—IV fluids and sodium bicarbonate to correct acidosis
- Chelation with IV desferrioxamine (5–15mg/kg/h—start at higher dose then reduce after 4–6h—max 80mg/kg/24h). Therapy should be stopped when the acidosis improves. It is rarely required for >24h. Use of desferrioxamine leads to orangey-red urine which demonstrates that free iron has been bound to the desferrioxamine. It is also associated with hypotension, rashes, pulmonary oedema and acute respiratory distress syndrome.
- Haemofiltration has been used in children, in combination with desferrioxamine to rapidly reduce iron levels.[607]

Paediatrics

The most common salicylate is acetylsalicylic acid, ie aspirin, which is not recommended in children <16y due to its association with Reye's syndrome (p652). Choline salicylate is found in Bonjela® for adults. Since 2009, Bonjela teething gel® in the UK has used lidocaine as its active ingredient, however Bonjela teething gel® in other countries (eg Australasia) continues to contain choline salicylate (8.7%) and there are reports of toxicity in children.[608] Methyl salicylate is found in oil of wintergreen (98%). As little as 3mL can be fatal in children.[609] Methyl salicylate is also found in muscle rubs such as Bengay®, Deep Heat®, and Tiger Balm® (~15–40%). *Presentation:* Toxicity occurs at ~100mg/kg aspirin. Early signs include tinnitus and hearing loss. Stimulation of respiratory centres leads to tachypnoea and a respiratory alkalosis. Interference with aerobic metabolism leads to the metabolic (lactic) acidosis which is characteristic of salicylate poisoning. GI irritation (nausea, vomiting, abdominal pain is common). Central effects lead to agitation, delirium and seizures. Rhabdomyolysis, pulmonary oedema and electrolyte disturbances may also occur. *Tests:* Blood gas; FBC; U&E, glucose. Salicylate levels are best obtained at 6 hours (reflects a peak level) however, do an initial level to confirm diagnosis, and then levels every 2h to confirm levels are decreasing—enteric coated (EC) preparations can lead to delayed absorption. Large bezoars of EC aspirin may be seen on radiograph. *Management:* Resuscitate with boluses of 10–20mL/kg of 0.9% saline. Correct hypoglycaemia. Potassium may be needed as hypokalaemia is common. Serious poisoning is indicated by levels >2.5–3.6mmol/L—consider urinary alkalinization with IV sodium bicarbonate to enhance elimination (under expert guidance in ITU). Activated charcoal is effective in adsorbing aspirin, but as patients are liable to vomit or experience ↓GCS consider intubating first and using a NGT. Repeat doses can be given. Haemodialysis is the definitive treatment: use when evidence of end organ injury[610] (seizures, severe acidosis, rhabdomyolysis, renal failure, pulmonary oedema). *Seek expert help.*

Paracetamol (acetaminophen) poisoning

The therapeutic dose is 15mg/kg. Hepatotoxicity can occur if ≥150mg/kg/24h ingested. The initial features are nausea and pallor. Hepatic enzymes rise after ~24h. Jaundice and an enlarged, tender liver occur after 48h. Hypoglycaemia, hypotension, encephalopathy, coagulopathy, coma may also occur.

Management of single oral paracetamol overdoses:
• If you are certain the ingested paracetamol is <150mg/kg in a child with no hepatic risk factors (below), then management may be safely done at home.[611]
• Admit those presenting within 8h of ingesting >150mg/kg (or an unknown amount or with high risk factors) and do a serum paracetamol concentration at ≥4h post ingestion. If presenting <1h, and >150mg/kg of tablets ingested, and no contra-indication (eg vomiting; ↓GCS), give activated charcoal—not beneficial if elixir has been ingested which is absorbed in ~15 mins.[612]
• Decide if the child has any high-risk factors, eg patients who are on enzyme-inducers (p300) or who are malnourished (eg anorexia, alcoholism, HIV +ve), or have febrile illness—in whom toxicity may occur at doses of >75mg/kg.[613]
• Consult the nomogram on the opposite page. If the child is high risk, use the lower treatment line, if not—use the upper line. If plasma paracetamol level is above the appropriate line, treat with acetylcysteine (NAC). The initial dose is 150mg/kg in up to 200mL (depending weight; see *BNF*) of 5% dextrose infused over 15min, followed by 50mg/kg IVI over the next 4h, and 100mg/kg IVI over next 16h. It is very effective in preventing liver damage if given in <8h.
• Patients with a delayed presentation (>8h) or in whom a level cannot be obtained within 8h, should have acetylcysteine started immediately if ingested dose is >150mg/kg, or dose is unknown. Check often for hypoglycaemia.

- Consider the cause: typically teenage girls seeking attention. All need psychiatric evaluation. Causes may be extremely complex and deep-seated: although the patient may claim a seemingly superficial cause this may be hiding deep social or psychiatric pathology.

Staggered overdose: Seek expert help: these patients are at potentially greater risk than those with single point overdoses, and may present with greater delays.[614] Paracetamol levels alone may not be reliable in staggered overdoses, so LFT and INR are also done. If >8h from 1st dose, treat with NAC; don't wait for levels as efficacy is waning fast. If <8h, do levels (see graph).

Paediatrics

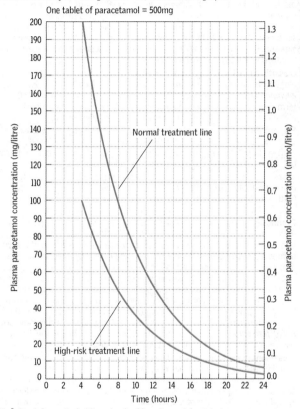

One tablet of paracetamol = 500mg

Normal treatment line

High-risk treatment line

Plasma paracetamol concentration (mg/litre)

Plasma paracetamol concentration (mmol/litre)

Time (hours)

Fig 1. Graph for use in deciding who should receive acetylcysteine.
©Dr Alun Hutchings (University of Wales).

▶This graph DOES NOT apply to IV paracetamol. If 4h level following IV paracetamol overdose is >50mg/L (below high-risk treatment line) or if a single IV overdose of >60mg/kg has been given, then treatment should be started.[615,616] This is because IV paracetamol plasma concentration peaks at the end of administration. By 4h levels may have dropped considerably. Consult with NPIS. Other countries use different nomograms. Australasian guidelines have a single treatment line which starts at 150mg/L—that is midway between the UK high risk and normal treatment lines.[617]

ALL is the commonest (80%) childhood leukaemia (~500 cases/yr); it is a malignant disorder of lymphoid progenitor cells. Other forms: OHCM p346–53. Peak age is 2–4years, with a second peak >50y. Incidence is greater in white children than in black children. *Causes:* Precise cause is unknown. There are genetic associations: ALL is concordant in ~25% of monozygotic twins; individuals with trisomy 21 have a 4-fold increased risk (also increased risk in Bloom's syndrome, ataxia-telangectasia). Chromosomal translocations such as t(12;21) resulting in the TEL-AML fusion gene are associated with 30% of cases (only present in 1% of the general population). t(9;22)—the Philadelphia chromosom—occurs in 15–30% (mostly adults) and is associated with a poor prognosis. Environmental risk factors which have been implicated include prenatal exposure to x-rays; *in utero* exposure to infection, delayed postnatal exposure to infection and environmental radiation.[618–620]

Classification The French-American-British (FAB) criteria of L1,L2,L3 morphology is obsolescent and is replaced by the WHO classification of ALL into either *B lymphoblastic leukaemia* or *T lymphoblastic leukaemia.*[614] Prior to 2008 the term pre-B cell ALL was used to distinguish *B lymphoblastic leukaemia* from mature B-cell ALL which is termed Burkitt lymphoma/leukaemia.

Presentation Pancytopenia (pallor, infection, bleeding), fatigue, anorexia, fever, bone pain. Painless lumps in neck, axilla, groin. The period before diagnosis is often brief (2–4 weeks). Cranial infiltration may lead to CNS effects, eg cranial palsies. Testicular infiltration can lead to orchidomegaly.

Tests *Bloods:* WCC↑, ↓ or ↔. Normochromic, normocytic anaemia ± platelets↓, urate↑, LDH↑. *Marrow:* 50–98% of nucleated cells will be blasts. *CSF:* Pleocytosis (with blast forms), protein ↑, glucose ↓. *Cytogenetic analysis:* 80% will have genetic abnormalities at diagnosis. *CXR:* May show mediastinal mass.

Prognosis depends on clinical signs, biologic features of lymphoblasts and response to induction chemotherapy. Based on these features patients can be stratified into 4 risk categories. *Standard risk:* Patients are aged 1–9.9yrs, have WCC of <50×10⁹/L; lack unfavourable cytogenetic features, show a good response to initial chemotherapy and have <5% bone marrow blasts by 14 days and <0.01% blasts by 28 days. *Low risk:* These patients meet the standard risk criteria and have favourable genetics, such as trisomy 4, 10 or 17. *High risk:* Patients do not meet standard criteria or have extra-medullary involvement (eg brain/testis). *Very high risk:* Have unfavourable genetics, such as the Philedelphia chromosme, hypodiploidy—or poor response to initial chemotherapy. *Event-free survival* at 5yr is 95% in the low risk group; 30% in the very high risk. Infant leukaemia has the worst outcome: 20%. Overall survival is 80%.

Treatment of ALL typically has 3 phases: *Induction therapy:* 3-drug induction over 4 weeks (eg **vincristine, dexamethasone,**[621] **L-asparaginase**) + intrathecal (IT) therapy (**methotrexate ± cytarabine + hydrocortisone**) results in remission of >95%. High-risk patients may get a further agent eg **daunorubicin.**[614] ~2% die of infection. *Consolidation phase:* Cranial irradiation if known CNS disease. Further chemotherapy (eg **cyclophosphamide; cytarabine; mercaptopurine**). *Continuation phase:* For ~2½yrs (daily **mercaptopurine** + weekly **methotrexate** ± **vincristine/steroid** pulses). 3-monthly intrathecal drugs.

Complications *Neutropenic sepsis:* See BOX. **Co-trimoxazole** prevents pneumocystosis. Revaccinate (1 dose of each type, p151) 6 months after chemotherapy (as vaccine-specific antibody↓).[622] *Hyperuricaemia:* From massive cell death at induction: pre-treat with ↑ fluid intake + **allopurinol.** *Poor growth:* Monitor carefully.[623] *Cancer elsewhere:* Risk of CNS tumours or a 2ⁿᵈ leukaemia is 3%.

Relapses: Consider FLAG¹, **clofarabine**[624] or marrow transplant; consider if risk ↑↑, eg WCC >200×10⁹/L, MLL gene rearrangement, B-cell ALL with t(8;14).[625,626] Tyrosine kinase inhibitors (eg **imatinib**) are used in children with t(9:22).

Pitfalls ▶Ignoring quality of life; eg most cytotoxics may be given at home. • Omitting to examine the testes (▶a common site for recurrence). • Thiopurine methyltransferase deficiency may cause fatal myelosuppression (?do pre-treatment pharmacogenomic analysis).[627] • Inappropriate transfusion (leukostasis, *OHCM* p346, if WCC >100×10⁹/L).[628] • SE of chemotherapy. NB: **ondansetron** is better than other anti-emetics.

▶▶Febrile neutropenic patients who may be septicaemic (eg from an infected venous catheter)

Suspect infection when untoward events happen in a neutropenic patient (WCC <2×10⁹/L, or neutrophils <1×10⁹/L). Do T° often; brief rises to ≤38°C *may* be ignored if lasting for <6h only if the child is well. Emphasize to the parents and child the importance of swift routes to hospital. Do blood cultures and MSU; swab all orifices. Do FBC, CRP & serology. Get help from your senior and a microbiologist; follow local protocols.

Likely organisms In one UK study, blood cultures were +ve in 30%. Gram-positive organisms predominated (80%) and most were coagulase-negative staphs. 6% were Gram-negative isolates and <1% fungal.[629]

Blind treatment Use local protocols, eg Tazocin®[630] ± gentamicin[631] OR imipenem (±teicoplanin)—the broadest-spectrum β-lactam[2] antibiotic, which may have advantages over cephalosporins if an anaerobe such as *Bacteroides* is suspected (NB: imipenem is not indicated in CNS infections).[632]

Tazocin® = piptazobactam = piperacillin + tazobactam IV over 3–5min or IVI: 1 month–18yrs: 90mg/kg/6h, max 4.5g/6h. (The neonatal dose is 90mg/kg/8h.)

Gentamicin Child 1 month–12yrs: 2.5 mg/kg/8h. 12–18yrs 2mg/kg/24h.

Imipenem—*Dose in children <40kg:* 15mg/kg/6h max 2g/24h. Heavier children have the adult dose: 250–500mg/6h (less sensitive organisms: up to 25mg/kg/6h IVI; max, eg 1g/6h). Do U&E. If creatinine clearance <70mL/min, ↓dose frequency (see *Data sheet*). NB: do not use IM formulations IV (IM formulations are not for use in children). If blood culture *does* prove +ve, either change imipenem after microbiological advice, or continue it for 5 days, if he has been afebrile for >24h. If blood cultures are –ve, give for a few days and send home when well and afebrile for >24h. SEs: (It is usually well-tolerated.) Thrombophlebitis, anuria, polyuria, seizures (eg in ~2%), confusion, psychic disturbance, encephalopathy, vertigo, tinnitus, transient hearing loss, BP↓, pruritus, taste perversion, pseudomembranous colitis; arthralgia; eosinophilia; WCC↓; Hb↓ LFT↑. There are few clinically important drug interactions, eg seizures if co-therapy with ganciclovir.[633]

Meropenem is preferred in some units (unlicensed; more active against most Gram –ves than imipenem but is less active against most Gram +ves).[634] Dose: 1 month to 12yrs: 10–20mg/kg/8h IVI over 5min. Over 50kg weight: adult dose (eg 1g/8h IVI). SE: D&V (eg antibiotic-associated colitis); abdominal pain; LFT↑; platelets↓; partial thromboplastin time↓; +ve Coombs' test; eosinophilia; WCC↓; headache; paraesthesiae; rash; pruritus; fits (rare).[635]

Teicoplanin For blind treatment of the worst infections, consider adding this to imipenem. Dose: 10mg/kg/12h IV for 3 doses, max 400mg, then 6mg/kg/24h (max 400mg); neonates: 16mg/kg on day 1, then 8mg/kg/day). SE: (few) headache; WCC↓; platelets ↓/↑; LFT↑; allergy (rare). No major interactions.[636]

If fever persists and blood cultures remain –ve ask: Is aciclovir indicated? Is a fungus possible? For **amphotericin** see SPC/*data sheet* & *OHCM* p168.

---

1 FLAG = **Fl**udarabine, cytarabine (**A**ra-C), and **G**-CSF (recombinant human granulocyte-colony stimulating factor); clofarabine; it is non-standard.[637,638] A novel alternative is myeloablative chemotherapy and radiation followed by infusion of umbilical cord blood saved after delivery for this kind of eventuality.[639]
2 Named for the β-lactam ring in their structure. Examples: penicillins, cephalosporins, etc.

The clinical problem You have the results of a full blood count, showing anaemia (Hb <11g/dL, p220, the WHO criterion). *How should you proceed?*

1 Take a history (include travel, diet, ethnic origin); examine the child.

2 MCV <70fL: ?IDA/iron deficiency anaemia (poor diet, poverty, bleeding, stomatitis, koilonychia) or *thalassaemia* (Mediterranean/SE Asia areas, short stature, muddy complexion, icteric sclerae, distended abdomen ∵ hepatosplenomegaly, bossed skull, prominent maxillae, from marrow hyperplasia).

3 MCV >100fL: suspect ↓folate (malabsorption; phenytoin), ↓B₁₂ (breast milk from a vegetarian, ↓intrinsic factor, malabsorption), or haemolysis. Signs of B₁₂↓: poor feeding, late milestones; odd movements; microcephaly, failure to thrive.

4 MCV 81–97fL (normocytic): suspect haemolysis, or marrow failure (transient, after infections, or thyroid, kidney, or liver failure, or malignancy). Causes of aplasia: chloramphenicol; Diamond–Blackfan (p640); Fanconi's anaemia (p644).

5 WCC/differential abnormal? Eosinophilia + anaemia + tropics ≈ hookworms.

6 Severe tropical anaemias (eg Hb <5): malaria; bacteraemia (eg nontyphoid salmonella[640]); worms; HIV; B₁₂↓; G6PD↓; iron deficiency; sickle cell anaemia.

7 Next look at the ESR and CRP. This may indicate some chronic disease.

8 Film + reticulocyte count ± thick film for malaria. Hypochromic microcytic RBCs ≈ IDA; target cells ≈ liver disease or thalassaemia; ferritin for IDA; sickling tests + Hb electrophoresis for thalassaemia & sickle-cell anaemia; B₁₂; red cell folate.

9 Prevention: no cows' milk if <1yr; if formula-fed, use iron-fortified; wean at 4–6 months. Adequate vitamin C intake; iron supplements if premature.

Iron deficiency anaemia (∼26% of infants, worldwide;[641] peak age ∼18 months) this is despite fortification of, formula, breakfast cereals and noodles etc.[642] The chief behavioural effect is that iron deficient babies are less happy than others, with ↓psychomotor development and poor cognition (?from altered myelination).[643] In the UK, dietary causes are common, eg poverty, lack of education, or coeliac disease. In recurrent IDA, suspect bleeding (eg Meckel's diverticulum, p651, or oesophagitis). ℞: Ferrous fumarate syrup (140mg/5mL), 0.25mL/kg/12h PO (if <12yrs old (max20mL), or Sytron®. Warn of the dangers of overdose, p191. Aim for a rise in Hb of >1g/month (do reticulocyte count after 2 months). In many places, the 1ˢᵗ step is de-worming.

Haemolysis Is malaria or sickle-cell disease possible? Get help, and try to provide the expert with sufficient information to answer these 4 questions:

1 Any evidence of ↑RBC production? (Polychromasia, reticulocytosis.)

2 Is there decreased RBC survival? (Bilirubin ↑, haptoglobins ↓.)

3 Is there intravascular haemolysis? (Haemoglobinuria.)

4 Is there an inborn error of metabolism (eg G6PD deficiency, spherocytosis, or is the defect acquired (usually with +ve Coombs' test?)

Hereditary spherocytosis is the main cause of haemolysis in north European children (mainly autosomal dominant; spontaneous mutations in 25%). It is often mild; parvovirus B19 infection can trigger transient severe anaemia. Flow cytometric analysis of eosin-5-maleimide (EMA) binding to red cells, and cryohaemolysis test have replaced osmotic fragility tests.[644] Splenectomy leads to ↑RBC survival and is sometimes indicated; gallstones may occur in the 1ˢᵗ decade, and if symptomatic cholecystectomy ± splenectomy may be needed.[645]

Sickle-cell disease: OHCM p334. Hydrate and give O₂. *Pain relief:* Warmth, hydration, ibuprofen 10mg/kg/8h PO,[ ] ± morphine sulphate solution, load with 0.4mg/kg PO,[646] then 0.3mg/kg/4h + MST® 1–1.5mg/kg/12h[ ] for background analgesia; this *may* be preferred to IVI morphine, eg 0.1mg/kg (+lactulose 2.5–10mL/12h PO ± senna). *Patient-controlled analgesia:* Morphine 1mg/kg[ ] in 50mL 5% glucose at 1mL/h with self-delivered extra boluses of 1mL as needed; do respiration & sedation score every ¼h + SₐO₂ if chest or abdominal pain.[647,648] Deferasirox (Exjade®) is a good but expensive oral iron chelator; needed if many transfusions are used.

Paediatrics

Iron deficiency without anaemia

▶Don't think that if a child is not anaemic he is not iron deficient. CNS iron levels fall *before* RBC mass. If in doubt, check ferritin. Treating low ferritins may improve: •Memory •Lassitude •Developmental delay •Mood •Cognition—in toddlers and adolescent girls, facing demands of puberty and menstruation. NB: pica (eating dirt, p210) is a sign of iron deficiency.

Purpura: 2 questions: is the child ill? what is the platelet count?

• *If ill & platelets ↓:* Meningococcaemia (↦ceftriaxone, p202), leukaemia, or disseminated intravascular coagulation (check a visual non-automated blood film & WCC, discuss with lab). Haemolytic uraemic syndrome (p176).
• *If ill & platelet count ↔ or t:* Viruses (measles; enteroviruses);[649] vasculitis (Kawasaki, p646; platelets↑);[650] SBE. Meningococcaemia less likely.
• *If well(ish) & platelet count ↔* and no history of trauma: HSP (below).
• *If well & platelet count↓* consider idiopathic thrombocytopenic purpura (rarely, Wiskott-Aldrich syndrome, p655, or aplastic anaemia). NB: vomiting or coughing can cause petechiae in superior vena cava distribution.

If in doubt, treat for meningococcaemia. NB: we can find no case of purpura for >48h being caused by meningococcal sepsis *in a child who is 100% well.*

Henoch-Schönlein purpura (HSP) is an acute immune complex-mediated vasculitis. Most patients have a antecedent upper respiratory tract infection. Purpura (purple spots/nodules not disappearing on palpation), arthritis/arthralgias (74%)—often knees/ankles—and abdominal pain (51%) are the classic triad. ♂:♀1.3:1.[651] *Other signs:* Renal involvement (54%; severe nephropathy in 7%, acute renal insufficiency in 2%), scrotal oedema (13%), and intussusception (0.6%). *Tests:* ESR↑ (57%), IgA↑ (37%), proteinuria (42%) ASO titres↑ (36%). Check U&E & BP. Steroids may help resolve abdo pain,[652] but role in prevention of chronic kidney disease is less clear.[653] Most recover in ≤2 months. Recurrences, verified in 35%, correlate with ↑ESR.

Complications (worse in adults): massive GI bleeds, ileus, haemoptysis (rare), and acute renal failure (rare). One option in HSP nephritis (not usually needed) is high-dose steroids + cyclophosphamide; this decreases proteinuria (a risk factor for renal insufficiency in HSP).[654] Chronic renal failure occurs in 5%.

Idiopathic (immune) thrombocytopenic purpura (ITP) is most chief acquired bleeding disorder in childhood. ITP has acute and chronic forms. *Presentation:* Acute bruising, purpura, and petechiae. Usually a history of recent URTI or gastroenteritis. May follow CMV, EBV, parvovirus, varicella-zoster, or live virus vaccine (eg MMR/rubella). If there is significant mucosal bleeding, or lymphadenopathy, hepatosplenomegaly, or pancytopenia, another diagnosis is likely. *Tests:* Isolated thrombocytopenia (<20×10⁹ in 80%); do a film to ensure no other abnormalities. Marrow is unnecessary, unless:[655]
• Unusual signs are present, eg abnormal cells on a film, lymphadenopathy.
• Platelet count is not rising after ~2 weeks.
• Treatment is contemplated with steroids or immunoglobulin—may decrease period of profound thrombocytopenia.
Intracranial haemorrhage occurs in <1% (mortality is 50%)[656]—do CT if there is headache or CNS signs. *Natural history:* Gradual resolution over ~3 months for 80% with or without therapy. 20% become chronic (>6 months); the chronic form is compatible with normal longevity, and normal activities, provided contact sports are avoided. ℞: Admit eg if: •Unusual features, eg excessive bleeding. •There are rowdy siblings who might engage in physical badinage. Life threatening bleeding requires platelet transfusion. Splenectomy is considered for chronic ITP and failure of treatment. Rituximab[1] and anti-D[2] (p9) reduce the need for splenectomy.

---

1 Rituximab can induce remission in ~30%.[657] SE: T°↑, pruritus, throat tightness, serum sickness.
2 Anti-D: a single dose of 50µ/kg IV ↑ platelet count to ≥20×10⁹/L in 70% of children within 3 days.[658]

Synonyms: *primary hypogammaglobulinae-mia* (not secondary to protein-losing enteropathy, chronic lymphatic leukaemia, or myeloma). Bruton's agammaglobulinaemia was the first immunodeficiency syndrome to be described.[659]

Essence Antibodies (that are produced by B lymphocytes) can kill pathogens by binding to target antigens and activating complement system or facilitating their uptake by phagocyte cells. They can also neutralize the toxins secreted by the pathogens. Disorders of B cells increase susceptibility to infections by encapsulated bacteria, but not (usually) viral or fungal infections. Most are recessive, eg caused by mutations in genes on autosomal or X chromosomes.[659]

Typical signs:
• Frequent infections
• Bronchiectasis
• Chronic sinusitis
• Failure to thrive
• Nodular lymphoid hyperplasia (gut)
• Absent tonsils
• Enteropathy
• Hepatosplenomegaly
• Anaemia
• Arthropathy
• Lymphopenia
• Serum total protein↓ (albumin; immunoglobulins are missing)[660]

The patient When the signs in the MINIBOX are unexplained, refer to an immunologist, to assess antibody responses to protein and carbohydrate antigens, measure IgG subclasses, specific antibodies to the immunized illnesses, and count lymphocytes involved in antibody production (CD4, CD8, CD19, CD23 +ve lymphocytes). Immunoglobulin levels are interpreted by age. There is a role for watching responses to test vaccinations. Primary immunodeficiency is more likely if there is a positive family history/parental consanguinity.[661]

Types of primary immunodeficiency See BOX.

Management Aim to include the patient and the family in the process. Treat intercurrent infections promptly. This may include postural physiotherapy, and bronchodilators as well as antibiotics. Immunoglobulin replacement obviates most complications and is best delivered by an immunologist, after detailed assessment. Many patients can join a self-infusion programme. Before infusions, exclude active infection (to minimize risk of adverse reactions), and a baseline check of transaminase enzymes, creatinine, and anti-IgA antibody titres should be done. The dose of IV immunoglobulin is determined by the severity and frequency of infections, and the plasma level of IgG. Most receive ~400mg/kg/month (see *data sheet/SPC*, usually as 2 doses, 2 weeks apart.[9][662] Have hydrocortisone and an antihistamine at the ready. SE: headaches, abdominal pain, anaphylaxis, transmission of hepatitis.[663] IM immunoglobulins are not favoured, but the subcutaneous route is being investigated and appears satisfactory.[664] N=40

Complications *Chest:* Bronchiectasis, granulomas, lymphoma. *Gut:* Malabsorption, giardia, cholangitis, atrophic gastritis, colitis. *Liver:* Acquired hepatitis, chronic active hepatitis, biliary cirrhosis. *Blood:* Autoimmune haemolysis, ITP (p197), anaemia of chronic disease, aplasia. *Eyes/CNS:* Keratoconjunctivitis, uveitis, granulomas, encephalitis. *Others:* Septic arthropathy, arthralgia, splenomegaly.

Gene therapy Autologous haematopoietic stem cells transduced with the γc gene can restore immune system in boys with severe combined immunodeficiency. A harmless retrovirus carries the replacement gene, and infects the stem cells *in vitro*. When these are replaced in the marrow an immune system develops within a few months[1]—obviating the need for intrusive anti-infection isolation measures and IV immunoglobulin. It is an alternative to marrow transplants (eg if no HLA match can be found). There is likely to be a limitation to initiation of normal thymopoiesis, so do it promptly.

---

1 T cells & repertoires of T-cell receptors were ~normal up to 2yrs post-op; thymopoiesis is shown by naive T cells. Antibody production is adequate.

Types of antibody deficiency

IgA deficiency (IgA↓ + normal or ↑ levels of other immunoglobulins). It is the most common primary antibody deficiency. Many are asymptomatic. It may accompany CVID (below). Patients tend to develop respiratory infections which may lead to bronchiectasis. Gastrointestinal infection (eg giardia) and disorders such as malabsorption, coeliac disease, ulcerative colitis are associated with IgA deficiency. Although rare, all blood products/IV immunoglobulin infusion can lead to severe, even fatal, anaphylaxis due to the presence of IgA. Ideally blood products if needed should be obtained from a IgA-deficient individual—or washed red cells given. Patients are recommended to wear a medical alert bracelet because of this. [665] *Prevalence:* Varies with ethnicity: 1 in 143 in Middle East; 1 in 875 in UK; 1 in 18,500 in Japan. [665]

Transient hypogammaglobulinaemia of infancy Temporary delay in antibody production. *Onset:* 3–6 months. It is more severe than normal antibody deficiency that happens at this age. Immunoglobulin levels become normal by 2–4 yrs. *Prevalence:* ~1 in 10,000. [666]

Common variable immunodeficiency (CVID) (IgG↓, IgA↓, IgM variable). *Onset:* Second to third decade of life. Enlarged tonsils, splenomegaly, gastrointestinal disease, liver dysfunction and cancer (esp lymphoma) may be present. *Prevalence:* ~1 in 10,000–50,000. [667]

Bruton x-linked agammaglobulinaemia Tyrosine kinase gene mutation (xq21) causes ↓ immunoglobulins and ↓mature B cells, [668] hence ↑ susceptibility to bacterial (but not viral) infections. Lymphocytes are unable to synthesize immunoglobulin. *Onset:* 3months–3years. [669] Also: arthropathy + absent Peyer's patches, tonsils and appendix. *Prevalence:* ~1 in 250,000 (the commonest inherited antibody deficiency). [668] R: Beware septicaemia and CNS infections (may require interferon-α and high-dose IV immunoglobulin). [670] After marrow transplantation serum immunoglobin rises to normal levels over ~3 months. [671]

IgG subclass deficiency There are ↓ levels of one or more of 4 subclasses of IgG. Total IgG levels may be normal. IgG_2↓ is the most common and often is associated with IgA↓, and ataxia-telangiectasia.

Severe combined immunodeficiency (SCID) T-cell dysfunction usually causes combined immunodeficiency as T cells are necessary for B-cell differentiation. *Onset:* 1–3 months. Patients are susceptible to all types of bacterial, viral, fungal, and protozoal infections. *Treatment:* Stem cell transplant. *Prevalence:* ~1 in 50,000–75,000. [672]

Paediatrics

Causes Meningoencephalitis; head injury; subdural/extradural bleeds (abused?); hypoxia (eg near-drowning); ketoacidosis; tumours; thrombosis;[1] Reye's (p652).

Signs Listless; irritable; drowsy; headache; diplopia; vomiting; tense fontanelle; ↓level of responsiveness (Children's Coma Scale if <4yrs, see OPPOSITE, or use the Glasgow Coma Scale if >4yrs (p722); If unconscious look for: pupil changes (ipsilateral dilatation); abnormal posturing (decorticate/decerebrate); Cushing's triad (slow pulse, raised BP and breathing pattern abnormalities) warns of imminent coning. Chronic: papilloedema and hydrocephalus.

Management Aim to prevent ischaemia. Help venous drainage by keeping head in the midline, elevated at ~25°. Give O_2. Fan/sponge (tepid water) if τ °>40°c. Treat hypoglycaemia. Control seizures (p208). ▶Don't do LP: this risks coning. If severe, take to ITU to monitor ICP & cerebral perfusion pressure (CPP=mean arterial pressure minus ICP; if CPP <40mmHg cerebral ischaemia is likely).
▶▶ Intubate. Hyperventilation is no longer recommended.
▶▶ Give mannitol 20% (check it is crystal-free), eg 2.5mL/kg IVI over 30min[673] or 3% hypertonic saline (5mL/kg bolus) which may have fewer side effects.[674]
▶▶ Dexamethasone: if <35kg, 16.7mg IV (20.8mg if >35kg) then as per BNF[c] §6.3.2.
▶▶ Fluid restriction & diuresis, avoiding hypovolaemia (keep Na^+ 145-150mmol/L, osmolarity to 300-310, and CVP to 2-5cmH₂O). ▶▶ Pulse & BP continuously.
▶▶ Send to neurosurgical centre now.

Herpes simplex encephalitis (HSE) is the most treatable encephalitis. ▶Think of it in any febrile child with focal or general seizures and CNS (esp. temporal lobe) signs ± ↓consciousness. Signs are often nonspecific.[675] Nasolabial herpes is often absent. CNS deficits may be mild or gross (eg hemiparesis). Tests: CT, EEG and CSF often nonspecific (do PCR). MRI is better than CT. R: ▶▶Start aciclovir. If >12yrs old: 10mg/kg[IBW]/8h by IVI over 1h eg for 3wks (20mg/kg/8h in neonates).[676] Monitor U&E & urine output; Mortality: ~7%. 60% survive intact. CNS sequelae: Kluver–Bucy syndrome (hypersexuality, rage, visual agnosia; aphasia;[677] amnesia; auditory agnosia; autism.[678]

Brain tumours ▶Arrange urgent referral if unexplained headache and/or focal symptoms, eg progressive weakness or numbness, unsteadiness, difficulty speaking, or vision changes/VI nerve palsy. ⅔ are in the posterior fossa. Consider brain tumours in children with lethargy, behavioural change, visual disturbances, diabetes insipidus (polyuria/polydipsia), growth disturbances (e.g. growth failure , delayed/arrested/precocious puberty), nausea ± vomiting.[679]

Medulloblastoma: Midline cerebellar embryonal tumour (inferior vermis) causing ICP↑, speech difficulty, truncal ataxia ± falls. ♂:♀=4:1. Peak age: 4yrs. Seeding is along CSF pathways. Rx: surgical resection + radio/chemo-therapy.

Brainstem astrocytoma: Most common brain tumour in children. Associated with neurofibromatosis 1) and prior radiation. Cranial nerve palsies; pyramidal tract signs (eg hemiparesis); cerebellar ataxia; signs of ICP↑ are rare.

Midbrain and third ventricle tumours may be astrocytomas, pinealomas or colloid cysts (cause posture-dependent drowsiness). Signs: behaviour change (early); pyramidal tract and cerebellar SIGNS; upward gaze defect.

Suprasellar gliomas: Visual field defects; optic atrophy; pituitary disorders (growth arrest, hypothyroidism, delayed puberty); diabetes insipidus (DI). Cranial DI is caused by ADH↓, so that there is polyuria and low urine osmolality (always <800mosmol/L) despite dehydration.

Cerebral hemispheres: Usually gliomas. Meningiomas are rare. Fits are common. Signs depend on the lobe involved (OHCM p503). Tests: MRI/CT ± EEG. Options: Excision if possible; CSF shunting; radiotherapy; chemotherapy alone.[680]

Other space-occupying lesions Aneurysms; haematomas; granulomas; tuberculomas; cysts (cysticercosis); ▶abscess: suspect if ICP↑; τ↑; WCC↑. Get help.

1 Venous sinus thrombosis risk↑ if: infection; perinatal problems; blood dyscrasias. Signs: ↓consciousness (50%), papilloedema (18%), cranial nerve palsy (33%), hemiparesis, hypotonia. Thrombolysis may be needed.[681]

Children's coma scale (An objective record of coma level to help quantify prognosis and monitor progress.) Use if <4yrs; if >4, use Glasgow scale, p720.

- **Best motor response** (6 grades, quantified in the *blue numbers below*)
  - 6 *Carrying out a request ('obeying command'):* Moves to your request.
  - 5 *Localizing response to pain:* Put pressure on the patient's finger nail bed with a pencil or sternal pressure: purposeful movements towards changing painful stimuli is a 'localizing' response.
  - 4 *Withdraws to pain:* Pulls limb away from painful stimulus.
  - 3 *Flexor response to pain:* Pressure on the nail bed causes abnormal flexion of limbs—decorticate posture.
  - 2 *Extensor posturing to pain:* The stimulus causes limb extension (adduction, internal rotation of shoulder, forearm pronation; decerebrate posture).
  - 1 *No response to pain.* Score best response of any limb.

- **Best verbal response** (5 grades) If intubated *can the patient grimace?*
  - 5 Orientated: Smiles, is orientated to sounds, fixes and follows objects.
  - 4 Crying but consolable (or interaction odd/inappropriate)
  - 3 Inconsistently consolable (or moaning)
  - 2 Inconsolable crying (or irritable)
  - 1 No response

- **Eye opening** (4 grades)
  - 4 *Spontaneous eye opening.*
  - 3 *Eye opening in response to speech:* Any, not just a request to open eyes.
  - 2 *Eye opening to response to pain:* Pain to limbs as above.
  - 1 *No eye opening.*

Add the score in the 3 areas. Eg: no response to pain + no verbalization + no eye opening = 3. As a rule of thumb, <8 ≈ intubation needed; 4–8 ≈ intermediate prognosis; 3 ≈ bad prognosis.

Migraine

(*OHCM* p462)

In children we modify migraine criteria to include *bilateral* or *frontal* headache lasting 1–72h with nausea/vomiting + any 2 of: photophobia, phonophobia, difficulty thinking, lightheadedness, or fatigue[682] (vertigo and abdo pain also occur) sometimes heralded by visual or sensory aura. Most children have to lie down during attacks; sleep resolves the attack. *Prevalence:* 5% (10% in adolescence). *Triggers:* School pressure, tantrums, excitement: upset, hypoglycaemia, sleep lack or excess (weekend migraine), sensory events (noise, light, heat/cold), sympathetic activity (sports). *Drugs:* (as early as possible in an attack); par-acetamol (p143); ibuprofen 10mg/kg PO (see p143).[683] If this fails and over 6yrs, try sumatriptan,[684] eg if weight >30kg.[683] If vomiting, use rectal (paracetamol suppositories) or nasal routes (**sumatriptan** dose: 12–18 years 10–20mg stat, repeated once after ≥2h if needed) or IV chlorpromazine (0.15mg/kg if >8y; max 10mg).[685] *Non-drug treatments:* Relaxation training, biofeedback, self-hypnosis, and guided imagery have a role.[686] *Prophylaxis:* Encourage regular sleep. Consider **propranolol** and **pizotifen**. **Amitriptyline** and **sodium valproate** are used, but note lack of robust evidence of efficacy.[687] Nimodipine, timolol, pa-paverine, trazodone, clonidine, metoclopramide, and domperidone are 'ineffec-tive'.[688] Signs for prompt referral:

- Headaches of increasing frequency or severity, or if aged <6yrs.
- Headache unrelieved by paracetamol or ibuprofen.
- Irritable; loss of interest/skills; slowing of physical or cognitive development.
- Head circumference above the 97th centile, or greatly out of line.

Other causes of headache Viruses; meningitis; sinusitis (frontal sinus not developed until >10yrs); hypertension (always do BP), stress, behavioural.

Signs Flu-like prodome, consciousness↓; odd behaviour; vomiting; fits; т°↑; meningism. *Infective causes:* include HSV (►►aciclovir, p200); mumps (ask about parotiditis/testicular pain); varicella zoster (recent chicken pox?); rabies (dog-bite abroad); parvovirus (slapped cheek syndrome), immunocompromise (CMV, EBV, HHV-6); influenza; toxoplasmosis; TB; mycoplasma; malaria (if a possibility do a thick blood film and enlist specialist help, OHCM p394); dengue; Rickettsia.[589] Do CSF PCR; test stool, urine, and blood. *Non-infective differential:* hypoglycaemia; DKA; kernicterus (p115), hepatic failure (eg Reye's syndrome), lead or other poisoning, subarachnoid haemorrhage, malignancy, lupus.[690]

Investigations: CSF MC&S and PCR; bloods, stool (enteroviruses), urine
▶*Prolonged fevers*—consider: endocarditis; Still's (p654); malignancy.

►►Meningitis   APLS, NICE

Suspect this in any ill baby or child. Symptoms may be subtle, especially in infants—irritability, abnormal cry, lethargy and difficulty feeding. Signs include fever, seizures, apnoea, bulging fontanelle. ▶*Get expert help from your senior.* If there is any hint of meningococcal disease, ►►GIVE IV CEFTRIAXONE *(50–80mg/kg; max 2–4g).* See BNF[c] §5.1.2. Sending blood/CSF cultures must not delay this.

Septic signs: commonly present before meningeal signs—include т°↑; cold hands/feet, limb/joint pain, abnormal skin colour, odd behaviour; rash (don't *expect* petechiae with meningococcus); DIC; pulse↑; BP↓; tachypnoea; WCC↑.

Meningeal signs: comparatively late, and less common in young children, they are neither sensitive nor specific[691]—include stiff neck ("unable to kiss knee"; often absent if <18 months); Kernig's sign (resistance to extending knee with hip flexed); Brudzinski's sign (hips flex on bending head forward); photophobia; opisthotonus

Other causes of stiff neck: Tonsillitis, pneumonia, subarachnoid bleed.

Lumbar puncture: Often inappropriate (see p200); contraindicated if: focal signs; DIC; purpura or *brain herniation* is near (odd posture or breathing; coma scale <13, p201; dilated pupils, doll's eye reflexes, BP↑, pulse↓, papilloedema). Preliminary CT cannot show LP will be safe. *Technique:* (OHCM p782) Learn from an expert. • Explain everything to mother. • Get IV access first: acute deterioration is possible. Ask an experienced nurse to position child fully flexed (knees to chin) on the side of a bed, with his back exactly at right angles with it. • Mark a point just above (cranial to) a line joining the spinous processes between the iliac crests. • Drape & sterilize the area; put on gloves. • Infiltrate 1mL of 1% lidocaine superficially in the older child. • Insert LP needle aiming towards umbilicus. Keep the needle perpendicular to the back at all times. • Catch 4 CSF drops in each of 3 bottles for: *urgent Gram stain, culture, virology, glucose, protein* (do blood glucose too). • Do CNS observations often. • Report to mother. *After LP:* FBC, U&E, culture blood, urine, nose swabs, stool virology. CRP: is it >20mg/L? CXR. Fluid balance, TPR & BP hourly. Is CSF lactate >3mg/L? (a more sensitive way to distinguish bacterial from aseptic meningitis than the blood/CSF glucose ratio.)

Treating pyogenic meningitis before the organism is known
▶▶ Protect airway; give high-flow O₂; set up IVI: if in shock give 0.9% saline in 20mL/kg boluses. If shock persists beyond 3 boluses—consider intubation and inotropic support. Call a paediatric intensivist early.
▶▶ Ceftriaxone 50–80mg/kg/day (max2–4g) IV infusion if >3months–18yrs.
▶▶ Cefotaxime 50mg/kg—/12h if <7d; /8h if 7-21d; /6h if <21 days-3months) PLUS amoxicillin/ampicillin p204.
▶▶ Dexamethasone (0.15mg/kg/6h IV eg for 4 days) with 1st antibiotic dose (in developed countries)[692] unless the organism is very likely to be *N. meningitidis*.[693]

➻ If pre-hernia signs, treat for ICP↑ (p200), eg **mannitol** 20%, 2.5–5mL/kg IVI.

Treat for cryptococcus if HIV+ve. After culture, check the minimum inhibitory concentration (MIC) of the antibiotics used to the organism *in vitro*.

Complications Disseminated sepsis, subdural effusion, hydrocephalus, ataxia, paralysis, deafness (steroids prevent this), IQ↓, epilepsy, brain abscess.

CSF in meningitis	Pyogenic:	Tubercular:	Aseptic:	Normal range if >1 month old
Appearance[694,695]	often turbid	may be fibrin web	usually clear	clear
Predominant cell	polymorphs eg 1000/mm³	mononuclear 10–350/mm³	mononuclear 50–1500/mm³	≤5 lymphocytes; ~0 neutrophils
Glucose level	<⅔ of blood	<⅔ of blood	>⅔ of blood	>⅔ of blood
Protein (mg/dL)	↑ (mean ≈300)	↑ >40 (mean ≈200)	≥40 and <1500	<40

Bacterial antigen detection for *N. meningitidis*, *H. influenzae* & streps helps in partially treated meningitis. CSF lactate typically rises before the CSF glucose falls in pyogenic meningitis.

Preventing deaths from meningococcal disease Because death is so swift, this can seem a hopeless task. Nevertheless, the following (and using your 6th sense) *can* save lives, and the meningococcus is not always *that* fast.
• Rapid skilled assessment of all febrile children. Nurse triage is unreliable.
• Don't expect meningeal signs; septicaemic signs are more fatal.
• Any rash (or none) will do for the meningococcus. If you wait for purpura, you may be waiting until the disease is untreatable.
• For any acutely unwell child *leave your consulting room door ajar.* Explain that a doctor can be contacted *at any time* if:
  –He seems to be worsening   –Cold hands or feet; odd skin colour
  –A rash develops   –Unrousable or crying in an odd way
  –Poor response to antipyretics   –Odd features eg limb/joint pain
• Beware fever + lethargy + vomiting, even if no headache or photophobia.
• Give parenteral penicillin *early* (p205), before admission to hospital.
• Monitor pulse, BP, respiratory rate, pupil size/reactivity, level of consciousness (AVPU, p103); WCC and platelets (both may be ↓).
• Urgent activation of and transfer to paediatric intensive care unit (PICU). Do blood gases to assess degree of acidosis. Get fresh frozen plasma to the bedside **now** to deal with coagulopathy. Intubation, ventilation and vigorous IV fluid resuscitation must be prompt. Monitor catheter urine output. Crossmatch blood. Continuously monitor ECG.
• Inotropes may be needed: dopamine or **dobutamine** (same dose) eg at 10µg/kg/min (put 15mg/kg in 50mL of 5% glucose and infuse at 2mL/h).[696] This is OK by peripheral vein, but if adrenaline is needed, use a central line (0.1µg/kg/min, ie 300µg/kg in 50mL of 0.9% saline at 1mL/h).[696]
• If plasma glucose <3, give 10% glucose 5mL/kg as a bolus, then as needed.

Heroic, non-standard ideas: Extracorporeal membrane oxygenation; terminal fragment of human bactericidal/permeability-increasing protein (rBPI21) to ↓cytokines; heparin with protein c concentrate to reverse coagulopathy; plasmapheresis to remove cytokines, and thrombolysis (rTPA) for limb reperfusion.[697]

Other issues Ensure immunization (protein–polysaccharide conjugate vaccine prevents type c but not the common type which is B; p151). Inform your local CDC (consultant in communicable diseases). ►Stop parents smoking! 37% of cases are put down to aerosolized spread via smokers coughs.[698]

Meningococcal prophylaxis for contacts with aerosolized meningococci (or *deep* kissing).[699] **Rifampicin**—12hrly for 4 doses PO: if <1yr, 5mg/kg; 1–12yrs: 10mg/kg (max 600mg); >12yrs: 600mg. It interacts with the contraceptive Pill, can stain contact lenses, and turns urine red. **Ceftriaxone** single IM dose: 125mg if <12yr; 250mg if >12yr. **Ciprofloxacin** 500mg PO is an option if ≥12yrs old (250mg if 5–12yrs).

Paediatrics

The meningococcus, the pneumococcus, and, in the unvaccinated, *Haemophilus influenzae* are the great killers. In the former, the interval between seeming well and coma may be counted in hours. If you suspect meningococcal disease, give benzyl-penicillin (BOX) before hospital admission[700]NICE (do not worry about ruining the chance of a positive blood or CSF culture later).

Neisseria meningitis Abrupt onset ± rash (purpuric or not, eg starting as pink macules on legs in 20%); septicaemia may occur with no meningitis (Waterhouse-Friderichsen, OHCM p707), so early LPS may be normal, giving false reassurance. Arthritis, conjunctivitis, myocarditis & DIC may coexist. *Typical age:* Any. *Film:* Gram −ve cocci in pairs (long axes parallel), often within polymorphs. *Drug of choice:* cefotaxime/ceftriaxone (p202) or benzylpenicillin (G) 50mg/kg/4h IV. If penicillin and cephalosporin-allergic, give chloramphenicol (below). Treat shock with colloid (± inotropes, p203). *Prevention:* p202.

Haemophilus influenzae (Rare if immunized). *Typical age:* <4yrs. *CSF:* Gram −ve rods. The lower the CSF glucose, the worse the infection. *Drugs:* Ceftriaxone (p202) or, where there is no resistance, chloramphenicol 12-25mg/kg/6h IVI (neonates: see *BNF*) + IV ampicillin—if ≤1wk old, 30-60mg/kg/12h (/8h if 1wk-3wks old; /6h if 3–4wks old). If >4wks old 25mg/kg/6h (max 1g), doubled in severe infections. **Rifampicin** (below) may also be needed. With **chloramphenicol**, monitor peak levels; aim for 20–25μg/mL; usual doses may be far exceeded to achieve this. (Trough level: <15μg/mL.) As soon as you can, switch to PO (more effective). **Steroids** (p202) prevent hearing loss.

Strep pneumoniae *Typical age:* Any. *Risk factors:* Respiratory infections, skull fracture (▶is this 'minor runny nose' CSF rhinorrhoea?), meningocele, HIV.[701] *Film:* Gram +ve cocci. *R̥:* Ceftriaxone, p202 or benzylpenicillin 50mg/kg/4h slow IV—or, if resistance likely (eg parts of Europe and USA) ± rifampicin. As an add-in or an alternative, consider vancomycin, if >1 month old: 15mg/kg/8h (max 2g/24h) IVI over 1h, but CSF penetration is unreliable.[702] Monitor U&E.

E. coli This is a major cause of meningitis in neonates (in whom signs may consist of feeding difficulties, apnoea, seizures, and shock). *Drug of choice:* cefotaxime (p202) or gentamicin (p175).

Group B haemolytic streptococcus eg *via* mother's vagina (so swab mothers whose infants suddenly fall ill at ~24h-old). Infection may be delayed a month. *Drug of choice:* benzylpenicillin 25-50mg/kg/8-12h slow IV.

Listeria monocytogenes presents soon after birth with meningitis or septicaemia (± pneumonia). It is rare unless immunocompromised. Microabscesses form in many organs (granulomatosis infantiseptica). *Δ:* Culture blood, CSF, placenta, amniotic fluid. *R̥:* IV ampicillin (above) + gentamicin (p175).[703]

TB can cause CNS infarcts, demyelination with cranial nerve lesions, and tuberculomas ± meningitis (long prodrome with lethargy, malaise, and anorexia). Photophobia and neck stiffness are likely to be absent. The 1st few CSFs may be normal, or show visible fibrin webs and widely varying cell counts. *Dose examples:* Isoniazid 10mg/kg/24h PO max 500mg (? with vit B_6) + rifampicin 10mg/kg/24h (≤600mg/day) for 1yr + (for 2 months) pyrazinamide 35mg/kg/day with eg streptomycin if >4wks old, eg 20-30mg/kg once daily (max 1g) IM adjusted to give a peak plasma level <40μg/mL and a trough of <3μg/mL; alternative: ethambutol 15mg/kg/day PO if old enough to report visual problems.[704,705] Adding dexamethasone improves survival (at least in those >14yrs old) but probably does not prevent disability.[706] Children <14 should be given prednisolone 4mg/kg/24h for 4 weeks then follow a reducing course.[705]

Other bacteria Leptospiral species (canicola); Brucella; Salmonella.

Causes of 'aseptic' meningitis Viruses (eg mumps, echo, herpes, polio), partially treated bacterial infections, cryptococcus (use ink stains).

Giving IM benzylpenicillin before hospital admission

- 300mg IM up to 1 year old.
- 600mg if 1–9yrs.
- 1.2g if >10yrs.
- When in doubt, give it: it may be negligent not to do so.
- If penicillin-allergic, **cefotaxime** may be used (50mg/kg IM stat; if >12yrs 1g).[707]

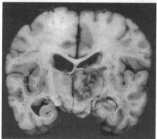

Fig 1. Image of glass test in purpuric rashes (eg meningitis). The rash has stained, and does not blanch. ©Dr Petter Brandtzaeg, and the Meningitis Trust.

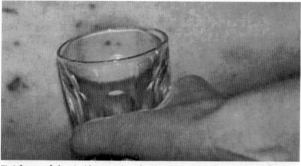

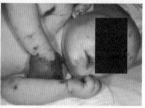

Fig 3. 4-month-old girl with gangrene of hands due to meningococcaemia. ©CDC.

Fig 2. Tuberculoma. Caseous (cheese-like) necrotic material is surrounded by epithelioid cell granulomas. Rupture releases mycobacteria into the subarachnoid space, hence causing TB meningitis. ©Prof. Dimitri Agamanolis.

EPILEPSY is a tendency to intermittent abnormal electrical brain activity. Classification depends on whether signs are referable to one part of a hemisphere (partial epilepsy) or not (generalized), and on whether consciousness is affected (complex) or not (simple). Seizures in *generalized epilepsy* may be:

- *Tonic/clonic (grand mal):* Limbs stiffen (the tonic phase) and then jerk forcefully (clonic phase), with loss of consciousness.
- *Absences (petit mal):* Brief (eg 10sec) pauses ('he stops in mid-sentence, and carries on where he left off'); eyes may roll up; he/she is *unaware of the attack.*
- *Infantile spasms/West syndrome:* Peak age: 5 months. Clusters of head nodding ('Salaam attack') and arm jerks, every 3–30sec. IQ↓ in ~70%.[708] EEG is characteristic (hypsarrhythmia). ℞: vigabatrin (SE: visual field defects);[709] ACTH.[710]
- *Myoclonic seizures:* 1–4yrs; eg 'thrown' suddenly to the ground. ℞: valproate.

Partial epilepsy Signs are referable to part of one hemisphere. Complex phenomena: (temporal lobe fits) consciousness↓; automatisms (lip smacking, rubbing face, running); fits of pure pleasure.[711,712]

Causes Often none is found. Infection (eg meningitis); U&E↑, glucose↓, Ca²⁺↓, Mg²⁺↓; Na⁺↓↑; toxins; trauma; metabolic defects; tuberous sclerosis; CNS tumour (<2%) or malformation; flickering lights, eg TV; exercise.[713]

ΔΔ: Arrhythmias, migraine, narcolepsy, night terrors, faints (reflex anoxic seizures, p207), tics, Münchausen's (eg by proxy, OHCM p720).

Tests Expert EEG; MRI is the preferred choice- it is more sensitive and has no exposure to radiation. CT may be more available and not require an anaesthetic—use in emergent situations to look for acute haemorrhage/lesions.[714]

A SIMPLE FEBRILE CONVULSION is a *single* tonic–clonic, symmetrical generalized seizure lasting <20min, occurring as T°↑ rises rapidly in a febrile illness—typically in a normally developing child (½–5yrs old). Think of meningo-encephalitis, CNS lesion, epilepsy, trauma, glucose↓, Ca²⁺↓, or Mg²⁺↓ if: •Focal CNS signs or CNS abnormality •Previous history of epilepsy •The seizure lasts >15min •There is >1 attack in 24h. *Lifetime prevalence:* ~3% of children have at least one febrile convulsion. *Examination:* Find any infection; if any neck stiffness consider meningitis. ℞: Put in recovery position; if fit is lasting >5min: lorazepam IV, buccal midazolam (p208), or diazepam PR. Tepid sponging if hot;[715] paracetamol syrup (p143). Consider FBC, U&E, Ca²⁺, glucose, MSU, CXR, ENT swabs.[716] **To LP or not LP?** Risk of pyogenic meningitis is as low (<1.3%) as the risk in a febrile child with no seizures[717] if *all* the above criteria are fulfilled. Avoid LP in the post ictal period as a CNS assessment will be impossible. If you suspect meningitis, then treat *now. Parental education:* Allay fear (a child is *not* dying during a fit). Febrile convulsions don't usually (≤3%) mean risk of epilepsy. For the 30% having recurrences, teach carers to use buccal midazolam or **rectal diazepam 0.5mg/kg**, eg with a 5mg tube (Stesolid®) if 1–3yrs,[1] or a 10mg tube if older only *during* seizures. *Further prevention:* Diazepam PR during fevers has a role;[718] other anticonvulsants are 'never' needed. Explain that all fevers (eg vaccination-associated) should prompt oral antipyretics (p142), but that this does not necessarily avoid another seizure, with diazepam PR to hand if needed. *Prognosis:* In typical febrile convulsions (defined above) there is no progress to epilepsy in 97%.[719] Risk is much higher if pre-existing CNS abnormality (50%), epilepsy in a first degree relative, or complex febrile seizures.

---

1 If <3yrs insert PR half-way to nozzle mark. ~2.5mL is expellable; don't worry about the bit left behind; it's allowed for by the manufacturer. Alternative: diazepam Rectubes®: its licence is for a 0.5mg/kg single dose (adults & children >10kg, a typical weight for a 1yr-old), which shouldn't be repeated until after 12h; very few reports of respiratory problems at this dose: all survived. Only insert half-way if <15kg, and always press the buttocks together after giving.[720] Dose example: 1 month–2yrs: 5mg; 2–12yrs: 5–10mg.

This is often a true dilemma, and it matters as epilepsy treatment can be toxic. Also, if it is harmful to label any child, it is doubly so to mislabel a child. So always get help with the diagnosis. Watching and waiting, repeat EEGs, and videos of attacks (eg on mobile phone) may be needed.[721] In one study of 22 babies <1yr old referred for '?epilepsy', 9 did have epilepsy. The other 13 showed one of five patterns of non-epileptic paroxysmal events (NEPE)—1 blinking 2 Head-shaking movements 3 Body posturing with head and arm jerk 4 Rhythmic masturbation movements ('gratification disorder', eg with grunts, leg-crossing, flushing etc—in the presence of a normal EEG) 5 Myoclonic head flexion. NEPE may be clinically indistinguishable from epilepsy. In the infants described above, ≥4 interictal EEGs were normal, the spells completely resolved after a fairly short period without anticonvulsants, and the infants continued to develop normally with no evidence of epilepsy at follow-up.[722]

Some specific types of seizure

Reflex anoxic attacks Paroxysmal, self-limited brief (eg 15sec) asystole triggered by pain, fear (eg at venepuncture) or anxiety, or an overwhelming confrontation with reality, perhaps in the form of a bath which is unexpectedly hot or cold. During this time the child is deathly pale—± hypotonia, rigidity, upward eye deviation, clonic movements, and urinary incontinence. Typical age: 6 months to 2 years (but may be much older). *Prevalence:* 0.8% of preschool children. ΔΔ: Epilepsy is often misdiagnosed, as the trigger aspect to the history is ignored or unwitnessed. When in difficulty, refer to a specialist for vagal excitation tests under continuous EEG & ECG monitoring (ocular compression induces the oculo-cardiac reflex; do not do this test if there is glaucoma, or known arrhythmia, or if you lack experience: it is uncomfortable). NB: tongue-biting is not described in reflex anoxic seizures. *Management:* Drugs are rarely, if ever, needed. Atropine has been tried, to reduce sensitivity to vagal influences. Anticonvulsants are not needed. Pacemakers might be an option. *What to tell parents:* Avoid the term 'seizure', as this is all that is likely to be remembered, *however* careful your explanation. *Pallid syncopal attack*, or *white breath-holding attacks* are useful synonyms. Emphasize its benign nature, and that the child usually grows out of it (but it may occur later in life, and in older siblings).[723]

Panayiotopoulos syndrome (6% of all epilepsies) A benign focal seizure disorder occurring in early and mid-childhood (peak age: 5yrs). Autonomic symptoms may predominate. EEG: shifting and/or multiple foci, often with occipital predominance. It occurs mainly at night, with vomiting and eye deviation with impaired consciousness before the convulsion starts. Many seizures last for 30 minutes (some may last hours)—but there is no permanent brain damage. Treatment: as remission often occurs within 2 years, antiepileptic medication is often not needed. Reassure.[724]

Age-dependent epileptic encephalopathy Ohtahara syndrome: tonic spasms ± clustering. EEG: suppression-burst.[725] Chloral hydrate may help.[725] This transforms over time into West syndrome, and thence to Lennox–Gastaut syndrome. Think of these as age-specific epileptic reactions to non-specific exogenous CNS insults, acting at specific developmental stages.[726]

Rolandic epilepsy (benign epilepsy with centrotemporal spikes, BECTS) 15% of all childhood epilepsy. Infrequent, brief partial fits with unilateral facial or oropharyngeal sensory-motor symptoms, speech arrest ± hypersalivation. Sulthiame may be used in some units.[727,728]

Mozart's sonata for 2 pianos, K448, has been found to reduce interictal epileptiform EEG discharges (compared with Beethoven's *Für Elise*) in a randomized, single-blind, crossover, placebo-controlled trial.[729]

Stepwise R of status epilepticus Supportive therapy: • Secure airway; give O_2. Set a clock in motion • Check t°; if ↑, give rectal paracetamol (it may be a febrile convulsion) • Do BP, pulse, glucose, Ca^{2+} (±Mg^{2+}). ► If hypoglycaemic, give glucose 5ml/kg IV of 10% solution, then 5–10mg/kg/min as 10% glucose IVI.

	►►Seizure control: proceed to the next step only if fits continue
0min	►►ABC. High flow O_2. Estimate weight. Check blood glucose. IV access
5min	►►Lorazepam 0.1mg/kg IV; slow bolus via a large vein OR buccal midazolam 0.3–0.5mg/kg; squirt half between lower gum and the cheek on each side.
15min	Repeat lorazepam. **Call for senior help. Prepare phenytoin.**
25min	►►Phenytoin 20mg/kg IVI; over 20mins. Monitor ECG OR (if on regular phenytoin) ►►Phenobarbital 20mg/kg over 5mins ►►Paraldehyde mixed with equal part of olive oil—0.8mL/kg of mixture (max 10mL) as a single dose PR; avoid contact with plastics/rubber may be given on direction of senior staff. *Call PICU & your anaesthetist—prepare for intubation* locate ET tube,etc p627
45min	►►Rapid sequence induction use ►►thiopental 4mg/kg. Transfer to PICU

► These times refer to elapsed time on the clock from the 1st drug, not gaps between each drug. Some authorities recommend starting ventilation earlier, and always be ready to do this to protect the airway.

Tests S_AO_2, ECG monitor, glucose, U&E, Ca^{2+}, Mg^{2+}, arterial gases, FBC, platelets, ECG. Consider anticonvulsant levels, toxicology screen, blood ammonia, lumbar puncture (after resolution), culture blood and urine, virology, EEG, MRI, CT, carbon monoxide level, lead level, amino acid levels, metabolic screen.

Once the crisis is over Refer to a specialist: is MRI or prophylaxis, eg with sodium valproate or carbamazepine (p209) needed? Aim to use one drug only. Increase dose until fits stop, or toxic level reached. Out of the context of status, prophylaxis is typically started after the 2nd seizure. Choice of anti-epileptic drug (AED) should be based on epilepsy syndrome/presenting seizure type.

Carbamazepine SE: Rash (± exfoliation); platelets↓, agranulocytosis, aplasia (all rare). It induces its own enzymes, so increasing doses may be needed.

Sodium valproate (200mg/5mL). SE: vomiting, appetite↑, drowsiness, platelets↓ (do FBC pre-R). Rare hepatotoxicity can be fatal (eg if coexisting unsuspected metabolic disorder). Monitor LFT, eg in 1st 6 months. When prescribing to girls of present and future childbearing potential, warn of teratogenic risk.

Ethosuximide The syrup is 250mg/5mL. SE: D&V, rashes, erythema multiforme, lupus syndromes, agitation, headache. Indication: absence epilepsy.

Lamotrigine Uses: absences and intractable epilepsy as an add-on. Dose when given with valproate if 2–12yrs: 0.15mg/kg/day PO for 2wks, then 0.3mg/kg daily for 2wks, then ↑ by up to 0.3mg/kg every 1–2 weeks. Usual maintenance: 1–5mg/kg/day (compare with if non-valproate anticonvulsants: ~2.5–7mg/kg/12h).

Vigabatrin (May be 1st choice in infantile spasms and tuberous sclerosis fits.) This blocks GABA transaminase. Consider adding it to regimens if partial seizures are uncontrolled. Starting dose: 15–20mg/kg/12h increased after 2wks to a typical dose of 30–40mg/kg/12h (max 150mg/kg/day). Blood levels do not help (but monitor concurrent phenytoin: it may fall by ~20%). SE: Drowsiness, depression, psychosis, amnesia, diplopia, and field defects (test every year).

Levetiracetam licensed for used as monotherapy for focal seizures—but thought not cost effective (NICE). SE: depression; lethargy; weakness

Diet Consider a high-fat ketogenic diet if 2 drugs fail to work (it can ↓ ↓ fits by ⅔).[730] It needs supervision. SE: constipation, vomiting, ↓energy, hunger.

Education If fits are few, educate teachers on lifting bans on supervised swimming, cycling etc. Showers are safer than baths. Emphasize compliance/concordance (one seizure may ↓the threshold for the next, ie kindling).[731]

Paediatrics

Newer anticonvulsants NICE reserves gabapentin, lamotrigine, oxcarbazepine, tiagabine, topiramate, and vigabatrin (as an adjunct for partial seizures) for children not benefiting from (or able to tolerate) older drugs (above) or older drugs have contraindications/interactions (the Pill)—or the child is of childbearing potential or is likely to need drugs into her childbearing years.[706]

Paediatrics

| Drug | Starting dose mg/kg/24h | Target dose for initial assessment of effect mg/kg/24h | Dose increment | | Usually effective dose mg/kg/24h | Doses per day | Target trough drug level in plasma | |
			Size mg/kg/24h	Interval in days			mg/L	µmol/L
Carbamazepine	5	12.5	2.5	7	10-25	2-3	4-12	
Valproate	10	20	10.0	10	15-40	1-2	Not helpful	
Phenytoin	5	7	1.0	10	5-15	2	10-20	40-80
Phenobarbital	3	6	0.5	1	4-8	1-2	15-40	60-180
Ethosuximide	10	15	5.0	5	10-20	1-2	40-99	280-700
Clonazepam	0.025	0.05	0.025	7	0.025-0.1	2-3	Not helpful	

Which drug?

Tonic–clonic fits: First try sodium valproate. If unsuitable try lamotrigine (may exacerbate myoclonic seizures) or carbamazepine (may exacerbate myoclonic and absence seizures).

Absences: First choice, ethosuximide; second, sodium valproate. If neither work, try lamotrigine, then try combinations. Carbamazepine, gabapentin, oxcarbazepine, phenytoin, tiagabine and vigabatrin are not recommended for absence seizures.

Myoclonic or akinetic fits: Sodium valproate is first line. Levetiracetam or topiramate are second line.

Infantile spasms: Vigabatrin (or corticosteroids).

Partial fits: First try carbamazepine or lamotrigine; then sodium valproate or oxcarbazepine.

If drugs fail Do not use ever more toxic combinations: ►refer for neurosurgical advice and MRI.[732] In drug-resistant epilepsy surgery or a ketogenic diet may help. See OPPOSITE and *Pediatr Neurol:* 2008;38(1):38-43.[733]

Stopping anticonvulsants See OHCM p497. The risk of seizure recurrence during the tapering down process is no greater if the tapering period is 6 weeks compared with 9 months. Source for table: J Engel 2007, Epilepsy, a comprehensive textbook, Solomon; and Brodie *NEJM* 1996; 334 168, 18.[734]

▶*Only enter battles you can win*. If the child can win, be more subtle, eg consistent rewards, not inconsistent punishments. Get a health visitor's advice; ensure everyone is encouraging the same response from the child.

Entrances *Food refusal* and *food fads* are common. Reducing pressure on the child, discouraging parental over-reaction, and gradual enlarging of tiny portions of attractive food are usually all that is needed. Check Hb. Keep a watchful eye on growth and weight gain. *Overeating:* Eating comforts, and if the child is short on comfort, or if mother feels inadequate, the scene is set for overeating and lifelong patterns are begun. Diets may fail until the child is hospitalized (p348). If obese (p226, p530), remember hypothalamic syndromes (eg Prader-Willi, p652), but the treatment remains the same.

Pica is eating things which are not food, eg plastic, or faeces (coprophagia); if persistent, look for other disturbed behaviours, autism, or ↓IQ. *Causes:* iron or other mineral deficiency; obsessive-compulsive disorder. *Complications:* lead poisoning; worm infestations.[735] Behaviour modification may help.[736]

Exits *Constipation* is difficulty in defecation; it may comprise of <3 stools per week; large hard stool; 'rabbit dropping' stool; distress/straining/bleeding with passage of stool. It may lead to abdominal pain, abdominal masses, overflow soiling ± 'lavatory-blocking' enormous stools (megarectum), and anorexia. Causes: diet, poor fluid, or fibre intake—or fear, eg as a result of a fissure. Rarely Hirschprung's disease (p130). Failure to pass meconium in first 48h? Ask about onset of constipation and precipitants (fissure/change in diet/timing of potty training/fears and phobias/moving house/acute infections/family upheavals).

Red flags include.

~Constipation from birth or first few weeks.
~Failure to pass meconium within 48h.
~Faltering growth (an amber flag really; consider coeliac disease/hypothyroid).
~New weakness/abnormal reflexes in legs, delayed locomotion.
~Abnormal appearance of anus / skin in sacral/gluteal region (look for sacral dimples/hairy patches/flattening of gluteal muscles/multiple fissures).
~Gross abdominal distension with vomiting.

Action: •Find out about pot refusal •Does defecation hurt? •Is there parental coercion? Break the vicious cycle of: large faeces → pain/fissure → fear of the pot→ rectum overstretched → call-to-stool sensation dulled → soiling → parental exasperation → coercion. ▶Exonerate the child to boost confidence for the main task of obeying calls-to-stool to keep the rectum empty. *Treat* faecal impaction with escalating dose regimen of polyethylene glycol 3350 + electrolytes eg 'Movicol® Paediatric Plain' as first line intervention (NICE suggests doses, which exceed those in the BNFᶜ, as follows: if <1y then ½–1 sachet daily; if aged 2–5y then 2 sachets on day 1; increase by 2 sachets every 2 days to max. of 8 sachets; if 5–12 start on 4 sachets and increase in steps of 2 to a maximum of 12 per day. If >12y use Movicol® (lacks electrolytes and contains a higher dose of polyethylene glycol 3350) at 4 sachets on day 1, escalating by 2 sachets/day to a maximum of 8. Follow this with maintenance 'Movicol® Paediatric Plain' (<12y)/Movicol® (>12y) ± lactulose ± prolonged alternate-day senna, adjusting dose to produce regular soft stools.

NB: behaviour therapy in combination with laxatives are effective,[738] but biofeedback methods are not.[739] Clinics run by nurse specialists can be more effective than those run by consultants.[740] Dietary modifications to ensure a balanced diet, with sufficient fluids and fibre are necessary but not sufficient by themselves. Encourage daily physical activity. Treat perianal cellulitis with co-amoxiclav (for example). Digital rectal examination and abdominal x-rays are rarely required. Do not use enemas until all attempts are oral medication have failed.

Soiling is the escape of stool into the underclothing.

Faecal incontinence is faecal soiling in the context of a physical/anatomical lesion (Hirschsprung's disease, anal malformation, anal trauma, meningomyelocele, muscle diseases).[741]

Encopresis is the repeated passage of solid faeces in the wrong place in those >4yrs old. ♂:♀≈5:1. It may be voluntary or non-voluntary. Is this due to chronic constipation, and a rectum which has lost its memory of what full and empty feels like? Treat retentive encopresis (80% of cases) with enemas, extra dietary fibre, stool softeners, and 'mandatory' daily toilet sittings ~15–30mins after eating). Try behaviour therapy for non-retentive soiling.[742] NB: this demarcation is not absolute: behavioural techniques such as differential attention, contingency management, and contracting are relevant to both forms of encopresis.[743] Rarely, encopresis signifies autoeroticism[1] or a defecation disorder or learning[2] difficulty.[744] Whatever the cause, ☺adopt a holistic stance and set the symptom in the family context. This is important because we know that encopresis is associated with anxiety, depression, attention difficulties, and environments with less expressiveness and poor organization, and social problems (disruptive behaviour, poorer school performance etc).[745] Aim to give the family time to air feelings that encopresis engenders (anger, shame, ridicule).

Enuresis: Infrequent bedwetting (<2 nights/week) occurs in ~20% at 4½yrs and 8% at 9½. 1-2% of >15y continue to wet the bed, usually from delayed maturation of bladder control (family history often +ve). Tests for diabetes, UTI and GU abnormality (p174) can occasionally yield surprises but are by no means compulsory unless there are clinical suspicions. The term 'secondary enuresis' implies wetness after >6 months' dryness, and raises concerns about worries, illness, or abuse. *History:* Ask about nights per week he wets the bed? Does it happen more than once per night? Severe bedwetting is less likely to resolve spontaneously. Are there any daytime symptoms? Frequency/urgency may indicate an overactive bladder. How much does he drink during the day? Is there constipation/soiling; history of recurrent UTI (underlying urological abnormality)? If the child was dry and recently started bedwetting consider systemic illness and the possibility of child abuse. *Treatment:* Start with advice and reassure parents than many children continue to wet the bed after achieving day-time dryness. Ensure that caffeine based drinks are avoided and the toilet is used regularly during the day (4-7 times is typical). Reassure that he is neither infantile nor dirty. A system of rewards for *agreed behaviours* (eg drinking recommended levels of fluid, using the toilet before bedtime, taking medicines, or helping change the sheets (*not for dry nights which the child can't control*) may be effective. Alarms (± vibrations) triggered by urine in the bed can make 56% dry at 1yr; relapses are preventable by continuing use after dryness. They are cheap or loanable from Child Guidance Services (or equivalent)—eg Drinite®[747] www.bedwetting.co.uk. **Desmopressin** sublingual dose (if >5yrs): 120µg at bedtime (max 240µg); fluid overload (Na⁺↓) is rare, eg after gulping in swimming pool water, or going to rave parties. Have 1 week 3-monthly with no drugs. CI: cystic fibrosis, uraemia, BP↑.

---

1 Anal erotic feelings reported by some encopretic children are intense, and some workers hold that the encopretic symptom, soiling, in these children is the result of a conscious form of anal masturbation in which the faecal mass is used for stimulation. Encopresis interventions may be over-simplistic unless they take into account what encopretic children know and say about their soiling.[748]
2 Behavioural treatment of non-retentive, nocturnal encopresis in those with learning disability involves waking prior to soiling, time-limited use of suppositories, and rewards for appropriate evacuation.[749]

Paediatrics

Attention deficit hyperactivity disorder (ADHD) is the most common neurobehavioral disorder of childhood. It has prevalence of 3–5% in Western nations.[750] ADHD is commoner in learning-disabled children, and if prenatal cannabis exposure.[751,752] The core diagnostic criteria are: *impulsivity, inattention* and *hyperactivity*. Not *all* those with ADD are hyperactive. *There is no diagnostic test* (but positron emission tomography may show ↓function of frontal lobes and nearby connections). Most parents first note hyperactivity at the toddler stage, but most locomotor hyperactivity at this stage abates with time, so the diagnosis is usually delayed until school entry or later. Signs often attenuate during adolescence, but may persist into mid-adulthood. There is a familial tendency, and families with ADD are more likely to have other diagnoses too, eg learning difficulties, mood, anxiety, and psychosocial disorders (DSM IV; p312). Associations: conduct disorder or other disruptive behaviour disorders (oppositional defiant disorder).[753] Children and adolescents with ADD are at risk of being victims of assaults, as well as suicide and self-harm.[754]

Attention deficit signs[DSM-IV]
Often unable to:
• Listen/attend closely to detail (∴ carelessness)
• To sustain attention in play activities
• Follow instructions
• Finish homework (when not due to defiance)
• Organize tasks needing sustained application
• Ignore extraneous stimuli
• Remember simple tasks

Hyperactivity signs
• Squirming/fidgeting
• 'On the go all the time'
• 'As if driven by a motor'
• Talks incessantly
• Climbs over everything
• Restless
• No quiet hobbies
• Impulsivity—ie:
• blurts out answers
• interrupts others
• too impatient to take turns or to queue

Treatment:[755 NICE] Diagnosis and drug treatment ought to be initiated by a specialist (eg pyschiatrist/paediatrician). Following diagnosis, time for explanation is required; offer a booklet to parents, give advice on **positive parenting** and **behavioural techniques**. 1st line treatment for pre-school children and school age children with moderate ADHD/moderate impairment is parent training/education programmes. Older children may benefit from cognitive behavioural therapy. Drugs may be useful in school age children if non-drug treatments fail (eg *methylphenidate* (Ritalin®): if 4–6y start at 2.5mg/12h, increasing weekly if needed by 2.5mg/day to a max of 1.4mg/kg/day; if >6 start at 5mg/12h increasing to a max of 2.1mg/kg/day (max 90mg daily); *atomoxetine*: 0.5mg/kg/day (if >6yrs old and <70kg) increasing after 7 days to 1.5mg/kg/day). Severe ADHD in school age children methylphenidate and atomoxetine are 1st line treatments so ensure referral. Evidence for long-term use is uncertain.[756,757] Parental training and behavioural modification techniques, eg **prolonged eye-contact** between parent and child should also be considered.[758] Hypoallergenic diets (eg no tartrazine) are controversial (may cause parental obsessions). Liaise with teachers: 30% of ADHD boys are excluded from school—this may violate their human rights.[759] *Other ideas:* Yoga,[760] **homeopathy** (probably no effect).[761]

School refusal *Setting:* Emotional overprotection; high social class; neurotic parents; schoolwork of high standard. In truancy, the reverse is true. *Treatment:* Confer with headteacher, parents, and an educational psychologist. Escort by an education welfare officer aids prompt return to school. Other methods: educational-support therapy, cognitive behaviour therapy, and parent-teacher interventions.[762] Hypnosis is a good alternative (the hypnotist maintains contact with the child on the way to school and during the stressful morning hours via a mobile phone).[763] Often anxiety (eg separation-anxiety or phobias) ± depression need treatment too.[764]

Babies usually learn to walk at ~14 months old. If this has not occurred by 20 months, ask yourself 2 questions: Is the child physically normal? Is development delayed in other areas too? The commonest causes reflect chronic illness, global delay, benign immaturity, and generalized joint hypermobility (BOX). In boys consider Duchenne muscular dystrophy early (genetic counselling *before* mother's next pregnancy). The major reason for identifying late walkers is to exclude cerebral palsy.

Typical causes:
Prenatal factors
• APH (with hypoxia)
• X-rays
• Alcohol
• CMV; rubella; HIV
• Toxoplasmosis
• Rhesus disease
Perinatal factors:
• Birth trauma
• Fetal distress
• Hypoglycaemia
• Hyperbilirubinaemia
Postnatal factors:
• Trauma/intraventricular haemorrhage
• Hypoxia
• Meningoencephalitis
• Cerebral vein thrombosis (from dehydration)

Cerebral palsy (CP) comprises chronic disorders of posture and movement caused by non-progressive CNS lesions sustained before 2yrs old, resulting in delayed motor development, evolving CNS signs, learning disability (35%), and epilepsy. Most are due to antenatal events unrelated to birth trauma. *Prevalence:* 9% if gestation 23–27wks; 6% if 28–30wks; 0.1% if term.[765] *Survival:* 20yrs if quadriplegic (much longer if less affected). ♀:♂≈1:1. *Signs:* Weakness, paralysis, delayed milestones, seizures, language/speech problems. *Classification:* There are four main types: Spastic; dyskinetic; ataxic and mixed CP. Spasticity suggests a pyramidal lesion; uncoordinated, involuntary movements and postures (dystonias) suggest basal ganglia involvement. Most have either a *spastic hemiplegia* (arm>leg; early development of hand preference—ie <12mth; delay in walking; increased deep reflexes of affected limb) or a *spastic diplegia* (both legs affected worse than the arms, so that the child looks normal until he is picked up, when the legs 'scissor'—hip flexion, adduction and internal rotation; with knee extension and feet plantar-flexed). *Spastic quadriplegia* is the most severe form and is associated with seizures and IQ↓. Swallowing difficulties (2° to retrobulbar palsy) may lead to aspiration pneumonia. *Dyskinetic (athetoid) cerebral palsy:* Unwanted actions; poor movement flow/posture control; spasticity; hypotonia; hearing↓; dysarthria. Association: kernicterus. *Ataxic palsies* are uncommon. There may be hypo- or hypertonia.

Management teams Children's views must be taken into account in all matters concerning them.[766] UN Convention on the Rights of the Child ▶*Assume that all disabled children are entitled to a 'full and decent life'.* The aim is quality of life and full integration into society. Because children have grown up hand-in-hand with disability and are often uncowed by it, they often score as high as anyone else on quality of life, if pain is treated.[766] Parents may find it a comfort to know this. Physio- and occupational therapists, orthopaedic surgeons, and orthoses experts aid holistic assessment: can he roll over (both ways)? Sit? Grasp? Transfer objects from hand to hand? Good head righting? Ability to shift weight when prone with forearm support. IQ. Is toileting possible? Can he hold a pen or a spoon? Muscle strengthening can help.[767] Callipers may prevent deformity (equinovarus, equinovalgus, hip dislocation from excessive flexion/adduction). Attempts to show benefits of neurophysiotherapy (to help equilibrium and righting) don't show benefit over simple motor stimulation. Some parents try the Hungarian *Petö approach*: ☸Here the 'conductor' devotes herself to the child, using interaction with peers to reinforce successes: eg manipulation, art, writing, fine movement, and social skills.[768] Treat co-morbidities such as epilepsy (p208). *Botulinum toxin* (p460) has an uncertain role.[769–771] *Epidural cord electrostimulation & intrathecal or oral baclofen* (benefits uncertain).[772,773]

Prognosis By 6yrs, 54% with quadriplegia (80% if hemiplegic or diplegic) gain urinary continence spontaneously. If IQ↓, 38% are dry at this age.[774] n=601

►When in doubt, ask the mother what she thinks is wrong. ►Always test the hearing. *Ensure the result is as reliable as possible.*

Speech development This dialogue portrays the mystery of language learning: *Daughter:* "I don't want to eat my ice cream yet" *Father:* "Don't procrastinate!" "Daddy, how can I understand you if you use words I don't understand?" "If I only ever used words you understood we could never have started talking." "Why?" "Well, to start with you never understood anything..." "Didn't I?—OK, wait a moment...I'll start my ice cream before it melts."

At ~1 year a few words may be used meaningfully.

At 1½yrs old 2-word utterances ("Daddy come").

At 2 years old... subject–verb–object sentences appear ("I want a pudding").

At 3½yrs old... the child has mastered thought, language, abstraction, and the elements of reason, having a 1000-word vocabulary at his or her disposal, enabling sentences such as: "I give her cake' cos she's hungry".

Words exist to give ideas currency, and so often that currency proves counterfeit—a process which so often starts with if, eg "If I hadn't thrown the cup on the ground, I might have got a pudding". The uttering of "If. . .", linked with an emotional response, is the most human of all constructions, opening up worlds divorced from reality, providing for the exercise of imagination, the validation of dreams, the understanding of motives, and the control of events. The rest of life holds nothing to match the intellectual and linguistic pace of these first years. Further linguistic development is devoted to seemingly conceptually minor tasks, such as expanding vocabulary.

There is much variation in speech timing: what is 'clearly abnormal'?

Vocabulary size: If <50 words at 3yrs old, suspect deafness—or:

Expressive dysphasia or speech dyspraxia (eg if there is a telegraphic quality to speech, poor clarity, and deteriorating behaviour, eg frustration).

Other causes of delayed talking
Congenital:
• Klinefelter's syn.
• Galactosaemia
• Histidinaemia
• Auditory agnosia
• Floating-harbor syn.
Acquired with or after:
• Meningoencephalitis
• Head injury
• Landau-Kleffner syn. (epilepsy + progressive loss of language)

• Audio-premotor syndrome (APM). The child cannot reflect sounds correctly heard into motor control of larynx and respiration. Instead of babbling, the child is quiet, unable to hum or sing.
• Respiro-laryngeal (RL) dysfunction (dysphonia from incorrect vocal fold vibration/air flow regulation). The voice is loud and rough.
• Congenital aphonia (thin effortful voice; it's rare).

Speech clarity: By 2½yrs, parents should understand most speech. If not, suspect deafness—or:
• Articulatory dyspraxia (easy consonants are *b* and *m* with the lips, and *d* with the tongue—the phonetic components of babbling). ♂:♀ ≈ 3:1. Tongue-tie is a possible cause (∴ poor sounds needing tongue elevation— *d* and *s*)—surgery to the frenum may be needed (+speech therapy). Distinguish from phonological causes (disordered *sound for speech processing*—may present as *sound awareness problems* (difficulty in analysing sound structure of words). Both are common.
• APM or RL dysfunction, as described above.

Understanding: By 2½ years a child should understand "Get your shoes" (if he has any), if not suspect: • Deafness—if the hearing is impaired (eg 25–40dB loss) secretory otitis media is likely to be the cause. Worse hearing loss is probably sensorineural • Cognitive impairment • Deprivation.

Speech therapy Refer early, before school starts. NB: randomized trials have not shown any clear benefits from this strategy.[175] N=159

WHO definitions *Impairment* entails a pathological process, eg spina bifida, which may cause certain *disabilities*, eg walking difficulty. Handicap is their social consequence (eg cannot walk to school).

Learning delay (mental handicap) *The mother often makes the first diagnosis.* An IQ <35 constitutes a severe learning disability (mental handicap, p314).

►Beware conflating IQ with intellect: the latter implies more than problem-solving and memory: intellect entails the ability to speculate, to learn from mistakes, to have a view of oneself and others, to see relationships between events in different domains of experience—as well as the ability to use language either to map the world, or to weave ironic webs of truth and deceit (and, on a good day, to do both simultaneously).

Causes: Severe mental impairment usually has a definable cause, whereas mild intellectual disability is often familial, with no well-defined cause. Be prepared to refer to an expert. *Congenital disorders* are legion: chromosomal (eg Down's; fragile X, p648); metabolic (eg PKU p183). *Acquired:* Perinatal infection p34–37, birth injury and cerebral palsy, trauma, meningitis.

Lead exposure: This is a leading preventable cause of mildly impaired IQ. For example in 2-yr-olds for each 0.48μmol/L plasma increment there is an associated 5–8 point fall in IQ as measured on the Wechsler Intelligence Scale for Children (revised). This defect is long-lasting.

Chemical defects associated with intellectual disability—eg: *Homocystinuria:* Paraplegia, fits, friable hair, emboli, cataracts; homocystine is found in the urine. Treat with a low-methionine, cystine-supplemented diet, with large doses of pyridoxine. *Maple syrup urine disease:* Hypoglycaemia, acidosis, fits, death. Urine smells of maple syrup, due to defective metabolism of branched chain keto acids. Treatment: high-calorie amino acid controlled diet. Thiamine has been tried. *Tryptophanuria:* Rough, pigmented skin. Treat with nicotinic acid.

Management: Refer to an expert, so that no treatable cause is missed. Would the family like help from group, such as MENCAP? Other members of the family may need special support (eg normal siblings, who now feel neglected). If the IQ is >35, life in the community is the aim.

Physical handicap *Sensory:* Deafness, see p548. Blindness: congenital defects are described on p454. Principal acquired causes of blindness are: retinopathy of prematurity, vitamin A deficiency, onchocerciasis (p450), eye injuries, cataract (eg Down's syndrome).

CNS & musculoskeletal problems: (Congenital or acquired) Causes: accidents (eg near-drowning), cerebral palsy (p214), spina bifida (p140), after meningitis, polio, congenital infections (above), tumours, syndromes (p638).

Wheelchairs:[1] For indoors or outdoors? Patient-operated, motorized or pushed? What sort of restraints to prevent falling out? If collapsible, how small must it be to get into the car? Are the sides removable to aid transfer from chair to bed? Can the child control the brakes? Are there adjustable elevated leg rests? Liaise with the physio and occupational therapist.

Callipers will allow some patients to stand and walk. Long-leg callipers are required for those with complete leg paralysis. The top should be constructed so that it does not induce pressure sores. A knee lock supports the knee in the standing position. An internal coil spring prevents foot drop.

---

1 Disabled Living Foundation, www.dlf.org.uk UK tel. 0845 130 9177 (local rate).[TM]

Check-list to guide management of handicap

In hospitals or the community, we should address each of these points:
- Screening and its documentation on local handicap registers.
- Communication with parents.
- Referring to/liaising with district handicap team+community paediatrician.
- Access to specialist services, including physiotherapy, orthopaedic surgery.
- Assessing special needs for schooling and housing.
- Co-ordinating neuropsychological/neurodevelopmental assessments.
- Co-ordinating measures of severity (eg electrophysiology ± CT/MRI).
- Liaison with dietician on special foods.
- Promotion of long-term concordance with treatment/education programmes.
- Education about the consequences of the illness.
- Encourage contact with family support groups.
- Offering family planning *before* patients become unintentionally pregnant.
- Pre-conception counselling (p2, with specialist in molecular genetics).
- Co-ordinating prenatal diagnostic tests and fetal assessment.

Society, paediatrics in the community, and family-oriented care

99.9% of paediatric care goes on in the community, provided by mothers, fathers, GPs, nurses, physios, community paediatricians, child-minders, special-needs teachers, sports/PE teachers, and their assistants. Inevitably if you are studying paediatrics within hospital you will have a biased view of what paediatrics is like—nowhere more at odds with reality than in the spheres of impairment, disability, and handicap. ▶ *If you really want to make a difference to children's lives, get out into the community at every chance.* Find out what is going on—and then start contributing.

Increasingly, this is being advocated by paediatric training programmes in the UK and abroad—eg the *Community Paediatrics Training Initiative*.[777]

Children's health and wellbeing are inextricably linked to their parents' physical, emotional and social health, social circumstances, and child-rearing practices.[778] These cannot be appreciated or moulded to the child's advantage without at least one foot in the community.

No paediatrician can work well without understanding the multicultural demographics and marriage statistics of the population from which her patients come. For example, in some areas the median income of families with married parents has increased by 146% since 1970, but female-headed households have had growth of 131% (less in inner city areas). In one study, the median income of female-headed households was only 47% of that of married-couple families and only 65% of that of families with 2 married parents in which the wife was not employed. The proportion of children who live in poverty is ~5-fold greater for female-headed families than for married-couple families.[778] In the UK, 1.4 million children live in poverty despite one parent having a job.[779] This has a greater effect on children's health than all the goings on in paediatric wards and hospitals. These problems seem resistant to socialism, the minimum wage, tax credits and benefits.

Most families with young children depend on child care, of varying quality. This causes ↑ costs (only partly mitigated by government funds), long days for children, with stress imposed by travel and exposure to infections.[778]

More and more parents are devoting time once available to their children to the care of their own parents. They won't tell you of this in brief ward encounters, but these facts become clear when working in the community.[778]

☼ Paediatricians have a key role in fostering interdisciplinary collaboration between schools, hospitals, and other child-related institutions, and they must feel able to refer parents for physical, emotional, or social problems, or health risk behaviours that can adversely affect the health or emotional or social wellbeing of their child.

Paediatrics

Families transmit the false values of materialism, and we pick up the pieces of childhood mental health problems when it all goes wrong.

Developmental disorders are a group of conditions leading to impairment in at least one functional area—eg cognition, motor skills (gross or fine), social-emotional or communication (speech, language, hearing or vision). Around 20-25% of children have at least one developmental delay, and as many as 50% of these will not be detected before starting primary school.[780] Conditions falling under the umbrella of developmental disorders include autism spectrum disorders, speech-language impairment, learning disabilities and psycho-social problems. *Biological risk factors* include: prematurity, low birth weight, birth asphyxia, chronic illness and hearing/vision impairment. *Environmental risk factors* include: poverty, low parental education, parental mental illness and social isolation.[781]

Developmental surveillance refers to an ongoing process of following a child over time with a view to contextualizing a child's development. It involves discussing concerns with parents, eliciting a perinatal history, identifying risk factors, as well as observing the child attempting different skills at different times and referring the child when appropriate to other health professionals (eg physiotherapists, speech therapists or audiometrists). Developmental surveillance can be incorporated into well-child checks, general physical examination and routine immunization visits.

Developmental screening refers to a brief assessment aimed at identifying those children who require further investigation and assessment. It is typically carried out using a developmental screening tool. Screening should be carried out within the broader undertaking of developmental surveillance. Repeating screening at different ages increases the accuracy of the test. Parental concern about a child's development may in itself constitute a reliable screening test.[782] The *Denver Developmental Screening Test (DDST)* and its successor the *Denver II* have largely been replaced with more sensitive tests. Screening may be based on parent report alone (parent completed tests) or through direct observation together with parent report (directly administered tests). Some of the most commonly used tests are discussed below—all are copyrighted products:

The *Parents' Evaluation of Developmental Status (PEDS)* tool is a parent completed test consisting of 10 questions (8 yes/no, 2 open ended). It can be given to parents to complete prior to attending health visits and takes less than 5 minutes to complete. It has a sensitivity of 74-80% and is suitable for children up to 8 years old.[780] It identifies children as low, moderate or high risk for various disabilities and identifies an optimal course of action. Available at www.pedtest.com

The *Ages and Stages Questionnaire (ASQ)*, another parent completed test, consists of 21 age specific questionnaires. It can be used to evaluate children aged 1 month to 5½ years old. It has a sensitivity of 85% and takes 10-20 minutes to complete.[780] It has a single cut-off score indicating which children need further referral. Available at: agesandstages.com

The *Modified Checklist for Autism in Toddlers (M-CHAT)* is a second-stage parent completed test that is more specific for autism spectrum disorders. It has a sensitivity of 90%. Available free online at: www.firstsigns.org.

The *Brigance Screens-II* is a directly administered test, combining parental observation and the eliciting of skills from children. It covers multiple domains of development including speech-language, motor, general knowledge as well as reading and maths at the older age groups. Available at: www.curriculumassociates.com

Whilst the American Association of Pediatrics recommends both developmental surveillance and screening,[783] the National Screening Committee (UK) doesn't recommend developmental screening.[784]

Developmental milestones

Average age	Milestone	Red flags
6 weeks	• smiles, • follow eyes past midline	
4–6 months	• sits with support • rolls • reaches out for objects • starts babbling	At 6 months if • no smile • no grasp • not rolling • poor head control
6–9 months	• crawls • sits without support • pulls to stand • gives toy on request • turns head to name • responds to 'bye-bye' • gestures with babbling • first tooth	At 9 months if • no response to words • lack of eye contact or facial expression • no gestures • no passing of toys from hand to hand • not sitting without support or crawling
7–12 months	• develops pincer grasp • plays 'peek-a-boo' • walks with a hand held • waves goodbye	At 12 months if • unable to pick up small items • not crawling / bottom shuffling • not standing holding on to furniture • no babbled phrases
12–15 months	• single words • listens to stories • drinks from cup	
18 months	• speaks 6 words • able to walk up steps • names pictures • walks independently • scribbles • builds with blocks	• uninterested in playing with others • no clear words • not walking without support • not able to hold crayon • unable to stack 2 blocks
1.5–2 years	• kicks/throws a ball • runs • 2-word sentences • follows a 2-step command • stacks 5–6 blocks • turns pages • uses a spoon • helps with dressing	At 2 years if • has <50 words • difficulty handling small objects • unable to climb stairs • no interest in feeding or dressing

Paediatrics

If there is regression, or loss of a previously developed skill, this should be considered a red flag requiring immediate investigation. Other red flags at any age include poor interaction with others, difference in strength between right and left sides of body, abnormal tone and strong parental concern.

Paediatrics

Biochemistry (1mmol = 1mEq/L)

Albumin^P	36-48g/dL
Alk phos^P	(depends on age) see below
α1-antitrypsin^P	1.3-3.4g/dL
Ammonium^P	2-25μmL/L; 3-35μg/dL
Amylase^P	70-300u/L
Aspartate aminotransferase^P	<40u/L
Bilirubin^P	2-16μmol/L; 0.1-0.8mg/dL
Blood gases, arterial	pH 7.36-7.42
P_aCO_2	4.3-6.1kPa; 32-46mmHg
P_aO_2	11.3-14.0kPa; 85-105mmHg
Bicarbonate^P	21-25mmol/L
Base excess	-2 to +2mmol/L
Calcium^P	2.25-2.75mmol/L; 9-11mg/dL
neonates:	1.72-2.47; 6.9-9.9mg/dL
Chloride^P	98-105mmol/L
Cholesterol^{P,F}	≤5.7mmol/L; 100-200mg/dL
Creatine kinase^P	<80u/L
Creatinine^P	25-115μmol/L; 0.3-1.3mg/dL
Glucose^P	2.5-5.3mmol/L; 45-95mg/dL
(lower in newborn; fluoride tube)	
IgA^S	0.8-4.5g/L (low at birth, Rising to adult levels slowly)
IgG^S	5-18g/L (high at birth, falls and then rises slowly to adult level)
IgM^S	0.2-2.0g/L (low at birth, rises to adult level by 1 year)
IgE^S	<500u/mL

Iron^S	9-36μmol/L; 50-200μg/dL
Lead^{EDTA}	<1.75μmol/L; <36μg/dL
Mg^{2+P}	0.6-1.0mmol/L
Osmolality^P	275-295mosmol/L
Phenylalanine^P	0.04-0.21mmol/L
Potassium^P mean mmol/L	3.5-5.5
Protein^P	63-81g/L; 6.3-8.1g/dL
Sodium^P	136-145mmol/L
Transferrin^S	2.5-4.5g/L
Triglyceride^{F,P}	0.34-1.92mmol/L (=30-170mg/dL)
Urate^P	0.12-0.36mmol/L; 2-6mg/dL
Urea^P	2.5-6.6mmol/L; 15-40mg/dL
Gamma-glutamyl transferase^P	<20u/L

Hormones—a guide. ▶ Consult lab

Cortisol^P	9am 200-700nmol/L midnight <140nmol/L, mean
Dehydroepiandrosterone sulfate^P:	
day 5-11	0.8-2.8μmol/L (range)
5-11yrs	0.1-3.6μmol/L
17α-Hydroxyprogesterone^P:	
days 5-11	1.6-7.5nmol/L (range)
4-15yrs	0.4-4.2nmol/L
T_4^P	60-135nmol/L (not neonates)
TSH^P	<5mu/L (higher on day 1-4)

B=boy; ^{EDTA}=edetic acid; ^{F}=fasting
G=girl; ^{P}=plasma; ^{S}=serum.

Alk phos^P u/L: 0-½yr 150-600; ½-2yr 250-1000; 2-5yr 250-850; 6-7yr 250-1000; 8-9yr 250-750; 10-11yr G = 259-950, B ≤ 730; 12-13yr G = 200-750, B ≤ 785; 14-15yr G = 170-460, B = 170-970; 16-18yr G = 75-270, B = 125-720; >18yr G = 60-250, B = 50-200.

Haematology mean ±~1 standard deviation. Range ×10^9/L (median in brackets)

Day	Hb *g/dL*	MCV *fl*	MCHC %	Retics %	WCC	Neutrophils	Eosins	Lymphs	Monos
1	19.0±2	119±9	31.6±2	3.2±1	9-30	6-26	(11) 0.02-0.8	2-11	0.4-3.1
4	18.6±2	114±7	32.6±2	1.8±1	9-40				
5	17.6±1	114±9	30.9±2	1.2±0.2					
Weeks									
1-2	17.3±2	112±19	32.1±3	0.5±0.03	5-21	1.5-10	(5) 0.07-0.1	2-17	0.3-2.7
2-3	15.6±3	111±8	33.9±2	0.8±0.6	6-15	1-9.5	(4) 0.07-0.1	2-17	0.2-2.4
4-5	12.7±6	101±8	34.9±2	0.9±0.8	6-15		(4)	(6)	
6-7	12.0±2	105±12	33.8±2	1.2±0.7	6-15		(4)	(6)	
8-9	10.7±1	93±12	34.1±2	1.8±1	6-15		(4)	(6)	
Months—all the following Hb values are Medians/Lower limit for normal									
3	11.5/9	88/88			6-15		(3)	(6)	
6	11.5/9	77/70			6-15		(3)	(6)	
12	11.5/9	78/72			6-15		(3)	(5)	
Year									
2	11.5/9	78/74			6-15		(3)	(5)	
4	12.2/10	80/75			6-15		(4)	(4)	
6	13/10.4	82/75			5-15		(4.2)	(3.8)	
12	13.8/11	83/76			4-13		(4.9)	(3.1)	
14B	14.2/12	84/77			4-13		(3)	(3)	
14G	14/11.5								
16B	14.8/12	85/78	30-36	0.8-2	4-13	2-7.5	(5) 0.04-4	1.3-3.5	0.2-.8
16G	14/11.5								
18B	15/13								

Note: *Basophil range*: 0-0.1×10^9/L; B$^S_{12}$ ≥150mg/L.
Red cell folate^{EDTA} 100-640ng/mL. B = boys; G = girls.
Platelet counts don't vary with age: 150-400×10^9/L.

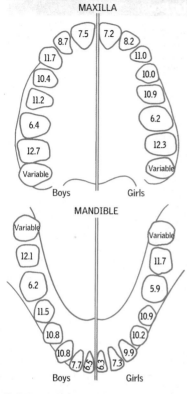

Fig 1. Mean times of eruption (in years) of the permanent teeth.

Deciduous teeth	Months		Months
Lower central incisors	5–9	First molars	10–16
Upper central incisors	8–12	Canines	16–20
Upper lateral incisors	10–12	Second molars	20–30
Lower lateral incisors	12–15		
A 1-year-old has ~6 teeth; 1½yrs ~12 teeth; 2yrs ~16 teeth; 2¼yrs ~20.			

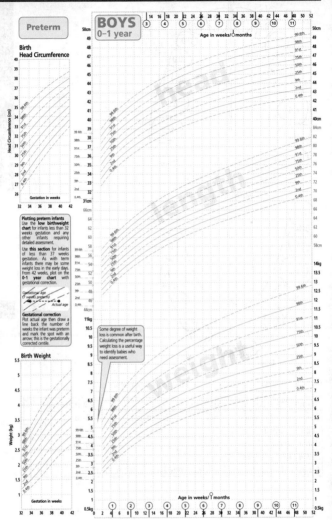

Fig 1. UK-WHO growth charts—boys aged 0–1 yrs

© 2009 Department of Health.

In 2006 the WHO introduced new growth standards which were adopted in the UK in 2009 (2010 in Scotland) for children 0–4y (UK-WHO charts). These growth standards were compiled from data from breast-fed babies (who grow slower than formula-fed infants)—from 6 different nations (the US, Norway, Oman, Brazil, India and Ghana). The linear growth patterns were similar between nations—so for this age group there aren't thought to be any ethnospecific differences in rate of growth. This rate of growth is taken to be an optimal growth rate for children, as opposed

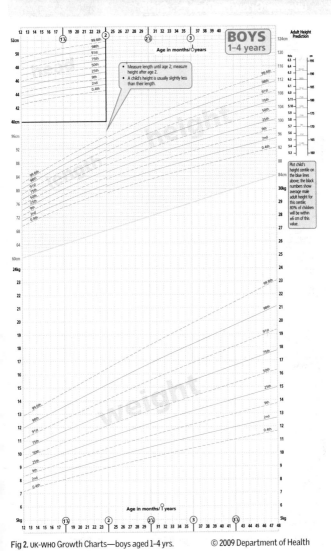

Fig 2. UK-WHO Growth Charts—boys aged 1–4 yrs. © 2009 Department of Health

to the previous growth charts (UK90) which described the prevailing growth patterns of UK children compiled from surveys done in the 1980s. As a result the UK-WHO charts have an increased number of overweight children and fewer underweight children, when compared with the UK90 charts. For <4yrs, the UK-WHO charts replace the UK90 charts. The UK90 charts are still used for children >4 (not reproduced here)

• Separate charts exist for children with Down's Syndrome, Turner's and achondroplasia

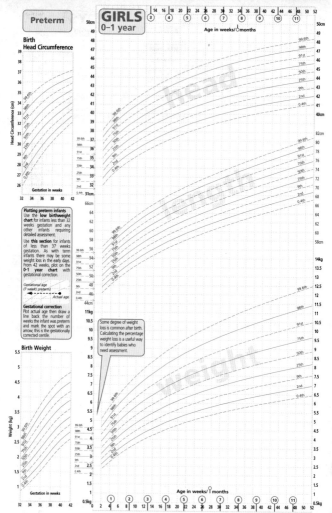

Fig 3. UK-WHO growth charts—girls aged 0–1 yrs.

©2009 Department of Health.

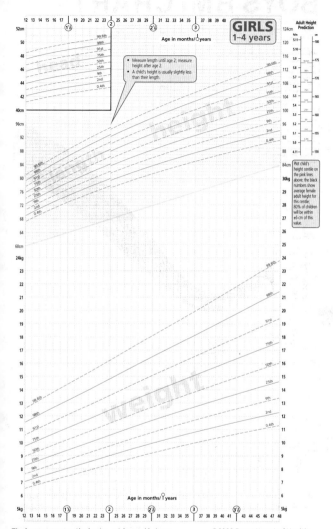

Fig 4. UK-WHO growth charts—girls aged 1–4 yrs. ©2009 Department of Health.

BOYS BMI CHART

(BIRTH - 20 YEARS): United Kingdom cross-sectional reference: 2002/1

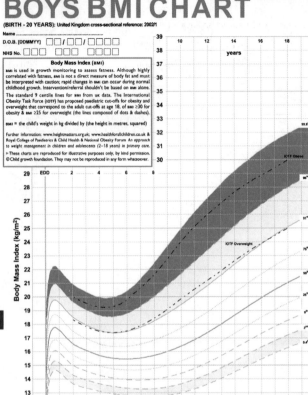

All rights are reserved. No part of this chart may be reproduced, stored in a retrieval system, or transmitted in any form or by any means, electronic, clockwork, magnetic tape, mechanical photocopying, recording or otherwise without permission in writing from the copyright owner. All enquiries should be addressed to the publishers

Designed and Published by
© CHILD GROWTH FOUNDATION 1997/1
(Charity Reg. No 274325)
2 Mayfield Avenue,
London W4 1PW

Printed and Supplied by
HARLOW PRINTING LIMITED
Maxwell Street · South Shields
Tyne & Wear · NE33 4PU

Risk factors for childhood obesity Changes in food availability and activity levels during the past 30 years are well known. Also: low socioeconomic status, maternal obesity, rapid infancy weight gain. *Obesity prevention programmes* have some success and show that changes in school and community environments can decrease childhood weight gain. In France, for example, children are weighed in school regularly, and regular exercise and healthy eating (not diets) are promoted in systematic ways. Input from a family healthy-eating coach has also been found to help.[785,786] Peer encouragement and feedback in the form of pedometer readings is one way of promoting more exercise.[787]

For *causes of obesity*, see p180. For other methods of preventing adult consequences of childhood obesity by intervening in childhood, see p156.

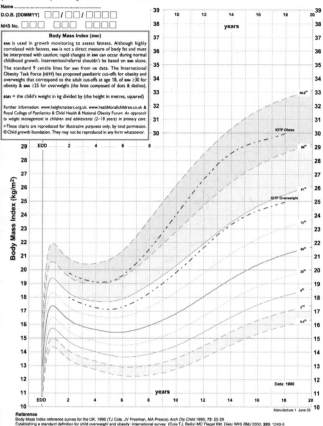

GIRLS BMI CHART

(BIRTH - 20 YEARS): United Kingdom cross-sectional reference: 2002/1

Name ....

D.O.B. [DDMMYY] □□ / □□ / □□

NHS No. □□□ □□□□

Body Mass Index (BMI)

BMI is used in growth monitoring to assess fatness. Although highly correlated with fatness, BMI is not a direct measure of body fat and must be interpreted with caution; rapid changes in BMI can occur during normal childhood growth. Intervention/referral shouldn't be based on BMI alone.

The standard 9 centile lines for BMI from UK data. The International Obesity Task Force (IOTF) has proposed paediatric cut-offs for obesity and overweight that correspond to the adult cut-offs at age 18, of BMI ≥30 for obesity & BMI ≥25 for overweight (the lines composed of dots & dashes).

BMI = the child's weight in kg divided by (the height in metres, squared)

Further information: www.heightmatters.org.uk; www.healthforallchildren.co.uk & Royal College of Paediatrics & Child Health & National Obesity Forum An approach to weight management in children and adolescents (2-18 years) in primary care.
▷These charts are reproduced for illustrative purposes only, by kind permission. © Child growth foundation. They may not be reproduced in any form whatsoever.

Reference
Body Mass Index reference curves for the UK, 1990 (TJ Cole, JV Freeman, MA Preece) Arch Dis Child 1995; 73: 25-29
Establishing a standard definition for child overweight and obesity: international survey (Cole TJ, Bellizzi MC Flegal KM, Dietz WH) BMJ 2000; 320: 1240-3

Designed and Published by
© CHILD GROWTH FOUNDATION 1997/1
(Charity Reg. No 274325)
2 Mayfield Avenue,
London W4 1PW

Printed and Supplied by
HARLOW PRINTING LIMITED
Maxwell Street · South Shields
Tyne & Wear · NE33 4PU

All rights are reserved. No part of this chart may be reproduced, stored in a retrieval system, or transmitted in any form or by any means, electronic, electrostatic, magnetic tape, mechanical photocopying, recording or otherwise without permission in writing from the copyright owner. All enquiries should be addressed to the publishers

z-scores for weight, height, and BMI: what do they mean? A z score (for weight-for-age) of –1 indicates that weight is 1 standard deviation (*OHCM* p737) below the median for that age/sex group. This means mildly underweight. z –2 (minus 2 standard deviations) is moderate, and z–3 is severe. Ditto for height. In the care of children with chronic diseases, eg HIV, monitoring and improving the BMI z-score is an important way of reducing morbidity and mortality.[788]

A BMI z-score of +2 to +2.5 counts as moderate obesity (severe if >2.5).[789,790] BMI z-score is chief determinant of metabolic syndrome in children;[791] a 1-point increase in BMI z-score yields a 2-fold increase in its prevalence (↑ from 27.6% to 60.7% if BMI z-score increases from 2.3 to 3.3).

BMI z-scores also help monitoring weight-intervention programmes.[792]

Dubowitz system for assessing gestational age

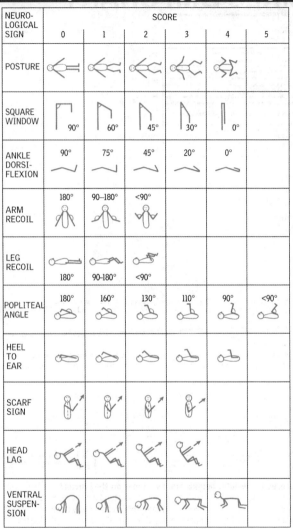

Fig 1. Neurological criteria for Dubowitz scoring (use in conjunction with table on p230–1).

Reproduced from Dubowitz, L. 'Assessment of gestational age: a practical scoring system' *Archives of Disease in Childhood* with permission from BMJ Publishing Ltd.

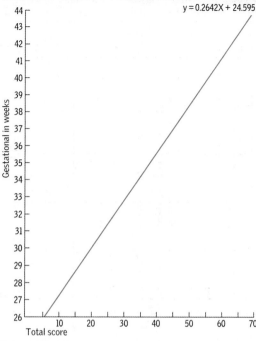

Fig 2. Assessment of gestational age: Dubowitz system. Graph for reading gestational age from total score.

Reproduced from Dubowitz, L. 'Assessment of gestational age: a practical scoring system' *Archives of Disease in Childhood* with permission from BMJ Publishing Ltd.

Paediatrics

Assessment of gestational age: Dubowitz system

Physical (external) criteria (for neurological criteria, see p228)

External sign	Score				
	0	1	2	3	4
Oedema	Obvious oedema hands and feet: pitting over tibia	No obvious oedema hands and feet: pitting over tibia	No oedema		
Skin texture	Very thin, gelatinous	Thin and smooth	Smooth: medium thickness Rash or superficial peeling	Slight thickening Superficial cracking and peeling, especially hands and feet	Thick and parchment-like superficial or deep cracking
Skin colour (infant not crying)	Dark red	Uniformly pink	Pale pink: variable over body	Pale Only pink over ears, lips, palms, or soles	

Skin opacity (trunk)	Numerous veins and venules clearly seen, especially over abdomen	Veins and tributaries seen	A few large vessels clearly seen over abdomen	A few large vessels seen indistinctly over abdomen	No blood vessels seen
Lanugo (over back)	No lanugo	Abundant long and thick over whole back	Hair thinning especially over lower back	Small amount of lanugo and bald areas	At least half of back devoid of lanugo
Plantar creases	No skin creases	Faint red marks over anterior half of sole	Definite red marks over more than anterior half, indentations over less than anterior third	Indentations over more than anterior third	Definite deep indentations over more than anterior third
Nipple formation	Nipple barely visible, no areola	Nipple well defined, areola smooth and flat diameter <0.75cm	Areola stippled, edge not raised, diameter <0.75cm	Areola stippled, edge raised diameter >0.75cm	
Breast size	No breast tissue palpable	Breast tissue on one or both sides <0.5cm diameter	Breast tissue both sides, one or both 0.5-1.0cm	Breast tissue both sides; one or both >1cm	

Paediatrics

Assessment of gestational age: Dubowitz system (continued)

Physical (external) criteria (for neurological criteria, see p228)

External sign	Score				
	0	1	2	3	4
Ear form	Pinna flat and shapeless, little or no incurving of edge	Incurving of part of edge of pinna	Partial incurving whole of upper pinna	Well-defined incurving whole of upper pinna	
Ear firmness	Pinna soft, easily folded, no recoil	Pinna, soft, easily folded, slow recoil places, ready recoil	Cartilage to edge of pinna, but soft in places, ready recoil	Pinna firm, cartilage to edge, instant recoil	
Genitalia • Male	Neither testis in scrotum	At least one testis high in scrotum	At least one testis right down		
• Female (with hips half abducted)	Labia majora widely separated, labia minora protruding	Labia majora almost cover labia minora	Labia majora completely cover labia minora		

Reproduced from Dubowitz, L. 'Assessment of gestational age: a practical scoring system' *Archives of Disease in Childhood* with permission from BMJ Publishing Ltd.

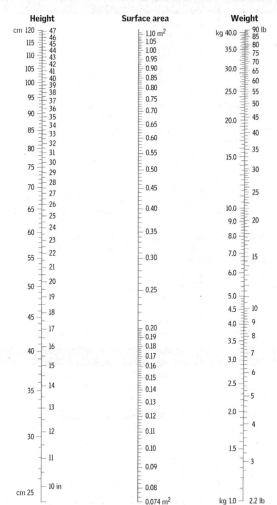

Fig 3. Nomogram for calculating the body surface area of children.

Reproduced from Dubowitz, L. 'Assessment of gestational age: a practical scoring system' *Archives of Disease in Childhood* with permission from BMJ Publishing Ltd.

Water See p235. An intake of 180mL/kg/day (range 150-200mL/kg/day) of human or formula milk meets the water needs of very low birthweight infants (VLBW; <1500g) under normal circumstances. In infants with heart failure water restriction is necessary (eg 130mL/kg/day).

Energy 130kcal/kg/day (range 110-165) meets the needs of the LBW infant in normal circumstances, and can be provided by formulas with similar energy density to human milk (65-70kcal/dL) in a volume of 180-200mL/kg/day. If a higher energy density is required keep it <85kcal/dL. The problems with energy densities above this are fat lactobezoars and U&E imbalance.

Protein Aim for between 2.25g/100kcal (2.9g/kg/day when fed at 130kcal/kg) and 3.1g/100kcal (4g/kg/day). Lysine should be as high as possible. Precise guidelines on taurine and whey:casein ratios cannot be given. At present LBW formulas are whey-predominant. Signs of protein deficiency: ↓urea; ↓prealbumin.

Fat Aim for 4.7-9g/kg (fat density 3.6-7.0g/100kcal). Longer-chain unsaturated fatty acids (>C12) are better absorbed than saturated fatty acids. Aim to have ≥4.5% of total calories as the essential fatty acid linoleic acid (500mg/100kcal).[793]

Carbohydrates Aim for 7-14g/100kcal, eg with lactose contributing 3.2-12g per 100kcal. Lactose is not essential; substitutes are glucose (but high osmolality may cause diarrhoea) or sucrose (± starch hydrolysates, eg corn syrup oils).

Vitamins See p123 & ESPGAN committee.[794]

Elements Na⁺: 6.5-15mmol/L. K⁺: 15-25.5mmol/L. Ca²⁺ 1.75-3.5mmol per 100kcal. PO₄³⁻: 1.6-2.9mmol/100kcal. Ca²⁺:PO₄³⁻ ratio: 1.4-2.0 : 1. Magnesium: 0.25-0.5mmol/ 100kcal. Iron: if breastfed, give 2-2.5mg Fe/kg/day (recommended total intake). Formula-fed infants may need a supplement to achieve this. Iodine: 10-45μg/100kcal. Manganese: 2.1μmol/100kcal. ►1cal=4.18 joules.

Fluid regimens to correct dehydration[APLS]

If tolerated, always use oral rehydration. Dioralyte® comes in sachets which contain glucose, Na⁺ and K⁺. Show mother how to make it up (water is the vital ingredient!). If breastfeeding, continue.

Daily IV water, Na, and K (mmol/kg/day) MAINTENANCE needs				
Age (yr)	Weight (kg)	Water (mL/kg/day)	Na⁺	K⁺
<0.5	<5	150	3	3
0.5-1	5-10	120	2.5	2.5
1-3	10-15	100	2.5	2.5
3-5	15-20	80	2	2
>5	>20	45-75	1.5-2	1.5-2

Use 0.45% saline with 5% glucose for these needs (contains few calories, but prevents ketosis). 0.9% saline is used for many conditions at risk from hyponatraemia (see NICE guidance). Pre-existing deficits and continuing loss must also be made good. Reliable input-output fluid balance charts are essential.

Calculating pre-existing deficit mL≈%dehydration×weight (kg)×10; give eg as 0.45% saline over 24h (eg 750mL for a 10kg child who is 7.5% dehydrated). Add in K⁺ (20mmol/500mL) once the child has passed urine. Don't forget the maintenance fluids for ongoing losses.

Estimating dehydration *Mild dehydration:* Decreased urine output.
5% dehydration: Dry mucous membranes; decreased urine output.
10% dehydration: The above + sunken fontanelle (but if crying, pressure↑), pulse↑; hoarse cry; skin turgor↓. *>10%:* The above, but worse, with: shock, drowsiness, and hypotension. If a recent weight is known, this is useful in quantifying dehydration. *Fluids for the first 24h in mild dehydration* This is best managed at home. Encourage parents to give little and often (ie 5mL every 5min by syringe). The patient will not need treatment until they are more dehydrated.

IV fluids for the first 24h in 5-10% dehydration
- Give maintenance water requirement (above) + the deficit over 24 hours. The most physiological method is Dioralyte® by NG tube, if tolerated. Some patients manage on oral fluids only. 'Rapid rehydration' involves 4 hours of 10mL/kg/h 0.9% NaCl then maintenance after if needed. Ensure the nurses are aware to drop the fluid rate after 4h, and change to 0.45%/5% glucose.
- Measure or estimate and replace ongoing losses (eg from the bowel).
- Monitor U&E on admission, and at least daily.

▸▸IV **fluid replacement in the first 24h in >10% dehydration** NB: Fluids should be given orally if possible—or by nasogastric tube, as above. Reserve IVI for those who are shocked (if IV access fails, use the intraosseous route, p236) or who do not tolerate NG rehydration.
- 0.9% saline 20mL/kg IVI bolus, while calculations are performed. Continuously monitor pulse, BP, ECG.
- Continue with boluses until the signs of shock ease.
- Then give the daily requirement + fluid deficit as above, making good continuing loss with 0.45% or 0.9% saline depending on type of dehydration.
- Measure plasma and urine creatinine and osmolality (p176), and plasma bicarbonate. Metabolic acidosis usually corrects itself.

Guidelines for success: Above all *be simple.* Complex regimens cause errors.
1 Stay at the bedside; use clinical state + lab results to adapt IVI.
2 Beware sudden changes in Na⁺ (↑ or ↓); may cause seizures or central pontine demyelinolysis.
3 Beware hidden loss (oedema, ascites, GI pools), and shifts of fluid from the intravascular space to the interstitial space ('third-spacing').
4 Measure U&E and urine electrolytes often.
5 Give potassium once you know that urine is flowing. The ready-prepared fluid '0.45% Saline With 5% glucose With Potassium Chloride 20mmol/L' is usually a good choice. Be guided by serum K⁺.[795]

Hypernatraemic dehydration: (greater water loss than salt, eg from wrongly made feeds, or rarely, if breastfed.) It causes intracellular dehydration (± fits, CNS thrombosis/haemorrhages on MRI).[796] Treatment: rehydrate slowly with 0.45% or 0.9% saline (which is hypotonic for a hypernatraemic patient): replace deficit over 48h, lowering Na⁺ by <12mmol/L/24h, and giving only 60% of maintenance volume, to avoid CNS oedema (p200). A big danger is too rapid rehydration. Hyperglycaemia is common, but self-correcting.[797,798]

Water balance in the preterm infant Water comprises 50-70% of weight gain (eg of 15g/day) in preterm babies. *Insensible water loss* (IWL) falls with increasing body weight, gestational age, and postnatal age; it increases with ↑T° (ambient & body) and low humidity. In a single-walled, thermoneutral incubator with a humidity of 50-80% IWL ≈30-60mL/kg/day (may double in infants on phototherapy under a radiant heater). *Faecal water loss* ≈5-10mL/kg/day (except during diarrhoea). *Urine loss:* If ~90mL/kg/day, there is no excessive renal stress.

Paediatrics

(APLS=advanced paediatric life support.)
Immediate vascular access is required in paediatric and neonatal practice in the following circumstances: cardiopulmonary arrest, severe burns, prolonged status epilepticus, hypovolaemic and septic shock. In many cases rapid intravenous access is not easily obtained. Intraosseous (IO) infusion is a rapid, safe, easy, and effective means of obtaining vascular access, and is recommended for life-threatening paediatric emergencies in which IV access cannot be obtained.[799] In such an emergency attempt an IV line but if unsuccessful within 60–90s, attempt an IO line. It is safe to administer all intravenous medicines via the IO. Bloods can be taken and sent to the lab for cross match, FBC, U&E.[800] Inform the haematology lab they will see blasts. A blood gas can be sent (if no fluids given already)—but it shouldn't be used on an autoanalyser as it may clog the machine. Send it to the lab and inform them that it is a marrow sample—they may be able to test it in a cartridge analyser.[800]

Contraindications Osteoporosis, osteogenesis imperfecta, and infection or fracture at the site of insertion.

Technical aspects *Learn from an expert.* The major choice is between a manual needle or a semi-automatic device such as an intraosseous gun or drill. The two major devices available are the Bone Injection Gun® (B.I.G.®)—a spring loaded device available for children and adults, and the EZ-IO ® device a reusable drill with a 15mm needle for children <39kg, and a 25mm needle for patients >40kg. A new 45mm needle is available for those with significant tissue/oedema overlying the site of injection. The EZ-IO may be faster than both manual needles and the B.I.G. and easier to place 1st time.[801]

Preparation Set trolley: Dressing pack, povidone iodine, needles, 10mL syringe, lidocaine (=lignocaine) 1% (5mL), scalpel, intraosseous needle, paediatric infusion set, 10mL 0.9% saline, adhesive tape.

Choosing the site of insertion The proximal tibia is the best site. Other sites are the proximal humerus, distal femur or distal tibia. Choose a point on the flat anteromedial surface of the tibia, 1-2 cm medial to and 1-2cm below the tibial tuberosity. The child's leg should be restrained, with a small support placed behind the knee.

Procedure
• Sterilize the skin with antiseptic, infiltrate with lidocaine as necessary. (Puncturing the skin with the scalpel is not usually necessary.)
• Insert the intraosseous needle at an angle of 90° to the skin; advance with a boring or screwing motion into the marrow cavity. Correct location of the needle is signified by a decrease in resistance on entering the marrow cavity.
• Stabilize the needle and verify the position by aspirating marrow, or by the easy flushing of 5-10mL of 0.9% saline, without any infiltration of surrounding tissue. The needle should stand upright without support, but should be secured with tape.
• Take samples for culture, U&E, FBC, group & save!
• Connect to IV infusion via an extension: better flow rates are often got by syringing in fluid boluses (standard bolus is 20mL/kg of crystalloid or colloid).

Complications (Infrequent) There may be extravasation of fluid, or cellulitis, fractures, osteomyelitis, pain, and fat or bone microemboli. These are more common with prolonged use—so intraosseous infusion should be discontinued as soon as conventional IV access is attained (should be within 24h).

NB: Intraosseous delivery may also be used in adults.[802] The position on the tibia in adults is 2cm medial to tibial tuberosity and 1cm above it (as opposed to below it in children).

▸▸ Never blame yourself for forgetting anything, except your humanity (and the dose of adrenaline).

▸▸ Call the resuscitation/cardiac arrest team (paramedics if in the community).

▸▸ Ideally place patient on back with legs raised. If they have significant respiratory distress allow the patient to put themselves in a position of comfort. Do not let them stand or sit up rapidly. If comatose, use left-lateral position (to prevent caval compression).

▸▸ ABCDE: Airway (any swelling, hoarseness, stridor?); breathing (rate↑, wheeze, fatigue, cyanosis, S_pO_2 <92%?); circulation (pale, clammy, BP↓, faints?); disability (conscious level, eg drowsy/coma?); exposure of skin (erythema/urticaria?).

▸▸ *The chief drug priority is adrenaline.* Give intra-muscularly (IM). Use a suitable syringe for measuring small volumes; absolute accuracy isn't essential.[803] Note strength! (1 : 1000 not 1 : 10,000.)

IM dose of 3 drugs:	Adrenaline 1:1000	Chlorphenamine	Hydrocortisone
If aged <6 months	0.15mL (150µg)[13]	25µg/kg	25mg
If aged 6 months–6yrs	0.15mL (150µg)	2.5mg	50mg
Dose if aged 6–12yrs	0.3mL (300µg)	5mg	100mg
Adolescent/adult dose	0.5mL (500µg)	10mg	200mg

▸▸ Repeat adrenaline dose after 5min if no improvement. Also: **high-flow O₂** (±IPPV) & **crystalloid** (20mL/kg IVI). *NB:* weight (kg)≈2(age in yrs+4). OK if 1–10yrs old.

▸▸ Remove the trigger, eg bee sting; turn off any drug or colloid IVI.

• *IV route:* This can be used for **hydrocortisone** and **chlorphenamine**, although there is little evidence these help much. Steroids are unlikely to be harmful, but antihistamines may worsen hypotension and cause somnolence which can cloud the picture with regards to the CNS effects of anaphylaxis so wait until initial resuscitation is complete prior to giving these. Don't use the IV route for adrenaline (unless on ITU with experienced user; special doses apply).

• *If bronchospasm is a feature:* give **salbutamol** 2.5mg nebulized too.

• *Continuously monitor:* pulse, BP, S_pO_2, and ECG. If cardiac arrest, start CPR.

• *Differential diagnosis:* asthma; septic shock; breath-holding or panic attack.

• *After the emergency:* if reaction is due to a drug, idiopathic or due to an envenomation, take blood as soon as possible after symptoms start; ideally 1–2h, but definitely within 4h for mast cell tryptase (>0.5mL in LFT bottle, ask lab to freeze); admit as an in-patient; refer to an allergist. Self-use of pre-loaded pen injectors may be needed (after training).[804] **EpiPen®** has 0.3mg of adrenaline (1:1000). This is suitable if weight >30kg. If 15–30kg, use Anapen Junior® or EpiPen Junior®, which both contain 0.15mg of adrenaline. Epipen Junior® (1:2000) delivers 0.15mg of adrenaline (1.7mL remains after using the autoinjector). It is suitable for a 15kg child (~4yrs).

Paediatrics

This algorithm assumes no equipment and that only 1 professional rescuer is present. Remove yourself and the child from danger. Phone for help at once.

How to give the rescue breaths *to a child:* Ensure head tilt and chin lift. Pinch the soft part of his nose. Open his mouth a little, but maintain chin up. Take a breath, and place your lips around his mouth (good seal). Blow steadily into his mouth over 1–1.5sec. Does his chest rise? Take your mouth away, and watch for the chest to fall. Take another breath, and repeat this sequence up to 5 times. *To an infant:* Do as above, but cover the nasal apertures and the mouth with your lips. The head should be in the neutral position. If the chest does not move, respiratory obstruction may exist ▶▶move on to 'Removing foreign body' sequence for obstructed airway—ie:

• If coughing, encourage to cough. Once unconscious or an ineffective cough:
• Remove any obvious obstructions. Recheck that there is adequate head tilt and chin lift, but do not overextend the neck.
• Do up to 5 back blows between the scapulae to dislodge hidden obstructions (hold on your lap whilst seated, positioning the head lower than chest).
• If this fails, do 5 chest thrusts: turn to supine; over 12sec, give 5 sternal thrusts (same position as for compressions, but be sharper and more vigorous). Remove any foreign bodies which have become visible.
• Tilt head upwards; lift chin to reopen the airway, and assess breathing.
• If not breathing; do 5 more rescue breaths: does the chest move now?
• If not, for a child >1 year, give 5 abdominal thrusts (directed towards diaphragm); use the upright position if the child is conscious; supine if not.
• Repeat these sequences until breathing is OK, alternating chest and abdominal thrusts. *Do not give abdominal thrusts to infants (risk of internal injury).*

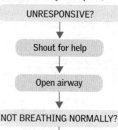

Paediatric Basic Life Support
(Healthcare professionals
with a duty to respond)

UNRESPONSIVE?

Shout for help

Open airway

NOT BREATHING NORMALLY?

5 rescue breaths

NO SIGNS OF LIFE?

15 chest compressions

2 rescue breaths
15 compressions

Call the resuscitation team

Fig 1. Paediatric basic life-support, applicable only to healthcare professionals with a duty to respond.
©Resuscitation Council UK
www.resus.org.uk

When breathing place in the recovery position—as near to the true lateral position as possible, with mouth dependent to aid draining of secretions. The position must be stable (eg use pillows placed behind back). The degree of movement is determined by risk of spinal injury.

How to give chest compressions: Compress lower half of sternum to ⅓ of the chest's depth; use the heel of one hand (or, in babies, with both your thumbs, with your hands encircling the thorax) If >8yrs, the adult 2-handed method is OK. For an infant, 2 fingers are sufficient, in the middle of a line joining the nipples. Perform resuscitation for ~1min before going for help. Remove the cause, if possible. Causes are: drowning; pulmonary embolism; trauma; electrocution; shock; hypoxia; hypercapnia; hypothermia; U&E imbalance; drugs/toxins, eg adrenaline (= epinephrine), digoxin, and blue-ringed octopi.[806]

Paediatrics

Neonates: see p107

Paediatrics

Paediatric Advanced Life Support

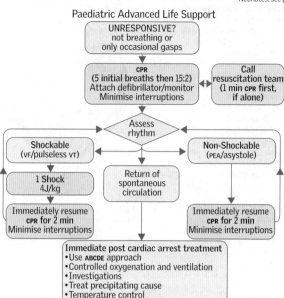

UNRESPONSIVE?
not breathing or
only occasional gasps

CPR
(5 initial breaths then 15:2)
Attach defibrillator/monitor
Minimise interruptions

Call
resuscitation team
(1 min CPR first,
if alone)

Assess
rhythm

Shockable
(VF/pulseless VT)

Non-Shockable
(PEA/asystole)

1 Shock
4J/kg

Return of
spontaneous
circulation

Immediately resume
CPR for 2 min
Minimise interruptions

Immediately resume
CPR for 2 min
Minimise interruptions

Immediate post cardiac arrest treatment
• Use ABCDE approach
• Controlled oxygenation and ventilation
• Investigations
• Treat precipitating cause
• Temperature control
• Therapeutic hypothermia?

During CPR
• Ensure high-quality CPR: rate, depth, recoil
• Plan actions before interrupting CPR
• Give oxygen
• Vascular access (intravenous, intraosseous)
• Give adrenaline every 3–5 min
• Consider advanced airway and capnography
• Continuous chest compressions when advanced airway in place
• Correct reversible causes

Reversible Causes
• Hypoxia
• Hypovolaemia
• Hypo-/hyperkalaemia/metabolic
• Hypothermia
• Tension pneumothorax
• Toxins
• Tamponade – cardiac
• Thromboembolism

Fig 1. Paediatric advanced life-support.   Resuscitation Council UK, © 2010.

Order of assessment and intervention for any seriously ill or injured child follows the ABCDE principles: Airway (AC for airway and cervical spine stabilization for the injured child); Breathing; Circulation (with haemorrhage control in injured child); Disability (level of consciousness and neurological status); Exposure to ensure full examination (while respecting dignity and temperature conservation). *Note:* 15:2 means 15 compressions (rate=100–120/min) to 2 ventilations.

In shockable VF/VT: ►►Give adrenaline (epinephrine) 10µg/kg IV/IO + amiodarone 5mg/kg IV over 3min after the 3rd shock, once compressions resumed. ►►Repeat adrenaline on alternate cycles until spontaneous circulation returns. ►►After 5th shock, give a last dose of amiodarone if still in a shockable rhythm. ►►Continue shocks every 2min, and continue compressions during defibrillator chargings.

Non-shockable rhythm: ►►Give adrenaline as soon as you have IV/IO access.

1 AED = Automated external defibrillator. IO = intraosseous (p236). PEA = Pulseless electrical activity.

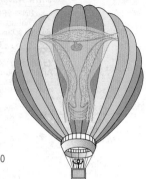

Fig 1. Caleb Parry (see OPPOSITE) is seen here unwisely mixing work and leisure: note the pedunculated fibroid within his balloon which, like his bedside manner, was made of varnished silk.[1]

We thank Ms Alison Peattie, our Specialist Reader, and Pooja Sakar, our Junior Reader, for their contribution to this chapter.

A holistic approach to gynaecology: Parry's dictum

'It is more important to know what sort of patient has the disease than what kind of disease the patient has.'

Caleb Parry (1755–1822; fig 2) was a doctor in Bath who was fascinated by events in his patients' lives, and their connection with their diseases, some of which he described for the first time. These early descriptions are notable for their effortless intertwining of psychological and physical phenomena.[1,2]

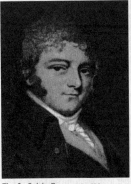

All this suggests a serious, one-sided doctor, but this is wrong. To get away from it all, he became a keen balloonist, lending ideas and materials to Edward Jenner, who dedicated his magnum opus on smallpox to him. From the Royal Crescent in Bath, he launched his great hydrogen balloon (see OPPOSITE).

His aphorism is particularly relevant to this chapter because many of its diseases are chronic, and the choices of treatment are many. Take endometriosis (p288), for example. If an examiner were to ask you 'what is the treatment for endometriosis'—you might well look at him thoughtfully, before replying that it all depends on who has got

Fig 2. Caleb Parry, MD FRS, was a Welshman who chose to peruse his medical studies at Edinburgh as the lectures there, by William Cullen, were given in English, not Latin (for the most part, the current edition of OHCS follows Cullen's practice).

Caleb Hillier Parry (1755–1822).
The James Lind Library.
© Roger Rolls, by kind permission.

it—where they are in their lives, how much the pain matters, what the plans are for future pregnancies, how these plans may be ambiguous and change, according to work, relationships, and the onset of friendships. What does the patient feel about long-term medication with agents that can change her sexuality, and hence the person who is suffering the disease? Some may tolerate doctor-induced hypoestrogenism (flushes, decreased libido, loss of bone density) thinking the price well worth paying for relief of endometriosis symptoms; others will take the opposite view; in a few, their ability to take a decision will be influenced by the drugs they are already taking.[3]

Sometimes rational choice is the hardest thing "How can you expect me to make a rational choice until you sort out these dreadful periods of mine: I cannot even think..."[4]

Be optimistic; discourage passive dependency; let the patient set the agenda. ►take time ►understand your patient ►offer all options, *then let her choose*.

Gynaecology

Let the patient do the driving.

History Let her tell the story. Note down her exact words. She may be reluctant to admit some problems, particularly if you are a man, so make sure you cover them in your questions. A frustration for the medical student is that the story you are told is different to the one elicited by the consultant or the GP. But sometimes the first telling is the most valid. ►It is also true that none of us (doctors and patients) can tell the same story twice.[1]

1 *Menstrual history:* ►Date of last menstrual period (LMP; 1ˢᵗ day of bleeding) or menopause. Was the last period normal? Cycles: number of days bleeding/number of days from day 1 of one period to day 1 of next (eg 5/26). Are they regular? If heavy, are there clots or floods? How many pads/tampons are needed (an unreliable guide)? Are periods painful? Is bleeding intermenstrual (IMB), postcoital (PCB) or postmenopausal (PMB)? Age at menarche?

2 *Obstetric history:* How many children? For each pregnancy: antenatal problems, delivery, gestation, outcome; weights of babies; puerperium? Terminations/miscarriages—at *what* stage, *why*, and (terminations) *how*?

3 *Symptoms:* If she has *pain* what is it like? Uterine pain may be colicky and felt in the sacrum and groins. Ovarian pain tends to be felt in the *iliac fossa* and radiates down front of the thigh to the knee. Ask about *dyspareunia* (painful intercourse). Is it superficial (at the entrance) or deep inside? If she has *vaginal discharge* what is it like (amount, colour, smell, itch)? When does she get it? Ask about *prolapse* and *incontinence*. When? How bad? Worse whilst standing? Ask about bowel symptoms (irritable bowel can cause pelvic pain), and faecal incontinence.

4 *Sex and contraception:* Is she sexually active? Are there physical or emotional problems with sex? What contraception is she using and is she happy with it? What has she tried previously? Has she had problems conceiving? If so, has she had treatment for subfertility? What about sexually transmitted infections? Date and result of last cervical smear?

5 *Other:* General health, smoking. Previous gynaecological treatment.

Examination ►Many women find pelvic examination painful, undignified, and embarrassing, especially if you are male. Explain what you are going to do. Be gentle. Use a chaperone. Royal Colleges and the General Medical Council (UK) recommend chaperones for all intimate examinations; use is increasing but not universal in general practice; training is needed, and they need to be friendly.[5]

General: Is she well or ill? Is she shocked? If so, treat it.

Abdomen: Palpate for tenderness and peritonism. If there is a mass, could it be a pregnancy? Listen for a fetal heart (p40).

Vaginal examination: (p246). Use your eyes to inspect the vulva, a *speculum* to examine the vagina and cervix and your *fingers* to assess the uterus and adnexae bimanually. Examination is usually done with the patient on her back or in the left lateral position (best for detecting prolapse). *Sims' speculum* has 2 right-angle bends, and is used for inspecting the vaginal walls, eg for prolapse and incontinence.

Cusco's (bivalve) speculum is used for inspecting the cervix with the aid of a light. Warm under the tap (unless it's plastic). Lubricate with jelly. Insert closed, with blades parallel to the labia, usually up to the hilt. When it is in, rotate it and open it and usually the cervix pops into view. If it does not, do a bimanual to check the position of the cervix, and try again. Do swabs (p284) and a cervical smear (p270) if needed. Close the speculum gradually, under direct vision, as you withdraw it, to avoid trapping the cervix.

---

1 The first telling awakes memories which colour or transform the next telling, which itself influences the next telling in an infinite regression in which one telling becomes the audience for the next.

Sexual health is the enjoyment of sexual activity of one's choice, without causing or suffering physical or mental harm.[6] Of course there is more to sex than enjoyment. 'Perhaps the sexual life is the great test. If we can survive it with charity to those we love, and affection to those we have betrayed, we needn't worry so much about the good and the bad in us. But jealousy, distrust, cruelty, revenge, recrimination... then we fail. The wrong is in that failure even if we are the victims and not the executioners. Virtue is no excuse...'

Graham Greene, *The Comedians*

Once one understands that human sexuality is infinitely complex, it is easier to appreciate statistics such as 'sexual dysfunction is a big health problem, affecting 43% of women and 31% of men'.[7]

Enemies of sexual health include:

• Disharmony in personal relationships, or simply *too many* relationships.
• Pain, or any medical or gynaecological condition.
• Anxiety (whether or not related to fear of failure); depression; fatigue.
• Drugs (eg tamoxifen; the Pill; cyproterone; antidepressants; narcotics).
• A multiplicity of irreconcilable roles (if your patient is trying to achieve ascendancy in her work, as well as being chief shopper, cook, housewife, mother, and friend, then the role of lover may be eclipsed—all the more if she also finds herself in the role of being chief person to blame if things go wrong—if the fridge is empty, if the money runs out, if the children do not get to school on time, or if her partner loses his job).
• Myths about sexual performance (eg that all physical contact must lead to sex, that sex equals intercourse, and that sexual relations should come naturally and easily).[8]

Gynaecology

The vulva comprises the entrances to the vagina and urethra, the structures which surround them (clitoris, labia minora, and fourchette), and the encircling labia majora and perineum. The hymen, when broken (by tampons or intercourse) leaves tags at the mouth of the vagina (*carunculae myrtiformes*).

Look for: Rashes; atrophy; ulcers; lumps (p266 & p268); deficient perineum (you can see the back wall of the vagina); incontinence.

The vagina is a potential space with distensible folded muscular walls. The contents of the rectum, which runs behind the posterior wall, are palpable through the vagina. The cervix projects into the vault at the top which forms a moat around it, deepest posteriorly, conventionally divided into anterior, posterior, and 2 lateral fornices. From puberty until the menopause lactobacilli in the vagina keep it acidic (pH 3.8–4.4), discouraging infection.

Look for: Inflammation; discharge (p284); prolapse (p290).

The cervix is mostly connective tissue. It feels firm, and has a dent in the centre (the opening, or os, of the cervical canal). Mucin-secreting glands of the endocervix lubricate the vagina. The os is circular in nulliparous women, but is a slit in the parous.

Look for: Pain on moving the cervix (excitation—p262 & p286); ectopy; cervicitis and discharge; polyps, carcinoma (p272).

The uterus has a thick muscular-walled *body* lined internally with columnar epithelium (the endometrium) connected to the cervix or neck. It is supported by the uterosacral ligaments. The peritoneum is draped over the uterus. The valley so formed between it and the rectum is the rectovaginal pouch (of Douglas), and the fold of peritoneum in which the Fallopian tubes lie is known as the broad ligament. The *size* of the uterus is by convention described by comparison with its size at different stages of pregnancy. Since that is variable, estimates are approximate, but the following is a guide: non-pregnant—plum-sized; 6 weeks—egg; 8 weeks—small orange; 10 weeks—large orange; 14 weeks—fills pelvis.

In most women the uterus is *anteverted*, ie its long axis is directed forward and the cervix points backwards. The body then flops forwards on the cervix—*anteflexed*. An anteverted uterus can be palpated between the hands on bimanual examination (unless she is obese, or tense, or the bladder is full).

In 20% it is retroverted and retroflexed (p246).

Look for: Position (important to know for practical procedures); mobility (especially if retroverted); size; tenderness (p262 & p286).

Adnexae These are the *Fallopian tubes, ovaries,* and associated connective tissue (parametria). They are palpated bimanually in the lateral fornices, and if normal may not be felt. The ovaries are the size of a large grape and may lie in the rectovaginal pouch.

Look for: Masses (p280) and tenderness (p286).

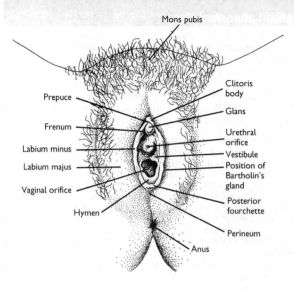

Fig 1. Gynaecological anatomy.

Vagina and uterus These are derived from the Müllerian duct system and formed by fusion of the right and left parts. Different degrees of failure to fuse lead to duplication of any or all parts of the system.

Vaginal septae are quite common (and often missed on examination).

Duplication of the cervix and/or uterus may also be missed, eg until the woman becomes pregnant in the uterus without the IUCD!

A partially divided (*bicornuate*) uterus or a uterus where one side has failed to develop (*unicornuate*) may present as recurrent miscarriage, particularly in the second trimester, or as difficulties in labour. Such abnormalities are diagnosed by *hysterosalpingogram*.

An absent uterus or a rudimentary uterus with absent endometrium is rare. They present with primary amenorrhoea.

An absent or short vagina is uncommon but can be corrected by plastic surgery. The membrane at the mouth of the vagina where the Müllerian and urogenital systems fuse (the hymen) may be imperforate. There is apparent primary amenorrhoea, with a history of monthly abdominal pain and swelling, and the membrane bulging under the pressure of dammed up menstrual blood (haematocolpos). It is relieved by a cruciate incision in the membrane. NB: in some communities, female 'circumcision' (p247) is still practised, and this is another cause of haematocolpos.

▶Renal system abnormalities often coexist with genital ones, so IVU and ultrasound should be performed.

Ovary Thin, rudimentary 'streak' ovaries are found in Turner's syndrome (p655). Ovaries are absent in testicular feminization syndrome, but primitive testes are present (p134). Remnants of developmental tissue (eg the Wolffian system) may result in cysts around the ovary and in the broad ligament.

Uterine retroversion

About 20% of women normally have a retroverted retroflexed uterus which is fully mobile. It is difficult to palpate bimanually unless you can push it into anteversion by pressure on the cervix. It causes no problems except (rarely) if it fails to lift out of the pelvis at 12 weeks of pregnancy, presenting with discomfort and retention of urine, eg at 14 weeks; catheterization and lying prone may relieve it.

Inflammation in the pelvis (due to infection or endometriosis) can cause adhesions which tether the uterus in a retroverted position. The patient may present with dysmenorrhoea, dyspareunia, or subfertility—problems which can only be relieved by treatment of the underlying disease.

Circumcision is a misnomer, as it implies a parallel with male circumcision, which is incorrect. Another term is female genital cutting/mutilation (affected women prefer the term genital cutting). 140 million women are believed to be affected (2 million/year). The female 'operation' is carried out later (at 5-7yrs) and may be much more damaging and extensive, eg as practised in Somalia. In the UK most affected women come from Somalia, Kenya, Eritrea, Ethiopia and the Yemen. It is common in Mali, Guinea and Egypt. Procedures include clitoridectomy ± infundibulation (removal of the clitoris, labia minora and labia majora, with oversewing or apposition by thorns). Even the milder Sunna entails removal of part of the clitoris, and more may be removed than intended. At betrothal, an attendant cuts the scar tissue to allow intercourse. Long-term problems include very slow urination, urinary tract infections, haematocolpos, dyspareunia or non-consummation, obstructed labour, increased susceptibility to HIV and other blood-borne diseases as well as emotional trauma. Social expectations are changing in countries that practice 'cutting' but parents believe the social harm of not cutting is greater than the physical, psychological and legal risk of 'cutting'.[10]

Defibulation may be performed before marriage; ideally electively at 20 weeks' gestation, or in the 1st stage of labour. If not corrected antenatally deliver in a unit with emergency obstetric care, having planned labour after expert advice. If vaginal examination is poorly tolerated, or anterior episiotomy anticipated, offer epidural. Only extreme anatomical distortion making defibulation impossible is an indication for caesarean section (but note that NICE guidelines 2011 allow for more patient choice).[11] Repair post-delivery should appose raw edges and control bleeding but must not result in a vaginal opening making intercourse difficult or impossible.[12] In 2003–5 female genital cutting affected 1.4% of UK maternities and was implicated in 4 maternal deaths.[9]

Labial cosmetic surgery is becoming more common in affluent countries and is comparable with more minor types of cutting, thereby posing ethical concerns.[13]

Gynaecology

Puberty is the development of adult sexual characteristics. The sequence: breast buds→growth of pubic hair→axillary hair→menses begin (**menarche**) from ~10yrs onwards (mean ~13yrs and falling—earlier if low birth weight; African; short & overweight in childhood; urban environment; various fascinating pheromone-related family events mediating anti-inbreeding strategies).[1][14]

Investigate if no periods by ~15yrs[15] (p250) or no signs of puberty by 14. A growth spurt (p184) is the 1st change in puberty and is usually completed 2yrs after menarche when the epiphyses fuse.

The menstrual cycle (fig 1). The cycle is controlled by the 'hypothalamic–pituitary–ovarian (HPO) axis'. Pulsatile production of gonadotrophin-releasing hormones by the hypothalamus stimulates the pituitary to produce the gonadotrophins: follicle-stimulating hormone (FSH) and luteinizing hormone (LH). These stimulate the ovary to produce oestrogen and progesterone. The ovarian hormones modulate the production of gonadotrophins by feeding back on the hypothalamus and pituitary.

Day 1 of the cycle is the first day of menstruation. Cycle lengths vary greatly (eg 20–45 days in adolescence); only 12% are 28 days. Cycles soon after menarche and before the menopause are most likely to be irregular and anovulatory. In the first 4 days of the cycle, FSH levels are high, stimulating the development of a primary follicle in the ovary. The follicle produces oestrogen, which stimulates the development of a glandular 'proliferative' endometrium and of cervical mucus which is receptive to sperm. The mucus becomes clear and stringy (like raw egg white) and if allowed to dry on a slide produces 'ferning patterns' due to its high salt content. Oestrogen also controls FSH and LH output by positive and negative feedback.

14 days before the onset of menstruation (on the 16th day of the cycle of a 30-day cycle) the oestrogen level becomes high enough to stimulate a surge of LH. This stimulates ovulation. Having released the ovum, the primary follicle then forms a corpus luteum and starts to produce progesterone. Under this influence, the endometrial lining is prepared for implantation: glands become convoluted ('secretory phase'). The cervical mucus becomes viscid and hostile to sperm and no longer ferns. If the ovum is not fertilized the corpus luteum breaks down, so hormone levels fall. This causes the spiral arteries in the uterine endothelial lining to constrict and the lining sloughs—hence menstruation.

Menstruation is the loss of blood and uterine epithelial slough; it lasts 2–7 days and is usually heaviest at the beginning. Normal loss is 20–80mL (median 28mL).

Climacteric The ovaries fail to develop follicles. Without hormonal feedback from the ovary, gonadotrophin levels rise. Periods cease (menopause), usually at ~50 years of age (p256).

Postponing menstruation (eg on holiday) Try norethisterone 5mg/8h PO from 3 days before the period is due until bleeding is acceptable, or take 2 packets of combined contraceptive Pills without a break.

Gynaecology

---

1 *The socioendocrinology of family life:* Presence in the household of the biological father *delays* sexual maturation—as does having a sister at home (esp. an elder sister). Brothers have no influence, but half- or step-brothers at home are associated with an *earlier* menarche. In addition, stressful life events such as immigration for adoption is associated with early menarche (risk of precocious puberty ↑×20, p184).

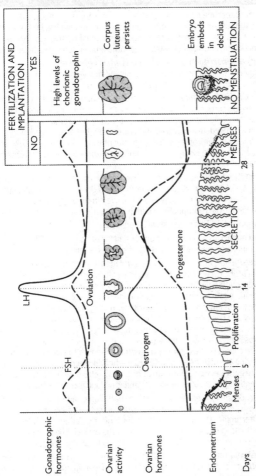

Fig 1. The menstrual cycle.

Primary amenorrhoea (see p251) This is failure to start menstruating. It needs investigation in a 15-year-old, or in a 14-year-old who has no breast development. For normal menstruation to occur she must be structurally normal with a functioning control mechanism (hypothalamic–pituitary–ovarian axis).

Secondary amenorrhoea (see p251) This is when periods stop for >6 months, other than due to pregnancy. Hypothalamic–pituitary–ovarian axis disorders are common, ovarian and endometrial causes are rare.

Ovarian insufficiency/failure This may be secondary to chemotherapy, radiotherapy or surgery. Many genetic disorders can cause ovarian follicle dysfunction or depletion-especially those affecting x chromosomes.[16] One X chromosome is needed for ovarian differentiation, but 2 are needed by oocytes. In Turner's syndrome (XO), oocyte apoptosis starts as 12 weeks and numbers deplete in the 1st 10yrs of life, mosaics 45X0/46XX may menstruate for several years after menarche.

Oligomenorrhoea This is infrequent periods. It is common at the extremes of reproductive life when regular ovulation often does not occur. Menstrual cycles in adolescents are typically <45 days, even in the 1st year.[17] A common cause throughout the reproductive years is polycystic ovary syndrome (p252).

Menorrhagia (p253) This is excessive blood loss.

Dysmenorrhoea This is painful periods (± nausea or vomiting). 50% of British women complain of moderate pain, 12% of severe disabling pain.

Primary dysmenorrhoea is pain without organ pathology—often starting with anovulatory cycles after the menarche. It is crampy with ache in the back or groin, worse during the first day or two. Excess prostaglandins cause painful uterine contractions, producing ischaemic pain. *R:* NSAIDs inhibit prostaglandins, eg **mefenamic acid** 500mg/8h PO during menstruation so reduce contractions and hence pain. No particular preparation seems superior.[18] **Paracetamol** is a good alternative to NSAIDs. In pain with ovulatory cycles, ovulation suppression with the **combined Pill** can help (thus dysmenorrhoea may be used as a covert request for contraception). Smooth muscle antispasmodics (eg **alverine** 60–120mg/8h PO) or **hyoscine butylbromide** (20mg/6h PO) give unreliable results. Cervical dilatation at birth may relieve it but surgical dilatation may render the cervix incompetent and is no longer used as therapy.

Secondary dysmenorrhoea: Associated pathology: adenomyosis (p288), endometriosis, chronic sepsis (eg chlamydial infection), fibroids—and so it appears later in life. It is more constant through the period, and may be associated with deep dyspareunia. Treatment of the cause is the best plan. IUCDs increase dysmenorrhoea, except the Mirena® which usually reduces it.

Intermenstrual bleeding This may follow a midcycle fall in oestrogen production. *Other causes:* Cervical polyps; ectropion; carcinoma; cervicitis/vaginitis; hormonal contraception (spotting); IUCD; chlamydia; pregnancy-related.

Postcoital bleeding *Causes:* Cervical trauma; polyps; cervical, endometrial and vaginal carcinoma; cervicitis and vaginitis of any cause. Screen for chlamydia and treat if positive. Refer all with persistent bleeding. Risk of cervical carcinoma in those with post-coital bleeding is 1 : 2400 aged 45–54; 1 : 44,000 aged 20–24.[19]

Postmenopausal bleeding This is bleeding occurring >1yr after the last period. It must be considered due to endometrial carcinoma until proved otherwise (p278). *Other causes:* Vaginitis (often atrophic); foreign bodies, eg pessaries; carcinoma of cervix or vulva; endometrial or cervical polyps; oestrogen withdrawal (hormone replacement therapy or ovarian tumour). She may confuse urethral, vaginal, and rectal bleeding.

▶ *Always ask yourself 'Could she be pregnant?'* See pregnancy tests (p6).

Primary amenorrhoea (see also p250). This may cause great anxiety. In most patients puberty is just late (often familial), and reassurance is all that is needed. In some, the cause is structural or genetic, so check:

- Has she got normal external secondary sexual characteristics? If so, are the internal genitalia normal (p246)?
- Causes can be the same as for secondary amenorrhoea: consider tests below.
- If she is not developing normally, examination and karyotyping may reveal Turner's syndrome (p655) or testicular feminization (p134). The aim of treatment is to help the patient to look normal, to function sexually, and, if possible, to enable her to reproduce if she wishes.

Causes of secondary amenorrhoea

- Hypothalamic–pituitary–ovarian causes are common (34% of cases) as control of the menstrual cycle is easily upset, eg by stress (emotions, exams), ↑exercise, weight loss. Up to 44% of competitive athletes have amenorrhoea.
- Hyperprolactinaemia (14%). (30% have galactorrhoea.) Other hormonal imbalances (hypo- or hyperthyroidism). Severe systemic disease, eg renal failure. Pituitary tumours and necrosis (Sheehan's syndrome) are rare.
- Ovarian causes: polycystic ovary syndrome (p252) is common (28%); tumours; ovarian insufficiency/failure (premature menopause: the cause in 12%, it affects ~1%[20] of women under 40 see p250).
- Uterine causes: pregnancy-related, Asherman's syndrome (uterine adhesions after a D&C: consider also TB, p274). 'Post-Pill amenorrhoea' is generally oligomenorrhoea/secondary amenorrhoea masked by regular withdrawal bleeds so, if need be, investigate as below.

Tests • βHCG (eg urinary) to exclude pregnancy. • Serum free androgen index (↑ in polycystic ovary syndrome). • FSH/LH (low if hypothalamic pituitary cause but may be normal if weight loss or excessive exercise the cause: raised eg FSH>20IU/L if premature menopause, in which case, if age <30 and concerns for future fertility, refer for karyotyping[21]). • Prolactin (↑by stress, hypothyroidism, prolactinomas and drugs, eg phenothiazines, domperidone, metoclopramide). If level >1000IU/L do MRI scan (p294). 40% of those with hyperprolactinaemia have a pituitary tumour. • TFT (4% of women with amenorrhoea have abnormal thyroid function). • Testosterone level: levels >5nmol/L may indicate androgen secreting tumour or late onset congenital adrenal hyperplasia so need more investigation, eg dehydroepiandrosterone sulfate level.

Treatment is related to cause. Premature ovarian failure cannot be reversed but hormone replacement (p256) is necessary to control symptoms of oestrogen deficiency and protect against osteoporosis. Pregnancy can be achieved with oocyte donation and *in vitro* fertilization techniques.

Hypothalamic–pituitary axis malfunction: If mild (eg stress, moderate weight loss) there is sufficient activity to stimulate enough ovarian oestrogen to produce an endometrium (which will be shed after a progesterone challenge, eg **medroxyprogesterone acetate** 10 mg/24h for 10 days),[22] but the timing is disordered so cycles are not initiated. If the disorder is more severe the axis shuts down (eg in severe weight loss). FSH and LH and hence oestrogen levels are low. Reassurance and advice on diet or stress management, or psychiatric help if appropriate (p348), and time may solve the problem. She should be advised to use contraception as ovulation may occur at any time. If she wants fertility restored now, or the reassurance of seeing a period, mild dysfunction will respond to **clomifene** but a shut-down axis will need stimulation by gonadotrophin-releasing hormone (see p294 for both).

Gynaecology

This would be better named polyfollicular ovary syndrome. It comprises hyperandrogenism, oligo-ovulation, and polycystic ovaries on ultrasound in the absence of other causes of polycystic ovaries, eg as seen with later onset adrenal hyperplasia and Cushing's. The cause is unknown. It is common (5–20% of premenopausal women). Acne, male pattern baldness and hirsutism can all be features. Darkened skin (acanthosis nigricans) on neck and skin flexures may reflect hyperinsulinaemia. LH is raised in 40%, testosterone in 30%. Subfertility may be a problem. The result appears to be a vicious circle of ovarian, hypothalamic– and adrenal dysfunction.

Insulin resistance and hyperinsulinaemia are features. There may be diabetes (40% have impaired glucose tolerance or diabetes by age 40: all are at risk, but if obese, especially so). During pregnancy do GTT by 20 weeks.[RCOG] Insulin resistance/metabolic syndrome is likely to be a problem in those with obesity—eg waist >80cm (p530)[24] + any 2 of: triglycerides >1.7mmol/L; HDL cholesterol <1.1mmol/L; BP >130/85; fasting glucose >5.6mmol/L. MI, stroke and transient ischaemic attack rate is↑ (eg ×3).

Hypertension may also be a problem. Hormonal cycling is disrupted, ovaries become enlarged by unruptured follicles, the endometrium hyperplastic. Ovarian and endometrial cancer risks are increased.

Stein–Leventhal syndrome eponymizes the subset of obese hirsute women with polycystic ovaries.

Diagnosis: Exclude thyroid dysfunction, hyperprolactinaemia, congenital adrenal hyperplasia, androgen secreting tumours, and Cushings syndrome (OHCM p217). If clinically hyperandrogenic and total testosterone >5nmol/L check 17-hydroxyprogesterone and exclude androgen secreting tumours. US scan shows ≥12 peripheral ovarian follicles, or ↑ ovarian volume (>10cm³).

Management: Advise smoking avoidance. Find and treat diabetes, hypertension, dyslipidaemia and sleep apnoea. Encourage weight loss and exercise to increase insulin sensitivity. **Metformin** improves insulin sensitivity, menstrual disturbance, and ovulatory function (as effective as clomiphene).[25] It is recommended by NICE for those of body mass index >25 trying to conceive.

Clomifene (best if with metformin)[26] usually induces ovulation (50–60% conceive in 1st 6 months of treatment; so offer before using other methods; use on specialist advice). Warn of risk of multiple pregnancy and ovarian cancer (p283). Monitor response by ultrasound in at least 1st cycle. Those not ovulating in response to clomifene are at ↑ risk of ovarian hyperstimulation (p311) with assisted conception so *in vitro* maturation (IVM p293) is a good alternative. **Ovarian drilling** (creating holes in ovaries by diathermy with the intent of reducing steroid production) is recommended by NICE[27] for those not responding to clomifene (though it may be useful as primary treatment).[28] RCOG recommends for those BMI <25. 65% conceive.[RCOG] It does not increase risk of multiple pregnancy. Pregnancy rates are similar to those with assisted conception.[29] Preterm birth, pre-eclampsia, gestational diabetes, and large babies complicate pregnancy so treat as high risk.[30]

The **combined Pill** will control bleeding and reduce risk of unopposed oestrogen on the endometrium (risk of endometrial carcinoma). Recommend regular withdrawal bleeds, eg 3-monthly, for example induced with **dydrogesterone** 10mg/12h PO on days 11–25 in those in whom oestrogen use is not wanted or is contraindicated.[31,23]

Hirsutism may be treated cosmetically, or with an anti-androgen, eg **cyproterone** 2mg/day, as in co-cyprindiol (avoid pregnancy). **Spironolactone** 25–200mg/24h/PO is also antiandrogenic (avoid pregnancy as teratogenic). **Finasteride** 5mg/24h/PO has also been used for hirsutism; again avoid pregnancy. Neither spironolactone nor finasteride is licensed for this use.

Gynaecology

Menorrhagia

This is increased menstrual blood loss (defined as >80mL/cycle); in reality loss is rarely measured, so management deals with those whose heavy menstrual bleeding interferes with life. What makes a woman consult may be a change in volume (clots, floods, etc), or a change in life (eg job change, or depression). Ask about both. Is she hypothyroid (eg constipation; weight↑; *oʜcм* p212) or anaemic? Examine with these in mind.

Causes In *girls*, pregnancy and dysfunctional uterine bleeding are likely. With increasing age, think also of IUCD, fibroids, endometriosis and adenomyosis, pelvic infection, polyps. Also hypothyroidism. In *perimenopausal women*, consider endometrial carcinoma. Ask about general bleeding problems as she may have a blood dyscrasia, eg von Willebrand's. Do abdominal and pelvic examination—which may reveal polyps, fibroids, or endometriosis.

Tests FBC; TFT; consider clotting studies; ultrasound or laparoscopy if pelvic pathology suspected; ultrasound + endometrial sampling, or hysteroscopy and directed biopsy if irregular bleeding or suspected cancer (eg persistent intermenstrual bleeding, >45yrs and failed/ineffective treatment).

Dysfunctional uterine bleeding (DUB) This is heavy and/or irregular bleeding in the absence of recognizable pelvic pathology. It is associated with anovulatory cycles, so is common at the extremes of reproductive life or it may be ovulatory (eg with inadequate luteal phase). Teenage menorrhagia generally settles without interference as cycles become ovulatory. If PV is normal and organic pathology is ruled out, this is the diagnosis, by exclusion.

Treating menorrhagiaₙᵢ꜀ₑ—**Drugs** *Progesterone-containing IUCDs*, eg **Mirena®** should be considered 1ˢᵗ line treatment for those wanting contraception. They reduce bleeding (by up to 86% at 3 months, 97% at 1yr), are effective in dysfunctional uterine bleeding and reduce fibroid volume after 6–18 months' use. 5-year follow-up gives satisfaction levels similar to hysterectomy (in the 58% still using this method).[33]

2ⁿᵈ line recommended drugs are antifibrinolytics, antiprostaglandins or the Pill. *Antifibrinolytics* Taken during bleeding these reduce loss (by 49%)—eg tranexamic acid 1g/6–8h PO (for up to 4 days). CI: thromboembolic disease—but this is no more common in those on tranexamic acid. *Antiprostaglandins*, eg mefenamic acid 500mg/8h PO pc (CI: peptic ulceration) taken during days of bleeding particularly help if there is also dysmenorrhoea. They reduce bleeding by 29%. *The combined Pill* is effective but see contraindications (p300).

3ʳᵈ line recommendation is *progestogens* IM (p304) or **norethisterone** 5mg/8h PO days 5–26 of menstrual cycle (also used to stop heavy bleeding).

Rarely *gonadotrophin (LHRH) releasing hormones* are used (p276).

Surgery *Endometrial resection* (p308) is suitable for women who have completed their families and who have <10wk size uterus and fibroids <3cm. Ablation is now commoner than hysterectomy in the UK for menorrhagia. About 30% become amenorrhoeic and a further 50% have reduced flow after any method of ablation. Contraception is still required. If not used pregnancy is commoner in those who bleed (3.2% vs 0.3%).[34] Treat as with uterus for HRT (p256).

For women wishing to retain fertility who have fibroids >3cm consider *uterine artery embolization* or *myomectomy* (p276).

Women not wishing to retain fertility, with a uterus >10wk size and fibroids >3cm may benefit from *hysterectomy* (p308), vaginal hysterectomy being the preferred route.

Gynaecology

Most women notice that their mood or physical state may be worse premenstrually. Symptoms may be mild one month and severe the next, eg depending on external events and tend to be worse in the 30s and 40s and improve on the combined Pill. 3% of women regularly have cyclical symptoms so severe that they cause major disruption to their lives: premenstrual syndrome (PMS) or tension (PMT). Causes: See BOX.

Symptoms Commonest symptom patterns are tension and irritability; depression; bloating and breast tenderness; carbohydrate craving and headache; clumsiness; libido↓. Almost any symptom may feature.

Diagnosis Suggest symptom diary. If she has PMS her symptoms are worst before periods, are relieved by menstruation, and there is at least one symptom-free week afterwards. Diaries may also reveal psychiatric disorders (which may be worse premenstrually) or menstrual disorders.

Treatment Simply to acknowledge her problem, listen, and reassure may be all that is needed to help her to cope. Are her partner and children understanding? Can she rearrange work schedules to reduce stress premenstrually? Some women find self-help groups supportive. Health measures, eg improved diet, reducing smoking and drinking, increased exercise and relaxation, often help. Herbal remedies are not scientifically tested but some find them helpful, eg sage and fennel for irritability. Any drug evokes a big placebo effect, improving 90% in some studies. Pyridoxine (vit B6) 10mg/24h PO for the symptomatic period or continuously, may help low mood and headache (DOH says higher, more effective doses cause neuropathy). For severe *cyclical mastalgia* consider:

1 Reduce saturated fats eaten: these increase the affinity of oestrogen-receptors for oestrogen.

2 Bromocriptine 2.5mg/12h PO days 10–26, even if prolactin normal.

3 Danazol 100–200mg/12h PO for 7 days before menstruation (see below).

Some benefit from suppression of ovulation with the combined Pill (Yasmin® may be especially suitable and seems to help reduce fluid retention[35]),[36] oestrogen patches or implants, with cyclical progesterone, or danazol 200mg/24h (SE nausea, weight gain, masculinization of the female fetus, so advise barrier contraception). Avoid diuretics unless fluid retention is severe (when spironolactone 25mg/6h PO days 18–26 of the cycle is the drug of choice).

SSRIs, eg fluoxetine 20mg/day PO help,[37] with ~30% experiencing remission (but the licence for use in PMS in UK has been withdrawn), and can be used just in the luteal phase.[38] Venlafaxine has also been shown to be beneficial. Cognitive behavioural therapy has been shown to be as effective at fluoxetine, effects possibly lasting longer when assessed at 12 months.

Alprazolam (0.25mg/day PO during the luteal phase) also helps, with apparently low risk of dependence. Buspirone has also been used as a anxiolytic, though SSRIs are felt to be more effective.[39] Agnus castus fruit extract helped symptoms in 50% of women in a placebo-controlled trial.[40]

Goserelin (p276) may help severe PMS but symptoms return when ovarian activity recommences and after 6 months' use bone thinning can be detected. Adding tibolone can ameliorate this effect. Goserelin is better used to predict the severely affected women who may benefit from hysterectomy with oophorectomy (results in 96% satisfaction rates[41]—these women can then have oestrogen replacement).

Follow-up: it is not 'cheating' to ensure that her next appointment will *not* be in the premenstrual phase—more objectivity may be forthcoming.

The Rapkin hypothesis and putative pathways in PMS[42,43]

Some physiological and pharmacological observations.

• There is no evidence that ovarian events cause premenstrual syndrome: models presupposing progesterone deficiency have not been confirmed (and progesterone suppositories are no panacea for the condition).

• Artificially altering circulating progesterone and estradiol (oestradiol) does not induce premenstrual symptoms in previously well women—only in those already prone to PMS.

• Studies with psychoactive compounds suggest that the key events are occurring in the brain, not the ovary—eg an abnormal CNS response to normal progesterone excursions occurring in the luteal phase.

• Allopregnanolone and pregnenolone (metabolites of progesterone) are psychoactive, interacting with γ-aminobutyric acid A (GABA-A) receptors.

• Allopregnanolone is anxiolytic, so lower levels may be associated with anxiety.

Putative conclusion: Neurons or glia in those with PMS preferentially metabolize progesterone to pregnenolone (which heightens anxiety) rather than allopregnanolone (which is anxiolytic and up-regulates serotonin receptors, so ameliorating depression). On this view, alprazolam, by augmenting GABA-A-receptor function, is a substitute for allopregnanolone.

Gynaecology

The climacteric is the time of waning fertility leading up to the last period (menopause). The menopause enables grandmothering—a unique institution, in humans (and whales). Problems are related to falling oestrogen levels.

- Menstrual irregularity as cycles become anovulatory, before stopping.
- Vasomotor disturbance—sweats, palpitations, and flushes (brief, nasty, and may occur every few minutes for >10yrs, disrupting life and sleep).
- Atrophy of oestrogen-dependent tissues (genitalia, breasts) and skin. Vaginal dryness can lead to vaginal and urinary infection, dyspareunia, traumatic bleeding, stress incontinence, and prolapse.
- Osteoporosis: the menopause accelerates bone loss which predisposes to fracture of femur neck, radius, and vertebrae in later life.
- Attitudes to the menopause vary widely, and partly depend on irritability, depression, 'empty nest syndrome'—all exacerbated by the menopause.

Management ≥20% of women seek medical help.

- Is it the menopause? Thyroid and psychiatric problems may present similarly. 2 FSH levels >30IU/L is suggestive of menopause: unreliable if on oestrogens.
- Counselling helps psychosocial *and* physical symptoms; enlist family's support.
- Menorrhagia may respond to treatment (p253). A D&C is required if irregular bleeding is abnormal (it may be difficult to decide).
- Use contraception until >1y amenorrhoea if >50y; 2y if <50y (55 if on hormones).
- Hot flushes may respond to **clonidine** 50–75µg/12h PO, HRT, or **tibolone** (NB: risk of endometrial cancer increased compared to non-users).
- Vaginal dryness responds to **oestrogen** (can be used locally).

Hormone replacement therapy (HRT) Oestrogen is not a panacea for all problems, but may help flushes and atrophic vaginitis. It postpones menopausal bone loss but is no longer recommended just for osteoporosis prevention. Trials show no cardiovascular benefits,●* no protection against dementia in the over-65s, and increased stroke and thromboembolism in users. HRT ↑breast cancer risk (p257), endometrial cancer (↑risk with unopposed oestrogen or sequential progesterone, possible ↓risk with continuous combined) and those using for >10yrs have double the risk of ovarian cancer of non-users.[44]

Women with a uterus should also receive cyclical **progestogens** to reduce incidence of endometrial carcinoma,—or use **tibolone** 2.5mg/day PO, a preparation which aims not to cause bleeds—or **continuous combined oestrogen/progestogen combinations**, eg Kliofem®, estradiol (=oestradiol) 2mg and norethisterone 1mg. For both these, start if >1yr after the last period, or, if changing from cyclical HRT, wait until after 54yrs of age; bleeding is common, in the 1st 4 months of use—reassure; if after 8 months, do endometrial biopsy. Kliofem® may be useful if cyclical HRT causes 'premenstrual' symptoms. There *may* be advantages in using 'lipid-friendly' progestogens, **dydrogesterone** (no androgenic, mineralocorticoid, or oestrogenic action), eg Femoston 2/10® but see p303 for possible SE (DVT). **Raloxifene**, a selective oestrogen receptor modulator (SERM) protects bones while *reducing* breast[45] and endometrial cancer risk. It is ineffective for flushes. For thromboembolism, see OPPOSITE.

HRT contraindications: • Oestrogen-dependent cancer • Past pulmonary embolus • Undiagnosed PV bleeding • LFT↑ • Pregnancy • Breastfeeding • Phlebitis. Avoid or monitor closely in Dubin–Johnson/Rotor syndromes (OHCM p712). If past spontaneous DVT/PE: *is there thrombophilia (OHCM p368)?*

Side-effects: Weight↑; 'premenstrual' syndrome; cholestasis; vomiting.

Alternative therapies[46] RCOL eg black cohosh (can cause hepatotoxicity)—p515.

Annual check-up: Breasts; BP (stop if BP >160/100 pending investigation and treatment). Weight; any abnormal bleeding?

Creams, pessaries, and rings are useful for vaginal symptoms, eg Ovestin®, ie **estriol 0.1%**, 1 applicator-full pv daily for 3 weeks, then twice weekly. They are absorbed but, if used intermittently, progestogens are probably unnecessary. If creams are unacceptable, consider an **oestrogen-containing vaginal ring** (eg Estring®), replaced every 3 months, for up to 2yrs. Vagifem® is an **estradiol (=oestradiol)** 25µg or 10µg vaginal tablet used daily for 2 weeks, and then twice weekly, with reassessment every 3 months.

Transdermal patches are less 'medical' but are expensive and women with a uterus still need progestogen, eg as tablets or Evorel® conti patches. **Estradiol (=oestradiol)** patches supply 25–100µg/24h for 3–4 days. SE: dermatitis.

Oestradiol gel 2 measures are applied daily to arms, shoulders, or inner thighs. Women with a uterus using gel also require progestogens for 12 days per cycle.

HRT and cancer The Women's Health Initiative[48] confirmed ↑breast cancer risk (and showed excess stroke and heart attack risk, and 2-fold increase in dementia[49] in users): the Million Women Study[50] showed that there is greater risk when combined oestrogen/progesterone preparations are used (relative risk=RR 2) compared to oestrogen alone (RR 1.3) or tibolone (RR 1.45). Risk increases with length of use. Ovarian cancer is increased in current users after 5 years' use (oestrogen component RR 1.2).[51] Endometrial cancer risk is ↑ with unopposed oestrogen use, ↔ with cyclical progesterone added, and possibly ↓ with continuous combined added progesterone.[52] Lung cancer mortality (but not incidence) is increased, (so stop, if lung cancer develops).[53] Hence our policy on HRT is:

- To discuss the risk of breast cancer with each patient considering HRT.
- To document this discussion in the patient's notes.
- Encourage breast awareness and to report breast change. Formal breast examination by nurses may give false reassurance (advice of the UK's Chief Medical Officer). Mammographic screening may be less effective in current users.[54] It is difficult if aged 40–50yrs (breast density↑).
- To use for symptomatic treatment (warn symptoms often return on stopping therapy however long it has been used for) at the lowest dose needed to control symptoms, for the shortest time possible.
- To be wary about HRT in those with a family history of breast cancer.
- To consider stopping HRT before 5 completed years of therapy.

HRT is no longer licensed for osteoporosis prevention: consider **raloxifene** (which ↓risk of breast cancer; it is related to tamoxifen),[55] or bisphosphonates.

HRT and venous thromboembolism (VTE) Overall HRT doubles risk (which ↑ with age). Consider other predisposing factors, such as prolonged immobility, surgery, obesity, *severe* varicose veins (others see p16). On starting explain risk and advise to seek urgent help if symptoms develop. Stop HRT if VTE develops. Before starting, elicit personal and family history of venous thromboembolism (VTE), discuss thrombophilia screen if history. Thrombophilia ↑ risk (×8 if Factor V Leiden or prothrombin 20210A mutation). If thrombophilic seek expert advice. Transdermal use has less risk, and oral HRT is contraindicated if past history of VTE. SERM therapy (OPPOSITE) carries same VTE risk as HRT. NICE[NICE] says stop 4 weeks pre-elective surgery; RCOG[RCOG] says consider cases individually and use thromboprophylactic measures for surgery.

▶Under British law, no one *has* to have an abortion, and no one *has* to do one. Worldwide, >20% of pregnancies are terminated and in the UK ⅓ of women have had a TOP by age 45. *Incidence:* >200,000 TOP/yr in Great Britain (GB).

Legal (GB) constraints The Abortion Act 1967 (amended 2002) and Human Fertilisation and Embryology Act 1990 allow termination if:

A There is risk to mother's life if pregnancy continues.

B Termination is necessary to prevent permanent grave injury to physical/ mental health of the woman.

C Continuance risks injury to the physical or mental health of the woman greater than if terminated (and fetus not >24 weeks).

D Continuance risks injury to physical/mental health of existing children of the woman greater than if terminated (and fetus not >24 weeks).

E There is substantial risk that if the child were born he/she would suffer such physical or mental abnormalities as to be seriously handicapped.

At present, two doctors must sign certificate HSA1. If <16yrs try to get patient's consent to involve her parents or other adult.[1] 97% are for ground C; 1% for D. <1% of TOPs are done after 20 weeks, usually after amniocentesis, or when very young or menopausal mothers have concealed, or not recognized, pregnancy. TOPs after 24 weeks may only be carried out in NHS hospitals.

Before TOP ▶She has to live with the decision for the rest of her life.

• Identify those needing support eg counselling. Not needed if sure of decision.

• Is she definitely pregnant (eg reliable urine test?). Give information on and choice of methods. If ultrasound needed (eg dates unsure) ask if she wishes to see images. Offer cytology screening if not up to date. If she chooses TOP:

• Screen for chlamydia: (± other STIs if relevant).

• Give antibiotic prophylaxis to reduce post-op infection rate (10% without) eg **metronidazole** 1g PR/800mg PO at TOP and **azithromycin** 1g PO same day.

• Discuss contraception (IUCD or sterilization at operation need plans).

• If RhD-ve she needs anti-D (all gestations, whatever method see p9). Bloods for Hb, ABO+RhD group and antibodies; ± HIV, hepatitis B & C, and haemoglobinopathies, if relevant.

• Assess venous thromboembolism risk.

Methods *Medical abortion* uses an antigestagen, eg **mifepristone** to disimplant the fetus followed by a prostaglandin eg **misoprostol** to complete abortion. It is highly effective from ≥6 weeks (98% effective at ≤7 weeks, 95% for weeks 7–9) and is also used for second trimester abortions. Misoprostol can be used orally or vaginally. For early abortions arrange follow-up (and scan) 2 weeks after procedure unless complete abortion confirmed on day of abortion. 5% will need surgical evacuation. Give NSAID pain relief during abortion; narcotic analgesia may also be needed, especially if gestation >13 weeks.

Surgical abortion (vacuum aspiration and dilatation). Consider need for pre-operative cervical priming (eg gestation >10 weeks, women <18 years of age) in all women eg with misoprostol 400µg PV 3h or sublingual 2–3h pre-op. Osmotic dilators provide superior dilatation from 14 weeks, but misoprostol can be used up to 18 weeks. Offer NSAID pain relief during abortion (paracetamol is ineffective). Bleeding and pain is less than with medical abortion.

Vacuum aspiration Used from 7 to 16 weeks. Local anaesthesia is safer than GA. If <7 weeks check for gestational sac in aspirate, follow-up with βHCG if not seen. If 14-16 weeks use wide-bore cannula. Access to US is desirable.

Dilatation & evacuation Surgical forceps may be used at 13^{+0}–24^{+0}wks after cervical priming. Experienced operators are required. Real-time ultrasound reduces uterine perforation rates and is recommended.

---

1 If the girl is a ward of court, the court has to approve abortion.[58]

Regimens for terminating intrauterine pregnancies[20][RCOL]

Early medical terminations ≤63 days' gestation
At ≤ 49 days' gestation use mifepristone 200mg PO + misoprostol 400µg orally 24–48h later. At ≤ 63 days' gestation mifepristone 200mg PO + misoprostol 800µg (4×200µg tablets) PV/buccal or sublingual 24–48h later. For women at 50–63 days' gestation, if no abortion 4h after misoprostol give a further 400µg PO/PV (route depending on preference and amount of bleeding).

Medical terminations 9–13 weeks' gestation
Mifepristone 200mg PO + misoprostol 800µg vaginally 36–48h later. A maximum of 4 further doses of misoprostol 400µg may then be given 3-hourly PV/PO.

Medical terminations 13–24 weeks' gestation
Mifepristone 200mg PO followed 36–48h later by misoprostol 800µg PV: then misoprostol 400µg PV/PO every 3h to a maximum of 4 further doses. If abortion does not occur mifepristone can be repeated 3h after the last dose of misoprostol and 12h later misoprostol recommenced. If there is clinical evidence that abortion is incomplete, surgical evacuation of the uterus will be needed.

Feticide
In terminations later than 21 weeks + 6 days (eg for abnormality) it is essential that the fetus is born dead (unless it is a lethal fetal abnormality). This may be achieved by use of 3mL intracardiac 15% potassium chloride (± anaesthetic and/or muscle relaxant instillation beforehand to abolish fetal movement). Confirm asystole with ultrasound. (Intra-amniotic digoxin is a less effective alternative requiring less expertise.) If born after 24 weeks the dead fetus is a stillbirth and needs registering (p83). If there are signs of life then a death certificate is required.[60][RCOL]

Complications of termination (terminology of risk)[1]
- Failure to abort (<1 : 100 medical TOP failure rate is higher than surgical).
- Infection post-abortion (~ 2 : 100); see screening and antibiotics OPPOSITE.
- Haemorrhage (<1 : 1000), (4 : 1000 if at ≥20 weeks).
- Uterine perforation (1–4 : 1000), surgical terminations only
- Uterine rupture (mid-trimester medical TOP): < 4 : 1000
- Cervical trauma (1 : 100). Risk less if early abortion: if experienced operator.
- Small risk of premature labour in future pregnancies (if surgical abortion).

After termination Has she had anti-D (p9)? (250iu if <20 weeks; 500iu +Kleihauer if later.) Is contraception arranged? (Can start Pill same day. Advise that long acting methods are more effective.) Give letter with sufficient information for practitioners elsewhere to manage complications. Give written and verbal information on symptoms to be expected, those requiring emergency care, and of symptoms of ongoing pregnancy. Give 24h telephone helpline number. Offer follow-up. Refer women requiring emotional support/ at mental health risk. Women having medical terminations not confirmed as successful at time of procedure need follow-up to ensure no ongoing pregnancy (rate 0.5–1%). Misoprostol risks teratogenicity. Decision to arrange uterine surgical evacuation is made on clinical signs and symptoms.

Worldwide it is estimated there are 210 million pregnancies at any one time, and 1 in 5 are terminated. Over three-quarters of women live in developing countries, where 97% of the estimated 20 million unsafe terminations are carried out. 68,000 women die annually after unsafe termination. Accessible contraception reduces need for termination. Legalization of termination reduces the number of unsafe terminations and subsequent maternal death.

---

1 **The language of risk:** 1:1–1:10 is very common; 1:10–1:100 is common; 1:100–1:1000 uncommon; 1:1000–1:10,000 is rare; <1:10,000 is very rare (modified from Calman *et al*).[8b]

Miscarriage is the loss of a pregnancy before 24 weeks' gestation. 20–40% of pregnancies miscarry, mostly in the first trimester. Most present with bleeding PV. Diagnosis may not be straightforward (consider ectopics p262): have a low threshold for doing an ultrasound scan. Pregnancy tests remain +ve for several days after fetal death. Heavy/persistent bleeding >2 weeks needs ERPC (p308).

Management of early pregnancy bleeding Consider the following.
• ►Is she shocked? There may be blood loss, or products of conception in the cervical canal (remove them with sponge forceps).
• Has pain and bleeding been worse than a period? Have products of conception been seen? (Clots may be mistaken for products.)
• Is the os open? The external os of a multigravida usually admits a fingertip.
• Is uterine size appropriate for dates?
• Is she bleeding from a cervical lesion and not from within the uterus?
• What is her blood group? If RhD –ve does she need anti-D (p9)?

If symptoms are mild and the cervical os is closed it is a *threatened miscarriage*. Rest is advised but probably does not help. 75% will settle. Threatened miscarriage (especially second trimester) is associated with risk of subsequent preterm rupture of membranes and preterm delivery—so book mother at a hospital with good neonatal facilities.

If symptoms are severe and the os is open it is an *inevitable miscarriage* or, if most of the products have already been passed, an *incomplete miscarriage*. If bleeding is profuse, consider ergometrine 0.5mg IM. If there is unacceptable pain or bleeding, or much retained tissue on ultrasound, arrange evacuation of retained products of conception (ERPC). Expectant management is used when the volume of retained products is small eg <15mm across on transvaginal scan; when 15–50mm, medical management eg with vaginal misoprostol may be offered (warn bleeding may last up to 3 weeks).

Missed miscarriage: The fetus dies but is retained. There has usually been bleeding and the uterus is small for dates. Confirm with ultrasound. Mifepristone and misoprostol may be used to induce uterine evacuation if the uterus is small but 50% will require surgical evacuation if uterine products are >5cm² in the transverse plane, >6cm² in the sagittal plane. Surgical evacuation is required for larger uteruses, if scar (previous caesar), by senior staff.

Mid-trimester miscarriage This is usually due to mechanical causes, eg cervical incompetence (rapid, painless delivery of a live fetus), uterine abnormalities, or chronic maternal disease (eg DM, SLE). An incompetent cervix can be strengthened by a cervical cerclage suture[62] at ~14 weeks of pregnancy (eg if 3+ premature deliveries/mid-trimester losses, or previous loss/preterm delivery and ultrasound proven cervical shortening). It is removed prior to labour.

After a miscarriage ►Miscarriage may be a bereavement. Give the parents space to grieve, to ask why it happened and if it will recur. Offer follow-up.[63] Fetal products should be incinerated but if the mother requests alternative disposal (to bury herself) respect her wishes. Give in opaque container.[64]

Most early pregnancy losses are due to aneuploidy and abnormal fetal development; 10% to maternal illness, eg pyrexia. 2nd trimester loss may be due to infection, eg CMV (p34). Bacterial vaginosis has been implicated. Most subsequent pregnancies are normal although at increased risk.

Recurrent miscarriage See OPPOSITE.

Miscarriage with infection Presents as acute salpingitis (p286) and is treated similarly. Start broad-spectrum antibiotics 1h prior to uterine curettage, eg co-amoxiclav (ampoules are 1.2g; 1g is amoxicillin and 200mg is clavulanic acid; give 1.2g/6h IV) + metronidazole (eg 1g by suppository/8h).

This is loss of 3 or more consecutive pregnancies before 24 weeks' gestation. It affects 1% of women. Prognosis for future successful pregnancy is affected by the previous number of miscarriages, and maternal age. (Rates of miscarriage are greatest when maternal age is ≥35 years, and paternal age ≥ 40 years.)

Possible causes

Endocrine: Polycystic ovaries are thought to be associated via insulin resistance. Metformin has been shown in small uncontrolled trials to reduce RSM. The role of progesterone in RSM is still being studied.

Infection: Bacterial vaginosis (p284) is associated with 2nd trimester loss. Screening (and treatment) was previously recommended for those with previous mid-trimester miscarriage or pre-term birth (benefit unproven).

Parental chromosome abnormality: 2–5% of those with RSM. It is usually a balanced reciprocal or Robertsonian translocation (p152). Refer to a clinical geneticist. Genetic counselling offers prognosis for future pregnancy, familial chromosome studies, and appropriate advice for subsequent pregnancy. Pre-implantation genetic diagnosis (p13—involving *in vitro* fertilization) has lower rates of achieving healthy pregnancy outcome compared to natural conception (30% *vs* 50%).

Uterine abnormality: It is uncertain how much abnormality is associated with RSM or if hysteroscopic correction of abnormality contributes to successful pregnancy outcome, though septum division may help.[65] It is known that open uterine surgery increases chance of uterine rupture in pregnancy.

Antiphospholipid antibodies: (lupus anticoagulant, phospholipid and anticardiolipin antibodies) These are present in 15% of women with RSM. Most women with antibodies miscarry in the first trimester. If they are present, giving aspirin eg 75mg/24h PO from the day of positive pregnancy test + low molecular weight heparin, eg enoxaparin 40mg/24h sc)[66] as soon as the fetal heart is seen (eg at 5 weeks on vaginal ultrasound) until 34 weeks' gestation helps.[67] Get expert advice. Resulting pregnancies are at high risk of repeated miscarriage, pre-eclampsia, fetal growth restriction, and pre-term birth so need special surveillance. Live birth rate is ~80%.

Thrombophilia: In those with inherited thrombophilia heparin helps those who suffer from 2nd trimester losses but evidence is less certain for 1st trimester losses.

Alloimmune causes: The theory is that these women share human leucocyte alleles (HLA) with their partners and do not mount the satisfactory protective response to the fetus. Immunotherapy has not been found to increase live birth rate, is potentially dangerous and should not be offered.

Recommendation

• Offer referral to specialist recurrent miscarriage clinic.
• Test all women for antiphospholipid antibodies: positive if 2 tests +ve, taken 12 weeks apart.
• Women with 2nd trimester losses test for thrombophilia.
• All women with recurrent 1st trimester losses, (or more than 1, 2nd trimester loss) should have pelvic ultrasound to assess uterus; further tests eg 3-D ultrasound/laparoscopy/hysteroscopy if anatomy abnormal.
• Karyotype fetal products (3rd and subsequent fetal losses). If an unbalanced chromosome abnormality is identified in the products of conception then karyotype the peripheral blood of both parents.

The fertilized ovum implants outside the uterine cavity. The UK incidence is 11.1 : 1000 pregnancies and rising; worldwide rates are higher. ~7% of maternal deaths are due to ectopics (1.8 deaths/1000 ectopic pregnancies).

Predisposing factors Anything slowing the ovum's passage to the uterus increases risk: damage to the tubes (salpingitis; previous surgery); previous ectopic; endometriosis; IUCD; the POP (p302); GIFT (p293). Pregnancy after tubal ligation is 9 times more likely to be ectopic.

Site 97% are tubal, mostly in ampulla; 25% in the narrow inextensible isthmus (presents early; risk of rupture↑). 3% implant on ovary, cervix, or peritoneum.

Natural history The trophoblast invades the tubal wall, weakening it and producing haemorrhage which dislodges the embryo. If the tube does not rupture, the blood and embryo are shed or converted into a tubal mole and absorbed. Rupture can be sudden and catastrophic, or gradual, giving increasing pain and blood loss. Peritoneal pregnancies may survive into the third trimester, and may present with failure to induce labour.

Clinical presentation ►Always think of an ectopic in a sexually active woman with abdominal pain; bleeding; fainting; or diarrhoea and vomiting.

There is generally ~8 weeks' *amenorrhoea* but an ectopic may present before a period is missed. An early sign is often dark blood loss ('prune juice', as the decidua is lost from the uterus) or fresh. In 10–20% there is no bleeding. Tubal colic causes *abdominal pain* which may precede *vaginal bleeding*. The ectopic may rupture the tube with sudden severe pain, peritonism, and shock. More often there is gradually increasing vaginal bleeding, and bleeding into the peritoneum producing shoulder-tip pain (diaphragmatic irritation) and pain on defecation and urination (due to pelvic blood). 10% report no pain. The patient may be faint, with a tender abdomen (95%), enlarged uterus (30%), cervical excitation (50%), adnexal mass (63%). Presentation may just be as diarrhoea and vomiting, or nausea and dizziness. Classical features may be absent. Examine gently, to reduce risk of rupture; preferably with an IVI *in situ*.

Management ►Remember to give anti-D prophylaxis (p9), if needed. Early diagnosis is vital. Dipstix testing for βHCG (human chorionic gonadotrophin) is sensitive to values of 25IU/L. Quantitate βHCG (blood); do ultrasound. If βHCG >6000IU/L and an intrauterine gestational sac is not seen, ectopic pregnancy is very likely, as is the case if βHCG 1000–1500IU/L and no sac is seen on *transvaginal* ultrasound. Normally βHCG doubles over 48h. The higher the index of suspicion, the quicker the diagnosis. Unless urgent laparotomy needed, consider type of treatment required in the light of the woman's future pregnancy wishes.

Immediate laparotomy: ►►Shock from a ruptured ectopic can be fatal. Immediate laparotomy is necessary as only clamping the bleeding artery will relieve it. If you suspect an ectopic, put up an IVI; if already shocked put up 2 (14 or 16G). Give crystalloid as fast as possible, then blood (group O Rhesus -ve if desperate, but usually better to wait for group compatible). Inform your consultant. Take immediately to theatre.

Laparoscopy vs laparotomy: Laparoscopy is preferred to laparotomy as recovery time is reduced and it is less costly. Rates of subsequent intrauterine pregnancy are similar but persisting trophoblast is more of a problem (12% *vs* 1.2%). Single-shot methotrexate use reduces this risk. Persistent trophoblast can cause later rupture and will need further treatment (surgical or methotrexate). See OPPOSITE. Repeat ectopic is slightly less common after laparoscopy.

Salpingotomy vs salpingectomy: If the contralateral tube is healthy, RCOG guidelines say there is no clear evidence that salpingotomy should be used rather than salpingectomy. Subsequent intrauterine pregnancy rates are higher after salpingotomy but so are rates of persisting trophoblast (8% *vs* 4%)

and subsequent ectopic pregnancy (18% *vs* 8%). Salpingotomy should be primary treatment if the other tube is not healthy to preserve chance of future intrauterine pregnancy (49%), but warn of risk of future ectopic pregnancy.[69][COI]

Methotrexate: **Methotrexate** (eg 50mg/m^2 IM or intratubal injection into the gestation sac) is sometimes used for small early ectopics (eg <3.5cm in greatest diameter; βHCG level <3000IU/L, minimal symptoms. Visualization of a fetal heart is a contraindication to treatment). ≥15% will require more than 1 dose, and 10% surgical intervention (rupture rate 7% despite methotrexate treatment). 75% of women will get some abdominal pain with treatment and admission for observation and ultrasound may be required to distinguish rupture from the pain of separation with tubal abortion). Variable systemic dose regimes have similar success to salpingotomy.[70] Advise avoidance of intercourse during treatment and use of effective contraception for the next 3 months (+ 12 weeks folate to restore levels once βHCG <5IU/L before attempting pregnancy). Multiple ovarian cysts, life-threatening neutropenia, pneumonitis, and late pelvic collections of blood have been reported with methotrexate treatment. Follow-up requires good compliance for repeat visits for serial βHCG until levels very low (usually <20IU/L). Fertility rates are no better with methotrexate or expectant management than with surgery.[71]

Expectant management: Some tubal pregnancies end themselves without any problem so conservative treatment *may* be an option in those without acute symptoms and with falling βHCG levels that are <1000IU/L initially. 88% successfully resolve if initial βHCG <1000IU/L. There should be no evidence of blood, and <100mL fluid in the pouch of Douglas. Follow-up twice weekly. Ideally βHCG drops by 50% and the adnexal mass is seen to be reducing in size by day 7. Follow-up until βHCG <20IU/L (as tubal rupture has been known to occur at low levels of βHCG). Expectant management may also be used for women with pregnancy of unknown origin (ie no ultrasound evidence of uterine or ectopic pregnancy). It may be used if initial βHCG 1000–1500IU/L. Actively intervene if symptoms develop, or βHCG levels plateau or rise at 48–72h (23–29%).

Management of persistent trophoblast: This occurs in 8.2% having laparoscopic salpingotomy; 4% after open salpingectomy. Diagnosis is by finding that βHCG does not drop according to the expected curve. Surveillance regimes vary: eg suspect if not fallen to <65% of pre-op value by 48h post-op, or to <10% by 10 days post-op. Treatment is with methotrexate IM as above.

Measures to reduce risk of missing ectopic pregnancies
• Always send uterine curettings at ERPC (p308) for histology.
• If histology does not confirm uterine failed pregnancy, recall the patient. (Ensure rapid return of histology results.)
• When ultrasound reports suggest an incomplete miscarriage but the fetus has not been seen—think: could this be an ectopic?

This comprises premalignant hydatidiform mole, and the malignant conditions of choriocarcinoma and the rare (0.23%) placental site trophoblastic tumour. Complete moles are diploid and androgenic, 75–80% following duplication of a single sperm after fertilization of an 'empty ovum', 20–25% after dispermic fertilization of an 'empty' ovum so no maternal nuclear DNA although mitochondrial DNA is maternal. Partial moles usually follow dispermic fertilization of an ovum and are triploid (2 sets paternal haploid genes, 1 haploid maternal set) but 10% are tetraploid or mosaic conceptions. Partial moles usually have evidence of fetal parts or red cells. They are 3 ×commoner, grow slower (so present later), and are less often malignant (1% vs 15%).

Hydatidiform moles (see fig 1) Tumours consist of proliferating chorionic villi which have swollen and degenerated. Derived from chorion, it makes lots of human chorionic gonadotrophin (HCG), giving rise to exaggerated pregnancy symptoms and strongly +ve pregnancy tests. *Incidence:* 1.54:1000 births (UK). It is commoner at extremes of child-bearing age, after a previous mole, and in Asians. A woman who has had a past mole is at ↑risk for future pregnancies; 0.8–2.9% after one mole, and 15–28% after 2 moles.

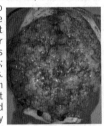

Fig 1. Hydatidiform mole
Courtesy of Prof. J. Carter.

<1% have familial recurrent moles (recessive) with <1:50 chance of normal pregnancy.[73] *Signs:* Most present with early pregnancy failure, eg failed miscarriage or signs on ultrasound. Bleeding may be heavy; aborted molar tissue may look like frogspawn. *Ultrasound* may show 'snowstorm effect' in a 'large-for-dates' uterus. Severe morning sickness or 1st trimester pre-eclampsia are rarer presentations. If accompanying twin pregnancy, proceed, if wished, (40% viable baby outcome without ↑ persisting neoplasia or adverse treatment results).

Abdominal pain may be due to huge theca-lutein cysts in both ovaries. These may rupture or tort. They take ~4 months to resolve after molar evacuation. HCG resembles TSH, and may cause hyperthyroidism. ►Tell the anaesthetist as thyrotoxic storm can occur at evacuation. *Treatment:* Molar tissue is removed from the soft, easily perforated uterus by gentle suction. Give anti-D if rhesus -ve (p 9). Pregnancy should be avoided for a year while HCG levels are monitored. Register the woman at specialist centre (below) for HCG monitoring. Levels should return to normal within 6 months. If levels drop rapidly to normal, oral contraceptives may be used after 6 months. If they do not, either the mole was invasive (myometrium penetrated) or has given rise to choriocarcinoma (10%). Invasive moles may metastasize, eg to lung, vagina, brain, liver, and skin. Both conditions respond to chemotherapy. See BOX p265.

Choriocarcinoma ►*Investigate all persistent post-pregnancy PV bleeding to exclude choriocarcinoma.* This highly malignant tumour occurs in 1 : 40,000 deliveries. The chief contexts are following a benign mole (50%), miscarriage (20%), or a normal pregnancy (10%). *Presentation: May be years after pregnancy,* with general malaise (due to 'malignancy' and ↑HCG) or uterine bleeding; signs and symptoms from metastases (may be very haemorrhagic, eg haematoperitoneum); nodules on CXR. Pulmonary artery obstruction via tumour emboli may cause pulmonary artery hypertension (haemoptysis; dyspnoea). *Treatment:* Choriocarcinoma in the UK is treated at 3 specialist centres; it is extremely responsive to combination chemotherapy based on **methotrex**ate. Outlook is good if non-metastatic and fertility is usually retained.

Placental site trophoblastic tumour These grow slower, present later, produce less HCG. Post chemotherapy residual disease is excised (eg womb and nodes).

Indications for chemotherapy[74]

- Plateauing or rising post evacuation HCG (taken days 1, 7, 14, 21)
- HCG ≥ 20,000 IU/L 4 weeks post evacuation
- ↑ HCG 6 months post evacuation, even if levels dropping
- Heavy vaginal bleeding, or gastrointestinal or intraperitoneal bleeding
- Evidence of brain, liver, or gastrointestinal metastases, or lung opacities >2cm (smaller lesions may regress spontaneously)
- Histology of choriocarcinoma

Gynaecology

Pruritus vulvae Vaginal itch is distressing and embarrassing. *Causes:* There may be a disorder causing general pruritus (p586) or skin disease (eg psoriasis, lichen planus). The cause may be local: infection and vaginal discharge (eg candida); infestation (eg scabies, pubic lice, threadworms); or vulval dystrophy (lichen sclerosis, leukoplakia, carcinoma). Symptoms may be psychogenic in origin. Psychosexual sequelae may ensue. Obesity and incontinence exacerbate symptoms. Postmenopausal atrophy does not cause itch.

The history may suggest the cause. Ask about autoimmune disorders and atopy. Examine general health and look for wider spread skin conditions. Examine the vulva and genital tract, under magnification if possible, and take a cervical smear, if due. Consider taking vaginal and vulval swabs and tests for diabetes and thyroid disease. If vulval dermatitis check serum ferritin and dermatology patch tests. Biopsy if diagnosis in doubt, if there is no response to treatment, or vulval intraepithelial neoplasia or carcinoma are suspected.

►Scratching and self-medication may have changed the appearance.

Treatment is often unsatisfactory.[1] Treat the cause if possible. Avoid sensitizers (patch testing may reveal sensitizing agents eg 26–80% in vulval dermatitis studies). Reassurance can be very important. Vulval care advice (OPPOSITE), may help. A short course of topical steroids, eg **betamethasone valerate** cream 0.1% may help. Avoid any topical preparation which may sensitize the skin, so give antipruritics orally if needed, eg **promethazine** 25mg/12–24h.

Lichen sclerosis Thought to be an autoimmune disorder (40% develop other autoimmune disorders), elastic tissue turns to collagen (usually after middle age—or, occasionally, before puberty). The 'bruised' red, purpuric signs may appear, to the unknowing, to suggest abuse—particularly if there are bullae, erosions, and ulcerations. The vulva gradually becomes white, flat, and shiny. There may be an hourglass shape around the vulva and anus. It is intensely itchy. It may be pre-malignant and long-term surveillance is desirable if unresponsive to treatment. *Treatment:* **Clobetasol proprionate** cream daily for 28 days, then alternate days for 14 doses, then twice weekly for 8 doses, then as needed;[75] vulval ablation may be needed to relieve itch. The 4–10% who are steroid unresponsive may respond to topical **tacrolimus** (off licence, use in specialist clinic only, for <2 years). In children, 50% resolve by menarche.

Leukoplakia (White vulval patches due to skin thickening and hypertrophy). It is itchy. It should be biopsied as it may be a pre-malignant lesion. *Treatment:* Topical corticosteroids (problems: mucosal thinning, absorption); **psoralens** with ultraviolet **phototherapy**; **methotrexate**; **ciclosporin**.

Lichen planus Of unknown cause, this is more likely to present with pain than pruritus. In mouth & genital area it can be erosive, appearing with a well demarcated glazed appearance around the introitus. It can affect all ages.

Lichen simplex This presents with chronic intractable itching, especially at night, in those with sensitive skin or eczema. There is non-specific inflammation of vulva, (±mons pubis and inner thighs). Stress, sensitizing chemicals an low body iron stores can exacerbate symptoms. Treatment is with vulval care (OPPOSITE), using steroids to break the itch/scratch cycle, if needed. Antihistamines or antipruritics (above) can help.

Vulvovaginitis Think of fixed drug reactions (NSAIDs, statins); stop for 2 weeks. Desquamative inflammatory vaginitis, of unknown cause, characterized by shiny erythematous patches ± petechiae. It responds to 2–4 weeks of intravaginal **clindamycin** cream with hydrocortisone to the vulva.[76]

---

1 As chronic vulval itch and chronic vulval pain are often recalcitrant (often ignored, or inappropriately diagnosed as candida)—and because of its effects on mood and sexuality, a patients' group (with professional input) has been set up in the UK (www.vul-pain.dircon.co.uk).

Vulval intraepithelial neoplasia

Vulval malignancy has a pre-invasive phase, vulval intra-epithelial neoplasia (VIN, fig 1, note white areas with surrounding inflammation). It may be itchy. Cause: often HPV, p269 (esp. HPV16); there may not be visible warts but 5% acetic acid stains affected areas white. If VIN is found on biopsy, examine cervix, anal canal if within 1.5cm,ᴿᴄᴼᴸ natal cleft skin and breasts (>10% have coexistent neoplasia elsewhere, most commonly cervical). *Treating VIN* Wide local excision is gold standard treatment of choice.ᴿᴄᴼᴸ Women should have access to reconstructive surgery afterwards, if needed. Histology reveals 12-17% unrecognized invasion in wide excision samples. There is higher response rates in women undergoing excision than in those undergoing medical treatment. Recurrences are

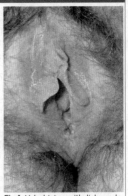

Fig 1. Vulval intra-epithelial neoplasia (VIN).

fewer if excision margins clear. Medical treatments have used 5% **imiquimod** cream with regression of grade 2–3 disease in 77%.[79] **Cidofovir** use is being studied. Laser therapy is useful for areas where surgery is contraindicated (eg in glans and clitoral hood). Laser treatment failures are ~40%. Therapeutic use of human papilloma virus vaccine, photodynamic therapy, interferon use, and cavitron ultrasonic surgical aspiration techniques have been tried but none are currently recommended treatments.ᴿᴄᴼᴸ Recurrence is common so follow-up regularly.

Vulval care for those with vulval disordersᴿᴄᴼᴸ

- Use soap substitute with water for washing (less drying than water alone).
- Shower, bath (with emollient), or clean vulva once daily only.
- Wash vulva with hand (not sponge/flannel); dab dry or blow dry with hair-dryer on cool setting held well away from the skin.
- Wear loose fitting silk or cotton white or light coloured underwear (blue/black dyes can be irritant). Sleep without underwear.
- Avoid tight jeans/cycling trousers but wear loose trousers, dresses or skirts. At home wearing skirts without underwear may be more comfortable.
- Avoid soap, bubble bath, shower gels, biological washing powders, fabric conditioners, vulval creams or douches, antiseptics, regular sanitary towel or panty liner wear, baby wipe use, coloured toilet paper, nail varnish.
- Regular emollient use (throughout day) can soothe and reduce flare ups.
- For irritated skin, dabbings of aqueous cream kept in the fridge can soothe.

Gynaecology

Causes of vulval lumps Local varicose veins; boils; sebaceous cysts; keratoacanthomata (rare); viral warts (condylomata acuminata); condylomata lata (syphilis); primary chancre; molluscum contagiosum; Bartholin's cyst or abscess; uterine prolapse or polyp; inguinal hernia; varicocele; carcinoma.

Vulval warts Human papilloma virus (HPV)—is usually spread by sexual contact. Incubation: weeks. Her partner may not have obvious penile warts. The vulva, perineum, anus, vagina, or cervix may be affected. Warts may be very florid in the pregnant and immunosuppressed. HPV types 16, 18, and 33 can cause vulval and cervical intra-epithelial neoplasia, so she needs annual cervical smears and observation of the vulva. Warts may also cause anal carcinoma (OHCM p633). Treat both partners. Exclude other genital infections. Warts may be destroyed by diathermy, cryocautery or laser. Vulval and anal warts (condylomata acuminata) may be treated weekly in surgeries and GU clinics with 15% podophyllin paint, washed off after 30min (CI: pregnancy). Only treat a few warts at once, to avoid toxicity. Self-application with 0.15% podophyllotoxin cream (Warticon® 5g tubes—enough for 4 treatment courses—is supplied with a mirror): use every 12h for 3 days, repeated up to 4 times at weekly intervals if the area covered is <4cm². Relapse is common. *HPV immunization and cervical cancer:* See p272. NB: HPV types 6 and 11 may cause laryngeal or respiratory papillomas in the offspring of affected mothers (risk 1 : 50–1 : 1500; 50% present at <5yrs old). Any warty lesion in a post-menopausal woman should be biopsied to exclude vulval cancer.[80][RCOL]

Exclude other genital infections. Treat both partners.

Urethral caruncle This is a small red swelling at the urethral orifice. It is caused by meatal prolapse. It may be tender and give pain on micturition. *Treatment:* Excision or diathermy.

Bartholin's cyst and abscess The Bartholin's glands and ducts lie under the labia minora. They secrete thin lubricating mucus during sexual excitation. If the duct blocks a painless cyst forms; if this becomes infected the resulting abscess is extremely painful (she cannot sit down) and a hugely swollen, hot red labium is seen. *Treatment:* The abscess should be incised, and permanent drainage ensured by marsupialization, ie inner cyst wall is folded back and stitched to the skin, or by balloon catheter insertion.[RICE] *Tests:* Exclude gonococcus.

Vulvitis Vulval inflammation may be due to infections, eg candida (p284), herpes simplex; chemicals (bubble-baths, detergents). It is often associated with, or may be due to, vaginal discharge.

Causes of vulval ulcers: Always consider syphilis. *Herpes simplex* is common in the young. Others: carcinoma; chancroid; lymphogranuloma venereum; granuloma inguinale; TB; Behçet's syndrome; aphthous ulcers; Crohn's disease.

Herpes simplex Herpes type II, sexually acquired, classically causes genital infection, but type I transferred from cold sores can be the cause. The vulva is ulcerated and exquisitely painful. Urinary retention may occur. *Treatment:* Strong analgesia, lidocaine gel 2%, salt baths (and micturating in the bath) help. Exclude coexistent infections. Aciclovir topically and orally shortens symptoms and infectivity. Oral dose: 200mg 5 times daily or 400mg/8h for 5 days (longer if new lesions appear during treatment or if healing is incomplete). If immunocompromized/HIV+ve: 400mg 5 times daily for 7–10 days during 1st episode or 400mg/8h for 5–10 days during recurrent infection.

Reassure that subsequent attacks are shorter and less painful. Prescribe aciclovir cream for use when symptoms start. For herpes in pregnancy, see p36.

Gynaecology

Carcinoma of the vulva ►Refer unexplained vulval lumps urgently.
90% are squamous. Others are melanoma, basal cell carcinomas or carcinoma of Bartholin's glands. They are rare and usually occur in the elderly (age 70–80).

Presentation may be as a lump; as an indurated ulcer which may not be noticed unless it causes pain and bleeding hence often presenting late (50% already have inguinal lymph node involvement). There may be a pre-invasive phase as VIN (for explanation and treatment see p267).

Treatment[80] If tumour <2cm width and <1mm deep node excision is not needed. If >1mm deep do 'triple incision surgery' =wide (>15mm margin) local excision + ipsilateral groin node biopsy (and, if affected, sample contralateral side too). More advanced disease may need radical vulvectomy (wide excision of the vulva + removal of inguinal glands). Skin grafts may be needed. Radiotherapy may be used pre-op to shrink tumours if sphincters may be affected. Chemoradiation is used if unsuitable for surgery, to shrink large tumours pre-operatively and for relapses. 5-yr survival is >80% for lesions <2cm with no node involvement; otherwise <50%.

This is the part of the uterus below the internal os. The endocervical canal is lined with mucous columnar epithelium, the vaginal cervix with squamous epithelium. The transition zone between them—the squamo–columnar junction—is the area which is predisposed to malignant change.

Cervical ectropion/erosion (see fig 1; an alarming term for a normal phenomenon). There is a red ring around the os because the endocervical epithelium has extended its territory over the paler epithelium of the ectocervix. Ectropions extend temporarily under hormonal influence during puberty, with the combined Pill, and during pregnancy. As columnar epithelium is soft and glandular, ectropion is prone to bleeding, to excess mucus production, and to infection. *Treatment:* Cryocautery will treat these if they are a nuisance; otherwise no treatment is required.

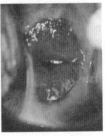
Fig 1. Cervical ectropion.
Courtesy of Mike Hughey.

Nabothian cysts These mucus retention cysts found on the cervix are harmless. *Treatment:* Cryocautery if they are discharging.

Cervical polyps These pedunculated benign tumours of endocervical epithelium may cause increased mucus discharge or postcoital bleeding. *Treatment:* In young women they may be simply avulsed, but in older women treatment usually includes D&C to exclude intrauterine pathology.

Cervicitis This may be follicular or mucopurulent, presenting with discharge. *Causes:* Chlamydia (up to 50%), gonococci, or herpes (look for vesicles). Chronic cervicitis (see fig 2) is usually a mixed infection and may respond to antibacterial cream. Cervicitis may mask neoplasia on a smear.

Cervical screening Cervical cancer has a preinvasive phase: cervical intra-epithelial neoplasia (CIN—not to be pronounced 'sin'). CIN 1 affects the lower basal third of cervical epithelium. Associated with oncogenic human papilloma viruses (HPV) 6 and 11, it commonly regresses (57%). CIN II and CIN III affect <⅔ and >⅔ or full thickness of epithelium respectively, are associated with the more oncogenic HPV viruses types 16, 18, (p272) are

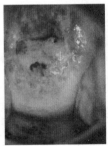
Fig 2. Chronic cervicitis.
Courtesy of Mike Hughey.

less likely to regress (43%, 32% respectively) and a significant number develop into invasive squamous carcinoma of the cervix. Papanicolaou smears collect cervical cells for microscopy for dyskaryosis (abnormalities which reflect CIN). A smear therefore identifies women who need cervical biopsy. The degree of dyskaryosis approximates to the severity of CIN (*Table*, p273). CIN III lesions tend to progress to invasive carcinoma. This may take ~10yrs, but may happen much faster in young women.

In the UK the 1st smear is taken at aged 25, then 3-yearly until 49, 5-yearly from 50 to 64 (only screen after 65 if one of the last 3 was abnormal). HIV +ve women should have annual smears. Those most at risk are the hardest to trace and persuade to have screening, eg older women, smokers, and those in inner cities. 83% of the eligible UK population is now screened, and mortality is 50% that of 1988 (the year screening started); this depends critically on being able to retain skilled lab staff.

- Explain the nature and purpose of the test, and how results will be conveyed. Warn that results are not always unequivocal.
- The cervix is visualized with a speculum (p242). Are there any suspicious areas? If so, carry on with the smear and indicate this on the referral form, but do not wait for its results before arranging further care.
- Cells are scraped from the squamo-columnar transformation zone with a special spatula or brush, then transferred to a slide and fixed at once.
- Liquid-based cytology (LBC)[82] involves rinsing the sampler or detaching its head into a vial of liquid creating a cell suspension from which slides are prepared which are quicker and easier to screen than conventional smears.
- Suspensions can also be tested for human papilloma virus (see p273) and chlamydia. Inadequate smear rates are reduced with LBC.
- Ensure regular training and supervision, and audit of numbers of 'inadequate sample' reports. Don't do smears on a one-off basis (in the UK NHS, professionalism mandates formal methods of quality control, and specifies an acceptable number of smears per year, etc).

Automatic analysers can identify areas of slides likely to be of interest to cytologists.[83] Good technique is needed (make sure that all 4 quadrants of the cervix are sampled): ►learn by instruction from an expert at the couch.

Gynaecology

𝕏𝕏𝕏 *Aim to detect pre-invasive disease.* ~1900 women die yearly of cervical cancer in the UK. The main cause is human papilloma virus (eg HPV 16, 18, 31, 33, 35, 39, 45, 51, 52, 56, 58, 59, 68). Vaccines work only against a subset, eg **Gardasil®**[1] covers HPV 16 & 18, the cause in 70% of cases. (99.7% of cervical cancers contain HPV DNA.)

Prolonged Pill use may be an important co-factor (may ↑risk 4-fold in those +ve for HPV DNA).[84] Other risk factors: high parity; many (>4) sexual partners or a partner with many other partners (especially if that male is uncircumcised);[85] early first coitus; HIV; other STDs; smoking.

Management of abnormal smears (See p273) the histology of cervical intra-epithelial neoplasia (CIN) is explained there.) Either a repeat smear or colposcopy and biopsy are needed, depending on likelihood of the smear reflecting CIN III or small-volume invasive disease (<3mm).

▶Abnormal smears may cause anxiety and guilt. Explain. Give support.

Treating pre-invasive cancer Examine the cervix by colposcope (×10 binocular microscope). Abnormal epithelium has characteristic blood vessel patterns and stains white with acetic acid. Take punch biopsies for histology. CIN is destroyed by cryotherapy, laser, cold coagulation, or large loop excision of transformation zone (LLETZ). These give ~90% cure rates with one treatment. She needs annual smears for at least 10yrs. If the squamo–columnar junction cannot be seen, or if small-volume invasive carcinoma is found on histology, the abnormal tissue is removed by cone biopsy, which may be curative. Colposcopy does not detect adenocarcinoma (it usually lies within endocervical canal).

Invasive disease Most are squamous cancers. 15–30% are adenocarcinomas (from endocervical epithelium), especially affecting women under 40. Spread is local and lymphatic.

Stage I tumours are confined to the cervix.
Stage II have extended locally to upper ⅔ of the vagina; *IIb* if to parametria.
Stage III have spread to lower ⅓ of vagina *IIIa*; or pelvic wall *IIIb*.
Stage IV have spread to bladder or rectum. *IVb* if spread to distant organs. Most present in stages I or II.

Diagnosis ▶Overt carcinoma is rarely detected on a smear. Non-menstrual bleeding is the classic symptom. The early tumour is firm. It grows as a friable mass which bleeds on contact. Use CT/MRI to stage; positron emission tomography if unsuitable for surgery detects para-aortic node metastases and may modify treatment regimes.[19]

Treating invasive cancers[86] Stage Ia1 (microscopic lesions, invasion <3mm) may be treated by cervical conization in those wishing to preserve fertility, extrafascial hysterectomy for those with completed families. Radical hysterectomy with pelvic lymphadenectomy or radiotherapy is used for stage Ia2 (microscopic, invasion 3–5mm depth <7mm horizontally) disease and some stage Ib1 (macroscopic, tumour <4cm). Chemoradiation is the 'gold standard' for most stage Ib, II or bulky stage II disease. It is also used for stage III and IV disease. Use of chemotherapy in advanced and recurrent disease is palliative. The main chemotherapy agent is **cisplatin**. Adding **topotecan** for recurrent, resistant or metastatic disease increases survival time, but with increased toxicity.[87] Pelvic exenteration (p309) is sometimes used in stage IVa disease. Cure rates for stages I (80% 5-yr survival) and II (60%). Radiotherapy causes vaginal stenosis, so encourage intercourse within 2 months of treatment (+lubricant). Follow-up: annual smears. Smears are of no value after radical radiotherapy. Terminal problems are pain, fistulae, and GI/GU obstruction.

---

1 Gardasil® targets HPV6, 11, 16 & 18. 3 IM does, 0.5mL (deltoid/lateral thigh). Age range: 9–18yrs (9–26♀♥). Dose 2 is ≥1 month after dose 1, and dose 3 ≥4 months after dose 1. CI: pregnancy, bleeding disorders. **Cervarix®** (bivalent; HPV16 & 18). Unanswered questions: How long does protection last? Should boys be vaccinated too? Will the ecospace created be populated by new carcinogenic strains of HPV?[88–90]

Histology of cervical pre-malignant disease		CIN=cervical intra-epithelial neoplasia
Papanicolaou class	**Action**	**Histology**
I Normal	Repeat in 3 years (Unless clinical suspicion)	0.1% CIN II–III
II Inflammatory	Take swab; treat infection Repeat in 6 months (Colposcopy after 3 abnormal)	6% CIN II–III
Mild atypia	Repeat in 4 months (Colposcopy after 2 abnormal)	20–37% CIN II–III
III Mild dyskaryosis	HPV test ± Colposcopy	20–30% CIN II–III
Moderate dyskaryosis	Colposcopy	50–75% CIN II–III
IV Severe dyskaryosis	Colposcopy	80–90% CIN II–III
'Positive'		5% invasion
'Malignant cells'		
V Invasion suspected	Urgent colposcopy	50% invasion
Abnormal glandular cells	Urgent colposcopy	?Adenoca cervix or endometrial ca

CIN I =mild dysplasia; CIN II=moderate dysplasia; CIN III=severe dysplasia/ *carcinoma-in-situ.*

The table above shows comparative terms and the recommended action. The third column, headed histology, shows the percentage of smears in each Papanicolaou (cytological) class which have more serious lesions (CIN II or III) on histology. With inflammatory smears, swabs should be taken and any infection treated. 6% of inflammatory smears have serious pathology, hence the recommendation for colposcopy if inflammation persists.

Borderline nuclear abnormality (BNA) implies doubt as to the neoplastic nature of any change.

Human papilloma virus (HPV) test From 2012 UK screening tests smears with borderline nuclear change and mild dyskaryosis for presence of oncogenic human papilloma viruses (HPV) This is referred to as HPV triage. The 20% that are HPV positive are then referred for colposcopy. Those negative for HPV return to normal screening (p270). For those having colposcopy, if CIN1 not requiring treatment is found, they will be resmeared (± colposcopy) after 1 year. If that smear has borderline nuclear change or mild dyskaryosis the sample will again be HPV triaged, and further colposcopy arranged if it is HPV positive; if that smear is HPV negative women return to routine follow-up. Women with CIN1, CIN2 or CIN3 requiring treatment are resmeared 6 months after treatment, and if the result is normal, or has borderline nuclear change and mild dyskaryosis, that sample is also HPV tested (this stage is referred to as test of cure). If HPV positive, further colposcopy is arranged and follow-up will follow national guidelines (eg annual smears for 10 years); if HPV negative, women will have a recall after 3 years. If that one is normal women over 50 years return to 5-year recall.

In the UK, 6×10^6 smears are done per year on women up to 65yrs old, and cervical cancer deaths have fallen by 15% in recent years to <1900/yr. The incidence of cervical cancer in England and Wales fell by 42% between 1988 and 1997. Cervical screening is thought to prevent 2000 deaths/year in the UK.[91.RCOL] 2.4% of smears show mild dyskaryosis, and 2.2% have BNA.

Terminology used in reporting smears changed in the 1980s, and different countries use different nomenclature—eg the Bethesda system.

Endometritis Uterine infection is uncommon unless the barrier to ascending infection (acid vaginal pH and cervical mucus) is broken, eg after miscarriage, TOP and childbirth, IUCD insertion, or surgery. Infection may involve Fallopian tubes and ovaries.

Presentation: Lower abdominal pain and fever; uterine tenderness on bimanual palpation. Low-grade infection is often due to chlamydia. *Tests:* Do cervical swabs and blood cultures. *Treatment:* Give antibiotics (eg **doxycycline** 100mg/12h PO with **metronidazole** 500mg/8h PO, eg for 7 days).

Endometrial proliferation Oestrogen stimulates endometrial proliferation in the first half of the menstrual cycle; it is then influenced by progesterone and is shed at menstruation. A particularly exuberant proliferation is associated with heavy menstrual bleeding and polyps.

Continuous high oestrogen levels (eg anovulatory cycles) make the endometrium hyperplastic ('cystic glandular hyperplasia'—a histological diagnosis after D&C). It eventually breaks down, causing irregular bleeding (dysfunctional uterine bleeding). *Treatment:* Cyclical progestogens (p253).

In older women proliferation may contain foci of atypical cells which may lead to endometrial carcinoma (p278).

Pyometra This is a uterus distended by pus eg associated with salpingitis or secondary to outflow blockage. *Treatment:* Drain the uterus, treat the cause.

Haematometra This is a uterus filled with blood due to outflow obstruction. It is rare. The blockage may be an imperforate hymen in the young (p246); carcinoma; or iatrogenic cervical stenosis, eg after cone biopsy.

Endometrial tuberculosis Genital tract tuberculosis is rare in Britain, except among high-risk groups (eg immigrants). It is blood-borne and usually affects first the Fallopian tubes, then the endometrium.

It may present with acute salpingitis if disease is very active, or with subfertility, pelvic pain, and menstrual disorders (40%) eg amenorrhoea, oligomenorrhoea. There may be pyosalpinx. Send peritoneal fluid at laparoscopy, and/ or endometrial curettings for culture and histology. Exclude lung disease by CXR. *Treatment* is medical with antituberculous therapy (OHCM p398–9). Repeat endometrial histology after 1 year. Total abdominal hysterectomy with bilateral salpingo-oophorectomy is treatment of choice if there are adnexal masses and the woman is >40yrs.[92]

Uterine ultrasound[93] Transvaginal ultrasound gives better resolution than transabdominal. Homogeneity, echoes of low intensity and presence of a linear central shadow are associated with absence of endometrial abnormality.

Normal cycle thickness: <5mm early cycle, 11mm in proliferative phase; 7-16mm late cycle. Endometrial cancer is suggested by endometrial thickness >20mm (>5mm if postmenopausal not on hormones), heterogeneous appearance, and hypoechoic areas. Polyps have cystic appearance (also with hyperechoic endometrium) and are most clearly seen in the early days of the cycle.

If postmenopausal and not on HRT, double-layer endometrial thickness should be <5mm (if perimenopausal <5mm on day 5 of cycle). Sequential hormone replacement ↑endometrial thickness (average 5–8.5mm); if on continuous combined replacement HRT thicknesses are ~4.5–7mm; tibolone treated endometrium <5mm; but tamoxifen thickens it to ~13mm (also associated with endometrial polyps, often large, usually benign). It thins down by 6 months after stopping tamoxifen, then stays thin.[94]

Ultrasound is useful for detecting fibroids and assessing cystic change in rapidly growing fibroids to assess risk of malignant change.

Gynaecology

These tumours are usually squamous. They are commonest in the upper third of the vagina. Presentation is usually with bleeding. Clear cell adenocarcinoma is associated with intrauterine exposure to diethylstilboestrol before 18 weeks' gestation but risk is low (0.1–1:1000). (Note: risk of invasive cervical carcinoma is also increased 3-fold, and structural abnormalities of the genital tract—uterine 69% and cervical 44%—are problems following past exposure).[95][RCOG] Spread is local and by lymphatics. Treatment is usually radiotherapy. Prognosis is poor eg 58% 5-yr survival for squamous vaginal carcinoma; 34% for adenocarcinoma.[96]

Fibroids are benign smooth muscle tumours of the uterus (leiomyomas) (fig 1. p240). They are often multiple, and vary in size from seedling size to tumours occupying a large part of the abdomen. They start as lumps in the wall of the uterus but may grow to bulge out of the wall so that they lie under the peritoneum (subserosal, 20%) or under the endometrium (submucosal, 5%), or become pedunculated. Fibroids are common (20% of women have fibroids), increasing in frequency with age and in non-Caucasians.

Associations Mutation in the gene for fumarate hydratase can cause fibroids and a rare association with skin & uterine leiomyomata, and renal cell cancer.[1][97]

Natural history Fibroids are oestrogen-dependent. Consequently they enlarge in pregnancy and on the combined Pill and atrophy after the menopause. They may degenerate gradually or suddenly (red degeneration). Occasionally they calcify ('womb stones'). Rarely, they undergo sarcomatous change—usually causing pain, malaise, bleeding, and increase in size in a postmenopausal woman.

Presentation Many are asymptomatic.
- *Menorrhagia:* Fibroids often produce heavy and prolonged periods (± anaemia, eg dyspnoea etc). They do not generally cause intermenstrual or post-menopausal bleeding.
- *Fertility problems:* Submucosal fibroids may interfere with implantation ('natural IUCD'). Large or multiple tumours which distort the uterine cavity may cause miscarriage should pregnancy occur.
- *Pain:* This may be due to torsion of a pedunculated fibroid, producing symptoms similar to that of a torted ovarian cyst. 'Red degeneration' following thrombosis of the fibroid blood supply: see OPPOSITE.
- *Mass:* Large fibroids may be felt abdominally. They may press on the bladder, causing frequency, or on the veins, causing oedematous legs and varicose veins. Pelvic fibroids may obstruct labour or cause retention of urine.

Treatment In many women, no treatment is needed.

Menorrhagia due to fibroids tends to respond poorly to anti-prostaglandins, progestogens, or danazol. If the uterine cavity is not too distorted a Mirena® intrauterine device can be used and may decrease fibroid size. Women who have completed their families may opt for *hysterectomy*. In younger women, a reversible menopausal state may be induced with analogues of LHRH (luteinizing hormone releasing hormone), eg **goserelin** (better than buserelin[2]). A single dose of 10.8mg sc reduces bulk by ≥50%.[98] Bone demineralization can occur, but is ameliorated by concurrent **raloxifene**[99] or **tibolone**.[100] They may be used pre-op to reduce fibroid bulk; in those unfit for surgery; or those desiring later pregnancy. Side effects are menopausal symptoms. Fertility (and fibroids) return when drugs are stopped.

Alternatively, fibroids may be surgically shelled out (*myomectomy*). Complications: torrential bleeding needing hysterectomy; post-op adhesions. Pregnancy rates can be ~50% post-op.[101] Laparoscopic surgery ± laser use is possible but needs much patience. Myomectomy is the treatment of choice in subfertility. *Embolizing fibroids* (interventional radiology) can shrink them, so resolving menorrhagia. This involves only a short hospital stay, but it is not widely available. It can be very painful. Fibroid bulk reduces by 30–46%.[102] 20–44% will require further surgery. Chance of successful pregnancy is better after myomectomy.[103]

Red degeneration requires only analgesia until symptoms settle.

Torsion may resemble an acute abdomen, requiring urgent surgery.

---

1 Gene location: 1q42.3–q43.
2 Buserelin nasal spray 100µg/4h is expensive and intermittent use may cause fibroid size to *increase*.

Fibroids in pregnancy

5:1000 Caucasian women have fibroids in pregnancy. They are commoner in Afro-Caribbean women. They may cause miscarriage. They increase in size in pregnancy—especially in the 2nd trimester. Ultrasound aids diagnosis. Colour flow Doppler distinguishes fibroids from myometrium.[104] If pedunculated they may tort. Red degeneration is when thrombosis of capsular vessels is followed by venous engorgement and inflammation, causing abdominal pain (± vomiting & low-grade fever), and localized peritoneal tenderness—usually in the last half of pregnancy or the puerperium. 'Here, a certain feverishness leads them to their final degeneration', and imitating the course of all grand passions, 'they grow big and tender, and then die' *D.H. Lawrence 'Sons & Lovers p324*

Treatment is expectant (bed rest, analgesia) with resolution over 4–7 days.

Most fibroids arise from the body of the uterus and do not therefore obstruct labour, as they tend to rise away from the pelvis throughout pregnancy. If large pelvic masses of fibroids are noted prior to labour, caesarean section should be planned. Obstruction of labour also needs caesarean section.

▶*Investigate postmenopausal vaginal bleeding
promptly as the cause may be endometrial cancer.*
Cancer of the uterine body is less common than
cancer of the cervix. It usually presents after the
menopause. Most are adenocarcinomas, and are
related to excessive exposure to oestrogen unopposed by progesterone. There is marked geographical variation: North American:Chinese ratio ≈7:1.

Risk factors
• Obesity[1]
• Unopposed oestrogen R_x
• Functioning ovarian tumour
• FH of breast, ovary, or colon cancer
• Nulliparity
• Late menopause
• Diabetes mellitus
• Tamoxifen,[2] tibolone[105]
• Pelvic irradiation
• Polycystic ovaries[106]

Presentation This is usually as postmenopausal
bleeding (PMB). A woman with a history of PMB
has a 10–20% risk of genital cancer. It is initially
scanty and occasional (± watery discharge). Then
bleeding gets heavy and frequent. Premenopausal
women may have intermenstrual bleeding, but 30% have only menorrhagia.

Diagnosis Postmenopausal bleeding is an early sign, and generally leads
a woman to see her doctor, and examination is usually normal. Endometrial
carcinoma can sometimes be seen on a smear. Uterine ultrasound may be suggestive (p274). The diagnosis is made by uterine sampling (p279) or curettage.
All parts of the uterine cavity must be sampled; send *all* material for histology. Hysteroscopy enables visualization of abnormal endometrium to improve
accuracy of sampling. Sceptics claim it may cause spread through the Fallopian tubes to the peritoneum. NB: hysteroscopy requires dilatation of the os
which may prove impossible (**misoprostol** 1mg PV self-administered the night
before surgery helps, but occasionally causes severe pelvic pain).[107]

Pathology Most tumours start in the fundus, and spread slowly to the uterine muscle, cervix and/or peritoneum. They may
metastasize to the vagina (5%), ovary (5%),
or any of the pelvic lymph nodes (7%).

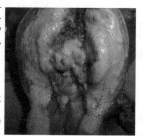

Staging (fig 1) The tumour is...
  I   in the body of the uterus only
  II in the body and cervix only
  III advancing beyond the uterus, but
      not beyond the pelvis
  IV extending outside the pelvis (eg to
      bowel and bladder).

Treatment Stages I and II may be cured
by total **hysterectomy** with bilateral **sal-
pingo-oophorectomy** and/or **radiotherapy** if unfit for surgery (5-yr survival:
stage I ≈72%, stage II ≈56%). Post-operative vault irradiation reduces vault
recurrence.[3] In advanced disease consider radiotherapy and/or high-dose
progestogens, eg **medroxyprogesterone** acetate 200mg/24h PO, which shrinks
the tumour (SE: fluid retention). Radiotherapy may be given either pre-operatively (caesium or radium rods inserted into the uterus and upper vagina) or
post-operatively (external radiation).

Fig 1. Uterine cancer (≥ stage II).
Courtesy of Prof. J. Carter.

Recurrent disease usually presents in the 1st 2–3yrs; common sites: pelvic
(in non-irradiated patients), lung, bone, inguinal/supraclavicular nodes, vagina,
liver, peritoneal cavity. **Medroxyprogesterone**, surgical exenteration ± radiotherapy may be tried. **Cytotoxics** may be used if unresponsive to the above.

---

1 BMI >25 doubles risk; BMI >30 trebles risk.
2 Note: **tamoxifen** 20mg daily ↓annual risk of breast cancer recurrence by 27%. Risk of endometrial
cancer from taking tamoxifen is 1.2 per 1000 person-yrs. Counsel to report abnormal vaginal bleeding.
3 NNT=16.8 to prevent 1 local recurrence; not needed if low risk type of stage 1 disease. Cochrane.[108]

Endometrial sampling in outpatients

This bedside investigation is used for postmenopausal bleeding, perimeno-pausal irregular bleeding, and unexpected bleeding patterns in women on hormone replacement therapy because it is cheap, reliable, and gives quick results without the need for anaesthesia. If transvaginal uterine ultrasound precedes the procedure, sample if endometrium >5mm thick. It is less useful in menorrhagia in women with regular cycles, as pathology is less common. It is not indicated if <35 years old.

A sample is obtained using a side-opening plastic cannula in which a vac-uum is created by withdrawal of a stopped central plunger mechanism. As the cannula is withdrawn and rotated in each quadrant of the uterine cav-ity, endometrial tissue is sucked into its interior, through the hole in its side (fig 1). Successful insertion is possible in 90–99% of women (D&C possible in 99%). Adequate samples will be obtained in 91% of these, and in 84% of those for whom postmenopausal bleeding (PMB) was the indication. Abandon the procedure if it is impossible to enter the uterus, or if it causes too much pain.

Technique

1 Bimanual examination to assess size and position of uterus (p242).
2 Bend cervical cannula to follow the curve of the uterus.
3 Insert device, watching the centimetre scale on the side; observe resist-ance on entering the internal os (at 3–4cm) and then as the tip reaches the fundus (eg at 6cm if postmenopausal or 8cm in an oestrogenized uterus).
4 When the tip is in the fundus, create a vacuum by withdrawing plunger until the stopper prevents further withdrawal. Then move sampler up and down in the uterus, rotate and repeat to sample whole cavity.
5 Remove cannula, and expel tissue into formalin. Send for histology. Vabra vacuum aspiration samples a greater area of tissue, and has higher cancer detection rates, but is more uncomfortable.[109]

Management Reassure those in whom the results show normal or atrophic endometrium and those in whom tissue was sufficient for diagnosis. If those with PMB re-bleed refer for hysteroscopy (polyps or a fibroid will be present in 20%). Those with simple hyperplasia on histology can be treated with cy-clical progesterones (but refer if >55yrs to search for exogenous oestrogen source). Refer those with polyps or necrotic tissue on histology for hyster-oscopy and curettage, and those with atypical hyperplasia or carcinoma for hysterectomy and bilateral salpingo-oophorectomy. If transvaginal uterine ultrasound is not already done, perform in those on whom the procedure was impossible or abandoned to establish endometrial thickness (<5mm normal in the postmenopausal; refer if >5mm thick or if polyps seen, for hysteroscopy and curettage).

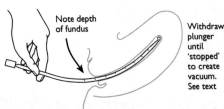

Note depth of fundus

Withdraw plunger until 'stopped' to create vacuum. See text

Fig 1. Endometrial sampling.[82]   Redrawn from information supplied by Genesis Medical.

Gynaecology

Any of the ovary's many tissue types may become neoplastic.

Benign tumours (94%). They are usually cystic. 24% of all ovarian tumours are functional cysts. Others: endometriotic cysts (5%—p288); theca-lutein cysts (p264); epithelial cell tumours (serous and mucinous cystadenomas—40%); mature teratomas (from germ cells—20%); fibromas (solid—5%).

Malignant tumours (6%). 5% are cystadenomas which have become malignant. 0.5% are a group of rare germ cell or sex cord malignancies (p281). 0.5% are secondaries, eg from the uterus or the stomach (Krukenberg tumours—in which spread is transcoelomic, ie in the case of the abdomen, via the peritoneum). *Risk markers of ovarian malignancy:* Nulliparity (risk↑ × 1.5); subfertility; early menarche; +ve family history (p283); no past use of the Pill (by 50%).

Presentations are varied, depending on size, form, and histological type:

Asymptomatic—chance finding (eg on doing a bimanual for a smear test).

Swollen abdomen—with palpable mass arising out of the pelvis which is dull to percussion (and does not disappear if the bladder is catheterized).

Pressure effects (eg on bladder, causing urinary frequency).

Infarction/haemorrhage—this mimics torsion (see below).

Rupture ± local peritonism. Rupture of a large cyst may cause peritonitis and shock. Rupture of a malignant cyst may disseminate malignant cells throughout the abdomen. Rupture of mucinous cystadenomas may disseminate cells which continue to secrete mucin and cause death by binding up the viscera (pseudomyxoma peritonei). See p281. Pseudomyxoma peritonei is treated by surgical debulking. 10-year survival is 30–50%.

Ascites—shifting dullness suggests malignancy or Meigs' syndrome (see BOX). If tense, ascites may be hard to distinguish from a mass.

Torsion—to twist, a tumour must be on a pedicle. Twisting occludes the venous return but the arterial supply continues to engorge the tumour, and causes great pain (with a high WBC). Tumours may twist and untwist, giving a history of intermittent pain. If the pain is not too severe, a firm tender adnexal swelling may be felt.

Endocrine or metastatic effects—Hormone-secreting tumours may cause virilization, menstrual irregularities, or postmenopausal bleeding.

Management *Ultrasound* may confirm the presence of a mass and may show whether it is cystic or solid.

Laparoscopy may distinguish a cyst from an ectopic pregnancy or appendicitis. Note: laparoscopy is not advised if malignancy is possible, due to seeding along the surgical tract. *Fine-needle aspiration* may be used to confirm the impression that a cyst is benign. Urgent *laparotomy* is required when a cyst problem presents as an acute abdomen.

Any cyst not positively identified as non-neoplastic should be removed, as seemingly benign tumours may be malignant. In younger women *cystectomy* may be preferable to oophorectomy. In postmenopausal women, if one ovary is pathological both ovaries and the uterus are removed. For guidelines for investigation and treatment of tumours in postmenopausal women see p282. For management in pregnancy see p282.

Functional cysts These are enlarged or persistent follicular or corpus lu-teum cysts. They are so common that they may be considered normal if they are small (<5cm). They may cause pain by rupture, failing to rupture at ovu-lation, or bleeding. If <5cm they usually resolve over 2-3 cycles.

Serous cystadenomas These develop papillary growths that may be so pro-lific that the cyst appears solid. They are commonest in women aged 30–40 years. About 30% are bilateral and about 30% are malignant.

Mucinous cystadenomas The commonest large ovarian tumours; these may become enormous. They are filled with mucinous material and rupture may rarely cause pseudomyxoma peritonei (p280). They may be multilocu-lar. They are commonest in the 30–50 age group. About 5% will be malig-nant. Remove the appendix at operation in those with suspected mucinous cystadenoma and send for histology. (Interestingly men can get pseudo-myxoma from intestinal or appendicular neoplasms; most women with pseu-domyxoma peritonei do not have overt rupture of ovarian tumours and 90% have concurrent intestinal or appendicular tumours and it is now thought that the ovarian tumours may be secondary to GI tumours.)

Fibromas These are small, solid, benign, fibrous tissue tumours. They are as-sociated with Meigs' syndrome: pleural effusion, often right sided + benign ovarian fibroma (or thecoma, cystadenoma, granulosa cell tumour) + ascites.

Teratomas These arise from primitive germ cells. A benign mature terato-ma (dermoid cyst) may contain well-differentiated tissue, eg hair, teeth. 20% are bilateral. They are most common in young women. Poorly differentiated malignant teratomas are rare.

Other germ cell tumours (all malignant and all rare) Non-gestational cho-riocarcinomas (secrete HCG); ectodermal sinus tumours (yolk sac tumours—secrete α-fetoprotein); dysgerminomas.

Sex-cord tumours (rare; usually of low-grade malignancy) These arise from cortical mesenchyme. Granulosa-cell and theca-cell tumours produce oes-trogen and may present with precocious puberty, menstrual problems, or postmenopausal bleeding. Arrhenoblastomas secrete androgens.

Symptoms suggestive of ovarian cancer[100][NICE]

- 'Bloating', abdominal distension
- Early satiety
- Loss of appetite
- Unexplained weight loss
- Change of bowel habit
- Fatigue
- Onset of 'irritable bowel' symptoms age >50 years
- Urinary frequency or urgency
- Abdominal or pelvic pain

Examine: if pelvic mass or ascites refer under 2-week rule to gynaecology. Check CA-125 (cancer antigen 125), (and α-fetoprotein (αFP), β-human chori-onic gonadotrophin (βHCG) if <40yrs to identify women who may not have ovarian epithelial cancer). See above. Ovarian epithelial cancers are ad-enocarcinomas. If CA-125 is >35 IU/mL arrange urgent abdominal and pelvic ultrasound. If ultrasound suggests ovarian cancer refer under 2-week rule to gynaecology. If ultrasound has suggested cancer arrange staging CT of abdomen (±chest) in secondary care.

These are found in ~1/1000 pregnancies. It is easier to distinguish them (lying as they do in the rectovaginal pouch) with an anteverted uterus than with a gravid retroverted uterus. Suspicion of presence of a tumour can be confirmed by ultrasound. Torsion of ovarian cysts is more common in pregnancy and the puerperium than at other times. Cyst rupture and haemorrhage into cysts may also occur, but not more commonly than at other times. Torsion may present with abdominal pain, nausea, vomiting, shock, local tenderness (usually at 8–16 weeks). 2–5% of tumours are malignant. Suspect malignancy with ruptures (then biopsy other ovary). ~25% of malignant tumours will be dysgerminomas.

Tumours can become necrotic due to pressure on them in labour. Tumours lying in the pelvis can obstruct labour so caesarean section will be needed unless they are cysts which can be aspirated under ultrasound control before labour.

Asymptomatic simple cysts <5cm across can be left until after delivery if watched by ultrasound. Those 5–10cm may be aspirated under ultrasound control (and the aspirate examined cytologically). Other tumours (those that are complex multilocular or with solid portions on ultrasound) should be removed at about 16 weeks' gestation (by which time the pregnancy is not dependent on the corpus luteum and miscarriage is less likely) to exclude carcinoma and prevent complications developing. If the diagnosis is made late in pregnancy and the tumour is not obstructing the pelvis, it is usual to let labour progress normally, and to remove the tumour in the early puerperium because of the risk of torsion then.

Postmenopausal ovarian tumours

The aim is to identify those with high risk of cancer for treatment at special cancer centres. 21% of postmenopausal women have cysts on screening ultrasound. Ultrasound is 89% sensitive and 73% specific for detecting cancer. CA-125 (p283) estimations 81% and 75% respectively. A CA-125 >30u/mL is +ve in 80% of malignancies (but in only 50% stage I). Risk of malignancy (RMI) can be calculated with the formula below. RMI <25 has a cancer risk <3%, risk is 75% if RMI > 250 (manage these high-risk women at a cancer centre).

RMI=U × M × CA-125 (M=3; CA-125 is the number for u/mL; U is 1 if ultrasound score=1, and 3 if ultrasound score 2–5.) To calculate ultrasound score add 1 for each of the following ultrasound features: multilocular cyst; solid area in cyst; bilateral lesions; evidence of metastases; ascites present.[RCOG][111]

Unilocular cysts <5cm with a normal CA-125 can be managed conservatively (ultrasound every 4 months for 1 year). Low-risk cysts may be removed at bilateral laparoscopic oophorectomy (if suitable for laparoscopic treatment). Postmenopausal cysts should not be aspirated. High-risk cysts need optimal surgical staging ie total abdominal hysterectomy + bilateral salpingo-oophorectomy + infracolic omentectomy at a cancer centre with cytology of ascites and washings, + biopsy of suspicious (eg peritoneal) areas/adhesions (random biopsy if none suspicious), + retroperitoneal lymph node assessment, (biopsy palpably abnormal para-aortic or pelvic wall nodes or random samples if none palpable).

This is rare, but more women die from it (it is the 5th commonest cause of cancer-related death in UK women) than from carcinoma of the cervix and uterine body combined because in ~80% it causes few symptoms until it has metastasized, often to the pelvis with omental and peritoneal seedlings (± lymphatic spread via the para-aortic nodes). Overall 5-yr survival <35%.

Incidence 1 in 2500 women >55yrs; 1 in 3800 if >25yrs. If *2 close relatives* affected lifetime ovarian cancer risk is 40% (liaise with a gynaecologist; see below). 10% of affected North American women carry mutations in *BRCA1* or *BRCA2* genes. Carrier risk of developing carcinoma is 40% for women with *BRCA1* mutation, 25% if *BRCA2*. It is commoner in those with many ovulations (*late menopause, nullipara*) and, possibly, after subfertility treatment (p294). Combined oral contraceptive Pill use (p300), breastfeeding, hysterectomy and tubal ligation reduce risk. Current HRT use increases risk.[1]

Presentation Symptoms are often vague. See page 281.

Screening & prevention There is really no good screening test. Transvaginal ultrasound with tumour blood flow measurement can differentiate between benign and malignant neoplasms at an early stage but does not seem to reduce mortality in high-risk women.[112] Plasma levels of cancer-associated antigen (CA-125) lack sufficient sensitivity or specificity for population screening.

Consider prophylactic oophorectomy when older women have hysterectomy. It is used for those with *BRCA1 & 2* mutations. The combined oral contraceptive Pill reduces the risk (up to 40%). Tubal ligation also reduces risk in those with *BRCA1* mutation.[113]

Diagnosis Histology. Ascites, ultrasound/CT, and CA-125↑ suggestive.

Staging at laparotomy

Stage I: Disease limited to 1 or both ovaries. *Stage Ic* if ruptured capsule, tumour on ovarian surface, or ascites/peritoneal washings +ve.

Stage II: Growth extends beyond the ovaries but confined to the pelvis.

Stage III: Growth involving ovary and peritoneal implants outside pelvis (eg superficial liver), or +ve retroperitoneal or inguinal nodes.

Stage IV: Those with distant metastases (including liver parenchyma).

80% present with stage III or IV disease. 5-yr survival: Stage I, 67%; Stage II, 42%; Stage III and IV, 14.4%.

Treatment Best carried out in specialist centres;[114] this depends on tumour type. Adenocarcinomas (89%, also called ovarian epithelial carcinomas) are treated with surgery and chemotherapy, which aims for cure. Surgery removes as much tumour as possible: the less left, the more effective is chemotherapy and the better the prognosis. In a young woman with early disease, the uterus and other ovary may be left for fertility. Ensure optimal surgical staging (OPPOSITE). NICE says low-risk stage 1a or b disease may not need chemotherapy.

Chemotherapy for ~6 months post-op is usual. Carboplatin with paclitaxel (from Pacific yew trees) produces higher response rates and longer survival both when used for initial treatment and for treatment of recurrences compared to use of carboplatin alone. Radiotherapy may be tried.

Further treatment may involve 'second look' laparotomy, with secondary cytoreduction if appropriate, further chemotherapy, or radiotherapy. Colloidal gold may control ascites.

Advanced or relapsed ovarian cancer: see NICE. Options include paclitaxel, pegylated liposomal doxorubicin, and topotecan. Palliative care involves relief of symptoms, which are generally due to extensive peritoneal disease.

---

1 NNT=1 extra cancer/2000 users, 1 extra death per 3300 users.[48]

Discharge may be physiological (eg pregnancy; sexual arousal; puberty; Pill). Most discharges are smelly, itchy, and due to infection. Foul discharge may be due to a foreign body (eg forgotten tampons, or beads in children). Note the details of the discharge. Has she a sexually transmitted disease (STD)? See *OHCM* p404. If so, refer to a genitourinary clinic. Do a speculum examination and take swabs: urine and endocervical samples for chlamydia (BOX); cervical swabs for gonorrhoea (*OHCM* p416). ►Discharges rarely resemble their classical descriptions.

Thrush (*Candida*) The 2nd commonest cause of discharge (1st is bacterial vaginosis), 95% is due to *C. albicans*, 5% *C. glabrata* (harder to treat). Vulva and vagina may be red, fissured, and sore, especially if allergic component; discharge is non-offensive, classically white curds. Her partner may be a carrier who is asymptomatic. Pregnancy, contraceptive and other steroids, immunodeficiencies, antibiotics, and diabetes are risk factors—check glucose. Candida elsewhere (eg mouth, natal cleft) in both partners may cause reinfection. Thrush is not necessarily sexually transmitted. *Diagnosis:* Microscopy (shows mycelia or spores) and culture. *Treatment:* Topical treatment (eg clotrimazole 500mg pessary + cream for the vulva) gives similar cure rates to oral fluconazole 150mg PO as a single dose. *C. glabrata* may require topical nystatin or 7–14-day course of an imidazole. Use topical regimen alone if pregnant or breastfeeding. Very recurrent infection may be treated by weekly maintenance doses of treatment (unlicensed).

Trichomoniasis *Trichomonas vaginalis* (TV; fig 1; sexually transmitted) produces vaginitis and a bubbly, thin, fish-smelling discharge. Exclude gonorrhoea (often coexists). Motile flagellates are seen on wet films (×400), or cultured. *R:* (treat partner too) metronidazole 2g PO stat or 400mg/12h PO for 5 days (eg if pregnant); if allergic or recalcitrant disease, vaginal acidification with boric acid can help.[115]

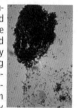

Fig 1. TV. © Prof S Upton; Kansas Univ.

Bacterial vaginosis Prevalence ~10% mostly asymptomatic. Any discharge has fishy odour, from cadaverine & putrescine. Vaginal pH is >4.5. The vagina is not inflamed and pruritus is uncommon. Mixed with 10% potassium hydroxide on a slide, a whiff of ammonia may be detected. Stippled vaginal epithelial 'clue cells' may be seen on wet microscopy (fig 2, top). There is altered bacterial flora—overgrowth, eg of *Gardnerella vaginalis*, *Mycoplasma hominis*, peptostreptococci, *Mobiluncus* and anaerobes, eg *Bacteroides* species—with too few lactobacillae. There is ↑risk of preterm labour, intra-amniotic infection in pregnancy, susceptibility to HIV,[116] and post-termination sepsis. Δ: By culture. *R:* Metronidazole 2g PO once, gel PV, or clindamycin 2% vaginal cream, 1 applicatorful/night PV 7 times. If recurrent, treating the partner may help. If pregnant, use metronidazole 400mg/12h PO for 5 days. Balance activ® vaginal acidic gel can be a useful (more natural) alternative.

Fig 2. Clue cells.© *Oxford Textbook of Medicine*, OUP

Discharge in children may reflect infection from *faecal flora*, associated with alkalinity from lack of vaginal oestrogen (prepubertal atrophic vaginitis). *Staphs* and *streps* may cause pus. *Threadworms* cause pruritus. Always consider *sexual abuse*. Gentle rectal examination may exclude a *foreign body*.

Tests: Vulval ± vaginal swab (hard to know if result is normal flora). MSU: *is there glycosuria?* For prolonged or bloody discharge, examine under anaesthesia (paediatric laryngoscopes can serve as specula) ± ultrasound or x-rays.

Management: Discuss hygiene. If an antibiotic is needed, erythromycin is a good choice. An oestrogen cream may be tried (≤1cm strip).

Gynaecology

Testing for chlamydia

Special swabs/kits exist for chlamydia transport to the lab and conventional enzyme immunoassay assay—but may be unreliable (sensitivity ~79%).[117] An example is the IDEIA chlamydia specimen collection kit® with a Dacron® tip supplied by some labs.

First-void (early morning) urine may be the single best diagnostic specimen (for *M. genitalium* and *C. trachomatis*) detection by PCR. An additional *endocervical specimen* may also be needed.[118] In one study, sensitivities for LCR (ligase chain reaction), PCR (polymerase chain reaction), gene probe, and EIA (enzyme immuno-assay) on urine were 96%, 86%, 92%, and 38%, respectively, while on cervical swabs the corresponding sensitivities of PCR, gene probe, and EIA were 89%, 84%, and 65%. DNA amplification methods may work best for urine and swabs in low-prevalence populations.[119]

One-stop test-and-treat: In an effort to decrease the number of chlamydial infections in the UK, the NHS is assessing over-the-counter availability of azithromycin for those visiting pharmacies (and their partners)—whose urine tests +ve for chlamydia.

Pelvic infection affects the Fallopian tubes (salpingitis) and may involve ovaries and parametria. 90% are sexually acquired, mostly chlamydia: 60% of these are asymptomatic (φ/σ=1 : 1) but subfertility or ectopic pregnancy may be the result, *which is why screening has been proposed*—eg by a urine ligase chain reaction DNA: *see* BOX. Other causes, eg the gonococcus, are rarer (14%—if found, retest after treatment). Organisms cultured from infected tubes are commonly different from those cultured from ectocervix, and are usually multiple. 10% follow childbirth or instrumentation (insertion of IUCD, TOP) and may be streptococcal. Infection can spread from the intestinal tract during appendicitis (Gram -ve and anaerobic organisms) or be blood-borne (tuberculosis).

Salpingitis Patients with *acute salpingitis* may be most unwell, with pain, fever, spasm of lower abdominal muscles (she may be most comfortable lying on her back with legs flexed) and cervicitis with profuse, purulent, or bloody vaginal discharge. Heavy menstrual loss suggests endometritis. Nausea and vomiting suggest peritonitis. Look for suprapubic tenderness or peritonism, cervical excitation, and tenderness in the fornices. It is usually bilateral, but may be worse on one side. *Subacute infection* can easily be missed, and laparoscopy may be needed to make either diagnosis.

Management ►Prompt treatment and contact-tracing minimizes complications. Take endocervical and urethral swabs if practicable. Remember to check for chlamydia. Admit for blood cultures and IV antibiotics if very unwell (eg **ceftriaxone** 2g/24h slow IV with **doxycycline** 100mg/12h PO) initially, then **doxycycline** 100mg/12h PO and **metronidazole** 400mg/12h PO until 14 days treated. Seek advice from microbiologist if gonorrhoea isolated. If less unwell give **ofloxacin** 400mg/12h PO and **metronidazole** 400mg/12h PO for 14 days. If infection is severe remove intrauterine contraceptive device (not needed if mild).[120]_{RCOG} Trace contacts (from within last 6 months and ensure they seek treatment—seek help of the genito-urinary clinic). Advise avoidance of intercourse until patient and partner treatments complete.

Complications If response to antibiotics is slow, consider laparoscopy. She may have an abscess (draining via the posterior fornix prevents perforation, peritonitis, and septicaemia—but laparotomy may be needed). Inadequate or delayed treatment leads to chronic infection and long-term tubal blockage (8% are subfertile after 1 episode, 19.5% after 2, 40% after 3). Advise that barrier contraception protects against infection. Ectopic pregnancy rate is increased 10-fold in those who do conceive.

Chronic salpingitis Unresolved, unrecognized, or inadequately treated infection may become chronic. Inflammation leads to fibrosis, so adhesions develop between pelvic organs. The tubes may be distended with pus (pyosalpinx) or fluid (hydrosalpinx).

Pelvic pain, menorrhagia, secondary dysmenorrhoea, discharge, and deep dyspareunia are some of the symptoms. She may be depressed. Look for tubal masses, tenderness, and fixed retroverted uterus. Laparoscopy differentiates infection from endometriosis.

Treatment is unsatisfactory. Consider long-term broad-spectrum antibiotics (eg **tetracycline** 250mg/6h PO 1h before food for 3 months), short-wave diathermy and analgesia for pain, and counselling. The only cures are the menopause or surgical removal of infected tissue.

Screening tests to prevent chlamydial pelvic infection

Opportunistic screening in family planning and TOP contexts, and routine GP appointments for all sexually active women aged up to 25yrs has been suggested. This might miss up to 20% of infections (increasing the age limit to 30 might miss just 7%). It is not clear how this screening is to be woven into routine appointments (which are already overfull), and whether patients will find screening acceptable. What is clear is that chlamydia is common in the young, with rates of 8.1% prevalence in under 20s reported as having infection from general practice settings, and 17.3% from genitourinary settings.[121] In Scotland prevalence was found to be 12.1% in under 20s at antenatal clinics, and 12.7% at abortion clinics, and cost-effectiveness studies suggest screening younger women attending these clinics and all attending colposcopy clinics as being the most cost effective.[122] Postal general population screening is not effective.[123] Infection is increasing annually, with 42,668 cases reported by UK GU clinics in 1997, and 113,585 cases in 2006, a 166% increase.

In the UK, some pharmacies offer free chlamydia tests funded by the NHS eg for those aged 16–24yrs (eg in London), and if +ve to their partners, whatever the age (± over-the-counter ℞ if +ve, p285). There is also a national screening programme that operates in colleges, prisons, and the armed forces.

Treatment of uncomplicated genital chlamydial infection is with **azithromycin** 1g PO as a single dose. Note: 80% of infections are asymptomatic. Unscheduled bleeding may be the only symptom.

Gynaecology

Foci of endometrial glandular tissue, looking like the head of a burnt match, occur beyond the uterine cavity, eg on an ovary (*chocolate cyst*), in the recto-vaginal pouch, uterosacral ligaments, on the pelvic peritoneum, and rarely in the umbilicus (fig 1), lower abdominal scars, and distant organs, eg lungs. If foci are found in uterine wall muscle, the term *adenomyosis* is used. Prevalence: ~10% of all women; 35–50% of those with subfertility.

Cause Possibly cell rests, or retrograde menstruation (Sampson's theory, explaining its association with age—typically 40–44yrs, long duration of IUCD and tampon use, its negative association with pregnancy and the Pill, and its pelvic distribution, but not its appearance elsewhere). There are genetic components, autoantibody associations, and environmental factors. Endometriotic foci are under hormonal influence with waning in pregnancy and (usually but not always[124]) at the menopause—and bleeding during menstruation. Free blood irritates, provoking fibrosis, adhesions and subfertility.

Presentation Asymptomatic (even in extensive disease)—or pelvic pain (classically cyclical, at the time of periods). It may be constant, eg if adhesions. Secondary dysmenorrhoea and deep dyspareunia are common. Thigh pain and pain on defecation may occur. ▶*Always think of endometriosis as an alternative to diagnosing irritable bowel syndrome.* Periods are often heavy and frequent, especially with adenomyosis. Patients may present with subfertility. Extra-pelvic endometriosis causes pain or bleeding at the time of menstruation at the site of the pathology, eg haematuria or haemothorax.

Diagnosis *Per vaginam:* fixed retroverted uterus or uterosacral ligament nodules and general tenderness suggest endometriosis. An enlarged, boggy, tender uterus is typical of adenomyosis. Laparoscopy reveals cysts, adhesions, peritoneal deposits, and differentiates it from chronic infection. Have low threshold for investigation of adolescents in whom it tends to be missed.

Treatment See p241. If asymptomatic, don't treat. Join an endometriosis society,[1] as treatment can be long and difficult: ▶*mutual support helps.* If analgesia/NSAIDs fail, consider the options below. Stress is a key exacerbating factor; address this too (p386).[125] Don't forget other pain management methods.[2]

Hormonal therapy aims to suppress ovulation for 6–12 months during which some (non-GI) lesions atrophy. Don't use if pregnant or lactating. The **combined Pill** helps some (low-dose monophasic, continuously). If insufficient, or contraindicated, or has bad side effects, consider **progestogens**—oral (eg continuous norethisterone), injected (p304), or intrauterine (eg Mirena®, p298—eg if adenomyosis), **danazol**, or **gonadorelin** analogues (eg **leuprorelin**. The latter are not recommended for adolescents as they ↓ bone density (up to 13% loss). Side effects are those of premature menopause. Oestrogen add-back is recommended with their use to protect bones.[126]

Surgery/laparoscopy Excision, fulguration (destruction by electric current) or laser ablation of peritoneal endometrial implants, endometrioma and rectovaginal nodule removals reduce pain. Alternative: total hysterectomy + bilateral salpingo-oophorectomy, depending on lesion site and wishes for fertility. Surgery may be best if symptoms seriously impinge on a patient's life, but relapse is common, and repeat surgery is often needed.

Complications Obstruction (GI; ureteric; fallopian). It is associated with ovarian endometrioid and clear cell cancers, Hodgkin's lymphoma and melanomas.

Prognosis Endometriosis is chronic or relapsing, being progressive in 50%. Surgery minimally helps fertility, but is recommended by NICE.

---

1 In the UK, 50 Artillery Road, London, tel. 0207 222 2776 endo.org.uk.
2 ▶Encourage optimism; discourage passive-dependency.[4] Biofeedback may ↓endometriosis pain.[127]

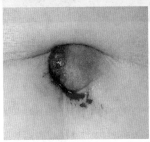

Fig 1. Endometriotic nodule in the umbilicus seen at menstruation.

A prolapse occurs when weakness of the supporting structures allows the pelvic organs to sag within the vagina. The weakness may be congenital, but it usually results from stretching during childbirth. Poor perineal repair reduces support (p92). Weakness is exacerbated by menopausal atrophy and by coughing and straining. They may cause distressing incontinence and be a nuisance but are not a danger to health—except for third-degree uterine prolapse with cystocele when ureteric obstruction can occur.

Types of prolapse are named by the structures sagging. Several types may coexist in the same patient.

Cystocele The upper front wall of the vagina, and the bladder attached to it, bulge. Residual urine within the cystocele may cause frequency and dysuria.

Urethrocele If the lower anterior vaginal wall bulges, this will displace the urethra and impair the sphincter mechanisms (p306), so leading to stress incontinence. Does she leak when she laughs?

Rectocele The middle posterior wall, which is attached to rectum, may bulge through weak levator ani. It is often symptomless, but she may have to reduce herniation prior to defecation by putting a finger in the vagina, or pressing on the perineum.

Enterocele Bulges of the upper posterior vaginal wall may contain loops of intestine from the pouch of Douglas.

Uterine prolapse With *first-degree prolapse* the cervix stays in the vagina. In *second-degree prolapse* it protrudes from the introitus when standing or straining. With *third-degree prolapse* (procidentia) the uterine fundus lies outside the vagina. The vagina becomes keratinized and the cervix may ulcerate.

Symptoms: 'Dragging' or 'something coming down' is worse by day. Cystitis, frequency, stress incontinence, and difficulty in defecation may occur depending on the type of prolapse. Examine vaginal walls in left lateral position with a Sims' speculum; ask the patient to bear down to demonstrate the prolapse. Do urodynamic studies (p307) to exclude detrusor overactivity and assess voiding.

Prevention: Lower parity; better obstetric practices, pelvic floor exercises.

Treatment: Mild disease may improve with reduction in intra-abdominal pressure, so encourage her to lose weight, stop smoking, and stop straining. Improve muscle tone with exercises or physiotherapy, and, if postmenopausal, topical oestrogens, eg **estriol cream 0.1%** as often as required (try twice weekly). **Estradiol** vaginal tablets used weekly provide a less messy vaginal alternative.

Severe symptomatic prolapse is best treated surgically. Incontinence needs to have the cause treated (so arrange urodynamic studies to plan the best type of surgery). Repair operations (p308) excise redundant tissue and strengthen supports, but reduce vaginal width. Is she sexually active? If so, surgery must compromise between reducing prolapse and maintaining width. Marked uterine prolapse is best treated by hysterectomy. Post-hysterectomy vault prolapse may be treated by sacrocolpopexy (eg with mesh). Transvaginal mesh repair for cystocoele may give fewer symptoms of recurrent prolapse at 1yr but higher rates of stress incontinence and serious operative complications (4%).[129]

Ring pessaries may be tried as a temporary measure or for the very frail. Select size by diameter of vagina at level of the fornices; it will only stay in if the vagina narrows nearer the introitus. Insert into the posterior fornix and tuck above the pubic bone (easier if the ring has been softened in hot water first). Problems: discomfort, infection, ulceration (change 6–12-monthly). For those in whom they keep falling out, try a shelf pessary.

Gynaecology

▶*This can be devastating to both partners* and its investigation a great strain. Sympathetic management is crucial. 84% of young couples having regular intercourse conceive within a year (92% by 2 years). Offer investigation after 1yr of trying (earlier if ♀ aged ≥35 years, amenorrhoea, oligomenorrhoea, or past pelvic inflammatory disease, undescended testes or cancer treatments which may affect fertility). Arrange counselling throughout. Fertility decreases with age: girls are born with ~300,000 potential eggs; by 30yrs, only 12% are left (by 40yrs, just 3%). In the 10% of subfertile couples consider:
• Is she producing ova? (Anovulation causes 21%.)
• Is he producing enough, healthy sperm? (Male factors cause 24%.)
• Are ova and sperm meeting? (Tubal cause 14%, hostile mucus 3%, sexual dysfunction 6%.) Aim for intercourse 3 times/week throughout the cycle.
• Is the embryo implanting?

Endometriosis is a cause in ~6% (laparoscopic surgery helps). The cause is 'unexplained' in 27% of couples: here, 60–70% achieve conception within 3yrs.

Initial management It takes 2 to be infertile (♀ causes ≈67%); see both partners; advise to stop smoking and lose weight if BMI >29. She should take 0.4mg folic acid/day from now on. Reducing stress and boosting wellbeing helps.[1]

Ask her about: Menstrual history; previous pregnancies (any miscarriages?); contraception; history of pelvic infections or abdominal surgery; drugs.

Ask him about: Puberty; previous fatherhood; previous surgery (hernias; orchidopexy; bladder neck surgery); illnesses (venereal, adult mumps); drugs; alcohol; job (is he home at ovulation time?) and erectile problems (seen in 4%).[130]

Ask both about: Mood; feelings about subfertility; technique; frequency/timing of intercourse (non-consummation is rare); parenthood; previous tests.

Examination Check the woman's general health and sexual development and examine the abdomen and pelvis. If the sperm count is abnormal, examine the man for endocrine and penile abnormalities, varicoceles; confirm there are 2 normal testes. What is his BMI? Obese men produce 60% less seminal fluid than men with a BMI ≤25, and have 40% higher levels of abnormal sperm.[131]

Tests for ovulation If cycles are regular ovulation is likely. Basal body temperature rises midcycle (but charting is difficult and may raise anxieties).

Blood tests Check rubella status; immunize if non-immune. If you suspect anovulation check: •Serum mid-luteal progesterone ie 7 days before expected period (>30nmol/L is indicative of ovulation) •Day 5 FSH (>10U/L indicates a poor response to ovarian stimulation; it may indicate primary ovarian failure—but FSH is pulsatile in release and one may get a high reading depending on the stage of the cycle) •Day 5 LH (for polycystic ovary syndrome) •TFT if symptomatic •Blood prolactin if anovulation or galactorrhoea (if high may be due to prolactinoma; MRI of brain and pituitary gland).

Semen analysis for: •Volume >2mL (mean 2.75mL now, formerly 3.4mL in the 1940s) •Sperm count/morphology •Infection. Normal count >20 million sperm/mL, >50% motile within 1h of ejaculate production (liquefaction also within 1h), and >30% normal form; WBC < 1 million/mL; mean sperm count=66 million/mL (113 million/mL in the 1940s; this average is falling—which may be due to an environmental influence—or more frequent ejaculations). Examine 2 specimens (ideally 3 months apart so spermatozoa cycle completed but soon if sperm severely deficient) as variation may be considerable. Transport sample fresh to lab (masturbated into a wide topped container). Avoid temperatures <15°C or >38°C. Reduced counts require specialist referral.

1 Each point on the 5-point *wellbeing index score* accounts for a 7% increase in sperm concentration[132]

Subfertility options: abbreviations, problems, and ethics

DI	Donor insemination (In some countries, children have no rights to information about their father: this can lead to problems—eg most children want their fathers to be proud of them, and with DI this is impossible.) The great questions such as *where do I come from?* become more opaque than ever. UK law *does* allow tracing of fathers.
FEC	Fetal egg child (offspring from an egg taken from an aborted fetus).
GIFT	Gamete intrafallopian transfer.
ICSI	Intracytoplasmic sperm injection (directly into an egg). Sperm may be taken surgically from the testis or epididymis. Such patients, with no exposure to their partner's sperm, are at increased risk of pre-eclampsia (p48): this supports a model of pre-eclampsia postulating absence of partner-specific immune tolerance as a causative factor.[133]
IMSI	Intra-cytoplasmic morphologically-selected sperm injection.[134] Pregnancy rate for IMSI is ~39% (vs 26% for ICSI).[135]
IUI	Intrauterine insemination with superovulation: a USA favourite. In 20%, this causes twins (in 10%, higher order pregnancies when pregnancy is achieved; a possibly unacceptable disadvantage).
IVF	*In vitro* fertilization: see p69 and p294.
IVM	*In vitro* maturation: immature eggs are collected from the ovaries, matured in the lab before sperm injection (ISCI). Avoids expensive ovulation-inducing drugs and risk of ovarian hyperstimulation, it may be especially suitable for women with polycystic ovaries.
MESA	Microepididymal sperm aspiration from testis, post-vasectomy
OT/NT(P)	Ooplasmic transfer/nuclear transfer procedure: the baby has 2 mothers: one (too old to conceive normally) gives a nucleus; the other gives fresher cytoplasm (+mitochondrial DNA) for the ovum. This is an example of human germline modification. 15 babies were born using this technique in the USA (2 had Turner's syndrome).
PESA	Percutaneous epididymal sperm aspiration (like MESA, but uses a needle inserted into the epididymis, so scrotal exploration is not needed).
PHC	Pregnancy by human cloning (illegal in many countries partly because of concern about premature ageing).
POST	Peritoneal oocyte sperm transfer.
POT	Pregnancy by ovary transplant has been reported (autologous transplant, 1 between identical twin sisters, another between sisters).

Various national embryology authorities exist and pronounce on the ethics of fertility options, and their edicts can appear to be set in stone (although being mutually contradictory with those from other countries). One problem with this approach is that fertility options are constantly changing, as are society's views on what is acceptable. It is not clear whether these views should lead, or simply be taken into account (an opaque phrase) or be trumped by appeal to some higher authority (God, or the conscience of a quango).

The above methods allow embryos to be sexed and screened for genetic diseases with implantation only for those with the desired characteristics, eg offering a perfect match for stem-cell trans-plantation to an older sibling, with Fanconi's anaemia. Controversies surrounding creating an individual expressly for the purposes of another might seem to be new, but mythology has, since before the dawn of time,[1] acclimatized us to this activity—which is why it is gaining acceptance.

---

1 According to *Paradise Lost*, the First Operator, in a controversial act of vivisection, 'opened my left side, and took from thence a rib, with cordial spirits warm, and life-blood streaming fresh: wide was the wound, but suddenly with flesh filled up and healed: the rib he formed and fashioned with his hands; under his forming hands a creature grew, manlike, but different sex, so lovely fair, that what seemed fair in all the world, seemed now mean, or in her summed up.' Thus was Eve made, not for herself, but simply to delight Adam and keep him company.[136] *Operators beware!* This sort of activity cannot now be done in your garden but only in clinics licensed by the Human Embryology Authority.

Tests of tubal patency (Screen for chlamydia first).

Unless damaged tubes are expected do hysterosalpingogram (or hysterosalpingo-contrast ultrasonography) first.

1 A hysterosalpingogram (contrast x-ray) demonstrates uterine anatomy and tubal 'fill and spill'. Unpleasant; it may require premedication. False positives may occur with tubal spasm. Give antibiotics, eg **cefradine** 500mg/6h PO with **metronidazole** 1g/12h PR for 24h before and eg 400mg/12h PO for 5 days after procedure to prevent pelvic infection.

2 Laparoscopy with dye. Pelvic organs are visualized and methylene blue dye injected through the cervix: if tubes are blocked proximally they do not fill with dye; with distal block there is no 'spill' into the peritoneal cavity.

Treatment of subfertility Treatment is directed at the cause.

• *Azoospermia* is unresponsive to simple treatment. A low sperm count may be improved by avoiding tobacco and alcohol. Avoiding tight pants does not change testis T° or semen parameters. Will they consider donor insemination (AID=artificial insemination by donor)? If so check ♀ ovulating; if tubal damage suspected, investigate. Give 3 cycles of intrauterine insemination (IUI) post ovulation; if unsuccessful do tubal investigations, then further 3 cycles. If still unsuccessful offer other treatment.

• *Problems of sperm deposition* (eg erectile dysfunction) can be circumvented by artificial insemination using the partner's sperm.

• *Hyperprolactinaemia* (OHCM p228) Remove the cause if one is found (eg pituitary microadenoma, drugs); if not, give **bromocriptine** 2mg/24h PO, increasing slowly until blood prolactin is normal. (Side effect: nausea.)

• *Anovulation* WHO classification: •Class 1 is hypothalamic pituitary failure (this responds to pulsed gonadotrophin releasing hormone or gonadotrophins with luteinizing hormone activity): •Class 2 is hypothalamic pituitary dysfunction (usually polycystic ovary syndrome, p252). Stimulate follicle development using **clomifene** 50–100mg/24h PO on days 2–6 inclusive. SE: flushes (10%), visual disturbance (1.5%), abdominal pain (5.5%, p311); warn about risk of multiple pregnancy ± excess risk of ovarian cancer (p280). Monitor response to clomifene with luteal phase progesterone (+ultrasound in at least 1st cycle). If *still* no ovulation, try gonadotrophins. After 6 months ovulating offer clomifene assisted IUI (p293) if not pregnant. •Class 3 is ovarian failure (treatment is IVF, *see below* using donated ova).

• *Tubal problems: Surgery may sometimes help.* Proximal blocks may respond to tubal catheterization or hysteroscopic cannulation. Endometriosis: p288. If amenorrhoeic with intrauterine adhesions, use hysteroscopic adhesiolysis.

In vitro fertilization Screen couple for HIV, hepatitis B & C. Women with hydrosalpinges should have salpingectomy prior to IVF to ↑chance of live birth. Psychological stability is required in the UK. Some non-UK clinics have given IVF to women >65yrs old.[1] 4 million IVF babies have been born worldwide, 200,000/yr.[137] Chance of live birth per treatment cycle is age dependent: 20% if ♀ age ≤35; 15% if 36–38; 10% if 39; 6% if ≥40. *In vitro* fertilization (IVF) is used for tubal (and other) problems. Ovaries are stimulated (see *hyperstimulation* p311), ova collected (by transvaginal aspiration under transvaginal ultrasound guidance), fertilized, and 2 embryos returned under ultrasound guidance to the uterus as an outpatient procedure. Single fresh ovary transfer with 2nd frozen embryo later, if needed, gives as good results.[138] For problems of offspring see (p69).

The possibility of adoption should not be forgotten. Those who remain childless may value counselling or a self-help group.

1 70-year-old Omkari Panwar is the world's oldest IVF mother. The oldest mother for natural conception is recorded as being 59.[139]

Spermatogenesis takes place in the seminiferous tubules. Undifferentiated diploid germ cells (spermatogonia) multiply and are then transformed into haploid spermatozoa, a process taking 74 days. FSH and LH are both important for initiation of spermatogenesis at puberty. LH stimulates Leydig cells to produce testosterone. Testosterone and FSH stimulate Sertoli cells to produce essential substances for metabolic support of germ cells and spermatogenesis.

Spermatozoa A spermatozoon has a dense oval head (containing the haploid chromosome complement) capped by an acrosome granule (contains enzymes essential for fertilization), and is propelled by the motile tail. Seminal fluid forms 90% of ejaculate volume and is alkaline to buffer vaginal acidity. Only ~200 sperm from any ejaculate reach the middle ⅓ of the Fallopian tube, the site of fertilization. Sperm counts are highest in spring and lowest in summer.[140]

Male subfertility Male factors are the cause of subfertility in ~24% of infertile couples. In reality, most are subfertile. Only a small number of men have an identifiable treatable cause. Causes include (% cited in one study):

- Idiopathic oligo/azoospermia (16%): testes are usually small and FSH ↑.
- Asthenozoospermia/teratozoospermia (17%): in asthenozoospermia sperm motility is reduced due to structural problems with the tails. Teratozoospermia indicates an excess of abnormal forms.
- Varicocele (17%): this is controversial for varicocele is found in 15% of males, most of whom have normal fertility.
- Genital tract infection (4%): gonococci, chlamydia, & Gram -ve enterococci cause adnexal infection (± painful ejaculation, urethral discharge, haematospermia, dysuria, tender epididymes, tender boggy prostate). Confirm by semen culture, urethral swab or finding >10^6 peroxidase +ve polymorphs/mL semen. Treatment has not been shown to restore fertility.
- Sperm autoimmunity (1.6%): *Risk factors for antibodies:* vasectomy, testis injury, genital tract obstruction, family history of autoimmunity. Most are on sperm membranes or in seminal fluid, but may occur in the woman.
- Congenital (cryptorchidism, chromosome disorders—2%): Klinefelter's account for 50% chromosome disorders. For optimal fertility undescended testes should be fixed in the scrotum before 2yrs of age.
- Obstructive azoospermia (1.8%): azoospermia, normal sized testes with normal or high FSH suggests this. It may follow infection, vasectomy, or be congenital (as in cystic fibrosis). It may be amenable to surgery, eg epididymo-vasostomy to bypass epididymal obstruction.
- Systemic—eg iatrogenic, or from drugs, eg cannabis (1.3%).[141]
- Coital disorders (1%).
- Gonadotrophin deficiency (0.6%): this is the only cause of testicular failure consistently treatable by hormone replacement.

Examination Look at body form and secondary sexual characteristics. Any gynaecomastia? Normal testicular volume is 15–35mL (compare with Prader orchidometer). Rectal examination may reveal prostatitis.

Tests *Semen analysis* (p292). *Plasma FSH* distinguishes primary from secondary testicular failure. *Testosterone and LH levels* are indicated if you suspect androgen deficiency. *Agglutination tests* to detect antibodies.

Treatment ICSI=intracytoplasmic sperm injection (direct into egg), the main tool for most male infertility. The source of sperm is the epididymis or testis in men with obstructive azoospermia; even if the problem is non-obstructive, sperm can be retrieved in ~50%. Check the man's chromosomes, and for cystic fibrosis carrier status before ICSI if azoospermic, oligospermic (not if postvasectomy). If they have Y chromosome AFZC deletions, so would offspring sons.[142]

Gynaecology

▶*Any method, even coitus interruptus, is better than none*. Without contraception about 85 of every 100 premenopausal sexually active women will become pregnant each year. Properly used, contraception reduces this rate (see OPPOSITE)..When dealing with under-16s use Fraser Guidelines (BOX 4).

Barrier methods ▶The main reason for failure is not using them. Condoms reduce transmission of most STDs but not those affecting the perineum. Caps give some protection against gonorrhoea and chlamydia but not syphilis or herpes. Some spermicides inactivate HIV *in vitro* but HIV not nonoxyl-9 impregnated sheaths (see below).[143] When failure is anticipated (eg 'split sheath'), remember post-coital emergency contraception (p299). Stop contraception at 55yrs (95.9% menopausal) unless regular menstruation.

- *Sheaths (condoms)* Effective when properly used, unroll onto the erect penis with the teat or end (if teatless) pinched to expel air. This prevents bursting at ejaculation. Method failure rate 5%, typical user failure rate 15%/yr.
- *Caps* come in several forms. Diaphragms stretch from pubic bone to posterior fornix. Check after insertion that the cervix is covered. Cervical caps fit over the cervix (so need a prominent cervix). Insert <2h before intercourse (keep in place >6h after sex). Use with a spermicide.* Problems: UTIs, rubber sensitivity. They need professional fitting. 92–99% effective if perfect use.**
- *Cervical sponges* Simple to use: spermicide* impregnated: unavailable UK.
- *The female condom* (eg Femidom®) Prescription and fitting are not needed. It has not proved popular. One reason for failure is that the penis goes alongside it, rather than in it; another, that it gets pushed up in the vagina or may fall out. They can be noisy. Uses lubricant, not spermicide. 95% effective.‡
- *Spermicide** Unreliable unless used with a barrier. **Nonoxinol-9**, the only spermicide available in UK is not recommended for those with or at high risk of HIV as it irritates vaginal epithelium and ↑ chance of HIV transmission.

Fertility awareness ('natural') methods involve physiological monitoring to find fertile times (6 days prior to ovulation; the life of a sperm) to 2 days afterwards (the life of the ovum). Cervical mucus becomes clear and sticky at the beginning of the fertile time and dry at ovulation (but is altered by semen and vaginal infections). Basal body temperature ↑∼0.3°C after ovulation (affected by fevers, drugs, recent food, or drink). Additional observations (mittelschmerz, p310 ± cervix changes) improve accuracy. Success is common if: • Regular cycles • Dedication • Self-control. UK teachers are available (tel. 01222 754628).

Lactational amenorrhoea See p95.

High-technology natural methods Devices eg Persona® use urine test sticks to measure oestrone-3-glucuronide (E3G—peaks 24h pre-ovulation) and luteinizing hormone (LH—ovulation occurs within 36h of LH surge and sperm penetration of cervical mucus drops after surge). Microtechnology builds a database of the woman's natural variability over time, to give her a green light (almost infertile), a red light (fertile—typically days 6–10) or an orange light (test early-morning urine for E3G and LH). Usually, only 8 urine tests are needed per cycle. She purchases sticks and monitor. A button is pressed the morning her period starts: she checks the monitor lights before passing urine each morning, in case a test is needed. *Reliability:* 93–95% (manufacturer's data, in motivated patients; it may be less in practice; results should be regarded as only preliminary; explain uncertainty). CI: Cycle <23 or >35 days or variation >10 days; breastfeeding; if already on hormones or tetracycline (minocycline is OK); menopausal; liver or kidney disease; polycystic ovaries, or if pregnancy is definitely undesired.

---

1 RCOG 2007 *FFPRHC Guidance* Female Barrier Methods.[144] This paper gives great detail of all caps, diaphragms etc available. ** but typical use failure rate (TUFR; user+method failure) = 16% in 1ˢᵗ year use of diaphragm, (TUFR) for cervical caps: 9% nullips, 20% parous ♀. ‡ (TUFR) 21%.

☼ Our future depends on contraception[145]

Unless we meet the huge unmet demand for contraception (especially in Asia) preventable starvation is inevitable.[146] A world population (~7 billion) growing at current rates (100×10^6/yr) is unsustainable, now the era of cheap food is over.

The ideal contraceptive—and the realities

An ideal contraceptive is: *100% effective*, with only desirable side effects (eg protection from sexually transmitted disease), and it must be *readily reversible*, and be usable *unsupervised by professionals*. Find the best compromise for each person depending on age, health, and beliefs. Methods available:

- 'Natural methods' (no intercourse near time of ovulation): acceptable to Catholic Church; also, the simplest are free, requiring no 'pollution of the body' with drugs: see OPPOSITE.
- Barrier methods (low health risk but need high user motivation & some protection from HIV). See page OPPOSITE.
- Hormonal (complex health interactions, but highly effective, p300–3).
- IUCD/IUS (convenient and effective—if not contraindicated—p298).
- Sterilization (very effective but effectively 'irreversible', p305).

Failure rates % in 1st year with typical (τ) and perfect (p) use[147]		
• No method	85 (τ)	85 (p)
• Cervical cap	16–32	9–20
• Natural methods	25	1–9
• Female condom	21	5
• Withdrawal	27	4
• Diaphragm +spermicide	16	6
• Male condom	15	2
• Pills (CoC+PoP)	8	0.3
• Copper coil (for τ-safe® Cu380A)	0.8	0.6
• Depo Provera®	3	0.3
• Tubal ligation	0.5	0.5
• Vasectomy	0.15	0.1
• Levonorgestrel IUS (Mirena®)	0.1	0.1

The Pill has given more people more freedom than any conceivable freedom fighter.

Gynaecology

"Is she pregnant already?"

This is a frequent question in family planning and other clinics. If a pregnancy test is not available, women who could be pregnant already will often be denied the contraception they need. Here, consider using this check list to see if the patient may be pregnant. If she answers Yes to *any* of these questions, and she is free from signs or symptoms of pregnancy, then pregnancy is very unlikely (negative predictive value >99%).

- Have you given birth in the past 4 weeks?
- Are you <6 months postpartum and fully breastfeeding, and free from menstrual bleeding since you had your child?
- Did you last menstrual period start within the last 7 days?
- Have you been using a reliable contraceptive consistently and correctly?
- Have you not had sex since your last period?[148]

Fraser guidelines (Gillick competence)

Those <16yrs may be prescribed contraception without parental consent if:
- They understand the doctor's advice.
- The young person cannot be persuaded to inform their parents that they are seeking contraceptive advice.
- They are likely to begin or continue intercourse with or without contraceptive treatment.
- Unless the young person receives contraceptive treatment their physical or mental health is likely to suffer.
- The young person's best interests require that the doctor gives advice and/ or treatment without parental consent.

IUCDs (coils) are plastic shapes ~3cm long with copper winding, and a plastic thread for a tail. They inhibit implantation and may impair sperm migration. Most need changing every 5–10 years. The larger, non-copper-bearing 'inert' types (eg Lippes loop®) caused more complications but did not need changing (still sometimes found *in situ*). Use those with ≥300mm² copper eg T-safe® copper T380A (the most effective),[149] for which pregnancy rate is 2.2 per 100 woman-years. The frameless device may be as effective. Most of those who choose the IUCD (5%) are older, parous women in stable relationships, in whom the problem rate is low. They can be used for emergency contraception (p299).

Problems with IUCDs 1 They may be expelled (5%) by a uterus which is nulliparous or distorted (eg by fibroids). 2 They are associated with pelvic infection and subfertility following sexually transmitted disease, or sometimes introduced at insertion. 3 They tend to produce heavy, painful periods. *Contraindications:* Pregnancy; current pelvic infection/STD (including TB); trophoblastic disease; cancer of ovary, endometrium or cervix; distorted uterine cavity.

Insertion Screen for STD prior to insertion or use prophylactic antibiotics. Skilled insertion minimizes complications. Each device has its own technique, so read the instructions carefully and practise beforehand.

An IUCD can be inserted any time (and as postcoital contraception), as long as she's not pregnant. Insert within 48h of, or >4 weeks after birth. Determine the position of the uterus. Then insert a uterine sound to assess the cavity length. Then insert the IUCD, placing it in the fundus. This may cause cramps. Uterine perforation rate is <1 : 1000. Once the coil is in place, cut threads to leave 3cm visible in the vagina. Teach her to feel the threads: ask her to check after each period. Misoprostol 400µg sublingually 1h before insertion dilates the cervix aiding insertion.[150] ▶Insertion of IUCDs may provoke 'cervical shock' (from increased vagal tone). Have IV atropine (and anti-epileptics if patient epileptic) and resuscitation equipment to hand.

Follow-up Most expulsions are in the first 3 months. Follow-up after 1st period. Threads may be easier to feel than to see. Expulsion rate <1 : 20 in 5 years.

Lost threads The IUCD may have been expelled, so advise extra contraception and exclude pregnancy. Seek coil on ultrasound; if missing arrange x-ray to exclude extra-uterine coils (surgical retrieval advised).

Infection Treat with the device in place, but if removed do not replace for 3 months. With symptomatic Actinomyces, remove coil, cut off threads and send for culture. If positive, seek expert advice on treatment.

Pregnancy >90% are intrauterine. Remove coil, if you can as soon as pregnancy is diagnosed to reduce risk of miscarriage (20% if removed early, 50% if left), and to prevent miscarriage with infection. Exclude ectopic.

Removal Alternative contraception should be started (if desired) prior to removal, or a fertilized ovum may be in the tubes. At the menopause, remove after 2 years' amenorrhoea if age <50yrs (1 years' amenorrhoea if age >50yrs).

IUCDs carrying hormones (IUS, intrauterine systems)—eg Mirena® (carries levonorgestrel). Local effect (reversible endometrial atrophy) makes implantation less likely, and periods lighter; perhaps 20% may experience reversible amenorrhoea (reliability equals sterilization, see p305). It lasts ~5 years. (If to protect endometrium with HRT (p256), change at 4 years.) There may be less risk of ectopic pregnancy. Risk of some sexually transmitted infections is reduced. Warn about spotting ± heavy bleeding (NB: bleeding may become *scanty* or *absent* after a few cycles). Pregnancy rate <1 : 1000 over 5 years. It may benefit women with endometriosis, adenomyosis, fibroids, or endometrial hyperplasia. Avoid if breast cancer. Minimally affected by enzyme inducers.

Gynaecology

Emergency contraception[151]

This is for use after isolated episodes of unprotected intercourse (UPSI), eg 'the split sheath' and should not be used regularly. Tablets cover that UPSI only. Although usually given after UPSI advance issue does not increase use and it may be sensible to 'be prepared'. ('Carrying an umbrella in the British climate is considered sensible, not a wish for rain.')[152] However, advance issue has not been shown to reduce pregnancy rates.[153]

Management History of LMP; normal cycle; number of hours since unprotected intercourse. Any CI to later Pill use (p300)? Check BP. Explain that teratogenicity has not been demonstrated. Discuss future contraception. Give supply of oral contraceptives if day 1 start at next period is planned; if started immediately advise extra precautions as below. Offer infection screen and to cover HIV. Offer follow-up at 3–6 weeks if coil inserted; or if pregnancy or STI tests desired, or if she has contraceptive concerns.

Emergency IUCD More effective than tablet contraception (prevents 99% of expected pregnancies); a copper IUCD can be inserted within 120h of unprotected sex. If exposure was >5 days previously it can be inserted up to 5 days after likely ovulation, so is useful in women who present later. Screen for infection. Insert under antibiotic cover, eg **azithromycin** 1g PO if screening results unavailable, or risk of IE. It is thought to inhibit fertilization by toxic effects and to inhibit implantation. If for long-term use, coils with 380mm² Cu have the lowest failure rates so should be used. Unaffected by enzyme inducers (p300), it is the method of choice for those taking them (but see below).

Ulipristal acetate Initiate within 120h of unprotected sex. Failure rate is ≤1.6% in non-inferiority (with levonorgestrel) trials. Efficacy is not reduced by obesity (levonorgestrel may be). It is thought to inhibit or delay ovulation. If vomiting ≤3h of taking the tablet, advise another (30mg). A progesterone receptor moderator, it is unsuitable for use if on, or within 28 days of taking, an enzyme inducer (p300), if on antacids or drugs raising gastric pH, for those with severe asthma uncontrolled by oral corticosteroids. Use with caution if liver dysfunction, hereditary galactose intolerance, Lapp lactase deficiency, glucose-galactose malabsorption. Avoid breastfeeding for 36h after use. Use only once per menstrual cycle. Periods average 2 days delay (7 days in ≤20%). Advise extra contraceptive precautions for 14 days for combined pills, 16 days for Qlaira®, 9 days for progesterone only pills , if started or continued. Starting oral contraceptive immediately after ulipristal acetate is off licence. Should pregnancy occur, though no harm known, register via manufacturer.

Levonorgestrel Initiate within 72h of unprotected sex. Failure rates are ≤2.6%. Suitable for those with focal migraine and past thromboembolism, there are no medical contraindications to its use. **Levonorgestrel** 1.5mg (1 Levonelle 1500® tablet or Levonelle® One Step over-the-counter) preferably within 12h and no later than 72h after unprotected sex. If on, or within 28 days of, taking an enzyme inducer (p300), or with post-sexual exposure HIV prophylaxis, the dose is 3mg. If vomiting occurs within 2h of taking the dose, take another immediately. The earlier taken after UPSI, the fewer the pregnancies which occur. It is believed to inhibit ovulation. It can be used more than once in 1 cycle; and can be used (but may be less effective) in same cycle after ulipristal acetate.

Warn that effective contraception should be used until the next period; and that she should return if she suffers any lower abdominal pain or the next period is abnormal. Advise pregnancy test if period >7 days late or unusually light, or after 21 days if 'quick start' contraception started. If immediate ('quick start') oral contraception started, or continuing extra contraceptive precautions are needed for 7 days for combined pills (avoid immediate co-cyprindiol start), 9 days for Qlaira®, 2 days for progesterone only pills.

Combined hormonal contraception (CHC) as vaginal ring, transdermal patch (p304) or pills (COC) contain oestrogen (eg ethinylestradiol) with a progestogen, either in fixed ratio or varying through the month (phased). Low-dose Pills (≤30µg oestrogen) are the norm. The combined Pill is taken daily for 3wks followed by a week's break. This inhibits ovulation, giving a withdrawal bleed in the Pill-free week. When prescribing CHCs, attend to the following areas.

History Why is Pill wanted? Does she know the risks? Explain risks. Alternatives considered? Contraindications? Ask about smoking (below) and drugs. Any anxieties, eg weight gain? (does not cause.) Offer help to stop smoking. If 1st degree relative with thromboembolism <45yrs, do thrombophilia screen. Weigh: check BP: calculate BMI annually. At age 50 advise alternative method.

Contraindications (ukmec4)[1,154] Diabetes with neuropathy, retinopathy, nephropathy, vasculopathy; BP ≥160/95; smoking ≥15/day if age ≥35; migraine with aura or (BOX p301); past stroke or venous or arterial thrombosis; thrombophilia (p33); heart disease with pulmonary hypertension or embolus risk; ischaemic heart disease; transient ischaemic attacks; liver adenoma, hepatoma, decompensated cirrhosis, active hepatitis, Dubin–Johnson or Rotor synd.; porphyria; SLE with unknown/+ve antiphospholipid antibodies; past haemolytic uraemic syndrome; pregnancy related pruritus, cholestatic jaundice, pemphigoid gestationis, chorea; hydatidiform mole (see p264); breast cancer in last 5yrs; breastfeeding (esp. 1st 6 weeks); immobility (in bed; leg in plaster cast).

Cautions (BNF) Hyperprolactinaemia (get expert help), BRCA gene carrier.
• *Venous risk factors:* Caution if *any* of these: (►avoid if ≥2 risks): 1st degree FH of thromboembolism age <45y;[2] BMI ≥30kg/m²; varicose veins (►avoid during sclerotherapy or past thrombosis); immobility (eg wheelchair).
• *Arterial risk factors:* Caution if *any* of the following (►avoid if ≥2 risk factors): smoker (or in last year); age ≥35yrs; BP >140/90 (►stop if ≥160/95); migraine without aura; BMI ≥30kg/m²; diabetes mellitus; 1st-degree relative with arterial disease <45yrs old (►avoid if she has dyslipidaemia too).

Drugs interfering with Pills (use condoms too) *Liver enzyme inducers*, eg some anticonvulsants,[3] aprepitant, bosentan, efavirenz, modafinil, nelfinavir, nevirapine, ritonavir, St John's wort, rifampicin and rifabutin ↓ efficacy by ↓ circulating hormones (see Nexplanon® p304). If short term, use extra precautions (p302) while used and for 28 days after (can cover with Depo-Provera® injection) and take only 4-day break. If long term, use 50–70µg ethinylestradiol, or Norinyl-1®, tricycled (3 packs in row) then 4-day break.[155] Use other contraception (IUCD/IUS/depot) with the potent enzyme inducers rifampicin, rifabutin. Beware lamotrigine (↓ fit control). Ulipristal: see p299. *Antibiotics:* p302.

Benefits of the Pill Very effective contraception; lighter, less painful periods; less PMS (p254) and benign breast disease, fewer menopausal symptoms, improved acne. In long-term users, reduced risk of endometrial carcinoma (↓ 50%) ovarian tumours (carcinoma ↓50% if 15-yr use) and colorectal cancer.

Serious disadvantages Risks of arterial and venous disease are increased, eg DVT and myocardial infarction. Use thromboprophylaxis (p16) if taking 4 weeks before major or leg surgery. Risk of death from the Pill increases sharply in those >40yrs: 1 : 2500 for nonsmokers; 1 : 500 for smokers. *Breast cancer:* there is slight increase in current users and in the 10 years after stopping. Duration of use is not thought to be a factor. The Pill acts as a co-factor with human papilloma virus to increase risk of invasive cervical cancer.[156]

---

1 ukmec4 category denotes that use poses unacceptable health risk: ukmec3=risk from use outweighs advantage; ukmec2=advantage of use outweighs risk; ukmec1=no restriction to use. ukmec 2009[1TM]
2 If family history of thromboembolism, avoid Pills with desogestrel or gestodene (or if prothrombotic coagulation abnormality, eg factor V Leiden or antiphospholipid antibodies, incl. lupus anticoagulant).
3 Eg: carbamazepine, esli/ox/carbazepine, phenobarbital, phenytoin, primidone, rufinamide,topiramate.

Migraine, ischaemic stroke, and the Pill

The problem is ischaemic stroke. The background annual incidence is 2 per 100,000 women aged 20, and 20 per 100,000 for those aged 40. Migraine itself is a risk factor. For those with migraine and CoC use, incidence of ischaemic stroke becomes 8:100,000 if aged 20; and 80:100,000 in those aged 40. Low-dose CoCs only should be used. Those with migraine with aura are known to be at special risk precluding use of combined Pills in these women (however, there is no problem with them using progesterone only or nonhormonal contraception). Other risk factors for ischaemic stroke include smoking, age >35yrs, ↑BP, obesity (body mass index >30), diabetes mellitus, dyslipidaemia and family history of arterial disease <45yrs. Women known to have migraine should be warned to stop Pills immediately if they develop aura or worsening of migraine. If a woman has 1st migraine attack on CoC, stop it, observe closely: restart cautiously only if there are no sequelae and if migraine attack was without aura and there are no other risk factors (above).[157]

Diagnosing migraine with aura (formerly called *classical/focal migraine*)
1 Slow evolution of symptoms (see below) over several minutes.
2 Duration of aura usually 10–30min, resolving within 1h, and typically before onset of headache.
3 Visual symptoms (99% of auras), eg:
   •Bilateral homonymous hemianopia.
   •Teichopsia and fortification spectra, eg a gradually enlarging C ℂ with scintillating edges.
   •Positive (bright) scotomata.
4 Sensory disturbance (31% of auras).
   •Usually associated with visual symptoms.
   •Usually in one arm spreading from fingers to face (leg rarely affected).
5 Speech disturbance (18% of auras): dysphasia; dysarthria; paraphasia.
6 Motor disturbances (6% of auras).

Both motor and speech disturbances are usually accompanied by visual and/or sensory disturbances.

Migraine without aura: (formerly called *simple* or *common* migraine) includes symptoms of blurred vision, photophobia, phonophobia, generalized flashing lights affecting the whole visual field in both eyes, associated with headache.

Absolute contraindications to CoC use
• Migraine with aura.
• Migraine without aura in women with >1 risk factor for stroke (above).
• Severe migraine or migraine lasting >72h (status migrainosus).
• Migraine treated with ergot derivatives.

Gynaecology

Check BP, BMI and health status after 3 months then annually. Do cervical smear if due (p271). Aim to use lowest-dose Pill to give good cycle control (ie no breakthrough bleeding). ▶If breakthrough bleeds screen for chlamydia.

Progesterone issues Norethisterone and levonorgestrel-containing COCs may cause breakthrough bleeding, acne, headaches, so prompted search for new progesterones, eg **gestodene** or **desogestrel** (Femodene®, Marvelon®, Mercilon®, Triadene®), but see problems with ↑ thrombosis (p303).

Drospirenone (DRSP) is a spironolactone-like progesterone with antiandrogenic/antimineralocorticoid action (said not to ↑weight; useful in those with acne or polycystic ovaries); thrombosis risk, see opposite.

Levonorgestrel containing pills seem safest (try first). Thrombotic risk of dienogest (Qlaira®), is currently unkown.

Switching from PoP: *If to a CHC,* start without gap. Use condoms for 7 days (9 if Qlaira®). *If to a progesterone-only Pill (PoP),* start as the old pack finishes.

Switching from CHC: *If to a CHC,* start immediately with no hormone-free interval. *If to a PoP,* start immediately the CHC preparation is finished.

Start CHCs/PoPs on day 1 of cycle, on day of TOP, ≥21 days postpartum, or ≥2wks after fully mobile post major surgery. If starting COC on day 1–5, cover is immediate, no other precautions (condoms) are needed. If later start (and not pregnant, p297), use condoms for 1wk. Qlaira:® start on day 1 (condoms for 9 days).

Stopping the Pill Tell to stop at once if she develops: •Sudden severe chest pain •Sudden breathlessness (±cough/bloody sputum) •Severe calf pain •Unexplained leg swelling •Severe stomach pain •Unusual severe prolonged headache; sudden visual loss; collapse; dysphasia; hemi-motor/sensory loss; 1st seizure •Hepatitis, jaundice, liver enlargement. •BP ≥160/95 •4 weeks before leg or major surgery (p300) •Any CI (p300). See cautions on p300; low-risk non-smokers may continue in their 40s. On stopping, 66% menstruate by 6 weeks, 98% by 6 months; women amenorrhoeic post-Pill usually were before.

Missed Pills (or severe diarrhoea): Consult package inserts; advice varies. In general, if the start delay is ≥48h, or >48h since last Pill continue Pills but use condoms too for 7 days (+ days of diarrhoea); if this includes Pill-free days, start next pack *without break* (omit inactive Pills in 'ED' formulations). If 2 pills of 1st 7 days in pack forgotten, use emergency contraception if unprotected intercourse since end of last pack. Vomiting <2h post-Pill: take another. Non-enzyme-inducing (p300) broad-spectrum antibiotics need extra precautions only if causing diarrhoea or vomiting. Postcoital options: p299.

Progestogen-only Pills (PoP=mini-Pill) Low-dose progestogen renders cervical mucus hostile to sperm. Desogestrel 75μg is more effective, inhibiting ovulation in 97%. Take at the same time of day (±3h), (±12h for desogestrel). PoPs can be used in most women with problems CI menorrhagia, PEG, migraine, past thrombosis, immobility, major surgery, ↑BP, (also if lactating). Avoid if on enzyme inducers (p300); breast cancer in last 5y; IHD, stroke or migraine with aura develop on R̲; GTD (p264); cirrhosis (metabolism problem); active viral hepatitis; liver tumours. Extra precautions are needed for 48h for late Pills, for time of use +28d if enzyme inducers given.

Postnatal Start 21 days after birth: eg COC if not breastfeeding; PoP, Depo-Provera® (or Nexplanon®) if breastfeeding. IUCD: fit ~4 weeks postpartum.

At the menopause Stop PoP if >50yrs old with >1 year's amenorrhoea (2yrs if <50yrs old)—as a rough guide. A spermicide and sponge may then be adequate in view of declining fertility. As COC masks the menopause, aim to stop at 50yrs, and replace with a nonhormonal method.

Flying and high altitude Avoid immobility if flight ≥3h. If trekking higher than 4500 metres for ≥1 week consider alternative.

Terminology

1st generation Pills are the original Pills containing 50µg oestrogen. *2nd generation Pills* are those containing ≤35µg oestrogen and levonorgestrel, norethisterone, norgestimate, or cyproterone acetate. *3rd generation Pills* contain desogestrel or gestodene as the progesterone. Although designed to be more lipid friendly 3rd generation Pills have not been proven to be better in those with cardiac risk factors and are more thrombogenic.[158]

Risk of venous thromboembolism

Risk of thromboembolism is increased by combined hormonal preparations; whether pill, ring or patch.[159] Figures are not well known for progesterone only preparations but they do not appear to be thrombogenic. Carriage of factor V Leiden mutation particularly increases risk of thrombosis (↑ risk

EURAS study 2007 [160]	
not on Pill	44:100,000
levonorgestrel	80:100,000
drospirenone	91:100,000
others	91:100,000
pregnant	291:100,000

×35). 3rd generation Pills particularly increase resistance to our natural anticoagulant (activated protein c, APC), so increasing thrombosis. With antithrombin 3, protein c or s deficiency have thrombosis rates ↑ ×5. Counsel those starting the Pill that it does increase the risk of thrombosis, particularly in 1st year of use, but it is still a rare event.

The Pill and travel: If immobile for >5h, the BNF recommends mid-journey exercises ± support stockings.

The Pill and surgery: Stop oestrogen containing contraception 4wks pre-op when immobilization expected and arrange alternative contraception.

When to use emergency contraception (eg missed-Pill)[161]

- CoC: if 3 or more 30–35µg pills or 2 or more 20µg pills forgotten in 1st 7 days of pack and unprotected sexual intercourse (UPSI) occurred in those 1st 7 days or pill-free week.
- PoP: if 1 or more PoPs have been missed or taken >3h late (>12h if Cerazette®) and UPSI has occurred in the 2 days following this.
- IUCD/IUS: if complete or partial expulsion identified or midcycle removal has been necessary and UPSI in the 7 days preceding this.
- Progesterone injection: if >14 weeks from last Depo-Provera® or >10 weeks from Noristerat® injection and UPSI occurred.

Barrier method: failure of method (eg splitting, slippage).

✚ **Depot progestogen ('the injection')** Simple, safe and effective, 2 preparations are available: **medroxy-progesterone acetate** 150mg given deep IM 12-weekly; start during the 1st 5 days of a cycle (postpartum see p95) or **norethisterone enanthate** (Noristerat®) 200mg into gluteus maximus 8-weekly—licensed for short-term use only, but can be used immediately postpartum (p95). Exclude pregnancy biochemically and use condoms for 7 days after late injections >2 weeks late. They inhibit ovulation and thicken cervical mucus. *ci:* Pregnancy; breast cancer; undiagnosed vaginal bleeding; acute liver disease; severe cardiac disease.

Advantages
• Secret
• No oestrogen content (no thrombosis risk, etc)
• OK if breastfeeding
• Fewer compliance problems
• Good when GI disease
• Protects against ectopics
• Fewer ovarian cysts
• Less endometriosis
• Less endometrial cancer (risk↓ 5-fold)
• Abolishes menor-rhagia eventually
• Reduces PMS (p254)
• Reduces PID (p286)

Problems: Irregular vaginal bleeding usually settles with time with amenorrhoea then supervening so encourage perseverance: eg 33% amenorrhoeic after 6-months' use; 50% for 1 year, and 60% for 18 months (14%, 27%, and 33% respectively for Noristerat®). If very heavy bleeding occurs, exclude pregnancy; give injection early (but >4 weeks from previous dose) and give oestrogen if not ci: (eg Premarin® 1.25mg/24h PO for 21 days or a CoC). Fears of osteoporosis in users prompted the Committee of Safety of Medicines to recommend review after 2 years' use in all users and avoidance in adolescents unless the only acceptable method. Bone mass density increases when stopped.[162] Other problems include weight gain (up to 2kg in 70% of women).

Special uses: Depot injections may be particularly useful:
• To cover major surgery. If given when stopping combined Pill 4 weeks before surgery it gives contraceptive cover for the next 8 or 12 weeks.
• Sickle-cell disease (reduces incidence of sickle-cell crises).
• Epileptics, fit frequency may be reduced. They are suitable for use with enzyme inducers (p300) without dose or interval change.[163]
• After vasectomy while awaiting partner's 'sperm-free' ejaculates.
• Where bowel disease may affect oral absorption.

There may be some delay in return of ovulation on stopping injections (median delay 10 months) but long-term fertility is not reduced.

Implants Progesterone implants give up to 3 years' contraception with one implantation. Nexplanon® is a radiopaque flexible rod containing **etonogestrel** 68mg which is implanted subdermally into the medial surface of the upper arm. It inhibits ovulation and thickens mucus. Contraceptive effect stops when the implant is removed. <23% of users become amenorrhoeic after 12 months' use. Infrequent bleeding occurs in 50% in the 1st 3 months' use; 30% at 6 months. Prolonged bleeding affects up to 33% in 1st 3 months; frequent bleeding affects <10%. Effective contraception may not occur in overweight women (BMI >35kg/m²) in the 3rd year, so consider earlier changing of implant. Liver enzyme inducers (p300) reduce efficacy, so use other eg barrier contraception if they are started. Avoid if breast cancer.

Patches Containing oestrogen and progesterone eg Evra® are similar to the combined Pill but breast discomfort and breakthrough bleeding is commoner in first 2 cycles. Relatively expensive, twice as many women discontinue due to side-effects, but compliance may be better.[164] Thrombotic risk is similar to the CoC.[165] They are affected by enzyme inducers (p300).

Vaginal rings Combined contraception (CHC p300) with better cycle control.[155]

Sterilization is popular. Each year ~47,000 women and ~64,000 men are sterilized (UK). ~25% of women rely on sterilization for contraception.

Ideally see both partners and consider the following:

- Alternative methods. Do they know about depot progesterone injections, coils, and implants? Give written information (in relevant language) about alternative contraception and ♂ and ♀ sterilization.
- Consent. Is it the wish of both partners? Legally only the consent of the partner to be sterilized is required but the agreement of both is desirable. Those lacking mental capacity to consent require High Court judgment.
- Who should be sterilized? Does she fear loss of femininity? Does he see it as being neutered? Does the ♀ really want or need hysterectomy? Examine the one to be sterilized.
- Irreversibility. Reversal is only 50% successful in either sex. Tubal surgery increases the risk of subsequent ectopics. Sterilization should be seen as an irreversible step. Sterilizations most regretted (3–10%) are those in the young (<30yrs), childless, at times of stress (especially relationship problems), or immediately after pregnancy (termination or delivery). Explain reversal or subsequent fertility treatment is rarely funded by the NHS.
- For sterilization at caesarean section, explain that it will only be done if the baby is normal and healthy. Counsel and agree ≥1 week pre-op.
- *Warn of failure rates*—10-year follow-up of 10,863 USA women gave pregnancy rates of 18.5:1000 procedures,[166] no better than new IUCDs (Copper T 380S®, Mirena®, GyneFIX®). Advise seeking medical confirmation if future pregnancy suspected or abnormal vaginal bleeding or abdominal pain. If pregnancy occurs there is ↑ risk of ectopic (4.3–76%).
- Side effects. A women who has been on the Pill for many years may find her periods unacceptably heavy after sterilization.

▶Record in the notes: *Knows it's irreversible; lifetime failure rate discussed*, eg 1 : 2000 for vasectomy, and 1 : 200 for ♀ sterilization; see above.

Female sterilization The more the tubes are damaged, the lower the failure rate and the more difficult reversal becomes. In the UK, most sterilizations are carried out laparoscopically under general anaesthesia. Filshie clip occlusion is recommended[167] with local anaesthetic applied to tubes (or modified Pomeroy operation at mini-laparotomy if postpartum or at caesarean). Do pregnancy test pre-op. Advise use of effective contraception until the operation and next period. Remove IUCD after the next period in case an already fertilized ovum is present. Alternatively, hysteroscopic sterilization using fallopian implants under local anaesthetic or IV sedation is endorsed by NICE.[168]

Vasectomy This is a simpler procedure than female sterilization and can be performed as an outpatient. The vas deferens is identified at the top of the scrotum and is ligated and excised or the lumen cauterized. Fascial interposition improves effectiveness.[169] Bruising and haematoma are complications. No-scalpel techniques reduce these complications.[170] Late pain affects 3% from sperm granulomata, which are less common if thermal cautery (rather than electrical cautery) is used. Warn of risk of chronic testicular pain.

The major disadvantage of vasectomy is that it takes up to 3 months before sperm stores are used up. Obtain 2 ejaculates 'negative' for sperm (the first 8 weeks post-op; 2nd 2–4 weeks later) before stopping other methods of contraception. Reversal is most successful if within 10 years of initial operation. *SE:* Evidence of ↑risk of prostate cancer post-vasectomy. Meta-analysis suggests a small risk which may be due to bias rather than causal.[171]

Control of bladder function Continence in women is maintained in the urethra by the external sphincter and pelvic floor muscles maintaining a urethral pressure higher than bladder pressure. Micturition occurs when these muscles relax and the bladder detrusor muscle contracts.

Incontinence or threat thereof dominates many people's lives. Ask about incontinence impact, role limitations, physical and social limitations, personal relationships, emotions, sleep/energy, and symptom severity. Ask patients to keep a diary of micturition for 3 days. Determine if symptoms indicate stress incontinence, urge, or mixed (NICE says this can be determined from history). If mixed, treat the detrusor overactivity (DOA) first (OPPOSITE) as this can be made worse by operations for stress incontinence. In all women exclude UTI and diabetes. Exclude pelvic mass (PV exam), and residual palpable bladder. In some postmenopausal women urgency, increased frequency, and nocturia is helped by estriol 0.1% cream PV or estradiol vaginal tablets used long term.

Urge incontinence "If I've got to go, I've got to go *now*". The bladder may be overactive, with high detrusor muscle activity. Treatment: see opposite.

Stress incontinence Small quantities of urine escape as intra-abdominal pressure rises, eg during sneezing. It is commoner in parous women (pregnancy, not mode of delivery is the risk factor).[173] Examination may reveal prolapse (p290) or incontinence (ask her to cough).

Overactive bladder (OAB) usually presents with *urge* incontinence, but in 25% presents as *stress* symptoms. It is a common cause of incontinence (33% of women; 50% of men, of the UK 3.5 million incontinent population).[174]

Management
- Exclude UTI and diabetes (dipstick urine; fasting glucose).
- Stress incontinence may respond well to pelvic floor exercises. Arrange supervised physiotherapy, (eg with weighted graduated vaginal cones)—8 contractions, 3 times daily for 3 months to improve muscle tone. A vaginal tampon supports the bladder neck, stopping leaks, eg while playing sport.
- Duloxetine (a serotonin/norepinephrine uptake inhibitor) 40mg/ 12h PO can reduce stress incontinence. Licensed for use in moderate to severe stress incontinence in the UK, NICE recommend it as an alternative to surgery, used in combination with physiotherapy.
- Surgery for severe stress symptoms aims to increase intraurethral pressure and reduce prolapse. NICE says cystometry is not needed before primary surgery[1] (but without it, incontinence from detrusor instability is missed in 5–10% so investigate if previous treatments have failed). Peri-urethral bulking may help, but effects may wear off after 1–2yrs. Mid-urethral tension free tape inserted under local anaesthetic, or synthetic slings can cure. If previous surgery has failed artificial sphincters may be needed.

True incontinence Continuous leakage may be due to congenital abnormality, eg ectopic ureters, or to acquired problems, eg vesicovaginal fistula due to trauma (eg post-abdominal hysterectomy in developed countries, after long labours, p90, in developing countries), malignancy, or radiotherapy. If surgery is impossible, seek the help of the continence adviser.

Interstitial cystitis Pathogenesis may involve loss of the bladder's glycosaminoglycan protective layer and a high number of activated bladder mast cells. Symptoms: frequency, urgency, bladder pain, and dyspareunia for >6 months. Symptoms are exacerbated by stress, ovulatory hormones, and certain foods. ℞: Dietary modification, bladder training, biofeedback, antidepressants, anticholinergics, NSAIDs, and bladder hydrodistension may be tried. Food diaries + ↓exposure to coffee, alcohol, tomatoes, vinegar, spicy foods, chocolate, and some fruits may help.[181]

1 Unless DOA clinically suspected, anterior prolapse, previous stress surgery, voiding difficulty.

Managing detrusor overactivity (overactive bladder)

- Refer if any neuropathy, prolapse, pelvic masses, or haematuria.
- Avoid caffeine (it is a mild diuretic and stimulates detrusor activity).
- Bladder training to increase time between voiding. Train for 6 weeks.
- Pelvic floor muscle physiotherapy if stress incontinence symptoms.
- Antimuscarinic drugs may be effective,[174] eg **oxybutynin**, starting with 2.5mg/12h, increasing slowly up to 5mg/6h (12 hourly if elderly; SE: dry mouth, blurred vision, nausea, headache, constipation, diarrhoea, abdo pain—SEs are less if modified-release once-daily tablets are used—20mg/day of Lyrinel XL® may be tolerated; approach this by weekly 5mg jumps). **Tolterodine** eg 2mg/12h is also effective; with lower side-effect profile. **Solifenacin** (5mg PO daily; up to 10mg as needed) is an alternative which may ↑ bladder capacity and ↓episodes of incontinence by 50%.[177]
- Nocturia may respond to **desmopressin** (unlicensed use).[174]
- Overactive bladders are occasionally treated with **botulinum toxin**, sacral nerve stimulation, augmentation cystoplasty, or urinary diversions.[172]

Voiding difficulty

Voiding difficulty is rarer in women than detrusor overactivity. ►*Remember faecal impaction as a cause of retention with overflow.*

Causes *CNS:* Suprapontine (eg stroke); cord lesions (cord injury, multiple sclerosis); peripheral nerve (prolapsed disc, diabetic or other neuropathy); or reflex, due to pain (eg herpes infections).

Obstructive: Early oedema after bladder neck repair is a common cause. Others: uterine prolapse, retroverted gravid uterus, fibroids, ovarian cysts, urethral foreign body, ureterocele, bladder polyp, or cancer.

Symptoms
• Poor flow
• Straining to void
• Hesitancy
• Intermittent stream
• Incontinence (eg overflow)
• Retention (acute or chronic)
• Incomplete emptying
• UTI from residual urine

Bladder overdistension—eg after epidural for childbirth.

Detrusor weakness or myopathy causes incomplete emptying + dribbling overflow incontinence. *Diagnosis:* cystometry; electromyography.[177] *Causes:* neurological conditions and interstitial cystitis (p306). It may lead to a contracted bladder, eg requiring substitution enterocystoplasty.[178]

Drugs: Especially epidural anaesthesia; also tricyclics, anticholinergics.

Tests: MSU (?UTI) + ultrasound for residual urine and bladder wall thickness: >6mm on transvaginal scan is associated with detrusor overactivity.[179] Then:
- Cystourethroscopy.
- Urodynamic studies: uroflowmetry (a rate of <15mL/sec for a volume of >150mL is abnormal). Do this before any surgery is contemplated.
- Subtraction cystometry is a subtraction of intra-abdominal pressure from measured intravesical pressure to give detrusor pressure (intravesical measure is a mix of bladder pressure and intra-abdominal pressure).

Treatment *Acute retention* may require catheterization (suprapubic if needed for several days). For persistent conditions (eg CNS conditions) self-catheterization may be learned, eg with a Lofric® gel coated catheter.

Detrusor weakness may respond to drugs to relax the urethral sphincter or stimulate detrusor: **α-blockers**, eg **tamsulosin** 400μg/24h, relax the bladder neck; **diazepam** relaxes the sphincter. Surgery may overcome obstructive causes, eg urethrotomy for distal urethral stenosis (uncommon).

Gynaecology

Gynaecology

Hysterectomy *Abdominal hysterectomy* is usually total (uterine body + cervix removed, but may be *Wertheim's* (extended to include local lymph nodes and a cuff of vagina)—used for malignancy. At *vaginal hysterectomy* the uterus is brought down through the vagina. Hospital stay is shorter but difficulties may arise at operation if the uterus is very bulky. Lower-segment caesarean section and nulliparity may also impede operation. Healthy ovaries are usually conserved, especially in young women, whichever route the uterus is removed by, unless the hysterectomy is for an oestrogen-dependent tumour. Complication: residual ovary syndrome (pain, deep dyspareunia, ovarian failure). *Laparoscopic hysterectomy* was developed for patients in whom problems with open surgery are anticipated (eg extensive adhesions with endometriosis), but most of these patients can have a vaginal hysterectomy—which is much quicker (77 minutes *vs* 131 minutes), with a similar complication rate. Hospital stays are shorter, but total recovery not quicker.

38,831 hysterectomies were performed in England in 2005–6, most for menorrhagia or fibroids, and rates vary widely. Femininity and sexuality are bound up with the uterus. *Subtotal hysterectomy* leaves the cervix behind so remember to go on smearing these cervices. The cervix is left in the belief that orgasm is less disrupted (controversial, and not borne out in systematic review)[182] but late cervical problems (including bleeding) are relatively common (11%). ▶Women who are counselled, and make their own decision about surgery, are less likely to have regrets. Operative mortality: ~0.06%. Severe complications occur in 3% and are commoner in younger women and with laparoscopically assisted surgery. Hysterectomy doesn't cause ↑psychological/sexual morbidity when compared with ablation (below) at 1yr post-op.

Manchester repair (Fothergill's operation) Pregnancy is still possible after this operation for uterine prolapse. The cervix is amputated and the uterus is supported by shortening the ligaments. It is an operation rarely performed.

Dilatation and curettage (D&C) The cervix is dilated sufficiently to admit a curette to scrape out a sample of endometrium for histology. D&C is a procedure for diagnosing abnormal bleeding (but outpatient endometrial sampling (p279) and hysteroscopy may make D&C unnecessary). Adequate sampling occurs in 75% but in 10% abnormal pathology may be missed. Evacuation of retained products of conception from the uterus after miscarriage (ERPC), or termination of early pregnancy, are carried out by **dilatation and suction**.

Hysteroscopy🔊 As an outpatient alternative to D&C, a hysteroscope can be inserted through the cervix into the uterus to visualize the endometrium. 'Blind' samples may then be taken using a sampler. Mainly used in the diagnosis of abnormal uterine bleeding or work up of infertility, it is also useful for some outpatient operative procedures: endometrial polypectomy, removal of small submucosal fibroids, endometrial ablation, removal of lost IUCDs, and transcervical sterilization. Use of saline distension medium gives better views, reduced vasovagal episodes, reduced procedure time and the ability to use cautery. Small scopes (2.7mm with 3–3.5mm sheath) reduce discomfort. NSAID taken 1h pre-procedure PO reduces post-procedure discomfort. Consider intracervical/paracervical local anaesthesia for postmenopausal women and if cervical stenosis (hence need for dilatation) anticipated: it is needed if large (>5mm) scopes used.

Endometrial ablation/resection by laser, diathermy, microwave, or other ablative method (under GA or spinal ± paracervical block) reduces bleeding by achieving a deliberate Asherman's syndrome (p251); as an alternative to hysterectomy, it has fewer complications. Endometrium may be thinned pre-op by leuprorelin or danazol. By 4 months 10% have menorrhagia again. Complications (major in 4% requiring further surgery in 1%): haemorrhage; infection (eg late necrotizing granulomatous endometritis); uterine perforation; haematometra, vesicovaginal fistula, fluid overload from irrigation fluid can cause ↑BP, ↓Na⁺, pulmonary oedema, CNS symptoms, and haemolysis. Some endometrium remains in most (so give progesterone-containing HRT later, if needed). Pregnancy and endometrial cancer can still occur after ablation: p253.

Laparoscopy The laparoscope is inserted umbilically. Instruments are inserted through ports in the *iliac fossae*. Occasionally a Verres needle is placed suprapubically to insufflate and aid manipulation of organs. This procedure allows visualization of the pelvic organs and is used for diagnosis of pelvic pain and ectopic pregnancy. The patient is spared a full laparotomy unless needed for treatment. A 'lap and dye' demonstrates tubal patency. Sterilization and hysterectomy may be laparoscopically carried out, and ectopic pregnancies treated.

Colporrhaphy or 'repair' The lack of support from the vaginal wall in cases of prolapse is rectified by excising redundant mucosa and doing a fascial repair. It is *not* an operation to correct urinary incontinence. The operation may be combined with Manchester repair or vaginal hysterectomy. The more mucosa is removed, the tighter the vagina. Enquire before surgery if she is sexually active. Catheterization circumvents post-operative retention of urine.

Cone biopsy A cone of tissue (point inwards) is cut out around the external cervical os, using knife or laser. This removes neoplastic tissue for histology, and may be curative. Complications: (immediate) bleeding, (long-term) cervical stenosis or incompetence.

Pelvic exenteration Consider this option when initial surgery fails to control neoplasia of the cervix, vulva, or vagina. It involves removal of the pelvic organs—ie ultra-radical surgery, which should only be contemplated if there is a chance of cure. Do your best to establish whether disease has spread to the pelvic sidewall or nodes, eg with MRI or CT scans and intra-operative biopsy with frozen section: if so, exenteration is probably not worthwhile. Only ~20% of possible candidates for surgery meet this criterion: in addition the patient should be quite fit, and ideally have a supportive partner. We know that palliative exenteration in those with unresectable disease is not worthwhile. 5-yr survival: ~50%. Operative mortality: ~5%. Complications: GI obstruction/fistulae; urinary fistulae. Remember to give full pre-operative counselling about colostomies, and sexual function (refashioning of the vagina *may* be possible).

Enhanced recovery This looks at patient pathways with a view to optimizing preoperative and postoperative care with the aim of minimizing inpatient length of stay. Measures adopted include admission on the day of operation, early removal of drips and catheters and early postoperative feeding. Daily ward rounds and good pain management are an integral part of care.

Gynaecology

This is intermittent or constant lower abdominal pain of >6 months' duration not associated exclusively with menstruation, intercourse, or pregnancy. Pain may cause, or be exacerbated by, emotional problems. She may be depressed. Adequate time needs to be given to allow women to tell their story, express their views as to the cause of pain, and explore psychological aspects and past abuse. A multidisciplinary approach effects most all round improvement.[184]

Laparoscopy may reveal a likely cause: chronic pelvic infection, endometriosis, adenomyosis, adhesions (eg residual ovarian syndrome and trapped ovarian syndrome),[185] or congested pelvic veins. Consider also irritable bowel syndrome (*OHCM* p268), and interstitial cystitis (p306).

If pain is quite cyclical ovarian suppression (Pill/Zoladex®) may help.

Pelvic congestion Congested lax pelvic veins (seen at laparoscopy) cause pain worse on standing, walking, and premenstrually. Typically variable in site and intensity, there may be unpleasant postcoital ache. Deep palpation reveals maximal tenderness over ovaries. Vagina and cervix may look blue as congestion. Look for associated posterior leg varicosities.

Remedies include explanation ('pelvic migraine'), ovarian supression, migraine remedies (*OHCM* p450) and relaxation techniques. For severe symptoms bilateral ovarian vein ligation, radiological embolization, or hysterectomy with salpingo-oophorectomy (±HRT) may cure.

Mittelschmerz This is mid-cycle menstrual pain which may occur in teenagers and older women around the time of ovulation—from the German *mittel* (=middle) and *Schmerz* (=pain).

Dyspareunia

This means pain during intercourse. There may be a vicious circle in which anticipation of pain leads to tense muscles and lack of lubrication, and so to further pain. ►*The patient may not volunteer the problem so ask about intercourse.* Her attitude to pelvic examination may tell you as much as the examination itself. Ask her to show you where the problem is. If the problem is actually vaginismus do not insist on examination and consider counselling and sex therapy (p384). Was there 'female circumcision' (p247)?

Dyspareunia may be superficial (introital) due so look for ulceration and discharge. Is she dry? If so is the problem oestrogen deficiency (p256) or lack of sexual stimulation? Has she had a recent postpartum perineal repair? A suture or scar can cause well-localized pain which is cured by massage or by removing the suture and injection of local anaesthetic. If the introitus has been rendered too narrow, she may need surgery.

Deep dyspareunia is felt internally (deep inside). It is associated with endometriosis and pelvic sepsis; treat the cause if possible. Ovaries lying in the rectovaginal pouch (or after hysterectomy) may be subject to coital thrusts; try other positions or ventrosuspension if a 'cure' can be obtained with trial use of a Hodge pessary.

Dermatographism is a rare cause of dyspareunia: look for itchy vulval wheals some minutes after calibrated dermatographometer application. It can occur on any surface. It is the commonest physical cause of urticaria, and the clue to its presence is linear wheals with a surrounding bright red flare (but no angio-oedema) elsewhere on the skin, in response to a firm stroke. Cause is unknown. Relief of dyspareunia in these cases has been achieved by 2% **adrenaline (epinephrine)** cream, and **cetirizine** 10mg/24h PO.

Gynaecology

This is a systemic disease resulting from vaso-active products released by hyperstimulated ovaries. The incidence for severe cases is 3–8% in women having ovarian stimulation (mild cases occur in 22–33% of treatment cycles). It is commoner in conception cycles, especially if multiple pregnancy. Other risk factors: see MINIBOX. Associated complications are ascites, reduced intra-vascular volume, pulmonary effusions and (rare) pericardial effusions. Thromboembolic complications may ensue (especially in upper limb and cerebral vessels).

Risk factors
• Age <30yrs
• Asthenic habitus
• Pregnancy
• Luteal phase HCG stimulation
• Polycystic ovarian syn
• Serum oestradiol >4000pg/mL
• Multiple follicles (>35)
• Previous hyperstimulation

Presentation Abdominal discomfort, nausea, vomiting, and abdominal distension ± dyspnoea. Presentation is usually 3–7 days after human chorionic gonadotrophin (HCG) administration, or 12–17 days, if pregnancy has ensued.

Prevention Note: *In vitro* maturation (IVM, p293) avoids the need for ovarian stimulation so is especially suitable for women with polycystic ovaries. In those in whom hyperstimulation is suspected (peak serum oestradiol >6000pg/mL and >30 follicles stimulated), the surest way to avoid hyperstimulation is to avoid administration of HCG so the stimulated follicles do not ovulate, thereby cancelling the cycle of treatment (or discontinue gonadotrophins and delay HCG injections until the serum oestradiol returns to 'safe' levels). Some selectively cryopreserve embryos for later transfer.

Management Admit to hospital unless just mild pain. Give adequate analgesia (opiates if necessary, avoid NSAIDs). Check FBC, U&E, creatinine, LFT, and coagulation profile. Do CXR if chest pathology suspected; ECG and echo if pericardial effusion suspected; blood gases if tachypnoeic or dyspnoeic. Chart urine output (if oliguria suspected catheterize and measure fluid output hourly). Measure abdominal girth and weigh daily. Ovarian size is a guide to severity unless oocytes have been harvested (eg, mild, ovarian size <8cm; moderate 8–12cm; severe >12cm). To avoid thromboembolism use antiembolic stockings, encourage leg mobility, and use heparin (p16) during inpatient stay[186] and possibly for 1st trimester if pregnancy ensues.[187]
.RCOL

Hyperstimulation is *severe* if haematocrit is >45%, WCC >15×10⁹/L, there is massive ascites, oliguria, mild renal, or liver dysfunction. Put up IVI, and consider CVP monitoring. Fluid replacement may be required, eg 500mL albumin over 2 hours. Paracentesis of ascites using ultrasound to avoid cysts may be needed to reduce discomfort, relieve breathing and for persistent oliguria (can improve renal function).

The situation is *critical* if the haematocrit is >55% and WCC >25×10⁹/L, there is tense ascites and renal failure, thromboembolic phenomena, and acute respiratory distress syndrome (*OHCM* p178). Admit to ITU. Symptomatic pleural effusions may need drainage. Use antiembolic measures as above. Pay meticulous attention to fluid balance. Aim to maintain intake at 3L/24h using normal saline if unable to tolerate oral fluids. Beware hyponatraemia.

The severity of effusions determines the time to recovery. In non-conception cycles with little ascites there will be resolution with menstruation. In conception cycles cysts may persist for weeks. Resolution usually occurs, but exceptionally termination of pregnancy may be needed. Deaths have been reported but are extremely rare (~1 : 500,000 stimulated cycles).

Gynaecology

Quite a few doctors hope to *make* patients better by taking responsibility for ordering the *mileau interieur*, and the credit when things go well. In psychiatry this approach is wrong. Mental health is about people (not patients) taking responsibility for themselves and their programme of change. The psychiatrist knows that his or her job is done, not when the patient is cured but when he becomes self-actuating, insightful, and interacting with the world in creative (not necessarily satisfactory) ways. So if you are hoping for a chapter dealing with mental disorders as if they were lung diseases with certain signs and agreed treatments this chapter will disappoint. A reader complained, to have pages on listening, dignity, etc? "Just tell me what to do." Well, here goes. Interpersonal problems: just do what you think you should do. Anxious? Get on with it: relax; try β-blockers. Depressed? SSRIs, tricyclics or get wired (ECT); think positive. Manic? Try lithium. Psychopathic? Tough luck. Schizophrenic? Antipsychotics; if dangerous, lock up. Psychotherapy for everything else. Phew! That's got it over with. Now sit back and rest. Or sit back and listen...if you listen, you may be able to help, rather than beat people over the head with formulaic solutions to problems they don't quite have.

 Read this chapter with *DSM-V*: a diagnostic and statistical manual that codifies all mental illness, but note that this flawed book ignores the social context of symptoms, and over-medicalizes them.[1]
We thank Dr Anish Patel, our Specialist Reader, and Dr Rashmi Singh, our Junior Reader, for their contribution to this chapter.

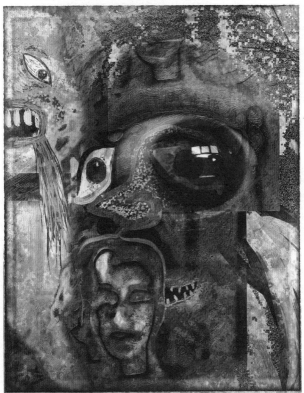

Doctors have never been very important because nothing that happens to our bodies ever really matters. In historical terms, what happens to our bodies rarely outlives our own times. Even the exceptions to this prove a different rule: we recall forever human images burnt on to stone at their moment of immolation in Nagasaki and Hiroshima. What happened to these people was important, and transcended their times. But it is all the more true that it isn't the way they lived, but the way they died that is important, and it is not the body or its image on stone which is important, but the image left on our minds. And so it is with psychiatrists, psychologists, and psychiatric nurses who play such vital roles in colouring our lives with hope or despair, who mitigate our madness, giving meaning, purpose, and dignity to the mental sufferings of so many of us. So when we think of them going about work, think of them burnishing humanizing images not on stone, but on the mind itself. How they do it is the subject of this chapter.

Fig 1. *Screaming but unheard: images born of paranoid schizophrenia.* Neil Houghton, the artist, says: "I was born in Bolton with a pencil in my hand. Always deep in thought and not mixing much with others. I have always been troubled with confusing and scary thoughts...diagnosed as schizophrenia. This painting is from a series chronicling a bad episode." ©Neil Houghton Gallery. When we asked him what message he would like to send doctors learning about mental illness, he replied "Patients can offer a valuable insight into their own illness." This value he points to is troubling, hard-won, but, ultimately, liberating.

"Terror grips when these things happen; the signs, the lights, the storm within: death by instalments... I'm a daily subscriber."

Psychiatry

Chaque homme porte la forme entière de l'humaine condition (Each of us bears the complete stamp of the human condition) This is the *first principle of psychiatry* and was proclaimed by Michel De Montaigne in 1580.[2] The *second principle* has yet to be agreed but will probably include reference to the idea that the bond between therapist and patient is unbreakable by any fact or revelation and exists entirely to foster growth and development.

A thought experiment Before reading further, cover the next paragraph with a card and write on it what you are trying to achieve as a mental health worker. Next, turn the card over and write down what was actually in your mind as unstated goals when you were last treating someone. So often our unconscious aim is just symptom control, obedience, or simply (simply!) normality. But if you were the patient (luck changes in a moment) what would you want? The aim of this page is to help you find out, by considering one person's answer.

The essence of mental health *Healthy (lucky!) humans are able:*... To love and be loved; without this asset, humans, more than all other mammals, fail to thrive.
... To embrace change—and face fear in a spirit of practical optimism.
... To take risks, free from endless worst-case-scenario-gazing.
... To satisfy the requirements of the group—if the person so desires.
... To deploy *joie de vivre*, and a wide range of emotional responses, including negative emotions, such as anger (pain's most motivating antidote).
... To make contact with reality: not too rarely or too often. *Human kind cannot bear very much reality.*
... To say "I was wrong" and learn from life and to have enough self-knowledge to heal the self and others, but not so much as to become demoralized.
... To inhabit fantasy worlds, enabling hope and creativity to flourish.
... To feel a sense of security, not always predicated on one's status in society.
... To enjoy self-expression—balanced by sensitivity to others' vulnerabilities.
... To feel a sense of awe and to risk enchantment (and hence disenchantment).
... To gratify bodily desires and eventually to be free from desire.[3] He who no longer desires anything for himself is both free and good, yet not superior.
... To have a sense of humour to compensate if the foregoing is unavailable.

> Go, go, go, said the bird: human kind
> Cannot bear very much reality.
> Time past and time future
> What might have been and what has been
> Point to one end, which is always present.
>   *Four Quartets,* TS Eliot

Happiness[1c] need not be an ingredient of mental health, as the merely happy are supremely vulnerable to events.

The essence of mental illness *Whenever a person's thoughts, feelings, or sensory impressions cause him objective or subjective harm that is more than transitory, a mental illness may be said to be present.* Often the harm is to society, but this is not part of the definition of mental illness, as to include it would open the door to saying that, for example, all rapists or all those opposing the society's aims are mentally ill. One feature of mental illness is that one cannot rely on patients' judgment, and the judgment of family, GP, or psychiatrist has a role. If there is disparity, let it be 'one person one vote', if voters are acting solely in the interests of the patient. Psychiatrists have no special voting rights (or else concepts of mental illness get too medicalized). Just because psychiatrists and GPs are not allowed more than one vote, this does not stop them from illuminating the debate by virtue of their special knowledge.

For convenience, English law saves others from the bother of specifying who has a mental illness by authorizing doctors to act for them. This is a healthy state of affairs only in so far as doctors remember that they have only a small duty to society, but a larger duty to their patient.

Learning disability (mental impairment) This is a condition of arrested or incomplete development of mind owing to low intelligence, p364.

 The external recipe for happiness ≈ stable family life + a good marriage + more wealth than your neighbours (absolute wealth is irrelevant)[4] + health + a cohesive trusting community.[5] The internal recipe is elusive.

Apart from showing sympathy, nothing is more to be desired than giving our patients dignity—not the dignity that they deserve (who among us would merit an ounce of dignity on this measure?) but the dignity that confirms to our patients that, mad, bad, or rambling, they are, root and branch, body and mind, just as human as their doctors—perhaps more so, because they are suffering.[1] *Let patients*

- Decide on modes of address, 'Miss Hudson' may be preferred to 'Amy, dear'. Dignity entails giving choices, and then respecting them.
- Know who we are (eg wear name badges). But don't label patients ("Go and see the new schizophrenic on Mary ward"). If you put a patient in a box the next thing you'll do is put a lid on it—and stop thinking.
- Wear their own clothes—and clothe them decently if they have none.
- Choose whether to take part in research—and whether to see students.
- Have personal space—both to stow their belongings, and to walk in, in private, whether alone, or with visitors.
- Participate in their treatment plans; explain about common side effects.
- Know what to do if a crisis develops. It's a great help to know that you will be seen in 4 hours rather than be left to moulder all weekend.

These 7 points are congruent with NICE (2012) and Human Rights law which lays out the right to life, freedom from inhuman or degrading treatment and torture, respect for privacy, the right to a fair hearing and freedom of expression. Some of these rights are inalienable, and unrevokable, even in time of war (on UK soil). So defences such as *'the ward was busy that day'* or *'there was no money to buy this service'* are unlikely to impress judges.

In practice, many mental health wards may do more harm than good (violence, verbal abuse, and sexual harassment eg from other patients).

Patients' other needs: Maslow's hierarchy and mental health

Maslow states that a healthy personality (ie fully functioning and self-actualizing) entails the meeting of a hierarchy of needs:

1 Biological needs (eg oxygen, food, water, warmth).
2 Safety needs (no present threats to safety); no pain. (Items 3–5 apply if this comfortable numbness, this 'stye of contentment'[6] is inadequate).
3 Love, affection, and 'belongingness' needs.
4 Esteem needs (self-respect, and need for respect from others: *see* top box). The latter is 2-fold: being valued for what you can do or bring to your community or family—and, above all, to be valued for who you are.
5 Self-actualization needs to follow one's calling and affirm "What I do is me: for that I came." Gerard Manley Hopkins If such needs are unmet, restlessness and anxiety result. To meet this need we might teach ourselves:
   - To be aware of the inner self and to understand our inner nature.
   - To transcend cultural conditioning.
   - To transcend the trifling and to grapple with life's serious problems.
   - To refresh consciousness by appreciating beauty and all good things.
   - To feel joy and the worth of living. www.connect.net/georgen/maslow.htm

Psychiatry

Uncomfortably numb on the lp ward... "Amy, dear, we are just going to put a tiny little needle in your back...you wont feel a thing."

---

1 Do our sufferings make us more human? Only if we can breathe meaning into them. Toothache doesn't make us more human because it has no meaning beyond the obvious and banal; but there is a kind of suffering 'which is a more effective key, a more rewarding principle for exploring the world in thought and action than personal good fortune'. (Deitrich Bonhoeffer). This suffering makes our souls. Not all our patients regret their psychological illnesses: sometimes, in retrospect, these patients refer to their break-*through*, not their break*down*. It is this power to grow and to transform experience which is human and humanizing. This is also why, paradoxically, illness is not the opposite of health. For humans, the true opposite to health is being stuck *In Status Quo*—that state which brooks no development. So if you find yourself writing ISQ (in status quo) in patients' notes you are invoking a kind of death.

It is important to decide if a patient has delusions, hallucinations (*that the patient believes are real*), or a major thought disorder (see below), because if present the diagnosis must be: schizophrenia, an affective disorder, an organic disorder, or a paranoid state (or a culturally determined visionary or spiritual experience), and not a neurosis or a personality disorder.

Patients may be reluctant to reveal odd ideas. Ask gently: "Have you ever had any thoughts which might now seem odd; perhaps that there is a conspiracy against you, or that you are controlled by outside voices or the radio?"

Hallucinations are auditory, visual, gustatory, or tactile sensations occurring without any stimulus. Common *hypnagogic/hypnopompic hallucinations* (on falling asleep or waking) do not indicate pathology. A *pseudo-hallucination* is one in which the person knows the stimulus is in the mind (eg a voice heard within him- or herself, rather than over the left shoulder). They are more common, and needn't indicate mental illness, but they may be a sign that a genuine hallucination is waning. Tactile or visual hallucinations (without auditory hallucinations) suggest an organic disorder (eg alcohol withdrawal, or Charles Bonnet syndrome, p438). NB: 2-4% of the general population experience auditory hallucinations, but only ~30% of these have a mental illness (more likely if associated with distressing delusions).[7]

Delusions are beliefs held unshakably, irrespective of counter-argument, that are unexpected, given the patient's cultural background. If the belief arrives fully formed, and with no antecedent events or experiences to account for it, it is said to be *primary*, and is suggestive of schizophrenia (or genius[1]). Such delusions form around a 'delusional perception', as illustrated by the patient who, on seeing the traffic lights go green (the delusional perception) knew that he had been sent to rid his home town of materialism. A careful history will reveal that delusions are often *secondary*—eg a person who is psychotically depressed may come to think of himself as being literally worthless. Delusions are especially relevant if they involve persecution and loss of control.[7]

Ideas of reference Sometimes we cannot help feeling that others are noticing the very thing we are ashamed of. If we know the thoughts come from ourselves, and are excessive, it is an obsession, not a delusion. NB: ideas of reference have poetic as well as pathological causes, as in dramatic storms, when thunder and lightning speak to us directly, in personal messages flashed onto to sky in some cosmic rendering of our own vision. *Chimes of Freedom* Bob Dylan; 1964

Ways to distinguish delusions/hallucinations from obsessional thoughts
1 Hearing the thought as a voice (a hallucination)—eg from a psychosis.
2 The voice is 'put into my head'—thought insertion (hallucination + delusion).
3 The voice is 'my own voice' but intrusively persistent (obsessional neurosis).

Major thought disorder This entails bizarre thoughts, or incongruent transition from one idea to another. (*Mania*—flight of ideas, p354; *schizophrenia*, p358). If hallucinations/delusions are present, ask: 1 What other evidence is there of mental illness? Hearing the voice of one's dead spouse is common, and does not mean pathology. 2 Could the odd ideas be adaptive, and the patient be better off 'ill'? A woman once believed she saw planes flying over her home, and that this data was taken from her head by the Ministry of Defence. She 'knew' she was playing a key role in defending Britain. When she was cured of her delusions (Ibsen's 'life-lie'[2]) she killed herself. An odd story; or is it so odd? According to the great poets, everything we cherish is an illusion, even our sense of distinctive self-hood, and without this primordial delusion, madness beckons.

1 'The moment I put my foot on the step the idea came to me without anything seeming to have paved the way for it, that the transformations I'd used to define the Fuchsian functions were identical with those of non-Euclidean geometry...the idea came with...suddenness, and immediate certainty.' *Act of Creation* A Koestler One

2 If psychiatrists have no authority to cure us of our life-lie (livslognen),[4] who has? Only dramatists who combine tragedy with comedy to awake us from our sleepwalking, and inoculate us against self-contempt. *Wild Duck* Ibsen

Some causes of odd ideas

A typical problem is trying to diagnose a young man presenting with hallucinations and/or delusions. The question often is: *Are these odd ideas due
to schizophrenia, drug abuse, or physical illness?*

1 Most auditory hallucinations not associated with falling asleep or waking up are caused by schizophrenia or depression.
2 In 90% of those with non-auditory hallucinations (eg seeing things), the
cause is substance abuse, drug withdrawal, or physical disease.
3 Evidence that substance abuse is to blame includes:
  • **The history:** Ask the patient, the family, and friends about abuse. Be
    precise about timing. If ≥4 weeks elapse between abuse and start-
    ing of odd ideas, substance abuse is an unlikely cause (but substance
    abuse may be an enabling factor promoting later psychosis).[1]
  • **Severity of symptoms:** If symptoms are severe, and the quantity of
    drug ingested is trivial, the drug is unlikely to be causative.
  • **Drug-seeking behaviour:** Be on the lookout for this.
  • **Physical examination:** This may reveal signs of drug abuse (eg injec-
    tion marks ± cellulitis), chronic alcohol abuse (eg spider naevi, liver
    palms, atrophic testes), or a physical medical illness (eg brain tumour).
  • **Blood or urine tests** may disclose the substance abused or give a hint
    of abuse (MCV↑ and gamma GT↑ in alcohol abuse).
  • **Imaging:** Consider CNS imaging if the patient is elderly with nothing to
    suggest substance abuse, or if there are CNS signs.
NB: middle-age is not a typical time for schizophrenia to present: alcohol
abuse or a primary CNS condition is more likely.

Diagnosing a *substance-induced psychotic disorder* implies that the
patient responds to the hallucinations or delusions as if they were real.
If the patient recognizes the hallucinatory nature of the experience, then
consider diagnosing *substance intoxication*, *substance withdrawal* or, if
there is past but no current exposure to hallucinogens, the diagnosis may
be 'flashbacks'—ie *hallucinogen persisting perception disorder*. This condition presents episodically up to 5 years after exposure to an hallucinogen, with flashback hallucinations—or phenomena such as geometric visual
hallucinations, seeing coloured flashes, or intensified colours, dots, spots,
or flashes, seeing trailing images or after-images, seeing complementary
coloured images of objects gone from view, seeing halos, seeing things too
small (micropsia), or seeing things too big (macropsia). These phenomena
may be self-induced or triggered by darkness, stress, or fatigue. DSM-IV 313

We all have odd ideas: it's our reactions to them and beliefs about them which are mad or sane or both.

Psychiatry

What's it like having hallucinations? Try virtual reality to find out

Doctors are always getting hung up on hallucinations, those tokens
used in games of clever diagnosis, without bothering to acquire real
knowledge of what it's like to have them. For doctors who have never experienced hallucinations, Professor Yellowlees has devised a virtual reality
experience on *Second Life*: a complex, unruly 3D world where we doctors
and our avatars get sucked into virtual clinics... Floors can fall away, leaving us walking riskily on stones above clouds. The eyes of a portrait flash
'shitface' as we pass, and a politician on an in-world TV might move in a single breath from platitudes to shouting "Go and kill yourself, you wretch!".
When it gets to the stage of our reflection in a mirror bleeding its eyes out
before expiring, most of us switch off.[9] But our patients cannot quit so easily. Virtual reality is just one way of sensitizing us to their struggles: other
ways are through blogs, painting (p313), and tragedy (the Ophelia effect).[10]

Voices in the margin are saying yet lost, ones.

---

1 Moderate cannabis use ↑ risk of psychotic symptoms in young people but has a much stronger
effect in those with a pre-existing predisposition to psychosis.[11,12] High-yield cannabis ('skunk') can
cause thought broadcasting, paranoia, depersonalization & visual/auditory hallucinations.[13]

Only people can change people: 'Alyosha's arrival seemed to have a sobering effect on him...as though something had awakened in this prematurely aged man that had long been smothered in his soul..."For you see, my dear boy, I feel that you are the only man in the world who has not condemned me" '. *Brothers Karamazof*, Dostoevsky; page 25

On starting psychiatry you may feel unskilled. A medical problem will come as a relief—you know what to do. Do not be discouraged: you already have plenty of skills (which you will take for granted). The aim of this chapter is to build on these. No one can live in the world very long without observing or feeling mood swings, and without devising ways to minimize what is uncomfortable, and maximize what is desirable. Anyone who has ever sat an important exam knows what anxiety is like, and anyone who has passed one knows how to master anxiety, at least to some extent. We have all survived periods of being 'down', and it is interesting to ask how we have done this. The first element is time. Simply waiting for time to go by is an important psychotherapeutic principle. (Voltaire teasingly remarked that the role of the doctor is to amuse the patient until nature effects a cure.) Of course, there are instances when waiting for time to go by leads to fatal consequences. But this does not prevent the principle from being useful.

Another skill with which we are all more or less adept is *listening*. One of the central tenets of psychiatry is that it helps our patients just to be listened to. Just as we all are helped by talking and sharing our problems, so this may in itself be of immense help to our patients, especially if they have been isolated, and feel alone—which is a very common experience.

Just as spontaneous regeneration and improvement are common occurrences in psychiatry, so is relapse. Looking through the admissions register of any acute psychiatric ward is likely to show that the same people keep on being re-admitted. In one sense this is a failure of the processes of psychiatry, but in another sense each (carefully planned) discharge is a success, and a complex infrastructure often exists for maintaining the patient in the community. These include group support meetings, group therapy sessions, and social trips out of the hospital. We all have skills in the simple aspects of daily living, and in re-teaching these skills to our patients we may enable them to take the first steps in rebuilding their lives after a serious mental illness.

So *time, listening,* and the *skills of daily living* are our chief tools, and with these simple devices much can be done to rebuild the bridges between the patient and his outside world. These skills are simple compared with the highly elaborate skills such as psychoanalysis and hypnosis for which psychiatry is famous. The point of bringing these to the fore is so that the newcomer to psychiatry need not feel that there is a great weight of theoretical work to get through before he starts doing psychiatry. You can engage in the central process of psychiatry from day 1. Use the knowledge and experience gained as a foundation on which to build the constructs required for the more specific and effective forms of psychotherapy.

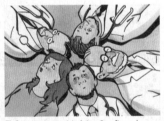

Fig 1. *Listening, not judging.* So often when we listen the fact that we are also judging leaks out in an unconscious disapproving gaze—and our patient clams up. This mythical ward round has adopted an extreme method to prevent this. Words waft up on thermals of hot air, unimpeded by cold or quizzical or uncomprehending gazes. So...don't let ward rounds descend into fact-based inquisitions. As one history-taker said, "They wanted facts. Facts! They demanded facts...as if facts could explain anything!" Joseph Conrad *Lord Jim*

Psychiatry

Thomas à Kempis.

If we knew more about ourselves, we would understand more about our fellow patients, bearing in mind that 'all gods and devils that have ever existed are within us as possibilities, desires, as ways of escape'. Herman Hesse 1919.[14] What we want our patients to achieve is insight. Our judging does not help this. Judgment turns patients away from us. We cannot expect our patients to be honest with us if they know that we are judging them.

- The good listener is *not* silent, but reflective—a mirror not a message. Mirrors do not judge but they enable self-judgment. Unless some criminal act is underway, it really does not matter what we think about our patients. What matters is how the patient thinks about him- or herself and his or her near-ones—and how these thoughts can be transformed.
- If we judge people they will not trust us. No trust ≈ no healing.
- If we judge, patients will leave us for others perhaps less well qualified.
- There is no evidence that judging improves outcomes. Worse outcomes are likely if the patient feels alienated.
- Patients know if we feel bad about them. They may internalize this, and assume that things will always be bad because *they themselves* are bad.

Despite these bullets, there is a problem that won't go away. If we find ourselves talking to perpetrators rather than victims, we may not be wise to suspend judgment forever. If a crime is afoot putting others at risk, you may need to break confidentiality. Discuss this with a colleague. Ask yourself whether Nazi and Rwandan doctors were *too* nonjudgmental with their fellow patients. If 'tout comprendre c'est tout pardonner'[1], then to pardon *all* actions is to abdicate our moral selves. What is the consequence of this—for us, and for our patients? Unless we exercise judgment, it might be thought, we may be condoning evil. 'For evil to flourish in the world, all that is required is for the good to remain silent'. If we remain silent long enough, then will our own moral sense sicken, and die? What human duties do doctors have which trump *anything* that goes on in the consulting room? Whenever you think the time may have come to judge, check with yourself that it is not from outrage, or disgust, or through the exercise of pride, or from a position of power that you are judging—but reluctantly, and from *duty*. The dreadful history of some doctors in the twentieth century teaches that we must be human first, and physician-scientists second.

Phosphorescent patients   *Dr. Quarrell's letter*—"My dear Elvet...

I am growing suspicious about the extent to which I need yr permission to have feelings about my patients. Clinical detachment is a profoundly unnatural state of mind and all sorts of evil can come of it...In Casualty amongst all that battered flesh...it was a survival tool. So it gets carried over into psychiatry. We offer our patients what appears to be human contact, human warmth—and we give them a calculated simulacrum of human contact, with no flesh, no blood, no love, no desire... I do not know how to proceed...help... this [patient] is slightly phosphorescent." AS Byatt 2003 p75 of *A Whistling Woman*

In judging others, we expend energy to no purpose...but if we judge ourselves, our labour is always to our profit.

Psychiatry

1 *Tout comprendre c'est tout pardoner*—'To understand all is to forgive all'. I have found it necessary to inscribe this phrase around the bell of my stethoscope. This bell then tolls in my mind's ear whenever my patient is making me angry or despairing—in other words whenever I have *not understood*. 'Tout comprendre c'est tout pardoner' is the most magnanimous phrase ever created, and was first promulgated by Madame Anne Louise Germaine de Staël: "tout comprendre rend très indulgent"—To understand all is to become very lenient."[15] The phrase was stolen by Tolstoy in the last chapter of Book 1 of *War & Peace*. Can we forgive this theft? Of course; not just because the theft gave anonymous immortality to Madame de Staël, but because Tolstoy probably needed to believe he had created it to sustain him in the illusion of his own infallible magnanimity,[16] without which his great literary enterprise would have been impossible.[17] *Vive nos illusions: Vive nos illusions magnifique!*

Some time ago, a child said "*To understand me you must swallow a world*".[18] Taking this quest for truthfulness about the inner life further, one of our most rigorous therapists has said that he must perform "the essential Jonah act of allowing himself to be swallowed, remaining passive, accepting..."[19] The sign that we are listening properly, from *within* the whale, so to speak, is that we are *immersed* in our patient and that what we are hearing could, perhaps, *change* us. Patients intuitively understand and respond to this level of listening. It takes great concentration. *Doing* something is always easier—hence Anthony Storr's aphorism: *Don't just do something—Listen!* [1]

Once we had the good luck to work on a psychiatric ward with a would-be surgeon, who, before he accustomed himself to psychiatry, would pace restlessly up and down the ward after clerking his patients, wondering when the main action would start, impatient to get his teeth into the business of curing people. What he was expecting was some sort of equivalent to an operating list, and not knowing where to find one he was at a loss, until it dawned that taking a history from a psychiatric patient is not a 'pre-op assessment', but the start of the operation itself—albeit a rather odd operation in which it is not the questions which are incisive but as often as not what happens in the silences. Even advanced textbooks of psychiatry appear to have missed this surgeon's insight, describing psychotherapy as something which should only happen after 'a full psychiatric history'.[20] There is no such thing as a full psychiatric history. In describing the salient psychological events of a single day even the best authors (eg James Joyce in *Ulysses*) need substantial volumes. This is why this chapter is starting so slowly: to give time for these notions of listening to take root. So swallow hard. Calm your restlessness. Stop. Reflect.

Taking a history sounds like an active, inquisitorial process, with lists of questions, and the tone of our page on this process (p322 & *mental state examination*, p324) seems to perpetuate this error. It isn't a question of *taking* anything. It's more about *receiving* the history, and *allowing* it to unfold. ▶If you only ask questions, you will get only answers as replies.

As the history unfolds, sit back and listen. This sounds easy, but during a busy or difficult day you will find your mind wandering (or galloping away)—over the last patient, the next patient, or some aspect of your own life. You may find yourself worrying about having to 'section' this patient or see the relatives afterwards. By an act of Zen, banish extraneous thought, and concentrate totally on the person in front of you—as if your life depended on it. Concentrate on the whole person—the language, the words, the nonverbal cues, and get drawn into their world. Initially don't even think of applying diagnostic labels. Open your mind and let everything flood in. Listening is hard. We wish we did it better. We all need to practise it more.

Avoid interruptions and seeming to be too purposeful, at least for the first few minutes (or days). Expect periods of silence. If prompts are needed try "and then how did you feel?" or just "and then..."; or repeat the last words the patient spoke. Don't be anxious if the patient is not covering major areas in the history. Lead on to these later, as the interview unfolds. Early in your career you will have to ask the relevant questions (p322) in a rather bald way (if the information is not forthcoming during the initial unstructured minutes), but it is important to go through this stage as a prelude to gaining information by less intrusive methods. Always keep in mind the chief aims of *making a diagnosis, defining problems,* and *establishing a therapeutic relationship.*

1 The converse of this aphorism is the Parris dictum: "*When people are anxious it isn't clever to make a virtue of listening. Sometimes our patients simply need to be told.*" Sometimes they need space for self-expression. Which approach is right—when? We only know this by knowing our patients: this entails listening—which is why, 9 times out of 10, Storr is right: but 9 out of 10 is not always.

What is the point of all this listening?

Listening enables patients to start to *trust* us. Depressed patients often believe they will never get better. To believe that they *can* get better, patients need to trust us, and this trust is often starts the therapeutic process. In general, the more we listen, the more we are trusted. Our patients' trust in us can be one of our chief motivations, at best inspiring us to pursue their benefit with all vigour. A story bears this out. One day, in 334 BC, Alexander the Great fell ill with fever. He saw his doctor, who gave him a medicine. Later he received a letter saying his doctor was poisoning him as part of a plot (it was an age of frequently fatal intrigues). Alexander went to his doctor and silently drank the medicine in front of him—then gave him the letter. His confidence was rewarded by a speedy recovery. We think it is unreasonable to expect *quite* this much trust from our patients, and one wonders what can have led Alexander to such undying trust in his doctor. We suspect that his doctor, above all else, must have been a good listener.

Lifeworlds, and how to keep them intact

Even if we all listen the same way, what we will hear will depend on our own expectations, anxieties, and past experience. Take this dialogue.[22]

> *Doctor:* "How long have you been drinking that heavily?"
>
> *Patient:* "Since I've been married."
>
> *Doctor:* [impatiently] "How long is that?"
>
> *Patient:* [giggling] "For years". Perhaps the doctor hears '4 years'.

If, prosaically, all we want to know is how long her liver was exposed to alcohol, we need facts in linear time. But she chooses to answer in event-time, or personal time. This is Mishler's great distinction between the *voice of medicine* and the *voice of the lifeworld*.[23] Sometimes we must set experiences not in linear time but in the order they first become significant to a lover or parent. *Justine, L Durrell 97* What would this patient have gone on to say if her doctor had swallowed her world? What did those giggles signify? We will never know, but they might have explained her coming death.

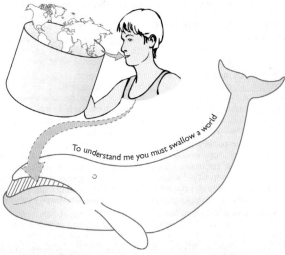

Fig 1. Swallowing a world.

To understand me you must swallow a world

Contrary to the one, Aristotle (Alexander's tutor) taught that love (not reward) is the foundation of trust.

Psychiatry

Introduce yourself; explain how long the interview may take. Describe its aim; emphasize that "here is a safe place to talk". Find out how the patient came to be referred, and what his expectations are. If the patient denies any problems or is reluctant to start talking, don't hurry. Try asking "How *are* you?" or "What has been *happening* to you?" or "What are the most important things?" "Does anyone *else* think there is a problem?" "Who does it effect most?" These are beautiful questions because they impose no categories, and seeing what categories your patients imposes, unprompted, will often tell you rich things. Listen, without interrupting, noting exact phrases. By inhabiting and using the categories your patient gives, you may enter his world. 2 minutes may be needed for this phase—or 2 years—depending on how unspeakable and distressing his or her thoughts are. Events surrounding war, torture, rape, and family dislocations may take years before they can be told.

Presenting symptoms Agree a problem list with the patient early on, and be sure it is comprehensive, eg by asking "If we were able to deal with all these, would things then be all right?" or "If I were able to help you, how would things be different?". Then take each problem in turn and find out about onset, duration, effects on life and family; events coinciding with onset; solutions tried; reasons why they failed. The next step is to enquire about mood and beliefs during the last weeks (this is different from the mental state examination, p324, which refers to the mental state at the time of interview). Specifically check for suicidal thoughts, plans, or actions—the more specific these are, the greater the danger. Discussing suicide does not increase the danger. Questions to consider: "Have you ever felt so low that you have considered harming yourself?" "Have you ever actually harmed yourself?" "What stopped you harming yourself any more than this?" "Have you made any detailed suicide plans?" "Have you bought tablets for that purpose?" Depression—ie low mood, anhedonia (unable to feel pleasure), self-denigration ("I am worthless"; "Oh that I had not been born!"), guilt ("It's all my fault"), lack of interest in hobbies and friends plus biological markers of depression (early morning waking, ↓appetite, ↓sexual activity, ↓weight); mania (p354); symptoms of psychosis (persecutory beliefs, delusions, hallucinations, p316); drug and alcohol use; obsessions; anxiety; eating disorders (eg in young women; often not volunteered, and important). Note compulsive behaviour, eg excessive hand-washing.

The present Housing, finance, work, friends, spouse/partners (negotiated or non-negotiated non-monogamy?).[24] Physical and mental health, job, and personality of family. Who is closest to whom? Any stillbirths, abortions?

Birth, growth, and development How has he spent his life? Ask about school, play (alone? with friends?) hobbies, further education, religion, job, sex, marriage. Has he always been shy and lonely, or does he make friends easily? Has he been in trouble with the law? What stress has he had and how has he coped with it? NB: noting early neurotic traits—nail-biting, thumb-sucking, food fads, stammering (not really a neurotic feature)—rarely helps.

Premorbid personality Before all this happened, how were you? Happy-go-lucky↔driven, gentle↔sadistic,[1] tense↔laid-back, happy↔depressed, social↔antisocial? Impulsive, selfish, fussy, irritable, rigid, insecure/schizotypal,[2] shy, hostile, competitive? ►Talk to whoever accompanies him, to illumine premorbid personality and current problems. But don't let her speak for the patient (at least make sure the patient has the first and last word).

Relevant medical history eg on retroviral drugs, or frequent asthma attacks. Next, examine the **mental state** (p324 & p353). You may now make a diagnosis, or decide that labelling is unwise. Ensure the areas above are covered in the light of any diagnosis so that the questions *"Why did he get ill in this way at this time?"* and *"What are the consequences of the illness?"* are answered.

Discussing childhood sexual abuse (CSA) with an adult who is currently experiencing psychological difficulties

A frequent question to arise is 'how far does past CSA account for current problems, and how much should this issue be explored now?' Each person is different: try to learn to use whatever your patient gives you, for their benefit. See p328 for how to talk about sexual issues. Sometimes it is possible to be optimistic, despite the fact that many patients and professionals believe that CSA causes intense, pervasive harm in the general population, regardless of gender. This issue has been examined in careful meta-analyses looking at 59 studies based on college data. These show that students with CSA were, on average, only slightly less well adjusted than controls. But this poorer adjustment cannot be attributed to CSA: family environment is consistently confounded with CSA and explains much more adjustment-variance than CSA. Self-reported reactions and effects from CSA indicate that negative effects are neither pervasive nor often intense. Also, men react much less negatively than women. Even though this college study is consistent with data from national samples, this optimistic meta-analysis should not blind you to the possibility that the patient sitting in front of you might be *very* damaged by CSA—but do not *assume* that CSA is the underlying reason for everything.[25]

▶When in doubt, get further help.

"I'm not going to be a victim all my life just because I was abused!"

Using whatever your patient gives you to make subjective but highly accurate, even valid maps of patients' worlds.

Doctor: "When you are like this, what's most difficult?"

Dawn: "Looking after the children—and going out to work".

Doctor: "Which is harder?"

Dawn: "Well, going out to work; sometimes the children help. Jo and Nick."

Doctor: "Anyone else?"

Dawn: "Well—my husband? Fat chance, even when he's sober."

Doctor: "So the children don't take after him, then?"

Dawn: "Lord no! Not yet, anyway—but all the blokes in his family drink like fish, so I'm worried for Nick when he gets that bit older."

Doctor: "You worry more about him than Jo?"

Dawn: "Yes—even though Jo cannot read yet, which is a worry. But she's got a way of looking after us somehow. She'll be all right—she's like her gran."

Doctor: "She still looks after you all sometimes?"

Dawn: "Well, she did, but she died last year, and then I went back on drugs."

All families evolve their own ways of communicating, and much goes on under the surface. In this dialogue, Dawn instigates a dozen categories or concepts. In an unconscious *tour d'horizon,* she draws a map for us, and as we impose none of our own suggestions, we can be fairly sure they represent some of the chief landmarks in her world. Don't place people and events on other people's maps: let them populate their own. Don't superimpose the quasi-objective platitudes and longitudes of time and place. It is better to let the map grow organically. **You yourself are on the map**, partly revealing and partly hiding the other elements. Move around a bit, and by a process of psychological parallax[3] you can estimate how far your patient is from the centre of her life.

---

1 *Narcissism + paranoia ≈ "authoritarian".* When paranoid, antisocial, narcissistic, schizoid, and schizotypal elements conjoin with sadism we have a perfect storm (Hitler, Stalin, Saddam Hussein, Kim Jong-il [etc] are such examples). As ever, if you identify this combination, get senior help (from the Royal Navy? or the Pope? or John Lennon?).

2 *Schizotypal ≈ the socially anxious, friendless loner with magical thinking, odd fantasies ± clairvoyance.*

3 *Parallax = apparent angular displacement of a celestial body due to a change in the position of the observer. With a baseline of known length between 2 observations, the distance to the object becomes known.*

This assesses state of mind at the time of interview. Take notes under the following headings.

- *Appearance and behaviour:* Eg signs of self-neglect; slowness, anxiety, or suspiciousness.
- *Mode of speech:* Speech rate, eg gabbling (pressure of speech), or slow/retarded. Note content.
- *Mood:* Note thoughts about harming self or others. Gauge your own response to the patient. The laughter and grand ideas of manic patients are contagious, as to a lesser extent is the expression of thoughts from a depressed person.
- *Beliefs:* Eg about himself, his own body, about other people and the future. Note abnormal beliefs (delusions) eg that thoughts are overheard, and ideas (eg persecutory, grandiose). See p316.
- *Unusual experiences or hallucinations:* "Sometimes when people are low they have unusual experiences; have you heard anything unusual recently?" Note modality, eg visual.
- *Orientation:* In time, place, and person. What year? What season? What month/day of week? Is it morning or afternoon? What is your name?
- *Short-term memory:* Recall a name & address 5min after learning it. Ensure he really has learned it before waiting for the 5min to elapse.
- *Concentration:* Months of the year backwards.
- Patient's *insight* and degree of your *rapport*.
- *Long-term memory:* Current affairs recall. Who is the monarch/head of state? This tests other functions, not just memory.

Psychiatry

Direct questions to try
• Any odd thoughts?
• Might your thoughts be being interfered with?
• Do you feel anyone is controlling you?
• Is anyone putting thoughts into your head?
• Do other people access or hear your thoughts?
• Is anyone harming you?
• Any plots against you?
• Do you hear voices when there's no one nearby? What do they say? Echoing you? Telling you off?
• Do you see things that others cannot see?
• Are you low/depressed?
• Is life worth living?
• Can anything give you pleasure?
• Sleep and appetite ok?
• Energy levels ↑ or ↓?
• Can you concentrate ok?
• Are you feeling guilty?
• Is your confidence low?
• Are you wanting to harm anyone? Yourself?
• Any worries/anxieties?

Non-verbal behaviour *Why are we annoyed when we blush, yet love it when our friends do so?* Part of the answer to this question is that non-verbal communication is less well controlled than verbal behaviour. This is why its study can yield valuable insights into our patients' minds, particularly when analysis of their spoken words has been unrevealing. For example, if a patient who consistently denies being depressed sits hugging himself in an attitude of self-pity, remaining in a glum silence for long periods of the interview, and when he does speak, using a monotonous slow whisper unadorned even by a flicker of a gesticulation or eye contact—we are likely to believe what we see and not what our patient would seem to be telling us.

Items of non-verbal behaviour:
- Gaze and mutual gaze
- Facial expression
- Smiling, blushing
- Body attitude (eg 'defensive').

Signs of auditory hallucinations:
- Inexplicable laughter
- Silent and distracted while listening to 'voices' (but could be an 'absence' seizure, p206)
- Random, meaningless gestures.

Signs of a depressed mood:
- Hunched, self-hugging posture
- Little eye contact

Dress:
('The apparel oft proclaims the man')[26]
- Hairstyle
- Make-up
- Ornament (ear-rings, tattoos, piercings).

Anxious behaviour:
- Fidgeting, trembling
- Nail-biting
- Shuffling feet
- Squirming in the chair
- Sits on edge of chair.

- Downcast eyes; tears
- Slow thought, speech, and movement.

What is a mental state?

A true description of mental states entails valid knowledge about current emotions plus their reactions to those emotions. These reactions are themselves emotional (eg being relieved that one's sense of remorse over x feels authentic), as well as being the bedrock out of which beliefs and attitudes are formed. These interactions make a picture to an observer which is complex, paradoxical, subjective, error-prone, contradictory—and fascinating.

Describing and communicating mental states is the central puzzle that confronts not just psychiatrists and our patients, but also artists. Poets and songwriters summon up diverse mental states (herein lies their genius) but none can control them or their infinite progeny (what happens next). This is the province of psychiatry. If we could control mental states at will at least half our job would be done (no doubt there would be unfortunate side effects). Drugs, psychotherapy, and behavioural methods are the tools available for this task, and they all, crucially, impinge on mental state. You cannot tell if these methods are helping if you cannot access your patient's mental state, which is why the page opposite is so important. If you think you can access mental states *just* by applying the formulaic regimen opposite, you will often fail, as any trip into the mind of another is not just a voyage without maps, it is ultimately a creative and metaphysical enterprise.

On this view, knowledge of mental states is doubtful, but often this is not so, eg a baby being put to the breast after separation from her mother, or an audience giving a standing ovation, or screaming fans waving at an idol, and we know *without doubt* that these mental states comprise unalloyed satisfaction, pleasure, and adulation. So often it's non-verbal behaviour that allows valid judgment about mental states: don't rely on words alone—those capricious (but indispensable) tokens of disguise and deception.

How many different selves are rolled up into your patient?

Here is an example: a person who happens to be black, who happens to be Muslim, who happens to be male, who happens to be questioning his sexual orientation while trying to be a good son and a good brother. He is trying on new identities and new relationships with Allah. How do these identities involving race, culture, religion, gender, and sexuality feed into his mental state now?[27] In the mental state examination, give space to find out about these roles, to get a feeling for what causes most turmoil, ambivalence, and introspection, the 3 'vital signs' of psychic life—TAI.[1] Aim to understand how good the patient is at articulating these roles. Try to understand from which platform the patient feels most comfortable in tackling his problems—and pay respect to each role separately, in order to gain trust.[28] Try to find out how plastic or rigid each identity is—the more plastic, the easier it is for the ego to function harmoniously (ie 'good identity integration').[29]

Lear: "Who is it that can tell me who I am?" Fool: "Lear's shadow".

Just as Shakespeare creates metaphysical places, such as Lear's[30] and Viola's Illyria, where answers to questions of identity can take shape, so psychiatrists create spaces in the silences of mental state examinations where our multiple personas can visit each other. Our masks shift and a few rays illumine our 'shadow selves', as we come to know the difference between who we are and who we think we are. Acknowledging that we have a shadow is hard, but vital.[31] Mental state examinations start this process leading to questions such as "Who knows most about who you are? Who else? How do their views differ? What truths about you do they acknowledge or hide?"

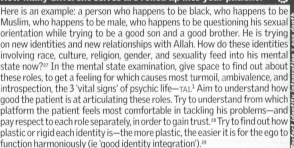

1 Tai Chi in Confucian philosophy is the mother of *yin* and *yang,* the *Supreme Ultimate Fist* which transcends and harmonizes those 'internal necessities in our our being' which forever drive us on. Herman Melville *Moby Dick* Ch 36

How to avoid doctor-dependency

A patient may become over-dependent on his or her doctor in many spheres of medicine. This is a particular danger in psychiatry because of the intimate and intense rather one-sided or asymmetrical relationship which may be built up between the patient and psychiatrist—who will often know more about a patient's hopes and fears than any close friend. This encourages the patient to transfer to the therapist thoughts and attitudes that are often directed to parent-figures. This process (known as **transference**) powerfully stimulates doctor-dependency, sometimes with serious consequences. *Other risk factors for doctor-dependency:* Chronic illness/prescribing; inability to achieve the sick role—eg if you have chronic back pain, your suffering is hidden from others (no scars, no bleeding, etc), and you may feel delegitimized in your sick role because you cannot be diagnosed or helped. But equally, because of this, you hold power over your doctor. It is difficult for her to challenge your ideas without damaging the therapeutic relationship. So the doctor is forced to collude with your definition of ill-health. This may harm you and society.[32]

Signs of non-therapeutic dependency Repeated phoning for advice, inability to initiate any plan without help from a therapist, and disallowing of your attempts to terminate treatment (eg by threatening relapse).

Assessing whether dependency is a problem Clearly, in the examples above, the patient's dependency on his doctor is non-therapeutic. At other times, for example, early in treatment, doctor-dependency may help. In these circumstances the danger is that the doctor will be flattered by his patient's dependency on him. Most therapists either want to be loved by their patients or want to dominate them (or both), and it is important to know, in each session with each patient, just where you lie within the space marked out by these axes. Ask yourself: "Why do I look forward to seeing this patient?" "Why do I dread seeing Mr X?" "Why do I mind if this patient likes me?"

▶When you feel good after seeing a patient always ask yourself why (it is so often because he is becoming dependent on you).

Avoiding dependency Planning and agreeing specific, limited goals with patients is one way of limiting dependency. If the patient agrees from the outset that it is not your job to provide him with a new job, wife, or family, he is more likely to have realistic expectations about therapy.

Planning discharge from the start of therapy helps limit doctor-dependency. Discharge is easy from the outpatient departments, but for the GP the concept of discharge is diluted by the fact of his contractual obligations. The patient is quite within his rights to turn up the day after being 'discharged' and demand that therapy be started all over again. The GP must have more subtle methods at his disposal to encourage the patient to discharge himself. For example, he can learn to appear completely ineffective, so that the dependency cycle (patient presents problem→doctor presents solution→patient sabotages solution→doctor presents new solution) is never started. Another method is to bore your patient by endlessly going over the same ground, so that the patient seizes control and walks out as if to say "I've had enough of this!".

The foregoing makes patients out to be perpetual seekers after succour and emotional support—and so they may be. But a great mystery of clinical medicine is that, spontaneously and miraculously, many apparently irremediably dependent patients *can* change, and start leading mature and independent lives. So don't be downcast when you are looking after such people: there is much to be said for simply offering a sympathetic ear, staying with your patient through thick and thin, and waiting for time to go by and for the wind to change. Of course, the wind may change back again, but, if it does, you will not be back at square one, for you will be able to inject the proceedings with the most powerful psychotherapeutic agent of all, namely hope.

How to improve quality of care

We have chosen *Psychiatry* for this universal topic because if the concept of quality can be made sense of here, despite Psychiatry's notorious lack of objectivity, then its applicability across the field medicine can be upheld. Quality is an important topic not just because it has political currency._{Lord Darzi 2008} _{NHS review} ³³ but because it has important personal relevance too, for your next patient.

Ancient principles for improving quality (derived from Hippocratic thought, онсм p1) Perpetually reaffirm and renew your commitment to put the patient first and do whatever it takes to make your patient better. Traditional approaches to quality in psychiatry stem from this: "We need better inpatient care, with better availability of psychotherapy and more highly motivated, energetic mental health professionals who aren't burnt out by overwhelming caseloads."³⁴

New principles In areas such as surgery, performance-management and quality centre around: •Efficacy •Safety •Equity (equal access to benefits) •Choice •Holistic patient experience/compassion. How do these precepts shape up in the world of psychiatry? Let's take a look, one at a time.

Efficacy: If agreed guidelines exist, we can compare care received with care advised, eg in schizophrenia, in one study ~50% had poor psychosocial care (note the need for patient interviews to unearth the extent of such problems)³⁵

But beware: how do you quantify success for people whose illness precludes them from seeing themselves as being ill? Patients may have their delusions and hallucinations treated so that none are left: but this does not equate with 100% quality of care if the problem is not the delusions and the hallucinations but rather urban alienation (p391), poverty, or unemployment. The hallucinations may be a way of coping with the latter. See p316.

Safety: Monitoring metabolic effects of new antipsychotics is a safety quality marker,³⁶ as is antipsychotic choice. See npsa.nhs.uk/patientsafety._{National Patients'} ^{37,38} _{Safety Agency}

Choice: Offering a choice as to which hospital to be compulsorily incarcerated in seems like tokenism. Also, sectorization (each team having its own geographical area) precludes choice. But because choice does not work in some areas it does not mean it has no role in others. It is legitimate to regard choice of psychotherapy, drugs, or both as a marker of quality of care in depression.

Equity: When this is looked for, ethnic minorities, children, and older people are often disadvantaged.³⁹,⁴⁰ (Obvious, perhaps, but ameliorable.)

Holistic patient experience/patient satisfaction. This is discussed on p510.

▶Some clinicians reject the new methodology: "What we have to do is get away from measurements and statistics and calculations and pieces of paper published by politicians and get back to what we know intuitively is the correct way to help people."³⁴ But what if our intuitions are wrong or contradictory? Is it possible to combine the best of the old and the new? Maybe...

Synthesis (old+new) Find out who wants what→If the patient's views are known, comply with them→make a commitment in your heart to put your patient first→do what it takes to make your patient better→attack all diseases with vigour→promote health where possible→palliate where cure is impossible→update care in the light of evidence→set yourself targets by all means, provided one target is *not to let targets skew the care you give*→take steps to find out if you have actually done what you intended (audit, p506).

Motivating professionals Only pay them if your quality goals are met? A favourite NHS tactic, but undermining of the notion of professionalism and prone to valuing the measurable over more important goals. If we had to select just one winning idea from this page to take forward to our next patient we would go with Hippocrates: make a commitment in your heart to put your patient first. This *is* very hard: just try it. (Did you notice how compassion got squeezed out of this page? How did that happen? Why does this *always* happen?)

Psychiatry

Sexual issues are easier when an overt part of consultations (contraception, fertility, and sexual diseases). More commonly they are a covert part of other emotional or behavioural problems. We may find sexual dialogue embarrassing and avoid it—with unpredictable or fatal consequences, eg for those made suicidal by abuse[41] or by confusing emotions relating to sexuality.

Language is important. It may be medical (eg 'coitus'); slang (eg 'fucking'); or socially acceptable (eg 'having sex'). It is not advisable to use slang as people think you are trying to be fashionable. Most will expect socially acceptable language; slang may shock and may put up barriers. But occasional mirroring of the patient's words can gain rapport. Ask if your words are acceptable.

• Ambiguity is a frequent pitfall—even for the most consummately articulate of all interlocutors:[42] "Ah!" said Mr. Woodhouse, shaking his head and fixing his eyes on her with tender concern.—The ejaculation in Emma's ear expressed, "Ah! there is no end of the sad consequences of your going..." Jane Austen Emma Ch 12 Make sure that you both know what the other is talking about! If a new phrase crops up (slang changes all the time), ask for an explanation right away (a little gentle helping on your part usually overcomes any embarrassment).

• Don't assume sexual knowledge. Not all young people know everything. Just as when we were younger, sex can be confusing and mysterious. There are still many myths, and it is just as hard as it ever was for young people to admit that they don't know something. Sex education in schools is uneven, and may be useless or non-existent (teachers may be too embarrassed to do it).[43]

• Don't *assume* a sexual orientation. It may be best to let these issues surface gradually rather than asking directly early on. Imply that it is safe to reveal feelings that are confused or non-standard. Your patient may be boxed in by societal, religious, or family views of what sexuality should be, so that suicide can seem the only way out.[44] Through your dialogue you may be able to show that there are other options, and that "there is no straight way through this world for any of us".[45] If orientation is causing distress, point out that there is more to a personhood than sexuality—roles they may be good at may include being a friend, colleague, brother, daughter, or son—as well as lover, now or in the future. "You don't need to have sex just to settle the issue of sexuality; feelings can be explored without sex acts, which can be left until you feel ready". In helping gay people decide when to 'come out' eg to parents, explain that reactions can be unpredictable.[46] "How well do you know your parents?" "How have they dealt with religious or sexual issues with your brothers and sisters?"; "Are you economically dependent on your parents?"; "Do you have a social support outside the home?".[47]

• Don't appear embarrassed. It is easier for people to open up if they think that you aren't going to blush, tell them off, or, worst of all, laugh. Don't act shocked and don't judge; give the wrong impression and they will stop being honest with you—see p319 for further discussion of this vital point.

• Act as if you have plenty of time to listen—all the time in the world.

The more you practise sexual dialogue, the easier it gets. If you avoid it, it will remain a problem to you. Also, your patients may learn techniques of sexual dialogue, helpful in their lives as a whole, augmenting self-esteem, enabling sexual negotiation (useful in negotiating safer sexual practices with partners).[48] Also, you may lay the foundation for honest sexual dialogue between this teenager and his or her offspring, 10–40 years from now.

Asking about sexual abuse Have you been in any relationships that made you feel uncomfortable? Has anyone touched you in a way that made you feel embarrassed? I am wondering if anyone has hurt you in a sexual way.

Confidentiality Young people need to know that you will only ever breach this if they (or someone else) is in mortal danger.[49,50]

How to perform a risk-assessment

This is a common problem: the courts, the GP, or the relatives want to know "Will he be violent again if he takes the medication?". A great deal—a man or woman's freedom, no less, may depend on our answers. The philosophical problems with giving a straight answer to these questions are given in the BOX below. Regression analysis shows that 4 factors are paramount: **1** Previous violence **2** Substance abuse **3** Lack of empathy and **4** Stress.[51] When in doubt, use a formal risk assessment tool (see BOX). Some of the advantages of these tools derive simply from having a well-structured approach, others from combining specific kinds of risk factors (static and dynamic).[52]

500, 995, 484, 682, 338, 672, 639

Imagine...there are only 24 people in the world, and each has only 2 types of moves: forward one step at a time, and, sometimes, alas, one step backwards. Surely we should be able to predict what will happen: it's as simple as a game of draughts (chequers). We win or lose at draughts by using rules of thumb (heuristics). In 2007, for the first time, there was sufficient computing power to replace these rules of thumb by *perfect knowledge*. In draughts, there are >500 billion billion play-positions (500,995,484,682,338,672,639), and now each has been analysed to decide what the next best move is. Well-programmed computers are right every time.[54] When we ask psychiatrists to do a risk assessment we want them to be right every time too. It is vital that they are. We blame them if they are wrong. Is this rational? Only if there are no more than 24 people in the world, and they only interact with each other in only one way—never moving sideways or forming attachments.

Psychiatrists do best using rules of thumb combined with validated risk assessment tools (*imperfect knowledge*), such as the *violence risk appraisal guide*.[55] Forensic risk-assessment models all stress risk factors, but often disregard the other side of the equation: protective factors. Mediating and moderating effects must also be considered.[56] We need to involve patients in the process of risk assessment and risk management. This may increase validity,[57] but it also adds unpredictability: the men and women on the board are now all kings and queens in our client-centred world.[53]

People are like icebergs, you only see the little bit on top.[53]

Psychiatry

How to use the full range of psychiatric services

Current UK community psychiatric services can be categorized as follows:
- Intensivist teams: Crisis and Home Treatment, eg with 24-h phone helpline.
- Support and recovery teams—Community mental health teams (CMHT); assertive outreach; rehabilitation.
- Drug and Alcohol teams: part of a wide range of substance abuse services.
- Inreach mental health services—residential care, acute hospital liaison, primary care liaison teams (PCL)—integrated CPNs/Psychiatrists with GP practices/Hospitals with good links into secondary community services.
- IAPT services (improved access to psychological therapies)—offer a wide range of community-based therapies eg CBT (p373), group therapy, etc.

Typically all these services are multidisciplinary (to a varying degree) with Nurses, OTs, Physios, Psychologist, Psychiatrists and Social workers.

Many of these community services are supported by 3rd-sector (voluntary) organizations eg MIND, Alzheimer's society, and other local organizations and charities that provide drop-in centres, group or individual therapy, homecare, advocacy, educational information etc.

PWD (patients with dementia) use more or less specialist Residential or Nursing homes; Social services input is very important as is close working with local councils, and health authorities. **Integrated care** has theoretical advantages—eg for a schizophrenic patient who is a substance abuser.[58,59]

How to help patients not to be manipulative

Fireships on the lagoon We have all been manipulated by our patients, and it is wrong to encourage in ourselves such stiffness of character and inflexibility of mind that all attempts by our patients to manipulate us inevitably fail. Nevertheless, a patient's manipulative behaviour is often counter-productive, and reinforces maladaptive behaviour. A small minority of patients are *very* manipulative, and take a disproportionate toll on your resources, and those of their family, friends, and colleagues. We are all familiar with these patients whom Ford Madox Ford describes as being like fireships on a crowded lagoon, causing conflagration in their wake.[60] After destroying their family and their home we watch these people cruise down the ward or into our surgeries with some trepidation. Can we stop them losing control, and causing meltdown of our own and our staff's equanimity? The first thing to appreciate is that, unlike an unmanned ship, these people *can* be communicated with, and you *can* help them without resorting to hosing them down with cold water.

Setting limits One way of avoiding becoming caught up in this web of maladaptive behaviour is to set limits, as soon as this behaviour starts. In a small minority of patients, the therapist may recognize that their needs for time, attention, sedation, and protection are, for all practical purposes, insatiable. Whatever a therapist gives, such patients come back for more and more, and yet in spite of all this 'input' they don't get any better. The next step is to realize that if inappropriate demands are not met, the patient will not become sicker (there may be vociferous complaints!). This realization paves the way for setting limits to behaviour, specifying just what is and is not allowed.

Take for example the patient who demands sedation, threatening to "lose control" if it is not given immediately, stating that he cannot bear living another day without sedation, and that the therapist will be responsible for any damage which ensues. If it is decided that drugs do not have a part to play in treatment, and that the long-term aim is for the patient to learn to be responsible for himself, then it can be simply stated to the patient that medication will not be given, and that he is free to engage in destructive acts, and that if he does so this is his responsibility.

The therapist explains that in demanding instant sedation he usurps her professional role, which is to decide these matters according to her own expert judgment, and that such usurpation will not be tolerated. If there is serious risk of real harm, admission to hospital may be indicated, where further limits may be set. If necessary, he is told that if he insists on 'going crazy' he will be put in a seclusion room, to protect others.

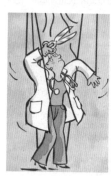

Fig 1. Drastic measures: sometimes you have to cut yourself free...discuss with a colleague first, and explain to the patient that continuing contact is not in their best interests as you are unable to make any headway. "Your case needs a fresh pair of eyes..." This may be safer than the kind of confrontations that Henrik Ibsen dangerously engineers: "When I look back on your long career, it's as if I saw a battlefield strewn at every turn with shattered lives." *The Wild Duck 1884*

Psychiatry

We live, as we dream—alone.
Conrad, *Heart of Darkness*

331

►Health entails harmonious membership of at least one social group. People who are unconnected get dementia (and die) sooner.[61] As the saying goes, it is healthier to eat a chocolate cake with a friend than to eat broccoli alone.

►Being unwanted is the worst disease that any human can experience. Mother Teresa

►Loneliness does not come from having no people about one, but from being unable to communicate the things that seem important to one.[62]

►Loneliness with depression is a predictor of suicide (eg in older women).[63]

A typical candidate for ameliorable loneliness is someone who is depressed after the loss of caregiving role—if a partner/spouse has died (p498)[64]—or if children have flown the parental nest. Loneliness is likely to be worse if the person is shy, has limited social skills, and poor self-esteem. Some people, of course, *like* to avoid their fellows. For them, intrusion into their private world may cause despair; but, for most, these intrusions are welcome, and necessary for health. Loneliness seriously affects 1 in 10 older people, and contributes to alcoholism, depression, and suicide. Suspect that loneliness is important when you find your hand being gripped for comfort after you thought that a social encounter was over—also whenever there is a verbal outpouring and a 'defeated demeanour.'

Do not assume that loneliness means social isolation. Someone who has brief visits 3 times a day, from, say, a nurse, a care assistant, and a 'meals on wheels lady' is not socially isolated, but may be very lonely. But if he or she gets on well with just one of these visitors, this can be enough to banish loneliness. So this is the first lesson: *be nice to people, and take trouble to find out their hopes and fears*. But more is possible: in general, it is depressing waiting for the doorbell to ring, so tailor your suggestions in the light of your patient's mobility. This needs initiative on your patient's part, but do not think you must treat your patient's depression *before* you tackle a lonely lifestyle: tackling this may be the route out of depression. Areas to think about include:

• What facilities already exist? Is there a local pub, day centre, or lunch club available? "God, I wouldn't be seen dead in one of those places!" we so often hear. But take time to point out that it does not matter initially whether they get anything out of a social interaction. After all, they may meet someone of like mind, so enabling these artificial crutches to be thrown away.

• Is the person religious? There may be activities and outings to plan and talk about, and reminisce over, even if not actually enjoyed at the time.

• Housing: if the person is planning a move, will they be near family, and other people who speak their own language (metaphorically and literally)?

• Alternative therapies, eg massage and aromatherapy, can relieve loneliness.

• Adult education is a good (expensive) way to make friends; as new skills are acquired, confidence improves, and socializing becomes more pleasurable.

• Involvement with community action groups may be a source of friends (and a source of frustration and disappointment—but do not expect your interventions to be without side effects: the thing is to plan for them).

• Details of local community activities can be found in the UK at the local *Council for Voluntary Services*. Other organizations advertise at libraries.

• While at the library, ask about joining a book club.

• Befriending schemes can be very helpful to those who are housebound.

• Technology forums such as the Internet may provide relief from boredom and loneliness—and for some this will offer the best chance of meeting with a kindred spirit, unlimited by the constraints of time and space.

• Befriending others, and offering phone support is an option, whether or not one is housebound. Ask local authorities to help to get suitable phones.

Psychiatry

Doctors have a higher than average incidence of suicide and alcoholism, and we must all be prepared to face (and try to prevent) these and other health risks of our professional and private lives. Our skill at looking after ourselves has never been as good as our skill at looking after others, but when the healer himself is wounded, is it clear that his ability to help others will be correspondingly reduced? Our own illnesses are invaluable in allowing us to understand our patients, what makes people go to the doctor (or avoid going to the doctor), and the barriers we may erect to resist his advice. But the idea of an ailing physician remains a paradox to the average mind, so that we may ask: ►Can true spiritual mastery over a power ever be won by someone who is counted among her slaves?[65] If the time comes when our mental state seriously reduces our ability to work, we must be able to recognize this and take appropriate action. The following may indicate that this point is approaching:

• Drinking alcohol before ward rounds or surgeries.
• The minimizing of every contact with patients, so that the doctor does the bare minimum which will suffice.
• Inability to concentrate on the matter in hand. Your thoughts are entirely taken up with the workload ahead.
• Irritability (defined as disagreeing with >1 nurse/24h).
• Inability to take time off without feeling guilty.
• Feelings of excessive shame or anger when reviewing past débâcles. To avoid mistakes it would be necessary for us all to give up medicine.
• Emotional exhaustion—eg knowing that you should be feeling pleased or cross with yourself or others, but on consulting your heart you draw a blank.
• Prospective studies suggest that introversion, masochism, and isolation are important risk factors for doctors' impairment.

The first step in countering these unfavourable states of mind is to recognize that one is present. The next step is to confide in someone you trust. Give your mind time to rejuvenate itself.

If these steps fail, various psychotherapeutic approaches may be relevant, eg cognitive behavioural therapy (p373), or you might try prescribing the symptom. For example, if you are plagued by recurring thoughts about how poorly you treated a patient, set time aside to deliberately ruminate on the affair, avoiding distractions. This is the first step in gaining control. You initiate the thought, rather than the thought initiating itself. The next step is to interpose some neutral topic, once the 'bad' series of thoughts is under way. After repeated practice, the mind automatically flows into the neutral channel once the bad thoughts begin, and the cycle of shame and rumination is broken. ►In addition...learn from the experience!

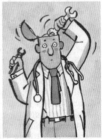

Fig 1. Hands-off! Don't get too drawn into treating your own mental illness without consulting a colleague.

If no progress is made, the time has come to consult an expert, such as your general practitioner. Our own confidential self-help group for addiction and other problems is the British Doctors' and Dentists' Group and may be contacted via the Medical Council on Alcohol (tel. 020 7487 4445[uk]). If you are the expert that another doctor has approached, do not be deceived by this honour into thinking that you must treat your new patient in any special way. Special treatment leads to special mistakes, and it is far better for doctor-patients to tread well-worn paths of referral, investigation, and treatment than to try illusory short cuts.

Burnout (running beyond empty)

Definition Falling performance and personal accomplishments, emotional exhaustion, negative affect, poor leadership, and depersonalization brought on by months or years of overexposure to emotionally demanding situations at work, on the battlefield, or at home.

Fig 2. Have you felt this way?

Measurement The Five minute speech sample and the Maslach burnout inventory.[68]

Risk factors *For doctors:* Lack of hobbies, lack of physical activity, and lack of enough time for vacations and religious activities are all important.[69] Pressure of work, conflict with colleagues,[70] less personal relationships with patients, overly formal hierarchies, and suboptimal income are put forward to explain the fact that some doctors (eg urologists) in the public sector are more at risk of burnout compared with private-service urologists.[71] Factors associated with emotional exhaustion: 'having to deaden one's conscience', lack of time to provide needed care, work being so demanding that it influences one's home life, and not being able to live up to others' expectations.[72]

Signs of burnout:
• Stress and depression
• Fatigue
• Non-restorative sleep[67]
• Emotional exhaustion
• Motivation↓; apathy↑
• Libido↓
• Insomnia
• Guilt or denial
• Paranoia/isolated
• Demoralization
• Amnesia
• Indecision
• Temper tantrums
• Low personal accomplishment
• Depersonalization
• Vicarious traumatization
• Irritability/impatience

Risk factors for psychiatric nurses: Unreciprocated giving, violent client population[73] leading to vicarious traumatization,[74] frequency of on-calls.[75] High expressed emotion (evidenced by critical comments ± negative relationships) predicts depersonalization elements of burnout.[68]

For medical students: Impulsivity, depression & money worries are predictive.[76]

For military personnel: Past history of physical trauma is predictive.

Management (Difficult) Some may respond to plans such as these:
• Diagnose and treat any depression (p336-7).
• Allow time for the person to recognize that there is a problem.
• More hobbies, and more nice holidays.
• Advice from wise colleagues in the specialty (regular follow-up). Mentoring consists in forming a supportive relationship with an independent colleague for the sole purpose of support.
• Return meaning and purpose to life via dialogue, self-transcendence and a sense of connectedness with others (meaning-centred psychotherapy).[77]
• Learn new professional skills—or consider early retirement.
• Set achievable goals in work and leisure (eg protected time with family).

Prevention Strategies such as career counselling are said to be effective but really do no more than point a lollipop at a furnace.[78][n=171] *Reducing stress* is one (unproven) way of avoiding burnout. Psychiatrists have found their own 'stress busting' groups helpful—these entail problem-solving with airing of stresses—ideally accompanied by talking to colleagues for support and catharsis. Having outside interests helps, as does getting support from family and friends, time management, and exercise.[79] On a more universal plane, ▶*we are all responsible for each other's burnout*. By being attentive to our own and others' feelings of troubled conscience we all have a role in preventing the burnout of our colleagues. We need opportunities to reflect on our troubled consciences. Appraisals (p508) and less formal routes to this awareness are becoming more accepted by professionals.[72]

Psychiatry

Speak up now or you will give in and burn out later — dialogue is the only remedy for your infarcted soul.[66]

Patients in disgrace: the fat-folder syndrome

The sorrow that has no vent in tears may make other organs weep.[80] Francis J Braceland

One role of the psychiatrist/GP is to act as the terminus for patients who have been shunted from hospital department to department. The aim is to reframe symptom-offering into problems that need solving. Start by accepting that the patient is troubled and looking for helpful responses from you that are yet to be defined. After establishing rapport, agree a contract with the patient, that we will give regular consultations for listening to how the patient feels and will try to offer help, if she acknowledges that past investigations haven't helped, that psychological factors play a part (somatization, p640), and that she agrees not to consult other doctors until a fixed number of sessions have elapsed.[81] Also, cognitive therapy (p374) examining the way that conscious thoughts and beliefs perpetuate disability, *can* lead to symptom reduction.[82]

Autosuggestion/dissociation (formerly 'hysteria')

Our stream of consciousness doesn't progress from cradle to grave as a single line: there are separations (dissociations) and confluences, for example, when we daydream, or drive to Porlock with no recollection of the scenery along the way, only of our inner landscape. Dissociation may be adaptive, eg by annihilating pain in near-death events (fig 1). Another example: a man who was homosexually raped had no conscious memory of this, but felt irresistible urges to write insulting letters about the perpetrator.

Types of dissociation *Amnesia* is the commonest type: see BOX. *Depersonalization:* Feeling of being detached from one's body or ideas, as if one were an outsider, observing the self; "*I'm in a dream*" or "*I'm an automaton*" (unrelated to drugs/alcohol) eg from stress.

Dissociative identity disorder: The patient has multiple personalities which interact in complex ways. It is present in 3% of acute psychiatric inpatients.

Fugue: Inability to recall one's past ± loss of identity or formation of a new identity, associated with unexpected, purposeful travel (lasts hours to months, and for which there is no me).

Follow-up (~6yrs) shows that ~5% of those referred to a CNS hospital who had hysteria/dissociation diagnosed turned out to have organic illness.

Treatment Exploring life stresses may help. Be ready to recognize psychological components of physical illness, and get expert psychiatric help, while leaving the door open for new diagnoses.

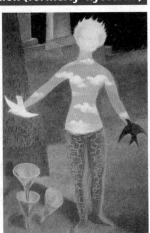

Fig 1. This lady has the knack of dissociating her body and replacing it with the airy nothingness of a summer sky. Roland Penrose, the artist, intuited this adaptive response to extreme events in her past: he did not know when he painted this that at aged 7 that Lee Miller, whose portrait this is, was raped, and had suffered traumatic douches to deal with the ensuing gonorrhoea. Nor could he have known that in 1945 she would be the first photographer to document the overflowing ovens of Nazi concentration camps, no doubt using her dissociative skills to keep her camera steady. How did she end up as the leading fashion photographer of her day? The nested funnels at the foot of the picture suggest an answer: the mind has an infinite capacity to distil one experience through another, and to channel experiences in new, creative ways.

Night & day, Roland Penrose, reproduced by permission of The Penrose Collection.

Is this amnesia dissociative?[1]

- Has a physical cause been carefully discounted? (Drugs, epilepsy, etc.)
- Is the patient young? Beware making the first diagnosis if >40yrs old.
- Have the symptoms been provoked by stress? Ask the family.
- Do related symptoms 'make sense' (eg aphonia in a news-reader)?
- What is the pattern of amnesia? If for distant *and* near memories, then dissociation is more likely (*vs* organic causes) than if the amnesia is for shorter-term memory.
- Indifference to major handicap, *la belle indifférence*, is of little diagnostic use, see fig 1.
- Is malingering likely? The answer is usually 'No', except in prisons and the military (when secondary gain is easy to identify).
- Is there a dissociative personality? The dissociative experiences scale (DES) screens for this: a 28-item visual analogue scale about the proportion of time spent on dissociative experiences (not those from drugs/alcohol) going from the normal, eg being so absorbed in TV that we are unaware of events around us, to severe forms, eg of having no memory of cardinal personal events, or feeling that our body belongs to another. In dissociative disorders, typical DES scores are ≥30; most others score nearer 0.[85]

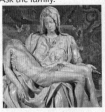

Fig 1. This Lady tells us why we must not place weight on *la belle indifférence*. She has her dead Son on her lap, yet her expression is of serene indifference, not overt sorrow. Michelangelo makes no error here, justly recognizing that dissociation is an adaptive reaction to calamity, be it 'hysterical' (21%) or real (29%).[84]

Detail from Pietà by Michelangelo, San Pietro, Vatican, © S Traykov, by permission.

Calibrating our sensitivity to psychosomatic events

Why do some doctors preferentially diagnose somatic illness? Why, when confronted by unexplained symptoms, do we often subconsciously try to fit them to a physical ailment? The reason is usually that prescribing a pill is easier than changing, or regulating, intrapsychic events. The patient and the doctor may collude with this approach, and then get angry when it yields nothing. Alternatively, some doctors are so used to diagnosing psychopathology that they are all too prone to launch into treating someone's depression and malaise, rather than their endocarditis or brucellosis. There is no single correct approach. We all make errors: the point is to find out in which direction you tend to make errors, then allow for this in your work.

Some patients are naively keen to name their condition, eg 'fibromyalgia', or 'somatization disorder'. Being able to name a disease or a condition is to start to control it. But it's only a start. In time, having named a condition may not prove all that helpful—and neither may seeing a string of experts. This paves the way for a cognitive shift that may allow progress—even healing—to come about. As one patient said "I stopped focusing on the specific diagnoses years ago, and switched to finding the best ways to increase my overall wellness. I use what I learned about my fibromyalgia to inform my choices, and have figured out what works best for me...Experts are just people, and are sometimes wrong...".[86]

Psychiatry

Doctors are wrong in 4%.[84] "They called my symptoms hysterical—until they understood my multiple sclerosis better".

---

1 Hypnotic phenomena share features with conversion (hysterical) symptoms, eg lack of concern, involuntariness with implicit knowledge, and a compliant tone (*la belle indifference*). Theories of consciousness postulate an altered relationship between self-awareness and the supervisory attentional system in both conditions (frontal and cingulate cortex are implicated).[87] Most subside spontaneously, but if they do not it is important to refer early to a psychiatrist, before associated behaviour becomes habitual.

Each year 40% of us have quite severe feelings of depression, unhappiness, and disappointment. Of these, 20% experience a clinical depression, in which low mood occurs with sleep difficulty, change in appetite, hopelessness, pessimism, or thoughts of suicide. *Diagnosis* of major depression:

1 Loss of interest or pleasure—*anhedonia* in daily life with dysphoric mood (ie 'down in the dumps') plus ≥4 of the following (the first 5 are 'biological' symptoms)—present nearly every day for at least 2 weeks:
2 *Poor appetite* with *weight loss* (or, rarely, increased appetite).
3 *Early waking*—with *diurnal mood variation* (worse in mornings).
4 *Psychomotor retardation* (ie a paucity of spontaneous movement, or sluggish thought processes), or *psychomotor agitation*.
5 Decrease in *sexual drive* and other appetites.
6 Evidence of (or complaints of) reduced *ability to concentrate*.
7 Ideas of *worthlessness*, inappropriate *guilt* or *self-reproach*.
8 Recurrent *thoughts of death* and *suicide*, or *suicide attempts*.

Why is depression often missed? • Ignorance • Preoccupation with physical disease • Psychiatric labels are hated • Doctors & patients collude "not to open that can of worms" • It's hard to spot depression coexisting with other illness.

Classification Classify as: • *Mild; moderate; severe.* • *With/without biological features.* • *With/without delusions or hallucinations.* • *With/without manic episodes* (ie bipolar not unipolar). These replace the old reactive/endogenous labels. *ΔΔ*: Cyclothymic disorder; substance-induced mood disorder; schizophrenia, dementia; mood disorder due to a general medical condition.

Why we get depressed: some ideas • Genetics: identical twins reared apart show 60% more concordance for depression than dizygotic twins (NB: these twin studies are suspect; see *Psychiatr* Q 2002 71[89] for the reasons why).
• Biochemistry: there are excess 5-hydroxytryptamine ($5HT_2$) receptors in the frontal cortex of brains taken from suicide victims. See *OHCM* p442.
• Endocrinology: ♀:♂ >1:1; dexamethasone suppression test (*OHCM* p217) is abnormal in ⅓. 17β-estradiol may help perimenopausal depression; risk rises 2-fold, in proportion to LH & FSH.[90] See also ghrelin (p530) & melatonin (SAD, p404).
• Stressful events (births, job loss, divorce, illness): seen in 60%.
• Freudian reasons: depression mirrors bereavement, but loss is of a valued 'object', not a person. There is ambivalence with hostility turned inwards.
• Learned helplessness: if punishment is unrelated to actions, but is perceived as random, the response is helplessness and depression.[91]
• Vulnerability factors: physical illness, pain, and lack of intimate relationships may allow depression to arise and be perpetuated.[92]

Management There is no clear distinction between the low moods we all get and illness needing vigorous treatment, but the lower the mood and the more marked the slowness, the more vigorous the treatment needs to be.
• **Psychological treatment** (eg cognitive therapy, p373) is part of the treatment of *all* depression; it may be all that is needed in milder depressions.
• Presence of biological features or stress predicts a good response to **antidepressants** (p340) especially if symptoms are severe. Not everyone wants drugs. Discuss all options. Herbalism can work: **hypericum** (St John's wort) may be useful in mild to moderately severe depression.[93] NB: omega 3 supplements may reduce suicidal behaviour.[94] 1.2g of eicosapentaenoic acid+ 0.9g decosahexaenoic acid/day
• Delusions or hallucinations prompt a physical treatment: **drugs** (antidepressants ±antipsychotic drugs, p360) or **ECT** (p342; beware: mania may result).
• Treat depression in bipolar illness as above (with SSRI, risk of mania is low[95]).
• **Lithium** or **valproate** prophylaxis may be needed (p354).[96]
• **Reasons to admit:** Social circumstances; high suicide drive; isolation.

Psychiatry

Who is likely to benefit from antidepressant drugs? (see p340)

Sometimes antidepressants need to be prescribed as a matter of urgency—eg if suicide is likely (see below) or, for example, if a mother's functioning is so impaired that she cannot look after her family. If you cannot persuade the patient to start therapy, enlist the help of his or her family, and of a colleague. They may be able to persuade the patient where you have failed.

Those who have had low mood or loss of desire for pleasure (anhedonia) most of the day for at least the last 2 weeks and who show ≥4 of the following 7 markers of severe depression are at especial risk of suicide.

Suicide plan or ideas of self-harm.
Unexplained guilt or worthlessness.
Inability to function (eg psycho-motor retardation or agitation).
Concentration impaired.
Impaired appetite.
Decreased sleep/early waking.
Energy low/unaccountable fatigue
►Enquire about these *whenever* depression is possible.

a moon swims out of a cloud
a clock strikes midnight
a finger pulls a trigger
a bird flies into a mirror
        e e cummings

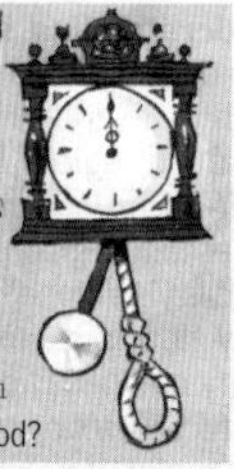

Fig 1.
Has he planned the time?[1]
Has he planned the method?

NB: treatment may still be needed if these criteria are not met: listen to the story. People often don't accept that they are depressed as "There is nothing to *make* me depressed". It helps to suggest that they could still be depressed, and that treatment could be very helpful. Give them time to go away and think about it, perhaps discussing it with someone they know (get consent). Try "Would your wife (or partner) say you were depressed? Please could you ask and let me know?" Such patients often return enriched by dialogue and reflection, and are successfully treated. This may not be over-medicalizing a patient's symptoms .There is evidence that such patients are simply inexperienced in understanding their depression: when they *next* become depressed, their views much more nearly match those of their doctor.

Over-diagnosing severe depression This is undesirable as patients lives are medicalized and drugs with significant side effects are needlessly given—as has been happening in the UK following NICE and QOF recommendation of use of the PHQ-9 diagnostic tool.

In some areas prescriptions for antidepressants have tripled from 1992-3 to 2006-7 without clear benefits.

Antidepressants for adjustment disorder and bereavement?

Adjustment disorder is one of the ways that stress causes psychopathology (other mechanisms reflect extraordinarily severe responses—**acute stress reaction** and **post-traumatic stress disorder**, p347). In adjustment disorder there is 'marked distress that is in excess of what would be expected given the nature of the stressor' (DSM-IV). In normal adaptive reactions to stress, functioning is less impaired. If there is an adjustment disorder and there are <5 signs of a major depression (above) antidepressants may not help much.[98]

Depressed mothers: do the needs of her children dictate the speed and risks of therapy? Drs have infinite ways to blackmail women...

Psychiatry

1 Poets, medical students (such as John Keats) and other harmless or immortal romantics tend to favour midnight as the proposed time for self-destruction: see p553 for Keats' midnight death wish "to cease upon the midnight with no pain." For once, Keats was wrong: just before lunch is in fact the favoured time for suicide (11am) in some communities.[99] The safest time is 4–8am. We should pay no attention to the phase of the moon: day of the week is much more important (Mondays are fatal).[100]

Distinguish suicide from non-suicidal self-harm (eg a cry for help—common, but *every non-fatal event may be fatal next time*,[1] hence treating both here; it is most prevalent in teenage girls; >1%/yr). Suicide is commoner in islands and east Europe, and rarer in Islamic peoples. Incidence: 10⁶/yr (~1/1000ᵘᵏ).[102]
Risk ↑ if:[103] bipolar disorder; depression; borderline personality disorder (p366); anorexia; substance abuse; past self-harm; farmers; vets; doctors and all other prisoners; poor problem-solving; recession/unemployment; serious illness; spring sunshine (affects serotonin neurotransmission and impulsivity).[104]ₙ₌₁₆,₆₇₃

Understanding suicide *Suicide* can be a form of protest,[2] or a way of avoiding pain or shame, and of keeping honour/autonomy,[105] the noble Roman in us preferring suicide to humiliation.[2] Other themes "Giving up an unequal struggle"; "I'm worthless"; "I'm invisible, disconnected from society".[106]
Self-harm may be a way of: Communicating a message, or gaining power by escalating conflict, often after an argument with a partner. Immaturity, inability to cope with stress, weak religious ties, and availability of drugs (psychotropics and alcohol are popular poisons) are also important, as is 'copy-cat' behaviour: when celebrities try suicide, others follow.
Antecedents of suicide: Disease, depression, bankruptcy; anything engendering rumination and hopelessness.[107,108] (esp. if psychiatric care is reduced).[109] Bullying, sexuality, intolerable stress to succeed, and falling behind in homework are also factors. If this mirrors your own state after trudging through endless handbook pages, shut this book, and take an immediate holiday.

Assessment[3] Think of a target with 3 concentric rings. *The inner ring* is the circumstances of the attempt: what happened that day; were things normal to start with? When did the feelings and events leading up to the act start? Get descriptions of these in detail. Was there any last act (eg a suicide note)? What happened after the event? Was this what he/she expected?
The middle ring is the background to the attempt: how things have been over the preceding months. Might the attempt have been made at any time over the last months? What relationships were important over this time?
The outer ring is the family and personal history (p322).
Now...come to the *bulls eye*, the intention lying behind the act, and the present feelings and intentions. Does the attempt reflect a wish to die (a grave, not-to-be-ignored sign); a wish to send a message to someone; or to change circumstances? Ask: "If you were to leave hospital today, how would you cope?" Examine the mental state (p324; is there is any mental illness?) *Summary:* •Any plan? What? When? Where? •Are the means available? •Ever tried before? How seriously? •Preparations (making a will, giving things away).
Before arranging hospital admission, ask what this is *for*. Is it only to make you feel happier?—or to gain something that cannot be gained outside hospital. Ask: *Why will discharge be safer in a few weeks rather than now?*

After the assessment, there are 3 stages in trying to help survivors
• Agree a contract offering help (p339), by negotiation. Discuss confidentiality, then talk with family as to how problems are to be tackled. Treat depression.
• Problem-solving therapy helps by pointing out how she coped with past problems.[110]ₙ₌₁₀₉₄ The aim is to engender a greater ability to cope in the future and to help with immediate personal or social problems.
• Follow-up, either alone or with the family, with **preventive strategies:**[111] ↑*Access to:* Samaritans & doctors; on-line help (Facebook is addressing this). ↓*Access to:* Guns/poisons.[112] *Less:* Poverty & dead-end work; alcohol/drugs; isolation; sexual coercion; suicide website availability. *More:* God;[113] family caring; shared meals;[114] justice; sexual equality;[115] poetry.[116]

---

1 Once a person has self-harmed, the risk of death by suicide rises by a factor of 50-100. *BMJ* 2011 1167
2 Suicide is powerful: Mohammed Bouazizi (a poor street vendor in Sidi Bouzid, Tunisia) set himself alight after humiliation by an official wanting a bribe, on Dec 17 2010, so sparking the demise of 4 Arab dictators.
3 Use clinical judgment and assessment tools: medscape.com/viewarticle/730857_5?src=emailthis

Nuclear confrontations "I'll kill myself if you leave me..."

339

The best approach is probably not to encourage patients to counter with "I hate you: if you go on threatening, it's *me* who'll commit suicide...". To avoid mutually assured destruction, explain that it's worth acknowledging close feelings (including negatives ones), emphasizing that a healthy relationship cannot be based on threats, and that there should be more to life than a single relationship, especially one based on coercion. It may be good to reflect aloud on past times when there was more range of things which made life worth living, and to explain that it's possible to get back to a balanced state through dialogue and giving and receiving pleasure. *Ellis & Newman, Choosing to Live*

The psychiatrist may become enmeshed in these webs of suicide threats, and may wrongly assume that because someone threatens suicide, they should be admitted to hospital (compulsorily if necessary) so that they can be kept under constant surveillance, and suicide prevented. This reasoning has 3 faults. The first is the idea that it is possible to prevent suicide by admission. There is no such thing as constant surveillance. Second, admission may achieve nothing if it removes us from the circumstances we need to learn to cope with. Third, we must distinguish between suicide gestures, which have the object of influencing others' behaviour, and a genuine wish to die.[3]

Before death, many suicide victims see a GP, and it is wise to be alert to undercurrents of suicide which only sometimes surface during consultations. Ask *unambiguously* about suicide plans (p322). On deciding that a threat is more manipulative than genuine, very experienced therapists may influence the person's use of suicide behaviour by forcing him to face the reality of his suicide talk, eg by asking: "When will you kill yourself?" "How will you do it?" "Who will discover the corpse?" "What sort of funeral do you want? Cremation, burial, with or without flowers?" "Who will come?"

See opposite for risk factors for suicide; they may be of no help in individual cases, so aim to think dynamically of risks and protective factors (eg family support), with suicide occurring after key events that accumulate risk.

▶*Take all suicide threats seriously*—but emphasis differs depending into which group the patient falls. Aim to form a *contract* with the patient, eg:
- The therapist will listen and help if the patient agrees to be frank, and to tell the therapist of any suicide thoughts or plans.
- Agreement about which problems are to be tackled is made explicit.
- Agree the type of change to aim for and who will be involved in treatment (eg family, friends, GP). Agree the timing and place of sessions.
- An agreement to collaborate with the therapist, and to do any homework.

Not all self-harm is suicidal Cutting can relieve stress; in helping people reduce the need to self-harm they may find addressing these questions helpful:

1 Have I got a solid support system I can call on if I feel like cutting?
2 Have I got 2-3 people I feel comfortable to talk to about cutting with?
3 Have I got a list of things I can do as an alternative to cutting?
4 Have I got a place to go if I need to leave home so as not to hurt myself?
5 Can I get rid of everything I might use to harm myself, without panicking?
6 Am I prepared to feel scared, frustrated while cutting down my cutting?

Psychiatry

"I was 7 years old the first time I brought a blade across my skin and watched the first trickle of blood streaming down my body..."

---

1 If in doubt about the energy with which we may pursue our own destruction, let us call in mind a notable Japanese pilot who, during World War II, persistently volunteered to be a Kamikazi pilot to run suicide missions against US ships, in the defence of Okinawa. The authorities just as persistently refused his request—he had a wife and 3 daughters. He kept on reapplying, determinedly. Not wanting to risk her husband's failure again, and not wanting to stand in Destiny's way, his wife killed their 3 daughters, and then herself, so removing the obstacle to her husband's mission—and on May 28, 1945, he finally took to the air, and achieved his end.

2 NICE says: 'the decision to discharge a person without follow-up after an act of self-harm shouldn't be based solely on the presence of low risk of repetition of self-harm and the absence of a mental illness, because many such people may have a range of other social and personal problems that may later increase risk. These problems may be amenable to interventions'.[118]

Psychiatry

Drugs improve mood and ↑synaptic availability of noradrenaline or 5HT. Your own personal qualities and psychotherapy (p370) are as important as drugs. Encourage socializing, exercising, and countering negative thoughts (p372).

- *Uncomplicated depression in middle age*—little suicide risk: If a cheap agent is essential, try **dosulepin**, ≤150mg at night (start with 25mg; max 225mg/day, in hospital).[119] Explain side effects (below); warn about driving/machinery use. Explain that benefits take weeks to develop. Avoid if arrhythmia risk (eg post MI). SSRI alternative: citalopram 20mg/day, unless QT is long (works fastest[120]); only use max dose of 40mg if LFT OK and <65yrs old; consider **sertraline** 50mg/day (if not responding in 2wks, switching to **paroxetine** 20–40mg/day is better than continuing sertraline).[121] N=132

- *Depression with intellectual disability:* Try SSRIs eg **fluoxetine**, 20mg/24h PO (doubled after 3wks if needed). t½≈3 days. If ♀, consider combining with 0.5mg/day **folic acid**: folate is low in major depression, and supplements may help.[121] N=127

- *Past history of good response to tricyclics, now suicidal:* Try **lofepramine**, 70mg/12h (less likely to be fatal in overdose; less risk of fatal arrhythmias).

- *Depression in an adolescent:* See p390; tricyclics/SSRI have problems. Unlicensed

- *Depression if elderly:* ?Avoid SSRI; halve dose of tricyclic (SES may be worse).

- *Depression + psychosis:* ECT (p342) ± antipsychotics (p360) may be needed.

- *Bipolar child:* Get help; **aripiprazole**, **olanzapine** & **risperidone** have a role.[123]

- *Depression in those insisting on driving:* Paroxetine (20mg each morning, increased by 10mg increments; max: 50mg/24h) is safer than tricyclics. It is the SSRI most associated with the unpleasant dystonias on withdrawal.

- *Depression + disordered sleep pattern:* Tricyclic, eg **dosulepin**, as above. If suicidal **mirtazapine** (blocks 5HT2, H1, and 5HT3—15mg at bedtime, max 45mg) *may* have a role. Warn not to rely on the 'fact' that daytime sleepiness usually wears off after a few weeks. NB: ordinary SSRIs can aggravate insomnia. Sleep is such a restorative for some patients, so give them the best chance.

- *Depression not responding to SSRI:* Venlafaxine (SNRI[1]) *may*●◆* have a role.[124]

- *Pregnancy/breastfeeding:* Tricyclics may be best; p408; get expert help.

- *Depression with obsessive-compulsive features:* Clomipramine or an SSRI.

- *Depression with Parkinson's disease:* SSRI (nortriptyline 2nd choice).

- *Post-stroke depression:* Nortriptyline is ?better than fluoxetine.[125]

- *Depression at menopause:* HRT may help but ↑ breast cancer risk, p256.

- *Depression+sexual dysfunction:* Mirtazapine or bupropion.

- *Depression + obesity:* Fluoxetine sometimes leads to weight↓.[126]

- *Worried about drug interactions:* Citalopram and sertraline have lowest risk. Most SSRIs inhibit CYP450 enzymes so can ↑levels of many drugs.

- *Depression in psychiatrists:* In a survey of psychiatrists, most said "I'd want citalopram, fluoxetine, or venlafaxine; in severe depression I'd want ECT."[127]

Side effects—*SSRI:* Citalopram & sertraline: •Nausea, vomiting, dyspepsia, diarrhoea, abdominal pain—also rash, sweats, agitation, headache, insomnia, tremor, anorgasmia♂♀/erectile dysfunction (sildenafil helps),[128] Na↓, GI bleeding.[129] Fluoxetine as above (insomnia & agitation commoner). Fluvoxamine as for citalopram but nausea more common. Paroxetine as for citalopram except more antimuscarinic effects and sedation, also extrapyramidal symptoms (rare). Sertraline may attenuate happiness, rapture, and love.[130] n=1

Tricyclics: Amitriptyline—common SE: sedation, dry mouth, urine retention, blurred vision, postural hypotension, tachycardia, constipation. *Other SE:* arrhythmias; convulsions (dose-related). Clomipramine, dosulepin, doxepin as for amitriptyline. Imipramine and lofepramine less sedating than amitriptyline. Trimipramine more sedating than amitriptyline.

---

1 SNRI = serotinin and noradrenaline reuptake inhibitor. Avoid if BP↑, U&E↑↓, or heart disease. **Specialist use only if >300mg;** monitor BP if on >200mg/day. Starting dose: 37.5mg/12h PO. SE: Constipation; nausea; dizziness; dry mouth; BP↑; ADH↑; Na↓; T°↑; dyspnoea, hallucinations, arthralgia etc: see BNF.

SSRI issues

SSRIs are under a cloud as a 2008 meta-analysis shows their effects in depression may be no greater than placebo.[131] Also, in one cohort study in *the elderly* (n=60,746) SSRIs had the highest hazard ratios for **falls** (1.66) and **hyponatraemia** (1.52). All-cause **mortality** was also higher *vs* tricyclics.[132] There is also the question of **suicidal behaviour**. *In adults*, research using the UK *GP research database* for 1993-9 found risk of suicidal behaviour wasn't significantly greater with SSRIs than *vs* tricyclics (but strong suicidal drive is reported).[133] Venlafaxine is also problematic.[134] In *teenagers*, the position is complex, and prescribing bodies tend to recommend that no antidepressants be used—but this is unworkable for those many teenagers with formidable mental health problems where there is lack of availability of cognitive therapies, or they are not working. Here the small risk of suicide (≤1 : 4000❋) may be the least bad option.[135] Before prescribing: get informed consent from the teenager and the parent/carer. Ensure meticulous follow-up, and ensure that it really is a major depression you are treating, using detailed questionnaires to aid diagnosis.

A patient-centred approach to depression

We can feel perplexed with antidepressants; it can feel like trial and error when prescribing them. What works well in one person may not help another. There seems to be an ever increasing choice of drugs and conflicting information on safety. In this context, the following may be helpful:

Advice to give a patient when treating depression
- Discuss choice of drug and non-pharmacological therapy. Cognitive therapy is known to be as effective as antidepressants in mild to moderate depression.[136] Combined use is better than either treatment alone.[137,138]
- Discuss side effects, not all side effects are undesirable (SSRIs may help premature ejaculation). Warn that there may be an initial worsening of symptoms in the first weeks so persevere before therapeutic effects are seen.
- Assess after 4-6 weeks. If effective continue for at least 4-6 months after recovery, if stopped too soon 50% relapse.[139] If no effect, increase dose and review in 2 weeks. If still no response, increase dose if it is safe to do so (unless poorly tolerated), review in 2 weeks. If no response or poor tolerability, switch to an alternative class of antidepressant (special method, p369).
- Recurrent depression: of those who have one episode of major depression 50-85% will have further episodes. Continuing antidepressants lowers the odds of relapse by ~65%, which is about half the absolute risk.[140]

Theories of antidepressant action 8 pharmacological actions are known, and over 20 antidepressants exist. How do all they lead to a similar response? Why is there a delay? 2 theories: The *neurotransmitter receptor hypothesis:* Postulates that a change in receptor sensitivity by desensitization and down-regulation of different receptors (not just ↑neurotransmitter at the synapse) leads to clinical effects after a few weeks. The *monoamine hypothesis of antidepressants on gene expression:* This suggests the effect of increased neurotransmitter at the synapse initiates a sequence of events to give the antidepressant response. This includes up and down regulation of various genes with subsequent varying expression of receptors and critical proteins.[141]

Have a non-pharmacological arm to every treatment plan...

Exercise (in wild Nature, eg on or near water❋), tai chi (p753), Yoga, social interaction, psychotherapy (p370), counselling (p380), reading clubs, meditation, poetry (reading/writing). Join a club, eg Ramblers. Rest from work. People may not want drugs, equating them with moral failure? If still unconvinced, an alternative therapy, eg St John's wort, may be acceptable?[142]

Mechanism There is MRI evidence for the idea that ECT interrupts the hyper-connectivity between the various areas of the brain that maintain depression.[143]

Indications NICE recommends ECT is used only to gain rapid (if short-term) improvement of severe symptoms after an adequate trial of other treatments has proven ineffective and/or when the condition is considered to be potentially life-threatening, in individuals with: •Severe depression •Catatonia (eg associated with schizophrenia).[144] •A prolonged or severe manic episode. Emergency ECT is possible, eg in some elderly patients, but rarely used (but the success rate is good, eg 80%)[145] Carry on antidepressants when ECT ends: this *may* prevent recurrences. ✦ *Typical course length:* 6 sessions (2 per week).

Contraindications Recent subdural/subarachnoid bleed; no consent (p402; involve relatives, but they cannot consent for an adult). **Cautions** Recent stroke MI, arrhythmia, CNS vascular anomalies. **SE:** Anaesthetic problems; amnesia; delirium/agitation (may respond to donepezil).[147] Parkinsonism may *improve*.[148]

Technique Check the patient's identity and that 'nil by mouth' for >8h.

• Ensure a detailed medical history and physical examination has been done, and any illnesses investigated and treated as far as possible. High anaesthetic risk?—See p614; seizure threshold ↑ if on concurrent benzodiazepines or anticonvulsants; also ↑risk of heart complications if on tricyclics. Liaise between psychiatric and anaesthetic staff. Do benefits outweigh risks?

• ECT is frightening; give calm reassurance away from the site where ECT is going on. (Patients should not witness other patients having ECT.[1])

• Are the consent forms in order (p402; see below)? In the rare instances in the UK where ECT is given without consent, a second opinion from the Mental Health Commission must state that the treatment is necessary (p402).

• Ensure that fully equipped resuscitation trolleys are present including a functioning defibrillator, suction apparatus, and pulse oximeter.

• Ensure anaesthetist (senior & ECT trained) knows of allergies ± drugs interfering with GA. For countering ECT-induced vagal stimulation, she may use **atropine** before using an ultra-short-acting anaesthetic agent with muscle relaxation (eg suxamethonium) to minimize the seizure's muscular component.

• The ECT machine: checked recently? Reserve machine to hand? What charge/energy is to be given? Which waveform will be used (bidirectional or modified sinusoidal, or unidirectional)? See manufacturer's information.

• Put jelly on the electrode sites (not enough to allow shorting). See fig 1.

• When the anaesthetist gives the word, give the shock. Be prepared to restrain the patient if paralysis is incomplete. While the current passes, the muscles will contract. This will cease as the current ceases. After ~10sec, further clonic spasms occur, lasting ~1min. The only sign may be lid fluttering. Clonus is probably needed for ECT to be fully effective.

• Then coma position and BP/pulse, until conscious. Ask the anaesthetist to try IV midazolam for those (few) who get very agitated during recovery.

Consent for today's shock is suspect if yesterday's ECT has made you unable to remember your basic biography (am I divorced?).[149] Reflect on the blogs OPPOSITE, and on Hay's paradox: *the organ giving consent is the organ affected.* As in all metaphysical paradoxes, don't get overly wound up by the lack of any way out: remember that humans are quite good at this sort of thing, yourself included. Start from the basic principle that **if your patient's wishes are known, comply with them.** Hay's paradox is partial because the organ giving consent is not uniformly affected, and decision-making may be rational. But if the deluded patient says "I want ECT because it fries the transmitter the Pope put in my head" you may need legal backing to endorse consent. But don't be too intellectually arrogant in dismissing a patient's reasoning: after all, none of us knows how ECT works, and all are entitled to an opinion.

What is the correct 'dose' of unilateral ECT?

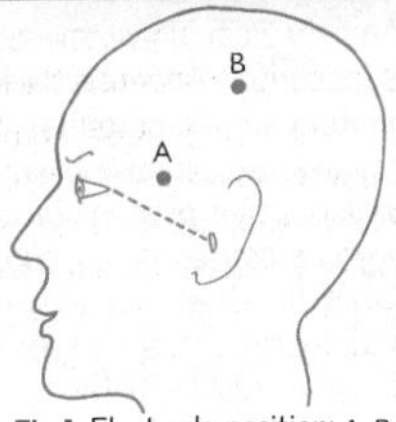

Fig 1. Electrode position: A–B =10cm; A is 4cm from the green dotted line.

There is no universal answer, but there is evidence that therapeutic effects of ECT are proportional to seizure length. Be sure that you have adequate training on this issue by the consultant in charge of the session. Dose is better measured in millicoulombs (mC) than milliamps. It depends on *seizure threshold*, which varies 40-fold among patients. A moderately 'suprathreshold' dose (eg 200% above seizure threshold) usually gives seizures of adequate duration, while aiming to minimize cognitive side effects—according to the Royal College of Psychiatrists *ECT Handbook*.

Doses need to change depending on response, and dose of propofol[150] in the anaesthetic: also, seizure threshold rises by ~80% as courses progress. A 'good' seizure is one which is of adequate duration (~15sec during early sessions; duration is less important later), with both a tonic and a clonic phase. Some machines allow EEG monitoring—useful as anaesthesia renders seizure analysis difficult. If the seizure lasts >2min, tell the anaesthetist, who will give a bolus of diazepam, or GA agent.

The frequency and speed of response of ECT varies according to indication, eg bipolar depression patients show more rapid improvement and need fewer treatments than unipolar patients.[151] N=228 One retrospective study has found that female patients respond better to ECT than male patients.[152]

Quotes from the blogsphere: *What's it like to have ECT?*

- "There is no treatment in psychiatry more frightening than ECT...There is also no treatment in psychiatry more effective than ECT."[153]
- "Nighty-night" says the blue mask with piercing green eyes, and an instant later, I feel myself falling into yummy unconsciousness. When I awake from the treatment, I am back in my hospital room. My brain feels very foggy. I can't remember what day it is or anything that happened that morning. I try to call my husband at home, but I can't remember my phone number and have to look it up in an address book I find in my nightstand. Waves of excruciating pain surge through my head, and I beg for pain medicine...This whole scenario repeats itself each day for the next week and a half. As the days pass, the headaches grow more and more unbearable, but life in general grows surprisingly more tolerable...Gone are the days filled with inescapable agony, misery, despair and a desperate determination to die. In short, I have my life back..."[154]
- "My memory seems pretty bad. I forget lots of common easy things that have no reason to be forgotten. This never happened prior to electroconvulsive treatment. My memory was picture perfect before. I have a mix of depression and anxiety. I find that with the ECT I also like 10mg Prozac... It's strange how these meds always did me a little bit of good by themselves, but that with ECT they work so much better."[155]
- "I've always had a super good memory. It is unreal how poor it is now. But I don't mind. It's almost comical."[155] "After you recover from depression, people encourage you to rebuild your life but...[after ECT] I couldn't even remember what my life was."[149] (≈↓retrograde autobiographical memory.)

"It's frightening, it's quick, and it works—and I might give it a go." (JML)

1 Had Rockland asylum banned witnessing ECT, the greatest poem extolling the humanity of mental illness *vs* military-industrial greed could not have arisen. Carl Solomon's post-ECT babble flowed directly into Allen Ginsberg's *Howl*: "I saw the best minds of my generation destroyed by madness, starving hysterical naked, dragging themselves through the negro streets at dawn looking for an angry fix, / Angelheaded hipsters burning for the ancient heavenly connection to the starry dynamo in the machinery of night... I'm with you in Rockland in my dreams you walk dripping from a sea-journey on the highway across America in tears."

Anxiety is a universal experience (♀:♂ ≈ 2:1); it is, according to some reckonings, the chief factor limiting human potential; it causes much suffering, costing the UK ≥£5 billion/yr. *Neurosis* refers to *maladaptive psychological symptoms not due to organic causes or psychosis, and usually precipitated by stress.* Apart from free-floating anxiety and depression, such symptoms are: fatigue (27%), insomnia (25%), irritability (22%), worry (20%), obsessions, compulsions, and somatization (p640)— all more intense than the stress precipitating them would warrant. Symptoms are not just part of a

> **Classifying anxiety**DSM-IV
> • Generalized anxiety disorder (GAD): anxiety +3 somatic symptoms and present for ≥6 months
> • Panic disorder
> • Phobia, eg agoraphobia
> • Post-traumatic stress disorder
> • Social anxiety disorder
> • Obsessive-compulsive disorder

patient's normal personality, but they may be an exaggeration of personality: a generally anxious person may become even more so, ie develop an anxiety neurosis, as a result of job loss. The *type* of neurosis is defined by the chief symptom (eg anxiety, obsessional, depressive). Before diagnosing neurosis, consider carefully if there is underlying depression needing antidepressants.[156]

Symptoms of anxiety: Tension, agitation; feelings of impending doom, trembling; a sense of collapse; insomnia; poor concentration; 'goose flesh'; 'butterflies in the stomach'; hyperventilation (so tinnitus, tetany, tingling, chest pains); headaches; sweating; palpitations; poor appetite; nausea; 'lump in the throat' unrelated to swallowing (globus hystericus); difficulty in getting to sleep; excessive concern about self and bodily functions; repetitive thoughts and activities (p346). *Children's symptoms:* Thumb-sucking; nail-biting; bed-wetting; foodfads.

Causes Genetic predisposition; stress (work, noise, hostile home), events (losing or gaining a spouse or job; moving house). *Others: Faulty learning* or *secondary gain* (a husband 'forced' to stay at home with agoraphobic wife).

Treatment *Symptom control:* Listening is a good way to ↓anxiety. Explain that headaches are not from a tumour, and that palpitations are harmless. Anything done to enrich patients' relationship with others may well help.

Regular (non-obsessive!) exercise: Beneficial effects appear to equal meditation or relaxation. Acute anxiety responds better than chronic anxiety.[157]

Meditation: Intensive but time-limited group stress reduction intervention based on 'mindfulness meditation' can have long-term beneficial effects.[158]

Cognitive-behavioural therapy (p373) and *relaxation* appear to be the best specific measures[159] with 50-60% recovering over 6 months.[160] N=404

Behavioural therapy employs *graded exposure* to anxiety-provoking stimuli.

Drugs augment psychotherapy: **1** Benzodiazepines (eg diazepam 5mg/8h PO for <4wks. SEs/withdrawal, p368, limit utility). **2** SSRI (p340, eg paroxetine in social anxiety).[161] **3** Azapirones (buspirone, 5HT1A partial agonist; 5mg/8-12h; ?less addictive/sedating than diazepam, and few withdrawal issues).[162] **4** Old-style antihistamines (eg hydroxyzine).[163] **5** β-blockers.[164] **6** Others: pregabalin and venlafaxine.[165]

Progressive relaxation training: Teach deep breathing using the diaphragm, and tensing and relaxation of muscle groups, eg starting with toes and working up the body. Practice is essential. CDs aid learning; in some contexts, eg stress, relaxation is not as good as cognitive restructuring.[166] N=87

Hypnosis Initially the therapist induces progressively deeper trances eg using guided fantasy and concentration on bodily sensations, such as breathing. Later, some patients will be able to induce their own trances. It powerfully reduces anxiety, and is useful, eg medical contexts (eg post-op).[167] N=32

Prognosis GAD often gets better by ~50yrs (often replaced by somatization).[168]

Some remarks on adolescent anxiety and mood swings

Anxiety is the engine in us, and also our steering wheel, weaving us in and out of the fast or slow lanes of our lives. Some of us seek out anxiety as a way of feeling alive (the tightrope walker, or the falconer, placing the meat for his bird between his own eyes). The lives of others are dominated by the imperative of minimizing anxiety, to the extent that some of us never leave home, either physically or metaphorically. Anxiety implies heightened awareness, which is why it is one of the dominant colours in the artist's metaphysical palette. The artist makes us anxious so that we see familiar objects differently. Anxiety, up to a point, makes us sit up, and take note; beyond a certain level (different in all of us, and different at different times) anxiety is counter-productive: we become preoccupied with the feeling itself, which chokes our ability to act (*angere* =to choke gives us *anxiety* and *angina*).

Anxiety is reduced by the chief CNS inhibitory neurotransmitter, GABA (gamma-amino-butyric-acid) which counteracts excitatory limbic system effects of glutamate. Stress releases allopregnanolone (THP) which increases GABA's calming effects in adults. But in adolescents (at least in adolescent mice), THP has the opposite effect. THP has 2 roles: 1 in the limbic system it tranquillizes; 2 in the hippocampus of adolescents THP does the opposite (the hippocampus is important for emotion regulation, as well as memory). This reflects adolescents' enhanced expression of $\alpha 4\beta_6$ GABA$_A$ receptors in the hippocampus. This may explain why, in some adolescents, and maybe other individuals, calmness is unattainable (activating the break also activates the accelerator, so responses are amplified into unpredictable mood swings).[169]

Quotes from the blogsphere: what's it like to have panic attacks?

- "I worry about everything: from the detergent I use to the war in Iraq. I am just completely ridiculous with it. To the point where I experience panic attacks, which are terrifying experiences. They feel like heart attacks. Worry steals every happy moment away. It takes away my drive, my ambition, my sense of adventure, my ability to relax, my ability to have fun. I'm aware of it, and I cannot seem to stop it, nor control it..."[170]
- "I woke up in my bed, in the middle of the night. I was sweating, but I was cold. I was so scared that I literally could not move—all my muscles were locked in position. My heart was racing, and I was breathing so hard that anyone listening would have thought I had just run a marathon..."[171]
- "I felt like I had a tennis ball wedged in the middle of my chest, below my breastbone and above my stomach. It was tight, made me breathe erratically...and caused me to panic... I couldn't drive like a normal human being—I had to stop every 20 minutes or so to let yet another panic attack pass. I usually had to get out of the car, walk around it a few times..."[172]
- "The dentist was in a hell of a hurry...I tried to tell him I was not having any reaction (to the anaesthetic). I had a panic attack...his hand, scrambled out of the chair trailing hoses & drills, scuttled across floor on hands and knees trying to escape. Then I had an asthma attack brought on by panic and it was touch and go for a while. Oh, did I mention that I wet myself?"[173]
- "It had been two years since my last panic attack (deep breathing, meditation, and generally better stress management eliminated even the tiniest hint of an attack) before I began to plan my trip home..."[174]

Immunizing ourselves against neurosis: one man's methodologies

• Bagpipes	• Surfing	• Self-hypnosis	• Pretending to be a tree
• Seneca (AD65)[1]	• Sea-bathing	• Exercise	• Playing with dolphins

1 ★"Men do not care how nobly they live, but only how long, but it is within the reach of every man to live nobly, but within no man's power to live long. ★Life without the courage for death is slavery. ★Most powerful is he who has himself in his own power. ★Toil to make yourself remarkable by some talent or other. ★Fire is the test of gold; adversity, of strong men. ★There is no great genius without some touch of madness."

Psychiatry

Phobic disorders involve anxiety in specific situations only, and leading to their avoidance. These are labelled according to specific circumstance: agoraphobia (*agora*, Greek for market place) is fear of crowds, travel, or situations away from home; social phobias (where we might be minutely observed, eg small dinner parties); simple phobias, eg to dentists, intercourse, Friday the 13th (triskaidecophobia), spiders (arachnophobia, p372), beetles (paint them red with black spots on and they are charming ladybirds). There may also be free-floating 'fear of fear', or fear of disgracing oneself by uncontrollable screaming.

Elicit the *exact* phobic stimulus. It may be specific, eg travelling by car, not bicycle. Why are some situations avoided? If deluded ("I'm being followed/persecuted"), paranoia rather than phobia is likely. For panic attacks, try cognitive-behaviour therapy[175] (p373, ± eg paroxetine 20–50mg/day PO).[176,177]

Obsessive-compulsive disorder (OCD) Compulsions are senseless, repeated rituals. Obsessions are stereotyped, purposeless words, ideas, or phrases that come into the mind. They are perceived by the patient as nonsensical (unlike delusional beliefs), and, although out of character, as originating from themselves (unlike hallucinations or thought insertion). They are often resisted by the patient, but if longstanding, the patient may have given up resisting them. An example of non-verbal compulsive behaviour is the rambler who can never do a long walk because every few paces he wonders if he has really locked the car, and has to return repeatedly to ensure that this has, in fact, been done. Cleaning (eg hand-washing), counting, and dressing rituals are other examples. *Pathophysiology:* CNS imaging implicates the orbitofrontal cortex[178] and the caudate nucleus. Successful treatment is reflected by some normalization of metabolism in these areas.[179] *Treatment:* Behavioural (or cognitive) therapy (p372). **Clomipramine** (start with 25mg/day PO) or SSRIs (eg **fluoxetine**, start with 20mg/day PO) really can help (even if patients are not depressed): see p340.

What's it like to have OCD? Quotations from the blogosphere: "That afternoon, I found that when I got home from school, I couldn't get around the house or do normal things without performing rituals to cancel out bad thoughts over and over again. It was weird and I didn't want to do it, but if I didn't I would feel a lot of anxiety and panic like something was very wrong. I kept having to enter and re-enter through the front door. I ended up spending about 3 or 4 hours in the bathroom because I couldn't get out of there because every time I tried to do the perfect ritual, my body would itch or something else would go wrong and I had to redo the rituals over again. After a few hours, I wanted to get out of there bad, I felt like a prisoner in my own bathroom!"[180]

Depersonalization This is an unpleasant state of disturbed perception in which people, or the self, or parts of the body are experienced as being changed ("as if made of cotton wool"), becoming unreal, remote, or automatized ("replaced by robots"). There is insight into its subjective nature, so it is not a psychosis, but the patient may think he is going mad. Depersonalization may be primary, or part of another neurosis. CNS imaging shows that it is associated with functional abnormalities in the sensory cortex in areas where visual, auditory, and somatosensory (cross-modal) data integrate.[181]

Derealization These are psychosensory feelings (akin to depersonalization) of detachment or estrangement from our surroundings. Objects appear altered: buildings may metamorphose in size and colour. The patient acknowledges the unreality of these ideas, but is made uneasy by them.

(Our isolation in an alien or unreal universe, and our estrangement from ourselves, are major themes of leading novelists such as Albert Camus.)[182]

Dissociation (formerly *hysteria*) *Clinical details:* p334. *Example of mass hysteria spread by TV*—Pokeman induced 'seizures': see '*the Pokeman contagion*'.[183] ℞: Behaviour therapy (p372 ± antidepressants) if he really wants to change.

Relieving stress Smoking, alcohol, and chattering are popular methods. If drugs must be used, **propranolol** 10mg/8h PO may ↓autonomic symptoms (CI: asthma; heart failure; heart block). Alternatives: exercise, singing, progressive relaxation (p344),counselling (p380).[185]

Post-traumatic stress disorder Suspect this if symptoms (BOX) become *chronic*, with these signs (may be delayed years): difficulty modulating arousal; isolated-avoidant modes of living; alcohol abuse; numb to emotions and relationships; survivor guilt; depression; altered world view in which fate is seen as untamable, capricious or absurd, and life can yield no meaning or pleasure.[185] NB: some people have this with no known stressor: DSM-IV wrongly calls this *adjustment disorder*, whereas it is a form of existentialism that only the healing power of story-telling can transform 'by serving as an axe for the frozen sea inside us.' [Franz Kafka]

Acute stress reactions
• Fearful; horrified; dazed
• Helpless; numb, detached
• Emotional responsiveness↓
• Intrusive thoughts
• Derealization (p346)
• Depersonalization
• Dissociative amnesia
• Reliving of events
• Avoidance of stimuli[184]
• Hypervigilance
• Concentration↓
• Restlessness
• Autonomic arousal: pulse↑; BP↑; sweating↑
• Headaches; abdo pains

MRI implicates the anterior cingulate area, with failure to inhibit amygdala activation ± lowered amygdala threshold[1] to fearful stimuli.[186,187]

Treatment: Debriefing may do more harm than good.[188] Macbeth's 'sweet oblivious antidote to cleanse the stuffed bosom of that perilous stuff which weighs upon the heart' has yet to be found. Is the best advice to try to forget or ignore the past? Macbeth's doctor asserts (*Act V*) that such a patient 'must minister to himself', when he had been unreasonably but royally commanded to 'raze out the written troubles of the brain'—and perhaps tragic literature *can* offer more than medicine here◆※ as demonstrated by the many soldiers who have benefitted from Jonathan Shay's book *Achilles in Vietnam*.[189] In *narrative exposure therapy*, adults or children are asked to describe what happened in great detail (what they saw, heard, smelled, felt, the movements they recall and how they felt and thought at the time). Initial distress is marked, but as sessions are long, habituation ensues as more and more details are recalled. Emphasize integrating emotional and sensory memory within a detailed autobiographic narrative. After 4 sessions, scores on intrusion and avoidance may drop markedly;[190] but don't expect depression to resolve.[191,N=28] *Eye movement desensitization and reprocessing* (EMDR) may also have a role.◆※

After the 2004 Indian Ocean tsunamis, psychopathology was as common as physical injury: WHO advised practical outreach help, and to avoid mental health labels (contrary to NICE's medicalizing approach to PTSD).[192]

Amitriptyline, mirtazapine, paroxetine, and **atypical anti-psychotics** (p360) can help (warn of SEs and withdrawal phenomena, p340).[193,194]

Prevention: Rehearse teamwork—and techniques of stress inoculation (by exposure), and desensitization (by helping real casualties, eg if preparing for war). Keeping combatants in tight-knit groups cemented by the ties of mutual interdependency is recommended by military strategists. NB: morphine use at the time of injury may be protective. www.killology.com

Logotherapy, Shakespeare, and healing through meaning... 'razing out the written troubles of the brain and other rooted sorrows'—Macbeth

Psychiatry

---

1 The Papez circuit of emotion runs from the hippocampus to the amygdala and thence to serotonergic pacemaker cells in the dorsal raphe nucleus (DRN).◆※ The DRN projects to the dentate gyrus directly and indirectly via pacemaker cells in the entorhinal cortex. The direct route promotes neurogenesis in the dentate; the indirect route has 2 purposes: to imprint ongoing moments of consciousness onto new dentate cells for retention as memory, and to provide -ve feedback for regulation. Pathologic overdrive of the DRN causes overdrive of the entorhinal cortex, which leads to excitotoxic cell death of neurons in the hippocampus involved in the -ve feedback loop. The disinhibited amygdala and DRN then orchestrate the syndromes of chronic stress. Recovery from chronic stress requires repopulating the dentate gyrus and restoring the feedback loop.[195]

Eating disorders are common—don't expect your patient to fit neatly into any category: 'Eating disorder not otherwise specified' is the commonest type; categories such as *purging disorder* and *non-fat-phobic anorexia nervosa* are newly proposed categories that may be appropriate to use.

Anorexia nervosa ►The most fatal of all mental illnesses (~20%, if severe). There is a compulsive need to control eating, as if worth equates with shape (a notorious western cult). Low self-worth is common and weight loss becomes an over-valued idea even when weight is very low. This is achieved by over-exercising, induced vomiting, laxative abuse, diuretics, or appetite suppressants. Many also have episodes of binge eating, followed by remorse, vomiting, and concealment. *Diagnostic criteria:*[196] 1 Weight <85% of predicted (taking into account height, sex, and ethnicity, p181), or BMI ≤17.5kg/m². 2 Fear of weight gain, even when underweight, leading to dieting, induced vomiting, or excessive exercise. 3 Feeling fat when thin. 4 Amenorrhoea: 6 consecutive menstrual cycles absent unless on the Pill (in women), or ↓libido♂.

Epidemiology: ♀:♂≥4:1[197] (men are more likely to be undiagnosed; don't assume that a fragile sexual identity exists in these men).[198] Typical age of onset is mid-adolescence—but may be older than 60yrs.[199] *Prevalence:* 0.7% in teenage girls and no restriction to a particular ethnic group. *Incidence in primary care:* 20:100,000 in females aged 10-39 (stable over the last 20 years).[200]

Cause: CRF hypothesis;[1] 55% concordance in monozygotic twins in some areas.

Comorbidity/risk factors: Depression; anxiety; obsessive compulsive features (=anankastic); perfectionism;[201] anxious-avoidant-dependent personality; substance abuse; TV (esp. soap-opera) watching; image-aware work (eg ballet);[202] past teasing or criticism for fatness.[203] Adverse life events and difficulties; most commonly in the area of close relationship with family or friends; low self-esteem; impulsivity; rarely dietary problems in early life; parents preoccupied with food; family relationships that leave the person without a sense of identity. There is scant evidence that the chief problem is psychosexual immaturity (antecedent sexual abuse is not a *specific* risk factor). *Other signs:* Fatigue; cognition↓ (cerebral atrophy) altered sleep cycle; sensitivity to cold; dizziness; psychosexual problems; dental caries; constipation; fullness after eating; subfertility/amenorrhoea; ↓WCC; anaemia; ↓platelets; glucose↑↓; ↓K⁺; ↓PO₄³⁻; ↑bicarbonate; ↑LFT; ↑amylase if binging/purging; ↑T₃/T₄ normal or ↑TSH; ↓LH; ↓oestrogen; ↑GH; ↑cortisol; ↑CCK; normal prolactin; ↓renal function; osteoporosis if malnourished; BP↓; ↑QT interval; amorphous ovaries. In early onset disease, functional MRI shows ↓blood flow to the temporal lobe unilaterally. Also: ↓visuo-spatial ability; ↓visual memory; ↑speed of information processing.

SCOFF questionnaire: (can be used for prevention)[1] Do you ever make yourself sick because you feel too full? Do you worry you've lost control over eating? Have you recently lost more than one stone in 3 months? Do you believe you are fat when others say you are thin? Does food dominate your life?[204]

ΔΔ: Depression, Crohn's/coeliac disease, hypothalamic tumours.

Red flags—risk↑↑ if: ✒ BMI <13 or below 2nd centile ✒ Wt loss >1kg/wk ✒ T°: <34.5° ✒ Vascular: BP <80/50; pulse <40; S₈O₂ <92%; limbs blue and cold ✒ Muscles: unable to get up without using arms for leverage. ✒ Skin: purpura ✒ Blood(mmol/L): K⁺<2.5; Na⁺<130; ↓PO₄³⁻<0.5. ✒ ECG: long QT; flat T waves.

Treatment:[2] Aim to restore nutritional balance (eg weight gain of 1.5kg/week; final BMI 20-25). Treat complications of starvation. Explore comorbidity. Involve family/carers. Address factors maintaining the illness. Severe anorexia

1 Anorexics possibly differ from others in being unable to adapt to corticotrophin releasing factor (CRF) elevations. Signs of CRF dysfunction and HPA-axis hyperactivity: ↑physical activity, ↓reproductive hormones, ↓sexual behaviour, amenorrhea, hypotension, bradycardia, anxiety, ↑social interaction, ↑vigilance, ↓immune system function, ↓food intake, impaired weight gain, affecting both energy intake and utilization.[205]
2 Screen if BMI↓; amenorrhoea; poor growth if >8yrs; unexplained vomiting; poorly-compliant type 1 DM.

(BMI <15kg/m², rapid weight loss + evidence of system failure) requires urgent referral to eating disorder unit (EDU), medical unit (MU) or paediatric medical wards (P). Re-feeding is considered 'treatment' under the Mental Health Act 1983/Children Act 1989, and it may be needed if insight is lacking. In moderate anorexia (BMI 15-17.5, no evidence of system failure) routine referral can be to the local community mental health team (CMHT)/adolescent unit or EDU if available. In mild anorexia (BMI >17.5) focus on building a trusting relationship and encouraging use of self-help books and a food diary.[206] If there is no response within 8wks, consider referral to secondary care. No drug treatments for anorexia nervosa are validated by good randomized trials. Fluoxetine (20-60mg/day) prevents relapse in open trials. ☛ Monitor Q-T interval. There is wide variability in the availability of psychological therapies and no uniform approach. Cognitive therapies (p372), analytic, interpersonal, supportive, or family therapy (±parent-to-parent consultations[3]) may be tried. In children and adolescents consider family therapy.[207] Olanzapine may help (unlicensed use).

Re-feeding syndrome: (On rapid intake of calories). Signs: rhabdomyolysis, respiratory or cardiac failure, BP↓, arrhythmias, seizures, coma, sudden death. Re-feeding syndrome is very rare when with home re-feeding. Acute gastric dilatation can occur if a poorly nourished patient binges. Monitor serum PO_4^{3-} (stop re-feeding if falling). Also watch for glucose↑, K⁺↓, and Mg²⁺↑.[200,208,209]

Prognosis: 43% recover completely, 36% improve and ~20% develop a chronic eating disorder. 5% die (mostly from suicide or direct medical complications, eg K⁺↓ and prolonged Q-T interval predisposing to arrhythmias). Mean time between diagnosis and death is ~11 years.[210] Mortality is higher if: aged 20-29 at presentation, delayed access to treatment, bingeing and vomiting.

Binge eating disorder/bulimia *Definition:* 1 Recurrent episodes of binge eating characterized by uncontrolled overeating; 2 Preoccupation with control of body weight 3 Regular use of mechanisms to overcome the fattening effects of binges, eg starvation, vomit-induction, laxatives, over-exercise 4 BMI >17.5.[211]

Epidemiology: ♀:♂≈9:1. Prevalence (rising in developed countries) ≈ 0.5-1.0% in young women. Social class distribution: even. In Britain, young Muslim Asian women are at ↑risk.[212] Homosexuality/bisexuality may be a specific risk factor for bulimia in males (asexuality is more typical in ♂ anorexia nervosa).[213]

Cause/associations: Urbanization (*not* a risk factor for anorexia); premorbid obesity. Commoner in ♀ relatives of anorectics, suggesting a shared familial liability. Genetic contribution of 54-83%. *Natural history: Age of onset:* ~18yrs.

Symptoms: Fatigue, lethargy,[4] feeling bloated, constipation, abdominal pain, oesophagitis, gastric dilatation with risk of gastric rupture, heart conduction abnormalities, cardiomyopathy (if laxative use), tetany, occasional swelling of hands and feet, irregular menstruation, erosion of dental enamel, enlarged parotid glands, calluses on the back of the hands (Russell's sign, from tooth marks due to induction of vomiting), oedema (use of laxatives and diuretics), metabolic alkalosis, hypochloraemia, hypokalaemia, metabolic acidosis (if laxative use), less commonly hyponatraemia, hypocalcaemia, hypophosphataemia, hypomagnesaemia, abnormal EEG, abnormal menstrual cycle, blunted response of TSH and growth hormone to thyroid releasing hormone.

Treatment: Mild symptoms: support, self-help books and food diary similarly to anorexia. Referral to CMHT or EDU (above) in case of no response, moderate or severe symptoms, and to a medical unit if medical complications.[214] Antidepressants have the most robust evidence at usual doses but fluoxetine may be needed at up to 60mg/day.[215] Cognitive therapy can help (p370-1).[216]

Prognosis: In 2-10yrs, 50% improve, 20% show no change.[217]

---

3 Parents describe parent-to-parent consultations as an intense emotional experience that helps them to feel less alone, to feel empowered to progress, and to reflect on changes in family interactions.

4 If hypersomnia, hyperphagia, and hypersexuality are features, suspect the Kleine–Levin syndrome.

Acute organic reactions (Acute confusion, delirium) The key feature is impaired consciousness with onset over hours or days. It is difficult to describe; take any opportunity to be shown it. You have the sense when trying to communicate that your patient is not with you. He is likely to be disoriented in time (doesn't know day or year) and, with greater impairment, in place. Sometimes he is quiet or drowsy; sometimes agitated, and you are called when he is disrupting the ward. Or he may be deluded (for example, accusing staff of plotting against him/her) or hallucinating. If there is no past psychiatric history, and in the setting of a physical illness or post-surgery, a confusional state is particularly likely—especially if symptoms are worse at the end of the day.

Differential diagnosis: If agitated, consider anxiety (usually readily distinguished on history-taking). If onset uncertain, consider dementia.

Causes: (BOX 1)Infection; drugs (benzodiazepines, opiates, anticonvulsants, digoxin, L-dopa); U&E↑↓; hypoglycaemia; P_aO_2↓; P_aCO_2↑; epilepsy; alcohol withdrawal; trauma; surgery (esp. if pre-op Na$^+$↓ or visual or hearing loss).[218]

Tests: U&E, FBC, blood gases, glucose, cultures (blood, MSU), LFT, ECG, CT, CXR±LP.

Management: Find the cause. Optimize surroundings and nursing care. Examine with above causes in mind; do tests; start relevant treatment, eg O_2.
• If agitation is distressing the patient, and non-drug methods fail, consider **haloperidol** 1-10mg IV/IM/PO[219] or **risperidone** 0.5-4mg/24h PO (smallest dose possible, esp. if elderly).[220] Monitor BP. Wait 20min to judge IM effects. Amnesia and cognition may *worsen*[221] (SE: BP↓↑, stroke,[220] insomnia, dyspepsia). Music, muscle relaxation, and massage (MMM) is a better approach to agitation.
• Nurse ideally in a *moderately lit* quiet room with same staff in attendance. Reassure and re-orientate often. A compromise between a quiet room and a place where staff can keep under surveillance has to be made. Monitor BP.

Chronic organic reactions (dementia) 6% of those ≥65yrs. *Cardinal signs:* Global intellectual deterioration without impairment of consciousness—plus memory loss. Get a history from friends/relatives. Exclude depression (may need a drug trial). Behaviour: restless; no initiative; repetitive, purposeless activity; sexual disinhibition; social gaffes; shoplifting; rigid routines.
• Speech: syntax errors; dysphasia; mutism.
• Thinking: slow, muddled; delusions. Poor memory. No insight.
• Perception: illusions, hallucinations (often visual).
• Mood: irritable, depressed; affect blunt; emotional incontinence (much crying).

Tests: •FBC; B_{12}; folate (MCV↑ suggests alcoholism, or low B_{12} or folate); ESR (malignancy); U&E, LFT, γGT, Ca^{2+} (renal/hepatic failure, alcoholism, malignancy, endocrinopathy (Ca^{2+} ↑ or ↓). TSH (hypothyroidism). • Serology: syphilis (OHCM p419)±HIV. •CT/MRI excludes tumours, hydrocephalus, subdural, stroke etc. Volumetric MRI to subtype the dementia, eg medial temporal (MTL) and hippocampal atrophy≈Alzheimer's disease (AD); in frontotemoral dementia temporal lobe atrophy is more inferior, and there may be marked asymmetry. In Lewy-body dementia, MTL is relatively spared.[222] DaT may help.[1] FLAIR MRI (fluid attenuated inversion recovery) for ischaemic damage (often co-exists with AD).

Management: ►*Involve the patient in her own therapy.* Exclude the treatable. Relatives may feel unable to look after the immobile, incontinent, aggressive, patient who keeps wandering. Good palliative care, walking frames, catheters, day care, holiday admission, an attendance allowance, electronic tagging♠*[2] ± an lasting power of attorney can help. If not, long-stay institutional care may be needed. Agitation: MMM before drugs, as above.[223]

Protective agents (possibly): Statins (relative risk 0.29); antioxidants.[224]$_{n=1364}$

---

1 DaTSCAN comprises ioflupane labelled with radioactive iodide. It is injected during SPECT imaging to detect loss of dopaminergic neuron terminals in the striatum. Specificity in Lewy body dementia: ~100%.
2 Supported by the Alzheimer's Soc. (if it's not a substitute for 1st class care); restraint is unacceptable.

Causes of organic reactions		
	Acute (delirium)	**Chronic (dementia)**
Degenera-tive		*Alzheimer's; Huntington's (OHCM p694); *Lewy-body (OHCM p478), CJD & Pick's (p650)
Other CNS	Cerebral tumour or abscess; subdural haematoma; epilepsy; acute post-trauma psychosis	Tumours; subdural haematoma; multiple sclerosis; Parkinson's; normal pressure hydrocephalus
Infective*	Many, eg meningoencephalitis; septicaemia; cerebral malaria; trypanosomiasis	Late syphilis; chronic or subacute encephalitis; CNS cysticercosis; cryptococcosis; HIV
Vascular	Stroke (or TIA); hypertensive encephalopathy; SLE	Thromboembolic multi-infarct (arteriosclerotic) dementia
Metabolic	*U&E↑↓; *hypoxia; *liver and kidney failure; non-metastatic cancer; porphyria; *alcohol withdrawal	Liver and kidney failure non-metastatic or metastatic cancer
Endocrine	Addisonian or hyperthyroid crisis; diabetic pre-coma; hypoglycaemia; hypo/hyperparathyroidism	T₄↓; Addison's; hypoglycaemia hypopituitarism; hypo-/hyper-parathyroidism[225]
Toxic	*Alcohol; many drugs (check datasheet/statement of product characteristics); lead; arsenic; mercury	*'Alcohol dementia'; barbiturate abuse; too much manganese or carbon disulfide
Deficiency	Thiamine; B₁₂; folate; nicotinic acid	Thiamine; B₁₂; folate; nicotinic acid

Don't exhaust your patient by ordering every possible test!

Psychiatry

* denotes a leading cause.

Example of advice addressed to relatives/carers of demented people

1 Alzheimer's disease is progressive, but some problems, eg aggression, *may* improve in time. Both rate of change and length of life vary greatly. *Should you try to explain to your relative what the diagnosis is?* There is no easy answer. The advantage of frank talking is that he can participate in his care (the vexed issue of stopping driving may be easier to handle). Also, in the early stages, he can consent to plans. Most *would* want to be informed if they got Alzheimer's.

2 Take opportunities to talk of your predicament with other people in the same position. This is often just as useful as talking to doctors. The Alzheimer's Disease Society exists to put you in touch: UK *tel:* 020 7306 0606.

3 Accept offers of help, eg with carer programmes, and of daycare and respite care:[1] you certainly deserve, and need, a break from time to time.

4 Help for carers:UK •Carers Allowance (>£58/wk[2]) •Attendance Allowance •Council tax rebate from Social Services •Local voluntary organizations •Annual health checks to look after the emotional/physical lives of carers •Direct payments •Help in balancing work and care. There are 6 million carers in the UK. ~50% give 20h care a week; >1 million give more than 50h/wk. We all need to be aware of this huge burden being carried by carers.[226]

5 Lock up any rooms in the house which you do not use. Your relative will not notice this restriction—and this may make your life much easier.

6 Lock drawers which contain important papers or easily spoiled items to prevent him storing odd things in them, such as compost, or worse.

7 Remove locks from the lavatory—so he/she cannot get locked in.

8 Sexual activities may stop; spouses should try not to fall into the trap of asking "What's the matter with me?" (NB: SSRI or **cyproterone acetate** titrated to 50mg/12h help ♂ hypersexuality[3] and other aggressive problems).[227]

9 Prepare yourself psychologically for the day when he/she no longer recognizes you. This can be a great blow, unless you prepare for it.

---

1 Social Services UK often refuse 24h help saying that needs aren't complex enough; Courts may reverse this.
2 Ineligible if: receiving state pension; <35h of care/wk; income >£95/wk after tax; a full-time student.
3 Real hypersexuality (libido↑) is rare. Most inappropriate sexual behaviors are related to disinhibition or lack of taking into account contextual environment and feelings of others.

A common scenario. "Doctor, I think my memory is failing. I go into a room full of people I know and cannot remember a single name: the only name to come is Alzheimer...." Is this mild cognitive impairment (and relatively static) or is it AD? (progressive). What most doctors do is some sort of memory test, but a better approach is to get a history from a friend/spouse ("Does he ever get lost in familiar territory/at home? trouble with shopping, and counting out cash etc) and then do some visuo-spacial tasks, eg "Draw a house with a door, a side, a chimney and a few windows" or "draw a clock face and put the numbers in and set to time to 2:30." A drawing is useful because it is a permanent snapshot of an unfolding process, and can be compared over time. Clock drawing is also part of systematic diagnostic methods—the TYM test (*Test Your Memory*, OHCM p85). See BOX 1 for a brief memory test.

Cause It is not clear if the problem is amyloid plaques and neurofibrillary tangles (are they epiphenomena?). Selective loss of temporal lobe synapses may be more important[228] ±loss of whole neurons in the hippocampus, amygdala, temporal lobe and subcortical nuclei (OHCM p492). Treatment doesn't focus on any of these areas, but assumes that what is important is loss of cholinergic function (?one reason why drugs often disappoint in AD). Vascular effects may trump any of the above (95% of AD patients show CNS ischaemia).

Risk factors 1st-degree relative with AD; Down's syndrome; homozygosity for the apolipoprotein (Apo) E e4 allele; PICALM, CL1 and CLU gene mutations; vascular risk factors such as ↑BP, diabetes, dyslipidaemia, ↑homocysteine,[1] atrial fibrillation; ↓physical and cognitive activity; depression. Evidence on smoking and alcohol is inconsistent: ≥2u/day of alcohol accelerated onset of AD by 5yrs in one study (others say red wine may be protective); ≥20 cigarettes/day≈2yrs; ApoE e4 genotype≈3yrs. ►Delaying onset by 5yrs would ↓prevalence by ~50%.

Presentation In STAGE I of AD there is amnesia and spatial disorientation. In STAGE II (some years later): personality disintegration, eg with aggression, psychosis, agitation, depression, and focal parietal signs, eg dysphasia, apraxia, agnosia, and acalculia. Parkinsonism may occur. She may use her mouth to examine objects (hyperorality). STAGE III Neurovegetative changes with apathy (or ceaselessly active—akathisia), wasting, immobility, and incontinence, ± seizures and spasticity. *Mean survival*: 7yrs from clinical (overt) onset.

Drugs Get expert help to increase CNS acetylcholine by inhibiting the enzyme causing its breakdown (**donepezil; rivastigmine; galantamine**). Memantine, a NMDA (N-methyl-D-aspartate) receptor antagonist, may help moderate to severe AD. *Cautions:* creatinine↑; epilepsy. SE: confusion, headache, hallucinations, tiredness; rarer: vomiting, anxiety, hypertonia, cystitis, ↑libido. *Dose:* initially 5mg each morning; ↑ in steps of 5mg at intervals of 1wk to 10mg/12h.

Practical help ►p351. Exclude treatable dementias (B₁₂, folate, syphilis serology, T₄, HIV). CT/MRI (p352). Treat concurrent illnesses (they worsen dementia). Avoid sedatives and neuroleptics (longevity, fluency, and cognition all suffer). In most, dementia progresses. Involve relatives and relevant agencies.

Prevention◆* B vitamins to lower homocysteine;[1] long-chain **omega-3 fatty acids/N-3 PUFAs**, eg eicosapentaenoic acid (EPA+DHA), in flax, walnuts, tuna, mackerel, and herring oil show promise.[229,230] More fruit (?risk↓ by ⅓);[231] **cognitively stimulating hobbies** (a 1-point ↑in cognitive activity score can ↓risk by ⅓).

A cohort study of 678 nuns showed that education and use of syntactically and imaginatively rich language at 18yrs old predicts onset of AD ~50yrs later.[232]

---

[1] 0.8mg folic acid, 0.5mg vit B₁₂+20mg vit B₆/day PO ↓mild cognitive impairment (MCI) if baseline homocysteine >11μmol/L. B vitamins also ↓ rates of MRI brain atrophy in MCI (Celeste de Jager's VITACOG trials).[233]

Check that he is fully awake and not in pain.

Present year and own age	2	Name of your country's ... 1
Time to nearest hour	1	president, ruler or premier
Recognition of people	1	Memorize address (42 West St, Hull) 1
Name of place	1	Date of world war (I or II) 1
Birthday (day & month)	1	Count backwards from 20 to 1 1

234Alternative: TYM test, OHCM p85; Mini-mental State cannot be printed for copyright reasons

Temporal lobe function is tested by memory tests (above); scores of ≤6 suggest confusion or dementia (correct in ~80%).[235] Serial changes mean more than a one-off value. Other illness can lower scores (eg ↓cardiac output).[236]

Other pointers to dementia Increasingly, do you find that...
• You forget what you are saying or reading in mid-sentence?
• You have to rely on lists whereas previously this was not necessary?
• Thought is slow or imprecise, harmonizing poorly with motor control?
• Mental agility is lacking, with powers of concentration declining?
• Is there difficulty executing fast movements of eyes or limbs, or difficulty in walking?—eg with spastic ataxic gait or quadriparesis of HIV-1 *associated cognitive/motor complex*, or psychomotor retardation, ± release reflexes such as a snout response, or hyperactive deep tendon reflexes.
NB: including an 'informant report questionnaire' improves the efficiency of the mental test score as a screening tool for dementia.[237]

Bedside tests of frontal lobe function (eg executive function).[238]
• *Verbal fluency and initiation:* Ask the patient to recall as many words as possible in 1 minute starting with 's'; fewer than 10 is abnormal.
• *Cognitive estimates:* Ask to give educated guesses to questions which they are unlikely to know the answer, eg "How old is the oldest person in the country?" "How many camels are there in Holland?"
• *Abstract thinking:* Proverb interpretation (however interpretation highly dependent on educational, cultural factors). Explain the linkage between pairs: eg poem & statue; praise & punishment; orange & banana.
• *Tests of 'response inhibition' and 'set shifting'*—eg a triangle and square test: draw an alternating sequence of triangles and squares—and ask the patient to copy what you are doing. Only the grossly impaired will keep drawing just one of the shapes (perseveration).
• *Clock drawing test:* 'draw a large clock face, put the numbers in, put the hands in to show ten past five'. Tests frontal (executive) and dominant parietal (praxis) function, and is an adjunct to mental test scores.

Quotes from the blogsphere.   *"My mother has Alzheimer's..."*

"Each morning she wakes up smiling and walks out not knowing she has soiled herself... She doesn't know why she is being stripped and washed. It's like a daily physical and emotional rape. Her cries echo in my ears even when she is not crying. In her lucid moments she says, "Anu, I don't know what I'm doing. Why is this happening to me?".

"My kids are petrified of old age and though they are very young, they keep asking me if I will become like my mother when I grow old. I have no time to spend with my husband...I can see my marriage getting affected, but after staying awake with my mother in her room for days and then dragging myself to work, not sleeping even four hours for weeks, I'm exhausted emotionally and physically. There are days I drive on the highway and wish a truck would crush me." Would Anu consider a nursing home? "My mother will die. Even though she is in an advanced stage of Alzheimer's she knows she is with family. In her lucid moments she asks, "Tum mujhe chod to nahin dogey na?" (You won't desert me will you?)".[239] Courtesy of Kavita Chhibber

This page is dedicated to Anu & her family.

Psychiatry

Quote from Zoë's mother:[240] "'There's been a fatality on the line...' Neither of us guessed it was you, even though you'd tried to kill yourself before. We called it a nervous breakdown when Bristol University sent you home for 'undisciplined behaviour.' As our memories faded and you seemed set for a brilliant career, no one spoke about this first episode. "I've been to the bottom," you used to say, "I'm strong." We put the horror behind us. It was over. Then when your charisma and enthusiasms grew wild again, and aggressive, we said "Zoë is just being Zoë". We were in denial and so were you. We followed your lead. You gave up your job and against everyone's advice, went to Morocco "to find myself". I loved the emails you sent in those first weeks, full of enthusiasm about Islamic culture, learning Arabic and meeting the love of your life. Then the emails grew wilder, your projects more farfetched, but we suspected nothing until we arrived to find you in full blown mania: attacking the hotel staff, knocking my glasses off my nose, refusing to eat, hectoring everyone in earshot with grandiloquent schemes to save the universe...Perhaps you were too fine for us? The beat of the drum you danced to didn't fit with our drab, calculating world; or was it random misfirings, turning your reactions from vivid to florid?" *Letter to a Lost Daughter* D. Schwarz; Chipmonka*

Prevalence may be increasing in those <19yrs old[241] (0.25% in 1994; 1% in 2003).

Signs of mania *Mood:* Irritability (80%), euphoria (71%), lability (69%).
• *Cognition:* Grandiosity (78%); flight of ideas/racing thoughts (71%); distractibility/poor concentration (71%); confusion (25%); many conflicting lines of thought urgently racing in contrary directions; lack of insight. *Behaviour:* Rapid speech (98%), hyperactivity (87%), ↓sleep (81%), hypersexuality (57%), extravagance (55%). *Psychotic symptoms:* Delusions (48%), hallucinations (15%). Less severe states are termed *hypomania*. If depression alternates with mania, the term *bipolar affective disorder* is used (esp. if there is a history of this). During mood swings, risk of suicide is high. Cyclical mood swings without the more florid features (as above) are termed *cyclothymia*.

Causes *Physical:* Infections, hyperthyroidism; SLE; thrombotic thrombocytopenic purpura; stroke; water dysregulation/Na⁺↓; ECT. *Drugs:* Amphetamines, cocaine, antidepressants (esp. venlafaxine[242]), captopril, steroids, procyclidine, L-dopa, baclofen. *Bipolar disorder:* (Age at onset: <25.)

In a 1ˢᵗ attack *Ask about:* Infections, drug use, and past or family history of psychiatric disorders. Do: CT of the head, EEG, and screen for drugs/toxins.[243]

Treating acute maniaᴺᴵᶜᴱ *Assess:* Psychotic symptoms (p316); cycling speed; suicide risk. *R* for acute moderate/severe mania: olanzapine 10mg PO, adjust to 5-20mg/day (SE: weight↑; glucose↑), or valproate semisodium, eg 250mg/8h PO (Depakote®; may be ↑ rapidly to 1-2g/24h). NB: some people are most fulfilled and creative when manic and don't want to change; others recognize, in retrospect, that use of mental health law (a last resort) was a turning point.

Prophylaxis Those who have bipolar affective disorder after successful treatment of the manic or depressive episode should have a mood stabilizer for longer-term control. If compliance is good, and U&E, ECG, and T₄ normal, give lithium carbonate 125mg-1g/12h PO. Adjust dose to give a plasma level of ~0.6-1mmol/L Li⁺, on day 4-7, ~12h post-dose. A range of 0.4-1 may be equally valid;• consider a tighter range if elderly (↑ sensitivity to Li⁺ neurotoxicity).[244]
• Check Li⁺ levels weekly (~12h post-dose) until the dose has been constant for 4wks; then monthly for 6 months; then 3-monthly, if stable; more often if on diuretic, NSAIDs, ACE-i (all ↑ Li⁺) or on a low-salt diet or if pregnant (?avoid Li⁺).
• If Li⁺ levels are progressively rising, suspect progressive nephrotoxicity.
• U&E + TSH 6-monthly; Li⁺ SE: hypothyroidism; nephrogenic diabetes insipidus.
▶Avoid changing brands [Li⁺↓↑]. ▶Ensure you can contact urgently if Li⁺ >1.4mmol/L. ▶Toxic signs: vision↓; D&V; K⁺↓; ataxia; tremor; dysarthria; coma.

Helping those with mania and a high risk of suicide

Risk of suicide is high if: •Previous suicide attempt •Family history of suicide •Early onset of bipolar disorder •Extent of depressive symptoms (eg hopelessness) •Increasingly bad affective signs •Mixed affective states •Rapid cycling •Abuse of alcohol or drugs.[245]

Lithium reduces risk of suicide.[245] If contraindicated, **olanzapine + fluoxetine** may be better than **lamotrigine** (below).[246] ►But don't rely on drugs. Often people with mania won't take them anyway. As one bipolar writer said "I do not believe that a complex problem can be solved simply by popping pills...I thrive in the extremes of my cycles, and the words pour from my mind and hand. All that evaporates in wellness,[1] so I imagine it would dissolve completely if I chemically alleviated my malady. I will not dilute my intensity and drain my writing. I feel dead in wellness, so I fear that I would feel just as lifeless if I was 'cured.' My identity is also still so blended with this disorder. It is a fundamental part of me and shapes my world. I accept this disorder as a forming force in my life and value how it has made me. It tested me; it made me stronger; it made me different; it gave me my creativity...It is not just a disease to be remedied; it is a real part of me that I need to learn to cope with and adapt to. I need to discover how to control it, rather than allow it to dominate me so that I can live with it as a vital aspect of my life."[247] **Cognitive therapy** (p373) is of great value in helping people (who retain some insight) ride their cycles without falling off.[246]

When lithium does not give good control

Note that abrupt cessation of lithium precipitates acute mania in up to 50% of patients. Discontinuation should be gradual over 2-4 weeks.

Anticonvulsants: Semisodium valproate (SE: hyperandrogenism if ♀) and **carbamazepine** (400mg/8h PO; swallow whole; do not chew) are next steps.[248]

Some authorities say most specific indication may be in rapid cyclers (≥4 acute mood swings/yr). **Lamotrigine** may be as good as **citalopram** in bipolar depressive states.[249] *Antipsychotics:* Olanzapine has a role.[250] In one meta-analysis, there was no difference in overall efficacy of treatment between haloperidol and olanzapine or risperidone. Some evidence suggests that haloperidol could be less effective than **aripiprazole**.[251]

Anticonvulsants such as **lamotrigine, gabapentin** and **topiramate** are potential mood stabilizers. Lamotrigine has the strongest evidence.[252]

Combination treatments: (Often tried). Lithium plus carbamazepine may be synergistic.[253] Lithium (or valpoate) plus an atypical antipsychotic, eg **risperidone** or **olanzapine** may help if unresponsive to monotherapy.[254,255]

Antidepressants with lithium Lithium (or an alternative mood stabilizer) reduces risk of mood fluctuations from mania to depression in people with bipolar affective disorder. For depression occurring during lithium treatment antidepressants can be used: selective serotonin reuptake inhibitors (SSRIs) **bupropion, venlafaxine**●✹ are said by expert committees to be best. Taper from 2 to 6 months after remission to minimize manic relapse.[256]

Consider **monoamine oxidase inhibitors** for anergic (=lacking in energy) bipolar depression.[257] ECT also has a role (p342),[258] and meta-analyses support use of omega 3 oils (only for when mood is low).[259]

---

1 A counter argument from the periodically depressed poet Thomas Krampf: "one can have a vision but no vision is worth anything if one is too sick to implement it"—and many writers have found their creativity flourish more when treatment is underway. M Berlin 2008 *Poets on Prozac*, Baltimore.

Psychiatry

Blogs subverts ideas of disease and cure: "I feel dead in wellness"

Schizophrenia is a common chronic/relapsing condition often presenting in late teens/early 20s with **psychotic symptoms** (hallucinations, delusions); **disorganization symptoms** (incongruous mood, abnormal speech and thought); **negative symptoms** (apathy, self-neglect, blunted mood, ↓motivation, withdrawal); and, sometimes, **cognitive impairment**.[260,261] It has major implications for patients, work and families. *Incidence:* ~0.15:1000/yr. *Prevalence:* ~1%.

What's in a name? Some experts hold that the term 'schizophrenia' has outlived its usefulness as it implies that all people with schizophrenia have the same pathology—and hence need antipsychotics. A more nuanced approach is to avoid diagnostic labels, certainly for the 1st 6 months, and not to use antipsychotics automatically. *Dopamine dysregulatory disorder* (BOX)[262] is a new name—without the pejorative overtones of violence, fear and unpredictability. *A word on 'psychosis':* In its florid form, psychosis is the archetype of the layman's 'madness' But, the *usual* picture is less obvious: the patient may be sitting alone, quietly attending to his or her voices. If hallucinations, delusions, or a thought disorder (defined on p358) are present, the cause 'must' be either schizophrenia and related disorders, a disorder of affect (mania or depression or both, p336), or be organic (eg drug misuse, head injury). So the term psychosis is not in itself a diagnosis, but is a useful term to employ, while the underlying diagnosis is being formulated. Beware labelling people; remember that even during the best of times, only a thin veil separates us from insanity.

Genes & environment Many genes implicated in schizophrenia also ↑ risk of bipolar disorder.[253–265 International Schizophrenia Consortium] Some are susceptibility genes (needing environmental triggers). Genome-wide studies point to a gene coding myosin on chromosome 22 and a region of >450 gene variants, in the major histocompatibility complex (MHC) region on 6p. The dysbindin gene on chromosome 6 is important too. Early use of cannabis is a trigger: those with vv homozygosity of the catechol-o-methyl-transferase gene (COMT; risk ↑×10 compared with mm variants). The timing of triggers is important.[266] Those starting cannabis at 15yrs old are 3× more likely to develop schizophreniform psychosis.[267,268]

Is schizophrenia a neurodevelopmental disorder? People with schizophrenia may suffer unusual neurodevelopment either through inheriting genes and/or some insult to the brain that impairs its development. This leads to subtle cognitive and behavioural effects in childhood[269] and then psychosis at or just after adolescence. Relevant prenatal/obstetric events: early rupture of membranes, gestational age <37 weeks, incubator use, winter births).[270]

MRI shows differences in the brains of those with schizophrenia (and their 1st degree relatives[271]): eg larger lateral ventricles, reduced frontal lobe and parahippocampal gyrus. Reduced (particularly on left) temporal lobe, hippocampus (subserves memory/emotion) and amygdala (involved in expression of emotion). MRI has shown diffuse reduction in cortical grey matter associated with poor premorbid function.[272] NB: use of psychotics may also cause brain shrinkage—eg up to 20%.[273] However, schizophrenia also has an onset later in life, particularly women over 30.[274] It has been estimated that about 40% of people who develop schizophrenia have a developmental problem, but the majority are not remarkably different from the general population and have no cognitive deficits. So what are the other pathways that lead to psychosis?

Social factors: Being brought up in cities increases the risk of schizophrenia (UK incidence is particularly high in London), and there are higher levels of schizophrenia in migrant groups such as Asians and African-Caribbeans (?mechanism through social adversity, racial discrimination, social isolation).[275] The associated 'stress' on the brain has been suggested to affect the morphology of the brain via hormonal influences as well as the stress of being psychotic resulting in high cortisol levels causing further brain changes.

Physical and metaphysical insights into schizophrenia

Auditory hallucinations One idea[275] is that there is misreading of inner speech. If you think of your favourite poem, you can produce its words in your mind, but you know that you produced them. A person with schizophrenia produces words in the mind in a similar way but then may misinterpret them as coming from an outside source. We know that during hallucinations, muscle activity resembling phonation is detectable in the tongue. Sub-vocal speech can be picked up from the larynx, and this may correspond to what the hallucinations are telling the patient to do. We know that during inner speech Broca's area is activated, and imaging studies show that auditory hallucinations activate Broca's area, indicating that they result from misattributing inner speech. But why do sufferers not realize it is their own inner speech? Shergill has shown that during auditory hallucinations there is *also* activation in the auditory cortex, temporal lobe and subcortical areas.[276] This reflects the activation of a system used when we are listening to external speech but not to our internal speech. This is why some minds are tricked into thinking the words come from outside.

Dopamine dysregulation and aberrant salience Whatever increases dopamine worsens psychosis, while blocking dopamine helps treat psychosis. Dysregulation of mesolimbic dopamine underlies the positive symptoms of psychosis. Dopamine mediates our attachment of salience or importance to ideas and objects hence excess mesolimbic dopamine leads to attaching salience to all sorts of unrelated phenomena. Sufferers cannot have a rational explanation and instead create what seems to them a convincing explanation: it is this we call a delusion. Note that the best philosophers (eg David Hume, 1711-76) show that the notion of causation is based on just such a delusion: there being no true or demonstrable connection between cause and effect—just a relationship that exists between ideas in our minds. Any being that has this power of making causal connections (attaching salience to unrelated events)[277] has adaptive advantage, but is a hair's breadth from psychosis. It is in this 'hair's breadth' (opposite) that we run our lives. Without our ability to attach salience there would be no such thing as love at first sight—maybe no love at all. Our humanity and our tendency to psychosis are two sides of one coin. This is why we owe the mentally ill an especial duty of care: they are suffering for what makes us human.

Antipsychotics reduce the underlying dopaminergic drive and this attenuates the abnormal attribution of salience. So people stop hallucinating or they stop thinking their neighbours are persecuting them, but they still believe that last week there really were voices telling them to do things.

How do patients explain what is happening? Mental illness may seem unfathomable; for others the turmoil of a 'mental breakdown' is later seen as a 'mental breakthrough': we need to see purpose in all things, including our mental illnesses. *Quote from a blog*, from a man with schizophrenia: "I was a passionate, devout Christian and believed I had found ultimate truth. A snowball of odd tragedies struck, which turned things around making life an inner hell. The powerlessness of not being able to cope with it all led to deep depression as well. I thought my life was truly over..." (an awful lot happened in these dot-dot-dots...but things did get better) "...I attained a level of transcendence and awareness that I never had before. My cognitive, writing, speaking, communication, insight and understanding abilities suddenly reached a level on their own. It was then that I was able to understand higher spiritual truths. So I was wondering then. Perhaps my soul or higher self wanted to evolve to a higher awareness level and when it was in the process of doing so, my physical brain had trouble adjusting to it, so it started misfiring and malfunctioning, which created those obsessions and delusions. Perhaps that is the reason behind some mental illnesses."[278,279]

When the voices take over I call it "getting possessed." Thephining is not the way out

3 millennia of failed explanations...from the blogosphere:

Schizophrenia entails distorted thinking and perception, eg delusions and hallucinations. These are common, eg in 1) Affective psychoses (depression; bipolar disorder); 2) Substance abuse psychotic disorders (eg alcohol, cannabis); 3) Psychosis due to a medical disorders (eg brain tumour); and 4) Schizophrenia-like non-affective disorders (brief psychotic disorder; delusional disorder; schizophreniform disorder).[280] When diagnosing schizophrenia look for:

1 *Thought insertion:* "He's is putting ideas into my head" *Thought broadcasting:* "People overhear my thoughts". *Thought withdrawal:* "Thoughts are being taken out of my head", or repeating of thoughts—*écho des pensées*.

2 Delusions of control, influence, or passivity, clearly referred to body or limb movements or thoughts, actions, sensations. Delusional perceptions (a rare non-ICD-10 example is *perception broadcasting*, eg "I am a webcam").[281]

3 Hallucinatory voices giving a running commentary on a patient's behaviour, or discussing the patient among themselves.

4 Persistent delusions of other kinds that are culturally inappropriate and completely impossible ("Rasputin has put a transmitter in my brain").

5 Persistent hallucinations in any modality (somatic, visual, tactile) which occur everyday for weeks on end.

6 Breaks or interpolations in the train of thought, resulting in incoherence or irrelevant speech—*knight's move thoughts* that change direction, flying off at tangents, with odd logic, or neologisms (made up words).

7 Catatonic behaviour, such as excitement, posturing, or waxy flexibility, negativism, mutism, echopraxia (involuntary imitation of the movements).

8 Negative symptoms (apathy, paucity of speech, blunting or incongruity of affect, eg laughing at bad news) usually resulting in social withdrawal.

(1-5 are co-extensive with Schneider's 1st rank symptoms of schizophrenia.)

Diagnostic guidelines for schizophrenia The main criterion is at least one very clear symptom (and usually two or more if less clear-cut) belonging to any of the groups 1-4 above, or symptoms from at least two of groups 5-8. Because many people have brief psychosis-like symptoms, do not diagnose schizophrenia unless symptoms last for ≥6 months and symptoms are present much of the time for at least one month, and there is marked impairment in work or home functioning. Also, 'rule out' other causes of psychosis (eg bipolar disorder, drugs/alcohol, CNS tumours, head injury).

ICD-10 distinguishes the following subtypes of schizophrenia: *Paranoid* (commonest subtype, here hallucinations and/or delusions are prominent). *Hebephrenic* (age of onset 15-25yrs, poor prognosis, changes in mood prominent with fleeting fragmented delusions and hallucinations). *Catatonic* (characterized by stupor, excitement, posturing, waxy flexibility, and negativism). In *simple* and *residual* types, negative symptoms predominate.

Frequent symptoms Lack of insight,[97%] auditory hallucinations,[74%] ideas of reference,[70%] paranoia,[66%] flat affect,[66%] persecutory delusions.[62%]

Frequent behaviours Social withdrawal,[74%] apathy,[56%] lack of conversation,[54%] anhedonia (inability to feel pleasure),[50%] psychomotor retardation,[48%] overactivity,[41%] self-neglect,[30%] posturing ± odd movements.[25%]

Better prognosis if: Sudden onset; no negative symptoms; supportive home; ♀ sex (better social integration[282]); later onset of illness; no CNS ventricular enlargement; no family history (data from WHO *disability assessment schedule*[283]). Overall, only 10% ever have one episode. With treatment, ≤7% need intensive input/hospital admission for >2yrs after 1st admission. 28% go >2yrs without needing further hospital admission. *Lifetime risk of schizophrenia:* ~1%. *Suicide rates:* 10% in acute phase; 4% in chronic.

Managing violence (after the Maudsley *Prescribing Guidelines*)

A person can be violent as a result of psychiatric illness, substance misuse, personality disorder, or physical illness. Or it may be the result of adverse ward environments: overcrowding, noise, alienation, and nowhere to go (no blue skies or green fields). This is the danger if sequestration on the ward is the result of withdrawal of privileges for 'bad behaviour'.

- Recognize early warning signs: tachypnoea, clenched fists, shouting, chanting, restlessness, repetitive movements, pacing, gesticulations. Your own intuition may be helpful here. At the first hint of violence, get help. If alone, make sure you are nearer the door than the patient.
- Do not be alone with the patient; summon the police if needed.
- Try calming and talking with the patient. Do not touch him. Use your body language to reassure (sitting back, open palms, attentive).
- Get his or her consent. If he does not consent to treatment, emergency treatment can still be given to save life, or if serious deterioration.
- Use minimum force possible. *Rapid tranquillization* (RT) is the use of medication in controlling behaviour. It should only be used as a last resort when non-pharmacological methods of behaviour control have failed.

>>De-escalation >>Time-out >>Placement, as appropriate.

- Offer **oral** treatment. If the patient is prescribed a regular antipsychotic, *lorazepam* 1-2mg or *promethazine* 25-50mg avoids risks associated with combining antipsychotics. Oral options if not already on regular oral or de-pot antipsychotic: (*olanzapine* 10mg, *quetiapine* 100-200mg, *risperidone* 1-2mg or *haloperidol* 5mg). Avoid using more than one antipsychotic to avoid QT prolongation (rapid tranquilization predisposes to arrhythmias).
- Repeat after 45-60min. Monotherapy with buccal *midazolam* 10-20mg may avoid the need for IM drugs (unlicensed).

If 2 doses fail or sooner if the patient is placing themselves or others at significant risk—consider IM treatment. Consider the patient's legal status and consider consulting a senior colleague. Options:

- *Lorazepam* 1-2mg IM (dilute with equal volume of water for injections) Have flumazenil to hand ∴ respiratory depression. Be cautious if very young or elderly, and those with pre-existing brain damage or impulse control problems, as disinhibition reactions are more likely.
- *Promethazine* 50mg IM is useful in a benzodiazepine-tolerant patient. Promethazine has slow onset, but is often effective. Dilution is not needed before IM injection. It may be repeated up to 100mg/day. Wait 1–2h to assess response. It is an extremely weak dopamine antagonist
- *Olanzapine* 10mg IM; don't combine olanzapine with IM benzodiazepine.
- *Aripiprazole* 9.75mg; *vs* olanzapine it's less hypotensive but ?less effective.
- *Haloperidol* 5mg is last-choice as incidence of acute dystonia is high; ensure IM procyclidine is to hand. Repeat after 30-60min if insufficient effect.
- Consider IV treatment if an immediate effect is needed: *Diazepam* up to 10mg as Diazemuls® over ≥5min. Repeat after 5-10mins if insufficient effect (up to 3 times). Have flumazenil to hand.

Seek expert advice from consultant or senior clinical pharmacist on call. Options are limited. IM amobarbital, paraldehyde & ECT have been tried.

>>Montor vital signs every 5-10min for 1h, and then half-hourly until ambulatory (if he refuses, observe for signs of pyrexia, hypotension, oversedation and wellbeing. If unconscious, monitor oximetry. A nurse must accompany until ambulatory. Monitor ECG, U&E & FBC if high-dose IM antipsychotics used.

Psychiatry

The liquid cosh creates perfect institutionalized zombies—or it may be no worse than padded cells or manacles?

Don't dawdle! Delaying antipsychotics worsens negative symptoms.[284] They can be dramatic, but managing schizophrenia is much more than drugs; it requires an individualized care plan that includes psychosocial interventions (eg supported employment with cognitive training)—and support for families.[28]

Advice and monitoring Before starting an antipsychotic ask about personal/family history of diabetes, hypertension, and cardiovascular disease. Give advice on diet, weight control and exercise. Perform BP, weight, fasting blood glucose, lipid profile, FBC, ECG if on clozapine or zotepine. Additional 6-monthly monitoring of LFT, U&E, prolactin, weight, Hb_{A1c} is recommended.[286]

Typical or atypical? *Typical antipsychotics* (chlorpromazine, haloperidol 0.5-3mg/8h PO) help symptoms in ~¾ of those with acute schizophrenia; they are less good for negative symptoms. Blockade of D2 receptors is the main reason for their antipsychotic effect—and the cause of side effects that often make people stop their tablets. *Treating extrapyramidal side effects* (EPSE) • Parkinsonism: ↓dose, change to atypical, or try procyclidine 2.5mg/8h PO; increase if necessary; max 30mg/24h • Acute dystonia can occur within hours of starting antipsychotics. ℞: Procyclidine 5-10mg IM or IV (may take ½h to work), repeat after 10min, max 30mg/24h • Akathisia—occurs within hours to weeks of starting antipsychotics, restlessness may be very distressing; so use lowest possible dose or change to atypical—treatment may be needed with propranolol ~20mg/8h PO ± cyproheptadine 4mg/6h PO • Tardive dyskinesia (chewing, grimaces, choreoathetosis) may be irreversible; but try tetrabenazine 12.5-50mg/6-24h PO.

Symptomatic hyperprolactinaemia: Galactorrhoea, amenorrhoea, oligomenorrhoea, female/male infertility. Reduce dose or switch to quetiapine. If not tolerated try amantadine 100mg/24h PO; max 200-300mg/24h PO.

Atypical antipsychotics are those causing no or minimal EPSE. They differ from one another significantly in pharmacodynamic and unwanted effects, which influences choice. Atypical antipsychotics relieve psychotic symptoms as effectively as typical drugs,[287,288] and may lower relapse rates.[289] NICE says to consider oral atypical antipsychotics 'in the choice of 1st-line treatments for individuals with newly diagnosed schizophrenia'.•❊ Not all trials agree.[290]

Which antipsychotic? Atypical antipsychotics: amisulpride, aripiprazole, clozapine, olanzapine, quetiapine, risperidone, sertindole, zotepine, paliperidone (a once-a-day drug). Risperidone recently came top of the list when psychiatrists were asked "If you become psychotic, what would you want?"[127, n=543] Clozapine is restricted to those resistant to, or intolerant of, other antipsychotics (agranulocytosis risk ≤0.8% in 1st yr of ℞; specialist monitoring is needed). Sertindole is only available on a named patient basis due to significant QTc prolongation and fatal arrhythmias.[291] Except for clozapine which definitely causes less EPSE,[292] there is no clear advantage for any one atypical antipsychotic over another, so side effects are important in tailoring treatment to the individual patient. Most unwanted effects are dose-related, so 'start low increase slow'. All antipsychotics ↓seizure threshold (esp. zotepine & clozapine).

Special patient groups Elderly, children and adolescents may get more side effects. In breastfeeding, most atypicals enter breast milk. Trials of use in pregnancy are few; weigh up potential benefits against harm to mother, fetus and neonate. Avoid breastfeeding. *Extrapyramidal side effects* (EPSE) are rare with quetiapine[293] and clozapine, and uncommon with aripiprazole and zotepine. Can occur at high doses with amisulpride, olanzapine and risperidone. *Hyperprolactinaemia:* Aripiprazole, clozapine and quetiapine have no or minimal effect on serum prolactin, olanzapine does at higher doses.[294]

Sexual dysfunction: All atypicals can cause sexual dysfunction, eg erectile dysfunction, ↓libido, ↓arousal, anorgasmia, eg from ↑prolactin (check level)[295] and ↓semen volume/viscosity;[296] retrograde ejaculation (α_1-receptor antagonism, eg with risperidone).[297] In one study, ~30% had stopped their drugs at some point owing to sexual side effects.[298] So ask about sex (p328; few will volunteer this information). If experiencing problems, adding cabergoline, bromocriptine, or amantadine, or switching to quetiapine may be appropriate.[299]

Weight gain is common, and ↓compliance and ↑risk of cardiovascular events and diabetes (greatest with olanzapine and clozapine, moderate with risperidone, sertindole, and zotepine; least with amisulpride and aripiprazole).[300]

Diabetes mellitus: Prevalence in schizophrenia is twice the expected rate;[301] antipsychotics further increase risk (esp. clozapine and olanzapine).

Cardiovascular effects: Olanzapine and risperidone ↑risk of stroke in the elderly when used to treat behavioural symptoms of dementia.[220] Postural hypotension is common (α_1 adrenoreceptor blockade). Long QTc on ECG with zotepine, sertindole; fatal myocarditis and cardiomyopathy (clozapine).

Daytime drowsiness: ~40% of those on clozapine (30% if on olanzapine or risperidone; 15% if on amisulpride, quetiapine, or sertindole).

Managing acute episodes of schizophrenia • If acutely disturbed use the *rapid tranquillization protocol* (p359) • Approach patients with optimism and empathy • Provide comprehensive information and consult any advance directive • Discuss antipsychotic choice with the patient and start promptly if distressed and symptoms not tolerable, otherwise refer to specialist in the mental health service (MHS). *Dose example:* Quetiapine 25mg/12h on day 1; 50mg/12h on day 2; 100mg/12h on day 3; 150mg/12h on day 4; then adjust according to response (eg 300–450mg daily in 2 doses; max 750mg/24h).

Add-on neuroprotection Case reports & 1 randomized trial give hope that *minocycline* (200mg/day, as early as possible) can ↓ negative symptoms.[302]

Managing risk and psychosocial aspects[303] Risk is divided into risk to self, others, and risk of self-neglect. Look at past psychiatric and forensic history. Is there past violence or suicidal or self-harming behaviour? Ask yourself *where is the patient to be treated? Do they have insight? Can they be managed at home?* (via early intervention/home treatment teams), or *do they need to be an in-patient* (Mental Health Act). Risk assessments are an important component of the management of a person with mental health problems: ▶p329.

Failure to respond Cross-taper (p369) to a new drug;[304] if all fail, combination therapy[305] is often tried, eg olanzapine with either amisulpride or risperidone, or quetiapine with risperidone. In theory, by acting on different receptors benefit may occur.[306] But often it doesn't go according to plan, and safety issues are opaque. Aripiprazole plus non-clozapine atypicals may *worsen* psychosis.

☯Psychological interventions towards the end of acute episodes look at treating residual symptoms, eg difficult thoughts, voices, negative symptoms. Aim for quick recovery and relapse prevention through education ± CBT, p372-4.

☯Enlist the family's support Address carers issues (embarrassment, self-blame, and shame are prevalent).[307] *Social support:* It is possible that particular social circumstances may result in alterations in dopamine that make relapse more likely. Addressing issues with housing, employment, support groups, benefits and social skills training are all just as important as being concordant with medication. *Aftercare:* Co-ordinate via an allocated key-worker and a multidisciplinary team (to look at biological, psychological, social and risk issues). It is performed through the Care Programme Approach (CPA). Family therapy may have a role.[308] If concordance with medication is an issue depots are useful, risperidone is now available as a long-acting injectable form (so less EP SEs compared to the older 'typical' depot preparations).

☯"I don't want to go on with the tablets..." Relapse is not always a disaster, and drug SE can be bad. Respect his decision, unless sectioning is needed. His life may become more meaningful. We tend to be over-impressed by +ve symptoms (eg hallucinations) which respond better to drugs than -ve symptoms.[309]

Essence "Visiting prostitutes is unfulfilling, empty, terrible...but I keep going."

Epidemiology of drug addiction Cannabis is commonly used by young people (33% men and 22% women), ecstasy is the commonest class A drug (9% of men and 4% of women aged 16-24).[310] Heroin users make up ~70% of Home Office[uk] notified addicts. For nicotine and alcohol addiction, see p512 & p363. Other drugs: hydrocarbons/glue sniffing, barbiturates, opiates, LSD, ecstasy.

Causes Individual factors (age, gender, personality, family background) and interact with external factors such as surrounding culture, price, availability, setting, advertising.[311] Inherited vulnerability is equally important.[312]

Suspect drug addiction if: • Arrests for larceny, to buy drugs • Odd behaviour, eg visual hallucinations, elation, mania • Unexplained nasal discharge (cocaine sniffing) • The results of injections: marked veins; abscesses; hepatitis; HIV • Repeated requests for analgesics, with only opiates acceptable.

Clinical presentation[313] *Acute intoxication:* Follows administration of alcohol or other psychoactive substances resulting in disturbances of level of consciousness, cognition, perception, affect, or behaviour. *Harmful use:* A pattern of psychoactive substance use that is causing actual damage to the mental or physical health of the user *Dependence syndrome:* 3 or more of the following:

1 Strong desire or sense of compulsion to take the substance (craving).
2 Difficulty in controlling substance use (onset, termination, level of use).
3 A physiological withdrawal state when reducing or ceasing substance use.
4 Tolerance: increased doses are required to produce the original effect.
5 Progressive neglect of alternative pleasures or interests.
6 Persisting use despite clear evidence of harmful consequences.

Opiate detoxification and methadone maintenance is ideally as part of a regimen in which a contract is made with the patient (p339), eg in a special clinic or in primary care, provided the GP has an interest and commitment.[rcgp.org.uk] *Daily observed methadone dosing* is the norm (NB: monthly supplies are not necessarily abused).[314] Drugs used: **methadone**, eg 20-70mg/12h PO, reducing by 20% every 2 days (caution: there is no reliable formula for heroin dose equivalence).[315] Cocaine use by patients on methadone is a big problem, and is associated with a poorer prognosis. **Disulfiram** has a role here.[315,N=67] A non-addictive alternative is **lofexidine** (α_2-noradrenergic agonist like clonidine)— eg 0.2mg/6h PO, increased by 0.4-0.8mg increments/day (max 0.8mg/8h); a 5-day regimen may be better than 10-day ones. SE: drowsiness, BP↓, pulse↓, dry mouth, rebound hypertension on withdrawal.[317] **Buprenorphine** is a synthetic partial agonist at μ-opioid receptors. It may be safer than methadone;[318] t½ ≈35h. Start at 0.8-4mg sublingnally per 24h, titrate by 2-4mg increments (max 32mg/day, maintenance: 12-24mg/day reached within ~1-2 weeks). Cautions: liver dysfunction; intoxication with other drugs (eg CNS depressants). **Naltrexone** is an opioid antagonist (blocks euphoria—useful in former addicts to prevent relapse, eg 25mg/24h PO after suitable opioid-free period). Warn patient of possible withdrawal reactions and monitor patient for 4h after 1st dose; monitor LFT.

Psychological support: Tailor to specific needs (residential or outpatient care, in groups or 1-to-1). Counselling, motivational therapy, cognitive therapy (p372), Alcoholics Anonymous, '12 steps programme', family therapy (p386) are all valuable ways to address triggers, motivation to change, and relapse prevention. Counsel about HIV & hepatitis C risk, needle exchange, and safe sex.

Relapse prevention As strong cravings precede relapse, anti-craving drugs seem to be a promising but unvalidated approach. See acamprosate, p363.

Barbiturate withdrawal may cause seizures±death; withdraw as an inpatient (⅓ of the previous daily dose as phenobarbital; lower the dose over 2wks).

Alcohol causes as much harm as smoking and hypertension. *Abuse* implies that repeated drinking harms a person's work or social life. *Addiction* implies:

- Difficulty or failure of abstinence
- Narrowing of drinking repertoire
- Increased tolerance to alcohol
- Often aware of compulsion to drink
- Priority is to maintain alcohol intake
- Sweats, nausea, or tremor on withdrawal.

Ask about tolerance, worry about drinking, 'eye opener' drinks used in the mornings, amnesia from alcohol use, and attempts to cut down. 2 points in TWEAK +ve (?more sensitive than CAGE questions).[319,320]

Alcohol & organ damage *Liver:* (normal in 50% of alcoholics). *Fatty liver:* Acute, reversible; hepatitis; 80% progress to cirrhosis (*liver failure* in 10%) *Cirrhosis:* 5yr survival 48% if alcohol intake continues (if it stops, 77%).

CNS: Poor memory/cognition; cortical/cerebellar atrophy; retrobulbar neuropathy; fits; falls; accidents; neuropathy; Korsakoff's/Wernicke's encephalopathy (*OHCM* p728; ➙urgent parenteral vitamins are needed).

Gut: D&V; peptic ulcer; erosions; varices; pancreatitis. *Marrow:* Hb↓; MCV↑. *Heart:* Arrhythmias; BP↑; cardiomyopathy; *fewer* MIs (?benefit only if ≥55yrs). *Skeleton:* Heavy drinking disrupts calcium metabolism (osteoporosis risk↑).[321] *Sperm:* Fertility↓; sperm motility↓ (in 34 precisely analysed medical students).[322] *Malignancy:* GI & breast. *Social:* Alcohol is related to violent crime and suicide. In medical students, alcohol correlates with events such as missing study, sexually escapades, fisticuffs, etc[n=194] ♀ and ♂ students are equally prone to use alcohol at high doses to relieve stress (this carries on into later years).[324]

Alcohol and drug levels Regular heavy drinking *induces* hepatic enzymes; binging *inhibits* enzymes; it's probably not a good idea to indulge in both and hope for the best. Be alert with phenytoin, warfarin, tolbutamide, etc. NB: paracetamol may cause ↑N-acetyl-*p*-benzoquinoneimine (it is hepatotoxic).

Withdrawal signs (Delirium tremens) Pulse↑; BP↓; tremor; fits; visual or tactile hallucinations, eg of insects crawling under the skin (formication). ℞:
- Admit; monitor vital signs (beware BP↓). • For the 1st 3 days give diazepam generously, eg 10mg/6h PO or PR if vomiting—or IVI during fits; chlordiazepoxide is an alternative. After a few days, ↓diazepam (eg 10mg/8h PO from day 4-6, then 5mg/12h PO for 2 more days). β-blockers, clonidine, carbamazepine, and neuroleptics (if no liver damage) are adjuncts (not advised as monotherapy).[325]

Treatment Does the patient want to change? If so, be optimistic, and augment his will to do so. Should **abstinence** or **controlled intake** be the aim? If the former, remarkable recovery of organs (eg hippocampus) is possible.[326]

Treat coexisting depression (p336). Refer to specialists. Self-help/group therapy (**Alcoholics Anonymous**) help, ± drugs which produce a nasty reaction if alcohol is taken (disulfiram 200mg/24h PO). Reducing the pleasure that alcohol brings (and craving on withdrawal) with naltrexone 25-50mg/24h PO (an opioid receptor antagonist) can halve relapse rates.[327,n=111] SE: vomiting, drowsiness, dizziness, joint pain. CI: hepatitis; liver failure; monitor LFT. Get expert help. Acamprosate (*OHCM* p445) can treble abstinence rates. CI: pregnancy, severe liver failure, creatinine >120μmol/L; SE: D&V, libido ↑ or ↓; dose example: 666mg/8h PO if >60kg and <65yrs old. Economic analysis supports its use, at least in some communities.[328,n=448]

Non-drug, physician-based brief interventions for problem drinkers: (Education, counselling, goal-setting + monitoring of γGT in those who have social or physical problems from alcohol, but who do not exhibit full dependency.) 50% of trials show that γGT falls in the intervention group, but none show clear improvement in alcohol-related morbidity. More costly regimens fare no better.

Homelessness is common; help with housing & rent, problem-solving, communication, drink refusal, and goal setting *can* help this desperate problem.[329,n=114]

Definition Below-average general intellectual functioning which originated during the development period and is associated with impairment in adaptive behaviour (Heber 1981). *People with learning difficulties are at ↑risk for mental illness.* Four subtypes: *Mild* (IQ 50-70): Accounts for 80% of people with learning disabilities. There is useful development of language, and learning difficulty only emerges as schooling gets under way. Most can lead an independent life. *Moderate* (IQ 35-49): most can talk and find their way about *Severe* (IQ 20-34) limited social activity is possible. *Profound* (IQ <20): simple speech may be unachievable. Special schooling and medical services are needed, as is adequate care and counselling for the families involved. In the UK, lack of resources and ambiguous community responsibilities are big problems.[331] *Further information:* ask MENCAP (tel.uk 020 7454 0454).[332]

Epidemiology 27 per 1000 (80% have IQ 50-70). People with learning difficulties are at ↑risk for mental illness compared to the general population.

The Patient *Physical:* Sensory and motor disabilities, epilepsy, incontinence. *Psychiatric:* All psychiatric disorders can occur but the *presentation* is modified by low intelligence. In the *diagnosis* of psychiatric disorder, emphasis is given to the behavioural manifestation of the disorder.

Causes *Physical causes* are found in 55-75% of severely learning disabled individuals. *Chromosomal abnormalities:* Down's syndrome, fragile X syndrome p648. *Antenatal causes:* Infections, alcohol, hypoxia, nutritional growth retardation, hypothyroidism. *Perinatal causes:* Cerebral palsy. *Post-natal causes:* Injury, infections, impoverished environment.

Forensic issues Arson and sexual offences (usually exhibitionism in males or, more rarely, 'public disrobing' in women)[333] are examples of offences. Care is needed in questioning learning-disabled people about an alleged offence, due to increased suggestibility and risk of making false confessions. Treatment may centre on issues of accepting that the offence took place, the taking responsibility for offences, accepting the intention of the offending behaviour, and on victim awareness.[334] Behavioural approaches might focus on masturbatory satiation, covert sensitization, and stimulus control procedures.[335]

Assessing learning-disabled people • Cause(s) of the learning disability • Associated medical conditions • Intellectual and social skills development • Psychological and social functioning • Dialogue with and support for carers.

Care of people with learning disability • Prevention and early detection is the aim—as is care in generic (eg NHS) services (minimized specialist care) unless there are complex physical, emotional and behavioural issues.[336] • Regular assessment of attainments and disabilities • Advice, support, and help for families—eg teaching parents how to be better 'tutors' can help[337] • Arrange special needs teaching at school and training/occupation • Housing and social support to enable self-care • Medical, nursing, and other services, as outpatients, day patients, or inpatients • Psychiatric and psychological services usually from a community-based multidisciplinary team.

Treatment of psychiatric disorders • Side effects of medication may not be apparent as learning-disabled patient may not be able to draw attention to them • Antipsychotics can lower seizure threshold and patients with learning disability are more likely to get seizures • Behavioural therapy is widely used.

The 14 *specific* rights below must be taken in the context of *general* psychiatric rights:[338] ★To have a professional skilled in dealing with your condition ★To receive treatment based on sound evidence ★To have treatment in a setting which is decent, humane, and non-abusive ★Regimes must promote a fulfilling social life ★Active participation in all decisions taken about care.

1 Ensure full assessment within the context of joint strategic needs assessment by Social Services, GPs, and other professionals fully trained in 'partnership working'.

2 Include the person in all decisions affecting him or her.

3 Promote enriching activity to counter idle humdrum impoverished living.

4 Listen to concerns of both the person and their carer.

5 Derive personalized care plans via dialogue with the person and carer(s).

6 Explain what the options are, ideally in terms that he/she understands.

7 Help him or her decide from a defined list of genuine choices.

8 Don't hurry through consultations "to get back to normal people"; spend *more* time; go *slowly*. Not being able to give a good history doesn't mean you can skip this bit: it means you must use other methods to get the information, eg discussions with carers or direct observation.

9 Don't be pleased because they are not complaining of anything. No reported symptoms and no complaints about circumstances does not let you off the hook! You may need to insist to carers that a nasty but apparently painless ulcer be treated—or that a fire-escape be unblocked.*etc etc*

10 Check for physical illnesses which may otherwise go unreported.

11 Watch for neglect/abuse from well-meaning under-trained over-worked staff (who may desperately crave your support and encouragement).[339]

12 Don't reach too readily for drugs to curb behaviour. Consider all options.

13 Be aware of local authority *Protection of Vulnerable Adults* protocols.

14 No tokenism! (paying lip service to the above without intending change).

Are all lives of equal value? We are better doctors if we believe so.

Psychiatry

Personality comprises lasting characteristics which make us who we are: easygoing or anxious; optimistic or pessimistic; placid or histrionic; ambitious or stay-at-home; fearless or timid; self-deprecatory or narcissistic[1] (self-love, founded on a grandiose belief in one's unique superiority).[340] Personality *can* change and develop quite quickly, eg after religious conversion in which a timid man is remoulded into a fearless activist. Personality is a spectrum lying between the above opposites. Statistical analysis reveals that all these distinctions overlap, and are describable in terms of a few orthogonal dimensions (eg neuroticism/psychoticism; introvert/extrovert). Those with abnormal personalities are defined as occupying the extremes of the spectrum. Abnormal personality only matters if it is maladaptive, causing suffering either to its possessor or his associates. In general, psychological symptoms which are part of a personality disorder are harder to treat than those arising from other causes.

DSM-IV classification of personality disorders[341]

Cluster	Description	Disorder
A	Odd or eccentric behaviour	Paranoid; schizoid; schizotypal (p323)
B	Dramatic or emotional behaviour	Antisocial (psychopathic); Borderline; histrionic; narcissistic[1]
C	Anxious or avoidant behaviour	Avoidant; dependent; obsessive-compulsive

Psychopathy *'He dislikes showing his feelings, and he'd rather be cruel than put his real feelings into words...he doesn't care for anyone and perhaps he never will'.* So says Dostoevsky; lesser psychologists dwell on reckless, antisocial acts, impulsivity, lack of guilt ± social and legal nonconformity. Dostoevsky's definition lasts because of its brevity—and that telling word *perhaps*. Can we change? *What* must change before psychopaths can love? This *perhaps* blowing in from 19th-century Russia sends a shiver down our 21st-century spines: perhaps all the psychopaths we lock up *might* be able to change. *What* needs to be unlocked? Read *Crime and Punishment* to find out.

Treatment is problematic unless there is a strong will to change. Peer pressure/group therapy (p376) may motivate. It is rarely wise to use drugs, but there is evidence that SSRIs (p341) may help aggressive personality disorder.

Borderline personality disorder There is unstable affect regulation, poor impulse control, and poor interpersonal relationships/self-image, eg with repeated self-injury, suicidality, and a difficult life-course trajectory.[342] Associations: ADHD;[2] learning difficulties. Genetics and adverse childhood events (eg abuse) are predispositions. Intervene (and refer) early with specific management plan, addressing work, Dialectical behaviour therapy, inpatient hospital programmes, and drugs can reduce depression, anxiety, and impulsive aggression. Eventually, supportive interpersonal dyads are achievable.[NICE 2011]

Other personalities *Obsessional personality:* The rigid, obstinate bigot who is preoccupied with unimportant (or vital) detail. *Emotionally unstable personality:* Tendency to form intense relationships and rapid fluctuations in mood, with impulsivity. *Histrionic personality:* The self-centred, sexually provocative (but frigid) person who enjoys (but does not feel) angry scenes. *Schizoid personality:* Cold, aloof, introspective, misanthropic.[343]

---

1 Narcissus was the 1st celebrity to be famous just for being beautiful. He carelessly spurned all lovers, including Echo. Mortified by his callousness, all but her voice was consumed by grief. This disembodied voice now repeats for us the 3 cardinal facts about narcissists: **1** They never understand others. **2** Loving a narcissist is a recipe for death. **3** If you manage to escape death, your narcissistic lover may blame you for his death; analysis of suicide notes reveals a class of suicides whose final act is to blame their lovers.[344] To help these characters outgrow narcissistic resentments, we may confront their illusions. This is powerful but dangerous. Narcissus discovered the torment of unrequited love only after falling in love with his own image as glimpsed in a pool. As often as he stoops to kiss it, so it fragments and vanishes. Dying of lovesickness, he gains insight into others' pain, whereupon he morphs into a handsome daffodil with a superb scent, which, to this day, blows to us each spring from Arcadia. See Ovid & J Holmes, *Narcissism* Icon Books [345]

Psychopathy seems to entail a genetically driven difference in connectivity (via the uncinate fasciculus) between the parts of the brain driving empathy, conscience (**free will**, or rather **free won't**) and impulse control (the orbito-prefrontal regions). It is not a fault necessarily, or a disease, or always a disadvantage (look at medical hierarchies!). This has serious ethical and legal implications, eg a defence of "my brain made me do it".[346]

Managing dangerous psychopathy: beyond medicine and the law

People with dangerous and severe personality disorder (DSPD[3]) and people with other psychopathic features form the bulk of forensic psychiatry. Therapeutic psychiatry is sometimes unfairly criticized for abandoning psychopaths—as if they were too much trouble. This easy criticism does not take into account civil liberties: patients must either want treatment, or they must have a *treatable* mental illness before they can be detained.

Renewable sentences and protective custody? It is against this background that the suggestion has arisen that those with a history of psychopathic violence should receive care outside penal and health set-ups. However, this is no guarantee against injustice: for example, a man without psychopathy who poisoned his wife might be free to marry again after 12 years in prison, but a man with psychopathy who had held hostages without harming them might never be free to rebuild his life. Hence considerations of natural justice make renewable sentencing hazardous.[341]

Methods of trying to treat DSPD include cognitive therapy and anti-libininal drugs (not always amounting to chemical castration).[4] **NB:** DSPD units at Broadmoor and Rampton hospitals have not chalked up successes matching their huge expense. Prof Peter Tyrer; 2010 As a leading DSPD psychotherapist says: "The only way that somebody with personality disorder is going to make progress is through their own efforts. They can be helped by professionals, but nobody else can do it for them in terms of arriving at that understanding of their own responsibility for what's happened." Tony Maden;2010 tinyurl.com/yeyvyyk

When patients' requests for anti-libidinal drugs[4] may be valid

• Hyperarousal (frequent sexual rumination/preoccupation, difficulties in controlling sexual arousal, high levels of sexual behaviour).
• Intrusive sexual fantasies or urges.
• Dangerous paraphilias (sadism; necrophilia). Highly repetitive paraphilic offending such as voyeurism or exhibitionism may also respond to drugs.

In the context of an offender in the community, the offender's manager must get prior authority to use anti-libidinal medication, and request the offender's GP to refer the offender to the 'approved psychiatrist'.

2 Attention deficit hyperactivity disorder (ADHD, p212) is increasingly recognized in adults, often with oppositional defiant disorder. Exercise regimens and methylphenidate may help.[347]

3 DSPD: give something an acronym and it half exists. Add an NNT (~5!) and the trick is done; we rush to memorize, categorize and research it. To study its causes perhaps we should confront our imagined worlds of myth, language, legalisms, and pure and impure invention, rather than value-free biological or mental health categories. But to be thoroughly sceptical about this scepticism: show us any value-free construct.

4 Antilibidinal drugs may ↓testosterone to young-boy levels—but risk liver damage, breast growth, hot flushes, depression and ↓bone density, eg oral cyproterone acetate (Androcur®). Long-acting drugs (leuprolide, goserelin, triptorelin) can be injected and may be better. SSRIs are sometimes used (unreliably) to ↓ libido and sexual preoccupation and compulsive re-offending.

Withdrawing benzodiazepines ▶*The withdrawal syndrome may well be worse than the condition for which the drug was originally prescribed.* So try to avoid benzodiazepine use, eg relaxation techniques for anxiety, or, for insomnia, a dull book, sexual intercourse, and avoiding night-time coffee may facilitate sleep. If not, limit hypnotics to alternate nights.

30% of those on benzodiazepines for 6 months experience withdrawal symptoms if treatment is stopped, and some will do so after only a few weeks of treatment. Symptoms appear sooner with rapidly eliminated benzodiazepines (eg lorazepam *vs* diazepam or chlordiazepoxide). It is not possible to predict which patients will become dependent, but 'passive dependent' or neurotic personality is partly predictive. Symptoms often start with anxiety or psychotic symptoms 1-2 weeks after withdrawal, followed by many months of gradually decreasing symptoms, such as insomnia, hyperactivity, panic, agoraphobia, and depression. Irritability, rage, feelings of unreality and depersonalization (p334, p346) are common; hallucinations less so. Multiple sclerosis may be misdiagnosed as there may be diplopia, paraesthesiae, fasciculation, and ataxia. Gut symptoms include D&v, abdominal pain, and dysphagia. There may also be palpitations, flushing, and hyperventilation symptoms. The problem is not so much how to stop benzodiazepine treatment, but how to avoid being manipulated into prescribing them unnecessarily. This is addressed on p330.

How to withdraw: • Augment the patient's will to give up (stress disadvantages of continuous R). • Withdrawal is harder for short-acting benzodiazepines, so change to diazepam. • Agree a contract to prescribe a weekly supply, and not to add to this if it is used up early. • Withdraw by ~2mg/week of diazepam. Warn to expect withdrawal symptoms, and not to be alarmed.

Withdrawing antidepressants: All antidepressants may cause a **discontinuation syndrome**. Distinguish between this and **withdrawal symptoms** (implies addiction). Patients often worry that they may get hooked on antidepressants which can affect compliance. Discontinuation symptoms are explained by the theory of *receptor rebound*, eg an antidepressant with potent anticholinergic effects may be associated with diarrhoea on withdrawal,[349] ~30% get the syndrome and it may mimic the original symptoms of the illness.[350] Withdrawal is best over ≥4 weeks unless fluoxetine is co-prescribed (it has a long t½, so no withdrawal regimen is needed, and it also helps reduce symptoms, see BOX).[351]

Fluoxetine may help withdrawal from paroxetine●※
• Days 1-3: 30mg paroxetine + 10mg fluoxetine
• Day 4: 20mg paroxetine+ 20mg fluoxetine
• Day 5: 10mg paroxetine + 20mg fluoxetine
• Days 6-9: 0mg paroxetine + 20mg fluoxetine
• Then stop fluoxetine.[348]

Discontinuation symptoms • Onset is within ~5 days of stopping, sometimes after cross-tapering or missing doses. Usually mild and self-limiting but can be prolonged and severe ("a dark frightening tunnel...I was that frayed I'd have killed").[348] Some symptoms are more likely with certain drugs. *MAOIs: Common:* • Agitation, irritability, ataxia, movement disorders, insomnia, cognition↓, slowed or pressured speech. *Occasionally:* • Hallucinations, paranoid delusions. *The most troublesome MAOIs:* tranylcypromine, when metabolized, has amphetamine-like properties so can have true withdrawal syndrome. *Tricyclics: Common:* •'Flu symptoms; insomnia; ↑dreaming. *Rarer:* • Movement disorders; mania; arrhythmias. *The most troublesome tricyclics:* amitriptyline; imipramine. *SSRIs: Common:* •'Flu-like symptoms; headaches; nasty shock-like sensations;[352] dizziness; insomnia; tears/irritability/fury; vivid dreams. *Occasionally:* • Movement disorders; poor concentration/memory; delirium. *The most troublesome SSRIs:* Paroxetine; venlafaxine (both have short half-lives). ▶Consider stopping alcohol before starting withdrawal, and starting meditation and an exercise programme.[348,353] Tell friends "I won't be myself for a while."

Swapping antidepressants: how to cross-taper

When an antidepressant has failed to work at an adequate dose, or is poorly tolerated, changing drug is appropriate. Avoid abrupt withdrawal when swapping antidepressants; cross-tapering is preferred. Speed of cross-tapering is best judged by patient tolerability. NB: co-administration of some anti-depressants is absolutely contraindicated, see below—dangers include precipitating the **serotonin syndrome**[354] (restlessness; diaphoresis, ie excessive sweating); tremor; shivering; myoclonus; confusion; convulsions; death).

Example of cross-tapering based on the Maudsley regimen[355]

	Week 1	Week 2	Week 3	Week 4
Withdrawing amitriptyline from 150mg/24h	100mg/24h	50mg/24h	25mg/24h	Nil
Introducing sertraline	25mg/24h	50mg/24h	75mg/24h	100mg/24h

Cautions When swapping from MAOIs or tranylcypromine to any other antidepressant, withdraw and wait for 2 weeks (the time taken for monoamine oxidase to be replenished); for moclobemide wait 24h. Do not co-administer clomipramine and SSRIs or venlafaxine. Beware fluoxetine interactions (may still occur for 5 weeks after stopping, due to long half-life).

Psychiatry

As usual, it was dialogue that combed out my muddle. Arthur Miller *Timebends* 88

Medicine has three great branches: *prevention*, *curing by technical means*, and *healing*—and psychotherapy is the embodiment of healing: a holistic approach in which systematic human dialogue becomes a humanizing enterprise for the relief of suffering and the advancement of self-esteem. Questions such as "What is the meaning of my life" and "what is significant?" are answered in a different way after exposure to a gifted psychotherapist. Changes occur in cognition, feelings, and behaviour. This is why psychotherapy is dangerous and exciting: it changes people. Hence the need for supervision and ongoing training and self-awareness on the part of the therapist.

Psychotherapy stands in stark contrast to the increasingly questioned technical, machine-based realm of medicine, and we accord it great prominence here, in the hope that our explicit descriptions, and their reverberations throughout our books will produce corresponding reverberations in our minds and in our daily work in *any* branch of medicine, to remind us that we are not machines delivering care according to automated formulae, but humans dealing with other humans. So, taken in this way, psychotherapy is the *essence* of psychiatry—and the essence of all psychotherapy is communication. The first step in communication is to open a channel. The vital role that listening plays has already been emphasized (p320).

It is not possible to teach the skills required for psychotherapy in a book, any more than it is possible to teach the art of painting in oils from a book. So what follows here (p372-5) is a highly selective tour round the gallery of psychotherapy, in an attempt to show the range of skills needed, and to whet the reader's appetite. It is not envisaged that the reader will try out the more complicated techniques without appropriate supervision.

The psychotherapies may be classified first in terms of *who is involved* in the treatment sessions: an individual, a couple, a family, or a whole group; and secondly they may be classified by their *content and methods* used: analytic, interpersonal, cognitive, behavioural.

Behavioural therapies (more details: p372) aim to change behaviour, eg if avoiding crowded shops (agoraphobia) is the issue, a behavioural approach focuses on the avoidance-behaviour. Such approaches will define behavioural tasks that the patient is expected to carry out between sessions.

Cognitive therapy (p374) focuses on thoughts and assumptions, promulgating the idea that we respond to cognitive representations of events, not to raw events alone. If this is so, cognitive change may be required to produce emotional and behavioural change. So in the above example of agoraphobia, the therapist would encourage articulation of thoughts associated with entering crowds. The patient might report that she becomes anxious that she might be about to faint—fearing that everyone will think her a fool. These thoughts would be looked at using a Socratic approach: "Have you in fact ever fainted? How likely would you be to faint? If someone fainted in front of you in a shop, what would you think? *Are* they foolish?"

Long-term psychoanalytical therapies (p382) are concerned with the origin and meaning of symptoms. They are based on the view that vulnerability arises from early experiences and unresolved issues, eg from childhood. The therapist adopts a non-dominant stance, encouraging the patient to talk without inhibitions. The therapist encourages change by suggesting interpretations for the content of the patient's talk.

Which psychotherapy is most successful? This is tackled on p388.

1 Further reading: I Levi *Basic Notes in Psychotherapy*, Petroc Press ISBN 1-900603-50-0

There are important differences in how people use the term psychotherapy. The first recorded definition states that

Psychotherapy includes every description of therapeutics that cures by...intervention of the psychical functions of the sufferer. F Eeden 1892 Med Mag

This definition is worth bearing in mind because, uniquely, it focuses on the content of the intervention made by the patient, not on the specifics of the therapist's intervention. The most general modern definition, and the one employed in this section, is summarized thus:

Psychotherapy denotes treatment of mental disorders and behavioural disturbances using...support, suggestion, persuasion, re-education, reassurance, and insight in order to alter maladaptive patterns of coping, and to encourage personality growth. Dorland's Medical Dictionary

Some commentators draw a distinction between counselling and psychotherapy—but using the above definition (or any definition that recognizes the great heterogeneity of psychotherapy) no valid distinction can be made, unless it is between the various types of psychotherapy. The main issue to bear in mind is that psychotherapy can be more or less specific, and more or less involved in, and driven by, theory.

So is 'just being nice to patients' in the course of one's medical activities an example of psychotherapy at work? The answer is 'no'—not because being nice is therapeutically neutral, but because one's attention is not focused on planning change through the systematic use of interpersonal techniques.

The issue of training is very important, and here are some questions that might usefully be addressed to anyone offering psychotherapy:

1 Is there proof of efficacy? Ask for evidence of long-term results.
2 What qualifications does the therapist hold? Is he or she supervised?
3 Is the recommended regimen tailored to the patient's unique needs?
4 How will progress be monitored?
5 Is confidentiality assured?
6 Is there support and follow-up after the formal programme ends?

Psychiatry

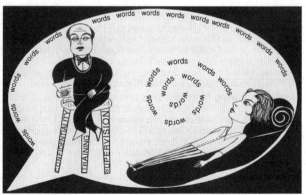

Fig 1. *Inside the speech-bubble:* The therapist is precariously supported by a tripod of *confidentiality*, *training* and peer-based *supervision*. The couch hardly ever exists in practice, but it stands for a place where anything can happen—where we sit side-by-side with our shadow selves and hear the stuff of dreams, nightmares, and realities, uncushioned by workaday self-deceptions. It contains its own labyrinth. ©Miriam Longmore

Behavioural therapy aims to change a person's behaviour using one of several techniques depending on the condition. When used in conjunction with cognitive therapies (see p374) the term cognitive-behavioural therapy is used (CBT).

Exposure/flooding/implosion *Indication:* Phobias. *Technique:* • The anxiety-provoking object or situation is presented *in vivo* or in imagination (prolonged *in vivo* in flooding). • Implosion involves imagined exposure to stimuli in a non-graded manner. • The patient then stays with the anxiety-provoking stimuli until there is habituation (ie he becomes accustomed to the anxiety by frequent exposure), and the avoidance response is extinguished.

Relaxation training *Indication:* Mild/moderate anxiety. *Technique:* • A system of exercises & regular breathing to progressively relax individual muscle groups. Aim to achieve relaxation in all postures: recumbency is easiest (?from ↓baroreceptor load).[356] • Link the relaxed state with pleasant, imagined scenes so that relaxation can be induced by recalling the imagined scene.

Systematic desensitization *Indications:* Phobic disorders. *Technique:* Patients form a hierarchy of fears about the phobic stimulus. Therapy uses graded exposure (least fearsome first) to real or imagined stimuli Joseph,Wolpe[357] while patients perform relaxation techniques until anxiety is extinguished. It is ethically less controversial than flooding[358] as progress up the hierarchy is only when patients are completely comfortable with the current level; eg fig 1 can be preceded by an almost neutral image, such as ψ.[359]

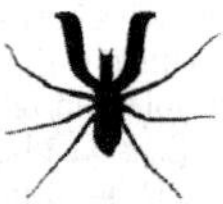

Fig 1.[366]   ©JML.

Response prevention *Technique:* • Involves exposure to an anxiety-provoking stimulus (eg a toilet seat for patients fearing contamination). • The patient is subsequently prevented from carrying out the usual compulsive behaviour or ritual until the urge to do so has passed *Indications:* Obsessions.

Thought stopping *Technique:* The patient is asked to ruminate and then taught to interrupt the obsessional thoughts by arranging a sudden intrusion, eg snapping an elastic band on the wrist. *Indications:* • Obsessional thoughts occurring without compulsive rituals. • Undesired sexually deviant thoughts.

Aversion therapy/covert sensitization *Technique:* • Aversive therapy involves producing an unpleasant sensation in the patient in association with an aversive or noxious stimulus (eg electric shocks, chemically induced nausea, pain) with the aim of eliminating unwanted behaviour. • Covert sensitization involves the use of aversive stimuli in imagination (eg the approach of a policeman to arrest him/her for his/her undesirable behaviour). *Indications:* • Alcohol dependence syndrome (disulfiram used to induce nausea if alcohol is consumed). • Sexual deviations. *Cautions:* • Punishment procedures are generally ineffective unless patients are taught more appropriate behaviours.

Social skills training *Technique:* • Aims to modify a patient's social behaviour in order to help overcome difficulties in forming/maintaining relationships. • Video is used to define and rate elements of a patient's behaviour in standard social encounters • The patient is then taught more appropriate behaviour by a combination of direct instruction, modelling, video-feedback and role play. *Indications:* Patients with social deficits due to a psychiatric disorder.

Token economy *Technique:* Positive reinforcement improves behaviour: tokens are given when desirable behaviour is displayed. These can later be exchanged for goods or privileges. *Indications:* • Children (p210) • Learning disabled patients • Addictive disorders • Chronic psychiatric disorders. *Problems:* • Patients become mercenary as they only behave well in exchange for tokens. • It does not prepare people for a world where rewards are subtle and delayed.

Modelling and role play *Technique:* The acquisition of new behaviours by the process of imitation. *Indications:* Lack of social skills and assertiveness.

Behaviour therapy in impulse control disorders (sex, shopping, gambling)
Hypersexuality after brain injury: Examples: two clients were troubled by inappropriate touching of the opposite sex, and a third involved exhibitionism. In one case of touching, feedback was used to decrease inappropriate touching. In the other case of touching, scheduled massage was used to shift stimulus control to an appropriate setting. In the case of exhibitionism, a combination of self-monitoring, private self-stimulation, and dating-skills training were used to suppress the behaviour.[360] Behaviour therapy also has a role in paraphilias such as voyeurism and masochism/sadism. It is controversial when consent is an issue (eg following a court's recommendation).

Cognitive elements can be added with the aim of minimizing self-deception regarding the effects of paraphilia behaviour.[361]

Exposure response therapy is used eg in obsessive-compulsive behaviour (eg obsessive cleaning of some putatively contaminated object). The therapist gradually exposes the client to contaminated objects, preventing the compulsion by reducing anxiety about contamination, eg by breathing techniques.

CBT (cognitive-behaviour therapy) helps change how we *think* and hence how we *feel*. Fig 2 is a vicious circle if thoughts are negative and lead to hostile, negative actions. By defining these relationships, CBT lets us see how thoughts and feelings interact; by changing thoughts, the cycle is broken or turned into a virtuous cycle—eg to prevent relapse after voluntary abstinence vis-à-vis impulse control disorders (eg bulimia). For purely cognitive therapy, see p374.

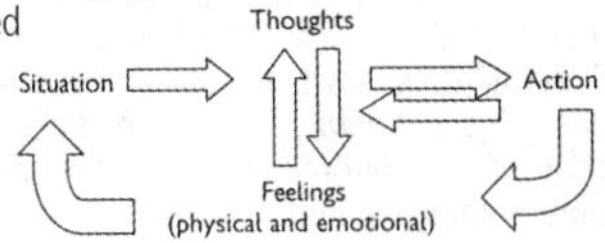

Fig 2. CBT.

The *abstinence violation effect* (AVE) is a pivotal construct describing our cognitive and affective response to re-engaging in self- or court-prohibited behaviour. AVE refers to the client's belief that abstinence, once broken, always leads to relapse ("Now I've eaten one chocolate the whole box must go—and I then I'll have to empty the fridge and now I'm on the slippery slope leading straight to the ice-cream in the freezer..."). The false creation of an all-or-none requirement, loss of feeling of control, and ensuing failure resulting in guilt, self-blame and lowered self-esteem can all be tackled by cognitive-behaviour therapy, eg by identifying high-risk situations and 'offence precursors'.[362] These may be feeling lonely and rejected, after a break-up with a partner—or stress at work. In the case of paedophilia, CBT can be combined with group therapy and one way to confront paedophiles with the reality of their offence yet which is helpful because it provides their first opportunity to express their feelings, sexual fantasies and thoughts about paedophilia.[363] In general, the effects of cognitive-behavioural treatment for the most serious forensic inpatients (arson, violence, rape) are sometimes quite good in terms of oppositional-defiant/egotistical behaviours—and there are also (unreliable) improvements in psychopathological symptoms, personality traits, and coping.[364]

Psychiatry

Psychiatry

Key concepts Beck suggests that a person who habitually adopts ways of thinking with depressed or anxious *cognitive distortions* will be more likely to become depressed or anxious when faced with minor problems. The cognitive distortions in cognitive theory include: *Arbitrary inference*—conclusions drawn with little or no evidence to support them. *Selective abstraction*—dwelling on insignificant (negative) detail while ignoring more important features or stimuli. *Overgeneralization*—drawing global conclusions about worth/ability/performance on the basis of single facts. *Magnification/minimization*—Gross errors of evaluation with small bad events magnified and large good events minimized. These mechanisms lead to distortions within the cognitive triad of the self, the world and the future.

• In cognitive therapy, the patient first learns to identify cognitive distortions from present or recent experiences with the use of daily records/diaries.
• The patient records such ideas and then learns to examine the evidence for and against them, ie tests out beliefs in real life.
• The patient is encouraged to undertake the pleasurable activities that were given up at the onset of depression or anxiety.
• In this way, cognitive restructuring takes place when the patient is able to identify, evaluate and change the distorted thoughts and associated behaviour.

Techniques • Patients are evaluated to get a good history and background information to better understand the nature of the difficulties for which treatment is being sought. • Assessment tools or questionnaires may be used. • Treatment usually takes place on a weekly basis and focuses on current issues. • A *treatment plan* is formulated with clear goals and objectives and progress is monitored. • The number of sessions varies with the type of difficulties being treated. • Patient's participate actively in their own therapy.

Indications[365] *General:* • The patient prefers to use psychological interventions, either alone or in addition to medication. • The target problems for CBT (extreme, unhelpful thinking; reduced activity; avoidant or unhelpful behaviours) are present. • No improvement or only partial improvement has occurred on medication. • Side effects prevent a sufficient dose of medication from being taken over an adequate period. • Significant psychosocial problems (eg relationship problems, difficulties at work or unhelpful behaviours such as self-cutting or alcohol misuse) are present that will not be adequately addressed by medication alone.

Specific: • Depression • Generalized anxiety or panic disorder • Phobias • Obsessive-compulsive disorder • Post-traumatic stress disorder • Hypochondriasis • Bulimia • Schizophrenia • Bipolar affective disorder • Sexual abuse.[366]

Cautions: It is difficult to carry out therapy if the patient is feeling severely depressed and has very poor concentration. There is a need to pace sessions so as not to disappoint or overwhelm the patient. Patients may have difficulty talking about their feelings of depression, anxiety, shame or anger.

Evidence is increasingly available that CBT is as effective as pharmacological therapy for mild to moderate depression, with the added advantage that relapses are less likely.[367] In one study, GPs' knowledge of depression, and attitudes towards its treatment showed no major difference between intervention and control groups at 6 months—ie training had no discernible impact on patients' outcomes.[368] One reason for this may be that skills were indeed learned, but that there was insufficient time to apply these skills in ordinary general practice, where depression may be only one of a series of problems presented to the GP in a single 10-minute consultation.

Applying cognitive therapy, using the example of depression

We respond to cognitive representations of events, not raw data. Mood and thoughts can form a vicious cycle. Using the example of depression: low mood leads to gloomy thoughts and memories (eg dwelling on exams you did badly in, rather than those in which you performed well). These gloomy thoughts make you feel more depressed (mood) and this lowering of mood makes your thoughts even more gloomy. Cognitive therapy tackles this circle by tackling the thoughts. Take, say, the thought: "I'm a failure, and all my friends are avoiding me". In cognitive therapy the process is to:
• Clarify the thought exactly; don't let it be just a vague negative belief.
• Look for evidence for and against the proposition in the thought.
• Look for other perspectives.
• Come to a conclusion. NB: 6 sessions are better than fewer.[369][N=104]

The therapist encourages the patient to find other explanations by challenging him, eg by examining what "I'm a failure" means. "What are the main areas in your life?" "What do you count as success or failure?" *Catastrophizing* denotes how we see disasters in small mishaps, eg "he didn't like my hat... he doesn't like me...nobody likes me". There are many kinds of biased thinking that cognitive therapy helps us to recognize: eg *black and white thinking*, *over-generalizing* (as when one failure as a symbol of everything).

Is it possible to apply these lessons in primary care? Yes; if full training is offered. Randomized trials of CBT in primary care with less extensive training (4 half-days) and hence with more realistic costs have been disappointing. The lesson is: if the benefits of CBT are to be brought to primary care, what is needed is *time*: time to learn a new skill, and, above all, time to exercise it.

The NHS has been recruiting cognitive therapists to meet the needs of all those with moderate and severe depression and anxiety who might benefit from it. Cost: £170 million. Projected savings (by getting people back to work) £12 billion/yr. Until access is improved computerized CBT is one option.

JML undergoes NICE-approved computerized cognitive therapy

Depression Relief® is a self-help, educational internet program for those feeling depressed. JML signed up for the course to bring readers a 1st -hand account. Initial assessment suggested he was significantly depressed as there was nowhere to say that his early-morning waking was not from depression but from eagerness to get on with authoring *OHCS* pages.[etc etc] Quite correctly, he was told "You may also wish to consider seeing your doctor or healthcare professional if your symptoms do not improve or become worse. You should definitely do this if you are feeling hopeless and don't want to go on...". Sections include: "Taking the 1st step to controlling your depression"; "You can move your mood"; "Actions speak louder than words"; "Focus on the positive"; "Redefine your problems"; "Don't go blaming yourself"; "Relax away your sorrows"; "Using your imagination"; "Get physical"; "Open up and share your feelings".

Here are some snippets to get the flavour: "After a week or two of writing down your positive thoughts in your mood log, you will be ready to learn how to use these positive thoughts to change your negative thinking."

Impression: professional; humorous (not too); surprisingly humanizing.

Groups are interactive microcosms in which the patient can be confronted by the effect his behaviour and beliefs have on others, and be protected during his first attempts at change.[1] This implies that group psychotherapy (as with all psychotherapies) is only practical for those who want to change.

General indications We know that the most suitable patients are: 1 Those who enter into the group voluntarily, not as a result of pressure from relatives or therapists; 2 Those who have a high expectation from the group, and do not view it as inferior to individual therapy; 3 Those who have adequate verbal and conceptual skills. See also psychodynamic psychotherapy p382.

Specific indications • Personality disorders • Addictions[370] Drug and alcohol dependence • Victims of childhood sexual abuse • People with difficulties in socialization • Major medical illnesses—eg breast cancer.[371 N=50]

Technique Clearly the selection procedure needs to be carried out by an experienced psychotherapist. He will aim for a group of, say, 6-8 members balanced for sex, and avoiding mixing the extremes of age. He will decide if the group is to be 'closed', or whether it will accept new patients during its life. He will usually take on a co-therapist of the opposite sex, and he will prepare the patients in detail before the group starts. The life of the group (eg 18 months) will develop through a number of phases ('*forming*'→'*norming*'→'*storming*'). First there is a settling-in period when members seem to be on their best behaviour, seeking to be loved by the therapist, and looking to him for directive counselling (which he rarely provides). Next is the stage of conflict, as the patient strives to find his place in the group other than through dependency on the leader. Frustration, anger, and other negative feelings are helpful by testing the group's trustworthiness. It is worth learning that expressing negative feelings need not lead to rejection—and this is a vital prelude to the next stage of intimacy, in which the group starts working together.

Typically the therapist steers the group away from outside crises and searches for antecedent causes towards the here and now—eg by asking "Who do you feel closest to in the group?" or "Who in the group is most like you?" "Who would you say is as passive (or aggressive) as you are?" He/she must avoid sacrificing spontaneity, and learn to use what the group gives, eg "You seem very angry that John stormed out just now". He avoids asking unanswerable questions, especially those beginning "Why?". He promotes interaction, observation, and learning. Special methods used to augment this process include written summaries of group activities, video, and psychodrama.

Intensive group cognitive therapy combines cognitive and group therapy (16 group sessions in 3 weeks). In social phobia, it's better than individual therapy.[372]

Cautions Those who are unlikely to benefit include those with severe depression, acute schizophrenia, or extreme schizoid personality (cold, aloof, hypersensitive introverts); hypochondriacs; narcissistic (self-admiring) or paranoid (suspicious and pessimistic about the role of others); sociopathic types (they have low thresholds for frustration and little sense of responsibility)—but sociopathy is difficult to treat by *any* means, and group therapy may be the least bad option, as other members of the group may provide the only valid mirror that can be held up to these people, and other people *may* provide the impetus for change. See psychodynamic psychotherapy, p382.

---

1 Miriam was the threshing-floor on which he threshed out all his beliefs. While he trampled his ideas upon her soul, the truth came out for him...because of her, he gradually realized where he was wrong. And what he realized, she realized 'DH Laurence p227 of *Sons and Lovers* But Lucy was mute. Can it be worth taking such a patient to group therapy? Mira accused her of not pulling her weight—this was unhelpful—but another group member piped up with something like "You can be in another world where there's too much space and meaning to speak...she can only hear your complaining like dead leaves rustling. What you say may have force here... not where she is...listen to her silence." AS Byatt 2003 p77 of *A Whistling Woman*

Psychiatry

▶*Through play a child becomes aware of what he or she knows.* When that knowledge is disturbing, play can re-form, recast and redeem that knowledge.[373] Parents hold the key cards for influencing a child's behaviour—love, mutually understood channels of communication, systems of rewards, and knowledge of right and wrong. It is the families without these, which are most likely to need the help of professionals. ▶Never underestimate a child's capacity for insight: *don't expect children's methods of communicating insight to mesh with adult's.*[374] *The 10 rules:*

1 Take time early on to make friends with the child. *Don't rush.*
2 Accept the child on his own terms—*exactly as he or she is.*
3 Avoid questioning, praising, or blaming. Be *totally permissive.*
4 *Don't say "Don't"*, and only restrain to prevent serious imminent harm.
5 Show the child that he or she is free to express *any* feeling openly.
6 The responsibility for making choices is *always* the child's *alone.*
7 Follow *wherever* the child leads: avoid directing the conversation.
8 Use *whatever he gives you*. Reflect his or her feelings back to him.
9 Encourage the child to move from acting-out his feelings in the real world, to *expressing them freely* in words and play.
10 Prepare the parents for change in the child.

Child and therapist play together to give the child a way to verbalize his innermost fantasies. As Virginia Axline explained to one of her 5-year-olds, play therapy is "a time when you can be the way you want to be. A time you can use any way you want to use it. A time when you can be you" Axline V: *Play Therapy* · *Dibs in Search of Self*

Evidence *vis-à-vis* 'activity-based interventions' (broader than Axline's play therapy) is mixed: no effect on war-torn children,[375] but good effects on social functioning after sexual abuse,[376] neglect,[377] and in autism.[378]

Art therapy

Art therapy is the use of art materials for self-expression and reflection in the presence of a trained art therapist. No previous experience or skill in art is needed as the art therapist is not primarily concerned with making an aesthetic or diagnostic assessment of the client's work. The chief aim is to effect change and growth in self-esteem through use of art materials in a safe and facilitating environment. Patients stop being patients, and take the initiative in externalizing pain and problems through self-expression.[379] ▶The person becomes his or her own therapeutic agent. What higher ideal is there in medicine? It is far ahead of our drug-based models of care, and taps into ancient ideas about health, self-healing, and the proper relationship among humans.[380]

As ever, the relationship between therapist and client is vital, but art therapy differs from other psychotherapies as it is a 3-way process between client, therapist and artefact. The therapist's evaluating of the art establishes the intellectual, spiritual, cultural, and emotional status of clients in ways that are helpful to those who find it hard to express thoughts and feelings verbally.[380] It can be a mistake for therapists to interpret the art: *leave this to the client.*[381]

Art therapists have good understanding of art processes with sound therapeutic knowledge. They work with individuals and groups in residential or community settings, eg mental health (eg anorexia and dementia, where art therapy can improve interactive and coping skills),[382] learning disabilities, child and family centres, palliative care, disaster zones,[381] and in prisons. baat. co.uk

NICE says we must always consider non-drug treatments for depression—so what are the experiences of UK primary care? In one setting with 3 artists in residence in Dursley (a ceramicist, a poet, and a painter) there was a reduction in anxiety, an increase in self-esteem, and fewer consultations from 'heartsink' patients.[383] Art therapy also helps coping in the context of cancer.[384]

Psychiatry

Occupying the interval between the spilling of our lives and their congealing into history, crisis intervention recognizes that moments of maximum change are times of greatest therapeutic opportunity.[1] Debate these questions:

• What events have led to these difficulties? Thoughts/actions in the last days.
• What is his mental state *now* (p324)? Depressed? Suicidal? Psychotic?
• In the past how has he been able to combat stress and to resolve crises?
• What solutions to this crisis have been tried? How have they failed?
• Who are the significant people in his life? Can you rely on any of them?

Therapeutic strategy

• If he has been very badly affected by the crisis, you may insist on postponing all normal obligations/responsibilities to allow concentrated contact ('intensive care') in a therapeutic environment—eg a hospital or crisis unit.

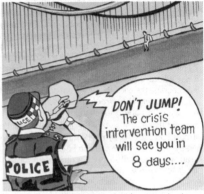

• Take practical steps to safeguard patient's commitments (eg transport of children to foster parents).

• Choose the best way of lowering arousal (time spent talking is

Fig 1. Crisis intervention teams must be responsive, immediate, accessible, and available out of hours—anywhere.

often preferable to administering anxiolytics, which may only serve to delay the natural process of adaptation). If the patient is shocked, stunned, or mute, take time to establish the normal channels of communication.

• As soon as the person is receptive, promote a sense of hope about the outcome of the crisis. If there is no hope (a mother, consumed by grief, after losing all her children in a fire), then this too must be addressed.

• The next step is to encourage creative thinking about ways whereby the patient might solve the problems. Start by helping him think through the consequences of all options open to him. Then help compartmentalize his proposed solutions into small, easily executed items of behaviour.

As the immediate crisis passes, and the patient has reasonable psychological functioning, it will be necessary to put him back in charge of his own life. A period of counselling is likely to be appropriate. This is described on p380. Making a contract about therapy is important in encouraging the patient to transfer from the 'sick role' to a self-dependent, adult role.

Crisis intervention often focuses on loss of face, loss of identity, or loss of faith—in oneself, in one's religion, one's goals, or one's roots.

Meta-analyses suggest that crisis intervention is a viable part of home-care, and can be used during the acute phase of any mental illness.[385]

▶*All home-care packages for severe mental illness need crisis management plans.* Where implemented, this keeps the vulnerable in contact with staff (NNT≈13 over 1yr) *and* reduces family burden (NNT≈3), *and* is a more satisfying form of care for patients and families. It is also said to be cheaper. In one trial,[386] availability of a crisis-resolution team reduced admission rates from 59% to 22% at 8 weeks—and was highly cost-effective.

---

1 See Sylvia Plath 1963 *A Birthday Present* in *Ariel*, Penguin, 50

►Are you afraid of uncomfortable questions? Here are some asked by a very experienced psychotherapist.[1]

❓Are you a saint? or have you ever...

❓Felt so bored and irritated by certain patients you want to quit?

❓Longed for the consultation to end, at any price?

❓Can you say you have *never* felt a flicker of sexual interest in a patient?

❓Have you never imagined the death of certain patients and the relief that would bring, not just to them but to us, their impotent carers?

❓Have you never resented the demands of people for whom illness seems to have become a way of life?

❓Whose thoughts have not sometimes drifted off towards their own concerns—to the need for sleep, food, or distraction or to some family, career, or future plans?

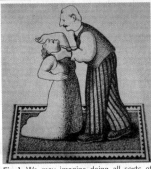

Fig 1. We may imagine doing all sorts of things to our patients. The crime is not the thought but the deed. The vital thing is to not to bury these things but to know that they are just that: imaginings. Perhaps we can use them in the service of our work? If the stressed, isolated doctor had been aware of and able to voice his fantasies maybe he would not have end up in custody or in bed with his sexually abused, vulnerable and depressed patient.

►The key to good doctoring is not regulation or revalidation, but fostering the ability to put ourselves in our patients' shoes. And we can use the feeling patients engender in us to understand how the patients nearest and dearest are frustrated, perplexed and deluded. For example, excessive worry about a patient may be the result of being infected by the patient's anxiety—beyond what is reasonable. This is know as *projective identification*.

Why does bad or harmful practice continue, despite GMC guidelines? It is because we are motivated by forces of which we are unaware.

1 *BMJ* 2002; 325: 722.1. Good doctor, bad doctor—a psychodynamic approach; Jeremy Holmes (whom we thank for permission to quote from his excellent article).

Good novelists (and counsellors) are somehow large enough to embody the world—so their characters (clients) are not just recreated in their own image. *Nothing* human is alien to them. Such exercise of the imagination is what enables virgins to counsel prostitutes—which they *can*, if they are submerged in and are fully aware of human affairs outside themselves.

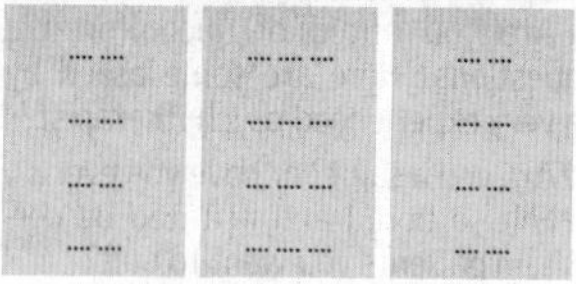

Fig 1. Nondirective counselling is a triptych of blanks: Where do you want to go? How will you get there? How will you know you have arrived? Just fill in the blanks....

After *Yellow Painting* by Barnett Newman.

Indications
• Current problems and stresses (eg experiencing acute psychological distress in response to life events or relationship problems).
• Brief anxiety disorders, especially when anxiolytic drugs not required.

Technique • Painting the triptych (fig 1) • Listening, understanding, and reflecting • Note how past stress has been coped with • Producing an agreed full list of problems • Redefining problems in terms of attainable goals • Use of therapeutic contracts to negotiate small behaviour changes • Aim for adult relationships between patient, family, and therapist, eg with a contract *vis à vis* duties, frequency, and duration of therapy, and what is expected of the client (*homework*), eg learning anxiety-reducing techniques, and carrying out *rewards,* eg cooking an extra-nice meal with the family if the client achieves an anxiety-provoking task such as shopping • *Talking* out (not *acting* out) anger in safe but cathartic ways • Reassurance. The therapist must not only give overt reassurance, but also by his demeanour he must reassure the patient that *whatever* he reveals (eg incest or baby battering), he will not be condemned.

Not all counselling is nondirective: problem-solving models of counselling (BOX) are sometimes directive, and *may* be appropriate if you know the client well.

Caution • 'Giving expert advice': patients may need medical, legal or financial advice. It may be best if this comes from a specialist agency not involved in the counselling • Patients with personality disorder, where the problems are too deep seated to be changed by counselling. Here there must be an awareness of the need to refer such patients for more formal psychotherapy.

Supportive psychotherapy

There are many people who seem to need continuous psychotherapy, as they that find daily activities pose unending stress. The smallest decisions are insurmountable problems, and the patient, lacking even a glimmer of insight, seeks support at every turn. What can we offer here?

Indication Relevant to all forms of psychiatric disorder.

Technique • Listening to what (s)he is saying, picking up verbal and nonverbal cues. Ensure a reasonably full account of the situation and problems • Reassurance: relieve fears, boost self-confidence and promote hope, • Explain to a patient why they are experiencing certain symptoms • Guidance and suggestion with regard to a particular problem • Expression of feelings eg anger, frustration and despair within a supportive setting.

Caution Patients can become dependent on the therapist and not be able to cope when therapy comes to an end—see p326 for how to deal with this.

Where tested against cognitive therapy, this less sophisticated therapy sometimes comes out well, eg in long-term schizophrenia care,[387] and also in care of adolescents with major depression—but not in minor depression.[388]

Counselling in primary care

Counselling has long been a central activity in primary care. Don't think of this as the expert handing down treatment to poor, benighted patients. It's more of a joint exploration between two humans who know each other reasonably well. On occasion, roles may be reversed—for example, following a medical disaster, a doctor, who may be blameless, may become so relentlessly and excoriatingly self-questioning that despair ensues. In these circumstances, it has been known for counselling and support from the original victim or one of his or her relatives to restore the doctor to health, and avert resignation.

Many UK general practices employ or have access to counsellors. This huge growth reflects the fact that people love to be listened to, and that GPs themselves may not have the time or inclination to satisfy this need. It is hard to prove the effectiveness of counselling, especially as skills and training vary markedly. But this does not mean it is ineffective.

There are 3 facets to counselling in general practice:

1 In some patients, problem-solving strategies are used, with the counsellor using a non-directive approach.
2 In fostering coping strategies, the therapist helps the patient to make the most of the position they are in (eg afflicted by a chronic disease).
3 In cognitive therapy, we concentrate on elucidating negative thinking, and help patients learn how to intervene in negative cycles of thinking.

Randomized trial evidence: Counselling and cognitive-behaviour therapy carried out in primary care are both more effective in treating depression than usual GP care in the short term. But in one study, there was no difference in outcome after 1 year.[389,N=197][390] NB: 'no difference' may indicate that too few counselling sessions were offered—or, perhaps that GPs were already effective counsellors—or maybe more focused counselling would be more effective.[391]

Therapeutic communities, and the example of substance misuse

Therapeutic communities (TCs) are a popular treatment for the rehabilitation of IV drug users and dealing with personality disorders—in both the USA and Europe. The rationale is that the benefits of peer-feedback (group therapy) can be magnified in the microcosm of a therapeutic community. Also these communities provide a safe environment for those with complex needs.

In trials of residential therapy *vs* therapeutic communities the latter can come out better *vis à vis* staying off drugs and not reoffending (eg if the 'residential' arm of the trial is prison).[392] Life in a community is more beneficial (*vis à vis* reoffending or reusing drugs) if it is for 12 months compared with 6 months. After the time in the community, aim to give continuing aftercare.[393] However, there is little evidence that TCs offer major benefits compared with other residential treatment, or that one type of TC is better than another.

European TCs adapt the early harsh behaviourism found in the US by concentrating more on milieu-therapy and social learning emphasizing dialogue and understanding. Either professionals or ex-addicts can provide input.[394]

Key concepts: 1 *The unconscious:* Individual dynamic psychotherapy is based on the premise that a person's behaviour is influenced by unconscious factors (thoughts, feelings, fantasies). Evidence for the existence of unconscious activity include • Dreams • Artistic and scientific creativity • Hysterical symptoms (p334) • Abreaction[1] • Parapraxes—'slips of the tongue'.

2 *Psychological defences:* Our immune system protects our physical integrity, and our psychological vulnerabilities are shielded by psychological defences. In both cases, overactive defences can lead to trouble, eg: *Psychotic defences:* • Delusional projection/paranoia • Denial • Distortion. *Immature defences:* • Projection[2] • Schizoid/autistic fantasy • Dissociation (p334) • Acting out (BOX) • Hypochondriasis • Passive aggression. *Neurotic defences:* • Repression • Displacement[3] • Reaction formation[4] • Intellectualization. *Mature defences.* • Altruism • Humour • Suppression • Anticipation • Sublimation[5].[395]

3 *Transference and countertransference:* The past patterns (transfers) our present reactions to people. If we have trusted our parents, we will be likely to trust our doctors, teachers, and friends. The intense psychotherapeutic relationship brings these assumptions to the fore where they can be examined, understood, and learned from. We in turn have unconscious reactions to patients based on our past, ie countertransference. Errors from countertransference arise when we react as though our patient were a significant person in our early life[396] (if our mother was an alcoholic we may be oversolicitous or rejecting with alcoholics). *Our reactions are also a key to our patient's feelings:* if a patient makes us feel rejected (as alcoholics often do), perhaps that person himself was rejected as a child and turned to the bottle in compensation.

Assessing suitability *Psychological understandibility:* The patient's difficulties must be understandable in psychological terms. *Psychological mindedness:* The capacity to think about problems in psychological terms. *Motivation:* There must be motivation for insight and change. *Intelligence and verbal fluency:* The ability to communicate thoughts and feelings through talking. *Introspectiveness:* The ability to reflect and think about their feelings. *Dreams:* The capacity to remember dreams. *Ego strength:* The ability to tolerate frustrating or distressful feelings without engaging in impulsive behaviour. *Capacity to form relationships:* There should be a history of at least one sustained relationship in the past or current life.

Specific indications • Dissociative/conversion disorders • Depression • Psychosomatic disorders • Personality disorders • Relationship problems • Grief.

Technique The therapist provides a secure *frame*—a regular time and place and her own consistency and acceptingness. The patient *narrates* vignettes about himself and his life (~3/session). The therapist *listens* carefully, to the stories and to her reactions to them. She then makes *linking hypotheses*, or *interpretations* that offer *meaning*. Previously inexplicable behaviour begins to make sense. Meanwhile, the patient forms a close relationship with the therapist based on *empathy*, *genuineness*, and *non-possessive warmth* (shown experimentally to be key factors) and sometimes *challenge*. These may be novel experiences for the patient that can be *internalized* as he *works through* difficulties safely. Reactions to *ending* will bring up past unprocessed losses.

Psychodynamic therapy can be *time-limited* (brief dynamic psychotherapy)—suitable for circumscribed problems, eg unmourned grief, or *open-ended* (BOX 3) eg if there are severe personality disorders or complex needs.[397].N=1053 In depression, 16 sessions seem to be no better than 8.[398]

---

1 *Abreaction:* cathartic reliving of buried traumas; repressed terrors are made conscious and *tamed.*[399]
2 *Projecting* our own undesirable impulses to another, so pretending that the subjective is objective.
3 *Displacement:* redirection of an undesired intense emotion towards someone neutral and harmless.
4 *Reaction formation:* doing the opposite of true desires (eg training to be a pilot to cover up fear of flying).
5 In sport, for example, we *sublimate* (and make safe) brutal urges into rituals of formal competition.

Acting out is making something happen or doing something instead of dealing with the corresponding feeling, eg when we unconsciously engage in actions or any non-verbal communication, or take on psychosomatic symptoms, instead of examining our true feelings. We fail to acknowledge to ourselves what we really feel and experience.[400] It is a kind of **unconscious self-destructive anger** and as such is the opposite to sublimation.[5] For example, a client may become accident-prone, attempt suicide, or commit unconscious self-sabotage (eg destroying his friends or work).

We also 'act out' desires forbidden by our Super ego but intensely desired by our Id. We cope with pressure to do what we think is wrong simply by siding with our Id. Immaturity, cognitive short-sightedness, counter-suggestibility, and 'contrarian tendencies' all play a role in acting out.[401]

Patients often act out with us as an expression of transference. Joyce is stamping her foot saying "You take such poor care of me. It shows you don't want me as a patient. Why not get rid of me?" A plea for love and a simultaneous self-destructive attempt to replicate past rejections?[402]

Sexual acting out is common too, eg in institutionalized (motherless) female adolescents, heterosexual acting out wards off regressive wishes, kindled by object loss, to reunite symbiotically with the cross-oedipal mother.[403]

Cautions: when dynamic psychotherapy might not be right

1 Repeated admissions, many suicide attempts, repeated risk-taking, and severe somatization suggest insufficient ego strength for psychotherapy.
2 A history of repeated failed ventures or dropping out of relationships.
3 In general, patients with acute psychosis are less amenable.
4 Severely depressed patients may be too slowed up and too unresponsive.
5 Over-sedation may hinder capacity to access feelings (?reduce doses).
6 Patients who are actively abusing alcohol or illicit drugs are problematic.
7 No real motivation to change or grossly unreal expectations of therapy.

Has psychoanalysis changed the world?

The world is no better than before psychoanalysis came along with its perceived promises of explaining us to ourselves and self-realization. Either the explanations are wrong or explaining things doesn't help—or we have missed the point of psychoanalysis. It may be charming to learn, for example, that the anorgasmia of a patient seen in today's clinic is explained by the specific psychodynamics of an 'anal-retentive defence against pre-oedipal fears of anal-sadistic impulses and fear of ego-loss'.[404] Likewise it is not clear that extended pre-orchidectomy counselling dwelling on anticipated narcissistic grief will actually improve outcomes.[405] But note that as soon as we learn about the concept of narcissistic grief we never forget it: it's like a promise of eternal love; it assumes its own truth, and if we dare to test it, it can only ever be us who are found to be wanting.

Joyce: the young mother's story Psychoanalysis took ages to get under way for a young mother happily named Joyce, who had inexplicably severe eczema. But things started happening by interview 236. Latent fears of being lesbian surfaced at this point and the psychiatrist was rewarded by the perfect sentence "It used to be if I just thought of her, I could start scratching".[406] But was the patient rewarded as well as the psychiatrist? It is impossible to know if any benefits were related to the specifics of the psychodynamic process—or just to the extraordinary input of time and attention. Either way, though, we must accept that psychoanalysis has more than entered and populated our consciousness: it's made it into our unconscious—so we cannot reject it, even if we want to.

What the hell! I'll do it now and repent tomorrow.

Psychiatry

After 236 sessions with Joyce the therapist strikes gold, but…oh boy! Joyce had to pay for it!

This is an example of *couple therapy*: often the problem is not specifically sexual, and sexual difficulties may recede once other aspects of the relationship improve. Here, specific sexual dysfunctions are considered in the light of a modernized *Masters & Johnson* approach using a model of sexual response entailing excitation, plateau, orgasm, and resolution.[407]

Start with a full (joint) description of the problem. This may be premature (or delayed) ejaculation, female frigidity (anorgasmia), erectile dysfunction, or dyspareunia (eg from spasm—vaginismus—or other physical causes). How did the problem start (eg after childbirth)? Was there ever a time when sex occurred as desired? Is the problem part of some wider problem? What does your partner expect from you? Are you self-conscious or anxious during sex? Are there medical problems, eg ischaemic heart disease,[408] or mastectomy; prosthesis use is discouraged at intercourse as it delays confrontation with and acceptance of mastectomy. Techniques of body imagery and sensate focus (below) have special roles here.[409,410]

Sexual history Early experiences; present practices; any hints pointing towards transexualism, commercial sex work, or drug abuse? Orientation to either or both sexes. Difficulties with other partners? When did you meet? What attracted you to each other?

Drugs Alcohol, hypotensives (erectile dysfunction, ED); SSRIs (delayed ejaculation); β-blockers, finasteride, the Pill, and phenothiazines (loss of libido). *Other causes of ED:* (OHCM p222): diabetes, cord pathology, prolactin↑, drugs.

Principles of behavioural therapy for sexual difficulties comprise:
1 Defining the task which the couple wishes to accomplish.
2 Reducing the task to a number of small, attainable steps.
3 Asking the couple to practise each small step in turn.
4 At the next session, discussing difficulties encountered.
5 Ameliorating maladaptive attitudes.
6 Setting the next task.

Example: premature ejaculation and vaginismus: (Both relate to performance anxiety, and vaginismus may be part of a *generalized* anxiety-defence mechanism).[411] One sequence to agree with the couple might be:
1 A ban on attempted sexual intercourse (to remove fear of performance failure). Education and 'permission' giving (ie to talk about and engage in 'safe' sexual fantasies) is vital.
2 Touching without genital contact, 'for your own pleasure', initially, with any non-genital part of the body, to explore the range of what pleases, and then to concentrate on whatever erogenous zones are found ('sensate focus').
3 Touching as above 'for your own and your partner's pleasure'.
4 'Homework' using a vaginal dilator and lubricating jelly.
5 Touching with genital contact, first in turn, later together. Problems in taking the initiative may now surface. In premature ejaculation, the partner stimulates the penis, and as orgasm approaches the man signals to his partner, who inhibits the reflex by squeezing his penis at the frenulum.
6 Concentrate on playing down the distinction between foreplay and intercourse, so that anxiety at penetration is reduced.
7 Vaginal containment in the female superior position so that she can stop or withdraw whenever she wants. She concentrates on the sensation of the vagina being filled.
8 Periods of pelvic thrusting, eg with a 'stop-start' technique.

NB: the evidence for such techniques is not all that good for premature ejaculation.[412] For vaginismus, success rates of >93% have been obtained.[413]
Drugs such as **sertraline** (unlicensed) can improve ejaculatory control.[414]

Psychiatry

There is much more to helping people with sexual difficulties than is outlined opposite: it is just one approach to one problem. Such behavioural approaches may not be suited to dealing with forbidden, haunting, and disturbing sexual feelings, fantasies, and urges. Experiential psychotherapy and psychodynamic approaches are valid alternatives.[415] Also, we should not focus on performance of acts at the expense of promoting the quality of erotic connection and the attainment of transcendent levels of intimacy.

Lust, romantic love, and attachment These are the 3 primary colours of the sexual realm—mixed in different proportions at different times in our lives to give millions of subtle or clashing tones. Each emotion-motivation system is associated with a specific constellation of neural correlates and a distinct behavioural repertoire.[416] Sex therapy has different tasks in each of these areas. In any therapy the following universals need to be addressed:

- Never assume that a patient is too old or too ill for sexual issues to be relevant. ▶Assume that everyone has a sex life, perhaps in fantasy only (fantasy is always found to be an important component of sexuality).[417]
- Treat sexual problems holistically—eg there may be relevant medical, drug, or other psychopathologies (depression is common).
- Psychological approaches are always important, whatever is offered by way of physical props or drugs such as sildenafil. Men randomized to receive group therapy + sildenafil had more successful intercourse than those receiving only sildenafil. Group psychotherapy also significantly improves erectile dysfunction compared to sildenafil alone.[418]
- Psychological events have physical sequelae, and physical events have psychological sequelae.
- All pleasure, including all erotic pleasure, is either purely sensory or arises from associations of ideas: this offers many points of intersection for negative operators, such as distraction, spectatoring, guilt, anxiety, fear of failure, pain, and inappropriate stimulation.
- As in all walks of life: ▶*when in doubt...communicate*. This is the basis of the salutogenesis approach to sexual health. Salutogenesis asks not what disease is present but how and individual or a couple stay healthy. And the answer is often 'through communication' and 'by being intimate'.[419] Intimacy may be a more powerful determinant of health than improved diet, stopping smoking, genetic vulnerabilities, and prescription drugs.[420]
- All humans have a need to give as well as to take. Reawakening this instinct may be an important part of therapy.[421] N=1

What used to be called *family therapy* is now better known as *systemic practice*, which is an evolving body of ideas and techniques focusing on a person's difficulties within the context of the people and culture that surround them. Therapy is based on the assumption that most people have the resources and potential for resolving life's difficulties. Therapists may work with individuals or families. Screening rooms may be used where co-therapists observe family interactions during therapy via a one-way screen.

Its origins began in *cybernetics*.[422] Behaviour maintains itself by feedback loops, eg disruptive behaviour in a son draws divorcing parents together. This led to *strategic therapy*—the paradoxical approach where the symptom is prescribed so interrupting the behaviour-problem cycle. *Structural therapy*[423,424] sought to be more objective. A family can be described in terms of dimensions. Research interviews have given rise to a measure of 'expressed emotion' (EE) which is associated with severity of chronic illness in many disorders (eg schizophrenia, anorexia nervosa, cystic fibrosis). Therapy includes prescribed exercises, eg parents may agree to go out for a meal at a secret location. In an over-involved family, this strengthens parental executive subsystems, providing opportunity for disengagement and management of concomitant anxiety. *Systemic family therapy* was pioneered by the Milan School, emphasizing family behaviour according to 'myths', 'scripts', and family secrets, which dominate the inter-generational transmission of repeating behaviours. Drawing a genogram (family tree) with the family is a good way to reveal this. Hypothesizing, maintaining a neutral stance and the use of circular questioning are important components.

Narrative therapies[425] consider that knowledge is developed by story-telling not through the logico-scientific method, working on the basis that there is no single truth about the reasons for problems but that 'truths' are constructed via conversations between therapist and therapee. People can be maintained in problem-saturated lives by 'viewing themselves in the context of a dominant knowledge'. By constructing an alternative knowledge, they can be liberated to challenge the problem. Narrative therapists help by restoring people's control over their problems via externalizing the problem. Faecal soiling is popularly viewed as an act committed by the child as a response to family dysfunction. But if it is viewed as a struggle between the family and the problem by identifying the 'sneaky poo' as the enemy, then the family can be engaged in a battle against it. The use of written letters is also considered a useful tool.

Brief solution focused therapy[426] makes use of a structured approach to draw on people's resilience, and motivate problem solving. It centres conversations on solutions, not problems. "If it works, do more of it. If it doesn't work do something different. No problem happens all the time."

Session 1	Session 2 and beyond
1 Why have you come?	1 What's got better?
2 How may we be of help?	2a Elicit: Ask about positive changes
3 The miracle question (below)	2b Amplify: Ask for details on +ve changes
4 Exception questions	2c Ensure he notices and values change
5 Spectograms	2d Start again. Ask what else is better.
6 Agreed achievable tasks	3 Ending. How can you get back on track?

'Miracle' question: "If you woke up and a miracle had occurred in the night, how would you know? How would your life be different?"

Exception question: Search with the client for possible exceptions.

Spectograms: "On a scale of 0 to 10, how much would you like your miracle to happen?" "What would have to happen/What would you have to do to make your score move from 3 to 4?"

Psychiatry (side margin)

Family structure is viewed by Minuchin[424] as an invisible set of functional demands that organize family interactions. These transactional patterns are self-regulating in a way that attempts to return a family to its habitual mode and minimize anxiety.

Dimensions of family functioning[428,429] (McMaster model) The 6 dimensions allowing any practitioner to describe family functioning are:

• *Problem solving:* Can the family act together to solve everyday emotional and practical problems? Can they identify a problem, develop, agree, and enact solutions, and evaluate their performance? Success may be dependent upon functioning in other dimensions.

• *Congruence of verbal and non-verbal communications:* Are communications clear and direct or are there hidden agendas or hidden meanings? Do people listen to one another?

• *Roles:* Who is in charge and how are executive decisions made? Who provides for the family? Who is concerned for the child's education and emotional development? Families may function most effectively when roles are appropriately allocated and responsibilities explicit.

• *Affective involvement:* Relationships in families tend to exist on a continuum from over-involved (enmeshed) to disinvolved (dis-engaged). Empathic involvement is ideal. This depends on development, as greater involvement is needed for babies than adolescents. Enmeshment may lead a child to be so anxious about a parent that they feel unable to leave them, and avoid school as a consequence.

• *Affective responsiveness:* How do individual family members respond emotionally to one another both by degree and quality? Welfare feelings would include love, tenderness, and sympathy. Emergency feelings would include fear, anger, and disappointment.

• *Behavioural control:* How is discipline maintained? Is there negotiation? Is it flexible? Chaotic? Absent? (depends on quality of communication).

Dysfunctional family patterns Triangulation: When parents are in conflict, each demands the child sides with them. When the child sides with one, they are automatically considered to be attacking the other. The child is paralysed in a no-win state where every movement is a perceived attack on a parent.

Scapegoating: When an individual is singled out by the family as the sole cause of the family troubles. This serves to temporarily bury conflicts that the family fear will overwhelm them.

†*Expressed emotion:* Derived from a family interview: reflects hostility, emotional over-involvement, critical comments, and contact time.

Psychiatry

Psychiatry

Westen's dictum Beware making false dichotomies into supported and unsupported therapies. Randomized trial methodologies don't suit all therapies. What follows does not entirely avoid the trap Westen alludes to. Also be aware of many different variations on a theme, eg cognitive and analytic therapy (CAT) and DBT (dialectical behaviour therapy).[1]

Principal recommendations and levels of evidence[2]

• Psychological therapy should be routinely considered as an option when assessing mental health problems.[B]

• Patients who are adjusting to life events, illnesses, disabilities or losses may benefit from brief therapies such as counselling.[B]

• Post-traumatic stress symptoms may be helped by psychological therapy, with most evidence for cognitive-behavioural methods. Routine debriefing following traumatic events is not recommended.[A]

• Depression may be helped (but is often not cured) by cognitive therapy or interpersonal therapy. A number of other brief structured therapies for depression may be of benefit, such as psychodynamic therapy.[A]

• Anxiety disorders with marked symptomatic anxiety (agoraphobia, panic disorder, social phobia, obsessive-compulsive disorders, generalized anxiety disorders) are likely to benefit from cognitive-behaviour therapy.[A]

• Psychological intervention should be considered for somatic complaints with a psychological component with most evidence for CBT in the treatment of chronic pain and chronic fatigue.[C]

• Eating disorders can be treated with psychological therapy. Best evidence in bulimia nervosa is for CBT, interpersonal therapy (IPT) and family therapy for teenagers. Treatment usually includes psycho-educational methods. There is little strong evidence on the best therapy type for anorexia.[C]

• Structured psychological therapies delivered by skilled practitioners can contribute to the longer-term treatment of personality disorders.[C]

Evidence • Psychological therapy shows benefits over no treatment for a wide range of mental health difficulties • There is evidence of counselling effectiveness in mixed anxiety/depression, most effective when used with specified client groups, eg postnatal mothers, bereaved groups • CBT has been found helpful. Some evidence of efficacy has been shown for other forms of psychological therapy. Single-session debriefing appears to be unhelpful in preventing later disorders • CBT and IPT (interpersonal psychotherapy) can effectively reduce symptoms of depression. Benefit has also been found for other forms of psychological therapy, including focal psychodynamic therapy, psychodynamic interpersonal therapy and counselling • CBT effectively reduces symptoms of panic and anxiety. Behaviour therapy and cognitive therapy both appear effective in treatment of obsessional problems • Psychological therapies have benefit in a range of somatic complaints including gastrointestinal and gynaecological problems. CBT has been found more effective than control therapies in improving functioning in chronic fatigue and chronic pain • Efficacy of CBT and IPT in bulimia has been established. Individual therapies have shown some benefit in anorexia, with little to distinguish treatment types. Early onset of anorexia may indicate family therapy, and later onset, broadly based individual therapy • A number of therapy approaches have shown some success with personality disorders, including dialectical behaviour therapy, psychoanalytic day hospital programme and therapeutic communities.

1 CAT is collaborative programme for looking at the way a person thinks, feels and acts, and the events and relationships that underlie these experiences (often from childhood or earlier in life). It combines understandings from cognitive psychotherapies and psychoanalytic approaches into an integrated whole. **2** A Based on a consistent finding in a majority of studies in high-quality systematic reviews or evidence from high-quality studies. B Based on ≥1 high-quality trial, a weak or inconsistent finding in high-quality reviews or a consistent finding in reviews that don't meet all the high-quality criteria. C Based on evidence from single studies that don't meet all the criteria of 'high-quality'. D Based on evidence from structured expert consensus.

Index on child mental health problems

This section (to p398) deals with some aspects of childhood mental health—but many issues in child psychiatry overlap with pages in the adult section of this chapter, and also with paediatrics. The psychiatry of attempted suicide is a good example. Many of these patients will be in the last phases of childhood, and it is unclear which service will suit them best. As ever, take a holistic view of your patient, and design a care plan which takes these facets into account.

Psychiatry

Mental health in adolescence

Adolescents face major mental health challenges owing to existential crises (p390), changing looks, emerging sexualities, identity problems, exam pressure, family break-up, ready availability of drugs and alcohol, media pressures, and the onset of adult responsibilities (eg when they get pregnant). Psychotic illness also often starts in adolescence, and may be partly related to urban stress (p391).

What can we do to help? Paediatricians, psychologists, psychiatrists, counsellors, GPs, and so on all have a role of course—but access to them depends on the fact that a problem has occurred. This is often a bit late—which is why teachers have such an important role in promoting mental health.

Some schools offer classroom-based workshops such as *MasterMind: Empower Yourself With Mental Health*. MasterMind-type initiatives work by creating a toolbox for mental health by making a safe place for discussion of mental health and emotionally charged topics. The aim is to increase student knowledge of mental health issues, and to provide the tools to develop and maintain mental health (eg techniques in de-stressing). Instructional materials address topics identified through needs assessment. These and other written exercises are combined with peer-teaching-peer group activities, individual assignments, and open discussion. Students can ask questions anonymously, and through interaction they build each other's self-esteem (provided they are not feeling totally negative). When these interventions have been evaluated, it is found that students' enthusiasm and participation increases throughout the course, and they give high satisfaction scores to the topics covered.[433]

Of course, we all want to know what mental illness is prevented—but this is to ask the wrong question. Mental health issues will never be cured or go away—they are part of what it means to be an adolescent. The question is more "How are these adolescents adjusting to their self-made world?" and "Is adolescence proving to be a humanizing or an alienating experience?" The answers to these questions are more metaphysical than quantitative.

We often have the impression that the incandescent adolescent sitting in front of us is burning too brightly within his sullen shell—and our foreknowledge of his impending death in a shoot-out, stabbing, or drug-overdose seems inevitable. ▸▸What is not inevitable is that he should go to his grave without anyone having tried to help. The following pages may serve as a first step.

Accepting that the big task of adolescence is forging new independent identities, it comes as no surprise that the main signs of depression in this group spell ERSATZ: a German word we use to mean *fake*.[1] Existential hopelessness related to dawning awareness of freedom to narrate one's own life and death; relationship & sexual problems; anger in the face of conflicting adult values; tearfulness when it all goes wrong, and overzealous attachment to false gods (eg causing body image dissatisfaction and self-harm).

Features as seen in adults:	*Features common in childhood:*
Low mood	Defiance; running away from home
Loss of interest and self-esteem	Separation anxiety ± school refusal
Socially withdrawn	Complaints of boredom; poor school work
Psychomotor retardation	Antisocial behaviour
Tearful; feelings of guilt	Insomnia (often initial, not early waking)
Anxiety	Hypersomnia
Lack of enjoyment in anything	Eating problems

One-to-one interviewing is usually best. Consider the possibility of concealed factors (eg past child abuse, bullying, p395). Parents can be interviewed separately (ask the child's permission, and see the child alone, again, if appropriate, *after* seeing the parents, to report back: this helps avoid seeming to collude with the parents). NB: parents are often unaware of depression in their children.

Assessment is often hard: questions may be answered by silence or a shrug. If not getting anywhere, keep listening, or offer silences—but do not give up.

Always ask about thoughts of suicide/self-harm. Any past attempts? 15-20% make further attempts (↑risk if: conduct disorder, ↑alcohol use, hopelessness, or in local authority care). Self-harm may be a form of communication—a message in a bottle; not always 'picked up' and sometimes it is difficult to decipher the teenager's exact intentions. Refer urgently if risk is considered significant. Adolescents with conduct disorders can be manipulative and extremely difficult to assess—an urgent second opinion is frequently of help.

Management Ideally this should be a combined approach:

1 Social: addressing sources of distress (eg bullying) and removing opportunities for self-harm (eg no paracetamol at home). Improve sense of belongingness, especially if he/she feels on the margins of society (eg for reasons of sexuality, or because of substance abuse).[434]

2 Psychological: encourage verbalizing of moods; explore the vocabulary of internal states. Counsellors, good teachers, and youth workers help here.

3 Cognitive therapy (CBT, p373) helps (often unavailable in primary care).[435]

4 If criminality and gang culture is at work, peer mentorship may help.[435]

5 Drugs: often disappointing (and dangerous); but as 1-4 above is often insufficient in major depression, drugs (eg **fluoxetine** or **escitalopram** 10mg/day[436] need to be considered. NICE exclude 1ˢᵗ-line use, even in severe depression, but this obsessively self-exculpating ban may do more harm than good.[437] If marked sleep disturbance, consider **mirtazapine**. If drugs are used:
   • Evaluate risk/benefit ratio (try to include parents in the discussion).
   • Monitor suicide ideation ≥weekly for 1ˢᵗ month, then ≥ every other week.
   • Before an antidepressant is initiated, a safety plan should be in place with an agreement with the patient and family that the patient will be kept safe and will contact a responsible adult if suicidal urges get too strong.
   • Ensure the availability of psychiatric help 24/7.[438]

Specific drugs to avoid if <18yrs old, if possible (BNF/CSM): citalopram, paroxetine, sertraline. Also tricyclics, venlafaxine, and fluvoxamine.[439,440]

---

1 All constructed identities are fakes, adult or adolescent, but in adulthood we have more time to reassemble our selected fakes into coherent patterns. For this reason adults are not *simply* burnt-out adolescents.

In many centres, early-onset schizophrenia is diagnosed with the same criteria as adults (p358) as it seems to be continuous with later-onset forms (eg more males being affected).[441] This is simplistic, as delusions and hearing voices are common in children and are essential to some forms of play.

- Visions may relate to folklore or religion, eg nocturnal hallucinations in up to 40% of teenage boys studying in stressful ultra-orthodox Yeshivas where there is a belief in demons and dead souls who visit at night.[442] n=302
- Another example is delusional erotomania (p640) which is commoner in adolescents living in places such as China where expressing sexual interest has to be indirect. There are many other examples where to equate delusions and hallucinations with psychopathology would be wrong.[443]
- Hearing unwanted tunes (earworms) is common: if there is any psychopathology, it will be more likely to be obsessions rather than psychosis.
- Hallucinations are more common in the isolated and withdrawn; here their importance may lie in alerting you to this fact.[444,445]

Some hallucinations should receive very serious attention:
»» Those which are imperative ("kill so-and-so") or exciting strong emotions.
»» Those heard unambiguously outside the head.
»» Those referring to ideas that the person feels are not their own.
»» Multiple voices talking at once, and especially voices talking to *each other*.

Sometimes hallucinations resist diagnosis. This is not in itself a problem as the diagnosis will sooner or later become clear. Meanwhile, ask yourself whether these odd ideas are likely to indicate that your patient is at increased risk of serious outcome, eg suicide.[446,447]

Causes of odd ideas Substance abuse; drugs; schizophrenia; anxiety/depression; hypomania; head injury; epileptic aura; migraine; Charles Bonnet syndrome (p438); SLE; encephalopathy (eg lead exposure); infections (herpes, EBV-associated Alice-in-Wonderland syndrome, OHCM p708); stress; abuse.

Tests MRI/CT may be indicated, eg in olfactory hallucination.[448]

Management ►Early intervention helps, and may reduce chances of later chronic schizophrenia, so refer promptly.[448] If you are the child's GP, ensure there is a treatment plan with a named worker, incorporating antipsychotics (if indicated, p360) with psycho-educational, psychotherapeutic, and social components. New antipsychotics (p361) are rarely *specifically* licensed for children, but their use in well-monitored environments is encouraging.[449] SEs are legion; they may not be as bad as older drugs see p361.[450,451]

Social interventions in deprived urban areas Risk of psychosis rises when young people with a genetic predisposition (expressed as poor social and cognitive functioning) have to cope with urban life,[452] poverty,[453] isolation,[454] crime,[455] and inequality.[456] What can be done to alleviate urban stress and gang culture? •Autonomy for housing estates (Housing Association[uk] may help) •Wardens drawn from the local community •Training schemes •Clubs (for art/self-expression) •Sport •Debates •Very local radio[457] •Skills/time banks (where those with skills deposit hours of help which others can 'cash') •Cycle repairs (if you learn to fix an unclaimed bike, you keep it)[458] •Children's centres •Saturday school/healthy living •Prostitution and drug abuse initiatives agreed with police •Avoid punishment/imprisonment.[459]

Prognosis Spontaneous improvement of psychotic-like symptoms occurs in the majority of children. In one follow-up study, many developed chronic mood disorders; <50% met diagnostic criteria for a major disorder (schizoaffective or bipolar disorder, depressive disorder, 'psychotic disorder not otherwise specified'). In those not developing a mood or psychotic disorder, disruptive behaviour disorders are very common.[460]

Psychiatry

Not falling asleep Try plenty of daytime activity (each hour of sitting ↑sleep latency by 3mins).[461] Insist on a routine wind-down 1 hour before bed→warm bath for 10min→a story→then straight into a darkened bedroom._{Gurney method}

Waking at 3am *(ready to play, or wanting entry to parent's bed)* For those not appreciating these visitations from the pure of heart, consider refusing to play and buy earplugs to lessen the impact of screaming—or let the child into the bed. Or try extinguishing the behaviour by attending to the child ever more distantly: cuddle in bed→cuddle on bed→sitting on child's bed→voice from doorway→distant voice. Try to avoid hypnotics. If essential, consider **Weldorm Elixir® (cloral betaine)**; dose if >2yrs: 30mg/kg, max 1g/day.

Other sleep disturbances Hunger/colic (infants); poor routines (preschool); worry (adolescence). Bedroom TV may be to blame. Try behavioural therapy before hypnotics. Day-time sleepiness: Causes: night sleep↓; depression; sleep apnoea (*OHCM* p186); narcolepsy;[1] encephalitis lethargicans (rare in children): suspect this whenever sleepiness occurs with extrapyramidal effects, oculo-gyric crises, myoclonus, inversion of diurnal rhythms, obsessions, and mood change. Possible causes: influenza; flu vaccination;● measles; Q fever; myco-plasma; hypothalamic lymphoma. MRI: subcortical involvement.

Sleepwalking & parasomnias[2] Of all our non-insane automatisms, somnam-bulism is the most familiar and striking, literally (rarely) as households may be endangered when the bloodiest dreams of junior somnambulists are enacted. The young are by far the best sleepwalkers (the old may emulate them eg if stress is augmented by excess alcohol or caffeine use, and lack of stage IV sleep—our deepest sleep). Any psychic event associated with sleep may be termed a parasomnia. *Parasomnias comprise:* •*Arousal disorders* (sleep-walking; night terrors; 'confusional arousal') •*Sleep-wake transition disor-ders* (rhythmic head-banging disorder) •*REM sleep parasomnias* (rapid eye movement sleep associated nightmares, sleep paralysis, hallucinations, and REM sleep behaviour disorder (box 1). •*Others.*[1]

Suffering from night terrors is often a familial problem. The child awakens frightened, hallucinated, and inaccessible—and is obviously alarmed.

It is common to observe movement in children during sleep: it is their *repeti-tive* nature which allows the diagnosis of rhythmic movement disorder. The movement may be body-rocking, leg-rolling, or head-banging (this 'jactatio capitis' may lead to subdurals, fractures, eye injuries, and false accusations of abuse). Tongue-biting may suggest epilepsy. But do not try to be too ob-sessive in differentiating parasomnias from nocturnal epilepsy, for 3 reasons: **1** Our definition of epilepsy is tested to destruction by the parasomnias ('epi-lepsy is intermittent abnormal brain activity manifesting as simple or complex seizures'). **2** Those with clearly defined parasomnias are at risk of developing tonic-clonic nocturnal seizures later in life. **3** Some parasomnias are signs of autosomal-dominant nocturnal frontal lobe epilepsy (ADNFLE). ADNFLE is associ-ated with abnormalities in genes coding nicotinic acetylcholine receptor α_4-subunit (chromosome 20). EEG: rhythmic slow anterior activity; video polysom-nography: sleep-related violent behaviour, sudden awakening and dyskinetic or dystonic movements, and complex behaviours ± enuresis.[462]

Antiparasomniacs: Bedtime **clonazepam; amitriptyline; carbamazepine**. If not working, consider self-hypnosis or waking ½h before the expected event.[463]

---

1 In narcolepsy we succumb to irresistible attacks of inappropriate sleep ± vivid hallucinations, cataplexy (sudden hypotonia), and sleep paralysis (BOX 2). Mutations lead to loss of hypothalamic hypocretin-contain-ing neurons, via autoimmune destruction. HLA DR2+ve. ℞: 1 Methylphenidate, 10–15mg PO after breakfast and lunch) may cause dependence and psychosis 2 Modafinil (~200mg/d PO, before noon; SE: anxiety, aggression, dry mouth, euphoria, insomnia, BP↑, dyskinesia, alk phos↑ 3 Gamma-hydroxybutyrate (GHB).[464]

2 Sleep-related dissociative disorder, sleep enuresis, exploding head syndrome, hypnagogic or hypnop-ompic hallucinations, catathrenia (end-inspiratory apnoea + groaning), sleep-related eating disorders, drug-induced parasomnias, myoclonus nocturnus; nocturnal bruxism, ie teeth grinding..

Sleep architecture and REM sleep behaviour disorder

We sleep in one of two states: rapid eye movement sleep (REM sleep ≈25% of all sleep) and non-rapid eye movement (NREM, which has 4 stages). In REM sleep, breathing is irregular, BP rises, and tone lapses (atonia; paralysis). EEG during REM sleep is similar to that in wakefulness and associates with dreaming. Tricyclics, SSRIs, and serotonin-norepinephrine reuptake inhibitors may all suppress REM.

In REM sleep behaviour disorder, REM paralysis is incomplete or absent, with acting out of dreams that are vivid and violent (with shouting, punching, kicking, flailing etc enough to endanger bed-partners). *Associations/causes:* Parkinson's disease, dementia (may be an early sign), alcohol and drug withdrawal (eg SSRI). *Polysomnography:* Muscle tone ↑ during REM sleep. *Treatment:* Sleep alone; remove all dangers from the sleep environment. Put the mattress on the floor. **Clonazepam 0.5mg** at bedtime may help.

Sleep paralysis

When we sleep we trawl forbidden seas, arranging and being rearranged by the flotsam and jetsam of our waking lives. As our nets descend through the various stages of sleep, our Sovereign Reason or Will usually remains quietly on deck, but if by chance it descends with the nets then, like the tail wagging the dog, it adopts and propagates a life of its own, which may be full of danger. Because our vessel has been vacated, Marie-Celeste-style, we are judged, in Law, to be not responsible for our actions while asleep—be they theft, arson, or homicide. Without will or wind, our vessel, like Coleridge's *Mariner's* (see poem below), is moved 'onward from beneath' by secret forces. So here we have the model of Reason and Will residing, during sleep, either upstairs or downstairs: but in sleep paralysis, neither is the case—the tail cannot wag the dog, nor the dog wag his tail. Sleep paralysis may involve complete paralysis of all voluntary muscles, even the diaphragm. For anyone who has experienced it, it is frightening, unforgettable, and difficult to describe—like being aware during anaesthesia with total neuromuscular blockade.

Sleep paralysis was first described by Ishmael during a reverie on deck, sleeping between Queequeg, the cannibal whaler from the South Seas, and his harpoon, before Herman Melville embarks them on the *Pequod's* voyage to track down Moby Dick: "At last I must have fallen into a troubled nightmare of a doze; and slowly waking from it—half steeped in dreams—I opened my eyes, and the before sunlit room was now wrapped in outer darkness. Instantly I felt a shock running through all my frame; nothing was to be seen, and nothing was to be heard; but a supernatural hand seemed placed in mine. My arm hung over the counterpane...for what seemed like ages piled on ages, I lay there frozen with the most awful fears ... thinking that if I could but stir it one single inch, the horrid spell would be broken." *Moby Dick* p44 Penguin

Till noon we quietly sailed on
    Yet never a breeze did breathe:
Slowly and smoothly went the ship,
Moved onward from beneath.
Under the keel nine fathom deep,
From the land of mist and snow,
The spirit slid: and it was he
That made the ship to go.   *The Rime of the Ancient Mariner*
Samuel Taylor Coleridge (*part v*)

Psychiatry

Autism spectrum disorders (ASDs)

ASDs are *the* lifelong pervasive developmental disorders of our times.[1] Prevalence: ≥1:200[465] ♂:♀ ≈ 4:1. Managing autism is a huge challenge. It is a triad of:

1 Impaired reciprocal social interaction.
2 Impaired imagination (±abnormal verbal and nonverbal communication).
3 Restricted repertoires of activities and interests.[466]

Cause Unknown; severity correlates with testosterone in amniotic fluid.♦
Genes (on chromosome 11p12 ± neurexin) play a part.[467] If one child is affected, risk of the next pregnancy being affected is ~5–10%. Blood glutathione levels are low and this may jeopardize CNS & GI antioxidant activity.[468] There is associated epilepsy in 30%. Any association with MMR vaccine (p151) is thought to be due to changing definition of autism at the time that MMR was introduced.[469]

Diagnosis ≳6 items, with ≳2 from '**A**' symptoms, and one each from '**B**' and '**C**'. Telling comments before the age of ~2yrs are: "he does not respond to his own name; he hates his routine being changed; he is not interested in toys."[470]

Impaired reciprocal social interaction ('A' symptoms)

- Unawareness of the existence and feelings of others (treating people as furniture; being oblivious to others' distress or need for privacy).
- Abnormal response to being hurt: he doesn't come for comfort; or makes a stereotyped response, eg just saying "Kiss it better kiss it better kiss it...".
- Impaired imitation (eg does not wave 'bye-bye' or copies/echoes without understanding, eg waves on passing a door when no one is in fact leaving).
- Repetitive play: eg solitary, or using others as mechanical aids.
- Bad at making friends (lack of empathy). If he tries at all, the effort will lack the social conventions, eg reading the phone directory to uninterested peers.

Impaired imagination ('B' symptoms; part of abnormal communication)

- Little babbling, few facial expressions or no gestures in infancy.
- Avoids mutual gaze; no smiles when making a social approach; does not greet his parents; stiffens when held.
- Does not act adult roles; no interest in stories; no fantasy/pretend play.
- Odd speech, eg echolalia (repetitions); odd use of words ("Go on green riding" for "I want a go on a swing"); odd use of pronouns ("You" instead of "I").
- Difficulty in initiating or sustaining reciprocal roles in conversations.

Poor range of activities and interests ('C' symptoms)

- Stereotyped movements (hand-flicking, spinning, head-banging).
- Preoccupation with parts of objects (sniffing or repetitive feeling of a textured object, spinning wheels of toys) or unusual attachments (eg to coal).
- Marked distress over changes in trivia (eg a vase's place).
- Insists on following routines in precise detail.
- Narrow fixations, eg lining up objects, or amassing facts about weather.

CHAT screening test: sensitivity 38%; specificity is 98% if done at 1½yrs old.[471, N=16,235]

Treatment *Early intensive behavioural intervention* (EIBI) ±*speech therapy*[472] ± *special schooling*. EIBI starting at 3yrs old can ↑IQ in >60% and enhance motor, social, and living skills.[473] *Selfhelp*:[uk] 020 81830 0999. *Parent training* helps communication, enriches parental knowledge of autism, enhances parent-child interaction, and ↓parental maternal depression.[465] Encourage parents to attend more to 'good' behaviours, and to have clear rules. *Social skills training/role-play* can help. *Get benefits*/Disability Living Allowance.
[uk] Other partly successful *behavioural approaches* include that of Lovaas.[474] *Drugs* have a small role: fish oils[475] (may help tantrums and self harm); atomoxetine[476] (hyperactivity); risperidone (irritability; repetition; social withdrawal; SE: weight↑).[477] *Diet*: Eliminating gluten & casein is popular but unproven.[478]

Outlook 70% remain badly handicapped; 50% have useful speech; 15% lead an independent life.

1 There is overlap with: Asperger's; multiple complex developmental disorder; schizoaffective disorder.[479]

▶*Every individual should have the right to be spared oppression and repeated, intentional humiliation, in school as in society at large.*[480] Bullying is important not just because it is unacceptable, but also because it leads to depression, somatization, withdrawal, submissive behaviour, school phobia,[481] vomiting, sleep disturbance, drug abuse, poor communication, and suicide.[482]

▶*Most parents don't know their offspring are bullies or being bullied.*[481]

▶*Bullying is bad for bullies:* antisocial behaviour persists into adulthood with impaired reciprocal diadic relationships (≈poor love life).[483]

Incidence 27% of primary and middle school children report bullying each term, and 10% of secondary pupils. In a study of prevalence, 4% were direct bullies, 10% bully/victims (both bully and victim), and 40% victims. Pure victims have poor health. Pure bullies have fewest↑health problems.[484]

Bullying behaviour Rumour-spreading→excluding others→racial abuse→hostile staring→punking¹→victimization→pushing→violence→torture→murder.

Risk factors Isolation, looking different, being small, or gay, or seeming gay.[485]

Interventions targeting bullying or emotional distress may reduce the severity of both problems.[486] *Liaise with the school.* School-wide policies *do* work.[487] Psychotherapy has a role. Ensure that the bully doesn't prosper from bullying, so learning to 'achieve dominance over others by the abuse of power'.[488]

The hardest task is to combat the ethos among bystanders, which allows bullying to continue as if it were 'none of my business'.[489]

This implies that we all have a role in minimizing bullying. Bullying in health services is well-documented,[490] and most of us have suffered from insecure people abusing positions of power. We fear to act when we are bullied as we might get a bad reference or because we don't think our own humiliation is important. It is easier to take a more rational view when we see others being bullied: we must not allow it. Remember that the bullier may not be able to stop the behaviour without help—which is available: see www.nhs-exposed.com.

School-based anti-bullying interventions are successful in primary schools but less so in secondary schools.[491] *Homosexual bullying:* Teachers are often aware of homophobic bullying but are confused, unable, or unwilling to help. Citizenship education programmes may be important here.[492] *When the teacher is the bully:* Problems may become *very* deep-rooted. Studies of bullying by teachers reveal the subtlety and complexity of teachers' strategies for distancing themselves from being held accountable for intimidation.[493]

On a universal level, we can recognize that we are all potential bullies, when stressed, frightened, overworked, or threatened by uncontrollable events (such as patient demand). We stop ourselves from being bullies, more or less successfully, by intrapsychic appeals to well-respected mentors who 'would never behave like that', and by communicating our feelings to our colleagues directly before they are forced underground only to resurface as bullying. Try: "I'm feeling rather stressed at the moment: tell me if I seem bullying or hectoring—but we've got to get this job done, and I suggest doing it like this..."

False accusations of bullying *You are trying to bully me* is a phrase which may be used correctly, or it may be an attempt to stop someone in authority from pursuing her proper role. The test is: "Is this action tyrannical, and is its purpose to belittle me, or is it that I am being asked to do something I don't want to do by someone who is honestly trying to make an institution work?" Professors of Organizational Behaviour emphasize that *everyone* suffers if dynamism and the promotion of change are mistaken for bullying.[494]

---

1 Punking is male-on-male violence, humiliation, and shaming to affirm masculinity, toughness, dominance and control.[495] When boys who believe they merit privilege are instead harassed or called gay, they can be driven to avenge 'wrongs', and assert a victorious masculinity. Mass shootings may result.[496]

Reading ability usually goes hand-in-hand with intelligence, but when this is not so, and someone with, say, an IQ of 130, finds reading difficult, the term dyslexia is often used. The term 'specific learning difficulty' is preferred by some people, as 'dyslexia' is often a term used by parents to help cope with having a child whose general intellectual skills, including reading, are less than hoped for. NB: dyslexia can be associated with other speech and language disorders: consider referral to a speech and language therapist (SALT).

Essence There is a problem with appreciating phonemes, eg that 'cat' comprises /c/, /a/, and /t/. Breaking up unfamiliar words into phonemes and having a go at stringing them together is the central act of learning to read. This is what needs to be taught, educationalists say, and children should not be made to rely on unstructured guesswork (the 'look and say' approach) which is now discredited as the sole means of equipping children for reading.

Quite often, distortion/jumbling of text during reading is reported. Visual aids have been used with some success to improve reading.[497][N=47]

Children with dyslexia also have difficulty in telling how many syllables there are in a word (don't we all? "How many syllables are there in *strength*?" analytical dyslexics may ask). They also have difficulty with verbal short-term memory—eg for meaningless strings such as phone numbers. There is also a problem with telling if two words rhyme or not, and in distinguishing phonemes which sound similar (eg /k/ and /g/). There may also be left/right muddle. *Genetics:* Boys are more afflicted than girls, and show stronger genetic effects (up to 50% of boys are dyslexic if their fathers are). Genes on chromosomes 1, 2, and 15 are implicated, and linkage on chromosome 6 near the HLA complex may explain associations between dyslexia and autoimmune diseases.[498]

Biology Boys learn language later than girls and are more prone to dyslexia. Finding candidate genes (eg DYX1C1)[499] seems easy, but remember: genes don't specify cognitive processes; they code regulatory factors, signalling molecules, receptors, and enzymes that interact in complex ways, modulated by environmental influences, in order to build and maintain a person's brain.

CNS examination shows left-sided cerebral lesions (rare) or changes may be seen *postmortem*, eg in perisylvian regions ± unusual asymmetry of the plenum temporale (Wernicke's area), with cortical dysplasia and scarring. *In vivo* characterization of this asymmetry is becoming possible.[500]

Perhaps dyslexia reflects weak connectivity between anterior and posterior parts of the language areas of the brain, and the angular gyrus. Positron emission images show that when dyslexic adults perform rhyme judgments and verbal short-term memory tasks they activate less than the full set of centres normally involved with these tasks. www.shianet.org/~reneenew/hist.html

Note that there is functional MRI observation of specific involvement of one subsystem of the visual pathways which prevents rapid processing of brief stimuli presented in quick temporal succession (*magnosystem hypothesis*).[501]

Tests The GAPS test aims to diagnose children before school starts.[502][503]

Management Make sure the 'dyslexia' is not from lack of teaching. The person may gain insight by discussing his or her problem with fellow sufferers, and by finding out about past dyslexics such as Leonardo da Vinci. Special educational programmes are available for addressing dyslexic problems, as the phonetic approach to learning to read usually presents problems. NB: 'wait-and-see' is not wise—studies support identification *before* school with exercises in sound categorization using rhyme and alliteration, with special teaching of letters.[504]

You may be asked about **dietary supplements** with highly unsaturated fatty acids (HUFA, eg Efalex®). These do play a role in neurodevelopment, but evidence of benefit in dyslexia from large randomized trials is sparse.[505] They appear to reduce dyslexia-associated delay in dark adaption.[506][n=10]

Patient pathways: descending the 'dark spiral'[1] of madness, as tweeted from a straightjacket in 1855

The next pages concern the psychiatrist as jailer. To reflect on this let us follow one patient's journey, along the edge of chaos, to his straightjacket via a series of verbatim tweets from the manic streets of Paris (with proposed timings).

3pm	Bought two velvet screens covered with hieroglyphic figures...to consecrate the forgiveness of heaven.
4pm	Met my friend George...wet through and tired out...laid on his bed.
6pm	Marvellous goddess appeared to me saying "I am the same as Mary, the same as your mother."
7pm	Said to George "Let's go out".
7.15pm	Crossing Pont des Arts explaining the transmigration of souls to him.
7.20pm	Told George...I have the soul of Napoleon in me commanding me to do great things.
7.30pm	In the Rue Du Coq I bought a hat. While George is waiting for my change I went to the Palais-Royal...everyone staring at me.
7.50pm	A persistent idea is fixing itself in my mind...there are no more dead.
8pm	Went through the Galerie de Foy saying "I have committed a sin...".
8.10pm	Somewhat interested in little girls dancing in rings.
8.15pm	Café de Foy...Dense crowd...nearly suffocated.
8.20pm	Extricated by 3 friends...into a cab...taken to Hospice De La Charité.
3.02am	Walking about various wards...I'm like a god with powers of healing.
3.05am	Laying my hands on some patients now.
3.20am	Going up to a statue of the Virgin Mary...
3.21am	Taking off its crown of flowers in order to test the power in me.
3.29am	Talking in an animated way of the ignorance of men who think they can be cured by science.
3.40am	Bottle of ether on the table...
3.42am	Drinking it in one gulp
3.43am	Hospital assistant with face like an angel trying to stop me
3.45am	Tell him he does not understand my mission.
3.55am	Doctors coming along.
4am	Harangue on the impotence of their art.
4.02am	Thrusting me into a straightjacket
6am	Am in an asylum outside Paris...

Gérard De Nerval
Aurélia 1855

Gérard De Nerval, whose tweets these are, was famous during his colourful life for extravagant orgies, eating ice-cream out of skulls[507] and for taking his pet lobster for walks in the gardens of the Palais Royal on a blue silk lead.

He hanged himself from a Paris street light in 1855.[508]

After his death his critics read and reread his masterpiece *Les Chimères* (a fragment of which appears below),[6] proclaiming it to be an infinite hall-ucination in a jewel of immense value.[509] We honour Gérard De Nerval here to remind ourselves that the next patient we imprison using mental health laws deserves our infinite respect, however rough their diamonds appear to be.

---

1 Un arc-en-ciel étrange entoure ce puits sombre,
Seuil de l'ancien chaos dont
le néant est l'ombre
Spirale engloutissant les Mondes et les Jours!

Around this tunnel plays a strange rainbow arc
On the edge of primeval chaos
whose hollow form is the spiral dark
That swallows up Worlds and Days!

Translation ©JML

AC	approved clinician	LSSA	local social services authority
AMHP	approved mental health professional	MCA	Mental Capacity Act 2005
ASW	approved social worker	MHAC	Mental Health Act Commission
CTO	community treatment order	MHRT	Mental Health Review Tribunal
ECHR	European Convention on Human Rights	NHSFT	NHS foundation trust
ECT	electro-convulsive therapy	PCT	primary care trust
GSCC	General Social Care Council	RC	responsible clinician
IMCA	independent mental capacity advocate	RMO	responsible medical officer
IMHA	independent mental health advocate	SCT	supervised community treatment
LHB	local health board	SOAD	Second Opinion Appointed Doctor

Before reading the subsequent pages which reflect the 1983 Mental Health Act it is vital to understand how the Act has been amended and added to by the 2007 Mental Health Act—which does not replace it—but rather sits beside it.

Imperatives governing use of Mental Health Acts (required in the 2007 act)
• Respect patients' past and present wishes and feelings.
• Minimize restrictions on liberty and involvement of patients in planning, developing and delivering care and treatment appropriate to them.
• Avoid unlawful discrimination.
• Pay due attention to the effectiveness of treatment.
• Respect the views of carers and other interested parties.
• Respect for diversity, including, in particular, diversity of religion, culture and sexual orientation (within the meaning of the Equality Act 2006).
• Patient wellbeing and safety, and public safety need balancing.

2007 Mental Health Act In 2007, three key measures were introduced:
1 Community treatment orders (CTOs) allow compulsory treatment in the community. As a safeguard, there is a duty to consider what risk there would be of a deterioration of the patient's condition if he were not detained (as a result, for example, of his refusing the treatment he requires for his mental disorder). CTOs have the same duration and renewal periods as section 3 (p400): 6 months initially, then renewed for 6 months, then renewed annually.
2 The criteria for a CTO is that the patient is detained after an application for admission for treatment, and it is necessary for his health and safety or for the protection of other persons that he receives treatment, which can be provided outside hospital (subject to a power of recall). CTO roles:
• Ensuring the patient receives the treatment stipulated.
• Preventing harm to the patient's health or safety. • Protection of others.
3 People diagnosed with severe antisocial personality disorders are now within the scope of mental health law and can be detained even if they have committed no crime, if they are deemed a danger to themselves or others.

Other provisions: A new statutory advocacy service for detained patients, and:
• Children are protected from being put in adult wards (section 140).
• 2 professionals from diverse disciplines must now agree to detention renewal.
• No ECT can be given in the face of capacitous refusal, other than in emergency. Emergency ECT can only be given if it is immediately necessary to save life or immediately necessary to prevent a serious deterioration.
• 16- and 17-year-olds' capacitous refusal of treatment cannot be overridden by parental authority; a SOAD is needed for ECT to be given; and there must be a referral for a MHR Tribunal annually for patients who do not request a hearing.
• There is a new 'treatability' test, ensuring compulsory treatment must be of 'therapeutic benefit'. The wording is: 'Any reference in the Act to medical treatment, in relation to mental disorder, shall be construed as a reference to medical treatment the purpose of which is to alleviate, or prevent a worsening of, the disorder or one or more of its symptoms or manifestations.'
• Patients may be transferred from one place of safety to another. The hope is that patients detained by police officers on section 136 will be quickly transferred from a police station to a therapeutic environment.[510]

Procedures governing use of compulsory powers (2007)[511]

Stage 1 *Preliminary examination:* Decisions to begin assessment and initial treatment of a patient under compulsory powers must be based on a preliminary opinion by two doctors and a social worker (or another suitably trained mental health professional) that a patient needs further assessment or urgent treatment by specialist mental health services and, without this, might be at risk of serious harm or pose a risk of serious harm to others.

Stage 2 *Formal assessment/initial treatment under compulsory powers:* A patient will be given a full assessment of his or her health and social care needs and receive a formal care plan; the initial period of assessment and treatment under compulsory powers is up to 28 days; after that, continuing use of compulsory powers must be authorized by a new independent decision making body, the Mental Health Tribunal, which gets advice from independent experts as well as taking evidence from the clinical team, the patient ± his or her representatives, and other agencies, as appropriate.

Stage 3 *Care and treatment order:* The Tribunal (or the Court in the case of mentally disordered offenders) can make a care and treatment order to authorize the care and treatment specified in a care plan recommended by the clinical team. This must be designed to give therapeutic benefit to the patient, or to manage behaviour associated with mental disorder that might lead to serious harm to other people. The 1st 2 orders can be up to 6 months each; subsequent orders may be for periods of up to 12 months.

NB: one new provision is that it is now possible for people with dangerous personality disorders to be detained before a crime has been committed.

Methodology/criteria for using CTOs (community treatment orders)

- A SOAD certificate must be issued authorizing the treatment. The SOAD is appointed in the normal way by the MHAC. The criteria for the SOAD authorization is simply that 'it is appropriate for the treatment to be given'. With SOADs, the certifying doctor has a duty to consult 2 statutory consultees but no duty to consult the patient or the responsible clinician.
- The treatment is immediately necessary and the patient has capacity and consents to its administration; or...
- The treatment is immediately necessary and the patient lacks capacity, but a deputy or the court of protection consents to it on his or her behalf.
- The patient lacks capacity and may resist the treatment, but force may be justified as proportionate response to the likelihood of serious harm to the patient, and the treatment is *either* immediately necessary to save the patient's life; *or* (not being irreversible) is immediately necessary to prevent serious deterioration; or (being neither irreversible nor hazardous) is immediately necessary to alleviate serious suffering; or (being neither irreversible nor hazardous, and the minimum interference necessary) is immediately necessary to prevent the patient from behaving violently or being a danger to her/himself or others.

Psychiatry

Provisions under the 1983 Act (in England)

▶The patient must have a mental disorder and need detention for treatment of it, or to protect himself or others, before compulsion may be used (if voluntary means have failed).

Admission for assessment (Mental Health Act[1] 1983, section 2)

- The period of assessment (and treatment) lapses after 28 days.
- Patient's appeals must be sent within 14 days to the Mental Health Tribunal (composed of a doctor, lay person, and lawyer).
- An approved social worker (or the nearest relative) makes the application on the recommendation of 2 doctors (not from the same hospital), one of whom is 'approved' under the Act (in practice a psychiatric consultant or senior registrar). The other doctor should ideally know the patient in a professional capacity. If this is not possible, the Code of Practice recommends that the second doctor should be an 'approved' doctor.

Section 3: admission for treatment (for ≤6 months)

- The exact mental disorder must be stated.
- Detention is renewable for a further 6 months (annually thereafter).
- 2 doctors must sign the appropriate forms and know why treatment in the community is contraindicated. They must have seen the patient within 24h. They must state that treatment is likely to benefit the patient, or prevent deterioration; or that it is necessary for the health or safety of the patient or the protection of others.

Section 4: emergency treatment (for ≤72h)

- The admission to hospital must be an urgent necessity.
- May be used if admission under section 2 would cause undesirable delay (admission must follow the recommendation rapidly).
- An approved social worker or the nearest relative makes the application after recommendation from one doctor (eg the GP).
- The GP should keep a supply of the relevant forms, as the social worker may be unobtainable (eg with another emergency).
- It is usually converted to a section 2 on arrival in hospital, following the recommendation of the duty psychiatrist. If the second recommendation is not completed, the patient should be discharged as soon as the decision not to is made. The Section should not be allowed to lapse.

Detention of a patient already in hospital: section 5(2) (≤72h)

- The doctor in charge (or, if a consultant psychiatrist, his or her deputy, applies to the hospital administrator, day or night.
- A patient in an A&E department is not in a ward, so cannot be detained under this section. Common law is all that is available, to provide temporary restraint 'on a lunatic who has run amok and is a manifest danger either to himself or to others'[512] while awaiting an assessment by a psychiatrist.[513]
- Plan where the patient is to go before the 72h has elapsed, eg by liaising with psychiatrists for admission under section 2.

Nurses' holding powers: section 5(4) (for ≤6h)

- Any authorized psychiatric nurse may forcibly detain a voluntary 'mental' patient who is taking his own discharge against advice, if such a discharge would be likely to involve serious harm to the patient (eg suicide) or others.
- During the 6h the nurse must find the necessary personnel to sign a section 5 application or allow the patient's discharge.

---

1 This Act operates in England; Scottish law is different. The situation in the UK is changing and these pages should be read along with current legislation in the area where you are working.

Psychiatry

Section 7: application for guardianship Enables patients to receive community care if it cannot be provided without using compulsory powers.
- Application is made by an 'approved social worker (ASW)' or 'nearest relative' and also needs two medical recommendations.
- The guardian, usually a social worker, can require the patient to live in a specified place, to attend at specified places for treatment and to allow authorized persons access.

Renewal of compulsory detention in hospital: section 20(4)
- The patient continues to suffer from a mental disorder and would benefit from continued hospital treatment.
- Further admission is needed for the health or safety of the patient—which cannot be achieved except by forced detention.

Section 25: supervised discharge This is as a result of the Mental Health (Patients in the Community) Act 1995—incorporated within the 1983 Act.
- It allows formal supervision to ensure that a patient who has been detained for treatment under the Act receives follow-up care.
- The application is made at the time of detention for treatment by the Responsible Medical Officer. It is supported by an ASW and a doctor involved in the patient's treatment in the community.
- A supervisor is appointed who can convey the patient to a place where treatment is given.

Section 117: Aftercare & the Care Programme Approach (CPA) Section 117 requires provision of after-care for patients who have been detained on the 'long sections' (3, 37, 47, or 48). The CPA is not part of the Act but stipulates that no patient should be discharged without planned aftercare: the systematic assessment of health and social needs, an agreed care plan, the allocation of a keyworker, and regular reviews of progress.

Section 136 (for ≥72h) allows police to arrest a person 'in a place to which the public have access' who is believed to be suffering from a mental disorder. The patient must be conveyed to a 'place of safety' (usually a designated A&E department—better than a police station; a police station is rarely a place of safety and most people dying in police custody will have mental health problems and will have been on the receiving end of excess force employed by undertrained officers). In a hospital there can be a full assessment by a doctor (usually a psychiatrist) and an approved social worker. The patient must be discharged after assessment or detained under section 2 or 3.

Section 135 This empowers an approved social worker who believes that someone is being ill-treated or is neglecting himself to apply to a magistrate to search for and admit such patients. The ASW or a registered medical practitioner must accompany the police.

Psychiatry

Capacity entails being able to grasp and retain information relevant to a decision, and to weigh it as part of a process of making that decision.[514] ^{Mental Capacity Act 2005}

Consent to treatment comes in Part 4 of the Mental Health Act; it applies to:
• Treatments for mental disorder.
• All formal patients unless detained under sections 4, 5, 35, 135 and 136. The Act doesn't apply to those subject to Guardianship or Supervised Discharge, who have the right to refuse treatment, except in emergencies.

Where a person is deemed to have given their consent to treatment under Section 57 or Section 58, the person can withdraw that consent at any time. The treatment must then stop and the appropriate procedures followed, unless discontinuing treatment would cause 'serious suffering' to the patient, in which case continued treatment *may* be justified.

Section 57: treatments requiring consent *and* a 2nd opinion Some treatments are deemed so restricting that patients cannot automatically have them even if they do consent. Also, 3 people (1 doctor and 2 others who cannot be doctors) must certify that the person concerned is capable of understanding the nature, purpose and likely effects of the treatment and has consented to it (**competence**). They are appointed by the Mental Health Act Commission. Treatments falling into this category are destruction of brain tissue, or functioning and implantation of hormones to reduce male sex drive.

Section 58: treatments requiring consent *or* a 2nd opinion Applies to people who are detained under certain Sections without consent, or where the person is not able to consent, eg to ECT or drugs for a mental disorder if 3 months since the person first had the drugs during their current period of detention under the Act. In the first 3 months the treatment can be given without consent. The 3-month period starts from when drugs are first given.

If the person is capable of understanding the nature, purpose and effects of the treatment and consents to it, the Responsible Medical Officer (RMO) must certify that understanding and consent are present. If the person is capable of understanding the nature, purpose and likely effects of the treatment and doesn't consent to it, or has ↓capacity so cannot consent, then a doctor is appointed by the Mental Health Act Commission to give a 2nd opinion. She must consult 2 professionals involved in the patient's treatment; one must be a nurse.

The certificates must state the treatment plan in precise terms, eg the number of ECT treatments. If the plan changes, new certificates are required.

The provisions of Section 58 don't prevent urgent treatment (sect 62).

Section 62: urgent treatment The requirements of Section 57 and Section 58 need not be followed for urgent treatment to save the patient's life or to...
• Prevent serious deterioration, so long as the treatment is not irreversible.
• Alleviate serious suffering (if the treatment isn't irreversible or hazardous).
• Prevent the patient behaving violently or endangering self or others, so long as the treatment is neither irreversible nor hazardous, and is not excessive.

Section 37: Hospital Orders made by Courts This allows a Court to send a person to hospital for treatment, or to make the person subject to Guardianship, when the outcome might otherwise have been a prison sentence. The Order is instead of imprisonment, a fine, or probation. The person concerned...
• Will have been convicted by a Magistrates Court or Crown Court of an offence punishable with imprisonment (except in the case of murder, where the Court has to impose a sentence of life imprisonment in all cases).
• May not have been convicted, but may be charged with an imprisonable offence. Without convicting the person, the Court can make a Hospital Order under Section 37 if there is mental illness or severe mental impairment.

The initial period is 6 months from the Order's date. It can be renewed under Section 20 for 6 months and then annually. The Court must be satisfied that...

- There really is a mental illness, as evidenced by 2 doctors who must agree at least in part as to the type of mental illness or impairment present...and...
- The nature and degree of the mental disorder makes it appropriate for the person to be detained in hospital for medical treatment (that the treatment is likely to alleviate or prevent a deterioration of the person's condition in the case of psychopathic disorder or mental impairment)...and...
- Making a Section 37 Order is the best way to deal with the person...and ...
- A specific hospital is willing and able to admit the person within 28 days.

Section 61: review of treatment Where a treatment plan is being carried out under Section 57 (or 58 without consent), the RMO must report to the Mental Health Act Commission if the period of detention is renewed under Section 20.
- The Commission may demand a report at any other time if it wishes.
- The Commission can cancel the certificate under which treatment is given.
- In the case of people subject to Restriction Orders a report on the treatment being given must be provided for the Commission:
  1 6 months after the restriction order or direction is made, and
  2 At times when the RMO reports to the Home Office on the person's condition.

Deprivation of liberty safeguards (DoLS) *Use:* eg after being admitted to a rest home during an infection when a patient lacked capacity, and the doctor 'acted in his best interests'. DoLS provide the person with a representative, and...
- DoLS allow a challenge in the Court of Protection against 'false imprisonment.'
- DoLS give a right for deprivation of liberty to be reviewed regularly.

Source: patient.co.uk/doctor/

Psychiatry

Enriching consent: making decisions truly informed (GMC advice)[515]

We mustn't assume that because a patient lacks capacity today for one issue that he will lack capacity on all issues. We must plan for changes in capacity. Extra support will be needed for those with dementia and learning difficulties. NB: where possible, use multimedia formats to explain issues: we know these are better at making difficult decisions *truly informed*.[516]

Children under 16 disagreeing with their parents[517]

Capacity matters, not age. Parents' wishes are *not* supreme if the child has capacity (above). If you take a decision for a patient, you must have a 'reasonable belief' that capacity is lacking and that the act is in his/her best interests.

Medicolegal issues—use of Common Law in clinical situations

Clinical situations *Deliberate self-harm* Adapted from Feldman 2000:[518] 'A 30 year old male is brought to A&E after an overdose. There is no history available and the patient refuses to say anything, other than he wants to be left alone to die. He refuses to give blood for a drug level and is refusing any treatment. What should we do?'* Should we assume he has full capacity? If so, he may die—but autonomy is maintained. Or should the clinician act in the patient's best interests (the doctrine of necessity) as part of their duty of care? Most people who self-harm are depressed—but this does not prove incapacity. However, in the acute setting, Feldman asserts that 'there are usually good grounds for reasonable doubt with respect to the patient's capacity to make a fully informed and reasoned choice, and to proceed with whatever action is necessary to save his life under the common law'.

Restraint: The Mental Health Act is an *enabling act* (it needn't be used in all valid situations). Its use gives certain legal safeguards for patients and staff. 'A 40 year old female with alcohol problems has been admitted to hospital following a head injury 2 days ago. She has shown fluctuating levels of confusion, agitation and is now trying to leave the ward.'* Here, due to refusal or lack of capacity, the transient nature of the disturbance, and the need for intervention, common law is applicable. If stronger measures are needed, or the situation persists, it is wise to use the Mental Health Act to detain a patient with delirium; however it is not commonly used.

Lying thus in the sun one is liberated from doubts and from misgivings; it is not that problems and difficulties are resolved, it is that they are banished. The sun's radiation penetrates the mind...anaesthetizing thought. AE Ellis, 1958 The Rack

Some people find that depressions start in winter, and remit in spring or summer. It is postulated that disordered secretion of the indole melatonin from the pineal gland is to blame in some patients with SAD. **Melatonin**, the hormone of darkness, is secreted by the pineal only at night, eg at 30μg/night.

Dysregulated circadian rhythms and novel antidepressants Sleep disturbance is often seen in depression, and manipulating the sleep-wake cycle is one methodology for treating depression, so maybe dysregulated circadian rhythms really are causal. Our circadian rhythms are regulated by a core biological clock in the hypothalamic suprachiasmatic nucleus. Its pacemaker activity is regulated by light (and nonphotic modulatory pathways) via serotonergic input from the raphe, and melatonin originating from the pineal gland. We note with interest that agomelatine, a new antidepressant, acts as an agonist at melatonergic MT1 and MT2 receptors and as an antagonist at 5-HT2C receptors. It is known to resynchronize the sleep-awake cycle (in animals).[519]

Treatment choices As a rule, the more that typical winter symptoms (hypersomnia, carbohydrate craving and weight gain) predominate, the more likely that light therapy should be a treatment of first choice. But if winter episodes are characterized by early morning wakening and weight loss, and especially if there are non-seasonal recurrences, traditional antidepressants are advised.

Light therapy
- The antidepressant effect of light is potentiated by early-morning administration in circadian time, optimally at ~8.5 hours after melatonin onset or 2.5 hours after a sleep's midpoint.[520] N=42
- A dose-response effect exists between the amount of light administered in phototherapy and the degree of improvement in depression (as measured on Hamilton ratings). 6h/day of increased light brought about a 53% decrease in scores, whereas treatments of 2h (or red-light treatment) produced only a 25% reduction. These effects were correlated with suppressed plasma melatonin concentrations at 23.00h. Variables of uncertain importance include: the type of light (device and spectrum), distance between patient and source, and the duration of treatment.[521]
- Therapy should stimulate the nasal retina, as retinal ganglion cells projecting to suprachiasmatic nuclei are unequally distributed.[522] N=8
- However, evidence in this area is often contradictory, and it is probably unwise to rush into recommending light for all patients whose recurrent depressions start in the autumn or winter. This might have the undesirable effect of enticing such patients to book unaffordable winter holidays to exotic locations—with inevitable disappointments and recriminations.

Antidepressants
Sedative antidepressants are usually avoided and selective serotonin reuptake inhibitors (SSRIs) are often 1st choice. Newer antidepessants to consider: agomelatine, an agonist of melatonergic MT1 & MT2 receptors and antagonist of 5-HT2 receptors. It appears to resynchronize disturbed circadian rhythms and to reduces depression.[523] It also causes less sexual dysfunction compared with SSRIs (5% vs 62%).[524] Venlafaxine and reboxetine may also have a role. In patients with established winter recurrences, it is usual to instigate treatment as soon as symptoms re-emerge in the autumn and to phase out treatment in spring. For patients who also experience non-seasonal episodes, year-round prophylaxis may be deployed, sometimes regularly increasing the antidepressant dose during the winter months.[525]

Community care

Since the early 1980s, most UK inpatients with psychosis have had the focus of their care moved from hospital to the community. The aim has been to save money and improve care, but in the UK this policy is now being partly reversed. Has community care failed, or have there been successes? Five questions keep recurring, each (ominously) prefixed by a 'Surely...'

1 *Surely hospitals will always be needed for severely affected people?* In general, the problem is not the severity of the mental illness, but its social context which determines if community care is appropriate.

2 *Surely community care, if it is done properly, will be more expensive than hospital care, where resources can be concentrated?* Not so—at least not necessarily so. Some concentration of resources *can* take place in the community in day hospitals and mental illness hostels. It is also true that the 'bed and breakfast' element of inpatient care is expensive, if the running and maintenance costs associated with deploying inpatient psychiatric services are taken into account. In most studies, costs of each type of service doesn't differ much, and sometimes good community care turns out cheaper.[526,527]

3 *Surely there will be more homicides and suicides if disturbed patients are not kept in hospital?* Offending by the mentally ill is of great public concern (60 homicides/yr in England). A cohort study however found rates of violent offending are low and the strongest association with offending was previous offending. Psychiatric variables were less important, with diagnosis and number of previous admissions showing no significant association. Substance misuse and sexual abuse are associated with increased offending risk.[528]

4 *Surely if inpatient psychiatric beds are not available, however good the daytime team is in the community, some patients will still need somewhere to go at night?* The implication is that the skills available in bed-and-breakfast accommodation may be inadequate at times of day when there is no other support, other than the general practitioner. Studies that have looked at this have certainly found an increase in non-hospital residential care in those selected for community care, and this increase may be as much as 280% over 5yrs. In the UK, new proposals guarantee 24-hour open access to skilled help, but it is not known what pressures this will put services under.

5 *Surely community care will involve a huge bureaucracy in pursuit of the unattainable goal of 100% safety?* This will be so if every patient has a lengthy care plan and repeated risk assessments. Concern for safety may also spawn a non-therapeutic custodial relationship.

Advantages reported for community care are: better social functioning, satisfaction with life, employment, and drug compliance—but in randomized studies in the UK these advantages are not always manifest. Furthermore, trends have been repeatedly found indicating that the longer studies go on for, the harder it is to maintain the initial advantages of community care. If it is hard for teams to keep up their enthusiasm during a trial, it will probably be even harder when the trial period has ended, or when team members are ill. These constraints may in part explain the observation that with inadequately funded and supervised community care, patients can fail to get essential services, and when hospitals are being run down, and a patient's condition worsens, so that 'sectioning' followed by admission becomes impossible, the patient is left in the community 'rotting with his rights on'. *Assertive community care and case management* is one way out of this impasse (here a key-worker has direct responsibility for care plans). This set-up helps ensure more people remain in contact with psychiatric services (NNT=15); this inevitably increases hospital admission rates.[529,530] When combined with family therapy and social skills training results are good.[531]

Social deprivation is positively associated with premature mortality, and poverty makes almost *all* diseases more likely (but not Hodgkin's disease, eczema, bulimia, or melanoma).[532] See *Health and social class*, p463. In the UK, the number of homeless people is 1-2 million. >30% suffer from mental illness (10% have schizophrenia), most do not know where to go for help, and most have no doctor. A 3-tier strategy may help. 1 Emergency shelters 2 Transitional accommodation 3 Long-term housing.

The cost in health terms to society and the individual is enormous. Diseases and symptoms such as diarrhoea, which may pass as a minor inconveniences to the well-housed, may be a major hurdle for the homeless, with severe social and psychological effects. Capture-recapture techniques show that the *unobserved* population of the homeless is about twice that observed. This method of enumeration collects samples (lists) and looks for tags (duplicates) in subsequent counts, and from this determines the degree of under-counting. If all in the subsequent count are duplicates, then there is no underestimate of the original count. Statistical techniques can allow for migration in and out of the population area.[533] These studies show that psychiatric morbidity is greatest in the observed homeless populations: the implication is that the psychiatric illness makes these people more 'visible'.

In the UK, as in many other Western countries, what started out as an enlightened policy of looking after people with mental health problems in the community (p405) has resulted in large numbers of psychiatric patients living on the street in grinding poverty—relieved by occasional admissions to often overcrowded acute units. This 'revolving door' model of care has failed many patients, not least because continuity of care is compromised.

One way to tackle poverty is to pay people not to be poor: in the 1990s, in Singapore, poor families were paid SP\$26,400 over 20yrs if they had ≤2 children. But economic success in Singapore evolved independently[534] from this idea which was perhaps *too* Quixotic (ie innocently impractical, see BOX).

Income Support[UK] is an income-related (means-tested) benefit paid to those who do not have enough money to live on. Income is subtracted from a standard fixed income level (the 'applicable amount'), and the difference is the amount of Income Support payable. The person's capital is also taken into account. Income Support is a non-contributory benefit. This means that a person does not have to have paid any National Insurance contributions in order to qualify for Income Support. The rates of Income Support are fixed each year by government and are usually increased every April. Income Support acts as a 'passport' to certain other help. A claimant and her/his partner will automatically qualify for: • Free school meals • Free prescriptions • Free dental care • Vouchers for spectacles • Free milk and vitamins for expectant mothers and children under 5 • Free vitamins for nursing mothers • Maximum housing benefit • Maximum council tax benefit.

Epidemiology There is no evidence that simply living in a deprived area makes a person more prone to illness and death. All the excess mortality and morbidity is explained by the person being poor.[535] Their immediate neighbours who are not poor do not share the same risk. So we need to target care at poor people wherever they live, not at poor areas.

Poverty, reoffending, and mentally ill offenders[536] *Two contrasting ideas:* 1 The economic arguments for keeping non-violent mentally ill criminals out of prison and rehabilitating them are self-evident. 2 Prison provides an ideal opportunity to treat people who are mentally ill who might otherwise be hard to reach. They should have optimum treatment to improve their quality of life, as well as to lessen the risk of reoffending.

Psychiatry

'The innkeeper acquainted all in the inn with the lunacy of his guest (Don Quixote), about his standing vigil over his armour and the knighting he expected. They marvelled at so odd a form of madness and went to watch him at a distance, and saw that with a serene expression he sometimes pranced to and fro; at other times, leaning on his lance, he turned his eyes to his armour without turning them away for a long time. Night had fallen; but the moon shone with such a lustre as might almost vie with the sun who lent it; so that everything our new knight did was seen clearly by everyone. Just then it occurred to one of the mule-drivers in the inn to water his pack of mules, and for this it was necessary to move Don Quixote's armour, which was on the trough; our knight, seeing them approach, called in a booming voice:

"Oh thou, whosoever thou art, reckless knight, who would touch the armour of the most valiant knight whoever took up arms! Take heed what thou doest, and touch it not, unless thou wouldst pay for thy audacity with thy life."

The muleteer cared not a jot for this reasoning—it would have been better for him if he had, for it meant caring for his health. Instead, picking the armour up by the straps, he tossed it a good distance. And seeing this, Don Quixote lifted his gaze to the skies and, turning his thoughts (as it seemed) to his lady Dulcinea, he said:

"Help me, my lady, in this the first insult aimed at this thy servant's breast; in this my first crisis let not thy grace and protection fail me."

And, continuing this line of argument, and dropping his shield, he raised his lance in both hands and gave the mule-driver such a clout on the head as to demolish him; if this first blow had been followed by a second, he would have had no need for a doctor ('*maestro*') to cure him. Having done this, Don Quixote picked up his armour and began to pace again with the same gravity as before. A short time later, unaware of what had happened—for the first mule driver lay stunned—a second approached, also intending to water his mules, and when he began to remove the armour so as to get to the trough, without so much as a by-your-leave or even a word, Don Quixote let slip his shield and raised his lance, and without quite reducing the second mule-driver's head to smithereens, he thrice sliced it, fracturing the skull in four places. When they heard the noise, all the people in the inn hurried over, among them the innkeeper. When he saw this, Don Quixote took up his shield, placed his hand on his sword, saying:

"Oh queen of beauty, whose spark and fire warms the sickness in my heart (*debilitado corazón mío*)! From your greatness, it is time that you do bend your eye on this thy slavish knight, who expects so vast an exploit."

And with this he acquired, it seemed to him, so much courage, that if all the mule-drivers in the world charged him he would never retreat one step. The wounded men's comrades, seeing their two fallen friends, began to rain stones down on Don Quixote, and he did all he could to deflect them with his shield, not daring to move away from the trough and leave his armour unprotected. The innkeeper implored them to stop as he had already told them the knight was mad, and whatever the number of deaths no wind of blame could ever extinguish his innocence.'[538]

Don Quijote de la Mancha[539] by Miguel de Cervantes[540] 1547-1616; see translations by Shelton (1605),[541] Grossman (2003, HarperCollins) & Jarvis (OUP) chapter 3 (p33-5).

We present the idealistic knight-errant who teaches us to value the very things he is deluded by: heroism and valour.[537]

Psychiatry

Postnatal depression

Risk of major depression is 3-fold that of those with no recent pregnancy. Causes: social circumstances; sleep deprivation; genetic; hormonal change.[542]

Natural history Although most postnatal depression resolves in ≤6 months, don't put off treatment, and just hope for the best. *Consider these facts:*
• For the patient, 6 months is a long, long time.
• For the infant, 6 months is more than a long time: it's literally an age.
• Suicide is a waste, but for a young family, a mother's suicide is especially destructive—unthinkable, indeed, for those who have not experienced it.
• Postnatal depression impairs infant cognitive and social skills.[543,544]

What's it like having postnatal depression? *Here is a blog:* "I had the normal baby blues in the 1st couple of weeks following his birth. I was weepy at the drop of a hat, recovering quickly after a good cry. Often I would gaze at my son, crying from pure joy. But then things changed...I began to look at him and feel absolutely nothing. An empty void. Then the visions started. I would be holding him and see, in my mind, him alone in the woods as it snowed around him, crying for help that never came. The vision was overpowering, and I wept for that baby lost in the woods. I swore that I would never do such a thing but it seemed a betrayal of him just to see that image, which haunted me endlessly. I had difficulties with breastfeeding and took it as a sign that I was failing as a mother. That, the awful vision, and anything that went the slightest bit wrong, only solidified my conviction that I should never have been given charge of this tiny, precious life. I would lie awake at night, listening to him breathe, afraid that if I nodded off he might die. But I also daydreamed endlessly about how nice life was before being a mother. Often I wished desperately that I could just give him back, then hated myself."[545]

Help ▶*Have a low threshold for referring to multidisciplinary teams in mother-and-baby units.* The first step is to try not to be caught unawares by a major depression that apparently strikes like a bolt from the blue, but which, in reality, has been building up over time. Pregnancy and infant-motherhood is supposed to be a time of unclouded joy. We often collude with this view. We are always hearing ourselves saying: "Oh Mrs Salt, what a lovely baby! You must be so pleased—and you always wanted a little boy. We are so delighted for you..." But what if *she* is not delighted? She hardly dares confess her traitorous thoughts saying that she is unaccountably sad, that she spends the nights crying, and that her exhausted days are filled with a sense of foreboding that she or some other agency will harm the child. The place to start to pre-empt these feelings is in the antenatal clinic. ▶Involve fathers;[546] explain: "When the baby comes you'll need help and rest—don't think you can do it all yourself: become a team—eg taking turns in getting the baby off to sleep".[547] In the puerperium give permission for the new mother to tell her woe. When this is revealed, counselling, and input from a health visitor and a psychiatrist is wise, as is close follow-up. You may need to arrange emergency admission under the Mental Health Act: but the point of being prepared for postnatal depression is to avoid things getting this bad. Interventions for persistent depression need to address relationship difficulties as well as depressive symptoms.[548]

Pharmacology Short-term, **fluoxetine** is as good as **cognitive-behaviour therapy**. More trials with longer follow-up are needed to compare drugs and psychotherapy.[549] Although all antidepressants are excreted in breast milk, tricyclics and SSRIs are rarely detectable by standard tests. Observe babies for possible SEs; it may be best to stop breastfeeding if large doses are used.

Adding **lithium** (p354) or ECT may help. Evidence on **oestrogen** is conflicting (use is non-standard)—*dose example:* 3 months of transdermal 17β-estradiol (200µg/day) for 3 months on its own, then with added dydrogesterone 10mg/day for 12 days each month for 3 more months. CI: uterine, cervical, or breast neoplasia; past thromboembolism/thrombophlebitis; breastfeeding.[550]

Edinburgh postnatal depression scale (EPDS)[562,563]

1 *I've been able to laugh & see the funny side of things:*	As much as always could
	Not quite so much now
	Definitely not so much
	Now not at all
2 *I've looked forward with enjoyment to things:*	As much as I ever did
	Rather less than before
	Definitely less than before
	Hardly at all
3 ★*I've blamed myself unnecessarily when things went wrong:*	Yes, most of the time
	Yes, some of the time
	Not very often
	No, never
4 *I've been anxious or worried for no good reason:*	No, not at all
	Hardly ever
	Yes, sometimes
	Yes, very often
5 *I've felt scared/panicky for no very good reason:*	Yes, quite a lot
	Yes, sometimes
	No, not much
	No, not at all
6 ★*Things have been getting on top of me:*	Yes, most of the time I haven't been able to cope at all
	Yes, sometimes I haven't been coping as well as usual
	No, most of the time I have coped quite well
	No, I have been coping as well as ever
7 ★*I've been so unhappy that it is difficult to sleep:*	Yes, most of the time
	Yes, sometimes
	Not very often
	No, not at all
8 ★*I've felt sad or miserable:*	Yes, most of the time
	Yes, quite often
	Not very often
	No, not at all
9 ★*I've been so unhappy that I've been crying:*	Yes, most of the time
	Yes, quite often
	Only occasionally
	No, never
10 ★*Thoughts of harming myself have occurred to me:*	Yes, quite often
	Sometimes
	Hardly ever
Instructions *Underline what comes closest to how you have felt in the last 7 days.*	Never

Never trust this sort of thing totally; ~40% lie on the form, being afraid that health visitors would call in social services (± removal of baby).

Ask to score answers 0, 1, 2, or 3 according to increased severity; some (★above) are reverse scored (3, 2, 1, 0). Add scores for 1–10 for the total. Let her complete the scale herself, eg at the 8-week check-up, unless literary difficulty. ►A score of 12/30 has a sensitivity of 77% for postnatal depression (specificity: 93%).

Validity is not very good; in one study;[552] face-to-face detection may be better.[1]

Prognosis of children whose mothers have postnatal depression A longitudinal study over 11 years shows that a good clinical interview (in contrast to the EPDS) can identify mothers whose children are at an ↑risk (4-fold) of developing psychiatric disorder in later childhood.[553]

---

1 High rates of postnatal relapse occur if past psychosis, perhaps ♦ triggered by postdelivery fall in estrogens, causing dysregulation of CNS dopaminergic systems. Oestrogens may not prevent this, but of the 40% of women relapsing, those on the high doses of estradiol (800µg/day) need less psychotropics, and are discharged sooner than those on low doses.[554] Methodological problems abound in this area.

410 **5 Ophthalmology**

What shall human optics know...?
my twenty six selves
bulging in immortal spring...
farthest becomes near (e e cummings)

*D*octors assume that our eyes are passive organs whose sole job is receiving and organizing photons. Philosophers and physiologists are less sure. Ludwig Wittgenstein said "we do not see the human eye as a receiver, it appears not to let anything in, but to send something out. The ear receives; the eye looks. (It casts glances, it flashes, radiates, gleams.) One can terrify with one's eyes, not with one's ear or nose. When you see the eye, you see something going out from it. You see the look in the eye. If you only shake free from your physiological prejudices, you will find nothing queer about the fact that the glance of the eye can be seen too. For I also say that I see the look that you cast at someone else."[1]

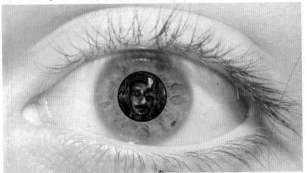

Fig 1. Between blinks.   Derived from image of an eye, ©Ken Banks.

⁞ If you were Wittgenstein's pupil[1] (fig1) and he cast you one of his notorious glances in a tutorial, would you meet his gaze? Choosing where to look can be perplexing. You might toy with the idea of looking him in the eye, but then back off. MRI shows different parts of the medial frontal cortex are active when we choose to make eye movements of our own free will, compared with when we face duress and conflicting choices.[2]

So studying eye movements teaches us about the seat of the soul, if we accept that appreciating and resolving ambiguities is the essence of consciousness.

1 *Pupilla* is Latin for doll. Pupils are named after our own doll-like reflections, seen on gazing into an eye, which perfectly mirror our movements.[3] (Wittgenstein's pupils were never so obedient.)

We thank Brinda Muthusamy MRCP, MRCOphth for masterminding this chapter, and Gillian Bennerson and the imaging department at the Bristol Eye Hospital for permission to reproduce images.

*A*ccommodation Changing of lens shape to focus near objects, using the ciliary muscle. Young lenses can go from furthest (a star) to nearest in 0.35 seconds (approaching kisses go out of focus at ~7cm: see p426).[4]

Acuity A measure of how well the eye sees a small or distant object (p415).

Amblyopia ↓Acuity uncorrectable by lenses, with no anatomic defect.[5]

Amsler grid Test chart of intersecting lines used for screening for macular disease. If present, lines may appear wavy and squares distorted.

Anisocoria Unequal pupil size.

Anisometropia Having different refractive errors in each eye.

Aphakia The state of having no lens (eg removed because of cataract).

Blepharitis Inflamed lids.

Canthus The medial or lateral angle made by the open lids.

Chemosis Oedema of the conjunctiva.

Choroid Vascular coat between the retina and the outer scleral coat.

Ciliary body Portion of uvea (uveal tract) between iris and choroid, containing ciliary processes and ciliary muscle (for accommodation).

Conjunctiva Mucous membrane on anterior sclera and posterior lid aspect.

Cycloplegia Ciliary muscle paralysis preventing accommodation.

Dacryocystitis Inflammation of the lacrimal sac.

Dioptre Units for measuring refractive power of lenses.

Ectropion The lids evert (especially lower lid).

Entropion The lids invert (so that the lashes may irritate the eyeball).

Epiphora Passive overflow of tears on to the cheek (p419).

Fornix Where bulbar (scleral) and palpebral (lid) conjunctivae meet.

Fovea Cone-rich area of macula capable of 6/6 vision, p447. Foveola: p445.

Fundus That part of retina normally visible through the ophthalmoscope.

Keratoconus The cornea is shaped like a cone. See p458.

Keratomalacia The cornea is softened.

Limbus The annular border between clear cornea and opaque sclera.

Macula Retinal area ~5mm across, lateral to optic disc (surrounds fovea),[p]445.

Miotic An agent causing pupil constriction (eg pilocarpine).

Mydriatic An agent causing pupil dilatation (eg tropicamide).

Near point Where the eye is looking when maximally accommodated.

Papillitis Inflammation of the optic nerve head.

Optic cup The cup-like depression in the centre of the optic disc (p441).

Optic disc That part of optic nerve seen ophthalmoscopically in the fundus.

Presbyopia Age-related reduced near-acuity from failing accommodation.

Pterygium Wing-shaped degenerative conjunctival condition (p416).

Ptosis Drooping lids.

Refraction Ray deviation on passing through media of different density; or determining refractive errors and correcting them with lenses.

Retinal detachment The sensory retina separates from the pigmented epithelial layer of retina.

Sclera The whites of the eyes starting from the corneal perimeter.

Scotoma A defect causing a part of the field of view to go missing.

Slit lamp A device which illuminates and magnifies structures in the eye.

Strabismus (squint) Eyes deviate (they are not looking at the same thing).

Tarsorrhaphy A surgical procedure for uniting upper and lower lids.

Tonometer A device for measuring intraocular pressure.

Uvea Iris, ciliary body and choroid.

Vitreous Jelly like substance filling the globe behind the lens.

Vitrectomy Surgical removal of the vitreous.

Ophthalmology

Medicine is a foreign language: learn it by using it—and don't be put off by the size of the task: remember...there are no native speakers!

Asking about trauma, symptoms of pain *vs* irritation, loss of vision, and pattern and speed of onset help direct examination towards visual acuity (never omit!), optic nerve function (pupil reaction; colour vision), visual fields, eye movements and ophthalmoscopy to assess the media and the retina (p455).

Acuity is a measure of the clarity or sharpness of vision; always test it carefully as any loss may be serious. Record it accurately, especially in a patient with eye injury. Examine the right eye first. Sit the patient 6 metres from the Snellen chart (p415); to get 6 metres in a 4-metre room, place the chart just above the patient, pointing towards a mirror 3 metres away. Obscure the left eye with a lollipop-shaped eye paddle or card, not *pressed* to the eye, but just enough to *occlude* the visual axis (more reliable than peepable through fingers or a slipping palm). Ask the patient to read the chart from the top using the right eye, then the left. Use glasses if worn. The last line completed indicates the acuity for distant vision. An objective test of vision? *Not quite!*[1]

The chart is designed so that the top line can be read by someone with normal vision at 60 metres, the next at 36 metres, the next at 24, the next at 18, the next at 12, the next at 9, and the next at 6 metres. Acuity is recorded as 6/60, 6/36, 6/24, 6/18, 6/12, 6/9, 6/6 to indicate the last line accurately read (6/6 vision is normal). For acuities <6/60 patients can be brought forward to 5, 4, 3, 2 and 1 metre from the chart to read the top line. If he can read it then acuity is expressed as that distance, eg 5/60, 4/60, 3/60, 2/60 or 1/60. If the vision is below 1/60 ask the patient to count your fingers at 50cm distance. This is recorded as CF (count fingers). If unable to count your fingers move your hand in front of the eye at a distance of 25cm. If he can detect movement, record HM (hand movement). If he cannot see this, dim the lights and shine a torch into the eye. If the patient perceives light, record PL. If there is no perception, record 'no PL' (the eye is blind). NB: in practice, if nothing on the Snellen chart can be read, it is common to go straight to finger counting.

If the patient sees less than 6/6 with or without glasses, examine again with a **pinhole** in front of the eye: a narrow beam removes the need for focus. In simple refractive errors, acuity will improve through the pinhole. This is an important test as it shows that refractive errors are the likely cause of reduced acuity. (Make a pin-hole with a 22G needle in a 10×10cm opaque card; check that you can see through the hole before giving it to the patient.)

If patients >40 years old complain of near-vision blurring, the cause may be presbyopia (p426). Test near vision using a near vision testing card (p414). If the patient can read N5 at 30cm, near vision is normal.

Visual field This is the area that can be seen with both eyes without shifting gaze. The uniocular field is smaller than the binocular field. Questions to address: does the defect affect one eye or both? Are there any clear boundaries to the defect? Does the boundary lie in the vertical or horizontal meridians? Is acuity affected? Confrontation tests: p428.

Extraocular movements It is vital to examine these in those with diplopia. Ask the patient to watch a pencil move diagonally: up left; up right; down left; down right; horizontally left; horizontally right. Ask which movement provokes most diplopia, and when looking in that direction, block each eye in turn and ask which one sees the *outer* image: that is the eye which is malfunctioning. NB: avoid extremes of movement as inability to maintain fixation stimulates nystagmus. For eye movements and squint, see p422.

Ophthalmoscopy This helps detect pathology in the lens, vitreous, and retina. Start with high + numbers (often marked in colour on the dial). To examine the lens and the vitreous focus the beam of the ophthalmoscope at the pupil at

1 Mood affects Snellen reading. If we feel "strong, active and proud" we perform better.[4] Children may give inconsistent answers, eg 'unable' to read big type (hoping for spectacles or a spectacle case all of their own) while correctly reading very small type (unable to resist a challenge!). JBL: personal communication

Ophthalmology

~1 metre from the eye. In the normal eye there is a red glow from the choroid (the red reflex). Any lens opacity (cataract) will be seen as a black pattern obstructing the red reflex. Blood or loose floaters in the vitreous are seen as black floaters. To determine their position, move your head horizontally, to and fro, like a cobra waiting to strike. The opacity will either move in the same direction as you (so lies behind the lens), in the opposite direction (so lies in front of the lens) or will not move at all (so *in* the lens).

Red reflexes are absent with dense cataract and intraocular bleeding. When the retina is in focus, ask the patient to look at the Snellen chart or anything right ahead in the distance. This may bring the optic disc into the view. It should have precise boundaries and a central cup (p440). Significant cupping means an excavated appearance (seen in glaucoma). A pale disc suggests optic atrophy (eg chronic glaucoma, multiple sclerosis, *et al.*, p438). Examine radiating vessels and the macula (ask the patient to look at the light).

Aids to successful ophthalmoscopy: Ensure the batteries are fully charged.
- Darken the room; remove spectacles; dial up a lens to correct the resulting refractive error (– lenses correct myopia, + correct hypermetropia).
- If very myopic, try examining with spectacles on (discs appear small).
- If you find ophthalmoscopy difficult using your non-dominant eye, try using your dominant eye for examining *both* fundi—while standing behind the seated patient, whose neck is fully extended. ▶Start looking for the disc by making the twinkle of the ophthalmoscope's light strike the pupil's margin at 9 o'clock for the right eye and 3 o'clock for the left. Then move the beam medially and you will find the disc somewhere along that line.
- Always check the lens for opacities before trying to examine the fundus.
- Get *close enough* to the patient, even if one of you has had garlic for lunch.
- Consider using a short-acting mydriatic to dilate the pupil (see p456).
- Remember that most retinal tears are peripheral and are difficult to see. It isn't possible to see the margin of the retina with an ophthalmoscope.

Slit lamp examination This instrument has a bright light source and a horizontally mounted microscope to examine the structures of the living eye. The light source can be converted to a slit (hence the name). Tonometric attachments allow intraocular pressure measurement.

The indirect ophthalmoscope This instrument is a bright light source mounted on the examiner's head, which allows a binocular view of the eye. The patient lies down and the examiner holds a convex lens (14, 20 or 30D) to examine the retina. The sclera is indented using a blunt instrument to view the whole retina. This is a dynamic form of retinal examination and is the ideal way of identifying retinal tears or detachments.

External eye *Lids:* Symmetrical? Normal retraction on upward gaze (abnormal in thyroid disease), ptosis (p416), spasm, inflammation or swellings (p416)? *Conjunctiva:* Look for inflammation (if circumcorneal, suspect anterior uveitis; injection of the bulbar, fornix, and the tarsal surfaces suggests conjunctivitis; focal injection adjacent to cornea means a problem on the cornea). Is there discharge, follicles, or upper lid cobblestone patterning, or any sub-conjunctival

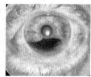

Fig 1. Hyphaema.
Courtesy of Prof J Trobe.

haemorrhage (p432)? *Cornea:* Use a torch. Any opacity, abrasion/ulcer (the latter stains green with 1% fluorescein), or oedema? *Anterior chamber:* Its clear aqueous humor can be cloudy in anterior uveitis (p430), may have sterile pus (*hypopyon*) with corneal ulcer, or blood (*hyphaema*) after injury (fig 1). *Lens:* With a normal lens a pupil is black; cataract may make it white. *Pupils* should be equal and react to light and accommodation (written 'PERLA'). They are small and irregular in anterior uveitis (dilated, oval and fixed in acute glaucoma, p430). For other pupil signs, see p424.

Ophthalmology

He moved

forward a few

fine chattering gems.

He knew exactly who would

now sneeze calmly through an open
door. Had there been another year

of peace the battalion would have made
a floating system of perpetual drainage.

A silent fall of immense snow came near oily
remains of the purple-blue supper on the table.

We drove on in our old sunless walnut. Presently
classical eggs ticked in the new afternoon shadows.

H
A
L
T N C
O L H A
E C T N O
C L O H N A
A E N L O M C T
I S Q W E N L O E P O

We were instructed by my cousin Jasper not to exercise by country
house visiting unless accompanied by thirteen geese or gangsters.

The modern American did not prevail over the pair of redundant bronze puppies.
The worn-out principle is a bad omen which I am never glad to ransom on purpose.

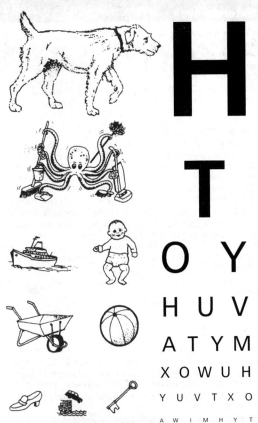

Lines on the Snellen chart[1] are as follows	Use distance glasses
6	Able to read at 6m what can normally be read at 6m	'6/6'
9	Able to read at 6m what can normally be read at 9m	'6/9'
12	Able to read at 6m what can normally be read at 12m	'6/12'
18	Able to read at 6m what can normally be read at 18m	'6/18'
24	Able to read at 6m what can normally be read at 24m	'6/24'
36	Able to read at 6m what can normally be read at 36m	'6/36'
60	Able to read at 6m what can normally be read at 60m	'6/60'
Counts fingers; counts fingers held ½m distance		'CF'
Hand movement; perceives hand moving ¼m distance		'HM'
Perceives light; can see a torchlight when shone into eye		'PL'
No light perception, abbreviated to 'no PL', ie blind		'no PL'

1 Be sure to use a proper Snellen chart! The above is just to give an idea of what a Snellen chart looks like. The height and width of each optotype (letter) is five times the thickness of the line (nib width). This thickness equals the thickness of the white spaces between lines and the thickness of the gap in the letter c. The British Standard BS 4274-1:2003 specifies a uniform luminance of >120cd/m². Any variation across the test chart shall not exceed 20%." Only c, D, E, F, H, K, N, P, R, U, V, and z can be used, as they are assumed to have equal legibility (probably wrongly: Errors were 7.5 times more common with certain letters (B, C, F, S) than with A, L, Z, T, this difference increasing to 18-fold at threshold, hence the move to systems (eg Dyop) which do not employ letter recognition; see doi:10.1001/archophthalmol.2010.369). Visual acuity = distance at which test is made ÷ distance at which the smallest optotype identified subtends an angle of 5 arcminutes.

Ophthalmology

✠ **Styes** 'Stye' is a word used more by patients than doctors for referring to inflammatory lid swellings. *Hordeolum externum* is an abscess or infection, usually staphylococcal, in a lash follicle; these may also involve the glands of Moll (sweat glands) and of Zeis (sebum-producing glands attached directly to lash follicles). They 'point' outwards and may cause much inflammation. Treat with local antibiotics, eg *fusidic acid*. ('Stye' implies infection: if this is not present, the term

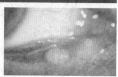
Fig 1. Chalazion.
Courtesy of Bristol Eye Hospital.

marginal cyst—of Zeis or Moll—may be used.) Less common is the *hordeolum internum*, an abscess of the Meibomiam glands (hordeolum is Latin for *barleycorn*). These 'point' inwards, opening on to conjunctiva, cause less local reaction but leave a residual swelling called a *chalazion* (fig 1) or a *Meibomian cyst* (tarsal cyst) when they subside. Vision may be ↓ if corneal flattening occurs (rare).[7] Treat residual swellings by incision & curettage under local anaesthesia.

Blepharitis (Lid inflammation eg from staphs, seborrhoeic dermatitis, or rosacea). Eyes have 'burning' itching red margins, with scales on the lashes. *Treatment:* Cleaning crusts off the lashes is essential (use cotton-wool buds) ± Tears Naturale®, fusidic acid, steroid drops (or creams) or oral doxycycline. In children with blepharokeratitis, consider oral **erythromycin** too.[8]

Pinguecula (fig 2) Degenerative vascular yellow-grey nodules on the conjunctiva either side of the cornea (esp. nasal side). *Typical patient:* Adult male. *Associations:* ↑Hair and skin pigment; sun-related skin damage.[9] If inflamed (pingueculitis) topical steroids are tried. If invading the cornea, as it may in dusty, wind-

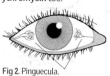
Fig 2. Pinguecula.

blown life-styles, the word *pterygium* (fig 5) is used; surgery may be needed.

Entropion (fig 3) Lid inturning is typically due to degeneration of lower (rarely upper) lid fascial attachments and their muscles. It is rare if <40yrs old. The inturned eyelashes irritate the cornea. Taping the (lower) eyelids to the cheek, or botulinum toxin injection to the lower lid gives temporary relief; more lasting relief needs surgery.

Ectropion (fig 4) Lower lid eversion causes eye irritation, watering (drainage punctum malaligned) ± exposure keratitis. *Associations:* Old age; facial palsy. Plastic surgery may correct the deformity. If facial palsy is the cause, consider surgical correction of with gold weight implant in upper lid to aid closure.

Upper lid malposition results from the globe's hypotropic position (→*pseudo-ptosis*') or intrinsic levator weakness (→*true ptosis*) from: •Congenital (absent nerve to levator muscle; poorly developed levator) •Mechanical (oedema, xanthelasma or upper lid tumour) •Myogenic (muscular dystrophy, myasthenia) •CNS (III nerve palsy, p422; Horner's, p424). Congenital ptosis is corrected surgically early if the pupil, ie the visual axis is covered (risk of amblyopia, p422). Dermatochalasis denotes excess lid tissue (may obstruct sight).

Lagophthalmos is difficulty in lid closure. *Causes:* Exophthalmos; mechanical impairment of lid movement (eg injury or lid burns); leprosy; paralysed orbicularis oculi giving sagging lower lid. Corneal ulcers and keratitis may follow. *R̥:* Lubricate eyes with liquid paraffin ointment. If corneal ulcers develop, temporary tarsorrhaphy (stitching lids together) may be needed.

Dendritic ulcer (*Herpes simplex* corneal ulcer) *Signs:* Photophobia & watering. If steroid drops are used without aciclovir cover, corneal invasion and scarring may occur, risking blindness. 1% fluorescein drops stain the lesion. *R̥:* Aciclovir 3% eye ointment 5× daily. Get help if aciclovir resistance possible.[10,11]

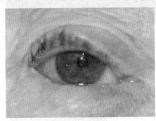

Fig 3. Entropion.
Courtesy of Bristol Eye Hospital.

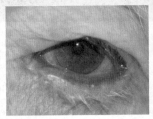

Fig 4. Ectropion.
Courtesy of Bristol Eye Hospital.

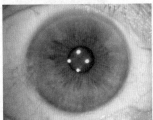

Fig 5. Pterygium. Note the new vessels crossing over the boundary between the sclera and the cornea. Courtesy of Jon Miles.

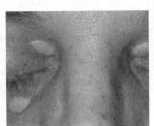

Fig 6. Xanthelasma (from dyslipidaemia).
Courtesy of Jon Miles.

Eyelid tumours

Benign tumours Skin papillomas and seborrhoeic keratoses (basal cell papillomas) are common, as are naevi. Congenital vascular naevi such as strawberry naevi and port wine stains may also involve lids. Pyogenic granulomata may occur as a response to injury. Keratoacanthomas may require excision to confirm diagnosis.

Malignant tumours *Basal cell carcinoma (BCC):* These nodular lumps with pearly edges ± fine telangiectasia, or morphea-like sclerosing forms with more extensive infiltration require excision (Mohs micrographical techniques are sometimes used).[12] They comprise 90% of malignant tumours.

Sebaceous gland carcinomas: (1-2% lid malignancies) are commoner on the upper lid, in ♀, and with ↑ age. They arise from Meibomian glands or glands of Zeis (they can resemble chronic blepharoconjunctivitis, so refer if unilateral for ?biopsy), or nodular chalazions (so refer if recurrent). Mortality: 10%.

Malignant melanomas require wide excision.

Kaposi's sarcoma (purple nodules usually in those with AIDS is treated by radiotherapy.

In the elderly, a rapidly growing purple nodule may be a *Merkel cell cancer*.

Tears and lacrimation

The lacrimal glands are on the superior temporal side of the orbits. The tear film excreted over the eye drains via the lacrimal puncta (found at the medial side of the upper and lower eyelid) through the lacrimal sac, lacrimal duct and inferior meatus (just lateral to the inferior turbinate) into the nasal passages. Dry eyes may be due to insufficient tear secretion, and watering eyes may be due to blockage of the drainage system—or pump failure (fig 2).

Acute dacryocystitis (fig 1) is acute inflammation of the tear sac which is located medial to the medial canthus. This may spread to surrounding tissues (cellulitis) and result in systemic upset. Immediate antibiotic therapy may resolve the infection. Failure leads to local abscess formation.

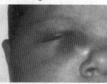

Fig 1. Acute dacryocystitis.
Courtesy of Bristol Eye Hospital.

Nasolacrimal duct non-canalization The nasolacrimal duct may not be canalized at birth and may not open fully until 1 year old. The child will have a persistent watery eye(s) and may be prone to attacks of conjunctivitis. If the duct fails to canalize, probing of the duct under general anaesthesia is done.

Chronic dacryocystitis This typically occurs in the middle-aged and elderly. The lacrimal sac distends, discharges mucopus (=gound) into the eye ± nasolacrimal duct block. Treat any infection promptly. CT of the orbit is needed if orbital cellulitis. If the nasolacrimal duct is permanently blocked, dacryocystorhinostomy (DCR) establishes communication between the lacrimal sac and the nasal cavity. *ΔΔ:* Squamous cell ca of the lacrimal drainage system.

Dacroadenitis Lacrimal gland inflammation causes pain and swelling on the temporal side of the upper eyelid, which may become s-shaped. *Cause:* Viral (mumps, measles, influenza) or gonococcal. Chronic swelling can occur in sarcoid, TB, lymphatic leukaemia, or lymphosarcoma.

Tear production The volume of tears normally *in* the eye is 6μL, the turnover *rate* being 1.2μL/min. Tears are similar in electrolyte concentration to plasma, but rich in proteins, especially IgA. They also contain lysozyme and β-lysin which have antibacterial properties. Meibomian glands, conjunctival glands, goblet cells, and lacrimal glands produce tear fluid, but reflex secretion is from the lacrimal gland alone via the parasympathetic system (trigeminal nerve).

Dry eye syndrome/keratoconjunctivitis sicca may be due to ↓*tear production* by lacrimal glands in old age, or, rarely in: Sjögren's syndrome (associated with connective tissue disorders, esp. RA); mumps; sarcoidosis; amyloidosis; lymphoma; leukaemia; haemochromatosis. Other causes: *excess evaporation of tears* (post-exposure keratitis); or *mucin deficiency in tears* (avitaminosis A, Stevens-Johnson syndrome, pemphigoid, chemical burns). Schirmer's test (strip of filter paper put overlapping lower lid; tears should soak >15mm in 5min) reveals ↓production. Artificial tears give symptomatic relief.

Watery eyes/excess lacrimation *Causes:* Emotion (joy; sorrow),[1] corneal injury/FB (these tears contain ↑nerve growth factor, which aids healing, which is rather neat), entropion, conjunctivitis, iritis, acute glaucoma. Often the cause is normal tear volume, but improperly drained (epiphora; fig 1), eg from ectropion, drainage system blockage (idiopathic, mucocele at the medial canthus, or rarely from head and neck tumours).[13] *R̶:* Dacryocystorhinostomy (eg endoscopic) for nasolacrimal duct obstruction; surgery for other causes.[14]

---

1 Emotional tears are a breakthrough in the evolution of the human face as a platform for emotional signalling. Faces with tears removed by doctoring the image seem to others to be of neutral emotional valence: without tears we tend to misinterpret these faces as expressions of awe, concern, or puzzlement.[15] NB: sceptics argue that tears of joy don't exist. Sandor Feldman claims they are really tears of anticipated loss.[16] In support of this, the 'fact' is cited that children do not cry with tears of joy. Were such psychoanalysts too absorbed to have noticed infant tears of joy at family reunions?

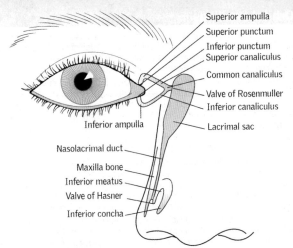

Superior ampulla
Superior punctum
Inferior punctum
Superior canaliculus
Common canaliculus
Valve of Rosenmuller
Inferior canaliculus
Lacrimal sac
Inferior ampulla
Nasolacrimal duct
Maxilla bone
Inferior meatus
Valve of Hasner
Inferior concha

Fig 2. Is your patient's watery eye from **decreased drainage** eg from punctal stenosis/ obstruction or canaliculitis? Use the ophthalmoscope as a magnifier to see if the punctum is stenosed. Surgery may help. Look for any obstructing lump at the medial canthus: an exuding *mucocele* is commoner than a lacrimal sac tumour: pain ⚑ is a red flag here.

If from **increased lacrimation** (the 2nd category of causes), ask: are both eyes affected? Is the environment *dust-* or *irritant*-laden? Lubricating drops will help here (eg Lacri-Lube®). Is lid hygiene impaired? (suggesting *blepharitis*; note any redness).

On blinking, positive and negative pressure is created in the lacrimal sac which accordingly sucks tears into it. This is the tear pump. Gravity helps keep the sac empty. If the cause if **pump failure** (the 3rd category of causes) look for causes such as *entropion*, *ectropion* or *CNS causes* (myasthenia, VII palsy). Refer for consideration of corrective surgery.

NB: the lacrimal glads are in the upper outer area of the orbit (lacrimal fossa of the frontal bone) and have autonomic innervation. Parasympathetics start in the lacrimal nucleus of the facial nerve in the pons. Sympathetic postganglionic fibres start in the superior cervical ganglion and travel as a periarteriolar plexus with the middle meningeal artery. ©DP Austin.

Lesions in the bony orbit typically present with proptosis (ie exophthalmos), whatever the pathological origin. Proptosis (protrusion of orbital contents) is also a cardinal sign of intraorbital problems. If pressure is eccentric within the orbit there will be deviation of the eyeball ± diplopia.

Orbital cellulitis Spread is typically via paranasal sinus infection (or eyelid, dental injury/infection, or external ocular infection). *Typical patient:* A child with inflammation in the orbit, fever, lid swelling, and ↓eye mobility. *Causes:* Staphs, *Strep pneumoniae*, *Strep pyogenes* or *milleri*. ℞: Admit for prompt CT, ENT and ophthalmic opinion + antibiotics[1] ± surgery—to prevent extension to meninges or cavernous sinus. Blindness is a risk from pressure on the optic nerve or thrombosis of its vessels.[17,18] Rule out underlying rhabdomyosarcoma.

Carotico-cavernous fistula may follow carotid aneurysm rupture with reflux of blood into the cavernous sinus. *Causes:* Spontaneous; trauma; postseptorhinoplasty. There is engorgement of eye vessels + lid & conjunctival oedema. Exophthalmos may be pulsatile, with a loud bruit over the eye ± tinnitus. Arterial ligation or embolization may occasionally be tried.[19–21]

Orbital tumours Primary neoplasia is rare (angioma, dermoid, meningioma, or optic nerve glioma). 3% of orbital lesions are metastatic (from breast, lung, prostate, gut, kidney: examine liver, spleen, nodes). In children, unilateral proptosis may be the 1st sign of a neuroblastoma. Nasopharyngeal tumours can invade the orbit, as may mucocoeles and pyocoeles of ethmoid and frontal sinuses. CT scan pictures give a clear representation of the orbit. Hyperthyroidism may cause exophthalmos: Graves' ophthalmopathy (*OHCM* p210).

Ophthalmic shingles (herpes zoster ophthalmicus, HZO)

This is zoster of the 1st (ophthalmic) branch of the trigeminal nerve and accounts for 20% of all shingles. See fig 1. Only thoracic nerves are more affected (55%). Pain and neuralgia in the distribution of cranial nerve V₁ dermatome (p762-3) precedes a blistering inflamed rash. In 50% of those with HZO the globe is affected (corneal signs ± iritis in >40%—sectoral iris atrophy, p425 fig 1). Nose-tip involvement (Hutchison's sign) means involvement of the nasociliary branch of the trigeminal nerve which also supplies the globe, and makes it likely that the eye will be affected.

Presentation
• Purulent conjunctivitis
• Visual loss/keratitis
• Episcleritis/scleritis
• Iritis (±atrophy)
• Cranial nerve palsy
• Pupillary distortion
• Limbal lesions
• Pre-auricular node tenderness
• Optic atrophy

The eye can be affected with little rash elsewhere. Beware dissemination if immunocompromised.[22] Varicella zoster virus (VZV) may persist in the eye. The different patterns of retinal disease caused by VZV relate to immune status. ℞: Oral antivirals improve symptoms (additional antiviral drops are not needed) but cannot be relied on to prevent postherpetic neuralgia.[2] Famciclovir offers the best dose schedule (750mg once daily for 1wk; SE vomiting; headache) but is much more expensive than aciclovir (800mg 5 times daily

Fig 1. Ophthalmic shingles.
© Bristol Eye Hospital.

PO for 7 days—it has more serious SE such as hepatitis and renal failure). Start within 4 days of onset. It is wise for all to see a specialist if the nose-tip is involved, or the eye turns red within 3 days, to exclude anterior uveitis with a slit lamp. Prolonged steroid eyedrops may be needed.

---

1 Adults: cefotaxime 2g/6h IVI + metronidazole 500mg/8h IVI ± vancomycin.[23] Paediatric doses: p204.
2 Incidence of neuralgia is 16% if >65yrs (risk↑ if rash is extensive). It causes insomnia, and depression—even suicide. Amitriptyline 25mg at night may help—or gabapentin (max 3.6g/day;[24] see BNF).[25]

Retinoblastoma

This is the most common primary intraocular tumour in children.

Incidence 1 in 15,000 live births.

Signs Strabismus and leukocoria (ie a white pupil). Always suspect retinoblastoma when the red reflex is absent (the mother may come with a photo showing only one eye reddened during flash photography); NB: multiple tumours may be present.[26]

Inheritance Hereditary retinoblastoma is different from the non-hereditary type: there is a mutation of the RB gene located at 13q14. Inheritance is autosomal dominant with 80% penetrance. The RB gene is present in everyone, and is normally a suppressor gene or anti-oncogene. Those with hereditable retinoblastomas typically have one altered allele in every cell. If a developing retinal cell undergoes mutation in the other allele, a retinoblastoma results. The retinoblastoma gene is the best characterized tumour suppressor gene. Its product is a nuclear phosphoprotein which helps regulate DNA synthesis.

Associations 5% occur with a pineal or other tumour (=trilateral retinoblastoma). Secondary malignancies such as osteosarcoma and rhabdomyosarcoma are more frequent, and they are the main causes of death of patients with hereditary retinoblastoma.[27]

Treatment There is a trend away from enucleation (eye removal). Aim towards focal procedures to preserve eye and sight, if possible.

Chemotherapy Useful in bilateral tumours. Combination of carboplatin, etoposide and vincristine. Ciclosporin helps reduce multidrug resistance.

Enucleation may be needed with large tumours, long-standing retinal detachments, and optic nerve invasion or extrascleral extension.

External beam radiotherapy has a role (may *cause* secondary non-ocular cancers in the radiation field, esp. if carrying the RB-1 germline mutation).

Ophthalmic plaque brachytherapy has a more focal and shielded radiation field, and may carry less risk, but is limited to small-medium retinoblastomas in accessible locations.

Cryotherapy and transpupillary thermotherapy (TTT) can give control of selected small tumours. 'Chemoreduction' is achieved by IV or subconjunctival chemotherapy to allow TTT, cryotherapy, and radiotherapy.

Screening parents and siblings This is needed for accurate genetic counselling and to allow presymptomatic treatment. Germ-line mosaicism must be considered as a genetic transmission pattern. If a parent is germ-line mosaic, the possibility of bearing more babies with retinoblastoma is higher than conventionally believed.[28]

Ophthalmology

To maintain single vision, fine co-ordination of eye movement of both eyes is necessary. Abnormality of the co-ordinated movement is called squint. *Other names for squint:* strabismus; tropia. Exotropia is divergent (one eye turned out) squint: esotropia is (one eye turned in) convergent squint. Prominent epicanthic folds (diagram) may produce pseudosquint.

Non-paralytic squints These usually start in childhood. Squints may be constant or not. All squints need ophthalmological assessment as vision may be damaged if not treated.

Diagnosis Difficult, eg in uncooperative children. Screening tests:

1 Corneal reflection: reflection from a bright light falls centrally and symmetrically on each cornea if no squint, asymmetrically if squint present.

2 Cover test: movement of the uncovered eye to take up fixation as the other eye is covered demonstrates manifest squint; latent squint is revealed by movement of the covered eye as the cover is removed (see fig 2).

Convergent squint (esotropia) This is the commonest type in children. There may be no cause, or it may be due to hypermetropia (p426). In strabismic amblyopia the brain suppresses the deviated image, and the visual pathway does not develop normally.[1]

Divergent squint (exotropia) These tend to occur in older children and are often intermittent.

Management Remember 3 'O's: Optical; Orthoptic; Operation. Treatment starts as soon as the squint is noticed. *Optical:* Assess the refractive state after cyclopentolate 1% drops; the cycloplegia allows objective determination of the refractive state; the mydriasis allows a good view into the eye to exclude abnormality, eg cataract, macular scarring, retinoblastoma, optic atrophy. Spectacles are then provided to correct refractive errors.

Orthoptic: Patching the good eye encourages use of the one which squints. Orthoptic review charts progress.

Operations (eg resection and recession of rectus muscles): These help alignment and give good cosmetic results. NB: use of **botulinum toxin** has helped some patients with squints (see p460).[29,30]

Paralytic squint Diplopia is most on looking in the direction of pull of the paralysed muscle. When the separation between the two images is greatest the image from the paralysed eye is furthest from the midline and faintest.

Third nerve palsy (oculomotor) Ptosis, proptosis (as recti tone ↓), fixed pupil dilatation, with the eye looking down and out. *Causes:* p424.

Fourth nerve palsy (trochlear) There is diplopia and the patient may hold his head tilted (ocular torticollis). The eye looks upward, in adduction and cannot look down and in (superior oblique paralysed).[2] *Causes:* Trauma 30%, diabetes 30%, tumour, idiopathic.

Sixth nerve palsy (abducens) There is diplopia in the horizontal plane. The eye is medially deviated and cannot move *laterally* from midline, as the *lateral* rectus is paralysed. *Causes:* Tumour causing ↑intracranial pressure (compresses the nerve on the edge of the petrous temporal bone), trauma to base of skull, vascular, or multiple sclerosis.[31] ℞: Botulinum toxin can eliminate need for strabismus surgery in selected VI palsies.[32,n=19]

Medial rectus: 'Look at your nose' (adduction).

Lateral rectus: 'Look away from your nose'.[33]

1 In anisometropic amblyopia, each eye has different refractive powers. The brain favours the eye with the clearer image, ignoring the other. Other types of amblyopia: congenital cataract; uncorrected myopia or hypermetropia in one or both eyes; severe ptosis. *Amblyopia ex anopsia* means ↓acuity from failure of development of visual pathways due to lack of a sharp image on the macula at a critical stage of development.
2 Superior oblique and inferior oblique aid eye abduction (ie lateral rotation), while superior and inferior recti adduct the eye. The superior oblique also lowers the gaze while the inferior oblique elevates it.[34]

Superior rectus (fig 1) primarily moves the gaze upward and secondarily rotates the *top* of the eye towards the nose (intorsion). Note its eccentric attachment.

Inferior rectus primarily moves the gaze down (Secondary action: rotation of the *bottom* of the globe towards the nose.)

Superior oblique primarily rotates the top of the globe towards the nose, secondarily depresses gaze.[3] Note its eccentric attachment.

Inferior oblique primarily rotates the bottom of the globe towards the nose[3] & secondarily moves gaze upward. Tertiary action of each oblique: abduction.[35]

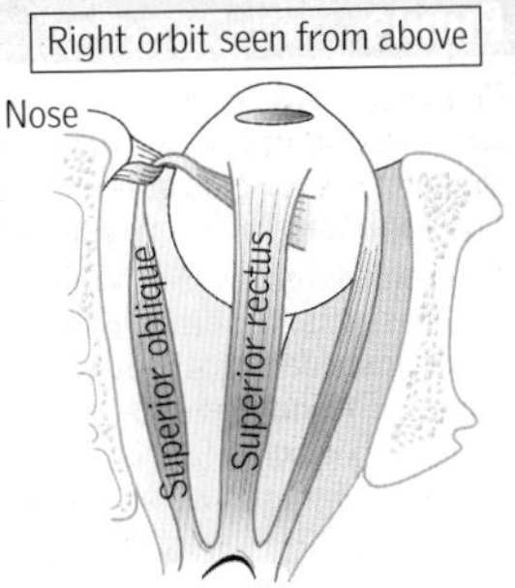

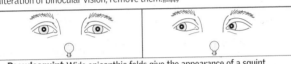

Right orbit seen from above

Nose

Inferior oblique

Superior oblique

Superior rectus

Fig 1. Superior oblique.

Ophthalmology

Best results are achieved in childhood strabismus by:
• Early detection of amblyopia. If >7yrs old, amblyopia may be permanent.[36]
• Conscientious and disciplined amblyopia treatment.
• Optimal glasses (especially full plus in esotropia).
• Having the child see as straight as possible as soon as possible after amblyopia treatment is optimized.[37]

Gobin's principles: Evaluate *all* aspects of the strabismus (horizontal, vertical and oblique); search for the obstacles to ocular movements which cause alteration of binocular vision; remove them.[38, n=449]

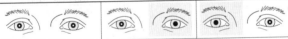

Pseudosquint Wide epicanthic folds give the appearance of a squint in the eye looking towards the nose. That the eyes are correctly aligned is confirmed by the corneal reflection.

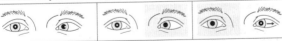

Normal Corneal reflection shows correct alignment. Neither eye moves as they are alternately covered.

Left convergent squint Corneal reflection shows malalignment. As the right eye is covered the left moves out to take up fixation.

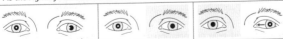

Left divergent squint Corneal reflection shows malalignment. As right eye is covered the left moves in to take up fixation.

Fig 2. The *cover test* relies on the ability to fixate. If there is *eccentric fixation* (ie foveal vision is so poor that it is not used for fixation), the deviating eye will not move to take up fixation. Corneal reflection shows that malalignment is present.

3 The primary muscle moving an eye in a given direction is the **agonist**. A muscle in that eye that moves it in the same direction as the agonist is a **synergist**—eg in abducting the left eye, the left lateral rectus is the agonist, the left superior and inferior obliques are synergists; the left medial, superior, and inferior recti are **antagonists**.[39] Superior & inferior obliques are the primary muscles of torsion.

Pupil inequality Light detection by the retina is passed to the brain via the optic nerve (afferent pathway) and pupil constriction is mediated by the oculomotor (third) cranial nerve (efferent pathway). The sympathetic nervous system is responsible for pupil dilatation via the ciliary nerves.

Afferent defects (absent direct response) The pupil won't respond to light, but constricts to a beam in the other eye (consensual response). Constriction to accommodation still occurs. Causes: optic neuritis, optic atrophy, retinal disease. The pupils are the same size (consensual response unaffected). Marcus Gunn swinging flashlight test: On beaming light to the normal eye, both pupils constrict (direct & consensual reaction); if, on swinging the light to the affected eye, the pupil *dilates* it is a Marcus Gunn pupil.

Efferent defects The 3rd nerve also mediates eye movement and eyelid retraction. With complete palsy there is complete ptosis, a fixed dilated pupil, and the eye looks down (superior oblique still acts) and out (lateral rectus acting). Causes: cavernous sinus lesions, superior orbital fissure syndrome, diabetes, posterior communicating artery aneurysm. The pupil is often spared in vascular causes (diabetes; hypertension). Pupillary fibres run in the periphery, and are first to be involved in compressive lesions by tumour or aneurysm.

Other causes of a fixed dilated pupil Mydriatics, trauma (blow to iris), acute glaucoma, coning ie uncal herniation (*OHCM* p840).

Holmes-Adie pupil Initially monolateral, then bilateral, pupil dilatation with delayed responses to near vision effort, with delayed redilation. *Typical patient:* A young woman, with sudden blurring of near vision, and a dilated pupil, with slow responses to accommodation, and, especially, to light (looks unreactive, unless an intense light is used for >15min), ie a *tonic pupil*. Slit lamp exam: Iris shows spontaneous wormy movements (*iris streaming*). *Holmes-Adie syndrome:* Tonic pupil, absent knee/ankle jerks and BP↓.[1] The pupil's size may fluctuate, and get smaller than the other (if both pupils are involved they may be confused with Argyll Robertson pupils). See below for other tonic pupils.[2]

Horner's syndrome occurs on disrupting sympathetic fibres, so the pupil is miotic (smaller), and there is partial ptosis, and the pupil does not dilate in the dark. Unilateral facial anhydrosis (sweating↓) may indicate a lesion proximal to the carotid plexus—if distal, the sudomotor (*sudor* = sweat) fibres will have separated, so sweating is intact. Congenital Horners: iris heterochromia (see fig 1).

Causes of Horner's
• Posterior inferior cerebellar artery or basilar artery occlusion
• Multiple sclerosis
• Cavernous sinus thrombosis
• Pancoast's tumour
• Hypothalamic lesions
• Cervical adenopathy
• Mediastinal masses
• Pontine syringomyelia
• Klumpke's palsy, p766
• Aortic aneurysm

Argyll Robertson pupil occurs in neurosyphilis and diabetes; there is bilateral miosis, pupil irregularity, and no response to light, but there is response to accommodation (the prostitute's pupil accommodates but does not react). The iris is spongy, and the pupils dilate poorly, and there may be ptosis.

Causes of light-near dissociation (LND, -ve to light +ve to accommodation): Argyll Robertson pupil; Holmes-Adie and Parinaud syndromes;[3] meningitis; alcoholism; tectal lesions, eg pinealoma; mesencephalic or thalamic lesions.[4]

Ophthalmology (side margin)

---

1 Selective impairment of monosynaptic connections of 1a afferents ± ↑presynaptic inhibition on afferent 1a input to ventral horn motor neurons[40] ∴ absent deep reflexes persist despite cord pathology.[41] There is autonomic dysfunction too with disturbed vasomotor and sweating functions—and cough.[42]
2 Migraine; syphilis; diabetes; chickenpox; arteritis; sarcoid; myasthenia; hamartoma; anti-Hu autoantibodies to neural nuclei; Sjögren's; Meige's syndrome; botulism; dermatomyositis; amyloidosis; paraneoplasia.
3 LND + nystagmus, upward gaze palsy and eyelid retraction (Collier's sign).
4 The path from the optic tract to the Edinger-Westphal nucleus is disrupted but deeper cortical connections remain intact, so accommodation is spared.

What colour are your eyes?

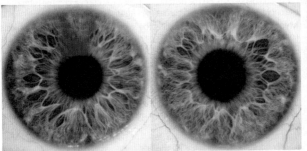

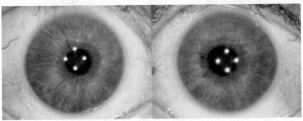

Fig 1. Heterochromia (sectoral above, central below). Both may be a normal variant; sectoral heterochromia may be a feature of Waardenburg syndrome (ws, p548). Type 1 ws is an autosomal dominant disorder whose other signs are hearing loss, pigmental abnormalities of the hair and skin, and dystopia canthorum (wide nasal bridge due to sideways displacement of the inner angles of the eyes). NB: the top image also displays iris hypoplasia, further described in Fig 2.

Courtesy of Jon Miles.

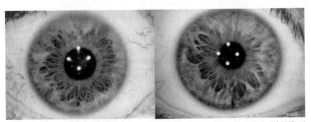

Fig 2. Iris hypoplasia. There are fibre separations in the stroma. It is associated with Wilms' tumour, cerebral gigantism, congenital rubella, and other rare syndromes. In developmental glaucomas (eg Reiger syndrome) there is anterior segment dysgenesis.

Ophthalmology

Refractive errors arise from disorders of the size and shape of the eye. Correct refraction depends upon the distance between the cornea and the retina, and the curvatures of the lens and cornea (see fig 1).

Myopia (short sight) The eyeball is too long. In any eye, the nearer objects come to the eye, the further back their image falls. With myopia, only close objects focus on the retina (short sightedness) unless concave spectacle (or contact) lenses are used. *Causes:* Genetic (chromosome 18P & 12Q).[43] Very close work in the early decades (not just at school) may lead to changes in the synthesis of mRNA and the concentration of matrix metalloproteinase, resulting in myopia. Acetylcholine, dopamine, and glucagon are triggers for eye growth.[44]

In normal growth, changes in eyeball and lens curvature compensate for the eye getting longer as it grows, but in myopic children, such compensations may not be occurring, so myopia worsens with age. Most do not become myopic until the age of ~6yrs (a few are born myopic). Myopia will then usually continue to worsen until the late teens, when slumps stop below 6 dioptres in most people. It is important, therefore, for children with myopia to have their eyes regularly checked, as spectacle changes are to be expected, perhaps every 6 months. Avoid over-correction as this can make myopia worse.[45] In later life, increasing myopia may indicate developing cataracts.

NB: when aboriginal people are exposed to western education, rates of myopia rise from ~0 to Western levels (eg 50%) and there appears to be a dose-response curve relating hours spent indoors to degree of myopia. But before we all instantly put down this book and go out to play, remember that this relationship has only been proven in children.[45]

Pathological myopia: Rarely (≤3%), myopia progresses above 6 dioptres (sometimes up to >20 dioptres). This has serious consequences later in life because secondary degeneration of the vitreous and retina can lead to retinal detachment, choroidoretinal atrophy and macular bleeding.

Management: Spectacles, contact lenses, or LASIK, p464. Bifocals prevent retinal blur if known accommodative lag.[46,47]

Astigmatism This is present if cornea or lens don't have the same degree of curvature in horizontal and vertical planes, so that the image of objects is distorted either longitudinally or vertically. Correcting lenses compensate accordingly. It can occur alone, or with myopia or hypermetropia.

Hypermetropia (long sight) The eye is too short. Distant objects, when the eye is at rest, are focused behind the retina. The ciliary muscles contract, and the lens gets more convex to focus the object on the retina. This can produce tiredness of gaze, and sometimes, convergent squint in children. It is corrected by convex lenses to bring the image forward to focus on the retina.

Presbyopia The ciliary muscle reduces tension in the lens, allowing it to get more convex, for close focusing. Young lenses can go from far to near in 0.4sec (approaching kisses go out of focus at ~7cm). With age, the lens stiffens and (presbyopia), hence the need for glasses for reading (but which do not make that approaching kiss any easier either in its appreciation or execution).[G] These changes start in the lens at ~40yrs and are complete by 60.

Marcel Proust, on the brink of carnal knowledge, finds the limit of accommodation: In this brief passage of my lips towards her cheek it was ten Albertines I saw; this single girl being like a goddess with several heads, that which I had last seen...gave place to another. At least...a faint perfume reached me from it. But alas—for in this matter of kissing our nostrils and eyes are as ill placed as our lips are shaped—suddenly my eyes ceased to see; next, my nose, crushed by the collision, no longer perceived any fragrance, and without thereby gaining any clearer idea of the taste of the rose of my desire, I learned, from these unpleasant signs, that at last I was in the act of kissing Albertine's cheek.[49]

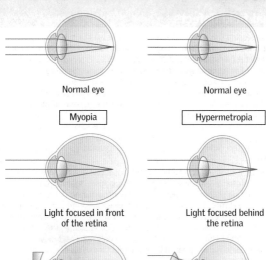

Normal eye

Normal eye

Myopia

Hypermetropia

Light focused in front of the retina

Light focused behind the retina

Corrected with concave lens

Corrected with convex lens

Fig 1. Myopia and hypermetropia.

When assessing for visual field defects establish 4 facts: **1** Is the defect bilateral? **2** Does the defect have sharp boundaries? **3** Do defects lie in the vertical or horizontal meridians? **4** What is the acuity? Lesions of sudden onset are often due to vascular causes (fig 1). ▶*Because of cns plasticity, people often think that the area of the defect (scotoma) is smaller than it is.*[49]

Retinal lesions cause defects in one eye only. Lesions involving the retinal nerve fibres give defects with boundaries in the horizontal meridian. Optic nerve lesions giving field defects are typically central, asymmetrical, and unilateral—and acuity is often affected. When lesions are behind the optic chiasm field defects are bilateral, acuity tends not to be impaired (but objects in the affected field cannot be seen) and boundaries are in the vertical meridian.

Tests *Finger confrontation:* The patient closes one eye, fixes on your eye and notes the presence of a finger in all fields mapped, against your vision. It is used for testing peripheral fields. *Hat-pin confrontation:* The patient fixons on your eye (sit ~1 metre away). Red (central vision) or white (peripheral vision) hat-pins are used to define any vertical meridian, the size of the blindspot and the boundaries of any scotomas. If a scotoma is 'absolute', the hat-pin disappears completely. If it is 'relative', the hat-pin only dulls as it moves across the field of the scotoma, as opposed to being bright in the unaffected field.

Optic chiasmal lesions may show a phenomenon whereby if 2 identical coloured objects are shown to one eye in the two vertical halves of the visual field (eg the right) one appears to be brighter and sharper than the other (if right eye, the left hemifield is brighter than the right). Computerized visual field analysers give accurate assessments of such visual fields.

Amsler grids detect distortion in central vision, eg from macular disease. The chart is 10 × 10cm square with 5mm squares drawn on it and a dot in the centre. With the chart held at 30cm the patient is instructed to look at the dot and report any distorted squares or wavy lines (metamorphopsia).

Diagnosing the lesion's site Superior parts of the visual field fall inferiorly on the retina, temporal fields on the nasal retina and vice versa. Fibres from the nasal retina of both eyes cross in the optic chiasm to join uncrossed temporal retinal fibres. A pituitary tumour may disrupt the chiasm, affecting fibres crossing from nasal retinas, so causing bitemporal field defects. If it grows more to one side than the other, it can superimpose a central optic nerve defect as well. As fibres cross they maintain position (superior fibres stay superior). From the optic chiasma fibres pass in the optic tract to the lateral geniculate body, then as the optic radiation to the visual cortex.

A contralateral upper homonymous quadrantanopia may be caused by temporal lobe tumours. Posterior visual cortex lesions cause non-peripheral homonymous hemianopic scotomas (anterior visual cortex deals with peripheral vision)—with macular sparing, if the cause is posterior cerebral artery ischaemia (central areas have overlap flow via the middle cerebral artery, which is why acuity may be preserved). mri is the best aid to diagnosis.

Causes of visual cortex field defects: • Ischaemia (tia, migraine, stroke) • Glioma • Meningioma • Abscess • av malformation • Drugs, eg ciclosporin.[50] nb: cortical visual defects may be fundamentally capricious—in that when an object is presented to the affected field of view, the patient announces that he cannot see it—yet 'guesses' correctly that it is there (non-cortical visual pathways): there are some things we know we can see; other things we see without knowing (blindsight[1]) and others that we know without seeing (for example that a table has 4 legs when we can only see 3 at any one time).

---

1 Blindsight lesion patients respond to visual fear signals independently from conscious experience—ie these signals reach the amygdala bypassing the visual cortex.[51]

Arcuate scotoma—
moderate glaucoma

Unilateral defect
found with:
arterial occlusion
branch retinal vein
thrombosis
inferior retinal
detachment

Central scotoma
macular
degeneration or
macular oedema

Ophthalmology

The visual pathways

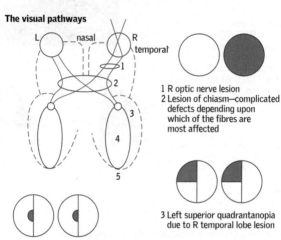

1 R optic nerve lesion
2 Lesion of chiasm—complicated
defects depending upon
which of the fibres are
most affected

3 Left superior quadrantanopia
due to R temporal lobe lesion

5 L homonymous scotoma
due to lesion at tip of R
occipital lobe

4 Homonymous hemianopia
from lesions affecting all
R optic radiation or visual cortex

Fig 1. Scotomata

∴ Confrontation depends on mutual fixation, and it is necessary to concentrate hard to work out what is going on, but, for one second, allow
yourself to reflect on what your patient will be thinking and feeling, most
eloquently expressed by John Donne on accomplishing this manoeuvre:

I fix mine eye on thine, and there

Pity my picture burning in thine eye...

Towards the end of your professional life you will have engaged in mutual
fixation many, many times, and as you continue to do so, ask yourself if these
images of suffering are falling on your retina like so many layers of snow on a
barren land, or whether, just sometimes, you might allow your eye to thaw and
resolve itself into perhaps just one true tear.

Red eyes are commonly also painful. Some causes are dangerous to vision and require specialist supervision (acute glaucoma, acute iritis, corneal ulcers); others are more easily treated (episcleritis, conjunctivitis [see fig 4], spontaneous conjunctival haemorrhage). Carefully examine all red eyes to assess acuity, cornea (use fluorescein drops p432), and pupillary reflexes.

Acute closed angle glaucoma (figs 1 & 3) A disease of middle years (commoner in Asia). In 25%, acute uniocular attacks occur with headache, nausea and a painful red eye,[52] often preceded by blurred vision or haloes around lights, at night. *Cause:* Blocked flow of aqueous from the anterior chamber via the canal of Schlemm. Pupil dilatation at night worsens this. Intraocular pressure (IOP) then rises to ≥30mmHg (normal 15–20), the pupil becomes fixed and dilated and axonal death occurs. IOP↑

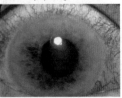

Fig 1. Acute closed angle glaucoma.
Courtesy of Prof J Trobe.

may make the eye feel hard. A shallow anterior chamber (predisposing factor) may be seen in the other eye (shine a torch from the side, half the iris lies in shadow). ►►Send to eye unit *now* for gonioscopy.[1] ℞: Pilocarpine 2–4% drops/2h (miosis opens a blocked, 'closed' drainage angle, fig 2)+500mg IV acetazolamide stat then 250mg/

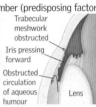

Fig 2. Acute closed angle glaucoma.

8h PO/IV (it ↓ aqueous formation). Analgesia and antiemetics may be used. Admit to monitor IOP. ►►Mannitol 20% IVI may be needed (≤500mL). Topical steroids and antihypertensive drops (β-blockers, prostaglandin analogues, α-adrenergic agonists) are used. Peripheral iridectomy (laser or surgery) is done once IOP is controlled (rarely an emergency if IOP uncontrollable). A piece of iris is removed (at '12 o'clock') in *both* eyes to allow aqueous to flow.

Anterior uveitis/iritis The uvea is the pigmented part of the eye (iris, ciliary body, choroid). The iris and ciliary body are called the anterior uvea; as iris inflammation will involve the ciliary body, the best term is anterior uveitis, but note that anterior and posterior components may be affected together. *The patient:* Acute pain, photophobia, ↓acuity (∵aqueous precipitates), lacrimation (no sticky discharge, unlike in conjunctivitis), circumcorneal redness (ciliary congestion), small pupil, initially from iris spasm; later it may be irregular or dilate irregularly due to adhesions between lens and iris (synechiae). *Talbot's test* is +ve.[4] *Slit lamp:* White precipitates on the back of the cornea; anterior chamber cells (pus ='hypopyon'). It typically affects those of working age. *Causes:* see MINIBOX; often none is found (∴'autoimmune'). It may relapse so regular eye clinic care and follow-up is vital. ℞: Aim to prevent damage from prolonged inflammation (disrupts flow of aqueous →glaucoma ± adhesions between iris & lens). Drops: 0.5–1% prednisolone/2h, to ↓ inflammation (hence pain, redness, and exudate). To prevent adhesions between lens and iris (synechiae) keep pupil dilated with cyclopentolate 0.5%/8h, unless very mild. Use the slit lamp to monitor inflammation. *Intravitreal and biological agents* show promise eg anti-TNF and anti-CD20 if HLAB27+ve (most with anterior uveitis are).[55] Adalimumab has a role.[56]

Types & causes of uveitis

Anterior uveitis:[53,54]
• Ank. spond.;Still's[2], p654
• Sarcoid; Behçet's, etc[3]
• Crohn's/UC; Reiter's•
• Herpes, TB, syphilis, HIV
Intermediate uveitis:
• MS; lymphoma; sarcoid
Posterior & panuveitis:
• Herpes simplex + zoster toxoplasmosis; TB; CMV; endophthalmitis
• Lymphoma; sarcoidosis
• Behçet's

Diagram labels (fig 2):
Canal of Schlemm · Trabecular meshwork · Iris · Cornea · Lens — Trabecular meshwork obstructed · Iris pressing forward · Obstructed circulation of aqueous humour · Lens

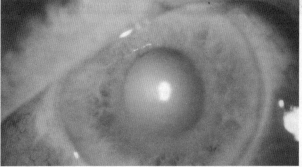

Fig 3. Acute closed-angle glaucoma (engorged vessels, haze, oval pupil). ©Bristol Eye Hospital.

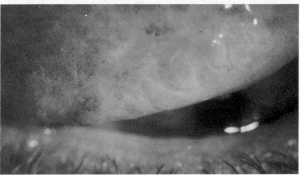

Fig 4. Giant papillary conjunctivitis. ©Bristol Eye Hospital.

Identifying dangerous red eyes: answer these questions:

1 Is acuity affected? A quick but sensitive test is the ability to read news-print with refractive errors corrected with glasses or a pin-hole. Reduced acuity suggests dangerous pathology.
2 Is the globe painful? Pain is potentially sinister, foreign body sensation may be so, irritation rarely is.
3 Does the pupil respond to light? Absent or sluggish response is sinister.
4 Is the cornea intact? Use fluorescein eyedrops, p432. Corneal damage may be due to trauma or ulcers.

Ask about trauma and discharge, general health and drugs; remember to check for raised pressure. ▶If in doubt, obtain a specialist opinion today.

	Conjunctivitis	Anterior uveitis	Acute glaucoma
Pain	±	++	++ to +++
Photophobia	+	++	–
Acuity	normal	↓	↓
Cornea	normal	normal	steamy or hazy
Pupil	normal	small	large
Intraocular pressure	normal	normal	↑

1 The Zeiss indirect goniolens employs prisms in the place of mirrors. Its 4 prisms allow visualization of the iridocorneal angle in 4 quadrants simultaneously; it is used with a slit lamp.
2 In juvenile arthritis, screen the child every 4 months until they are old enough to report symptoms.
3 This is one of the few occasions when the Sherlock Holmes's among us can properly ask "Have you been handling tarantulas recently?" (Their hairs cause uveitis.)
4 Pain increases on convergence (and pupils constrict) as patients watch a finger approach their nose.

Ophthalmology

Corneal problems Keratitis is corneal inflammation (identified by a white area on the cornea—indicating a collection of white cells in corneal tissue).

Corneal abrasion is an epithelial breach; it occurs without keratitis, eg in trauma, when prophylactic antibiotic ointment (eg **chloramphenicol**) may be used. Ulceration with keratitis is more serious: treat as an emergency, as below. Loss of corneal epithelium causes pain, photophobia ± ↓vision. Uninfective corneal ulcers may result from scratches from sharp objects, trauma, chemical injury or previous corneal disease. Use fluorescein drops and a (blue) bright light (shone tangentially across the globe) to aid diagnosis. Corneal lesions stain green (drops are orange and become more yellow on contact with the eye).

Corneal ulcers may be bacterial (beware pseudomonas: may progress rapidly), herpetic (simplex; zoster), fungal (candida; aspergillus), protozoal (acanthamoeba) or from vasculitis, eg in rheumatoid arthritis. Don't try treating ulcerative keratitis on your own: scarring and visual loss may occur. Except for a simple abrasion (℞: chloramphenicol ointment ± cyloplegia) get help ***today*** for urgent diagnostic smear/Gram stain and scrape. Liaise with microbiologist. ℞: p433. In early stages of ophthalmic shingles, use oral aciclovir (p420). *H. simplex* dendritic ulcers: p416. Cycloplegics (p456) ease photophobia. See BOX.

Episcleritis (fig 1) Inflammation below the conjunctiva in the episclera is often seen with an inflammatory nodule. Bilateral in 30%. The sclera may look blue below a focal, cone-shaped wedge (thin end towards pupil) of engorged vessels that can be moved over the area, unlike in scleritis, where engorged vessels run deeper. The eye aches dully and is tender (esp. over inflamed area). Acuity is usually OK. No cause is found in 70%,[53] but it may complicate rheumatic fever, PAN or SLE. ℞: Topical or systemic NSAIDs.[57,58]

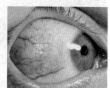

Fig 1. Episcleritis.

Scleritis (Vasculitis of the sclera.)[59] Rarely, the sclera itself is inflamed and pain is significant. There is generalized inflammation with oedema of the conjunctiva and scleral thinning (if necrotizing, globe perforation is a risk). Association: connective tissue disorders; infections. Refer to a specialist. Acuity may be ↓ (esp. if associated with ocular hypertension, a systemic disease, uveitis, or there is posterior scleritis). Tests: ESR, ANCA for AAV antineutrophil cytoplasmic antibody-associated vasculitis (Wegener's ➡polyangiitis). Most need oral steroids/immunosuppresion (ciprofloxacin, topical fortified amikacin, and vancomycin drops if staphylococcal).[60,61]

Conjunctivitis The conjunctiva is red and inflamed, and the hyperaemic vessels may be moved over the sclera, by gentle pressure on the globe. Acuity, pupillary responses, and corneal lustre are unaffected. Eyes itch, burn, and lacrimate. There may be photophobia. It is often bilateral with discharge sticking lids together. Causes: adenoviruses (small lymphoid aggregates appear as follicles on conjunctiva), bacteria (purulent discharge more prominent), or allergic. **Chloramphenicol** 0.5% drops/4-6h is often used (or **fusidic acid** drops). Staphs are common causes—and resistance to **ciprofloxacin** is spreading, and, to a lesser extent, to **gentamicin**.[62] It is usually self-limiting (more prolonged if allergic). In prolonged conjunctivitis, esp. in young adults or those with sexual diseases, consider chlamydial infection (get expert help; see ophthalmia neonatorum, p36). *℞ for allergic conjunctivitis:* Try antihistamine drops, and **emedastine** or **olopatadine** refer if not settling in a few days. **Sodium cromoglicate** and **steroid drops** (after advice from an ophthalmologist) may help.[63]

Subconjunctival haemorrhage This harmless but alarming pool of blood behind the conjunctiva is from a small bleed ("are you on warfarin?etc; your INR is...?"); check BP. It often occurs in frail old ladies who you can make laugh by asking "have you been white-water rafting recently?" (leptospira in sewage).

Refer to a specialist today. What appears below is so that one can have intelligent conversations with specialists, and should not be regarded as a blueprint for therapy by the inexperienced. Herpetic ulcers: see p416.

Smears and cultures Liaise with microbiologist. Specialists may take:
1 Smear for Gram stain—if chronic ulcer Giemsa, PAS (periodic acid Schiff) for fungi, ZN (Ziehl-Neelsen) or auromine for TB.
2 Conjunctival swab to blood agar for tear film contaminants.
3 Multiple corneal scrapes (by experienced person) from ulcer edge with needle for direct inoculation and PCR/other molecular methods.
4 Request the cultures detailed below.

Acute ulcers: Presume bacterial, so culture with blood agar (grows most organisms), chocolate agar (for *Haemophilus* and *Neisseria*), nutrient broth (anaerobes), cooked meat broth (aerobes/anaerobes). *Chronic history:* Consider rarities; culture as above + BHI (brain heart infusion broth for fastidious organisms & fungi, ie kertomycosis), Sabouraud's plate for fungi, anaerobic blood agar (peptococcus, proprionobacteria) + thioglycollate (anaerobes).

Unusual features: Use also viral transport medium, Lowenstein-Jensen agar slope for TB, *E. coli* seeded agar for acanthamoeba. PCR for fungi.[64]

Management: Do smears & culture. Get help. Remove contact lenses. Test cranial nerve v. Is he/she HIV +ve? Until cultures are known, alternate chloramphenicol drops (for Gram +ve bacteria) with ofloxacin drops (for Gram -ve bacteria)[65] or 0.3% cefuroxime drops with gentamicin drops. Adapt in the light of cultures.[2] Admit, eg if diabetes, immunosuppression, or you doubt that the patient will manage the drops. Ofloxacin is given up to a drop every 15min to start with, reduced as necessary (most eye departments have their own protocol). Steroid drops can be added once recovery starts.

Ophthalmology

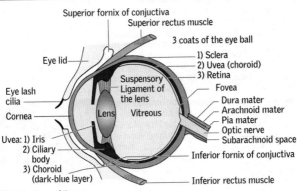

Fig 2. Anatomy of the eye.

Superior fornix of conjuctiva
Superior rectus muscle
3 coats of the eye ball
Eye lid
1) Sclera
2) Uvea (choroid)
3) Retina
Suspensory Ligament of the lens
Fovea
Eye lash cilia
Lens
Vitreous
Dura mater
Arachnoid mater
Pia mater
Optic nerve
Subarachnoid space
Cornea
Uvea: 1) Iris
2) Ciliary body
3) Choroid (dark-blue layer)
Inferior fornix of conjunctiva
Inferior rectus muscle

1 Mooren's ulcer is a chronic, painful peripheral corneal ulcer of unknown cause that easily leads to loss of vision. Severe pain is common and eye(s) may be very red, photophobic, and tearing. It is more common in southern and central Africa, China, and India. Treatments tried: steroidal and non-steroidal anti-inflammatory drops, cytotoxics (topical and systemic), conjunctivectomy, and cornea debridement (superficial keratectomy). None is known to be superior. COCHRANE
2 In one study, the chief Gram +ve bacteria were coagulase -ve staphs (19%) & corynebacteria (16%). The chief Gram -ve organisms were *Moraxella* (19%) and *Pseudomonas aeruginosa* (PA; 3%). PA may be sensitive to ceftazidime and ciprofloxacin. Amikacin, imipenem, and gentamicin are 2nd-line.[65,67]

Ophthalmology

▶▶Urgent help is needed in: retinal artery occlusion of <6h; any sudden visual loss of <6h if the cause is unknown, or giant cell arteritis (GCA). *5 questions:* • Headache associated? (GCA, ESR↑ (▶do this test urgently in all cases ≥50yrs old) • Eye movements hurt? (optic neuritis) • Lights/flashes preceding visual loss? (detached retina) • Like a curtain descending? amaurosis fugax may precede permanent visual loss, eg from emboli/GCA • Poorly controlled DM: fig1 shows vitreous haemorrhage (bottom left) from new vessels (top right). *Check:* Acuity, pupil reaction, fundi. Then refer. See BOX.

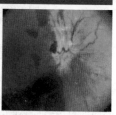
Fig 1. Vitreous haemorrhage.

Anterior ischaemic optic neuropathy (AION) The optic nerve is damaged if posterior ciliary arteries are blocked by inflammation or atheroma. *Fundoscopy:* pale/swollen optic disc. *Arteritic AION (giant cell arteritis): The other eye is at risk* until steroids are given. *Symptoms:* malaise, jaw claudication (chewing pain) ± tender scalp and temporal arteries (thickened ± absent pulses), neck pain. *Tests:* ESR (>47) & CRP (>2.45mg/dL) preferably before steroids; temporal artery biopsy within 1 week of starting prednisolone; may miss affected sections of artery (skip lesions). ℞: ▶▶Start prednisolone 80mg/24h PO promptly (some advocate higher IV doses if visual failure is occurring). Tailing off steroids as ESR and symptoms settle may take >1yr.[67,68] *Nonarteritic AION:* Associations: BP↑; lipids↑; DM, smoking. Treating these protects vision in the other eye. Histology: necrosis & apoptosis at the photoreceptor level.[69]

Vitreous haemorrhage (VH) Source from retinal new vessels (diabetes, branch or central retinal vein occlusion; see BOX), retinal tears, retinal detachment or trauma. Small extravasations of blood produce vitreous floaters, (seen by the patient as small black dots or tiny ring-like forms with clear centres) which may not greatly obscure vision. With a large enough bleed to obscure vision, there is no red reflex and the retina may not be seen. A B-scan ultrasound is needed to identify a cause in this situation. VH undergoes spontaneous absorption. In dense VH a vitrectomy is done to remove the blood in the vitreous if the retina is torn/detached or the patient needs treatment of new vessels. In diabetic patients who have previously had photocoagulation for new vessels with recurrent VH, it is acceptable to wait 3 months for resolution.

Subacute loss of vision *Optic neuritis* (fig2) Unilateral loss of acuity occurs over hours or days. Colour vision is affected (dyschromatopsia): reds appear less red, 'red desaturation'—and eye movements hurt. The pupil shows an afferent defect (p424). The disc is normal in ~60%, swollen (papillitis) in 23%, blurred and/or hyperaemic in 18% (+haemorrhages in 2%). Temporal pallor occurs in 10% suggesting a past attack of optic neuritis in the same eye.

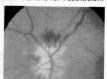
Fig 2. Optic neuritis

Recovery is usual over 2-6 weeks, but 45-80% develop multiple sclerosis (MS) in the next 15yrs. Other causes: syphilis, Devic's demyelination, Leber's optic atrophy, diabetes, vitamin deficiency. ℞: High-dose methylprednisolone• for 72h (250mg/6h IV), then prednisolone (1mg/kg/d PO) for 11 days may briefly delay onset of MS (no change to long-term disability).[70]

Transient visual loss ▶Always think of vascular causes, such as platelet-fibrin/cholesterol microemboli from atherosclerotic plaques in the heart or carotid arteries (any stenosis or bruit?).[71] Be cautious in diagnosing migraine for the 1st time if aged >50yrs.

Typical causes:
• Vascular; TIA; migraine
• Multiple sclerosis
• Subacute glaucoma (not always painful)
• Papilloedema

Central retinal artery occlusion

There is dramatic visual loss within seconds of occlusion. In 90% acuity is finger counting or worse. An afferent pupil defect (p424) appears within seconds and may precede retinal changes by 1h. The retina appears white, with a cherry red spot at the macula (figs 1-2, p436). Exclude temporal arteritis. Occlusion is often thrombo-embolic (clot, tumour, infective etc). Look for signs of atherosclerosis (bruits; BP↑), heart valve disease, diabetes, smoking, or lipids↑.[72] ▶▶If seen within 6h of onset aim is to increase retinal blood flow by reducing intraocular pressure by ocular massage, surgical removal of aqueous from the anterior chamber or the use of antihypertensive treatment. NB: fluorescein angiography may show branch retinal artery occlusion.[73] Hyperbaric oxygen has been tried (~70% get improved acuity).[74]

If a single branch of the retinal artery is occluded, the retinal and visual changes relate only to the part of the retina supplied.

Retinal vein occlusions: central or branch vein?

Central retinal vein occlusion (CRVO) Incidence increases with age. It is commoner than arterial occlusion. Causes/associations: arteriosclerosis, BP↑, diabetes and polycythaemia; glaucoma (all types). If the whole central retinal vein is thrombosed, there is visual loss (eg acuity reduced to finger counting). It is less sudden than central retinal artery occlusion. Visual loss may be perceived as sudden by the patient but the mechanism is of visual loss is due to the development of ischaemia and macular oedema.

CRVO is divided into non-ischaemic and ischaemic (with cotton wool spots, swollen optic nerve, macular oedema, and risk of neovascularization; hence need for follow-up). Non-ischaemic forms have better acuity (even 6/6) and prognosis (signs are less dramatic too). But this can convert to the ischaemic form in 30%; hence the need for follow-up. A fundus fluorescein angiogram is used to determine the degree of ischaemia and pan-retinal photocoagulation is given to prevent or treat neovascularization. Unfortunately even if the macular oedema resolves anatomically visual prognosis is poor. Aim to prevent rubeotic glaucoma and a painful eye (beracizumab and ranbizumab (Lucentis®) (p439))[75] can treat the macular oedema), as can lasers and dexamethasone intravitreal implants.NICE 2011

Branch retinal vein occlusion Signs: Unilateral visual loss and fundal appearances in the corresponding area. Retinal ischaemia leads to release of vascular endothelial growth factor (VEGF) and retinal new vessel formation. Treatment of neovascularization is with laser photocoagulation. Macular oedema persisting for months without improvement may receive grid pattern argon laser photocoagulation (± arterial crimping).[76, n=72]

Diagnosis and differential diagnosis Other causes of sudden loss of vision: • Retinal detachment (p444) • Acute glaucoma (painful, p430) • Migraine.

Stroke patients may complain of monocular blindness but visual field testing will usually reveal a homonymous hemianopia. Sudden bilateral visual loss is unusual (may be CMV infection in HIV patients, p448).

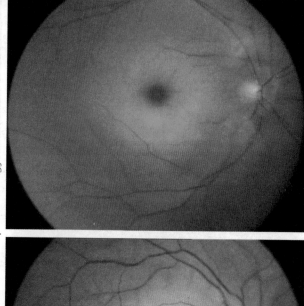

Figs 1-5. Retinal artery occlusion (both the above images) and central retinal vein occlusion (right).[1] With arterial occlusion note retinal pallor and the cherry-red macula. With central retinal vein occlusion note hyperaemia and haemorrhages—known as the stormy sunset appearance (last figure).

1 We thank Dr R K Reddy, Dr Badrinath, and Dr Ravishankar (Sankara Nethralya, Chennai, India) for their help with this page, and for permission to reproduce these images.

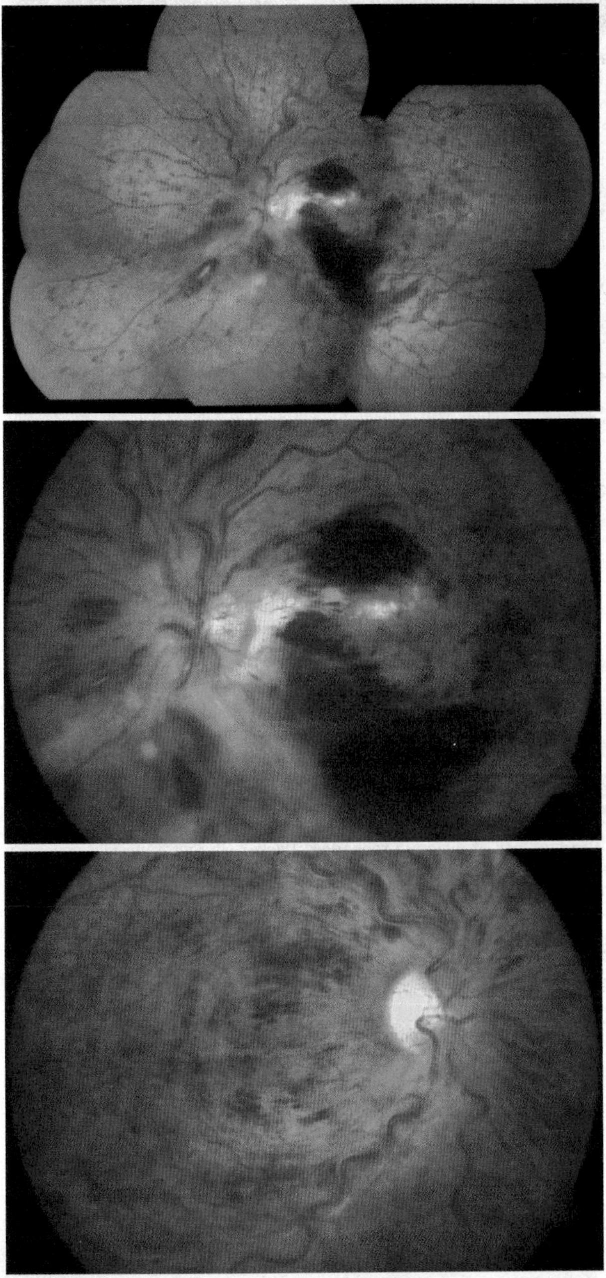

Be aware that for many, the chief question is likely to be "will I go blind?": be optimistic where possible. Patients may *not* tell you that they also fear they are going mad, having complex visual hallucinations, often of faces. These occur without psychiatric signs and are often related to failing vision in the elderly: the Charles Bonnet syndrome (p463).[77]

Typical causes
• Cataract
• Macular degeneration
• Glaucoma (p440)
• Diabetic retinopathy
• Hypertension (p448)
• Optic atrophy (below)
• Slow retinal detachment

Choroiditis (choroidoretinitis) The choroid is part of the uvea (iris, ciliary body and choroid), and inflammatory disorders affecting the uvea may also affect the choroid. The retina may be invaded by organisms which set up a granulomatous reaction (which can be mistaken for a retinoblastoma). Toxoplasmosis and toxocara are more common than TB. Sarcoidosis is another cause. *Tests:* CXR; Mantoux; serology. In the acute phase, vision may be blurred, a grey-white raised patch is seen on the retina, vitreous opacities occur, and there may be cells in the anterior chamber. Later, a choroidoretinal scar (white patch with pigmentation around) will be seen, these being symptomless unless involving the macula. Treat the cause.

Choroid melanomas are the commonest malignant tumour of the eye. Appearing as mottled grey/black on the fundus, they can cause retinal detachment over the growth. Spread is haematogenous or by local orbit invasion. *Treatment:* Enucleation, plaque radiotherapy, local tumour irradiation, photocoagulation, transpupillary thermotherapy & microsurgical resection.

Age-related macular degeneration (ARMD) is the chief cause of registrable blindness.[UK] Cause: behavioural/nutritional factors (eg ↓B_{12})[78] and (epi)genetic mechanisms.[2] It occurs in the elderly who present with deteriorating central vision. There is pigment, drusen (BOX & fig 2) and sometimes bleeding at the macula. ARMD is categorized as dry or wet. Dry ARMD shows mainly drusen and degenerative changes at the macular. It progresses slowly. Wet ARMD occurs when aberrant vessels grow from the choroid into the neuro-sensory retina and leak (choroidal new vessels: CNV): Vision deteriorates rapidly and distortion is a key feature. Ophthalmoscopy shows fluid exudation, localized detachment of the pigment. Treatment is available for wet ARMD (BOX). Be prompt as substantial visual loss may occur while the patient waits.[79] Patients are advised to stop smoking and have a diet rich in green vegetable.

Gradual loss of vision in teenagers Think of Stargardt macular degeneration and look for prominent yellow flecks in the retina. This condition was the first to be treated with embryonal stem cells.

Tobacco-alcohol amblyopia From cyanide radicals, when smoking and alcohol excess are combined. Signs: optic atrophy (fig 1); loss of red/green discrimination (early) scotomata. Vitamins *may* help (B_1, B_2, B_6, B_{12}, folic acid).[80]

Optic atrophy Discs are pale (degree doesn't correlate with visual loss). It may be from ↑intraocular pressure (glaucoma), or retinal damage (choroiditis, retinitis pigmentosa, cerebromacular degeneration), or be due to ischaemia (retinal artery occlusion). *Causative toxins:* Tobacco; methanol; lead; arsenic; quinine; carbon bisulfide.

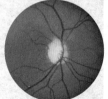

Fig 1. Optic atrophy.

Other causes: Leber's optic atrophy (p648), multiple sclerosis (MS), syphilis, external pressure on the nerve (intraorbital or intracranial tumours, Paget's disease affecting the skull). Examine the cerebellum and eye movements: nystagmus in the abducting eye suggests MS (or stroke or DM); in the elderly look for temporal artery pulselessness (or a scar from a previous biopsy).

Ophthalmology

Use of services by older patients with failing vision

There is good evidence in the UK of under-use of services by older people. Population-based cross-sectional studies in primary care show that prevalence of bilateral visual impairment (acuity <6/12) is ~30%. Most of these are not in touch with ophthalmic services. ▶*Three-quarters of these have remediable problems.* In one study, 20% had acuity in one or both eyes of <6/60 ('blind'). Typical causes were found to be cataract (30%), macular degeneration (8%), and undiagnosed chronic glaucoma.[81][n=1547]

Optic nerve drusen

Drusen signify optic nerve-head axonal degeneration. Abnormal axonal metabolism leads to intracellular mitochondrial calcification. Some axons rupture and mitochondria are extruded into the extra-cellular space.[82] Calcium is deposited here, and drusen form. The optic disc edge is made irregular by the lumpy, yellow matter. The optic cup is absent and vessels show abnormal branching patterns.[83]

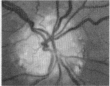

Fig 2. Optic drusen. ©Mr C Chau.

Managing age-related macular degeneration (ARMD)

Arrange a fluorescein angiogram at the outset and then 4-6-weekly reviews with a photograph and an OCT (optical coherence tomography).

Intravitreal vascular endothelial growth factor (VEGF) inhibitors: Benefits: ↑acuity; ↓cell proliferation, ↓formation of new blood vessels, ↓vascular leaks.[84] Monthly bevacizumab (Avastin®) and ranibizumab (Lucentis®; NICE approved) injections for 1yr give the same acuity benefit (~8 more letters seen on the chart). Avastin® is *far* cheaper but may have more SE (24% vs 19%).[85][CATT study][N=1208]

Laser photocoagulation: May be used in eyes with specific signs on fluorescein angiography and juxtafoveal or extrafoveal lesions only. Persistent or recurrent CNV occurs in ~50% of treated eyes within 3 years of therapy.

Intravitreal steroids: Triamcinolone is an adjunct to PDT & VEGF inhibitors.[86]

Screening: Once signs of ARMD are seen, patients explain about reporting signs of neovascularization: a good self-test is "do straight lines on graph paper appear straight?". Refer if distortions or sudden blank spots.[87]

If these measures are inapplicable: Most must rely on visual aids (eg magnifiers) to read. Advise a diet rich in fruit and leafy green vegetables, with supplements if this diet causes problems.[88]

Antioxidants/vitamins: AREDS ([Age-Related Eye Disease Study][89]) 'established' that supplementing diets with zinc, β-carotene, and vitamin C & E slowed AMD progression.[1] Recently lutein, zeaxanthin, B vitamins, and omega-3 fatty acids are also reported to ↓progression, while vitamin E and β-carotene where found to ↑risk of late AMD, so more trials are under way (AREDS2).[89,90] NB: antioxidants may have unintended, even fatal consequences:[91] so...be cautious!

---

1 Studies of monozygotic AMD-discordant twins: the twin with more advanced AMD, larger drusen, and pigment area tended to be the heavier smoker. The twin with the earlier stage tended to have ↑dietary vitamin D, betaine, and methionine intake.[92]

Ophthalmology

Glaucoma implies optic neuropathy with death of many retinal ganglion cells and their optic nerve axons. It is asymptomatic until visual fields are badly impaired; hence the need for screening. If ↑intraocular pressure (IOP) is found, lifelong follow-up is needed (≥yearly; more often early on). It accounts for 7% of new blind registrations. Visual field loss may manifest as dangerous difficulty dodging cars while crossing busy roads.[93]

Definition/pathogenesis Glaucoma is present when, on field testing, 3 or more locations are outside normal limits, and the cup-to-disc ratio[1] is greater than that seen in 97.5% of the population. IOP may be raised, *but this is not part of the definition*. Susceptibility of a patients retina and optic nerve to IOP related damage is very variable. IOP ≥21mmHg may or may not correlate with cupping (deepening and excavation), nerve damage, with scotomata (sausage-shaped field defects near the blind spot, which may coalesce to form big defects). Nasal and superior fields are lost first (temporal last). Normal cups are similar in shape and occupy <50% of the disc. In glaucoma these enlarge (esp. along vertical axis). As damage progresses the disc pales (atrophy), and the cup widens and deepens, so vessels emerging from the disc appear to have breaks as they disappear into the cup and are then seen at the base again (figs 1-2). Notching of the cup and haemorrhage at the disc may occur. Since the central field is intact, good acuity is maintained, so presentation is often delayed until irreversible optic nerve damage. Control of IOP *does* stop visual field loss but does not reverse it.[94] Some get glaucoma with *normal* IOP (eg if retrobulbar blood flow↓).[95]

Screen if at high-risk >35yrs old (typical age at detection: 60yrs) with +ve family history (esp. siblings); African-Caribbean; myopia; diabetic/thyroid eye disease. Technology is making primary prevention cost-effective. *Tests must be combined*, as follows, in order of effectiveness: •Multiple stimulus static visual field screening •Documenting optic disc cupping •IOPs↑.[96,97] Follow-up of ↑IOP.[98] Accredited community-based optometrists with a special interest (OSIS) in glaucoma may reduce what is a *huge* task for hospitals.[2012]

Drugs treatment Reduce IOP by 30% of baseline. Surgery is used if drugs fail.
• *Prostaglandin analogues* (latanoprost 50µg/mL; travoprost) ↑uveoscleral outflow. *Dose:* once daily (evenings). SE: red eye, iris colour change, periocular skin pigmentation, eyelash growth.
• *β-blockers* (timolol 0.25–0.5% or betaxolol 0.5%) use twice daily (/24h for Timoptol LA®) to ↓production of aqueous. They are β-blockers. (∴ caution in asthma or heart failure; systemic absorption occurs with no 1st-pass liver metabolism.) SE: dry eyes, corneal anaesthesia, allergy, ↓exercise tolerance.[99]
• *α-adrenergic agonists* (brimonidine, apraclonidine) ↓production of aqueous and ↑uveoscleral outflow. SE: lethargy dry mouth.
• *Carbonic anhydrase inhibitors* (dorzolamide & brinzolamide drops, acetazolamide PO) ↓production of aqueous. SE of acetazolamide: lassitude, dyspepsia, K+↓, paraesthesiae. Avoid if pregnant.
• *Miotics* (pilocarpine 0.5–4% drops) ↓resistance to aqueous outflow. It causes miosis, acuity↓, and brow ache from ciliary muscle spasm. Use 4 times daily.
• *Sympathomimetic* (dipivefrine 0.1% drops). Caution if heart disease, BP↑, and closed angle glaucoma. SE: sore, smarting, red eyes/vision↓. Use 12-hourly.
• *Fixed-dose combination drops*: Can give the best 24h efficacy NB: dorzolamide + timolol is better than brimonidine + timolol.[100]

Surgery: Trabeculectomy is a filtration surgery that establishes a pressure valve at the limbus so aqueous can flow into a conjunctival bleb. Problems include early failure, hypotony, bleb leakage, infection (normal healing can cause bleb failure, but this can be delayed by topical cytotoxics, eg fluorouracil). Effects of *argon laser trabeculoplasty* are often brief: its role may be in the elderly.

Follow-up Equipment and regimens are complex, and must conform to NICE advice; 4-6-monthly visits may be needed if IOP is off target and risk of developing chronic open angle glaucoma is high (take into account age, IOP, corneal thickness, appearance and size of the optic nerve head). If favourable, monitor every 1-2yrs.

Optic disc cupping is characterized by loss of disc substance—hence enlargement of the cup. Normal cup:disc ratio 0.4-0.7.[101] This depends on the size of the disc: ▶a large cup in a small disc is probably pathological.[1] As cupping develops, the disc vessels are displaced nasally. Asymmetric cupping suggests glaucoma. The cup:disc ratio is increased to >0.4 (fig 1). If the cup:disc ratio is >0.9, cupping is said to be severe.[102] Notching at the neuroretinal rim is usually inferior, and best seen where the vessels enter the disc. The sharp turning of the vessels is called bayoneting.[103] Progression is more related to the size of the neuro-retinal rim than to lack of disc size.[104] Glaucoma affects the anterior visual pathway at least up to the optic chiasm, to an extent that correlates with glaucomatous optic nerve damage.

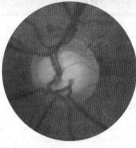

Fig 1. Cupped disc. ©Mr C Chau.

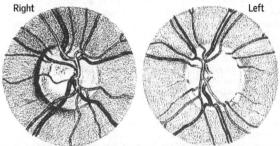

Fig 2. This patient has open angle glaucoma which hasn't yet damaged the right disc. The left optic disc is grossly cupped and atrophic.
Reproduced from Parr, Introduction to Ophthalmology, with permission from University of Otago Press.

Educating people about their glaucoma

It is common for people to be seen regularly for years in the glaucoma clinic and yet understand almost nothing about their condition. "This is their fault—if they asked, we'd be delighted to tell..." But it's really our fault and we should do better, as lack of knowledge is dangerous and demoralizing. In one study 80% thought that glaucoma drops could have no systemic effects, and 48% believed symptoms would warn them of disease progression. 30% of new patients believe that blindness is likely.[105]

So try to explain what happens in glaucoma, and give printed details (check that the patient can read them), and stress that they should let their doctors know that they are on glaucoma treatment.

"Can I do anything to help myself?" Possibly: reducing oxidative stress in mitochondria can be protective, eg with gingko, dark chocolate, polyphenolic flavonoids (in tea, coffee, red wine), melatonin, and anthocyanosides[2] eg in bilberries[uk] (*Vaccinium myrtillus*) and blueberries[usa] (*V. corymbosum*).v[106,107]

There is more to glaucoma than just...

1 Normal small discs (1.0-1.3mm) have small cups and normal big discs (>1.8) have large cups, so large normal discs may be misnamed glaucomatous. Mean disc diameter: 1.5mm. Mean cup:disc ratio is ~0.35, 0.45, & 0.55 for small, medium and big discs (95th centiles for upper limit of normal are 0.59, 0.66, & 0.74).[108]

2 Anthocyanosides (eg from fresh or dried blueberries[109]) have interesting eye effects: they ↓problems from retinal inflammation and help night vision in myopes,●[98] eg with asthenopia (eye strain/pain, blurred vision, headache and occasional double vision on reading, computer work, or tedious visual tasks).

▶When a cataract is found, measure fasting plasma glucose (to exclude DM). ▶Any opacity in the lens is called a cataract. ▶The 4 major causes of blindness in the world are cataract, vitamin A deficiency, trachoma, and onchocerciasis. Cataracts are found in 75% of over 65s but in only 20% of 45-65-year-olds.

Ophthalmoscopic classification is by lens appearance. With immature cataracts the red reflex still occurs; if dense cataract there is no red reflex, or visible fundus. Nuclear cataracts change the lens refractive index and are common in old age, as are cortical spoke-like wedge-shaped opacities. Anterior and posterior polar cataracts are localized, commonly inherited, and lie in the visual axis. Subcapsular opacities (eg from steroid use) are just deep to the lens capsule—in the visual axis. Dot opacities are common in normal lenses but are also seen in fast-developing cataracts in diabetes or dystrophia myotonica.

Presentation Blurred vision; unilateral cataracts are often unnoticed, but loss of stereopsis affects distance judgment. Bilateral cataracts cause gradual loss of vision (frequent spectacle changes as refraction changes) ± dazzle (esp. in sunlight) ± monocular diplopia. In children they may present as squint, loss of binocular function, or a white pupil, or as nystagmus (infants)/amblyopia.

Surgery Mydriatic drops, sunshades/sunglasses help a bit, but if symptoms are troubling, lifestyle is restricted, or if unable to read a number-plate at 67 feet (and they need to drive) offer surgery.[1] Explain risks: 2% get serious complications; even if surgery may vastly improves vision, eyes may not be entirely normal after (dazzle/glare often remains). Distant spectacles are often needed too. >30% have co-existing macular degeneration,[et al] which limits outcome.

The ideal is day-case surgery using local anaesthesia with small-incision surgery and phacoemulsion + a intraocular lens (IOL) implant. This applies to the vast majority of patients. Younger people, high myopes, and the squeamish may prefer general anaesthesia. An incision of ~3mm is made, and the lens is removed by phacoemulsion (ultrasound breaks it up: it is then aspirated into a cannula). The incision is fractionally enlarged and an artificial lens (eg of Perspex, acrylic, or silicon) implanted. Lenses are foldable so they can be put through a smaller incision. The patient can usually return home immediately afterwards. A dressing may be needed for a few hours. With phacoemulsification, full activities can be resumed next day. With complicated surgery or extracapsular extraction, a larger incision is needed and there may be more limitations. Patients use antibiotic and anti-inflammatory drops for 3-6 weeks post-op. Then they need to change spectacles to get the full benefit of surgery. Multifocal IOLs exist and in appropriately selected patients they can be helpful.

Post-op complications: Post-op posterior *capsule thickening* is common. It is deliberately left at surgery to make surgery safer. It opacifies in ~20%, over months or years post-op; it seems "like my cataract returning". It is easily treated by capsulotomy with a Yag laser as an outpatient.

As refraction is corrected, *astigmatism* is more noticed. This can be corrected during surgery (eg by toric intraocular lens or eyeball shape change by placing the incision in the exact right place) in the light of pre-op biometry.

Some *eye irritation* needing additional or altered drops post-op is common. Some may have *anterior uveitis* requiring new medication. Rarely, there may be vitreous haemorrhage, retinal detachment, or glaucoma (± permanent visual loss), and endophthalmitis (<3/10,000; but pseudomonal clusters may occur).

Prevention/photoprotection● 1 Use sunglasses (UV-B↓).[111] 2 ↓Oxidative stress (esp. in smokers, with antioxidants, eg vitamin C and caffeine[etc]).[112,113]

---

1 Don't support arbitrary thresholds of acuity, eg 'both eyes <6/12', adopted by some cash-poor NHS PCTs.

Cataract risk factors

Most cataracts are age related. In children, many are genetic (?some genetic influence in adults too). Cataracts occur early in: diabetes mellitus; with topical, oral, or inhaled steroid use; with high myopia; dystrophia myotonica.

Pre- and post-operative care

Prior to surgery *ocular biometry* must be done. This is a measurement of the curvature of the cornea and the length of the eye which enables prediction of the suitable intraocular lens implant for the patient (fig 1). In most cases it is aimed to leave the patient emmetropic (in focus for distance), or just slightly myopic, but this may vary considerably depending on patient preference and pre-existing refraction. It is not an exact science as the clinical measurements vary and many people do continue to wear spectacles post-operatively for a remaining refractive error—but heightened patient expectations for precise post-operative refractive results make biometry vital.[114]

On obtaining new spectacles many experience symptoms of imbalance; these should settle in 2-3 weeks. If they do not, recommend return to the optometrist to check the correct spectacles have been dispensed. If there is still a continuing problem they should return to the ophthalmologist.

If patients develop a painful red eye or loss of vision post-operatively they should be referred back to the ophthalmologist urgently to deal with possible complications. Many experience awareness of the eye or dry, or gritty sensations and lubricants such as **Viscotears**® may help. If vision deteriorates with time they should initially visit the optometrist to see if they need a new prescription change; and thereafter the ophthalmologist to consider Yag laser capsulotomy or exclusion of other problems.

Ophthalmology

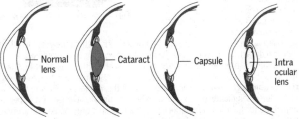

Normal lens — Cataract — Capsule — Intra ocular lens

Fig 1. Position of the intraocular lens after cataract surgery.

Cataracts at birth: ▶act within 4 weeks!

If there is a congenital cataract the patient needs to be referred urgently to ophthalmology for surgical consideration. Intervention needs to be done within the latent period of visual development (1st 6 weeks of life) to prevent significant deprivation amblyopia. Do a TORCH screen too (p35).[115]

The retina consists of an outer pigmented layer (in contact with the choroid), and an inner sensory layer (in contact with the vitreous). At the centre of the posterior part lies the macula: at its centre lies the fovea (fig 1, p447). This has many cones, so acuity is greatest here. ~3mm medial to the fovea is the optic disc, which contains no rods or cones (the visual field's blind spot).

Optic disc Think *colour; contour; cup. Colour* should be a pale pink. It is more pallid in optic atrophy (p438). *Contour:* the disc may appear oval in astigmatic eyes, and appear abnormally large in myopic eyes. Disc margins are blurred in papilloedema (eg from raised intracranial pressure, malignant hypertension, cavernous sinus thrombosis), and optic neuritis. Blood vessels radiate away from the disc. The normal arterial/venous width ratio is 2:3. Venous engorgement appears in retinal vein thrombosis; abnormal retinal pallor with artery occlusion; and haemorrhages + exudates in hypertension and DM. *Cup:* the disc has a physiological cup which lies centrally and should occupy ~⅓ of the disc diameter. Cup widening and deepening occurs in glaucoma (p440).

Retinal detachment (RD, fig 1)[116] may be rhegmatogenous,[1] following separation of the vitreous leading to a retinal tear then detachment; secondary to some intraocular problem (eg melanoma, or fibrous bands in the vitreous in diabetes), occur after cataract surgery and trauma (retinal dialysis). Myopic eyes are more prone to detachment, the higher the myopia, the greater the risk—and cataract surgery for myopia carries ↑risk of detachment.

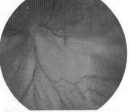

Fig 1. RD; note retinal folds (1-3 o'clock) & distorted disc.   ©Bristol Eye Hospital.

In retinal detachments, holes/tears in the retina allow fluid to separate the sensory retina from the retinal pigment epithelium. If a retinal break is identified before a detachment occurs, cryo/laser retinopexy may be preventive.

Detachment presents with 4 'F's: floaters, flashes (in ~50%), field loss, and fall in acuity—painless and may be as a curtain falling over the vision (eg the curtain falls down as the lower half of the retina detaches upwards). Field defects indicate position and extent of the detachment (in superior detachments field loss is inferior). Ophthalmoscopy: grey opalescent retina, ballooning forward. Extensive detachment of the retina will pull off the macular. If it does detach, central vision is lost and doesn't always recover completely even if the retina is successfully fixed. Rate of detachment varies: upper halves are quicker. ►►Refer urgently, for surgery: vitrectomy and gas tamponade (or silicone oil), scleral silicone implants. Cryotherapy or laser coagulation is used to secure the retina. Post-op re-detachment occurs in 5-10%.

Retinitis pigmentosa This is the most prevalent inherited degeneration in the retina. Sporadic types are more common (mostly autosomal recessive—but autosomal dominant types have better prognosis; x-linked is the rarest form, with poorest prognosis). Through life, 25% retain ability to read, with reduced visual fields. Only a few have acuity ≤6/60 at aged 20yrs; but by 50, many are reduced to this level.[117] Novel non-standard therapies: neural prosthetics (artificial vision by stimulating retinal ganglion cells electrically).[118]

Toxoplasma This intracellular protozoan may cause 'punched-out' pigmented chorioretinal scars (seen on fundoscopy; may cause acuity↓↓). R: OHCM p404.

---

1 *Rhegmatogenous* derives from Greek *rhegma*, a discontinuity or a break.[119] Rhegmatogenous retinal detachments (RRD) occur when a retinal tear leads to fluid accumulation with a separation of the neurosensory retina from the underlying retinal pigment epithelium. It is the commonest type.

Glasgow's nomenclature [120] The macula is an area ~5.5mm across, just lateral to the optic disc. Its carotenoid pigments give it its colour. It nearly corresponds to the histological *area centralis* (>1 layer of ganglion cells). In its middle is a 1.5mm pit, the fovea (≈*fovea centralis*; no ganglion cells). This has a tiny area (350µm[121]), the foveola (overlapped by the *capillary-free zone*, 400µm across), where cones are narrow, long and densely packed (300,000/mm²) compared with cones on the foveal rim (fig 1, p447), which in turn, are narrower and longer than perifoveal cones.[122] This cone gradient correlates with acuity.[123]

A macular hole (fig 1) is a full-thickness defect of retinal tissue. It involves the fovea (visual acuity↓). Prevalence: 3.3/1000 in persons >55yrs. There is an approximately 12% chance of a similar hole developing in the other eye.

Presentation Distorted vision with visual loss. Look for a tiny punched-out area in the centre of the macula: there may be yellow-white deposits at the base. Slit lamp exam (with a convex lens, 78D) shows a round excavation with well-defined borders interrupting the slit lamp beam. Often there is semi-translucent tissue suspended over the hole—the hole is typically surrounded by a grey halo of detached retina. ►Refer to a specialist vitreo-retinal surgeon.

Pathogenesis Idiopathic focal age-related perifoveal vitreous cortex shrinkage→tangential traction on the fovea→detachment→macular holes. Displacement of the fovea reveals the underlying xanthophyll pigment.

Stages:

1a Impending hole seen as a yellow spot at the fovea. There is loss of the characteristic foveal depression due to anterior traction from the vitreous.

2b Occult hole: donut-shaped yellow ring (~200-300µm) centred on the foveola. Vision is usually good at this stage. ~50% of holes progress to stage 2—when treatment is needed.

3 Full thickness macular hole (<400µm). with a surrounding cuff of subretinal fluid. The cortical vitreous is still attached to the fovea. Vision is reduced with image distortion.

4 Holes >400µm with localized separation of the vitreous cortex at the macula.

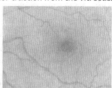

Fig 1. Macular hole.

Tests Amsler grids (p428) reveal visual distortion; optical coherence tomography (OCT, fig 2) diagnoses and stages macular holes. Fluorescein angiography (FA) helps differentiate macular holes from cystoid macular oedema and choroidal neovascularization (CNV).

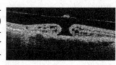

Fig 2. Stage 4 hole (optical coherence tomography).
©Quresh Mohamed FCROphth.

Treatment In stage 1, see what happens (no treatment if there is spontaneous resolution or no progression). Surgery: a vitrectomy is done to remove the vitreous and the internal limiting membrane over the hole is peeled. An air bubble is introduced to nudge (tamponade) the macula back into position. The patient spends 1-2 post-op weeks face down. Series of patients have been variously reported, with hole closure rates of ≤95% (~67% improve by ≥2 lines of visual acuity). Success is also possible if the hole is long-standing (>6 months).

However, in some patients, more than one operation is needed to close the hole, and adverse effects may occur: macular retinal pigment epithelium changes, retinal detachments, iatrogenic retinal tears, enlargement of the hole, macular light toxicity, postoperative intraocular pressure spikes. Many patients develop cataracts (76% of cases requiring extraction within 2 years). Patients not suitable or not wishing for this need visual aids (eg to read).

▶Keep BP <150/85mmHg and all the major diabetic retinopathies are less common.[1] Diabetes can be bloody and blinding—the leading cause of blindness in those aged 20-65 (UK). Almost any part of the eye can be affected: mainly cataract and retinopathy. 30% of adults have ocular problems when diabetes presents. At presentation, the lens may have a higher refractive index producing relative myopia. On treatment, the refractive index reduces, and vision is more hypermetropic, so don't correct refractive errors until diabetes is controlled.

Structural changes Diabetes accelerates formation and progress of age-related cataract. Typically this is premature senile cataract, but young diabetics can also be affected at presentation; here the lens has taken up a lot of glucose which is converted by aldolase reductase to sorbitol. Diabetes causes ocular ischaemia, which can cause new blood vessel forming on the iris (rubeosis), and, if these block the drainage of aqueous fluid, glaucoma may result.

Retinopathy Pathogenesis: microangiopathy in capillaries, precapillary arterioles and venules causes occlusion ± leakage. *Vascular occlusion* causes ischaemia ± new vessels in the retina, optic disc, and iris, ie *proliferative retinopathy*. New vessels can bleed (vitreous haemorrhage). Retraction of fibrous tissue running with new vessels heightens risk of retinal detachment. Occlusion also causes *cotton wool spots* (ischaemic nerve fibres). *Vascular leakage:* As pericytes are lost, capillaries bulge (microaneurysms) and there is oedema & hard exudates (lipoprotein & lipid filled macrophages). Rupture of microaneurysms at the nerve fibre level causes flame shaped haemorrhages; when deep in the retina, *blot haemorrhages* form.

▶Presymptomatic screening enables timely laser photocoagulation. Screen by regular eye exam or retinal photography. Screen all diabetic patients annually in the community, by dilated fundus photography which is then reviewed by a trained screening service. Referrals are then made accordingly. Lesions are mostly at the posterior pole and can be easily seen by ophthalmoscope. *Non-proliferative diabetic retinopathy (NPDR)* is rated as mild, moderate or severe depending on the degree of ischaemia. Signs comprise microaneurysms (seen as 'dots'), haemorrhages (flame shaped or 'blots') hard exudates (yellow patches), engorged tortuous veins, cotton wool spots, large blot haemorrhages (the latter 3 are signs of significant ischaemia). NPDR can progress to sight-threatening proliferative retinopathy. *Proliferative diabetic retinopathy (PDR):* Fine new vessels appear on the optic disc, retina and can cause vitreous haemorrhage. *Maculopathy:* Leakage from the vessels close to the macula cause oedema and can significantly threaten vision (clinically significant macular oedema). It can exist with otherwise mild retinopathy.

▶Refer those with maculopathy, severe NPDR, or proliferative retinopathy *urgently* for assessment[2] and treatment (eg photocoagulation) to protect vision.

Treatment Good control of diabetes prevents new vessels forming. 'Metabolic memory' effects mean that early good control of diabetes with insulin pays dividends later.[124] Pregnancy, dyslipidaemia, BP↑, renal disease, smoking, and anaemia may accelerate retinopathy. Photocoagulation by laser is used to treat both maculopathy (focal or grid) and proliferative retinopathy (panretinal). Intravitreal **triamcinolone** and anti-VEGF drugs (p439) are used with laser to treat diabetic macular oedema. See figs 1 & 2. If vitreous haemorrhage is massive and does not clear, vitrectomy may be needed.

CNS effects Ocular palsies may occur, typically nerves III and VI. In diabetic third nerve palsy the pupil may be spared as fibres to the pupil run peripherally in the nerve, receiving blood supply from the pial vessels. Argyll Robertson pupils and Horner's syndrome may also occur (p424).

1 UKPDS data: N=1148. Absolute risk for blindness was 3.1 per 1000 patient-years if control was tight vs 4.1 for others. There was no difference if the BP was lowered by ACE-i or β-blockers.[125]
2 Fluorescein angiography and optical coherence tomography OCT imaging are important tools here.

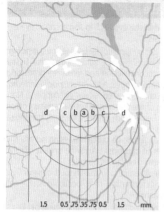

Fig 1. In this diagram of the retina that is depicted in **fig 2**, where are the lesions? In this image of the macular region, **a** is the *foveola*, **b** is the *fovea centralis*, **c** is the *parafoveal area*, and **d** is the *perifoveal area*.[126] See p445 for anatomical/histological nomenclature.[127] In day-to-day clinical parlance the word fovea is often used (confusingly) to refer to fovea centralis and/or the foveola.

The macula is a circle centred on the foveola whose diameter is the distance between the temporal border of the optic disc and the foveola.[128] NICE

Results of retinal screening in diabetes: when to refer to a surgeon:

1 Maculopathy:
  - If screening shows exudate or retinal thickening within one optic disc diameter of the centre of the fovea
  - Circinate or other group of exudates within the macula
  - Any microaneurysm or haemorrhage within 1 disc-diameter of the centre of the fovea, if best visual acuity is <6/12.

2 There are features of pre-proliferative retinopathy (venous beading; venous loops or reduplications; multiple deep, round or blot haemorrhages).

3 Any unexplained drop in visual acuity.[128] NICE

4 *Proliferative diabetic retinopathy* This is treated with panretinal (scatter) laser photo-coagulation (PRP). This type involves treating the peripheral retina which is not receiving adequate blood flow. By treating these areas, the stimulus driving the neovascular process may be halted. As this treatment involves many laser applications (eg >1000) it may be divided into ≥2 sessions. **NB:** panretinal photocoagulation does not improve vision. It is intended to help prevent blindness. It may cause some loss of peripheral, colour, and night vision. Some patients get generalized blurring of vision which is usually transient but may persist indefinitely.

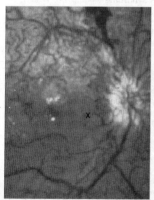

Fig 2. Retinopathy before the laser.

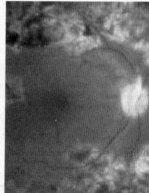

Fig 3. After the laser.   Figs 2 & 3 ©Prof J Trobe.

Systemic disease often manifests itself in the eye and, in some cases, eye examination will first suggest the diagnosis.

Vascular retinopathy This may be *arteriopathic* (arteriovenous *nipping*: arteries nip veins where they cross—they share the same connective tissue sheath) or *hypertensive*—arteriolar vasoconstriction and leakage—producing *hard exudates, macular oedema, haemorrhages*, and, rarely, *papilloedema*. Thick, shiny arterial walls appear like wiring (called 'silver' or 'copper'). Narrowing of arterioles leads to infarction of the superficial retina seen as cotton wool spots and flame haemorrhages. Leaks from these appear as hard exudates ± macular oedema/papilloedema (rare).

Emboli to the retina cause *amaurosis fugax* ('a curtain passing across the eyes'). *Typical cause:* atheroma (listen to carotids).[1] Arrange urgent carotid Doppler; treat eg by aspirin, statin ± carotid endarterectomy.

Retinal haemorrhages are seen in leukaemia; comma-shaped conjunctival haemorrhages and retinal new vessel formation may occur in sickle-cell disease; optic atrophy in pernicious anaemia.

Note also Roth spots (retinal infarcts) of infective endocarditis (*онсм* p144).

Metabolic disease Diabetes: p446. Wilson's disease (Kayser-Fleischer ring, fig 1). Hyperthyroidism, and exophthalmos: *онсм* p211. In myxoedema, eyelid and periorbital oedema is quite common. Lens opacities may occur in hypoparathyroidism. Conjunctival and corneal calcification may occur in hyperparathyroidism. In gout, monosodium urate deposited in the conjunctiva may give sore eyes.

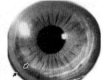
Fig 1. Kayser-Fleischer ring.
Courtesy of Jon Miles.

Granulomatous disorders (TB, sarcoid, leprosy, brucellosis, toxoplasmosis) all produce inflammation in the eye (uveitis). TB, congenital syphilis, sarcoid, CMV, and toxoplasmosis may all produce chorioretinitis. In sarcoid there may be cranial nerve palsies and lacrimal gland swelling.

Collagen and vasculitic diseases These also cause inflammation. Conjunctivitis is found in SLE and Reiter's syndrome; episcleritis in polyarteritis nodosa and SLE; scleritis in rheumatoid arthritis; and uveitis in ankylosing spondylitis and Reiter's syndrome (*онсм* p552). In dermatomyositis there is orbital oedema with retinal haemorrhages. Behçet's syndrome causes uveitis & retinopathies. Temporal arteritis leads to ischaemic damage to the optic nerve.

Keratoconjunctivitis sicca/Sjögren's syndrome (*онсм* p724). There is reduced tear formation (Schirmer filter paper test), producing a gritty feeling in the eyes. Decreased salivation also gives a dry mouth (xerostomia). It occurs in association with collagen diseases. **Pilocarpine** and **cevimeline** help sicca features and topical **ciclosporin** helps moderate or severe dry eye.[129] Silicone nasolacrimal punctal plugs help maintain tears on the eye surface for longer

HIV/AIDS Those who are HIV +ve may get CMV retinitis (often despite highly active antiretroviral **R**),[130] with retinal spots ('pizza pie' fundus, signifying superficial retinal infarction) + flame haemorrhages involving ever more of the retina. This may be asymptomatic or cause blindness; it implies AIDS and ↓CD4 count. IV **ganciclovir** or its prodrug (oral **valganciclovir**) are used.[131] Cotton wool spots may indicate HIV retinopathy (may present before full AIDS); it is a microvasculopathy, not a retinitis. Candidiasis of the aqueous and vitreous is hard to treat. Kaposi's sarcoma (fig 1 p607) may affect the lids or conjunctiva.

Other causes of retinopathy (*haemorrhages, microaneurysms, hard exudates*)[132] radiation; carotid artery disease; central or branch retinal vein occlusion; retinal telangiectasia/Coats' disease; Leber's miliary aneurysms.

1 Causes of amaurosis fugax: giant cell arteritis, orbital schwannomas, meningiomas, ocular small vessel disease, Churg-Strauss vasculitis, antiphospholipid syndrome, arrhythmias, dysfibrinogenemia, uveitis-glaucoma-hyphaema syndrome post-cataract extraction.[48,133–138]

Ophthalmology

A swollen optic nerve head is called *papillitis* (there are many causes). *Papilloedema* is swelling of the optic disc that is non-inflammatory and caused by raised intracranial pressure. Papilloedema is usually though not always bilateral. In figs **2** & **3**, the discs are swollen forwards and also outwards into the surrounding retina. Disc margins are hidden and in places retinal vessels are concealed, because oedema has impaired the translucency of the disc tissues. The retinal veins are congested and there are a few haemorrhages at 9 o'clock in fig **2**. ►Whenever you see these appearances, get help. Measure the *BP*, and look in the other eye. Any hypertensive changes or haemorrhages? Or signs of central retinal vein occlusion? (p435). *Bilateral disc changes* suggest intracranial hypertension (ICP↑). Is there *headache*—worse in the mornings, centred in the frontal region, and are aggravated by bending down? In young obese women, think of benign intra-cranial hypertension.

Fig 2. Papilloedema.

Fig 3. Papilloedema.

Pseudopapilloedema (=pseudoneuritis =pseudopapillitis; see fig **4**) is usually associated with hypermetropia ± astigmatism or tilted discs, as in this patient below (from a 12-yr-old boy referred for '?brain tumour'). The disc margins are blurred and the disc appears elevated. Its cup may be absent but there is no true oedema and veins are of normal size and pulsate (transmitted from a nearby artery). It is usually bilateral and symmetrical and does not change over time. Fluorescence angiography (FA) distinguishes it from papilloedema or optic neuritis/papillitis (there is no contrast leakage).

Fig 4. Pseudopapilloedema.

Opaque myelinated nerve fibres may be confused with papilloedema (fig **5**). Other causes of swollen discs include *optic neuritis* (p434) and disorders of the nerve sheath (eg a *meningioma*, as seen in the MRI image, fig **6**).

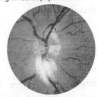

Fig 5. Nerve fibres mimicking papilloedema.

Optic nerve head drusen (fig **7**) are multiple hyaline bodies extending beyond the disc margins. Abnormal branching of the retinal vessels is often present. The nerve head is usually small (bilateral 'crowded disc'). If the hyaline material is buried in the disc substance, diagnosis is confusing, especially if a field defect is also present. *NB:* optic atrophy in the contralateral eye is the Foster-Kennedy syndrome (eg from meningioma of the optic canal in the eye with optic atrophy; in practice, the usual cause is consequential ischaemic optic neuropathy).

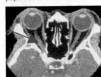

Fig 6. Meningioma of left optic nerve sheath.

Nystagmus suggests a lesion in the posterior fossa; *Sixth nerve palsy* may be a false localizing sign. *Homonymous field defects* may accompany compression of the supra-geniculate or posterior visual pathway by a glioma, meningioma, or AV malformation.

We thank Mr J F Cullen FRCS for permission to use the images. Fig 4 Reproduced from Brain's Diseases of the Nervous System, OUP.

Fig 7. Optic drusen.

Ophthalmology

Xerophthalmia & keratomalacia These indicate vitamin A lack, eg if poor, weaned early on to vitamin A deficient milk products, alcohol abuse, steatorrhoea or a food-fad or intolerance ("dairy products make me sick...").

Peak incidence: 2-5yrs; 40 million children worldwide.

Signs: Night blindness (nyctalopia), tunnel vision, poor acuity, and dry conjunctivae (xerosis). The cornea is unwettable and loses transparency. Small foamy plaques (Bitôt's spots, **fig 1**) occur, raised from interpalpebral conjunctiva. Vitamin A reverses these changes. Early corneal xerosis is reversible. Corneal ulceration and perforation can occur. In keratomalacia there is massive softening of the cornea ± perforation and extrusion of the intraocular contents.

Tests: Visual fields tests; dark-adapted electroretinography (bilateral ↓amplitudes≈diminished rod function);[139] plasma vitamin A↓.

℞: Just hand out the vitamins?[1] It's not so simple. Every Bitôt spot is a stain on the soul of the body politic, and as each represents a failure of education and politics, we are all implicated. ►Examine the cultural web that led to the deficiency, and try to take ***whatever*** steps are necessary to correct it.

Trachoma Caused by *Chlamydia trachomatis* (serotypes A, B, or C). It is spread mainly by flies, where it is hot, dry, and dusty and the people are poor, living near their cattle. 400 million people are affected; 100,000,000 are children.

Staging: 1 There is lacrimation. Follicles under the upper lid give a fine granular appearance (**fig 2-3**). 2 There is intense erythema. The follicles are larger and underneath both lids. A fine pannus and capillaries grow down towards the cornea. 3 The follicles rupture and are replaced by scar tissue. The pannus is more advanced. The cornea may ulcerate. 4 Scar tissue distorts the lids and causes entropion. Eyelashes scratch the cornea, which ulcerates.

*Drugs: **Mass anti-trachoma treatment:*** tetracycline 1% eye ointment 12-hrly for 5 days each month for 6 months. In active disease use 8-hrly for 6 weeks + **tetracycline** 250mg/6h PO for 14 days. **Azithromycin** (20mg/kg stat) is 78% effective in children and is a preventive that can be repeated 6-12 monthly.[141,142]

Lid surgery: Eg lid margin splitting + tarsal plate fracture + everting sutures.

Prevention: Good water; wash face often; **azithromycin**.

Onchocerciasis (river blindness) This is caused by nematode microfilariae (*Onchocerca volvulus*), transmitted by black flies of the Simulium species. Of the 20-50 million people affected, 95% live in Africa. It may cause blindness in 40% of some populations. Unless the eye is affected, problems are mostly in the skin. Fly bites result in nodules from which microfilariae are released, to invade conjunctiva, cornea, ciliary body, and iris (rarely retina or optic nerve, **fig 4**). Sometimes they may be seen swimming in the aqueous or dying in the anterior chamber. Microfilariae initially excite inflammation; fibrosis then occurs around them; if in the cornea, corneal opacities (nummular keratitis) occurs. Chronic iritis causes synechiae ± cataracts and a fixed pupil.

Tests: Skin snip tests, triple-antigen serology; PCR.

℞: Get expert help. **Ivermectin**[2] is the chief microfilaricide, ~150μg/kg PO stat every 6-12 months, until adult worms die (*OHCM* p443). In lightly infected expatriates, the first 3 doses are advised to be monthly, with observation in hospital after dose 1 (reactions are common in expatriates). Macrofilaricides: **doxycycline** 200mg/day for 4wks (or for 2wks if with rifampicin) is under trial.[139,140] Macrofilariae are adults living in lymphatics. Steroids: *OHCM* p443.

1 For children: **retinol palmitate** 50,000U IM monthly until eyes are normal (adult dose 100,000U, weekly to start with); or oral **retinyl palmitate** 200,000U PO. β-carotene (a pro-vitamin) 1.2×10^6U PO, is as effective, and cheaper. Avoid ↑vitamin A in pregnancy (vitamin A embryopathy).

2 A problem with ivermectin is that it's a monotherapy microfilaricide that has limited effect on adult worms, and so needs continuing for the life span of the adult worm (up to 15yrs).[143]

Fig 1. Bitôt's spots.
Reproduced from the British Journal of Ophthalmology, with permission from BMJ Publishing Ltd.

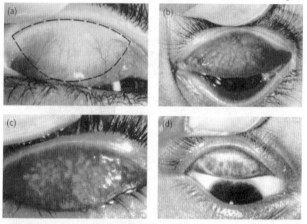

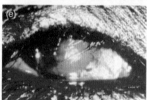

Fig 3. Trachoma: (a) dots outline the area to be examined; (b) follicular trachomatous inflammation (>5 follicles in upper tarsal conjunctiva); (c) intense trachomatous inflammation (inflammatory thickening partially obscures numerous follicles; (d) trachomatous scars (white bands or sheets in the tarsal conjunctiva); (e) trachomatous trichiasis and corneal opacity (lashes rub the cornea, which eventually clouds).

Fig 3. Reproduced from the Oxford Textbook of Medicine, with permission from OUP.

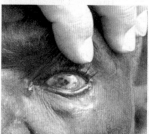
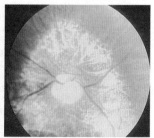

Fig 4. Left: sclerosing keratitis in a man blinded by onchocerciasis in Nigeria © Prof. Anthony Bryceson. Right: Hissette-Ridley fundus & optic atrophy; some central keyhole vision remains. Reproduced from the Oxford Textbook of Medicine, with permission from OUP.

►Prevention is the key, eg wearing goggles, or plastic glasses when near small moving objects or using tools (avoids splinters, fish-hooks, and squash-ball injuries). *Always record acuity* (both eyes; if the uninjured one is blind take all injuries *very* seriously). Take a detailed history of the event.

If unable to open the injured eye, instil a few drops of local anaesthetic (tetracaine 1%): after a few mins, comfortable opening may be possible. Examine lids, conjunctiva, cornea, sclera, anterior chamber, pupil, iris, lens, vitreous, fundus, and eye movement. An irregular pupil may mean globe rupture. Afferent pupil defects (p424) do not augur well for sight recovery. Note pain, discharge, or squint. CT may be very useful (foreign bodies may be magnetic, so avoid MRI).

Penetrating trauma Refer urgently: delays risk of ocular extrusion or infection. Uveal injury risks of sympathetic ophthalmia in the other eye. ►A history of flying objects (eg work with lathes, hammers, and chisels) prompts careful examination + x-ray to exclude intraocular foreign bodies (±skull x-ray or CT to exclude intracranial involvement). ►*Don't* try to remove a large foreign body (knife; dart). Support the object with padding. Transport supine. Pad the *unaffected* eye to prevent damage from conjugate movement.

Foreign bodies (FB) (fig 1) *Have a low threshold for getting help*; FBs often hide, so examine *all* the eye; for lid eversion *see* tinyurl.com/5jbt7v. FBs cause chemosis, subconjunctival bleeds, irregular pupils, iris prolapse, hyphaema, vitreous haemorrhage, and retinal tears. If you suspect a metal FB, x-ray the orbit. With high-velocity FBs, consider orbital ultrasound: pick-up rate is 90% *vs* 40% for x-rays; skill is needed (not always to hand in busy A&E departments). Removal of superficial foreign bodies may be possible with a triangle of clean card (chloramphenicol 0.5% drops after, to prevent infection.)

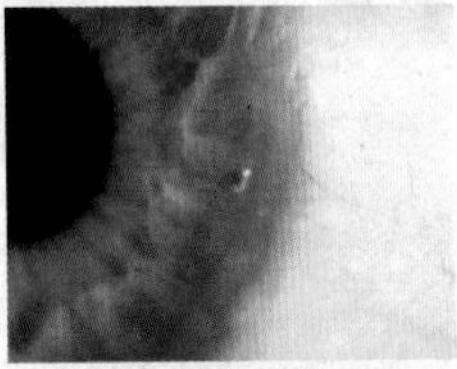

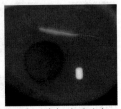
Fig 1. Corneal FB (centre).
Courtesy of Bristol Eye Hospital.

Corneal abrasions (fig 2; often from small fast-moving objects, eg children's finger-nails; twigs.) They may cause intense pain. Apply a drop of local anaesthetic, eg 1% tetracaine before examination. They stain with fluorescein and should show sign of healing within 48h. Apply chloramphenicol eye ointment and dilate the pupil. Send the patient home with analgesics. Re-examine after 24h. If still having a foreign body sensation after removing the pad, stain again with fluorescein. If the cornea stains, repeat the procedure for another 24h.

Fig 2. Corneal abrasion just above the pupil. ©Bristol Eye Hospital.

If it still stains after 48h, refer. NB: meta-analyses of small corneal abrasions do not favour using pads.[145-147]

Burns Treat chemical burns promptly: instil anaesthetic drops (tetracaine) every 2min till the patient is comfortable. Then hold lids open and bathe the eyes in copious clean water while the specific antidote is sought. Often the lids close tight from severe pain. Late serious sequelae: eg corneal scarring, opacification, and lid damage. Alkali burns are more serious than acid. Refer promptly.

Arc eye Welders and sunbed users who don't use UV protection may damage the cornea (FB sensation, watering, blepharospasm). ℞: Local anaesthetic drops every 2min. After dose 2, excruciating pain can vanish. Apply an antibiotic ointment and it will recover in 24h. It is very painful; be generous with analgesia.

Finally, remember **fat embolus** in trauma patients with visual problems.

Ophthalmology

Contusions and intraocular haemorrhage

Our eyes are protected by our bony orbital ridges. Severe contusions from large objects may damage the eye, but smaller objects such as champagne corks, squash balls, and airgun pellets (p720) cause local contusion, eg resulting in lid bruises and subconjunctival haemorrhage (if the posterior limit of such a haemorrhage cannot be seen, consider fracture of the orbit). Both usually settle in 2 weeks. ▶Get expert help with all injuries penetrating the eyeball.

Intraocular bleeds: ▶Get expert help: acuity may be affected. Blood is often found in the anterior chamber (hyphaema, fig 1, p413): small amounts clear spontaneously but if filling the anterior chamber, evacuation may be needed. It is often recognizable by pen-torch examination. Even small hyphaemas must be carefully evaluated (so refer): it may signify serious injury. *Late complications:* Glaucoma; corneal staining. Pain suggests glaucoma or re-bleeding.

Secondary haemorrhage: This may occur within 5 days and may produce sight-threatening secondary glaucoma. Sometimes the iris is paralysed and dilated due to injury (called traumatic mydriasis). This usually recovers in a few days but sometimes it is permanent. Vitreous haemorrhage will cause dramatic fall in acuity. There will be no red reflex on ophthalmoscopy. Lens dislocation, tearing of the iris root, splitting of the choroid, detachment of the retina, and damage to the optic nerve may be other sequelae; they are more common if contusion is caused by smaller objects rather than large.

Blows to the orbit: Blunt injury (eg from a football) can cause sudden ↑ in pressure within the orbit, and may cause blowout fractures with the orbital contents herniating into the maxillary sinus. Tethering of the inferior rectus and inferior oblique muscles causes diplopia. Test the sensation over the lower lid skin. Loss of sensation indicates infra-orbital nerve injury, confirming a blowout fracture. CT may show the depressed fracture of the posterior orbital floor. Fracture reduction and muscle release is necessary.[148]

Types of major injury, and prognosis

The ocular trauma score (OTS) gives prognostic information: to get the score, assign a point value for initial visual acuity from row 1 of the table. Then subtract the appropriate points for each diagnosis from subsequent rows. A patient with an initial visual acuity of <6/60, scleral rupture, and retinal detachment has a score of 80-23-11= 46. Higher OTS scores indicate a better prognosis. For exact details of how, see asotonline.org/ots.html; but note that some 2008 data suggest that OTS may be over-pessimistic.[149]

Visual acuity (p412)	No light perception	60
	Light perception/hand movement only	70
	<6/60	80
	6/50–6/15	90
	>6/12	100
Globe rupture		-23
Endophthalmitis		-17
Perforating injury		-14
Retinal detachment		-11
Afferent pupillary defect (Marcus Gunn pupil)		-10

In one series, the chief injuries were corneal wounds (68%), lens injury (50%), retinal lesions (50%), vitreous haemorrhage (25%), and endophthalmitis (14%). Multiple foreign bodies causing perforating injury with retained posterior segment foreign body occurred in 7%. Outcome was worse if acuity was affected, presence of a large foreign body, or there was bacterial endophthalmitis or proliferative vitreo-retinopathy.[149]

Ophthalmology

The pattern of blindness around the world differs considerably, depending on local nutrition and economic factors. 90% of the world's blind live in developing countries—and 80% would not be blind if trained eye personnel, medicines, ophthalmic equipment, and patient referral systems were optimized. The diseases responsible for most of the blindness in the world are trachoma, cataract (50% of the world's blindness), glaucoma, keratomalacia, onchocerciasis, and diabetic retinopathy (see BOX). In the past smallpox, gonorrhoea, syphilis, and leprosy (10% of those affected were blind) were also common causes of blindness.

Rates of blindness are higher than 10/1000 in some parts of Africa and Asia, but in the UK and the USA rates are 2/1000. Blindness may be voluntarily registered in England, registration making one eligible for certain concessions. Although the word blind suggests inability to perceive light, a person is eligible for registration if their acuity is less than 3/60, or if >3/60 but with substantial visual field loss (as in glaucoma). There are ~350,000 people registered blind in the UK. *Criteria for partial sighted registration:* acuity is <6/60 (or >6/60 with visual field restrictions).

Causes of blindness These have changed considerably in the UK over the last 70 years. Whereas in the 1920s ophthalmia neonatorum (p36) was responsible for 30% of blindness in English blind schools, this is now a rare but treatable disease. Retrolental fibroplasia was common in the 1950s, mostly affecting premature infants: monitoring of intra-arterial oxygen in premature babies tries to prevent this. With an ever-aging population, the diseases particularly afflicting this population are the common causes of blindness. Nearly two-thirds of the blind population are over 65 years of age, and nearly half over 75. Macular degeneration, cataract, and glaucoma are the three commonest causes of blindness.

Registration In England, responsibility for blind registration lies with the local authority. Application is made by a consultant ophthalmologist and is voluntary, not statutory. Registration as blind entitles one to extra tax allowances, reduced TV licence fees, some travel concessions, and access to talking books. Special certification from an ophthalmologist is necessary for the partially sighted to receive talking books. At one time it was statutory that the registered blind should receive a visit from a social worker but this is no longer the case, although the social services employ social workers who specialize in care of the blind. The Royal National Institute for the Blind[1] will advise on aids, such as guide dogs (available if required for employment). It sells talking mobile phones and other helpful gadgets on its website.[150]

Special educational facilities These provide for visually handicapped children. Special schools have a higher staff/pupil ratio, specialized equipment, and many have a visiting ophthalmologist. The disadvantage is that the children may not mix much with other children—especially if they board.

---

1 Royal National Institute for the Blind, 224 Great Portland St, London W1N 6AA (UK 0845 766 9999).

Common causes of blindness in the world

1 Trachoma
2 Cataract
3 Glaucoma
4 Keratomalacia
5 Onchocerciasis
6 Diabetic retinopathy

The most common cause of irreversible blindness and partial sight in developed countries is age-related macular degeneration. In patients of working age, diabetic retinopathy is the leading cause in the West. In a recent survey in Taipei City, the leading causes of registrable blindness and low vision were glaucoma, optic neuropathy, diabetic retinopathy, retinitis pigmentosa, and age-related macular degeneration.[151]

Colour vision and colour blindness

For normal colour vision we require cone photopigments sensitive to blue, green, and red light. The commonest hereditary colour vision defect is x-linked failure of red-green discrimination (8% ♂ and 0.5% ♀ affected—so those with Turner's syndrome have ♂ incidence and those with Klinefelter's have ♀ incidence). Blue-yellow discriminatory failure is more commonly acquired and sexes are affected equally.

Diagnosis: This is by use of coloured pattern discrimination charts (eg Ishihara plates, see endpapers). Depressed colour vision may be a sensitive indicator of acquired macular or optic nerve disease.

Monochromatism This may be due to being born without cones (resulting in low visual acuity, absent colour vision, photophobia, and nystagmus), or, very rarely, due to cone monochromacy where all cones contain the same visual pigment, when there is only failure to distinguish colour.

The eye does not retain drops for as long as ointments and 2-hourly applications may be needed. Eye ointments are well-suited for use at night and when crusting and sticking of the lids occurs. Allow 5min between doses of drops to prevent overspill. The antibiotic drops most used are not those generally used systemically, eg fusidic acid, chloramphenicol, neomycin, and framycetin. All eye preparations have warnings not to use for more than one month.

Mydriatics (=cycloplegics) These dilate the pupil. They also cause cycloplegia and hence blur vision (warn not to drive). Pupil dilatation prior to examination is best achieved using 0.5% or 1% **tropicamide** which lasts for 3h. 1% **cyclopentolate** has an action of 24h and is preferred for producing cycloplegia (paralysis of the ciliary muscle) for refraction of children. These drugs may be used to prevent synechiae formation in anterior uveitis. ►Over-60s with shallow anterior chambers (especially if a family history of glaucoma) may have acute glaucoma triggered, so only use on ophthalmological advice.

Miotics These constrict the pupil and increase drainage of aqueous. They are used in the treatment of acute glaucoma (p430).

Local anaesthetic Tetracaine (0.5% drops) is an example, used to permit examination of a painful eye where reflex blepharospasm is a problem, and to facilitate removal of a foreign body. ►It abolishes the corneal reflex so use to treat pain is to risk corneal damage. To relieve pain, give an eye pad, and be generous with oral analgesia. In children use proxymetacaine (it stings less).

Steroid and NSAID drops ►Steroids are very useful in managing ophthalmic inflammation. They are dangerous as they may induce catastrophic progression of dendritic ulcers (p416). Ophthalmoscopy may miss dendritic ulcers, and slit lamp inspection is essential if steroid drops are being considered, eg for allergy, episcleritis, scleritis, or iritis. Steroid drops ↑intraocular pressure (newer drops less so: eg **rimexolone** has a low IOP-elevating potential, comparable to **fluorometholone** and < **dexamethasone** & **prednisolone** acetate).[152] NSAID drops, eg **ketorolac**, may obviate the need for some steroid drops.[153]

Iatrogenic eye disease Allergic reactions may damage conjunctiva & cornea, eg toxic epidermal necrolysis (fig 2, p601) in aspirin allergy (Lyell's syndrome). Another type of toxic reaction is nystagmus indicating phenytoin toxicity.

Dry eyes: Propranolol and oxprenolol are typical culprits.

Corneal deposits: Amiodarone, chloroquine, chlorpromazine, and gold.

Lens opacities: Steroids (including high-dose inhaled) are the typical culprits.

Glaucoma: Typical culprit: steroid drops (above), mydriatics and anticholinergics (some antiparkinson drugs and tricyclics).

Papilloedema: Tetracyclines; nalidixic acid; steroids; the Pill.

Retinopathy: The drugs below are culprits if used chronically. • *Vigabatrin.*

• *Ethambutol:* Warn patients to report *any* visual side-effects (loss of acuity, colour blindness). ~10% report new visual problems, and in 10% of these the cause is optic neuropathy (which may be irreversible).[1]

• *Isoniazid:* ↓Red-green perception; pyridoxine co-administration prevents this.

• *Chloroquine (CQ)/hydroxychloroquine (HCQ)* can cause (untreatable) retinopathy if high doses are used. Risk of toxicity increases sharply towards 1% after 6yrs of use, or a cumulative dose of 1000g of HCQ. Risk increases with continued use. Most patients are routinely given 400mg of HCQ daily (or 250mg CQ). This is OK unless short stature (then dose by ideal body weight). *Screening schedule:* Baseline exam on starting (maculopathy would be a contraindication). Start annual screening 5yrs (or sooner if there are unusual risk factors). Newer objective tests, such as multifocal electroretinogram, spectral domain optical coherence tomography, and fundus autofluorescence, can be more sensitive than visual fields (which remain useful).[154]

Fortified guttate gentamicin is 15mg/mL (the normal commercial gentamicin is 3mg/mL); penicillin 5000u/mL, meticillin 20mg/mL, and antifungals can be obtained from the Chief Pharmacist, Moorfields Eye Hospital (tel. 020 725 33411). Antibiotics can be home-made as follows: Gentamicin forte: Add 2mL of 40mg/mL IV **gentamicin** to a 5mL bottle of commercial guttate gentamicin (3mg/mL).[2]

Other antibiotics can be made up using IV preparations to the required concentration using water or normal saline. These are stable for the time recommended for IV solutions in the manufacturers *Data sheets*. Penicillin G can be used up to 500,000u/mL.

Eyedrops as a cause of systemic symptoms

Drugs applied to the eye may be absorbed through the cornea and produce systemic side-effects—eg bronchospasm or bradycardia in susceptible individuals using antiglaucoma β-blocking drops, eg **timolol, carteolol, betaxolol**—which is cardioselective. ▶Symptoms may be subtle and insidious—eg gradually decreasing exercise tolerance, or falls from arrhythmias. Serious problems are more likely if there is co-morbidity (eg respiratory infection).

Other anti-glaucoma drops (p440) cause headaches, and a bitter taste in the mouth; urolithiasis is reported with **dorzolamide**.

Pilocarpine may cause parasympathetic sweating. Accommodation spasm may lead to brow-ache (worse if <40 years old, or just starting treatment). Other SE: 'flu-like syndrome, sweating, urinary frequency; more rarely: urinary urgency, D&V (or constipation ±flatulence), dyspepsia, flushes, BP↑, palpitations, rhinitis, dizziness, lacrimation, conjunctivitis, visual disturbances, ocular pain, rash, pruritus.

Even highly selective α$_2$-receptor agonists used in glaucoma, eg **brimonidine**, can cause effects such as dry mouth (in 33% of patients), headache, hypertension, fatigue, and drowsiness.[155]

---

1 Ethambutol eye problems: ↓acuity (65%), ↓ visual fields (65%), abnormal colour vision (61%), optic disc pallor (38%), ↑latency on visual evoked potential (65%). ~30% showed improved vision on stopping ethambutol in one Korean study; latency for recovery: 5.4±1.7 months. No one with optic disc pallor at the time of diagnosis of optic neuropathy showed visual function improvement.[@19145123]
2 Mr J Dart FRCS, Moorfields Eye Hospital; see also ncbi.nlm.nih.gov/pmc/articles/PMC2417514/?page=1

80% of contact lenses are worn for cosmetic reasons. Only 20% are worn because lenses are better for the eye condition than spectacles. Among this 20% a minority wear the lenses to hide disfiguring inoperable eye conditions, a greater proportion have them for very high refractive errors. Myopia above -12 dioptres and hypermetropia above +10 dioptres are indications for lenses because equivalent spectacles produce quite distorted visual fields. Lenses are used for ocular reasons, eg after corneal ulceration or trauma when a new front surface of the cornea is needed to see through, and in keratoconus.[1]

Types of lens Hard lenses are 8.5-9mm in diameter and are made of polymethylmethacrylate (PMMA). Gas-permeable hard lenses are about 0.5cm larger and are designed to allow gas to permeate through to the underlying cornea. They can only be made to cope with a limited degree of astigmatism and do not wet as well as standard hard lenses, so may mist up in the day. With the advent of the larger (13-15mm diameter) soft contact lenses it was hoped that many of the problems with hard lenses could be circumvented. Soft disposable lenses can be worn during the day for up to 4 weeks and then disposed of. Special contact lenses called toric lenses can be used to correct astigmatism of up to 2 dioptres. With more astigmatism, correction is not achieved because the lens fits the astigmatic cornea taking on its shape. They are more delicate than hard lenses and need meticulous cleaning. Extended wear-lenses can be worn for up to 4 months. Sometimes coloured lenses are used simply to change eye colour. Disposable contact lenses are now more common.

Patients may suffer from keratoconjunctivitis or giant papillary change in the upper tarsal conjunctiva, possibly due to sensitization to the cleansing materials used or to the mucus which forms on the lens.

Cleaning lenses Cleaning solutions made by different manufacturers should not be mixed. With hard lenses 2 solutions are usually used, one for rinsing and cleaning, and one for storage. The storage solution should be washed off before the lens is inserted. Soft contact lenses, being permeable, tend to absorb chemicals, so weaker solutions for cleaning are used (also, lenses are usually intermittently cleaned with another system, eg enzyme tablets, to remove mucoprotein on their surface). *Sensitivity to cleaning agents* usually presents as redness, stinging, increased lens movement, increased mucus production, and thickened lids. It may be necessary to stop wearing lenses for several months. When restarting, use a preservative-free cleansing system.

Can I reuse my daily disposable contact lenses (DDCL)? No! Overnight storage in blister-pack saline results in contaminated lenses and infections (esp. staphs and esp. in men). We *must* educate patients in correct use of DDCL.

Complications

1 Despite a shift to using of frequent-replacement daily-wear contact lenses, corneal ulcer is still a real problem, eg from *Pseudomonas aeruginosa*; ofloxacin drops have a role when suspected.

2 Corneal abrasion is common early while adjusting to wear. Pain ± lacrimation occurs some hours after removing the lens.

3 Sensitization to cleaning agents ± staining, eg by rifampicin or fluorescein. Eye ointments must not be used, nor eye-drying drugs. See BNF.

4 Losing the lens within the eye. Hard lenses may be lost in any fornix, soft lenses are usually in upper outer fornix.

5 Keratitis and risk of acanthamoeba infection (see BOX).

iContacts Futuristic contact lenses with a tiny aerial and embedded pixels have already been tested in Finland.[156] Whether these will enable you to read constantly updated pages from *OHCS* while you jog remains to be seen.

Ophthalmology

Hygiene and wear tips

►Pay attention to contact lens containers, as well as lenses.

►Do not assume that because a person uses disposable lenses there can be no nasty acanthamoebae infections. These free-living protozoa (found in soil and water, including bathroom tap water) may cause devastating keratitis even with disposable lenses.

• Scrub container's inside with cotton wool bud moistened with lens fluid.

• Disinfect the container with hot water (≥80°C); leave to dry in open air.

• Wash your hands before handling the contact lens container.

• Replace the container at least every year.

• Protozoa may survive new '1-step' solutions of 3% hydrogen peroxide. Amoebae are difficult to treat, and there is current interest in salicylate's potential to reduce microbial attachment when used in contact lens care solutions.[157]

• Follow instructions about getting used to extended wear. Most corneal ulcers from contact lenses are in people who are not used to extended wear and sleep overnight with their contact lenses in, or napped with them on a plane, or elsewhere for as little as 2-3 hours.

---

1 In keratoconus the cornea bulges and is somewhat conical on lateral viewing. Vision is distorted. Multiple images and sensitivity to light can greatly impact on life, even if acuity is unaffected.[158] Other causes apart from ill-fitting contact lenses: UV exposure; LASIK complications (p464) compulsive eye-rubbing;[159] Down's syndrome. NB: idiopathic keratoconus entails chronic, noninflammatory, degenerative thinning of the cornea starting in young adulthood. Atopy and oxidative stress in the cornea may be important Susceptibility locus: SNP rs4954218, near RAB3GAP1 gene. Treatment: rigid gas permeable contact lenses are employed to vault over the cornea, replacing irregularities with a smooth, uniform refracting surface. This is often insufficient, and keratoconus is a leading reason for corneal transplantation.

Blepharospasm is involuntary contraction of orbicularis oculi. It commonly occurs in response to ocular pain. Repetitive blepharospasm, which may have a serious impact on quality of life, or make the patient effectively blind, is a focal dystonia (*онсм* p473). If the condition is not recognized, it is all too easy to dismiss the patient as hysterical and to think that screwing up of the eyes is deliberate—especially, the more the sceptical doctor questions and probes the afflicted patient, the worse the blepharospasm may become (stress is an important exacerbating factor). It is important to understand that it may have a serious negative impact on patients' lives.[160]

Presentation ♀:♂ × 1.8 : 1. Blepharospasm is often preceded by exaggerated blinking. Other dystonias may be present (eg oro-mandibular). It usually starts unilaterally, becoming bilateral. Patients may develop tricks to reduce it such as touching or pulling the eyelids—a variation of *geste antagoniste* seen in other forms of dystonia. *Causes:* (Mostly unknown.) Neuroleptic drugs, Parkinson's disease, progressive supranuclear palsy, paraneoplastic (p589, eg from lung ca).

Treatment Drugs: *Botulinum neurotoxin:* Palliation is achieved with small doses injected to orbicularis oculi; here it produces a temporary flaccid paralysis. It can help some people recover effective vision. It binds to peripheral nerve terminals and inhibits release of acetylcholine. 3-monthly treatments are needed. Response is variable; good effects may wear off. Other options: anticholinergics (**trihexyphenidyl**, eg 1mg/day PO, max 5mg/6h; tablets are 2mg or 5mg). Dopamine agonists (L-dopa, bromocriptine) may help. *Supportive treatment:* If the cause is compensation for apraxia of lid opening, wearing goggles may help.[161] See also the UK Dystonia Society, tel: 0207 329 0797.

Allergic eye disease

Seasonal allergic conjunctivitis and perennial allergic conjunctivitis head the list (BOX 2), followed by atopic keratoconjunctivitis (AKC), giant papillary conjunctivitis and other rarer conditions. Sight-threatening vernal keratoconjunctivitis is described below.

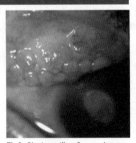

Vernal keratoconjunctivitis (VKC) comprises 0.5% of allergic eye disease. It begins as a type I hypersensitivity reaction; later there are infiltrates and a type IV reaction. *Typical patient:* An atopic boy (<14yrs old) from warmer climes with severe bilateral symptoms in spring: itchy eyes, blepharospasm, foreign body sensation, photophobia, tearing (lid skin is spared, unlike in AKC, see

Fig 1. Giant papillae & superior grey oval corneal ulcer ('shield' ulcer) in VKC.   Courtesy of Mr D Tole FRCOphth.

BOX). ♂:♀ × 2 : 1. VKC often resolves spontaneously soon after puberty. *Signs:* Thick mucoid discharge from large conjunctival papillae, eg under the upper lid (fig 1) and enough to cause ptosis; when flattened they look like cobblestones. Corneal perilimbal papillae may occur. Conjunctival scarring and plaques occur. The cornea can erode, forming sight-threatening shield ulcers (fig 1).[162] *℞:* Start with drops, eg olopatadine or lodoxamide (BOX 1). If uncontrolled or if corneal disease develops, steroid drops are needed (eg 1% prednisolone acetate/2h; taper rapidly). Ciclosporin drops (1-2%) also help VKC.[163] Corneal involvement needs careful eye clinic review and often coverage with steroids, antibiotic drops and lid hygiene to limit staphylococcal colonization. If severe blepharitis, oral **erythromycin** or **doxycycline** (in adults) can help. Topical lubricants also help soothe eyes and washout allergens.

Ophthalmology

3 principles for successfully managing allergic eye disorders[164]

1 Remove the allergen responsible where possible ("don't travel to places which make your symptoms worse").

2 General measures: •Cold compresses •Artificial tears to wash out allergens and ↓itch •Oral antihistamines for symptom relief, eg loratadine 10mg/d PO •Nasal steroid sprays may help even if no nasal symptoms.[165,166]

3 Eye-drop specifics (rapid action + fewer SEs , being topical)—eg antihistamines (eg azelastine), drugs inhibiting mast cell degranulation (cromoglicate; lodoxamide), and accessory drugs, eg steroids (eg dexamethasone; beware inducing glaucoma), ± NSAIDs (eg diclofenac),[167] immunosuppressants (ciclosporin, specialist use only), and vasoconstrictors (eg xylometazoline—not very effective and may cause rebound hyperaemia).

Allergic conjunctivitis and associated conditions

Acute allergic conjunctivitis is caused by an IgE mediated type 1 hypersensitivity, triggering release of inflammatory mediators by mast cells.[168] Most have a history or family history of atopy (eg asthma or eczema).

Chronic allergic disorders are characterized by an increase in the number of the local conjunctival T-cell population with a mixed cellular infiltrate of mast cells, eosinophils, neutrophils and macrophages.

Seasonal allergic conjunctivitis (SAC) Up to 50% of allergic eye disease. Symptoms are seasonal and mild—but may continue long after allergen exposure.[166] Examination shows small papillae on the tarsal conjunctiva. It is self limiting and not sight threatening. ℞: Antihistamine drops, eg ketotifen, azelastine, epinastine, emedastine, or olopatadine. 2nd line: diclofenac 0.1% drops.[169] Mast cell stabilizers may be used prophylactically.[170]

Perennial allergic conjunctivitis (PAC) Symptoms are mild and may persist all year with seasonal exacerbations. Small papillae are found on the tarsal conjunctiva. *Management: Prescription drops:* olopatadine (antihistamine and mast cell stabilizer), lodoxamide and nedocromil (mast cell stabilizer). *Over-the-counter drops:* sodium cromoglicate 2% (/6h).[171,172]

Atopic keratoconjunctivitis (AKC) affects 1.5% of the population and is potentially sight threatening. Symptoms are severe with pain, redness, and reduced vision. Signs include conjunctival papillae and eventual conjunctival scarring which can lead to corneal opacification and neovascularization.

Atopic blepharoconjunctivitis (ABC) is similar to AKC but with associated blepharitis (lid margin inflammation) and limited corneal involvement.

Giant papillary conjunctivitis Giant papillae on the tarsal conjunctiva is an iatrogenic condition related to foreign bodies, eg contact lenses, ocular prosthesis and sutures. *Management:* Involves removal of the foreign body and treatment with topical mast cell stabilizers or steroids.

Contact dermatitis This describes erythema of the skin surrounding the eye. It is a reaction to a particular antigen. This is not sight threatening.

Phlyctenular keratoconjunctivitis This may be a delayed response to mycobacteria, staphs, yeasts, or chlamydia. The conjunctival phlyctenule begins as a hard, red, 1-3mm diameter papule surrounded by hyperaemia. At the limbus, it is triangular (apex points to cornea). It ulcerates, and then subsides within 12 days. Corneal phlyctenules develop as an amorphous grey infiltrate, and leave a scar. They may cause intense photophobia. *Management:* Get help. Steroid drops may help. Treat any bacterial cause.[173]

Lots of flashes may indicate the moment of a retinal tear or detachment; lots of floaters suggest blood or pigment released into the vitreous.

'Halo' refers to a circle of light, white or coloured, seen around *any* luminous body (not just saints). Also call to mind Monet, his cataracts (a cause of haloes) and his paintings and their 'investments in light' (another meaning of halo). In the poem, Monet refuses surgery for his cataracts: how differently doctors and artists see the world (BOX 1)! So before we advise surgery it's wise to get to know our patients, and to keep a eye on posterity.

> *D*octor, you say there are no haloes around the streetlights in Paris and what I see is an aberration caused by old age, an affliction. I tell you it has taken me all my life to arrive at the vision of gas lamps as angels.
>
> Lisel Mueller: Monet Refuses the Operation
> M Faith McLellan 1996. *Lancet* 1996 348 1641

Floaters they are often caused by RBCs (anything that causes new vessesl to form on the retina can lead to vitreous haemorrhage and perceived floaters (diabetic retinopathy; vein occlusions) trauma/retinal detachment (often with blood in the vitreous). White cells are the other main cause, eg from inflammatory/infective causes, posterior choroiditis (p438). Sinister causes are secondary to tumour seeding—either primary as in melanoma or retinoblastoma (patients often too young to complain of symptoms) or secondary metastasis. Also think of endophthalmitis (eg fungal). Degenerative causes include opacities in the vitreous: *asteroid hyalosis* (like stars in the night sky) and *syneresis* (here, each floater is a shadow of a mobile vitreous opacity cast on the retina. After the eye comes to rest, they continue to move—they are common in myopes, after cataract surgery or after trauma.

Floaters present as small dark spots in the visual field, particularly noticeable against a bright background. Often, they are just annoying (if central), but harmless, and may settle with time. Examine the vitreous and retina before reassuring. *Sudden showers* of floaters in one eye (±flashing lights) may be due to blood. ▶*Refer immediately* (for specialist assessment within 48h or sooner): the cause may be retinal detachment (p444).

Flashing lights (photopsia) Either from intraocular or cerebral pathology (migraine). Is there headache, nausea, or previous migraine? Detachment of a shrinking vitreous from the retina gives flashes and floaters. 5% go on to retinal tears and detachment. Retinal damage is usually peripheral and hard to see—refer immediately for specialist help.

4 'F's of retinal detachment • Floaters (numerous, acute onset, constant, and described as 'spider's web' • Flashes • Field loss (acute, progressive) • Falling acuity. See p444.

Posterior vitreous detachment (PVD) Degenerative changes in the vitreous lead to its eventual separation from the retina. This is part of normal aging. Patients describe monochromatic photopsia in the peripheral temporal field. This is more obvious in dim light and with eye movements. There is an increase in floaters but vision remains unchanged and there are no field defects. Refer for fundus check as retinal tears can happen as a consequence of the PVD.

Haloes Smooth, coloured haloes around lights are diffractive phenomena, being seen when a white light is inside a steamed-up window (street lights have haloes when seen through misted windscreens), or through scratched spectacles. Hazy ocular media may also be the cause (cataract; corneal oedema). In *acute angle closure glaucoma* it is corneal oedema that causes them as intraocular pressure rises with pupillary dilatation. If haloes are accompanied by eye pain consider this diagnosis and refer immediately. Jagged haloes which change shape are usually due to migraine. Beware labelling haloes as migrainous in those >50yrs who have not previously suffered from migraine.

"The greatest thing a human soul ever does in this world is to see something, and tell what it saw in a plain way. Hundreds of people can talk for one who can think, but thousands can think for one who can see." *John Ruskin Modern Painters; vol. III*

Interpreting but not over-interpreting our visual sensations entails the almost impossible task of seeing the indifferent pixels as well their patterns. Is it a stone or a frog (genus *Batrachus*)? Is it a leafless (*aphyllous*) branch or a snake? As Eliot knew, when *"the eye adjusts itself to the twilight, the dead stone is seen to be batrachian, the aphyllous branch ophidian"*.

When a classicist, revising for her exams, says "I'm preparing for my Unseen" she means "I'm preparing for a surprise. I'm going to have to translate, without warning, some unknown ancient passage (our primordial unconscious) into modern parlance (current sensations)." To do well, she (and we) have to expect the unexpected, or else the snake will bite us. More deeply, all visual experience is ambiguous, yet we believe and act on it all the time. Seers, philosophers, and, above all, poets know that the issue here is the role our imagination plays in seeing. *"I have seen sometimes what men imagine they see."* (J'ai vu quelquefois ce que l'homme a cru voir!) *The Drunken Boat Arthur Rimbaud*

How is this important clinically? Just as we are born expecting to hear each other's voices, so we are born expecting to see each other's faces. If in later life we lose our vision, then the brain, with exaggerated zeal, compensates by creating fictive visual percepts, almost always involving faces—a surprisingly common non-psychotic hallucination named after Charles Bonnet, who first described it in his 89-year-old grandfather in 1769.

Charles Bonnet's grandfather might say with insight: *"I have imagined sometimes what other men know they see"*—ie the mirror-image of Arthur Rimbaud's formulation. The point is that neither Rimbaud nor Bonnet can pinch themselves to see if their hallucinatory state is real. By their systematic derangement of their senses they teach us something universal about our place in our external and internal worlds, namely that we can never fully disentangle what we see from what we expect to see. It is as if our propensity for illusions validates and authenticates our experience of being us.

So don't get too annoyed with your patients when they give ambiguous answers to your questions about floaters, flashes and more complex fictive visual percepts. Just smile to yourself and to Rimbaud in his embodiment as a drunken, waterlogged boat (*Le bateau ivre*) and remember that *the boat is in the drink and the drink is in the boat*.

Ophthalmology

Refractive procedures are increasingly undertaken as an alternative to wearing spectacles; mostly for cosmetic reasons. Occasionally they are undertaken for anisometropia (imbalance of prescriptions); for astigmatism after surgery; or for intolerance of spectacles or contact lenses. A variation of PRK (photorefractive keratotomy) may be undertaken for some corneal diseases. LASIK (see below) is now the commonest procedure. It is well researched and in terms of surgical procedures is extremely safe but there are possible complications. It should be noted that most ophthalmologists wear spectacles!

Photorefractive keratotomy (PRK) This is an entirely laser treatment where the curved front of the cornea is altered by laser ablation. It is only done for low degrees of myopia and is less predictable than LASIK with some people having under-correction and others over-correction. Corneal haze with reduced vision, glare, and haloes are occasional problems. In most low myopes it gives good outcome but it is very painful for a few days.

LASIK (laser assisted *in situ* keratomileusis) This is a combination of minor surgery where the cornea is incised and an extremely thin trapdoor-shaped flap hinged away and then excimer laser is applied to the bare corneal stroma underneath. Thereafter the flap is pushed back into position and adheres naturally. It is, surprisingly, virtually painless, settles very quickly, and is fairly predictable in its outcome. Corneal sensitivity recovers after ~6 months. A thin flap with a nasally placed hinge is associated with the most rapid recovery of corneal sensitivity.[174] It is possible to undertake surgery on much greater degrees of refractive error; with up to 5 dioptres of hypermetropia; 5 dioptres of astigmatism; and 15 dioptres of myopia (if >15, risk ↑↑).[175] Serious complications are rare but due to trauma to or infection of the flap may result in permanent corneal scarring. In one series of 779 eyes no serious, vision-threatening, irreversible complication such as keratectasia or progressive endothelial cell loss was observed (follow-up: 5yrs). Warn that improved acuity tends to wane over time.[176] Intraocular pressure often falls (eg by 4mmHg). Note that LASIK tourism to find cheap surgery abroad is associated with problems such as corneal ectasia, flap problems, keratitis, and under- and over-correction.[177]

LASEK (laser epithelial keratomileusis) This is different from LASIK in that the corneal epithelium is softened with an alcohol solution and lifted off. Laser is then applied to reshape the cornea and the epithelium is carefully replaced.

Epi-LASIK tries to give the best of both LASIK and LASEK. A blunt blade is used to lift a 9mm-diameter flap of epithelium as a single sheet with a nasal hinge. It retains its integrity as a properly-viable entity. In this 'on-flap' method, the flap is repositioned and acts as a bandage while the underlying cornea heals. So far it looks as though 'off-flap' methods (complete removal of all the flap as in LASEK) and 'on-flap' epi-LASIK have equal visual and refractive outcomes in myopia, but other differences may declare themselves over time.[178]

Lens surgery Altering refraction by clear lens extraction with intraocular lens implantation with the appropriate corrective power is another option. Accommodation is lost, so reading needs correction. Another option is an intraocular lens implanted in front of the human lens (phakic implant).

Radial keratotomy This is historical and should no longer be done. It involved surgical incisions of the peripheral cornea to alter the curvature.

Other procedures These are much less commonly undertaken. They include insertion of perspex rings into the cornea; other laser techniques to alter corneal curvature; and surgery to the sclera to attempt to correct presbyopia. They are much less certain in outcome and are best regarded as experimental.

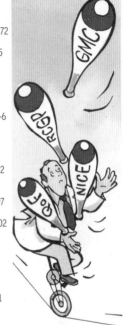

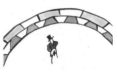

Fig 1. The correct method for conducting morning surgery: don't look down; don't stop pedalling. "How do I do it?...If I *did* know what I'm doing I wouldn't be able to do it."[1]
Is conducting morning surgery a performing art?...There is no shortage of farce (or tragedy).

Relevant pages elsewhere ►*Every page in all chapters.* This is why the above contents list is oddly starved of nice meaty clinical topics: don't worry: they all figure hugely in primary care, but not here because just the list would overwhelm you. See also *RCGP GP curriculum* rcgp-curriculum.org.uk/extras/curriculum/index.aspx

Because of the huge and undefined range of primary care, it is said that GPs 'need to be the most comprehensively educated of any kind of doctor'.

We thank Dr Konstantinos Kritikos, our Junior Reader, for his contribution to this chapter.

Primary care doctors are specialists in six areas: **1)** Diagnosis **2)** Health philosophy **3)** Disease in its earliest phases **4)** Prioritizing conflicting advice from organ-based specialists **5)** Families and their interactions with disease **6)** Prevention, and balancing of conflicting preventive duties. They are personal doctors, responsible for giving comprehensive and continuing generalist care to those seeking medical help, irrespective of age, sex and state of health. They are the only doctors qualified to diagnose health and they have special knowledge and experience of disease in its earliest phases. They can answer such questions as *"Why doesn't Miss Phelps ever attend the antenatal clinic?"* and *"What must change for her to do so?"*. There are few instances where GPs can offer more skill and expertise than all other doctors, but there are many times when her understanding of her patient is what counts, and for which no amount of expertise can substitute. So when, Miss Phelps's baby dies, to whom does she turn in her distress? She isn't a medical or obstetric problem; she isn't even a psychiatric problem: she is Miss Phelps; and the doctor who specializes in her is her GP.

Knowledge of the patient and *knowledge of disease* (from its earliest to its terminal phases) coupled with the *ability to diagnose health* (p470) is what comprises this unique discipline. If a patient is asking "Am I well, or could I have cancer" the doctor who is always responding by saying "Well, I'm not sure ... let's do one more test" is often a bad doctor, and always an expensive one. Some doctors have the gift of appraising a patient and knowing instinctively, when to treat, investigate, refer, or reassure. Nowhere is this instinct more used than in primary care. A chest physician may tell a person that his lungs are healthy, but if, on your way out, he says "Oh, and I've also got this pain in my leg..." she may feel out of her territory. This new symptom undermines her and she is likely to end up saying "Go and see your GP", who must then somehow decide whether to reassure, treat, or refer to another specialist.

Coming to primary care after hospital medicine This may be your first experience of taking *sole* responsibility for an episode of care. This may seem isolating, so take steps to make clinical friendships with likeminded staff. Ensure your plans make sense to your patient. Does he know to return if there are unexpected developments? You may need to use time itself rather than some complex scan to make the diagnosis. If tests are needed, they can be done in logical order, rather than all at once which tends to happen in hospital. *Cargoes of gold:* Hospital medicine often deals with a single problem using overwhelming, awesome force (eg shocks, IV antibiotics, scalpels *etc*) and delights in eliminating problem number one *now*. But primary care takes the long view, sometimes over generations, and wont always try to solve a pressing problem, rather seeking to preempt its complications, to set it in context, and to arrange for patients and families to have a psychological advantage when dealing with illnesses that may be interacting in enigmatic ways. We may not say to man with a chest infection "here's an antibiotic...and stop smoking 40 a day, you idiot..." when we realise he is the partner of last week's exotic self-harming patient whose psychosis is now mysteriously improving. Instead you may hear yourself saying to her: "I think it's marvellous how you look after each other...here are some tips on helping him when his chest is bad..." Will she find her new role as reciprocal carer humanizing, and over time, will she realize that if she self-harms less he will smoke less? Maybe. Let's see. ☺Primary care is full of such excitements, delayed fuses, ☀ exploding and unexploding bombs, and collateral blast injury (and delayed rewards, but only when done over years: keep at it, and today's dull surgery may one day deliver its cargo of gold into your lap.) This example embodies the ancient idea that your diagnoses *must* be social, spiritual, and psychological, as well as physical.

The whole earth is our hospital endowed by the ruined millionaire, wherein, if we do well, we shall die of the absolute paternal care...TS Eliot, Four Quartets.

A healthy man is, above all, a man of this earth, and he must, therefore, only live the life of this earth for the sake of order and completeness. But as soon as he falls ill, as soon as the normal earthly order of his organism is disturbed, the possibility of another world begins to become more apparent, and the more ill he is, the more closely does he come into touch with the other world. Dostoevsky *Crime & Punishment*

Apart from us health professionals, most people under the age of 40 have no commerce with this 'other world'. But from 40 to 50, most people have at least one illness which will not go away: their passport to Dostoevsky's world, that never expires. Illnesses multiply with each passing decade, until the day comes when we are full-time citizens of Dostoevsky's realm.

INTO my heart an air that kills
From yon far country blows:
What are those blue remembered hills,
What spires, what farms are those?

This is the land of lost content,
I see it shining plain.
The happy highways where I went
And cannot come again. A.E. Houseman, *A Shropshire Lad*

This explains why young doctors with their exaggerated good-looks and shining health so intoxicate some older patients. We are rare visitors blowing in from their 'land of lost content': rare, because, given our training and special knowledge, we might *understand*.

However many such passports we have, none gives us total access to our patients' worlds: each is unique. But don't assume that our patients must travel alone. Taking time to find out what it's like for our patients is the first step in forging an enduring doctor-patient relationship. When patients know we travel with them, and that we will not abandon them, they will accept our foibles, even our errors. How can we cope with this big commitment—big enough for one person, let alone a few thousand of our dependent patients? How can we do this without destroying ourselves? ▶*Do we give in to the highest bidder?* Here are some insights from a woman in a crisis with too many conflicting roles: daughter, mother, lover, and so on: 'There is a battle going on for my soul...and I cannot just give it to the highest bidder. I have an interest in it too... I have a duty to many people and somehow I will discharge it. I have a duty also to some continuing part of myself. I have...ripped open my self-protective layers. I see now what I am. It's not a question of "happiness". I don't value my own more—or much less than anyone else's. It's something more lasting: it's a question of being faithful to an essence'. Sebastian Faulks *On Green Dolphin Street*

If we spend day after day in surgery without attending to our other roles we are not necessarily better than a person who leaves work on time, so enabling a visit to a grandparent, or a dialogue with a son, or time for recreation. The medical world encourages the dangerous delusion that we are somehow inadequate if we do not give our all. What gives rise to this is the delusion that the best unit of measurement of our medical lives is the single consultation. This is how we are assessed, as if there were no valid distractions during consultations—as if our own needs were non-existent, and 100% of the focus is placed on the patient sitting in front of us. But what if you should not really be seeing this patient at all, but should be out on a visit which might or might not be urgent? Or would it be better to be on the phone, talking to a possibly suicidal patient who has missed their appointment? Perhaps you need to do all three. Then you will do none of them well. If we are going to be successful in primary care, with its unending responsibilities, we have to recognize that the best doctors may not do anything *very* well.[1] The best doctors just make the least bad decisions on how to spend their time, and themselves. As with the woman above, they do not simply give their soul to the highest bidder. Don't feel guilty about this. To give yourself to the highest bidder would be a betrayal: not even saints do this.

---

1 Most days it is possible to achieve excellence in encounters with at least one patient—try to do so to prevent a drift into mediocrity, provided doing so does not undermine your other encounters.

An English or quasi-English dictionary of primary care acronyms

►*If you speak the language, you may eventually come to understand it.*

ACBS Advisory committee on borderline substances; prescriptions thus endorsed reclassify special foods (eg without gluten) as a free 'drug'.

AGMS Alternative general medical services (non-NHS, purchased by PCTs).

AIS Associate in training (category of membership of the RCGP; may become a full member when training is successfully completed and MRCGP passed).

AKT Applied knowledge test (part of the MRCGP exam)

CHI Commission for health improvement—aims to improve standards by: assessing NHS organizations and publicly investigates failure—and checks that the NHS is following national guidelines. It advises on best practice.

CPN Community psychiatric nurse.

DES Directed enhanced services (see LES and NES).

DoH/DSS Government department of health/department of social services.

DNA Did not attend (for a booked appointment ≈ waste of NHS resources).

EBM Evidence-based medicine (p489) or the journal of the same name.

ECR Extracontractual referral, ie no existing contract exists (∴ costly).

EHR Electronic health record accessible anywhere in the NHS.

FMED3 Form for sick pay, p522. *FP10* NHS prescription form.

GMC General medical council (a lay-dominated statutory regulatory body).

IM&T Information management and technology.

LES Locally agreed enhanced service (see NES and DES).

LIS Local implementation strategy, eg for IM&T

LMC Local medical committee (blesses or curses central non-statutory policies).

MASTA Medical advisory service for travellers abroad. www.masta.org

MCP Male chauvinist pig; medical care practitioner, ½-way between nurse & GP.

MDU/MPS Medical defence union and the medical protection society.

MESH Medical subheadings used in medline searches, see p504.

MRCGP Member of the Royal College of General Practitioners (a kind of GP club)

NELH National electronic library for health. www.nelh.nhs.uk

NES National enhanced service, eg payment for specified (non-contractual) nationally-agreed activity.

NHS UK national health service: a system for providing universal health care free at the point of use, funded from taxation; the 20th century's best invention●

NICE National institute for health and clinical excellence. www.nice.org.uk

NMC Nursing and midwifery council (replaces UKCC).

NPSA National patient safety agency for reporting critical incidents.

NSF National service framework (eg for diabetes, heart disease etc, p523).

OTC Over the counter medicine; *POM* is a prescription-only medicine.

PACT® Trademark of the prescription pricing authority (PPA).

PALS Patient Advice and Liaison Service (NHS complaints body etc, p497).

PCO Primary care organization (usually a Trust—PCT).

PDP Personal development plan (see *appraisals*, p508) www.emispdp.com

QMAS Quality management analysis system (nationally agreed way of extracting data from GP computer systems to quantify quality points for QOF).

QOF Quality and outcomes framework (in the UK, getting paid by results, eg if 74% of diabetic patients have an Hb_{A1c} <7.4% and BP <145/85mmHg).

RCT Randomized controlled trial.

SAFF Service and financial framework—a financial plan.

SFE Statement of financial entitlement (NHS).

SLS Selected list scheme; written on an FP10, this makes Viagra*etc* free, eg if DM, MS, parkinsonism, prostate ca, spina bifida, cord injury, or polio.

SMR Standardized mortality ratios.

SPN Supplementary prescribing nurse (p474).

TQM Total quality management www.eiro.eurofound.ie/1997/05/feature/uk9705113f.html

DVLA Driving vehicle licensing authority www.dvla.gov.uk/medical/ataglance.aspx

Primary care

⚕️ **Primary care and distributive justice** WHO *Alma-Ata statement:*[3] Primary care should 'be made universally accessible to individuals and families in the community, by means acceptable to them, through their full participation, and at the cost that the community and country can afford to maintain in the spirit of self-reliance...[and] addresses the main health problems in the community, providing promotive, preventative, curative and rehabilitative services accordingly'. Factors affecting access to health include finance, ideology, and education.

Six GP job descriptions (Compare triage clinics with 'normal surgery'.)
• To clear the waiting room *efficiently* (*kindly* if possible) only spending yourself *et al* to gain specified worthwhile health gains. (*No time wasters, please!*)
• "Get me better, doctor, so I can go on doing the things that made me ill..."
• To do whatever the patient wants, within the law, usually. (*I'm a nice guy.*)
• To deal with local realities (loneliness, addiction, poverty, and mental illness) rather than hoping for diagnostic wonders to test your brilliance.
• To be skilled in: prioritization; delegation; health-need measurement; rationing.
• To care for people irrespective of age, sex, sexual orientation, race, illness, or status. To make early diagnoses, framed in physical, psychological, and social terms. To make initial decisions about all problems presented or unearthed. To arrange continuing care of chronic, recurrent, or terminal illness. To practise in co-operation with colleagues. To treat via physical and psychosocial interventions[4] (eg augmenting problem-solving in depression), to prevent disease, and to educate to promote health, reconciling our responsibility to the community.

Health ►*If you haven't had a dialogue with a patient about what counts as health for them, and where they are in their lives, you haven't started to do medicine yet.* 7 definitions to juggle with: **1** Health is the absence of disease—or:
2 A state of complete physical, mental, and social wellbeing. WHO 1946 definition
3 A process of adaptation, to changing environments, to growing up and ageing, to healing when damaged, to suffering, and death. Health embraces the future so includes anguish and the inner resources to live with it. Ivan Illich 1974 Medical Nemesis [6]
4 Any process enabling the giving, promoting, or engendering of life.
5 Restoring integrity, equilibrium & wellbeing through self-management. BMJ 2011 M Huber [7]
6 Acquiring and allocating resources to enhance survival and reproduction.
7 Health is whatever works, and for as long. J Stone 1980 All This Rain [8]

All the above have limitations, eg on definition 1, everyone is unhealthy all the time, except during coitus... Was Charles I healthy as he laid his head on the executioner's block? •What about a priest in the act of losing his celibacy? •Can a heart with a prosthetic valve that is gradually wearing out be healthy? •Was Gandhi healthy at the end of a hunger strike? •Can animals or babies be healthy? •What about death in childbirth? 'Answers' below:

Healthy according to definition: ☙	1	2	3	4	5	6	7
King Charles on the scaffold	NO	NO	YES	NO	NO	NO	YES
Fasting Gandhi	NO	NO	YES	YES	NO	NO	YES
Babies and animals	YES	YES	NO	YES	YES	YES	YES
Heart with failing valve	NO	NO	NO	NO	NO	NO	YES
Priest losing his celibacy	NO	NO	YES	YES	YES	YES	YES
Death in childbirth	NO	NO	YES	YES ☙	NO	NO	NO

Measuring health Scores on the health survey Short Form 36 (SF36) are reproducible quantifiable and valid when combined with a patient-generated index of quality of life ('name the 5 chief activities/areas affected by your condition ... and rank importance of improvements to them') and a daily time trade-off calculation (how much time would you give up to be in perfect health?). By combining instruments, defects in one can be mitigated (eg the SF36 asks if health limits your ability to walk a mile—irrelevant if you do not need or want to walk much). *Health need* is the difference between the state now and a goal. Needs may be ranked by the distances between states and goals.

Primary care

Why does health matter?

Health is one of the few unqualified, self-evident goods (although it is rather pointless if it brings no pleasure). One person's health cannot be achieved at the expense of another's: if it seems to be, we end up substituting one problem for many others (eg global insecurity, through creation of an underclass). This is why health achieves a confluence of foreign and domestic policies of all enlightened government ministers, who at least in the UK state unequivocally that health improves **global security**, enhances **development**, **trade**, and **human rights**.[9] Health creates a **standard** against which any action can be judged. If you are in a quandary, ask yourself "Which of my competing actions will promote health among those who have least access to health?" ►If we followed the answer just 1% of the time, a benign revolution would be born.

What are the determinants of health?

One answer is *wealth*. With wealth come more stable political systems, and these are what are necessary for literacy and education to flourish, which in turn lead to easy access to clean water (the key issue, as more than 1 billion people have no such access) and the possibility of developing equitable health delivery systems. After clean water, the next steps focus on better nutrition, smaller families, more self-help, and anti-HIV strategies. ►*How do you move a Western post-industrial population from a low level of health to a higher level of health?* Since 2004, UK NHS primary care has been a vast multi-million pound test-bed of a payment-by-results system. Targets can only ever be partially successful, for targets *always* distort clinical priorities (p490).

Future determinants of health are thought to rest on:
• Controlling climate change and reducing health inequalities.
• Decline in tobacco consumption in all age groups.
• Better health services with more effective, more acceptable treatments.
• Fewer under-doctored areas (currently defined as populations where there are fewer than 52.695 GPs per 100,000—ie a list size of >1898 per whole-time GP)—and more GPs in deprived areas. Funding more GPs has been calculated as one of the most efficient ways of reducing mortality.
• Education capable of influencing behaviour to ↓exposure to risk factors.
• Better protection of the environment and better housing.
• More patient-centred health care, so that patients are not passive recipients of care, but well-educated partners in the struggle against disease.

Core competencies European Academy of Teachers in General Practice[EURACT]

• Dealing with unselected problems covering *all* health issues, co-ordinating care with other professionals in primary care and with other specialists.
• Adopting a person-centred approach, seeing people in their social realities; using consultations to augment doctor-patient relationships, with respect for autonomy; to communicate, set priorities, and act together; to provide continuity of care[10] as determined by the needs of the patient.[11]
• Investigating *incrementally*; using time as a tool; tolerating uncertainty.
• Being able to manage many simultaneous complaints and pathologies—acute and chronic—while promoting health and wellbeing—by applying and prioritizing health promotion and disease prevention strategies.
• Community orientation includes the ability to reconcile health needs of individual patients and those of the community in which they live.
• Holistic modelling:[1] the ability to use a bio-psycho-social model, taking into account cultural and existential[2] dimensions of non-reductionist thinking.

---

1 *Holism*: (holon is Greek for *entity*) the tendency in nature to form wholes, that are greater than the sum of the parts, through creative evolution (Jan Smuts 1926). This process is called 'emergence'.
2 *Existential* implies more than just spiritual; it means that 'everything affects health' (p653).[12] Existential needn't always mean wearing black jeans and black polo-neck jerseys and singing about one's angst. "The song is sung, not after it has come to be, but rather: in the singing the song begins to be a song."—an example of *non-reductionist thinking*; see Heidegger.[13]

Primary care is the 1st contact with health services. 6 models: 1) *General practice* 2) *Phone* advice (NHS direct) 3) *Walk-in centres* run by enhanced nurses 4) *A&E* 5) *Pharmacies* 6) *Large clinics* (covering populations of >40,000 with a range of skills: GPs, trauma staff, imaging, simple surgery/endoscopy, with on-site labs, physio, and pharmacy).

Primary care core activities
• Ensuring freedom from want: safe food, water etc
• Basic illness treatment
• Provision of drugs
• Preventive care (p482)
• Enabling Maslow's hierarchy (p315)

Where needed, referrals are made from primary care (in ~10% of UK patients) to secondary care, eg district hospitals. Tertiary referral to regional centres may then occur. This seductively simple model misses out entirely on the cornerstone of primary health care: the responsibility that individuals and families have for their own physical and mental well-being. ▶90% of health problems are taken care of outside formal health systems. Unless individuals and families act on their own initiative to promote their health, no amount of medical care is going to make them healthy. In assessing how good a community is at primary health care, one needs to look not just at medical care, but also at social, political, and cultural aspects. Ask questions such as: *Is society making it easy for individuals to choose a healthy lifestyle?* and *How is society targeting health education?* and *Is this 'education' in fact indoctrination?* What you are being taught is an amalgam of current prejudice and the choices of this particular culture. The slightest look at history will show how impermanent these must be.

Primary health care defined as a strategy No country is rich enough to give its citizens (and illegal immigrants) everything that medicine can offer. Hence the need for efficient use of limited resource. This presupposes an effective system of primary health care. To be effective, this must be accessible; relevant to people's needs; properly integrated; have full community participation; be cost-effective, and characterized by collaboration between sectors of society.

UK facts • GP care costs <10% of total NHS costs (£20/consultation *vs* £60 in A&E).
• 90% of illnesses known to the NHS are handled entirely in primary care.
• ~26,000 GP Principals in England (GPs with PCT contract)[14,15] + ~7000 salaried GPs (paid by Principals) + ~1700 locums + ~2000 Drs doing foundation-year and specialist GP training (FY1, ST1-3)[16] Supporting staff: ≥3/whole-time GP.

Intermediate care[17]

This type of care lies between traditional primary care and secondary care. It integrates facilities from many areas to address complex health needs which do not require use of district general hospital services. Examples include preadmission assessment units; early and supported discharge schemes; community (cottage) hospitals; domiciliary stroke units; hospitals-at-home schemes; rehabilitation units. It is one of the mechanisms by which health and social services mesh to allow patients to receive the most appropriate care. Its main advantages are that it is said to allow:

1 Care close to home. 2 Best use of new technology, eg information technology, near-patient testing, and phone-activated devices to summon help. 3 Cost-effective use of resources. 4 Less rigidly demarcated professional roles. 5 Creative integration of working practices. Don't think of it simply as reducing bed-blocking, but it can.[18] It may also be more expensive than standard care.[19] NB: intermediate care also offers GPs a route to developing a special interest (GPSI). This option needs careful economic scrutiny: it's not obvious that such care will be cheaper, as someone else has to do the work of the GP while she is doing the special interest.[20] Reducing waiting times is a key policy driver behind GPSI services, but this is not the chief issue for patients. The thoroughness of the consultation and the expertise of the clinician are higher priorities.[21]

Simple self-care constitutes the health activities which we do on our own and within family, eg brushing our teeth, or going to bed with aspirins during flu. Empowered self-care is what can happen when primary, secondary (district general hospital), and tertiary care (eg regional burns units and cancer specialisms) work together with social services within the context of the family life cycle. Crucially, it uses the principles of intermediate care (see OPPOSITE). ▶*Of any health care system, ask how rich and deep are its community roots?* How many options are there for the care of this sick old lady who has a bad chest and is temporarily off her feet? If your health care system lacks depth, and if ties of religion and family are loose, the only option may be an emergency admission to a high-technology hospital. Emergency admissions in the UK and many other areas have been climbing inexorably. One important reason is lack of options in primary care.

Whenever you think of admitting a patient to hospital, ask ▶*What are the other options?* Do this not just to save the hospital work, but to force you to find out what your patient really wants, and to ensure that the most appropriate level of care is found. When you think of these options, don't think *doctors or nurses?*—think *universal health worker*. Universal health workers have various skills: find out about them, and judge them not according to historic professional codes but according to how good

Options without admitting:
• Neighbourly help
• Hospice
• Sheltered housing
• Hospital at home
• Nursing/rest home
• Social services home
• Twilight home nurses
• Domiciliary physio/OT
• Admission avoidance team
• Fast-response nursing

they are at empowering self-care. No health service can look after most patients most of the time. Empowered self-care in the context of interdependent social and medical services is not some new option that may or may not be used: it is the *only* option for health services which aim to look after more than one patient. Without this idea of empowered self-care, hospitals become places of passive dependency, they get too full, you cannot get people in, and you cannot get people out. NB: if you think that empowered self-care is a cliché, try doing your diabetic clinic without it: *you will always fail.*

Empowered self-care entails choice (p315), dialogue (p370), knowledge of mental states (p324), informed consent (p402), literacy/education (p494), participation in planning and respect by professionals for lifeworlds other than their own (p321). We have to harmonize our care-plans with patients' belief systems. So if a man takes strength from meditation, this should feed into the dialogues which inform his empowered self-care. This yields more patient satisfaction *and* improved outcomes (such as improved health, reduced prescribing, fewer side effects, etc): see p517.[22-25]

Barriers to this type of care
- People who are rendered helpless and hopeless by unemployment, poverty, and family strife. Others who have difficulty accessing care include: the homeless, refugees, drug abusers, ethnic minority groups, and patients living in rural areas without public transport.
- Professionals who want to monopolize and medicalize health.
- Nations which are keener to take up arms than to vaccinate them.
- A world which behaves as if it does not know the meaning of social justice and equality, and in which rich and poor fail to share common objectives—or simply fail to share anything.

Primary care

Whenever a task can be successfully delegated, delegate it. The antithesis is: *If you want a job done properly, do it yourself.* Nature favours the first maxim: when we die all our tasks are either forgotten or delegated, often by default. So the question is not *whether* to delegate, but *when*, and *to whom*. The principle of team work is: *No member is indispensable; all can contribute.* Teams may be small and close-knit, or large—for example the NHS 'super surgery', with doctors, dentists, opticians, a pharmacy, and heart clinics.[et al]

Doctors *Principals/partners:* GPs holding contracts with a Primary Care Organization (PCO) and consortia; some may specialize (eg endoscopy), or have a role in the PCO, eg in commissioning care;[1] *GP non-principals, sessional GPs locums; FY1, ST3 registrars.* Medical and other students may also be present.

A good question for any partnership to ask is "What is our range of skills, and is postgraduate training being arranged to fill in any lacunae?" GPs with special interests need not undermine the central role of being a generalist.

Community nurses (employed in England by Primary Care Trusts). Activities: post-op visits for dressings and the removal of sutures, dressing leg ulcers, and giving 'all care' to the dying, giving injections (eg to blind diabetic patients), and supplying incontinence and other aids ± catheterizations. *Nurse prescribers* have additional training and are termed *Independent* or *Supplementary Nurse Prescribers* (SNP). SNPs only prescribe according to protocols once a diagnosis has been made.[26]

Midwives They do antenatal classes, clinics, home visits, and home deliveries. They have a statutory obligation to visit in the puerperium for the 1st 10 days (she has right of access). At 10 days the health visitor takes over.

Health visitors have nursing and midwifery backgrounds, plus health visiting qualifications. Roles: developmental testing of children; immunization advice; breastfeeding; minor illness in children; handicap; advice to adults about diet & smoking; implementing health education officer (p495) strategies; screening of the elderly in their homes; bereavement visits.

Practice nurses activities include: •*Tests:* Urine; blood (best delegated to a phlebotomy-trained receptionist, with a 'health assistant' role); audiometry; ECGs; peak flow. •*Advice:* Diet; travel. •*Treatment:* Ear syringing; injections. •*Prevention & audit:* Vaccinations; BP; cervical smears; family planning/IUCDs (eg holding an English National Board Certificate). •*Chronic disease:* Diabetes, asthma, COPD, heart disease, etc. •*Chaperoning:* Usually she is too busy.

Nurse practitioners diagnose and initiate treatment. Patient satisfaction is high. No increase in adverse outcomes has been found; consultations are longer by 3-4 minutes, and more tests are done.[27,28] *Community matrons* have case-loads of ~60 vulnerable patients, eg with multiple pathologies such as CCF and falls. She gives home care (*active case management*) aiming to ↓emergency admissions (which fall by 6% on the most optimistic forecasts).[29]

Counsellors 30% of GP patients have psychological conditions, and to help with these, counsellors may be employed; their role is uncertain (p381).

Receptionists and secretaries Receptionists may take on a *health assistant role* taking blood, testing urines, doing BPs, capillary glucose, ECGs, or audits (have they had their hepatitis B vaccinations?)

Practice managers lead on: finance; employment law; tax; risk assessment/ reduction; health & safety; audit; commissioning care contracts. *Others:* Social worker, psychologist, physiotherapist. *Beyond the surgery:* NHS Direct; NHS walk-in services; nurse-led personal medical services; community pharmacists, health education officers (p495), community physicians.

---

1 Commissioning care may seem something you are not engaged in, but every time we sign a prescription we are commissioning care, and we all need to take responsibility for how money is spent.

Small practices *vs* huge commercial companies

Commercial primary care companies (eg The Practice®, under contract to the NHS,[30] with loyalties to shareholders, not the communities they serve) are new in UK primary care, but polyclinics have long existed in India, Germany, Russia, France, and USA). 40 or more primary care doctors work with dentists, midwives, nurses, physios, radiologists, chiropodists, endoscopists, and consultants. They aim to do half the work now done in hospital. Their champions say they are: •Cheap •More integrated (easy to refer across the corridor) •Better equipped •Available out-of-hours (24/7). But continuity of care suffers; this is highly valued by patients,[10] and gives much job satisfaction to GPs.

An example shows the value of continuity of care. One of us (JML) was called to an unrousable sweating 60-year-old man, whom we admitted to hospital with suspected septicaemia—which, years later, turned out to be the presenting symptom of an occult, indolent malignancy. We looked after him until his death at home. The continuity of care, not the clinical details, made the job interesting. But the continuity doesn't stop at the end of one life. Now, whenever we see his wife, on trivial and grave problems, we have this shared bond. When she refused hospital admission for pneumonia and hypoxia, we could use this shared bond to induce her, over a day or so, to change her mind.

The dangers of exhaustion and isolation are not solved by larger practices or polyclinics (which could add to professional isolation). NB: single-handed doctors are more likely to compensate for isolation from colleagues by identifying more with patients, which may well help patient centred care.

I am now about to start a day of single-handed general practice as my partner is away. The day is unplanned, the appointments book empty. People just turn up, bringing their infarcts, their sorrows, their trivia, and their life events to me. Some of the people who will come have not yet even fallen ill. There are the coronary artery plaques on the point of rupturing, the dizziness before the fall, the hallucination before its enactment, and someone is now writing a note to explain the impending suicide or the fact that they are leaving home forever, and taking the kids with them. All this is in the future; but for now, none of this has happened yet. I am completely up to date, and I command my general practice sitting behind an empty desk. I saw the last person who wanted to see me yesterday. There is no waiting list. Just the unknown. When the patient's dizziness *does* lead to the fall in the village shop, as it did yesterday, I will be on hand to patch up the old lady, and the receptionist will kindly finish off the patient's shopping for her, and escort her home.

Problems with large clinics Think-tanks (eg the King's Fund[31]) focus on:
- Access problems, not just in rural areas. People don't want to go 20 miles to see any old doctor rather than 'my doctor down the road'. ►But big clinics might be just what's needed in inner city areas if current premises are poor.
- Planned economies of scale cannot be relied upon. Consultants travelling time are much increased, and demand on hospital services may rise, not fall.
- Studies show that benefits of one-stop care often fail to materialize, eg the diabetologist is too busy to see Mrs Salt's foot today. Tomorrow is worse, and there is no vascular surgeon on site, so admission is needed anyway.
- Smaller establishments do better, generally, in terms of quality of care.
- Problems with leadership which make working together harder not easier.
- Co-location doesn't necessarily lead to co-working and good team dynamics.
- Efficiencies in the USA where specialists work from isolated offices will not accrue in the UK where specialists already work together in hospital teams.

A compromise... Less pure models of polyclinics have been toyed with in some countries, and in the UK allow GPs to retain their premises and share extra facilities for diagnosis/treatment. This model meshes with the RCGP *Roadmap*,[32] but funding issues are unresolved.

Primary care

3 views:

1 *No one is busier than a GP:* the busy GP is a typical role model and stereotype.

2 This 'busy' thing isn't a commitment: it's an evasion. Sebastian Faulks Engleby page 155

3 *Patients are busy too:* The DoH calculates that 3.5×10^6 working days are lost queuing to see GPs (this assumes queuing patients were well enough to work). Hence the move to walk-in supermarket health centres: see p507.

As the list of tasks to do in consultations lengthens, patient's own needs get crowded out. Depressed patients, for example, frequently hold back information they would like to discuss, as the doctor seems too busy. Does this matter? It does if your aim is patient-centred care (p478). One study shows that far from doctors having a patient-centred approach it's usually the other way around—the patient has a doctor-centred approach, and is altruistically keen to conserve scarce resources.[33] This concern about "not worrying the doctor" can be counterproductive. So every so often try saying "Take your time—I'm not in any hurry. Let's try to get to the bottom of what's going on ... [pause]"

Time and the consultation Consultation times have risen by 40% since 1992 (now ~12min).[34] Short consultations are riskier than longer ones (eg less time to look things up[35] and for safety netting "If x, y, or z develops, come back sooner..."), but they are frequently unavoidable. ▶Does heavy demand produce short consultations, or do short consultations produce heavy demand by failing to meet patients' needs? GPs' average consultation time is ~7min (with some consultations lasting ~½hr). This seems short, but remember that over a year the time spent with each patient is nearer 1h. The consultation time influences the degree of patient satisfaction, and may influence the consultation rate (in the UK, ~5.5 consultations/person/yr, rising by ~4%/yr),[36] with lower return visit rates for longer consultations (not shown in all studies),[37] lower rates of prescription issue (esp. antibiotics), and more preventive activities. Mean face-to-face consultation time is 8min for 10min appointments but only 9.2min for 15min appointments, suggesting extra time may not be well used by doctors when booking intervals are long. Running late is stressful for doctors (and patients): it is easier keeping to time for 10min (rather than shorter) bookings. Other factors apart from season, distance to the GP, and sex (women consult more than men) which increase (↑) or decrease (↓) consultation rates:

• Low frequency of contact associates with ↑educational status,[38] paid employment in the health sector, and low expectations of GP care for minor illness.
• The cheaper the housing (council tax band[UK]) the higher the consultation rate.[39]
• List size, and having personal lists (consultation rate ↓ by 7%—ie patients are encouraged to consult with only one doctor decreases overall attendance).
• Not prescribing for minor ailments—see p517 (?↓).
• New patients (for their 1st yr with a new GP), and patients over 65yrs (↑).[2]
• If the GP is extrovert (↑) he or she recalls more, and his rate is higher than others (eg 6/yr vs 2/yr). GP age and sex also influence rates.
• High latitudes—within the UK (↑). The South-East has lowest rates.
• Social deprivation (↑) and morbidity (↑).[40] Increasing requirements to monitor almost all diseases and drugs, eg shared care of rheumatoid arthritis (↑).
• Preventive activities (↑; but this can reduce need to invite people to clinics).

There is some evidence[37] for the Howie hypothesis[41] that consultation duration is a valid and measurable marker of quality (effectiveness, safety, equity, and holistic patient experience, p327 & p517). It is certainly not true that extending consultation times will *automatically* increase health and satisfaction.[37]

1 34% by nurses; 62% by GPs; 82% are in surgery; 12% by phone; 4% home visits (9% in 1995); few by email. **2** If ♀ the UK consultation rate at 10yrs old is ~2.4/yr; at 20 it is ~5/yr, at 80 it is 7/yr. If ♂ the consultation rate at 10yrs is 2/yr, at 20 it is 1.7/yr, at 50yr it is 2.7, at 70 it is 5.6, at 80 it is 6.7/yr. A GP with a list of 2000 with 300 patients >65yrs will have provided 210 more consultations to this group in 1998 than in 1992. This trend continues beyond 2002, it is believed.[4,2]

Phone consultations: saving time or creating problems?

Phone consultations/triage (p797) seem a tempting way to reduce need for precious appointments, and hence improve access (max wait ≤2 working days). What is the evidence? During phone consultations, most non-verbal cues are missing. To explore this issue in a practical way, try consultations with friends or actors with whom you are sitting back-to-back. One way to improve these consultations is to do more 'explicit categorization', eg 'First I am going to find out more about how you are now, then I'll ask about your drugs, then I'll go over what I can do to help, then what to do if things get worse.'

Research shows that use of phone consultations in place of same-day, face-to-face consultations does save time, but is often offset by higher re-consultation rates and less use of opportunistic health promotion.[43]

Safety of phone triage by nurses may be poor; urgency was correctly assessed in 69%, and underestimated in 19%.[44] Results may be better with computer-aided decision support: in one study, advice was considered OK in 97.6%. Patients' compliance: *Self-care*—81%. "*Go and see your GP*"—91%. "*Go to A&E*"—100%. Saving per call: €70, €24, and €22 respectively.[45]

Phone counselling of non-treatment-seeking primary care patients with alcohol abuse works: the higher the number of calls, the less risky the pattern of drinking.[46] *Mobile phones* offer greater flexibility, and are a valid method in treating school refusal (p212) and in telemanagement of difficult hypertension and diabetes (Blue Tooth® transmission of ambulatory data).[47]

From medical certification to living wills: all the GP forms

Incapacity/sick pay We despatch the metaphysical job of deciding who is well and who is sick, and for how long, with amazing (but spurious) precision: appendicectomy ≈ 2-3 weeks; CABG ≈ 6 weeks; MI ≈ 5 weeks; cholecystectomy ≈ 2 weeks (5 weeks if open); laparoscopic inguinal hernia ≤2 weeks (with driving; longer with older techniques). Form med3: see p522.

Form *MatB1* gives a pregnant woman time off work once she is 20 weeks before the expected date of delivery (signed by a GP or midwife).

Lasting power of attorney[48] This passes legal authority over financial, health, and welfare affairs to a named person, who can then sign cheques etc for another person. It holds good, eg if the patient has a stroke or dementia if the patient had capacity (p403) at the time it was made.[49]

Living wills Practices may keep advance directives limiting care a patient will accept after a mentally incapacitating illness, eg stroke. They have clauses such as 'If I have a stroke and there is little prospect of recovery, I decline to be tube fed, even if this hastens death. I understand what tube feeding is; it has been explained to me by my GP, Dr... on [date], and it is my considered, enduring wish that...' These documents have legal force. We must record their existence in the notes, and act on them. Patients don't have to be dying for the will to be triggered, and they may prohibit life-saving treatments. Patients send copies to the family and solicitor.[50] Knowing a person's wishes makes it easier for relatives to make difficult decisions.[51]

The consultation is the central act of medicine: all else derives from it. We must acquire flair for telling which part of which model is vital or dangerous at any time, so that in busy surgeries with urgent visits mounting up, both the doctor and his or her patients can survive.

Medical model History→examination→tests→diagnosis→treatment→review.

A patient-centred model[52] ≤9 stages (▶*depending on the patient's wish*)

1 The GP encourages patient contributions and communication. Preconsultation leaflets encouraging questioning and airing of concerns help here.[52]
2 The GP elicits patient's desire for information; knowing this, the GP decides to be brief & authoritative or reflective. ▶The patient leads this process.[53]
3 The GP may set the patient's complaint in social or psychological context while exploring and testing his or her ideas, concerns, expectations, and health beliefs. These beliefs are used to explain diagnosis and treatment.
4 The GP gets sufficient information for no serious condition to be missed.
5 Physical exam either addresses patient's concerns, or confirms or refutes hypotheses generated by the history, leading to shared working diagnosis.
6 The patient participates in the planning of treatment in the light of EBM.
7 Concordance (p519) discussions; patient sets his own target BP, Hb_{A1c} etc.[54]
8 The medical record entry may be something the patient wants to agree.
9 Establish rapport with the patient at all stages—and arrange follow-up.

The Stott & Davis model[55]   (other models: www.skillscascade.com/models.htm)

Managing presenting problems	Modifying help-seeking behaviour
Managing continuing problems	Opportunistic health promotion

A hypothesis-testing model Information is collected and its validity is ascertained by generating and testing hypotheses.

Goal models (ie ends matter, not means) Aim to:
• Cure; comfort; calm; counsel; prevent; anticipate; explain.
• Enable the patient to put himself back in control of his life.
• Manipulate society to the patient's advantage.
• Facilitate change where change is what the patient desires.
• Increase patients' stature—by tapping the sources of richness in their lives, so freeing them from the shadow of insoluble problems.

The inner consultation   Roger Neighbour
                                              ISBN 0-7462-0040-4
1 **Connecting** is the process of establishing rapport.
2 **Summarizing** marks the point at which the patient's reasons for attending, his hopes, feelings, concerns, and expectations have been well enough explored, acknowledged, and summarized for the consultation to progress.
3 **Handing over** follows the doctor's assessment and diagnosis of the presenting problems and entails an explained, negotiated, and agreed management plan.
4 **Safety netting** allows the doctor the security of knowing that she has prepared, or could prepare for, contingency plans to deal with an unexpected event and some departures from the intended management plan: see p532.
5 **Housekeeping** allows the GP to deal with any internal stresses and strains.

The hidden consultation Doctor-drivers that we may prefer to hide:
1 Keep to time at all costs: I *must* engineer an exit in the next 2 minutes.
2 Keep control: eliminate *any* space for undisciplined squads of emotions.
3 Defensive medicine: do tests/refer onwards to lessen the risk of a complaint.
4 Reframe/retell/lie to make the history fit criteria of a service you can refer to.
5 Don't rock the boat: do whatever a patient asks. "Refer me for MRI" "Yes sir!"
6 Make money: more income-generating tasks irrespective of health gains.

How to avoid these? Don't practise medicine in the 21st-century; don't cede control to large organizations; and above all, don't worry. ▶Doctor-neurosis is the single biggest obstacle to health in almost every consultation.[56-58]

In consultations that are going wrong...

Ask yourself "Am I granting as much space to the patient's agenda as to mine?" This is a particular problem with GP contracts which demand attention to background diseases—eg patient: "I'm worried about my husband ..."; GP: "OK, I'm going to test your vibration sense and pulses..."

• "Have I discovered his hopes and expectations, and his fears?" Does this matter? Yes! Congruence of illness representation leads to better communication, better adherence to advice, and better patient satisfaction.[59-60]
• "Am I negotiating openly with the patient over our clashing ideas?"
• "What are my feelings, and how can they be used positively?"
• Try saying: "Things aren't going very well. Can we start again?"

Perceptual filters, decision analysis, and unconscious consulting

When decision-analysts started work observing consultations they were amazed at the number of decisions per minute, and the wide range of possible outcomes, such as 'no action; review next week' or 'blue-light ambulance direct to tertiary referral centre' or 'refer for EEG' or 'prescribe x, y, and z, and stop Q in a week if the blood-level is such-and-such'. The average decision-analyst is disorientated by the sheer pace and apparent effortlessness of these decisions—so much so that doctors were often suspected of choosing plans almost randomly, until the idea of a 'perceptual filter' was developed.

Perceptual filters[61] This is the internal architecture of our mind—unique to each doctor—into which we receive the patient's history. It comprises our:
• Unconscious mental set: *tired/uninterested* to *alert, engaged, responsive.*
• Entire education, from school to last night's postgraduate lecture.
• Sum of all our encounters with patients. Ignore the fact that we can recall very few of these: this does not stop them influencing us strongly: does the rock recall each of those many, many waves which have sculpted it into extraordinary shapes, or which have entirely worn it away?
• Past specific, personal experience with this particular patient.
• Past specific, personal experience with the disease(s) in question.
• Non-personal subjective (eg 'endocarditis is the most dangerous and stealthy disease...') or objective ideas (eg evidence-based medicine, p489).

The mind's working space (random access memory, RAM)[62] The perceptual filter achieves nothing on its own. What is needed is interpretation, rearrangement, comparison, and planning of executive action.

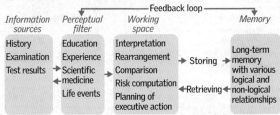

Fig 1. Consultation flowchart. After Sullivan.[61]

▶The abilities of our mental working space are determined by the number of items of data that can be integrated into a decision. There is evidence[63] that this vital number is 3-8. The interesting experimental point here is that if we overload our RAM in the consultation by recourse to a drawer full of guidelines, or unfiltered information—eg looking things up in an unstructured textbook, performance may decline.[63] As one juggler said (with 6 balls in the air) "How do I do it? ... If I did know what I'm doing I would not be able to do it."[64]

It is a sad fact that we lose some of our innate skills in communicating while at medical school. Consultation analysis aims to revive and extend this art, and we know it brings permanent improvement in those who participate. But do not conclude from this that research into the perceptible surface of behaviour can ever fully show us what is happening in the consultation.[165]

Methods The first step is to gain the patient's consent. The method which gives the most information and the most scope for learning employs an observer/director sitting behind a 2-way mirror, who can pass verbal instructions to the doctor through an earphone which is worn unobtrusively. The activity is videoed for later analysis. By directing the verbal and non-verbal behaviour, the observer can demonstrate the potential of a consultation in ways that the doctor may not have imagined possible. Other methods include simple video or audio recording, and joint consultations, in which the second doctor either participates in or observes the first doctor's consultations.

Consultation analysis is likely to be a somewhat threatening activity, so rules have been evolved to minimize this.[66] For example, facts are discussed before opinions, the consulting doctor says what he did well, and then the group discusses what he did well. Then the consulting doctor says what he thinks he could have done better, and finally the group says what he could have done better. In practice, these constraints are occasionally stultifying, but it is better to be stultified than hurt.

Mapping the consultation and scoring its effectiveness In the consultation mapped below, the patient's inferior myocardial infarction (sudden chest pains on swallowing hot fluids) was mistaken by the doctor (JML) for indigestion, illustrating that there is no point in being a good communicator if you communicate the wrong message. It also shows how misleading it is to add the scores (50/84, but the patient nearly died).

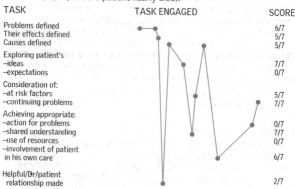

TASK	TASK ENGAGED	SCORE
Problems defined		6/7
Their effects defined		5/7
Causes defined		5/7
Exploring patient's		
–ideas		7/7
–expectations		0/7
Consideration of:		
–at risk factors		5/7
–continuing problems		7/7
Achieving appropriate:		
–action for problems		0/7
–shared understanding		7/7
–use of resources		0/7
–involvement of patient in his own care		6/7
Helpful/Dr/patient relationship made		2/7

Fig 1. Mapping a consultation.

Primary care

1 This paper uses concordances of serial consultations to investigate such things as the play of power in doctor/patient relationships, and shows that the old schools of behaviour-based and meaning-based analysis need not be mutually antagonistic.[67]

☼ On the impossibility of being a good doctor

Here is a list of some of the things pundits tell us we should be doing when we meet patients[68] (don't get depressed yet: we promise there *is* a solution).

1 *Listen*—no interrupting or taking control of the agenda (how often are we guilty of implying: "Don't talk to me when I am interrupting you")?

2 Examine the patient thoroughly (a nonsensical idea, or at least, so it would seem to the average patient with sciatica when you ask them to name the parts of a clock, or to pronounce 'The British Constitution').

3 Arrange cost-effective investigation (via Google or a trip to the library if needed).

4 Formulate a differential diagnosis in social, psychological, and physical terms (a famous triad, no doubt, but why exclude spiritual, allegorical, materialistic, metaphysical, and poetic dimensions of the consultation?).

5 Explain the diagnosis to the patient in simple terms (then re-explain it all to relatives waiting anxiously outside, and then try re-explaining it to the computer in terms *it* understands—ie 5-digit Read codes).

6 Consider additional problems and risk factors for promoting health.

7 List all the treatment options, and seek out relevant systematic reviews, guidelines, clinical trials, etc (evidence-based bedside medicine).

8 Incorporate the patient's view on the balance of risks and benefits, harmonizing his view of priorities, with your own assessment of urgency.

9 Arrange follow-up and communicate with all of the health care team.

10 Arrange for purchase of all necessary care, weighing up cost implications for your other patients and the community, welcoming accountability for all acts and omissions, and for the efficient use of resources—with justifications based on explicit criteria, transparency, and principles of autonomy, non-maleficence, beneficence, and distributive justice.

The alternative Look the patient in the eye. Look the disease in the eye, and then do your best.

The synthesis The alternative looks promising—even attractive, when compared with the 10 impossibilities above. But note that the alternative only looks attractive because it is vague. 'Do your best' is not very helpful advice—and once we start unpacking this 'best' we start to get a list like the 10 impossibilities. '*Professionalism*' sums up *part* of what being a good doctor entails—ie • Self-regulation • Self-actuating and self-monitoring of standards of care. • Altruism • Commitment to service • Specialist knowledge and technical skills reflecting but not determined by society's values • Consistently working to high standards of probity and quality (no bribes, no favouritism, but a dynamic concern for distributive justice). • Self-determination *vis à vis* the range and pattern of the kinds of problems it is right for it to attempt to solve. For a further discussion, see *On Being a Doctor: Redefining Medical Professionalism for Better Patient Care* (King's Fund).

Trying to achieve authenticity is a meta-goal, and may be a better mast to nail your colours to than the 10 impossibilities above not because it is easier but because paying attention to authenticity may make you a better doctor, whereas striving for all 10 of the impossibilities may make you perform less well (too many conflicting ideals). With *inauthentic consultations* you may be chasing remunerative activities, quality points, protocols, or simply be trying to clear the waiting room, at any cost, while the patient is trying to twist your arm into giving antibiotics or a medical certificate. *Authentic consultations* are those where there are no barriers; just 2 humans without status exploring and sharing hypotheses and beliefs and deciding what to do for the best (along the lines described in detail on p531)—with no ulterior motives and no conflicts of interest. Authentic consultations know and tell the truth where possible, and where this is not possible, the truth is worked towards—diligently and fearlessly.

The benefits of preventive activities are often uncertain: *the only certainty is that harm will be caused to some people.* The discipline of quaternary prevention (BOX) aims to minimize this.

Prevention through the human life cycle
Pre-conception (p2). Is she using folic acid supplements? Is she rubella immune? If not, vaccinate, and ensure effective contraception for 1 month after vaccination. Is she diabetic? If so, optimize glycaemic control as early as possible (p3, 24).

Child: Vaccination (p151); hearing; safety lessons; developmental tests (p218); heart disease, p156.

Preventing myocardial infarcts: See the UK National Service Framework for heart disease.[69] Smoking trebles risk above the rate for men who have never smoked. Systolic BP >148mmHg (40% of men) doubles risk,[1] and if serum cholesterol is in top 20% of the observed range, risk trebles. Help to stop smoking (p512), and treating hypertension (*OHCM* p134) & dyslipidaemia (*OHCM* p704) are the main interventions. GPs/practice nurses have a central role in preventing cardiac deaths, eg by screening for ↑BP, and encouraging less smoking—and giving statins (not based on a particular cholesterol level, but according to overall risk of MI and stroke).[2]

Preventing breast cancer deaths: Education and 'breast awareness'. Mammography ('negligible' radiation): cancer pick-up rate ≈ 5/1000 'healthy' women. Yearly 2-view images in postmenopausal women might ↓mortality by 40%, but the price is serious but needless alarm caused: (~10 false +ve results for each true +ve result). The NHS offers 3-yrly single views to those between 47 and 73 years old (older women may be screened too).

Preventing in the reproductive years (p488): Safe sex education (start at puberty; teaching to use condoms need not increase rates of sexual activity); family planning (p296-306), antenatal/prenatal care (p2, eg folic acid), screening for cervical cancer (p270), blood pressure, rubella serology.

Preventing oxidative damage by free radicals: Antioxidants, eg vitamin E, C, carotenoids, flavenoids, and selenium (*OHCM* p693) may have a role.[71]

Old age: 'Keep fit', pre-retirement classes, bereavement counselling, falls clinic. The main aim is to adopt the measures above, to ensure that there *is* an old age.

Side effects No intervention is without side effects, and when carried out in large populations the problems may outweigh the benefits.

Smoking and prevention: p512. **Seat belts and prevention:** p791

Examples of prevention
Primary prevention: (preventing occurrence)
• Vaccination
• Quit smoking advice
• Binge drinking advice
• Healthy eating advice
• Safe(r) sex advice (HIV)
• Hypertension screening
• Preconception folic acid to prevent spina bifida
• Fluoride in water (caries)
Secondary prevention: (screening for 1st stages)
• Cervical cytology
• Mammography
• Proteinuria in pre-eclampsia
• Microalbuminuria in DM
• Colonoscopy for polyps
• Densitometry (osteoporosis)
• Diet advice in impaired fasting glycaemia
Tertiary prevention: (preventing complications)
• Aspirin after a stroke
• Retinal photography in DM
• Hip protectors after falls
• 'Don't go barefoot' (diabetes)
• Vitamin D in osteoporosis
Metaprevention (or quaternary prevention):
⚬ Preventing medicalization
⚬ Prioritizing preventive options
⚬ Shielding from over-zealous prevention, eg no ACE-i for heart protection if prone to postural hypotension/falls.[70]

---

1 Reversible with antihypertensives and a statin (even if cholesterol 'normal or low'; ASCOT study.[72]
2 The Heart Protection Study (HPS) indicates that if a patient has vascular risk factors, eg family history, obesity, sedentary life, smoking, ↑BP, DM) statins can be of benefit even if lipid levels are considered OK. In HPS (N=20,000) overall risk of MI & stroke was ↓ by 30% in those on simvastatin 40mg/24h. Statins also ↓ risk of getting angina, the need for angioplasty/bypass, and amputations. Advantages hold good for women and men, and those over 70.[73] The AFCAPS/TEXCAPS study shows that treatment can ↓ adverse coronary events even in the primary prevention of patients with normal cholesterol levels and no risk factors (past MI etc).[74-76]

Genetic barriers Not everyone responds to preventive measures. Some of us, because of our genes, are 'immune' to the benefits of exercise, for example. As genetic advances occur, our habitual blanket advice of "take more exercise" looks increasingly old fashioned. What we should really do is get to know our patients psychologically and genetically, and tailor advice such as "for you, diet advice is more important than exercise". In one study, in the 8 exercising people showing the largest ↑ in insulin sensitivity, 51 genes were expressed in muscles at double the levels of the 8 people who showed the least improvement after exercise.[77]

Cognitive barriers (See BOX.) When, if ever, we contemplate cataclysmic but preventable ill health in ourselves, we may either believe that "*It won't happen to me*" or we deliberately dare fate to *make* it happen to us. To some people, over-zealous and sanctimonious-sounding hectoring from bodies such as the UK Health Development Agency creates barriers to prevention, inciting anger and rejection by those who resent their taxes being spent by some State Nanny who assumes that all her charges are 'backward 5-year-olds' who cannot be trusted to think for themselves.[78] So people are now proud to announce that "... I eat everything, as much butter and fried foods as I can get ... I smoke 40-60 cigarettes a day ... To eat cornflakes, you've got to have sugar on them, and lots of cream, otherwise there is no point in eating them ... As long as you keep smoking cigarettes, and drink plenty of whisky, you'll go on for ever".[79]

Psychological barriers All of us at times are prone to promote our own destruction as keenly as we promote our own survival. Knowing that alcohol may bring about our own destruction gives the substance a certain appeal, when we are in certain frames of mind—particularly if we do not know the sordid details of what death by alcohol entails. It provides an alluring means of escape without entailing too headlong a rush into the seductive arms of death. Gambling and taking risks are all part of this ethos.

Logistic barriers A general practice needs to be highly organized to be in a state of perpetual readiness to answer questions like "Who has not had their BP checked for 3 years"? or "Who has not turned up to their request to attend for screening"? or "Who has stopped sending in for their repeat prescriptions for antihypertensives?". UK IT systems have advanced a lot in the last years, enabling patient alerts to pop-up, allowing for opportunistic preventive activities. The price of this is that patient-centred activities are crowded out, and that, with many preventive activities offered, no guidance on prioritizing individual intervention is forthcoming. See quaternary prevention, p482.

Another example of logistical barriers is providing a sequence of working fridges in the distribution of vaccines to rural tropical areas.

Political barriers It is not unknown for governments to back out of preventive obligations as if influenced by groups who would lose if prevention were successful. Some countries are keener to buy tanks than vaccines.

Ethical barriers If child benefits were available only to those children who had had MMR vaccine, more mumps would be prevented (an unpopular approach!).

Financial barriers Practices must pay for extra staff to do effective screening. Angioplasty (for example) prevents some consequences of heart disease, but is too expensive to use on everybody whom it might benefit.

Motivation barriers As we rush out of morning surgery to attend the latest vascular disaster we use up energy which might have been spent on studying patients' notes in the evening to screen to prevent the next one. Changing from a crisis-led work pattern to strategic prevention is one way that practice nurses can lead the way. They are particularly successful at the meticulous, repetitive tasks on which all good prevention depends.

Primary care

We often find ourselves sitting on beds trying to persuade wayward people to courses of preventive action which will clearly benefit them, usually at some distant time in the future. We think this very clarity should be enough to persuade the person to act. But, as we dismally stamp our feet on the bare boards of our impatience, we resign ourselves to the fact that action will not follow. *Why is this so often the case?*

The best answer to this question comes from the world's worst patient and our own greatest poet: great not because of his mastery of his world, but because, as the world used him, often cruelly, and as his London doctors gave him up as a hopeless addict, he took on all our petty confusions and made them human, compelling, and universal. Samuel Taylor Coleridge answers our question thus: R Holmes *Coleridge* volume 2; page 225

> *'To love our future Self is almost as hard as to love our Neighbour—it is indeed only a difference of Space & Time. My Neighbour is my other Self, 'othered' by Space—my old age is to my youth an other Self, 'othered' by Time...'*

By being consumed by the fires of his addictions this poet becomes the wick in the lamp we can now use to illuminate our patients' frailties, and hence our own.

Russian roulette Coleridge accurately reveals us to ourselves when we are indifferent to our other selves, whether 'othered' by space or time. He also understood a deeper problem: those who go beyond indifference, ambivalently seeking their own destruction—as if playing Russian roulette with the barrel full every time while at the same time not wanting to die. Some people's attitude to HIV is like this—when safe sex messages are not so much ignored as trounced, or one person offers HIV to another as an erotic gift.[77] This exemplifies a phenomenon which is a human universal: *to know what is good, healthy, and sensible—and do the opposite*. We note that both Dostoevsky and Graham Greene are said to have played Russian roulette—and we conclude that this is a way of living as much as a way of dying: one lives while the barrel spins. Unless one understands something of this mentality, our preventive activities will always tend to smack of Girl Guide piety.

So when we catch ourselves trying to inculcate the principles of preventive medicine into the surly, silent, and self-destructive adolescent sitting beside us we should stop what we are doing and try to tap into the volcano.

This entails systematic testing of a population or a sub-group for signs of illness—which may be of established disease (pre-symptomatic, eg small breast cancers), or symptomatic (eg unreported hearing loss in the elderly).

Modified Wilson criteria for screening (1-10 spells IATROGENIC**)**[1]

(Summary: screening tests must be cost-effective.)

1 The condition screened for should be an important one.
2 There should be an acceptable treatment for the disease.
3 Diagnostic and treatment facilities should be available.
4 A recognizable latent or early symptomatic stage is required.
5 Opinions on who to treat as patients must be agreed.
6 The test must be of *high discriminatory power* (below), *valid* (measuring what it purports to measure, not surrogate markers which might not correlate with reality) and be *reproducible*—with safety guaranteed (see BOX).
7 The examination must be acceptable to the patient.
8 The untreated natural history of the disease must be known.
9 A simple inexpensive test should be all that is required.
10 Screening must be continuous (ie not a 'one-off' affair).

Informed consent: Rees' rule Before offering screening, we have a duty to quantify for patients the chance of being disadvantaged by it;—from anxiety (may be devastating, while waiting for a false +ve result to be sorted out) and the effects of subsequent tests (eg bleeding after biopsy after an abnormal cervical smear), as well as the chances of benefit. We are all guilty of exaggerating benefits and avoiding discussion of controversial areas with patients.

Comparing a test with some gold standard		Patients with condition	Patients without condition
TEST RESULT	Subjects appear to have the condition	True +ve (A)	False +ve (B)
	Subjects appear not to have the condition	False -ve (C)	True -ve (D)

Sensitivity: How reliably is the test +ve in the disease? A/A+C
Specificity: How reliably is the test -ve in health? D/D+B

Partly effective screening
Cervical smears (if ≥25yrs, p270)
Mammography (after menopause)[80]
Finding smokers (+quitting advice)
Looking for malignant hypertension (lesser hypertension is problematic)
Faecal occult bloods (colorectal ca)

Unproven/ineffective screening[2]
Mental test score (dementia, p353)
Urine stix (diabetes; kidney disease)
Antenatal procedures (p8)
PSA screening for prostate ca (detects too many harmless cancers?)●✱
Elderly visiting to detect disease[3]

Why screen in primary care? If screening is to be done at all, it makes economic sense to do it in primary care. In the UK, ≥1 million people see GPs each weekday, providing great facilities for opportunistic 'case-finding' (90% of patients consult over a 5 yrs). Provided the GP's records are adequate, the last 10% are then asked to attend for special screening sessions. Private clinics do limited work, but there is no evidence that their multiphasic biochemical analyses are effective procedures, and NHS resources are wasted chasing false +ves.

1 ▶For an excellent critique of the Wilson criteria, see Gray J 2004 *Br J Gen Pract* 501:292-8.
2 There is evidence that some screening causes morbidity (mortality-awareness and hypochondriasis**t**)—so why is screening promulgated? Because it is easier for governments to be optimistic than to be rigorous!
3 In one study (N=43,000 patients >75yrs old) neither in-depth assessment nor a targeted approach focused on those with ≥3 problems offered gains in survival or quality of life.[81]

Why should safety be guaranteed?

▶Nothing in this world is guaranteed—least of all the data on which statements about safety are made. It is only an ill-educated population who would demand this impossible criterion. In mammography the dose of radiation is tiny—but one of the reasons for doing it at intervals of >1yr is to reduce radiation exposure. Safety is not guaranteed.[82,83] Also, each population of women contains a very radiosensitive subgroup: those bearing a mutation of the gene BRCA1 or BRCA2. In these, repeated x-ray use must definitely be avoided.[84] But if genetic testing and counselling were to be a prequel to mammography, then counselling would be needed. There are some people who definitely should not have this can of worms opened—to find these may need psychological screening....thus safety issues can lead to a an infinite regress—and what started out as a good idea gets swamped. A better approach is to accept some risk—and try to limit it, where practicable.

▶The great thing is to teach people how to evaluate risk, and how to handle dangerous things safely—rather than just shun them.

Problems with screening

Take a healthy person, screen them, turn them into a patient, and then kill them. From a report on cervical screening: "By offering screening to 250,000 we have helped a few, harmed thousands, disappointed many, used £1.5m each year, and kept a few lawyers in work." Typical problems are:

• Those most at risk do not present for screening, thus increasing the gap between the healthy and the unhealthy—the *inverse care law*.
• The 'worried well' overload services by seeking repeat screening.
• Services for investigating those testing positive are inadequate.
• Those who are false positives suffer stress while awaiting investigation, and remain anxious about their health despite reassurance.
• A negative result may be regarded as a licence to take risks.
• True positives, though treated, may begin to see themselves as of lower worth than hitherto.

▶Remember: with some screening programmes of dubious value, *it may be* healthier not to know.

Deconstructing screening platitudes.

Primary care

Iatrogenic medicine at its best.

Examples of single-issue clinics which are conducted in primary care

- Well-woman/well-man clinic
- Elderly 'non-attending' patients
- Giving-up-smoking clinic (p512)
- Joint clinics with a consultant who shares care (eg orthopaedics: see polyclinics[et al], p475)
- Antenatal clinic
- Cardiac[1] and hypertension clinic
- Citizen's advice clinic[85]
- Diabetes clinic
- Asthma[86] and COPD clinics.

Advantages of single-issue clinics	Disadvantages
• Management protocol + action plan for self-care	• Extra time needed
• Check-lists prevent omissions	• Extra training needed
• Co-operation cards allow shared care	• Not holistic
• Flow charts to identify trends	• Not flexible
• Help from specialist practice nurse	• Value often unproven
• Fewer outpatient referrals (eg ↓by ~20%)	• Access to hospital technology↓
• GPs can improve clinical skills[87]	• Travelling time by consultants to outreach clinics is wasteful
• Better co-operation with hospitals	
• Improved dialogue with specialists[87]	• Untargeted diseases get ignored

Activities in well-woman clinics
- Cervical smear; breast awareness/mammograms
- Screening: osteoporosis; DM; atrial fibrillation[88]
- Antenatal/postnatal care (+pre-conception, p2)
- Protecting skin from sun; regular skin self-exam★
- MMR and tetanus vaccination★ (p151)
- Smoking and alcohol advice★
- Safer sex advice for HIV★
- Family planning/sterilization★
- Diet, weight & blood pressure★
- Discussion of HRT issues.

Breast examination/teaching breast self-examination in nurse clinics
There is disagreement about whether this is desirable, and, if so, whether we can delegate this to nurses. Some (but not all) studies report that cancers in those having this protocol are detected earlier, with improved survival, compared with mammography alone. But UK DoH advice is against breast palpation in asymptomatic women, even if on the Pill/HRT. The DoH advises against delegation to nurses, but in some practices it may *only* be nurses whom women find acceptable—so validating nurse training is a key issue.

Well-men Women live longer, so why should they get all the prevention? Nurses can do all the well-woman activities ★starred above in well-man clinics (substitute testicular self-examination ± PSA (prostate specific antigen) tests for breast awareness). One such clinic yielded ≥25% obese, 14% with diastolic BP ≥100mmHg, 66% needing tetanus vaccination, and 29% needing smoking advice; see the OXCHECK study, p495 and the National Service Framework for ischaemic heart disease (OHCM p79).[89]

Diabetes *Education/encouragement is the most important activity.* Group sessions are best: passive dependency is minimized and people (patients) help and motivate each other. Traditional one-to-one care *even when optimized*, is associated with progressive decline in knowledge, problem-solving ability, and quality of life. Group-engendered cognitive and psychosocial skills associate with more favourable clinical outcomes—including falling BMI and Hb_{A1c}.[90 n=120]

Advantages over outpatient clinics: patients see the same person each time; weekly appointments are possible if needed; telephone advice is easily available. Mini-clinics are cheaper and ?better than outpatient clinics.[91]

Even insulin-dependent diabetics can be managed *wholly* in primary care from presentation (p490). There are dangers if no ketoacidosis. However, the vital test is retinal photography or dilated fundoscopy (p412 & p446). Other vital areas are BP control (<145/85, lower if microalbuminuria), diet, exercise, and smoking advice, statins (for all) and round-the-clock blood glucose monitoring, with checks on U&E and Hb_{A1c}. *Liaison with community consultant-services:* May prevent hospital admission.

---

1 To check if on β-blocker & ACE-i post-MI + up-titration of β-blocker dose & ACE-i in heart failure.[92]

Evidence-based medicine (EBM)

This is the conscientious and judicious use of current best evidence from clinical care research in the management of individual patients—taking into account their values. *The problem* 2,000,000 papers are published each year. Patients may benefit from a tiny fraction of these. How do we find them?

A partial solution 50 journals are scanned not by experts in neonatal nephrology or the left nostril, but by searchers trained to spot papers which have a direct message for practice, and meet predefined criteria of rigour (below). Summaries are then published in *Evidence-based Medicine*.

Questions used to evaluate papers: **1** Are the results *valid*? (Randomized? Blinded? Were all patients accounted for who entered the trial? Was follow-up complete? Were the groups similar at the start? Were the groups treated equally, apart from the experimental intervention?) **2** What *are* the results? (How large was the treatment effect? How precise was the treatment effect?) **3** Will the results help *my* patients (cost-benefit sum).

Problems with the solution *The concept of scientific rigour is opaque.* What do we want? The science, the rigour, the truth, or what will be most useful to our patients? These may overlap, but they are not the same.

- Will the best be the enemy of the good? Are useful papers rejected due to some blemish? Answer: *all* evidence needs appraising (often impossible!).
- By reformulating patients in terms of answerable questions, EBM risks missing the point of the patient's consultation. He might simply want to express his fears, rather than be used as a substrate for an intellectual exercise.
- Is the standard the same for the evidence for *all* changes to our practice? We might not want to prescribe drug x for constipation if there is even a slim chance that it might cause colon cancer. There are many other drugs to choose from. We might need far more robust evidence than a remote chance to persuade us to do something rather counter-intuitive, such as giving heparin in DIC. How robust do the data need to be? There is no science to tell us the answer: we decide off the top of our head (albeit a wise head, we hope).
- EBM is a lucky dip if gathering *all* the evidence on a topic proves impossible.
- What of journal letter columns? It may be ages before fatal flaws are aired.
- There is a danger that by always asking "What's the evidence ..." we divert resources from hard-to-prove areas that may be very valuable, eg physiotherapy for cerebral palsy, to easy-to-prove ones. The unique personal attributes of therapists are as important as the objective regimen. It is all too easy to transfer resources to easy-to-quantify activity, eg neonatal screening.
- "My increased knowledge gradually permeated or repressed the world of intuitive premonitions ..."[Carl Jung] These premonitions may be vital! ▶See p505.
- Evidence-based medicine is rarely 100% up to date. Reworking meta-analyses in the light of new trials takes time—if it is ever done at all.
- EBM contributes to the problem of data overload by churning out endless guidelines that don't quite apply to the patient sitting in front of you.

Advantages of evidence-based medicine • It improves our reading habits.
- It leads us to ask questions, and then to be sceptical of the answers.
- As taxpayers, we should like it (wasteful practices can be abandoned).
- Evidence-based medicine presupposes that we keep up to date, and makes it worthwhile to take trips around the perimeter of our knowledge.
- Evidence-based medicine opens decision-making processes to patients.

Conclusion There is little doubt that, *where available*, EBM is better than what it is superseding. It may not have much impact, as gaining evidence is time-consuming and expensive. Despite these caveats, evidence-based medicine is one of the most rational recent medical developments. Let's all join in by subscribing to ideals and its journal (http://ebm.bmj.com).

Primary care

▶Freedom from only doing ordained tasks is essential for mental health.

▶There is nothing better (for the doctor and the patient) than doing a job for the love of it—and not many people love targets set by other people—so the target has to entail great benefits to outweigh its unintended consequences.

▶Beware accepting a protocol without knowing if it will affect your sympathy and time to communicate.

▶Is the protocol independently validated. What is its *hidden objective*, eg cost-containment, conformity, self-advertisement, empire-building, or care?

▶Reject protocols that don't specify conflicts of interest: most protocols (87%) are written by people with financial links to drug companies or public bodies wishing to curtail expense.[54,93-96]

Sympathy is a flower which has often withered before the end of morning surgery. If a protocol says that you must do 9 things to Mrs James who has diabetes, both of you may be irritated by item 5: the doctor is running out of time, and the patient is running out of goodwill. She is worrying about her husband's dementia, having long since stopped worrying about her own illnesses. She does not mind being assailed by forks, stix, and lancets, if this is the price for a portion of her doctor's sympathy. But if she finds that this sympathy has withered, who knows how she will view her doctor?

Guidelines are seen as friendly, if flexible, allowing for the frailties of clinical science as it meets bedside reality; they can also be interactive, if computer programming is skilful. Protocols, particularly if they have been handed down from some supposedly higher authority, have a reputation for being strict, sinister, and stultifying instruments for thought control. How well do these stereotypes stand up in practice? It is known that doctors working in highly regulated environments with strict protocols perform suboptimally.[97] It is also worth noting that very few laws define their own exceptions. You could say that patients have a right to be asked if they want to participate in a protocol, and if so, that it should be done properly. But what if it is the child's birthday today, and he really does not want to have his finger pricked for a glucose test, but he is most willing to go along with all other aspects of a protocol? If you are flexible, the price may be ketoacidosis after the party. Herein lies the paradox of protocols. They are designed to remove the many indefensible inconsistencies found in clinical medicine, yet protocols depend on the individual doctor's own flair and instinctive judgment so that they are applied in the best way.

The best approach is to welcome good protocols, and develop meta-protocols to be answered whenever (or almost whenever) such protocols are not adhered to. Why did you not adhere to the protocol? Please tick the appropriate box:
❏ My own convenience, eg if too many other more important tasks to do.
❏ My patient's preference (well-informed or otherwise).
❏ Evidence is shaky and may not apply to my practice population.
❏ Inefficient use of resources, eg scarce consultations are used up in follow-up.
❏ My instinct warned me not to apply the protocol in this case.[1]

To get round the problems of non-implementation of guidelines, some NHS primary care trusts send in visits from *pharmaceutical advisers* who have trained in outreach visiting (it is unfair to call them *thought-police*). But when this has been evaluated in randomized trials, no impact could be detected.[98]

Can we square guidelines & targets with patient-centred care? (p478) Answer: *No*; discussing this issue with purveyors of guidelines is a good way reveal the hidden agendas described above. Point out that leading authorities are now saying patients must decide their own target BP, Hb_{A1c}, etc.[99]

---

1 Understandably, many GPs don't follow protocols despite high awareness of them: other reasons include the fact that precise targets (eg for BP control) are always arbitrary, and should allow for some variation.

Placebo effects are very powerful and are important not just in research, but also in demonstrating to us how our demeanour may be just as important as the drugs we give. Both doctors and patients are susceptible to placebo effects—and unintentionally we use the placebo effect every day—as so few of our therapies are validated for the exact individual patient in front of us. In one placebo-controlled study of antihypertensives the partners of the enthusiastic doctor broke the code, and told him that his experimental treatment appeared similar to existing treatments without telling him who was having the active drug and who was having the placebo. ►From this point, there was an immediate, marked increase in BP in both groups, although the difference between the drug and the placebo was maintained.[100,101]

►Our beliefs and our behaviour sometimes matter more than our drugs.

What is the mechanism of the placebo effect? *Psychological:* Expectancy, anxiety reduction, and Pavlovian conditioning may operate. *Psychosomatic linkages:* Endorphins, catecholamines, cortisol, and psychoneuroimmunulogy play a part.[102] *Functional neuroanatomy:* Placebos have real effects on brain and body: ►they are not just response biases.[103] The nucleus accumbens (NAC), a CNS region involved in reward expectation, may mediate placebo responses. Dopamine release is seen during placebo administration, and is related to its anticipated effects. Individual variations in NAC response to reward expectation account for 28% of the variance in the formation of placebo analgesia.[104]

Don't conclude that we should give placebos to all our patients. This book is founded on the idea that we must be honest and straightforward with patients. Nevertheless, it may be unwise to share too many doubts: one GP randomly assigned his consulting style in those with apparently minor illness to a 'positive encounter' or a 'negative encounter'. In the former, patients were given a diagnosis and told they would be better in a few days; the latter group were told that it was not certain what the matter was. ⅓ of patients having negative encounters got better in 2 weeks, but over ⅔ of the positive group did so.

We conclude that in medicine *context matters*, and we must all take steps to optimize context and expectation in holistic, positive, and optimistic ways.[103]

Mandatory placebos? Some practitioners use evidence-based medicine (EBM) as a rationale for using placebos—*intentionally*. The argument goes like this: if there isn't a gold-standard treatment for the condition, and if EBM shows that a placebo has above-baseline effects, and if a placebo response wouldn't mask serious pathology, and if the patient gives informed consent and is told about other options, then a placebo is warranted—or even mandated.[105] There is one problem with this neat argument. The patient may well need to know that he or she has a chance of having an active drug for the placebo effect to work.

Nocebos Pharmacists often 'leaflet' customers with long lists of their drugs' side effects, that, like voodoo death, may be self-fulfilling prophesies. We often underplay side effects like impotence on the grounds that in such a sensitive area, the mere mention of impotence might bring it about. Too paternalistic?

The Hawthorne effect What is the optimal level of lighting for making circuit boards? Whatever level the experimenter tried (in the Hawthorne plant near Chicago in the 1930s), there was an increase in productivity, even at very low levels, showing that the act of doing an experiment changes people's behaviour. Special attention leads to special results. Similarly, in a trial of *Ginkgo biloba* in dementia, the placebo arm had two levels of follow-up, intensive and minimal: patients showed better cognitive function in the former group.[106] We conclude that because of these effects, generalizing from research is fraught with danger.

▶*Your patient is assessing you as much as you are assessing your patient.* We come to this enterprise in a spirit of humility. There are no culturally neutral or coherent encounters: all cultures have oddities and inconsistencies. Use cross-cultural encounters as a metaphor for exploring your own prejudices, fears, and ideas of selfhood,[107] and come to accept that mastery here is counter-productive, for mastery implies a supremacy which ultimately stifles dialogue.

Eastern manners ▶Do not expect an African-Asian person to answer intimate questions, without first explaining about confidentiality.
• Avoid prolonged eye contact and slow speech (indicates lack of respect).
• Control your gesticulations (the 'thumbs up' sign is considered rude).
• A psychiatric referral may destroy eligibility for marriage.

Sikh names Some Sikhs have no family name. Singh and Kaur indicate only sex and religion, so that extra identification is needed on the notes.

Muslims (The largest non-Christian UK sect) Sometimes the last name is not a family name, and the 1st name is not the personal name. There may be no shared family name. The 1st name is often religious (eg Mohammed). Common female 2nd names (eg Banu, Begum, Bi, Bibi, and Sultana) are of as little help in identification as the title 'Ms'. Writing the father's name can give extra identification.[108]
• Shoes are to be taken off before entering the house (for any purpose).
• Some Muslims do not shake hands with the opposite sex after puberty.
• Most Muslims do not drink alcohol (so do not offer tonics).
• Some Muslims may refuse to take their medication in Ramadan. If prescribing drugs once or twice daily (before sunrise; after sunset) is not OK, explain the disease; according to Islamic rules, ill people must not fast.
• Do not offer pork insulin to Muslims.

Muslims and death: Religious observance requires prompt burial, not cremation. Washing and shrouding is an important ceremony traditionally done by elders of the same sex and only relatives and friends may do it
• The dead body is sacred and never abandoned by relatives, so it is rare for undertakers to be involved. Bereavement lasts for 3–7 days (prayers in the home may be said almost continuously).
• In some cultures, wives may stay at home for several weeks after death of a spouse and they cannot re-marry for up to 3–4 months.
• Some cultures have restrictions for transplantation or autopsy.

How to avoid offending Western manners Western manners expect 'please', 'thank you', 'after you', and 'I'd love to ...' rather than 'I don't mind if I do ...' Westerners are notoriously sensitive to gaze and mutual gaze: not enough, and they think you are shifty; too much, and you are making unwelcome advances. The same goes with interpersonal distance: too close, and invasion is threatened.

Clinical Centile charts are different (p181). Bilateral cervical/inguinal lymphadenopathy may be normal in Asian and African children (but remember TB).
• BMI >23 carries ↑risk in Asian (vs Caucasian) men; give diet etc advice earlier.
• Bangladeshis are at greatest risk of heart disease, then Pakistanis, then Indians.
• Hypertension (and renal failure) is more prevalent in African-Caribbeans[109] who respond better to thiazides and Ca²⁺ channel blockers than to ACE-i/A2A.
• Most heart disease risk assessment tools underestimate risk in south Asians.
• Genetic disease prevalence↑—for example sickle-cell anaemia (eg in Africans and West Indians); haemoglobin E disease (eg in Chinese).
• Unusual malignancies (oesophagus in Japan, tongue from betel nuts).
• The length of gestation for Black infants averages 9 days shorter than that of White infants and they weigh 180–240g less than white infants at birth. However, at a similar gestational duration, Black infants are more mature than White infants and related to this increased maturity, premature Black infants also have a better survival rate than premature White infants.

Hindu names and some other customs

- First names (eg Lalita) are often male and female, but middle names (eg Devi) always denote sex and they are often written together (Lalitadevi).
- A Hindu is likely to give only his first 2 names, withholding his family name, to be polite. This can cause great confusion in registration.
- Some have dietary restrictions (no beef/veal); some are strict vegetarians.

Language, interpretation, and health

100 million people live outside their country of birth. All too often interpreters, if available, are only on hand during office hours. Friends and relatives may be available, but confidentiality issues are important. The interpreter's own cultural prejudices may distort your questions, and even make them vacuous.[110]

When a child interprets for his mother's or father's mortal illness, many other unknowable issues are raised.[111] Alternatives include telephone interpretation (eg with a hands-off conference phone). Although non-verbal signs are lost, there may be advantages as some patients may say things to a phone which they would be unhappy to say face-to-face.[112] Ask for these services from Health Authorities/Primary Care Trusts—and then the services are more likely to be in place, and the wheels well oiled when the real emergency arises.

The Phelan-Parkman 'rules' for interviewing with an interpreter
- Address patient in the second person; talk directly to your patient.
- Keep control of the consultation; make full use of written material.[113]
- Pause often, looking for non-verbal clues signalling misunderstanding.
- Be attentive when patient responds; check your patient's understanding.

Advice to consider before a Hajj journey to Mecca[114]

Hajj is a 5-day Muslim pilgrimage to Mecca to mark Abraham's readiness to sacrifice Ishmael. Its date varies. Pilgrims renew their faith shoulder to shoulder, as a sacred duty, with 2 million Muslims from all over the world. 20,000 travel from the UK, and another 29,000 also make a lesser pilgrimage to Mecca called Umrah. Hajj is physically taxing (but often exhilarating) involving walking and camping in the desert with little sanitation. Hajj is not required for those in poor health, and your role may be to advise on this.

- Meningococcal vaccination is mandatory (2 doses ACWY-VAX® conjugate meningitis vaccination, 3 months apart). Immunity is thought to last 3 years. Hepatitis A, influenza, and malaria prophylaxis are important.[115] Consider also polio, typhoid and diphtheria vaccines and hepatitis B vaccines.
- Women should not menstruate during Hajj. Menstrual delay by norethisterone (p248) or contraceptive pill may be requested.
- Sun stroke and heat exhaustion are major hazards. Advise acclimatization (so arrive 1 week before Hajj to enable optimum sweating), drink 5L/day (with up to half a teaspoonful of salt/L). Keep a bottle with you at all times. Take an umbrella (preferably white) as sun shade. Avoid travel in middle of day and on open top buses. Use liberal sun block if fair skinned.
- Much walking is needed so advise comfortable shoes and carrying a shoe bag to carry them in when removed for prayers (so as not to lose them). Sand is so hot that barefoot walking may cause sole burns.
- Male head-shaving by shared razor blades risks blood-borne infections. Advise using new razor blades (hair trimming may be acceptable).
- Take an adequate supply of medications and a list of them in generic names. Also take simple analgesics. Most injuries are to feet.
- Being crushed by crowds is a danger if laminar flow becomes 'stop-and-go' then turbulent.[116] Try avoiding the most popular times (eg travel at night).
- Temporary ITUs deal with ~140 patients/Hajj: heart disease (63%); infections (26%). ~10% of these patients die. 30% need referral to tertiary centres.[117]
- Post-Hajj diagnoses to consider: meningitis, hepatitis, hydatid, TB, malaria.

Health education: what's the point?

Health education presumes that people are rational and want to promote their own survival. It begs the question: what should we live for? Unless an individual has an optimistic answer, health education will fail. For 60% of UK people, death is an attractive option compared with doing more exercise.[118] Alcohol and drugs—anything that achieves oblivion as soon as possible—is an ever more popular approach to life, despite years of health education. So society needs to ask itself 2 questions: *are we making it easy for people to make wise health choices*—and, more importantly, *are we making it easy for people to find something worth living for?* In city after city, country after country, the answer is *No* and *No*. Britain is the worst place to live in the developed world, based on UNICEF measures of childhood wellbeing, so there is a long way to go before we get to the starting line where most people are amenable to health education. With this proviso, the following may make (a little) sense.

What is education?—five partial answers

1 Education is the way we pass down, from one generation to the next, society's values, attitudes, and culture. Thus crime, duplicity, double standards (and, on a good day, idealism) are perpetuated in a kind of cultural inheritance.

2 Education is an activity carried out on ignoramuses by people who assume they know best[119] (but who should know better). We don't need no education. Pink Floyd *Another brick in the wall*

3 Education is about changing people. It ends up implying "mend your ways... or else". In some countries, non-vaccination leads to imprisonment.[120]

4 Education performed on one mind by another, under duress, is indoctrination. This is a problem with some forms of religious education.

5 Education is *self*-education: the method by which we touch the great minds of the dead and come to know we are not alone in our confusions and questionings: the only remedy for the spiral of disconnectedness figured on p99.

Health education messages These must be *specific* and *direct*, eg in getting people to sign on for help for drinking problems, it is of little use saying "If you don't stop drinking you'll get these diseases ..." (~25% respond); saying "Signing on is good for you because of these benefits ..." (~50% respond); saying "If you don't sign here, you've had it" brings the biggest response. Optimum messages must be specific about dates, times, and places of help. Well-chosen images and a degree of 'fear' in the message helps: in enlisting patients for tetanus vaccine a 'low fear' message gets a 30% response, while more fear can double this. Graphic images depicting the effects of smoking are mandatory on UK cigarette packets (evidence is rather flimsy, so far)[121] and it is possible that too high a level of fear is counter-productive. A gruesome film about the worst effects of caries produces petrified immobility, not self-help or trips to dentists. A better approach is **professional teaching**. Compared with parents, teacher-based oral health education has a better effect on oral health (at least in middle-school Chinese students).[122]

Changing attitudes The following paradigm holds sway: knowledge→attitudes→intentions→behaviour. As Chinese thought reformers knew so well, attitude changes depend on a high level of emotional involvement. In questions of belief, as in so many other questions, emotion trumps reason '*people don't demand that a thing be reasonable if their emotions are touched. Lovers aren't reasonable, are they?*' Graham Green p115 *The End of the Affair* Only resort to applying reason to attitudes if emotions are too hot to handle. NB: the arrows in the model above may be reversed: if our behaviour is inconsistent with our ideas (cognitive dissonance), it is often our ideas, not our behaviour which change.

Objective feedback Giving standard written advice about physical activity helps promote exercise. But to make big strides, it helps to give quantifiable feedback—ie a pedometer.[123] This sort of feedback also improves quality of life.

Traditional approaches Leaflets and multimedia programmes can slightly increase knowledge, eg of breast self-examination (which is associated with smaller tumours and less spread in those presenting with breast cáncer). But effects are often disappointing. *Health education officers* (eg from a nursing, teaching, or health-visiting background) may do better when teamed up with a graphic artist to provide emotionally charged, slick messages.

Peer-to-peer methods Leaflets are authoritative, but this authority is itself a problem. Risk-takers are unlikely to listen to the prim and proper. So peer-education has been developed as a tool to reach certain groups, and evidence suggests that this is a promising way forward.[124] Peers may be better than authority figures (eg in stop smoking messages). A message about breast feeding will come best from a mother. Dramas with HIV and health issues reaching millions, eg *Soul City* in South Africa is another way of side-stepping these authority issues.[125]

However, if the issues are not well understood, authority may be helpful (the *BMJ* is more effective than *Woman's Own* in suggesting to mothers that a new formulation of aspirin should not be taken).

Health promotion by nurses Nurses are experts in this field, but even they are not very effective in reducing coronary risk (without recourse to drugs). In the community-based OXCHECK randomized trial ($N = 6124$, aged 35–64) serum cholesterol fell by only 0.08–0.2mmol/L—and there was no significant difference in rates of giving up smoking or in body mass index. Systolic (and diastolic) BP fell by ~2.5% in the intervention group receiving dietary and lifestyle advice. Blanket health promotion may not be a complete waste of resources, but it is expensive for rather limited gains. Similar results were obtained by the *Family Heart Study Group*. Depending on the assumed duration of risk reduction, the programme cost per discounted life year gained ranges from £34,800 if interventional benefits last for 1 year, to £1500 for 20-year duration. Corresponding OXCHECK figures are £29,300 and £900. These figures exclude broader long-term cost effects other than coronary mortality.[126]

The conclusion may be that energies are best spent on those with highest risk as determined in routine consultations by a few 'simple questions' about smoking, family history, etc. One trouble is that these questions are not always innocuous. It is not a good thing to bring up 'strokes and heart attacks in the family' in, for example, consultations about tension headaches. OXCHECK is not the last word—and there is evidence that if lipid-lowering drugs were used very much more extensively, cholesterol (and cardiac events) could fall by 30%.[127]

The Internet and health education

In well-connected European populations, 60% of adults use the Internet for health information—more in these subgroups: high education, women, people with poor health, people with children. 25% experience feelings of reassurance or relief after having read about an illness on the Internet (3-fold higher than those experiencing concern and anxiety). 3% say that they have changed their medication after reading information on the Internet—and this is done without prior contact with their doctor.[128]

A common occurrence is for a GP who knows little about a rare disease to be confronted by a patient with with reams of internet print-outs or who knows in great detail about a disease he or she may or may not have. What do you do? The key lies in the the sentence above, in the word 'confront'. Don't let it happen! Sit *side-by-side* with your patient as if collaborating on a joint enterprise. The product of this collaboration should be health (including a healthy relationship with possibly fatal symptoms) and a reduction in obsessive searching and and an acceptance that some uncertainty is inevitable.

Primary care

Mother-and-baby groups These are best set up in the first weeks after the birth of four or five babies. The health visitor encourages the group to form. A doctor may attend the group—regularly to start with, then less often as the group becomes self-sufficient. After a year or two a large practice will have a number of groups running. One aim is to increase motivation (through discussion) to enhance the uptake of health education and preventative medicine. Another aim is to ease the stresses involved in becoming a responsible parent by providing a social support network. A mother, noting for the first time her beautiful baby's ability to hate, to destroy, and to hurt, may find it a relief to know that other babies are much the same.

Patient participation groups (PPGs) ►Working *with* your patients is as important as working *for* them. The health care team meets with patients' representatives to discuss some of the following:

- Dealing with complaints (less adversarial than with formal methods—and independent of the NHS and doctors—hence reasonably credible).
- Harmonizing the 'consumer's' and the 'provider's' aims.
- Feedback to aid planning, implementation, and evaluation of services.
- Identifying unmet needs (eg among the isolated elderly).
- Improving links between the practice and other helpers.
- Health promotion in the light of local beliefs (p472).
- Pressurizing government institutions over inadequate services.

Owing to lack of interest, or to there being no clear leader or task, up to 25% of groups close over time. The complaint that participation mechanisms lead to tokenism (ie the democratic ideal has been exercised, but what has been created is just a platform for validating the *status quo*) does not turn out to be true if a group has power over funds which it has raised. Here, our experience is that analysis may be penetrating and decision swift, in a way that makes even the best-run health authorities/Trusts look pedestrian.

Another role for PPGs is to have dialogues with primary care organizations (PCOs) on proposed changes to services—eg whether practices are to be amalgamated or services withdrawn or replaced by provision via non-NHS private companies. PCOs have a statutory responsibility to consult, and patient participation groups have a valid role in bringing PCOs to account.[129]

The Patients' Association This group represents and furthers the interests of patients by giving assistance, advice, and information. It aims to promote understanding between patients and the medical world. Publications: *Patient Voice* and a directory of self-help organizations. See also the *Contact-a-Family* Directory: cafamily.org.uk/gap.html

Self-help organizations Many thousands of these groups have been set up worldwide for sufferers of specific rare or common diseases. They offer information, companionship, comfort, and a lifeline to patients and their families, eg for sharing techniques and self-remedies. A danger is that they share nightmares as well, for example, unnecessarily graphic descriptions of their children dying of cystic fibrosis may be spread, causing unneeded despondency. They raise funds for research, providing a 'welcome alternative to the expensive services of professionals'. Full directories exist (see above).

Groups as a way out of passive dependency If people learn in groups they take more control of their lives and they are more optimistic about being able to change things in their lives (such as their weight); self-esteem improves—and also objective measures of health (such as HbA_{1c} in diabetics, as we have already mentioned).[90] N=120

Who should I complain to? Tell someone close to the cause of your complaint, eg a doctor, nurse, receptionist, or practice manager *as soon as possible* (within 6 months of the incident, or within 6 months of discovering that you have a problem). It is often possible to sort out the problem at once. This is called Local Resolution.[1] You can phone or write to the practice complaints officer or to the individual concerned. If Local Resolution fails, you may ask the Health Care Commission to consider the complaint. Such a request must be made within 2 months (or as soon as practicable) following any response provided by the practice. *GP out-of-hours-service:* Complain to your Primary Care Organization (PCO) or your own GP. If your complaint is about *availability* or *organization of health care services*, contact the Complaints Officer of your local PCO. NB: every NHS trust/PCO in England has a *Patient Advice and Liaison Service (PALS)* which provides a named person to whom service users can turn for help and support, eg: • Information • Listening • Messenger (passing on information from service users to staff) • Go-between (passing information forward and back) • Supporter (helping service users to present their own views) • Mediator (when there are disputes). • Resource mobilizer.[130] (Although we welcome an alternative to adversarial approaches, PALS tends to be underused, and is not independent).[131]

How quickly will the complaint be dealt with? Within 2 working days is the aim. For written complaints and cases where more detailed investigation is required, your complaint will be acknowledged in writing within 3 working days and the aim is to respond fully in 20 working days.

What do I do if I am unhappy with the reply? You may request an Independent Review. You must ask for this within 28 calendar days from the date of the letter responding to your complaint. You will be asked to write a letter to the Convener of the NHS Trust responsible for the service saying why you are still dissatisfied. You will be advised of the Convener's decision within 20 working days of your request (10 working days if about GPs, chemists, or opticians).

Should an Independent Review Panel be set up, this will consist of the Convener, an Independent Lay Chairperson, and one other person nominated by the NHS Trust. The Panel will investigate the complaint and talk to everyone involved, seeking the specialist advice it needs. You will then be sent a report, including the Panel's conclusions.

What do I do if I am still unhappy? You may request an investigation by the Health Service Commissioner (ombudsman) who is independent of the NHS and the Government. NB: the General Medical Council can be involved with a complaint whether or not it relates to an NHS patient.

Clinical governance and **quality improvement** Complaint systems are only a part of clinical governance, a system which links continuing professional development, multidisciplinary learning, audit, risk management, and critical incident reporting. It is a 'framework through which the NHS is accountable for continuously improving the quality and safeguarding high standards of care by creating an environment in which excellence will flourish'. The sequence is: defining quality→assuring accountability→improving quality.[132]

It is one mechanism by which the Commission for Health Improvement (CHI) operates. Its areas of priority are partly set by the National Institute for Health and Clinical Excellence (NICE) and health improvement programmes (HImP).

---

1 It is the practice manager's duty to log each complaint with its outcome, to acknowledge written complaints within 3 days, and to send a copy of the Practice's Complaints Procedure leaflet. She ensures that the internal investigation takes ≤10 days (if longer, she must give reasons). She will take advice from any relevant medical defence organizations.

Don't touch me! Don't question me! Don't speak to me! Stay with me! Estragon: Waiting for Godot

The UK death rate is ~12:1000/yr, or ~30 deaths/GP/yr. 65% die in hospital, 10% in hospices, public places, or on the street, and 25% die at home. Of these deaths at home over half will be sudden. In the remainder, the GP and the palliative care team has a central role to play in enabling a dignified death in the way the patient chooses. Pain relief and symptom control are the central preoccupations of death

Helping agencies
• Family
• Community nurse
• Hospice/night nurses
• Friends/neighbours
• GP/health visitor
• Pain clinic
• CRUSE (self-help group)

in hospices, where death has already been somewhat medicalized, but in those who choose to die at home there runs a fierce streak of independence, so that their main aim is to carry on with the activities of normal living, come what may. This may cause distress to relatives who feel that the dying person is putting up with unnecessary pain. An open discussion is often helpful in harmonizing the family's aims. A key step is to find out what a patient wants—and then to enable him to do it. Be aware that aims change over time. The next step is to find out about his hopes and fears and how they interact with those of the family.

Is your patient dying? This is a key question. Failure to ask it, and to discuss with the mulidisciplinary palliative care team, may consign your patient to a painful unplanned death. Break this question into 6 parts:

1 Is there a fatal disease that is advancing? Check histology; any rising LFTs etc?
2 Is the patient's response weakening? Comatose? Obtunded? Cachexia? Unresponsive? Unable to swallow? Laboured breathing? Assess over time (minutes, hours or days). Don't base decisions on a single snapshot.
3 Have reversible causes been fixed? (eg drug overdose Ca^{2+}, *онсм* p690).
4 Is he in 'do not resuscitate' territory? Dialogue (family & patient) is wise. This helps stop inappropriate monitoring, such as blood glucose tests.
5 What does your instinct say? Spend time with the dying to hone our instincts.
6 What do other members of the palliative care team (and the family) think?

Pain See p500. Morphine is the standard choice. **Fentanyl** has a role (good in renal failure; doses don't accumulate). Skin patches last 72h. It may cause less sedation and constipation than morphine. Trans-mucosal lozenge forms exist.[133]

Bereavement is the process of adapting to a loss which is causing sorrow. When trying to help bereaved people bear in mind where they are on *Worden's journey:* 1 Numbness and denial until the fact of loss is accepted 2 Experiencing grief, yearning, and pain[1] (± somatization)[134] 3 Adapting to a new environment without the deceased 4 Redirecting the positive feelings towards the deceased in building a brighter future. It is often tempting to try and 'do something' by giving psychotropics, but it is known that most bereaved people do not want this, and there is no evidence that drugs reduce problems. Empathy and helping the patient to shed tears is probably the most valuable approach, especially when losses are covert or hard to acknowledge. Counselling after bereavement is effective.[135] After bereavement, risk of death in spouses rises in the 1st 6 months (men) or in the 2nd year (women). Men and younger bereaved are at greatest risk. It is not known whether this is due to shared unfavourable environments or to psychological causes (eg mediated by the immune system). The main causes of death are vascular, cancer, accidents, and suicide.[136]

---

1 'There is in this world in which everything wears out, everything perishes, one thing that crumbles into dust, that destroys itself still more completely, leaving behind still fewer traces of itself than Beauty: namely Grief.'[137] M Proust 1925 *Albertine Disparue*. NB: Proust's view is clear enough for grief surviving down generations—which it does not. But what of one person's grief? Surely this can last a lifetime, and Proust is wrong? No: we must assume that Proust had in mind an image from Gérard de Nerval (p397, the man with the pet lobster) who describes grief as being carved into us, not like lettering on stone, which may be worn away by time, but like those initials we carve into the bark of a living tree. As the tree grows, the lettering sinks ever deeper, so that it seems to disappear, but really it has been embodied (Richard Holmes on Gérard de Nerval in *Footsteps* 1996 HarperCollins, p222).

Activities which we should try to avoid[138]

- Distancing tactics: "Everyone feels upset when there is bad news, but you'll soon get used to it."
- False reassurance: "I am sure you will feel better; we have good antiemetics these days."
- Selective attention: "What is going to happen to me? I'm beginning to think I'm not going to get better this time. The pain in my hip is getting worse." Doctor: "Tell me more about your hip."

Breaking bad news

Bad news is any information that drastically alters a patient's view of their future for the worse. Patients have a right to such knowledge, but not a duty to receive it, so negotiation is needed to agree the type of information and the amount they want to hear at any moment. The advantages of patients being aware of bad news are:

- It helps maintain trust in those caring for them. Trust is what the bedside manner is all about. "Trust is necessary precisely where we cannot be certain. If we had certainty, we wouldn't need to trust." Onora O'Neill Reith lecture
- To reduce uncertainty.
- To prevent inappropriate hope.
- To allow appropriate adjustment.
- To prevent a conspiracy of silence.

The central activities in the breaking of bad news are:[139]

1 Preparation—choose a quiet place where you will not be disturbed.
2 Find out what the patient already knows or surmises.
3 Find out how much the person wants to know. You can be surprisingly direct about this. "Are you the sort of person who, if anything were amiss, would want to know all the details?"
4 Fire a warning shot. "I am afraid I have bad news."
5 Allow denial.
6 Explain (if requested). Share information about diagnosis, treatments, prognosis, and specifically list supporting people (eg nurses) and institutions (eg hospices). Ask "Is there anything else you want me to explain?".
7 Listen to concerns.
8 Recognize and encourage ventilation of the patient's feelings.
9 Summarize and make a plan.
10 Offer availability. The most important thing here is to leave the patient with the strong impression that, come what may, you are with him or her *whatever*, and that this unwritten contract will not be broken.

Useful agents: 1) GI problems *Diarrhoea (post radiation):* Low-residue diet.

Constipation: Co-danthramer capsules or liquid±bisacodyl 5-10mg at night.

Cachexia: Prednisolone 15-30mg/day or dexamethasone 2-4mg/day PO may help by ↑ appetite.

Gastric irritation eg associated with gastric carcinoma—proton pump inhibitors (omeprazole 20mg/24h PO) or H₂ antagonists (eg ranitidine 150mg/12h PO).

Itch in jaundice—Ondansetron 4mg/14h PO.

Pain with dysphagia or *vomiting:* Buprenorphine sublingual 0.2-0.4mg/8h. Not a pure agonist. 'Ceiling' effects negate dose increases.

Foul rectal discharges: Metronidazole 500mg/8h PR.

Vomiting: Cyclizine 50mg/8h PO, IM, SC. Haloperidol (p360) 0.5-2mg PO. If this fails, try levomepromazine, below *If from inoperable GI obstruction,* try hyoscine hydrobromide 0.4-0.6mg SC/8h or 0.3mg sublingual. Octreotide, max 600µg/24h SC via a syringe driver may avoid the need for palliative surgery, IVIs and NGTs. *If from gastric stasis:* Metoclopramide 10mg/8h PO/SC. If this fails, try domperidone 60mg/12h PR. Herbal remedies (eg ginger) may be tried.

2) Lung problems Optimize COPD care (eg tiotropium 18µg/d via Handihaler®)

Air hunger: Chlorpromazine (eg 12.5mg IV).

Rattles: Hyoscine 0.4-0.6mg/8h SC or 1mg/72h as Scopoderm TTS® patch. Glycopyrronium 0.6-1.2mg per 24h by syringe driver ↓ secretions and helps colic.

Dyspnoea: (hypoxic)—Table fans ± supplemental humidified oxygen.

Haemoptysis: Diamorphine, above; IV if massive.

Pleural effusion: Thoracocentesis (bleomycin pleurodesis).

Pleural pain: Intercostal nerve blocks may bring lasting relief.

3) Cardiovascular problems Distension from ascites often causes distressing symptoms. Try spironolactone 100-200mg/24h PO + bumetanide 1-5mg/24h PO.

4) GU problems Foul vaginal discharges: metronidazole vaginal gel.

5) Psychological problems *Agitation*—Try lorazepam half a 1mg tablet sublingually, or haloperidol (p360) 1-3mg PO (may help nightmares, hallucinations, and vomiting too). Or midazolam in syringe drivers (eg 20-100mg/24h SC)—or levomepromazine 12.5-50mg IM stat or 12.5-200mg/24h SC via a syringe driver. NB: some drugs cause local skin irritation when used with a syringe driver: avoid chlorpromazine, prochlorperazine, and diazepam.

6) Others—*Coated tongues* may be cleaned by 6% hydrogen peroxide, chewing pineapple chunks to release proteolytic enzymes, sucking ice, or butter. If oral thrush use fluconazole 50mg/24h for 7 days.

Superior vena cava or *bronchial obstruction, or lymphangitis carcinomatosa* —Steroids; dexamethasone is most useful: give 8mg IV stat. Tabs are 2mg (≈15mg prednisolone) NB: dexamethasone given at night can prevent sleep.

Appetite low, or headache due to ↑ICP—Steroids; most useful is dexamethasone, eg 4mg/12-24h PO to stimulate appetite, reduce ICP, and in some patients induce a satisfactory sense of euphoria.

►**Before leaving the bedside...** Have I diagnosed all symptoms? Are the bowels working? Is hypercalcaemia present? What is plan B, eg if he cannot absorb MST, are patches (eg fentanyl) in the house? Are parenteral anti-emetics available (eg cyclizine 50mg)? Have you asked for hospice and district nurse help?

---

1 UK patients and relatives may get much support via BACUP (Brit Ass" of Cancer United Patients, 3 Bath Place, Rivington St, London, EC2A 3JR, tel. 020 7613 2121). cancerbacup.org.uk/home. In the UK, *Social Services* can fast-track applications for financial help in the form if prognosis <6 months..

Pain has physical, emotional, and spiritual components: all aspects need addressing. What follows assumes that the patient is dying from an incurable disease, and that they want to be at peace, with no suffering, and that total sedation is preferred. Know your patient's desired place of death well in advance.

- Prescribe within established guidelines (such as the Liverpool Care Pathway Gold Standard).

- Document that each dose increase is proportionate, and plans have been discussed with an experienced colleague, and take into account GMC guidance.

- Be proactive: diagnose and monitor each pain separately. The prescriber (you?!) must take charge, and be responsible for complying with patients' wishes, the law, and making judgments about patients' capacity to take informed decisions.

- To comply with patients' wishes to be kept peaceful, doses may need to be at least doubled every 12h (if on a pump, increased by 5–50% every few hours).[140] Active management of death may need these geometric increments to avoid suffering. If you start with 10mg morphine/12h, and the need is for 200mg/12h, you are consigning your patient to weeks of misery if you use 5–10mg increments, but if you double doses every 12h while your patient remains distressed, control takes a few days at most. Your prescription must allow for this, and nursing staff must be brought in on decisions, with the rationale agreed at each handover. "This is what the patient wants" not "This is what the doctor says".

- Don't be frightened to use big or very big doses if smaller doses are not working. It's whatever is needed; this is very variable. While finding avoid transdermal drugs (dose escalation is slow and inefficient.[141]

- *Non-opiate analgesia* may especially help *bone pain* (ibuprofen 400mg/8h PO or diclofenac + misoprostol (Arthrotec®), 1 tablet/12h PO.) Pamidronate may also relieve pain from bony secondaries (*OHCM* p672). *Nerve destruction pain:* Amitriptyline 25mg PO at night ± clonazepam 0.5mg/24h, increased to 1-2mg/8h. Resistant pain: nerve blocks may help.

- *Opiate dose equivalence:* Diamorphine PO: 2mg≈3mg morphine. SC: 1mg diamorphine ≈ 1.5mg morphine. Sustained release morphine is available, eg MST-30® or MXL (lasts 24h). Use syringe drivers SC or suppositories if dysphagia or vomiting make oral drugs useless. If crystallization occurs with drugs mixed in syringe drivers, either ↑ dilution, or use 2 syringe drivers.

- *Transdermal patches* are also useful, eg fentanyl (last 72h: typical starting dose for someone needing the equivalent of 90mg morphine/day would be one fentanyl-25® patch (the 25 means 25µg fentanyl/h; 50 ≈ 135-224mg MST, 75 ≈ 225-314mg morphine/day and 100 ≈ 315-404mg morphine/day). Use non-irritated, non-irradiated, non-hairy skin on trunk or upper arm; remove after 72h and replace by another patch at another site.

- *Modified-release morphine sulfate:* 10–260mg/12h.[140,142,143] Oxycodone is an alternative, eg Oxycontin®. In one study, the mean daily OxyContin® dose was ~80mg/d. 20% need at least 3 times as much.[144]

- *Parenteral morphine:* 2.5–100mg/1–4h SC. For larger doses use a pump or diamorphine (very soluble, so volumes can be very small). If the problem is distress or dyspnoea, midazolam (5mg/4h SC) + morphine rescue doses may be best.[145] On demand doses are typically 25% of the background dose. If many rescue doses are needed, increase background analgesia by ≥50%.[146] In one study, 91% needed 5–299mg of morphine/day, 7% needed 300–599mg/day, and 2% needed ≥600mg of morphine/day.[147,148] Morphine doses SC via a syringe driver range from 0.5/h to 300mg/h.[149] Example of dose escalation: if 10mg/h is not working, give a bolus of 10mg, and then increase the rate by ≥50% (15mg/h). If distress continues, re-bolus with 15mg, and ↑background to 22mg/h and so on until full comfort is achieved.[150] It often helps to add midazolam 0.8–8mg/h;[151,152] the buccal route works too:[153] Buccolam® 5mg/mL. NB: validated protocols for dose escalation are absent.[154]

▶We cannot make ourselves better people by using a system or a machine: reflection, dialogue, and action are more likely routes to self-improvement.

From 2015 all UK patients will have the right to view their primary care records on-line.

Problem-orientated records—List problems as 'active' or 'inactive' Eg 'breathlessness' (not '?bronchitis'—or 'Down's syndrome', which may be unproblematic to the individual, but a problem to us 'normals'. Use 'SOAP':

Subjective interpretation: How the patient and/or carer sees the problems.
Objective: Physical examination and results of tests (not always objective!).
Assessment: Social, psychological, and physical interpretation.
Plan: Do the following tests ...' or 'Wait on events'; treatment: eg 'Start psychotherapy' and explanation—note what the patient has been told.

Internet records Could our health records be like Facebook? Yes. We allow various specialists to be friends and join in conversations, so that our records are under our control and always available. See www.patientsknowbest.com.

Computers with limited connectivity These give faster links (lab, hospital, GP). Computers automatically scan patients' records so that we are alerted via pop-up boxes, eg 'No BP in last 3yrs' or 'Has heart disease & chol. >5 & not on statin' etc.[155] This development, linked to payment by results/quality markers in the GP contract[uk] of 2004, has improved care in asthma, diabetes, and heart disease (MI rates are is falling faster in the UK than in any other European country).[156-158]

NHS extranet/summary care record (SCR) The idea is that NHS staff anywhere can access data held centrally on the 'NHS spine' to find out about current drugs, allergies ± major illnesses. These are updated nightly via GP and other sources.

• *Security* is untested—a major problem. Record access is logged, and NHS staff using smartcards to access records without need may be fired.
• Consent is presumed: opt-out is by discussion with the GP who adds code 93C3 to the record.

Decision support[35] *webmentorlibrary.com* (WML) is part of EMIS systems, with >25,000 key-worded facts connected by an intelligent index[160] linked to the medical record via Read/SNOMED codes to enable explanation of apparently unrelated phenomena—such as RASH & DEPRESSION & CONSTIPATION. See BOX below.

SCR may be good if you are:
• Needing emergency care
• On complex treatments
• Being seen out-of-hours
• Demented/confused/deaf
• Fed up with repeating name, date of birth.[etc, etc]
• Disbelieved by doctors
• Wanting 2nd opinion (you can print off your records)

Public unease with SCR
• Malicious access
• Mistaken identity
• Blackmail
• Staff errors could lead to gross inaccuracies
• NHS may sell data for cash
• Incomplete if secret items omitted (eg HIV status[etc])
• Expensive to maintain
• No tangible health benefit
• Bias against those who don't register with a GP

Mentor gives this reasoning to explain why sarcoidosis is one match
• Sarcoidosis frequently results in rash.
• **Depression** is commonly a feature of sarcoidosis. *WML explanation:* sarcoidosis can result in neuropathic pain neuropathic pain can result in depression.
• **Constipation** is commonly a feature of sarcoidosis. *WML explanation:* sarcoidosis can result in hypercalcaemia hypercalcaemia can result in constipation.

Other matches HIV, Whipple's disease, adrenal metastases, Cockayne syn...
To support or 'refute' these, *look for:* arthritis, dactylitis, ptosis, ascites, dementia, premature aging, splenomegaly, failure to thrive, weight loss...
(If one is present, click it to add it to the search, and so narrow the field.)

We all need to know about Medline—it's a skill as basic as taking blood—but easier. The **lucky-dip method** is good, but undiscriminating: just enter anything in the search box, and press the 'go' button. A natural-language interface (AskMEDLINE) also exists at www.askmedline.nlm.nih.gov/ask/ask.php.[161] If this is all you want and you want full-text, the best site is www.highwire.stanford.edu.

This page aims to help if you want to be sure you are not missing something (and want to cut down irrelevant hits). If Medline is new to you, find an Internet connection and an experienced friend and try the searches below in GREEN CAPITALS. When you click the 'go' button, the system tries to match your search to a nomenclature of medical subheadings (MESH terms). To explore alternative therapies for angina: type ANGINA AND THERAPY (use capitals; ►check your sfzpelling!); click 'go', then the 'details' button to show that this is mapped to (('angina pectoris'[MESH Terms] OR angina[Text Word]) AND (('therapy'[Subheading] OR 'therapeutics'[MESH Terms]) OR therapy[Text Word]). There are >45,000 hits. Adding AND RANDOM* to the search phrase (a star gets *randomized, randomised*, etc but also authors whose name starts with Random...) narrows these to <7000; adding COMPLEMENTARY before the word THERAPY gives <400 hits.

Square brackets The contents of these limit or expand the search. Mostly, let Medline do this for you, as in the above example. But there are some square brackets it's useful to add to the search yourself. For example, ANGINA AND BMJ gives (('angina pectoris'[MESH Terms] OR angina[Text Word]) AND BMJ [All Fields]). There are <90 hits; but searching on ANGINA AND BMJ [JOURNAL NAME] (*exactly* like that) automatically maps to (('angina pectoris'[MeSH Terms] OR angina[Text Word]) AND ((("BMJ"[Journal Name] OR "Br Med J" [Journal Name]) OR 'Br Med J (Clin Res Ed)'[Journal Name]) OR 'BMJ'[Journal Name])) This yields >500 matches, ie MESH expands as well as limit your search.

Other useful things to put in square brackets relate to authors [AUTHOR], publication dates [PDAT] and publication types [PTYP]—eg entering ANGINA AND RANDOMIZED CONTROLLED TRIAL [PTYP] AND BLACK DM [AUTHOR] 1996:2013[PDAT] gives a search which doesn't include articles using common words such as black, and goes from 1996 to now. Using Random* may be more inclusive than using RANDOMIZED CONTROLLED TRIAL [PTYP], but will include sentences such as 'there are no randomized trials'.

Finding MESH headings You can make search terms more certain by selecting them via the MESH browser button—look carefully: it's in the left-hand blue margin, half way down. Typing into the search box yields MESH terms which need no mapping. If no exact term is found, choose a likely one from the list offered, and press the 'browse term' button. Click the 'Add' button to add this to your search. Try this with SMALL VESSEL ANGINA. This is not a MESH term, but the MESH browser offers angina, microvascular, among a host of other less helpful possibilities. Confirm this for yourself. *Other ways of limiting searches:* Click the 'Limits' button to explore this, or add a word such as HASABSTRACT (one word, no space, added to the search phrase) to retrieve only articles having abstracts (this excludes editorials and correspondence items). "HUMANS" [MESH] excludes animal research. An example of Boolean logic: try NIFEDIPINE AND (AMLODIPINE OR FELODIPINE) NOT PRINZMETAL ANGINA [MESH]. This excludes studies of Prinzmetal's angina.

EBM Try ANGINA AND COCHRANE NOT COCHRANE[AUTHOR] or ANGINA AND META-ANALYSIS , or try the *clinical queries button*. Choose 'sensitive' to avoid missing possible hits, or 'specific' if you are getting too many hits.

Exercises Now you've got the idea, recall your last 6 patients and find meta-analyses relevant to them. *Why are my searches going wrong?* •Mis-spellings? •Not using capitals (AND, OR, NOT)? •Using the wrong search box?

Primary care

In the limelight we have the world of evidence-based medicine (p489), Medline, and the whole enterprise of objective science. In the shadows we have our premonitions. It is absurd that we spend so little time thinking about them, when they govern and control so much of what we do as clinicians. Carl Jung said "My increased knowledge gradually permeated or repressed the world of intuitive premonitions ..."—and so it often seems. The more we know, the more we have to use our premonitions, in deciding how to use that knowledge and on whom. Often the objective world yields conflicting instructions such as "Get this patient's blood pressure down" or "Falls here might be fatal—we must avoid falls at all costs, and reduce blood pressure treatment". Our premonitions tell us which of the voices from the objective world to listen to.

What is a premonition? Premonitions are warnings or foreknowledge of as yet unspecified events. They are the means whereby our subconscious notifies us of danger. Listening to one's premonitions is an example of intuitive thinking. Intuition is a non-linear process of knowing, perceived through physical and emotional awareness, and its methodologies entail making subconscious physical or spiritual

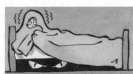

Fig 1. Subclinical premonitions. *Clinos* is Greek for bed, so *subclinical* means, literally, *under the bed.*

connections.[162] Some premonitions we are born with (such as our expectation of monsters under the bed); others we acquire slowly during our clinical lives. These premonitions are worth £billions to health services, which could not operate without them. Without them we would have to be guided by blind pessimism. We would have to think: this pain in the toe could be due to malignancy, and we must investigate accordingly. But if we grant our premonitions full play, and combine this with statistical probability, we can become much more useful physicians. The above thinking can be reformulated as: it's very rare for toe pain to be the presenting sign of cancer so we can default to never thinking about this (so our minds remain uncluttered)—until our premonitions send us a warning message: "I don't like the look of this—I've got a bad feeling...let's analyse this more..." There is nothing occult or paranormal about this: think of it simply as being effortless learning from experience.

How can we hone our premonitions? Some people object that this is like asking how we can sleepwalk more effectively; but consider these methods.
• Take every opportunity for feedback. What happened to Mr Jones with non-cardiac chest pain which you thought might be cardiac after all, after seeing him smother his fist with his dominant hand while describing the pain?
• Ask yourself "What did he mean...'I've never had pain like that before'?"
• Take time after every dozen consultations and ask yourself "What clues did I respond to; which did I ignore? Am I feeling uneasy? If you are, go back over the patients—find out what it is that is making you uneasy, and consider re-contacting the patient for further exploration.
• Don't stick to your guns—come what may. Be flexible in revising your opinions. Have a low threshold for admitting the possibility of error when you are detecting something moving in the shadows.
• Don't shun silences in consultations: this may be when we hear our premonitions best. Try "Let me reflect on what you have said for a few moments".
• Figuratively speaking, turn out the lights on all the workaday world of collecting and assembling data, so you can adapt to darker, less defined areas.
• You can give yourself thinking time or time for reflection by taking longer than strictly necessary during auscultation, say. By catching up with your feelings, you give your premonitions a chance to declare themselves.

Primary care

Audit comes from the Latin *audire*—to hear; and the term was once used for verbally presented verified financial accounts. Audit in clinical practice involves quality control by systematic review of an aspect of practice, implementing change and verifying that the desired effect was produced. Its purpose is as a tool to achieve best quality clinical care. Audit means asking questions such as: "Have we any agreed aims in medical practice?" and "Are we falling short of these aims?" and "What can we do to improve performance?" Audit is a part of the Summative Assessment required for all UK GP registrars/ST3 to pass before they can be principals. An 8-point audit is required. *[See examples]*

1 *Title:* When selecting a topic think: is it relevant; common or important; measurable; amenable to change? For a registrar audit, is it simple? For other audits, is it worth the investment (of time and money)? Say why you chose the particular topic. *[Does exercise improve diabetic control?]*

2 *What criteria were chosen:* State why the criterion/criteria were chosen. *[HbA1c will be used as a marker of diabetic care]*

3 *Setting standards* A standard is a statement of a criterion of good quality care. A target should be set (the degree to which the criterion will be met). Choose a realistic and obtainable target. Aim for standards to be evidence based. *[HbA1c <7.5% reflects adequate control. Target to have >50% patients with HbA1c <7.5%]*

4 *Planning and preparation* What have you done? For example, what literature has been consulted (essential). *[Consulted NSF (p523) for diabetes (literature): put all HbA1c results on computer as they came in]*

5 *First Data Collection* Gather the evidence. Observe current practice. Compare this with the standard. *[40% HbA1c <7.5%]*

6 *Implement changes* [Implement vigorous exercise programme]

7 *Second Data Collection* Compare with the standard and the first data collection. *[Check patients received intervention? 45% HbA1c <7.5%]*

8 *Conclusions [Exercise works; target not reached]* Use these to formulate your next title to complete the audit cycle. *[Better exercise intervention]*

Other people's audits can seem boring. It is only when a practice engages in audit itself that interest is aroused, and it can be satisfying to watch one's practice develop through a series of audits. With computers, audits can be done on many aspects of care, to answer questions such as—Is our care of diabetics adequate? Are all our fertile female patients rubella-immune?

The practice manager can have a central role in running an audit exercise—eg by relieving doctors of the burden of data collection and is able to communicate the results of the audit in a practice's annual report.

Possible dangers of audit (No intervention is without side effects.)

• It takes time away from eye-to-eye contact with patients.

• In becoming the province of professional enthusiasts, it can alienate some practice members, who can then ignore the results of the audit.

• There is no guarantee that audit will improve outcomes.

• It may limit our horizons—from the consideration of the vast imponderables of our patients' lives in a world of death, decay, and rebirth—to a preoccupation with attaining tiny, specific, and very limited goals.

• Some doctors fear that in espousing audit they risk transforming themselves from approachable but rather bumbling carers and curers who perhaps don't know *exactly* where they are going, into minor administrative prophets, with too much of a gleam in their eyes and zeal in their hearts.

As we move away from providing care in expensive high-technology hospitals, more is expected of primary care, with implications for capital expenditure, acquiring new skills, and local access to procedures needing expensive equipment, eg endoscopy or ultrasound. Whole specialisms such as dermatology and day-case surgery may move out of the secondary sphere, as the distinction between primary and secondary care becomes redundant. Anticoagulant clinics are another example of a hospital service which 'might as well be done in the community'. How are these developments to be structured (taking the NHS as an example)? What are the dangers and opportunities?

Market-led models Well-capitalized companies take over running general practices, after winning provider contracts from primary care trusts. Such companies create free-standing polyclinics (eg the Riverside Medical Centre[1]). Alternatively, large supermarkets/pharmacies create in-store health centres. In both, GPs become salaried employees of the company providing services.

Federated GP-led models General practices club together to purchase equipment and consolidate the new skills required. This is the model favoured by the Royal College of General Practitioners (*Roadmap*)—as providing the most flexible model which can rapidly adapt to local priorities[32]—and cause the least disruption to existing services—and maintain continuity of care.[163] Under this model GPs develop special interests and 'portfolio careers' playing to their strengths in both the clinical and administrative spheres in an increasingly complex health environment—in which they both commission and provide care.

Various kinds of federated GP models exist, from informal alliances to limited companies owned and run by GPs, who hold shares in the company.[164] One thing held in common is that they are part of the NHS family, and share core NHS values of inclusivity, fairness and distributive justice. The primary motive for their creation is to maintain general-practice-based primary care—and the system whereby patients can see the doctor of their choice near where they live who stands a good chance of having known them for years.

Pros and cons The RCGP cautions against developing polyclinics that focus on diseases and technical care—but it commend the value of co-location of services to reduce fragmentation. Whatever models are adopted, the cardinal values of general practice such as interpersonal care and continuity of care based on defined populations must be given full weight.

Support for registration of patients at multiple primary care outlets—or even registration at A&E clinics or urgent care centres is occasionally favoured by some NHS and other governmental bodies. This may be desirable for some patients working away from their practice based location—but such arrangements are bound to lead to expensive and fragmented care (this is why it is not RCGP policy). Also, registering patients with a single general practice allows longitudinal care, lifelong medical records, confidentiality, and team-based care to feed into a viable gate-keeping role. This gate-keeping role keeps costs down and protects patients from over-medicalization.

Quality control[2] If a service such as INR testing is taken out of the lab and fragmented to a number of smaller community-based clinics, quality control becomes problematic. Ditto for the validation of GPs with special interests.

Conflicts of interest If a GP federation is a for-profit organization (with funds flowing from the NHS) and if the doctors are sitting on boards deciding on which services are to be commissioned, there is a conflict of interest. The NHS is establishing procedures to minimize risk from this possibility—but nevertheless, probity is a vital issue, for doctors as well as other NHS staff.

1 Clinics may share with 'sister surgeries' and provide on-site gynae, mental health, surgical, and other clinics.
2 If a batch of reagents is faulty, the lab will be onto this at once, but who would know in the community if a batch of INR test strips was faulty? Perhaps only after a series of bloody deaths was investigated.

▶*Appraisal isn't the same as assessment.* For NHS doctors (yearly appraisal is required) peer appraisal is moving beyond a chat about one's professional development. 5 areas to address (with data) are: How do I know my clinical care is good? Do I keep up to date? How do I come across to my colleagues and patients? Am I in dialogue with my peers to ensure good use of resources (eg prescribing; referrals)? What have I *done* about what I have *learned*?

What form does UK appraisal take for GPs? There are 2 administrative forms (*Forms 1& 2*); then there is *Form 3*, needing thought and data gathering (in protected time)—with a commentary on your work, an account of how it has developed since last year, your view of your developmental needs, and cataloguing of factors that constrain you in achieving your aims, eg:

- What are the main strengths and weaknesses of your clinical practice?
- How has the clinical care you provide improved since your last appraisal?
- What do you think are the clinical care development needs for the future?
- What factors constrain you in achieving your aims for your clinical work?
- What steps have you taken to improve your knowledge and skills?
- What have you found successful or otherwise about these steps?
- What professional or personal factors constrain your skills and knowledge?
- How do you see your job and career developing over the next few years?
- What are your main strengths and weaknesses in your relationships with patients? How have these improved? What would you like to do better? What factors in the workplace (or more widely) constrain this?
- What are your main strengths and weaknesses in your relationships with colleagues? How have these improved? What would you like to do better? What factors in the workplace or more widely constrain this?
- Do you have any health-related issues which might put patients at risk?

Other areas: Teaching; financial probity; research; management activities.

During the appraisal *Form 4* is completed and signed by both parties. Form 4 feeds through to Clinical Governance Leads, who identify trends and make reports to the Trust's chief executive. *Form 5* is a non-obligatory form containing background ideas supporting Form 4 which may be used to inform other appraisals. Finally there is supportive follow-up (eg a further visit or phone call).

Appraisal is a supportive developmental process, a constructive dialogue, to reflect on our work, to consider developmental needs, to assess our career, and to consider how we might gain more job satisfaction. 'By giving feedback on performance it provides the opportunity to identify any factors that adversely affect performance, and to consider how to minimize or eliminate their effects. It is an important building block in a clinical governance culture that *ensures* high standards and the best possible patient care.'Chief Medical [165] Officer

There is a big question-mark over 'ensures', above. The effect of appraisal on patient care is unknown—but appraisal, it is hoped (and it only is a hope), can offer opportunities for interdependent support, self-education, self-motivation, and career development in the wider medical world. It may also be a catalyst for change and even a tonic against complacency.[166]

One criticism is that if appraisals are all about 'me' not 'us', opportunities for team-building are lost.[167] They may also destabilize by raising unrealizable hopes.

Appraisal assumes GPs aim to be professional, life-long learners (the 'move-&-grow' aspect of challenging appraisals). If this is not the case, the less cosy revalidation, performance management, assessment, and mediation will bite.

Revalidation (4-5yrly) aims to guarantee public safety. Appraisals feed into this. Its 2 core components are 5-yrly *relicensure* (a function of Royal Colleges to ensure objective assurance of continuing fitness to practise) and *specialist recertification* (affirmation of maintenance of particular standards that apply to a speciality, eg general practice). patient.co.uk/showdoc/40000773.

It would be nice for the public and the 'leaders' of our profession if there were a small number of under-performing doctors who could be retrained or struck off. Things are rarely so simple, and we may have to accept that, for many reasons, including chance, training, and resilience, the performance of *all doctors* will, at times, be, or appear to be, suboptimal. If all doctors were the same, and there was a valid yardstick for measuring quality (a big 'if'), then there would be, by chance, a large under-performing group, with a corresponding apparently 'over-performing' group. Anyone assessing performance data needs to take into account these questions.

What counts as data? Usually only what can be *quantified*; quality differs.

Are the data stratified for risk? Doctors' case-mixes can vary markedly.

Is our personal data's accuracy validated? Data entry is often unreliable.

Has the accuracy of the data we are being compared to been validated?

Could the differences between our data and others have arisen by chance? This is the most revealing question. Imagine a thought-experiment in which 4 equal doctors use different strategies for predicting whether a tossed coin will land heads or tails. One always chooses heads, one always chooses tails, and the other two alternate their choices out of synchrony with each other. When I did this experiment for a pre-decided 14 throws each (56 throws in total), the best doctor only had 2 errors, whereas the worst had 7 errors—over 3 times the rate for post-operative deaths (or whatever). The public would demand that this doctor be retrained or struck off, and the General Medical Council might feel obliged to comply, simply to keep public confidence (it is under great pressure to 'do something'). So must we all be prepared to be sacrificial lambs? The answer is Yes, but there are certain steps that can be taken to mitigate our own and our patients' risk exposure.

• When we encounter doctors who are clearly underperforming (eg due to addictions) we must speak out. This will encourage belief in the system.

• For statistical reasons any series with <16 failures might be best ignored. Such series simply do not have enough power to detect real effects.

• We must strive to be both kind and honest with our patients. The best response to "I'd like a home-delivery" might be to say "I haven't done one for 5 years—and that one went wrong: are you sure you want my services?"—rather than "The UK perinatal death-rate is the same for home and hospital".

• It might be the case that, contrary to the GMC, we should *not* always be on the look-out for colleagues who might be under-performing so that we can report them to the proper authorities: rather we should be encouraging an atmosphere of mutual support and trust—the sort of environment in which doctors feel safe to say "All my cases of X seem to be going wrong—can anyone think why?" To stop this trust turning into cronyism we must be prepared to engage in, or be subjected to, audit (p506). The alternative is for clinicians to develop into secret police, informers, and counter-informers. No one would benefit from this. We note that malicious informing is not an isolated occurrence in the UK; 80% of those suspended for presumed underperformance are exonerated, but few return to their previous job owing to the stresses enquiries always engender.

Typical areas in which doctors are seen to be under-performing Local Medical Committees (LMCs), complaints bodies, and NHS commissioners have all been systematically questioned about doctors whose performance they are reviewing. In the case of LMCs, for example, clinical skills were the chief worry, followed, in order, by communication problems, management problems, prescribing problems, and record-keeping problems. NHS Trusts have more concern over referral patterns.

Satisfaction is one of the few measures of outcome (not process) which is measurable. What patients mostly want is a personal service from a sympathetic doctor or nurse who is nearby and easy to get to see. A £13 million NHS GP survey in 2007 showed that 86% were satisfied on such measures as opening hours etc.[168] The following questionnaire[1] further quantifies satisfaction.[169]

1 I am totally satisfied with my visit to this doctor.
2 Some things about my visit to the doctor could have been better.
3 I am not completely satisfied with my visit to the doctor.
4 Professional care:
  • This doctor examined me very thoroughly.
  • This doctor told me everything about my treatment.
  • I thought this doctor took notice of me as a person.
  • I will follow the doctor's advice because I think he/she is right.
  • I understand my illness much better after seeing this doctor.
5 Relationships:
  • This doctor knows all about me.
  • I felt this doctor really knew what I was thinking.
  • I felt able to tell this doctor about very personal things.
6 Perceived time:
  • The time I was allowed with the doctor was not long enough to deal with everything I wanted.
  • I wish I could have spent a bit longer with the doctor.

Why do patients change their doctor? The most common reasons are that either the patient has moved, or the doctor has retired or is perceived to be too far away. Additional reasons are described in the table.[170]

Patient needs		Organizational problems		Problems with doctor	
One doctor for all the family	5%	Long waits	13%	Lost confidence in	21%
		No continuity of care	6%	Uninterested/rude	20%
Wants woman GP	4%	Rude receptionist	6%	Prescriptions criticized	5%
Wants alternative medicine	2%	Wants appointments	1%	Doctor too hurried	4%
Obstetric needs	1%	Wants open surgeries	1%	Visits problematic	4%
		Other staff rude	0%	Communication poor	4%

A USA study found that a *participatory decision-making style* leads to patient satisfaction. Participation was found to depend, in part, on the *degree of autonomy* perceived to be enjoyed by the GP, and on the volume of work.[171]

Another approach to gaining satisfaction is to agree and publish standards of care patients can expect, with performance figures for how well these standards are met in practice. This is the philosophy behind the UK government-led *Patient's Charter*/British Standards Kitemark BS5750, which aims to:

• Set standards, eg by agreement with patient participation groups (p496).
• Monitor progress towards these standards, and publish progress locally.
• Provide information about how services are organized. Maximize choice.
• Let users know who is in charge of what, and what their roles are.
• Explain to users what is done when things go wrong, and how services are improved, and what the complaints procedure is.
• Show that taxpayers' money is being used efficiently.
• Demonstrate customer satisfaction.

This culture has proved alien to some GPs, perhaps due to a very necessary preoccupation with illness and curing, rather than service and its glorification.

---

1 The only merit of this questionnaire is its brevity: validity is not assured. The best validated is EUROPEP.[172] The UK QoF system has relied on less well validated *Improving Practices Questionnaire* (IPQ) or the *GP Assessment Questionnaire*—GPAQ. It asks about *the practice* (eg 48h access) and *staff* (respect, confidentiality) as well as *individual doctors*. Formal evaluation (2007) shows they are unreliable.[173]

The term expert patient was coined to denote a well-informed patient in full possession of the facts about his or her case, and contributing to decisions in a valid way. Doctors often fear the expert patient, as so much time has to be spent investigating whether their viewpoints really are valid. This may lead to lack of harmony in the consulting room.

The inherent contradictions and strengths in the idea of expert patients are revealed through *reductio ad absurdum* (a logical technique beloved of Socrates).[174] Imagine a urologist consulting his GP about whether to have a radical prostatectomy or radiotherapy for his newly diagnosed prostate cancer. The GP might say to himself: "Why on earth is he consulting me? He knows far more about the options than I do." But let us imagine that his GP is, in fact, Socrates, who proceeds to ask various questions to reveal his inner fears (incontinence, erectile problems), and what he hopes to achieve by the various treatments on offer (to live long enough to see his disabled son through school). Socrates-the-GP is not adding any new facts. He is twisting the kaleidoscope, so that new patterns come into view. When a coherent pattern emerges he shows the urologist the door—saying "Let me know what you decide". The urologist sincerely thanks him. The man who leaves such a consultation is not the same as the one who entered. ▶ *The expert patient has met a different sort of expert.*

Greater patient involvement in health issues and in the decisions relating to patients' own illnesses may lead to greater satisfaction, and better health. The more the patient knows about his or her own set of diseases, the better he or she will be able to decide what treatments to opt for. This is the rationale behind the expert patient programmes (BOX). These are congruent with Bandura's social-cognitive theory of behaviour, which says that the main predictors of successful behaviour change are confidence (**self-efficacy**) in the ability to execute an action and expectation that a specific goal will be achieved (**outcome expectancy**). Expert patients (who are confident and assertive) are said to live longer, be healthier, and have a better quality of life,[175] and are exemplars of what health is all about (in chronic disease, health is not the absence of decay but an optimum, dynamic adaptation to it, p472).

Nonetheless, there is a group of expert patients who tend to be middle-class know-alls who consult at great length about various maladies, arriving with sheaves of Internet printouts about treatments you have never heard of. Don't reject these patients out of hand. And don't assume any sort of superiority or inferiority. Just give your advice as best you can. You may get better results than Socrates—whose last attempt at *reductio ad absurdum* (during his famous trial) ended fatally when he was forced to drink hemlock. He was right—but it didn't do him much good. And so with you: you don't always have to be right. And by not insisting on this you may live to consult another d...

A 6-week course in self-management, eg in arthritis self-care
1 Course overview; acute and chronic conditions compared; cognitive symptom management; better breathing; introduction to action plans.
2 Feedback; dealing with anger, fear & frustration; introduction to exercise; making an action plan.
3 Feedback; distraction; muscle relaxation; fatigue management; monitoring exercise; action plans.
4 Feedback; action plans; healthy eating; communication; problem-solving.
5 Feedback; making an action plan; use of drugs; depression management; self-talk; treatment decisions; guided imagery.
6 Feedback; informing the health care team; working with your health care professional; looking forward.

Stopping smoking tobacco

NHS targets aim to decrease smoking from 26% to <21% by 2010 and to <15% by 2018: rate of progress was only ~0.3%/yr,[177] until the smoking in public places ban in England in 2007. This has helped ≥400,000 people quit.[178]

Epidemiologists say that ~50% of smokers will die of smoking if they don't quit, losing ~25 years. Stopping smoking diminishes excess risk from tobacco, so that after 10-15yrs the risk of lung cancer approaches that of lifelong non-smokers (but a few genes involved in DNA repair may never return to normal functioning).[179] A similar but quicker decrease of excess risk (halved in 1st year) is found for deaths from coronary disease and, to a lesser extent, risk of stroke.[180] ►*60% of smokers want to give up*, and giving help achieves more QALYs/£ than any other intervention (£221-£9515/QALY).[181][182]

Annual UK health costs of smoking
- GP prescriptions: >£52 million
- GP consultations: >£89 million
- Hospital episodes: >£470 million

Advantages of stopping smoking Saving of life (110,000/yr in UK).
- Larger babies (smokers' babies weigh on average 250g less than expected, and their physical and mental development may be less than optimal).
- Less bronchitis (accounts for millions of lost working days).
- Less risk from the Pill: cardiovascular risk↑ ×20 if uses >30 cigarettes/day.
- Less risk from passive smoking (cot deaths, bronchitis, lung cancers).
- Return of the sense of taste and smell—and relative wealth.

To quit (AAMAA=ask, advise, motivate, assist, arrange follow-up.)[183]
1 Ask about smoking in all consultations (not just where relevant; be subtle; patients won't listen if agendas clash). Greet *any* success with enthusiasm!
2 Advise according to need. Ensure that advice is congruent with beliefs.
3 Motivate patients by getting *them* to list the advantages of quitting.
4 Assist in practical ways, eg negotiate a commitment to a 'quit date' when there will be few stresses; agree on jettisoning all smoking junk (cigarettes, ash trays, lighters, matches) in advance. Inform friends of new change.
  - **Nicotine gum**, chewed intermittently; ≥ten 2mg sticks may be needed/day. **Transdermal nicotine patches** may be easier. Written advice offers no added benefit to advice from nurses/GPs. Review at 2 weeks; people sense (and act on) your commitment. Only re-prescribe if abstinent.[184]
  - **Varenicline** is a selective nicotine receptor partial agonist, which NICE recommends as an adjunct to behavioural modification. Start 1 week before target stop date: initially 0.5mg/24h PO for 3 days, then 0.5mg/12h for 4 days, then 1mg/12h for 11 weeks (↓ to 0.5mg/12h if not tolerated). SE: appetite change; dry mouth; taste odd; headache; drowsiness; dizziness; sleep disorders; odd dreams; panic; dysarthria; acne; dysuria. Advise to stop if agitated, depressed or suicidal. **Bupropion:** see *BNF*.
5 Arrange follow up—until that date consider texting patients (get consent) to send messages of encouragement (can ↑quitting from 13 to 28%).[185][N=1705]

For those who do not want to give up Give them a health education leaflet, record this fact in the record, and try again later.

►25% of school leavers smoke regularly. The Health Education Council has a ˙moking education project for schools. It has been commented that smok-˙g rates may not be rising too fast in children owing to cost, and to mobile ˙nes, which are cheaper, and just as good a fashion accessory.

˙y health 'outlet' should have a policy on promoting non-smoking and ˙g practical advice: primary health care teams; hospitals; midwives; ˙acies—and also, perhaps, schools and employers. Health commissioners ˙d to promote knowledge and training in this area.[186]

The problem isn't alcohol, it's life—lives in which sobriety poses insuperable problems: consciousness of futility, debt, responsibility, and social inhibitions. Alcohol obliterates all these, and will continue to do so, until other methods are more attractive. Cheap alcohol and peer pressure matter too ("if I don't get pissed every Saturday and play sex games, I'd seem like a freak...").[188]

With the toll that excess alcohol takes in terms of personal misery and the national purse (>£1.6 billion/yr[UK]), the need to reduce alcohol use and its root causes intake should be almost top of government's social policy goals. But a powerful industry ensures that alcohol is cheaper (relatively) and more readily available than ever before—so that its use on an individually moderate scale arouses no comment. It is assumed to be safe, provided one is not actually an alcoholic. It is more helpful to view alcohol risks and benefits as a spectrum (see OHCM p236 for the *benefits* of alcohol). Problems are listed on p363.

▶A strategy to reduce bad effects of alcohol in your patients might comprise:
• If a symptom could be alcohol-related, ask *in detail* about consumption.
• Question any patient with 'alerting factors'—accidents, driving offences, child neglect, assault, attempted suicide, depression, obesity. Question others as they register, consult, or attend for any health check.

Helping people to cut down ▶Time interventions for when motivation is maximal, eg as (or before) pregnancy starts. Small reductions *do* matter.[189]
• Take more non-alcoholic drinks; reduce the sip frequency, eg by shadowing a slow drinker in the group. Don't pick up your glass until he does (and don't hold your glass for long: put it down to avoid unconscious sipping).
• Limit opening hours; don't drink alone or with habitual drinkers; sip, don't gulp.
• Don't buy yourself a drink when it is your turn to buy a drinks' round.
• Go out to the pub later (but some pubs now open all night).
• Take 'days of rest' when no alcohol is used. Try "No more for me please, I expect I'll have to drive Jack home" or "I'm seeing what it's like to cut down".

Agree goals to maintaining ↓drinking An alcohol diary helps get facts right.
• Teach him to estimate his alcohol intake (u/week, see below).
• Consider an 'Alcohol Card' which the patient can bring to each visit to show: units/week; pattern of drinking; reasons for misuse; each alcohol-related problem (and whether a solution has been agreed and action implemented); job record; family events; biochemical markers (GGT, MCV); weight.
• Give feedback about how he is doing—eg if GGT (γ-glutamyl transpeptidase) falls are discussed at feedback, there is much lower mortality, morbidity and hospitalization compared with randomized control subjects.
• Enlist family support; agree a system of 'rewards' for sobriety.
• Group therapy, self-help groups, disulfiram, local councils on alcohol, community alcohol teams and treatment units may also help (p363).

Setting limits for low-risk drinking eg ≤20u/week if ♂; ≤14u/week if ♀—there are no absolutes: risk is a continuum. NB: higher limits are proposed, on scant evidence (eg 4u/day; 3u for women). One unit is 9g ethanol, ie 1 measure of spirits, 1 glass of wine, or half a pint of ordinary-strength beer.[190] ▶*Primary care is a good setting for prevention*: intervention leads to less alcohol consumption by ~15%, reducing the proportion of heavy drinkers by 20%—at one-twentieth the cost of specialist services.[191] There is no evidence that GP intervention has to include more time-consuming advice such as compressed cognitive/behavioural strategies.[192] Simple advice works fine as judged by falling GGT levels, at least for men. After interventions, women may report drinking less, but this is not reflected in a falling GTT.[192]

Does education work? Rarely: as medical students, we do drink less in the final year, compared with year 2; but, overall, 27% are problem drinkers.[193] Should we all write and implement a personal alcohol policy? ▶'No doctor should practise after even 1 glass of wine.[194]

This is common but often unreported. It includes physical, sexual, emotional, and psychological abuse. It is rarely isolated, and often escalates in severity and frequency and involves children in 50-70%.[195] ►Ask directly about this, eg in antenatal clinics (risk is ↑ during pregnancy, and the life of the mother and baby are more at risk).[196] Distinguish between *generalized aggressors, family-only aggressors*, and *non-family-only aggressors*. Once violent always violent? This unfair generalization is less likely to be true for family-only aggressors.[197] This an important, as with each subsequent act of violence, guilt is less, at least when women are perpetrators[198] (violence is not male only, and same-sex partnerships are equally or more violence-prone).[199] 'To respond to violence only as a crime of a single party is a near guarantee of failure to reduce future violence. Violence can be reduced only by treating each incident as an opportunity for all parties...to explore their own involvement in and responsibilities for violence. Arbitrary 'punishment' of individuals for collective violence is, like most punishment, itself a form of violence. Arbitrary assignment of blame is an evasion of responsibility on the part of the blamer...Most strategies are primarily focused on blame and criminalization, are thus inherently counter-productive, resulting in the observed high rates of recidivism.'[200]

A model of violence?❋ Think of a 3-stranded noose: past patterns of *mutual violence* twisting in and out of known family and personal *psychopathology*, shot through by the central problem of *power imbalance*.[201] What tightens this noose (and around whose neck) depends on random dyadic events and loosened inhibitions, related to drugs, alcohol, or sexual jealousy. How to untie this knot? There is only one way: *dialogue* (humour, honesty, and hope).

Epidemiology 35% women experience domestic violence at some time; ~1 : 10 in the last year. 30% of domestic violence starts in pregnancy.[202] Police record >1 million incidents of domestic violence/yr (1 in 4 of UK assaults). Of women murdered, 40% are killed by a current or ex-partner. *Those who are abused are:* Likely to get PTSD (≥42-27%; p347);[203] 5-9 × more likely to abuse alcohol/drugs; 3 × more likely to be psychotic/depressed; 5 × more likely to commit suicide; and 15 × more likely to miscarry than non-abused women. Their partners are more likely to have many sexual partners without using condoms, ↑risk of HIV;[204] fear of violence may inhibit disclosing serology to partners.[205]

The abused may attend frequently with trivial or non-existent complaints. They may minimize signs of violence; be evasive or reluctant to speak in front of partners, and partners tend to be ever-present, so that it is difficult to talk to the client alone. This can be most difficult if the partner is needed for translation purposes (find another translator who is not from the family).

Social Services can help women disclose violence (eg after unexplained injury etc). Ask about abuse in antenatal clinics so that issues can be addressed *before* injury. Involve social services if children are involved (p146).

Refuge The Women's Aid Federation (0345 023468[UK]) can provide legal advice, emotional support, refuge, and police liaison. **Court orders** are obtainable quickly, and may be the only way to stop men going near previous victims.[206] They may also require someone to leave home, or let the victim return home. They are not long-term solutions, but can save life. In the UK, Law Centres give access to legal protection: to find the nearest, phone 0207 387 8570—or the patient's solicitor may be available. The police may also need calling.

Prevention Lack of full-time employment is a leading predictor of who is going to get abused,[207] but simply saying "Go out and get a job" rarely helps.

See also *Child abuse*, p146. *Parent-child interaction therapy* (PCIT)[1] is one validated way of reducing family violence.[208] This offers practical help in recognizing antecedent events which tend to trigger violence.

---

1 Through a one-way mirror, the therapist watches parents interact with the child. The parent wears a device in the ear to receive help & real-time feedback from the therapist next door.

Primary care

We need to know about alternative medicine to understand our patients'-undeclared distress, which use of these treatments is so often a sign of. We can also advise on the safety of various therapies. We must also learn from therapists about patient-centred care, and the sustainability of healthcare. This entails systems of interacting methods to restore and optimize health that have an ecological foundation, that are environmentally, economically and socially viable indefinitely, and that function harmoniously both with the human body and our wider environment, and that do not result in unfair or disproportionate impact on any ecosystem. *Alliance for Natural Health www.anh-europe.org*

Some alternative therapies are the orthodoxies of a different time (eg *herbalism*) or place (the *Ayurvedic medicine* of India), some are mainly diagnostic (*iridology*), some therapeutic (*aromatherapy*). Some doctors are suspicious of unorthodox medicine, and feel that its practitioners should not be 'let loose' on patients. But in many places the law is that, however unorthodox a practitioner may be, he or she cannot be convicted of unethical practice in the absence of clear harm. Many people (~5 million/yr in the UK) consult alternative practitioners, often as a supplement to orthodox treatment. Some will feel unable to tell their doctor about trips to alternative therapists, unless asked.

Modern medicine is criticized for sacrificing humanity to technology, and with little benefit for many people. In contrast to the orthodox doctor, alternative therapists is seen as taking time to listen, laying on hands rather than instruments, and giving medicines free (not always!) from side effects.

Acupuncture: Can treat many ailments; increasingly used in orthodox practice for pain relief, control of nausea and treatment of addiction. For these, endorphin release provides a scientific rationale.

Homeopathy: is based on the idea that 'like cures like', and that remedies are improved ('potentiated') by increasing dilution. Randomized trials show no greater efficacy than placebo, or suggest real (small) benefits, eg in asthma.

Manipulative therapies (osteopathy; chiropracty) are widely used and may help musculoskeletal and other problems, eg asthma.

Yoga: This is an ancient Indian discipline with physical, mental, and spiritual components which aims to achieve a state of spiritual insight and tranquility. Randomized trials show that yoga can produce worthwhile benefit.[209]

Clinical ecology: Starting from the fact that atmospheric pollutants, toxins, and xenobiotic chemicals (from other organisms) are known to be harmful, a system is built up around techniques (using intradermal injections) for provoking and neutralizing symptoms related to foods.

Holism: Holism entails a broad view: of the patient as a person, of the role of the therapist, of the therapies used. The patient's autonomy is encouraged through involvement in decisions, and nurturing of self-reliance. ►*Specialism doesn't exclude holism:* nephrologists can be as holistic as naturopaths. As shown on p478, most models of the GP consultation are based on a patient-centred holistic approach. Compare the sequence 'bronchitis→antibiotic' with 'bronchitis→smoker→stressed→redundancy-counselling→?antibiotic'.

"Doctor, can I use alternative therapy for HRT?" One answer might be: "Extracts from red clover (*Trifolium pratense*), soybean (*Glycine max*) and black cohosh (*Cimicifuga racemosa*; eg 8mg of standardized extract PO/24h) are often used. Some trials support their use,[210,211] but these are active agents that might have the same SEs as HRT. Finding out might cost £millions. You could try them, and you might well be lucky. ►Beware advertising influences."[212]

Integrative medicine: This is a patient-centred, interdisciplinary, non-hierarchical mix of conventional and complementary solutions to case management of patients with complex problems, eg chronic low back or neck pain.[213]

Years ago a patient had a seminoma successfully treated, and in the year that follow-up stopped, he had a myocardial infarction, followed by a good recovery. But the patient became morbid, self-centred, and depressed, perhaps because of the dawning appreciation of his mortality, his residual breathlessness, and his inability to do carpentry. His GP tried hard to cheer him up and rehabilitate him by encouraging exercise, sex, a positive self-image, and alternative hobbies. Rehabilitation was working when he began to develop headaches and kept asking forlornly whether these were a sign that his cancer had spread to his brain. There were no signs to suggest this. His GP knew that there *was* a chance that the tumour was resurfacing, but judged that starting a pointless chain of investigations would be disastrous to the patient's mental health. So instead of arranging CT scans the GP interpreted the forlorn questions "You are only asking questions like this because you are in a negative frame of mind...", and the patient and his GP developed strategies to avoid negative cognitions. The headaches improved, and the pressure to investigate was resisted, and a state of augmented trust was established between the patient and his GP: a marvellous asset in an uncertain, litigious world.

Primary care

Home visits

Friedrich Nietzsche 1886 *Beyond Good and Evil*; aphorisms 220-226

Glory or drudge? We hate home visits while in consulting rooms and acting up to images of the busy GP who must dispense precious time in miserly but fair aliquots. But when we are *doing* home visits, we love them. We are less often interrupted, and the possibilities of practising holistically are much enhanced. We see the family in their own context, and new diagnoses and treatment options tumble out of cupboards, bathrooms and larders as we wonder about lost corridors hoping for inspiration or a cup of tea. One colleague maintains that no home visit is complete without going through the bins on the way out: "what we discard tells us more about ourselves than what we keep". This is probably taking garbology too far, but the point is well-made. ►Home visits are greatly valued by patients, and are a good way to avoid 999 calls.[214]

Night visit with Nietzsche[215] (What follows will seem hard to follow in certain moods, but give yourself time in your profession and you will come across many mysterious motivations which will trump any hereinafter enacted.)

In a small car on an open road, I am heading to a sick child, aged 10. Nietzsche is sitting beside me, it seems, and muttering in the dark: "Why bother with all this medicine? It gives you no pleasure, and I see you feel no compassion. Be a free spirit like me! Let me to say to you: 'You are entangled in an unyielding snare and straightjacket of duties and cannot get free.' You think you are making a sacrifice to a noble cause. But listen: 'Anyone who has truly offered a sacrifice knows he wanted something for it and got it—perhaps something of himself in return for something of himself—that he gave up something here in order to have more there, perhaps just to be more, or at least to feel as if he were more'."

I drive on, obediently strapped to my straightjacket of duties. Then, on my right, I see, between the shadows of two houses, a huge moon, rising between them, low and red. It's far too big to believe, but I know I have seen this once before—aged 10—a huge harvest moon rising over the river Cherwell. Nietzsche cannot see it. He's too high. But I'm slumped over the wheel; I can see it just as it was a few decades ago. I wax. I wane. Ideals come and go, and will return. I do my night visit in a strange calm, sailing on my Sea of Tranquillity.

On my way back I look for my moon, to show it to Nietzsche. But Nietzsche has gone, and the moon is shining on someone else's night visit. Your night visit perhaps? I will wear your straightjacket and you can wear mine. I've got my moonlight inside me now; enough for a few more decades, I wonder?

GPs may not want to spend much time on minor conditions, but this may become unavoidable if he issues a prescription each time (rather pointless if all the patient wanted was reassurance). This reinforces attendance, as a proportion of patients will come to assume that a prescription is necessary. GPs rate ~14% of their consultations as being for minor illness (mild gastroenteritis, upper respiratory problems, presumed viral infections, flu, and childhood rashes).[216] In some studies, 80% are likely to receive a prescription (but this number may be falling), and >10% are asked to return for a further consultation. Why does this great investment of time and money occur? Desire to please, genuine concern, defensive medicine, prescribing as a way to end a consultation, and therapeutic uncertainty all play a part.

Positive correlations with low prescribing rates include a young doctor, practising in affluent areas and long consultation times. Patients in social classes I and II are more likely to get a home visit for minor ailments than those in other social classes. Membership of the Royal College of General Practitioners does not influence prescribing rates.[217] Not everyone wants to reduce prescribing, but advice is available for those who do.

- Encourage **belief in one's own health** and innate powers of recuperation.
- Using a **self-care manual** explaining about minor illness.[218]
- Using **self-medication** (eg paracetamol for fever).
- Using the **larder** (eg lemon and honey for sore throats).
- Using **time** (eg pink ear drums—follow-up if symptoms worsen).
- Using **deferred prescribing** "He'll get over it, I predict, in a few days; but here is a prescription if I am wrong: it's good for him to learn to deal with these infections himself, but if this doesn't happen, this is plan B." The use of Cates plots (ntonline.net/visualrx/examples) is one way (with a nice visual impact) for communicating NNTs to interested patients and colleagues. These smiley-faced plots can be a bit simplistic, eg the one for antibiotic prescribing for otitis media (NNT≈20) omits quantifying rare but serious complications (mastoiditis, p544).
- Using **pharmacists**,[219] or **granny** (a more experienced member of the family).
- **Pre-empting requests** for antibiotics (eg for sore throat): "I'll need to examine your throat to see if you need an antibiotic, but first let me ask you some questions ... From what you say, it sounds as if you are going to get over this on your own, but let me have a look to see." [GP inspects to exclude a quinsy.] "Yes, I think you'll get over this on your own. Is that all right?"

Empowering patients Any illness, minor or otherwise, is an opportunity to empower patients. Use the time to enable patients to improve their ability to:
- Cope with life and to understand their illness.
- Cope with specific illnesses.
- Feel able to keep themselves healthy.
- Feel confident on handling health issues.
- Be confident about the ability to help themselves.

We know that time spent this way improves patient satisfaction and clinical outcome[220] (although simply extending consultation times in the hope that this will happen is not enough).[37] This may be better than delegating minor illness to nurse-led triage clinics—which have no continuity of care as well as running the risk of increasing demand and augmenting medicalization of human events.[23,24,221] In some communities attendance for minor illness is falling, except in older males of low educational status.[38] Also, drug costs are falling in England in primary care (£8.81 billion in 2011 vs £8.83 billion in 2010).[222]

Equipment: Airway; stethoscope; auroscope; ophthalmoscope; patella hammer; scalpel; BP device; FeverScan® (or similar, for T°; no mercury); pulse oximeter; dipstix/capillary glucose; needles; syringes; gloves/KY jelly®; antiseptic fluid; sutures; specimen bottles/forms; sharps tin. Some drugs to have: *see* TABLE.

Drugs for your black bag (keep in date!—contents depend on local needs)		
IM/IV agents	*Oral/topical agents*	*Administrative items*
• Ceftriaxone	• Pain killers; antibiotics	• Mental Health Act forms
• Cyclimorph®; naloxone	• Prednisolone (soluble)	• Headed notepaper [etc]
• Prochlorperazine	• Lofepramine or SSRI	• Phone N°: chemists, ambu-
• Furosemide/bumetanide	• Ranitidine or similar	lance, police, hospitals [etc]
• Atropine; adrenaline	• Aspirin 75 & 300mg	• Certificates; nurse forms
• Chlorphenamine	• Paracetamol mixture	authorizing drugs for IV
• Benzylpenicillin (IM)	• Rehydration sachets	pumps; prescriptions
• Water for injections	• Inhalers; GTN spray	• Book to record batch
• Buccal midazolam (p208)	• Enemas/suppositories*	numbers for ampoules and
• Glucagon	• Fusidic acid viscous	narcotic use[223]
• 50% glucose	eyedrops	• Prescriptions; temporary
• Haloperidol	• Glucogel® glucose gel	resident and other forms
	• Diazepam± temazepam	

*Suppositories: diclofenac 100mg (for renal colic); paracetamol 60 or 125mg for vomiting feverish children.

For the pocket Phone (charged!). Try a *smart-phone device* eg incorporating this book, *OHCM* (we declare an interest!) & *BNF*; see Dr Companion (Med-Hand®) and oup.co.uk/academic/medicine/handbooks/pda. **NB:** the trouble with relying on books is that there is no room for more than one in a bag, and the danger is that if you keep them in your car, they are not to hand for easy reference. No-one wants to get to the top of a block of flats only to have to descend to see if *x* interacts with *y* or to find out the incubation time for scarlet fever. *Permanently on Internet access* means that as well as loaded books, everything else is available too, eg decision support and access to patients' notes—eg web EMIS/NHS spine/records; decision support.

For the car Maps, torches, nebulizer, spare batteries, speculum, defibrillator, ECG, dressings, peak flow meter; O₂, sat nav, chauffeur.

For the mind We have a duty to be fully conscious and reasonably healthy. Take opportunities to sleep before and after night duties. We know that on-call night work induces sleep debt with prolonged impairment of awake activities, sleep quality, and performance. Not working the following day after an on-call night only allows for *partial* recovery of sleep quality to begin.[224]

We have all been in the position of visiting patients who are less sick than we are—and we tend to carry on until we drop (see p689). This is bad for us and bad for patients. If you are sick, and no locum is to hand, phone your local Primary Care Organization or out-of-hours co-operative.

Open surgeries: riding the chaos With many simultaneous demands, and the waiting room filling up faster and faster with insoluble problems, panic may strike unless we get into the mood of our juggler (p466 fig 1). On his forehead is stamped *I am here for you.* The easier but doomed alternative is *Keep the patients at bay at any cost*—the stereotype of the unapproachable doctor behind a glass wall. To thrive in tumultuous open surgeries, don't hide behind anything: ride the torrent. Most of your patients will understand what you are trying to do, and will somehow support you.

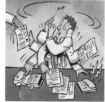

Fig 1. Riding the chaos...

On any day ~60% of people take drugs, only half of which are prescribed. The others are sold over the counter (OTC). The commonest OTCs are analgesics, cough medicines, and vitamins; for prescribed drugs the common groups are CNS and cardiovascular drugs, and antibiotics. On average, 6-7 NHS prescriptions are issued/person/year (21 in Italy and 11 in France).

GPs account for 75% of NHS annual prescribing costs (~10% of the total cost of the NHS), although many of these 'GP drugs' will have been initiated in hospital. The cost of these prescriptions has rises faster than inflation and is ~£300,000/GP/year. Positive correlations with low prescribing include a young doctor, practising in an affluent area, and longer consultation times (is extra time is spent explaining about minor illness (p517) may be given, so that expectation for a prescription is replaced by belief in one's own health).

Formularies aim is to make prescribing more cost-effective, by compiling an agreed list of favoured drugs. This voluntary restriction can work in tandem with compulsory NHS restricted lists, and lead to substantial savings (eg 18%). Developing formularies at individual practice level has been recommended, but this is time-consuming and may be better achieved by adapting an existing formulary. *ScripSwitch* is an alternative, using software to flag up more cost-effective solutions, which can be swapped in with one click if the GP so desires (eg valaciclovir→aciclovir). The problem of denying GPs drug choice leading increase referral to secondary care[225] is obviated by this method.

Dispensing doctors Where there is no chemist's shop (eg rural areas) UK GPs are paid to dispense to their patients. Their annual prescribing rate can be as low as 70% of their non-dispensing fellow GPs.

Compliance (Does the patient take the medicine?) ▸*There is no point in being a brilliant diagnostician if nobody can be persuaded to take your treatments.* Even in life-threatening conditions, compliance is a major problem occurring in up to 56% of patients (eg adolescents with acute lymphatic leukaemia). The following are associated with increased compliance.
• Being able to identify with a personal doctor.
• Patient's overall satisfaction with the doctor.
• Simple therapeutic regimens.
• Written information (use short words—Flesch formula >70, *OHCM* p3).
• Longer consultation times or prescribing on home visits.
• Prescribing in association with giving health education.
• Continuity of care, coupled with belief in efficacy of the treatment.
• Short waiting time for appointments.
• The encouragement of self-monitoring by the patient.

Monitoring compliance: Monitoring plasma drug levels is the most reliable way of doing this, but it is cheaper to ask patients to return with their tablets, so that you can count them (or to count during a phone contact)[226]—or, better still, establish a basis of trust so that the patient can check for him- or herself.

Compliance or concordance? *Compliance* suggests that you know best and patients who lapse are foolish. But it is known that adapting GP advice to their needs leads to fewer side effects, eg GI bleeding: your prescription may read 'ibuprofen 400mg/8h', but the patient may, sensibly, only take the drug when his joints are bad. Don't think of this as the patient failing to do something. It is you who have failed to reach a shared understanding of the pros and cons of drug-taking. Concordance denotes more than this: think of it as a liberating concept, promoting egalitarianism in medicine. ▸*There is no healthier ideal.*[227] Are you nodding in the direction of concordance while still covertly believing in compliance? Then let us put the boot on the other foot and await the time *you* are monitored for compliance with some marvellous guidelines: we predict that concordance will now seem more rational and desirable!

Since Neolithic times, healing has had a central place in our culture, and is recognized as 'mor bettir and mor precious pan any medicyne' (*OED* v 152.1). Recently medicines have improved greatly, so that the role of doctors as the purveyor of medicines has eclipsed their more ancient roles. We all recognize the limits of our role as prescribers, and we would all like to heal more and engage in repetitive tasks less often. But what, we might ask, *is* healing? How is it different for from curing? Healing is, at one level, something mysterious that happens to wounds, see p731.

On another level, healing involves transforming through communication: a kind of hands-on hypnosis. We can cure with scalpels and needles, but these are not instruments of communication. Here is an example of healing (an all too rare event in our own practice). On a rainy February evening, after a long surgery, I visited a stooped man at the fag-end of life, with something the matter with his lung. "I suppose it's rotting, like the rest of me—it's gradually dying." I reply: "Do you think you're dying?" "Aren't we all?" "Green and dying" I reply for some reason, half remembering a poem by Dylan Thomas (*Fern Hill*). The patient looks mystified: he thinks he misheard, and asks me to repeat. "Green *and* dying" I say, feeling stupid. There is a pause, and then he rises to his full height, puffs out his chest, and completes, in a magnificent baritone, the lines: "... Time held me green and dying, though I sang in my chains like the sea." bigeye.com/fernhill.htm By chance I had revealed a new meaning to a favourite poem of his which perhaps he thought was about childhood, not the rigours of his old age. Both our eyes shone more brightly as we passed to the more prosaic aspects of the visit. This illustrates the nature of healing: its unpredictability, its ability to allow us to rise to our full height, to sing, rather than mumble, and how externally nothing may be changed by healing, just our internal landscape, transformed and illuminated. It also shows how healing depends on communication, and is bound up with art. Healing may be mysterious, but it is not rare. We have so often kissed the grazed knees of our daughters that we expect the healing balm of kisses to wear out, but, while they are young, it never will, because children know how to receive—but not how to doubt, and the kiss is the paradigm of healing: contact between two humans, wordless service of the lips.

Our central task of sifting of symptoms, deciding what is wrong, and prescribing treatment are all tasks which, according to the editor of the *Lancet* are destined for delegation to microchips.[228] This implies that our chief role will be as healers and teachers. Meta-analyses of randomized healing trials (prayer, mental/spiritual healing, therapeutic touching) bear this out to some extent: 57% of randomized trials show a positive effect.[228]

There will always be some way to go before healing, the central ideal of medicine, becomes its central activity. After all, the last thing any of us wants during appendicitis, is a poet or a healer—but last things will always retain their power to set us thinking. We should also be able to combine healing paradigms with mechanical neuropsychological approaches to consultations. This is the aim of spiritually orientated group therapy.[1]

The healing effect of laughter and tears are never far away in significant consultations, as the latent becomes manifest: as one patient said "There had been latent feelings bottled inside me for years; after every teary session I felt better".[229] It's too glib to say what's broken gets mended, but tears *can* liquefy something in the soul that can then resolve itself, helped by the hugs that tears induce.[230]

---

1 Group prayer, yoga breathing, and spiritual readings with severely ill women can improve mood, affect, motivation, interpersonal bonding, and sense of self, and can succeed in reaching patients and promoting recovery in new ways.[231]

Primary care

Unemployment in families uk data show a link between child deaths and unemployment, lower social class and overcrowding. Babies whose fathers are employed are heavier at birth (by 150g) than unemployed fathers' babies, after adjusting for other factors. Accidents and infection are more rife among children of the unemployed compared with selected controls, and their mothers may be more prone to depression. As unemployment rises, so does child abuse. Other factors identified with this rise are marital discord, debt, and parents' lack of self-esteem, as affected families reveal: "When he lost his job he went bonkers. He changed completely. He became depressed and snappy. Frustrated."

Marital breakdown heads the list of problems of women with neurosis, coming 2nd (to job difficulties) in men, and is a leading factor in >60% of suicide attempts. In the usa, divorced men have the highest mortality. The greater incidence of cardiac deaths is in young divorced males. Being divorced and a non-smoker is nearly as dangerous as smoking a pack a day and staying married. Marital harmony (eg cuddling) protects from cardiac death, as shown in one prospective study of 10,000 Israeli hearts. Parental behaviours predicting problematic marriages among offspring included jealousy, being domineering, getting angry easily, being critical, moody, or taciturn.[232]

uk social security benefits For *England*, see dss.gov.uk/lifeevent/benefits. The *Disability Rights Handbook*, 36e, 2012 explains how the *Personal independence payment (PIP)* is replacing the *disability living allowance (DLA)*.

Statements of fitness for work (Med3)uk says how long a person is off work for. Self-certification occurs during the 1st 7 days of illness. If a patient asks for a sick note during this period, it has to be private and is chargeable. The GP can indicate whether modification to the workplace or amended duties would allow work to take place; a phased return to work can also be specified.

Med3s can only be backdated when based on a previous assessment. An assessment is defined as the date you either had a face-to-face or phone consultation or considered a report from another doctor or professional. GPs can issue a Statement on or after this date, but not before. If a patient asks for medical evidence to cover a backdated period for which there has not been a previous assessment a GP cannot issue a Med3 for the backdated period but in the comments box he can advise that the patient was not fit for work for an earlier period (if he has evidence to justify this advice).

Why are further reports (IB113/ESA113) sometimes needed from a GP? People suffering from specified severe disabilities may be treated as incapable of work without being tested. So uk Jobcentres take steps to identify such people before applying the Personal Capability Assessment (Incapacity Benefit) or Work Capability Assessment (Employment and Support Allowance). GPs help by giving a precise diagnosis and factual clinical details where a person may have a severe condition that, under Regulations, allows them to be treated as incapable of work without needing to undergo a benefit-related examination.

Advise people with more than one job to submit the statement to their main employer, who can note the details of the advice you have given. They can then present the form to their 2nd employer.   dwp.gov.uk/docs/fitnote-gp-guide.pdf

Social class and inequalities in health

With the introduction of the British NHS, with its ideal of each according to need and equal access we assumed that differences in the health of different social classes would go. The reverse has happened![233] *The Black Report: Inequalities in Health*

National Service Frameworks (eg NSFs for heart disease, diabetes, mental health, and older people) aim to redress inequalities, but increase inequalities (rich people make more use of new resources). This is compounded by the fact that the South-East is becoming ever richer while in some of our great Northern cities over 50% of households are 'breadline poor'.[234] *Joseph Rowntree Foundation 2007*

p53 genes and the locus and post-codes of poverty How does poverty cause ill-health? In breast cancer, relapse is more likely in deprived post-codes, where smoking, drinking and an unhealthy diet make p53 mutations more likely,[235] so its cancer-protecting protein is less abundant (see p649). The big way to remove health inequality is to ↓smoking in poorer people. And if some wealthy people quit too, so what? So health inequalities don't matter as long as overall health is improving? Not quite. Justice matters too. It is the lack of justice which led to the NHS—which would have been the best invention of the 20th century, if only it **had** removed inequalities.

UK Registrar General's scale of 5 social or occupational classes		
Class I	Professional	eg lawyer, doctor, accountant
Class II	Intermediate	eg teacher, nurse, manager
Class III^N	Skilled non-manual	eg typist, shop assistant
Class III^M	Skilled manual	eg miner, bus-driver, cook
Class IV	Partly skilled (manual)	eg farmworker, bus-conductor
Class V	Unskilled manual	eg cleaner, labourer

▶Poor people living in North London (eg Tottenham Green) live ~17yrs less than rich people (in Chelsea); their life expectancy (71yrs) is < that in Ecuador, China and Belize (none has a national health service!).[236] **Mortality rates are higher in social class V vs class I:** In stillbirths, perinatal deaths, infant deaths, deaths in men aged 15-64 and women aged 20-59 this factor is 1.8, 2, 2.1, 2, and 1.95. Ditto for lung cancer (SMR^1=1.98), heart disease (1.3) and stroke (1.9). Melanoma and Hodgkin's disease are exceptions.

Effects of social class and geography are hard to tease apart: in the UK, city dwellers' mortality rates are ~22% (95% confidence interval: 19%-25%) higher than those in the most rural areas (especially for lung cancer and respiratory disease—and pollution is a likely cause of this).[237]

Within occupations the effect of social class is seen in a 'purer' way than when groups of many occupations are compared: in a study of >17,000 Whitehall civil servants there was a >3-fold difference in mortality from all causes of death (except genitourinary disease) comparing those in high grades with those in low grades. Similarly in the army, there is a 5-fold difference in mortality from heart disease between highest and lowest ranks.

We know that illness makes us descend the social scale, but this effect is probably not big enough to account for the observed differences between classes. It is more likely that the differences are due to **smoking behaviour**, **education**, **diet**,[2] **poverty**, **stress**, and **overcrowding**. Cognitive ability can partly explain socio-economic inequalities in health ('intelligent people look after themselves'—has some truth). Note that smoking is 3-fold more common in nurses than in doctors[238] and cognitive factors must play some part in this. This need not imply pessimism about attempts to break the chain that links socio-economic status and cognitive ability with health. During some life stages, environmental factors may be able to influence cognitive skills. Interventions can be targeted in order to optimize these effects.[239]

1 The SMR (standard mortality ratio) is the ratio of mortality rates in one class compared with the average for the whole population. The whole population has an SMR of 1.00.

2 Low earners consume only a bit less wholemeal bread and more sugary drinks, processed meat and sugar than average, eg 2.5 portions of fresh fruit and vegetables, compared with the average of 2.8.[240]

By removing smoking you may have removed someone's only pleasure: their life will certainly seem longer!

Two sets of contrasting principles 1a He who pays the piper, calls the tune. 1b Priceless therapeutic assets cannot be bought or sold: compassion, continuity of care, and commitment. 2a My job is to spend, spend, spend, until all my patients are healthy. 2b The job of the Treasury is to squeeze, squeeze, squeeze, until all spending is within government targets. (The clarity of this dichotomy becomes turbid when the doctor is asked to do the squeezing.)

Never just ask how good a structure is without also asking how good it is at transforming itself: that which cannot transform, dies. The UK National Health Service is the largest employer in the Western world and for years the search has been on to find ways to control and transform this dear, mighty thing. The purchaser-provider split is the most powerful lever yet developed for this purpose. *Purchasers* commission care by drawing up contracts with competing *providers*, who deliver the care. The better the provider delivers secondary care (do *not* pause to ask what 'better' means: speculation on this point might ruin the argument) the more likely they are to get the contract next year. The catch is that all the extra effort the provider makes to out-perform a contract this year will probably be taken for granted next year. The same may hold true if purchasing is used for the imposition of guidelines ('evidence-based purchasing'). What has been created is a treadmill which goes faster and faster, while taking less and less account of individual patients' and doctors' legitimate but varying needs. Unless the market is rigged, natural selection ensures that the fittest and fastest providers survive. Patients and taxpayers benefit—until the point where cynicism and exhaustion set in. There is no evidence that once the purchaser-provider path is chosen, then cynicism and exhaustion *inevitably* follow, and there is evidence at local level that benefits accrue, and services become more tuned to consumers' desires. (Consumers are not infallible judges of what constitutes health—but they are the best judges we have.) ▶If the State runs both *supply* (money from general taxation) and *demand* (control of waiting lists etc), the rules of the market cannot operate and efficiency is hard to achieve—which is why NHS trusts are being freed from central NHS control.

Controlling change from on top: *an historical example from maternity:*
1 Government sets up an expert group (mothers, midwives, ministers, obstetricians, and general practitioners—these are jokers in the pack, because they are simultaneously consumers, purchasers *and* providers).
2 Issuing of objectives and indicators of success—eg by 5 years:
   •Women should have a named midwife to ensure continuity of care.
   •Women should be able to choose their place of delivery. Aim to achieve the outcome that she believes is best for her baby and herself.
   •≥75% of women should know the person who is to deliver them in labour.
   •Midwives should have direct access to some beds in all maternity units.
   •≥30% of women should have a midwife as the lead professional.
3 Fanfare phase: the group's attractive-looking report is issued (at great expense to taxpayers) to all groups and personnel involved (except mothers).
4 Lack of finance is blamed when no improvements are detected at 5 years.
5 Later, the units are marked for closure and the cycle of hope, rising expectations followed by despair and cynicism becomes complete as the consultation exercise proves to be a derisory exercise in making glossy reports.[241]

Anatomy of change Ideals (woman-centred care)→Specific policy objective (all women to have the chance to discuss their care)→Purchasers' action point (set up maternity services liaison committee with lay chairperson)→Providers' action point (provide link-workers, and advocacy schemes for women whose first language is not English). This type of activity may or may not lead to increased accountability and quality of services.[242]

There is great variability in individual GPs' referral statistics, which leads purveyors of government strategy to the error of saying "Why is there a 4-fold difference in referral rates between GPs? Such variation is insupportable; some doctors must be referring too much ..." An advance is made when this issue is reframed as: "*There is information contained in this variability*". This information can guide service development.[243]

Understanding the intricacies of purchasing health care depends on understanding referral patterns. If high-referring GPs refer needlessly, then the proportion of their referrals resulting in further action will be smaller than that of practices with low-referring GPs. Usually, this is not the case. Those with high referral rates have high rates of intervention. If I refer an ever-increasing number of my patients to a geriatric clinic, must a time come when admissions level off? The idea of a 'levelling-off effect' is important. If the consultant is 'correct', and the GP's expectation as to the outcome of referral are uniform (probably never true) then when a levelling-off effect is observed, it may be true that the *average* referral rate is optimal, and that low-referrers are under-treating, and high-referrers are wasting money. In fact, levelling-off effects are rarely seen, except in general surgery. Other specialists may admit a fixed proportion of patients referred to them. There is evidence that this was true for ENT consultants and tonsillectomy. Another possibility is the Coulter-Seagroatt hypothesis—that consultants have a threshold of severity for admission (eg a claudication distance of 50 metres) and even the majority of patients from the high-referrers fulfil this criterion. In this case (assuming the consultant is right), even the high-referrers are not referring enough. This may be true for angiography. But if the consultant is over-enthusiastic, and overstates treatment benefits, then the lower referrers are to be applauded for limiting the excesses of the consultant. ▶*In general, only agree that a referral is inappropriate if the patient, the GP, and the consultant concur on its lack of utility*. Each of these parties has different motivations—eg reassurance/explanation, medicolegal, as well as providing therapy. Despite the rhetoric, secondary care can be preoccupied by its own agendas and may have little interest in the unique needs of referred patients.[244]

Overall, referral rates are no more variable than admission rates, even in populations with similar morbidity. The reason may be that there is still a great deal of uncertainty underlying very many clinical decisions. We don't know who *exactly* should have knee replacements, cholecystectomy, etc.[245]

▶There is no known relationship between high or low referral rates and quality of care. Here are 3 cautions in interpreting referrals.

1 Don't accept GP list size as a denominator (takes no account of differing workloads in a practice). Consultations/yr is a better denominator.
2 If a GP has a special interest, this will influence referral patterns. More knowledge may lead to more referrals as partial knowledge leads to greater, not less, uncertainty. For example after a while all GPs with a special interest (GPSI) in dermatology will have been tricked by melanomas masquerading as seborrhoeic warts—so their referrals for histology will be higher than GPs who have less experience and have never been so tricked.
3 Years of data are needed to compare referrals to rarely used units.

Referral incentive schemes The foregoing shows that this is a complex and uncertain way to influence referrals.[246,247] But it is true that local educational interventions with secondary care specialists and structured referral sheets can impact on referral rates.[248] 'In-house' 2nd opinions and other primary care based alternatives to outpatient referral are promising.[248] In 2011 referrals in England fell by 5% (to 3.7×10^6) after a long period of rising.[249] The foregoing shows that there are many ways to interpret this statistic (rationing is biting; patients are less demanding; GPs are more realistic about hospital benefits).

Primary care

Ordinary UK driving licences issued by DVLA (driver & vehicle licensing agency) imply that *You are required by law to inform Drivers Medical Branch, DVLA, Swansea SA99 1AT at once if you have any physical or medical condition), that is, or may affect your fitness as a driver, unless you don't expect it to last more than 3 months.* It is the responsibility of the driver to inform DVLA. It is the responsibility of doctors to advise patients that medical conditions (and drugs) may affect their ability to drive and for which conditions patients should inform the DVLA. Drivers should also inform their insurance company of any condition disclosed to DVLA. ►If in doubt, ask your defence union.

Vascular disease *Uncomplicated MI:* don't drive for 4wks. *Angioplasty or pacemaker:* don't drive for 1wk post-op. *Angina:* no driving if symptoms occur at the wheel; DVLA need not be informed. *Arrhythmias:* driving may be OK if the cause is found, and controlled for >1 month if low risk of ↓consciousness & ↓motor power. Syncope: OK to drive 1wk after, if cause identified and treated. If no cause is found, stop for ≥6 months. *TIA/stroke:* stop for ≥1 month; no need to inform DVLA unless there is residual deficit for >1 month. *Abdominal aortic aneurysm >6.5cm:* Disqualification (if 6-6.4cm: inform DVLA; do annual review).

Diabetes All on *oral hypoglycaemics* or *insulin* must inform DVLA (in general, stop driving for 1 month after starting insulin, to get stable; drivers must show satisfactory control, and must recognize hypoglycaemia). Check vision conforms to required standard (BOX). Avoid driving if hypoglycaemic risk ↑ (eg meal delay; or after excess exercise). Carry rapidly absorbed sugar in vehicle and stop, turn off ignition and eat it if any warning signs. A card should be carried to say which drugs they are using, to aid resuscitation if needed. If an accident is due to hypoglycaemia a diabetic driver may be charged with driving under the influence of drugs. Advise patients to notify DVLA (±'stop driving' advice) if limb or visual problems or impaired awareness of hypoglycaemia.[250]

CNS disorders Disabling giddiness, vertigo, and problems with movements preclude driving. DVLA need to know about unexplained blackouts, multiple sclerosis, Parkinson's (any 'freezing' or on-off effects), motor neuron disease, recurrent TIAs and strokes. In the latter the licence is usually withheld for 3 months depending on an examination by an independent doctor, and sometimes a driving test. Those with dementia should only drive if the condition is very mild (do not rely on armchair judgments: on-the-road trials are better). Encourage relatives to contact DVLA if a dementing relative should not be driving. GPs may desire to breach confidentiality (the GMC approves) and inform DVLA of demented or psychotic patients (tel. 01792 783686^{UK}). Many elderly drivers (~1 in 3) who die in accidents are found to have Alzheimer's.

Epilepsy and brain surgery: If a seizure while awake, he must not drive for 1yr. If attacks are occurring only when asleep, driving may be possible, eg if after 3yrs no seizure has ever occurred while awake. Contact DVLA. *In any event, the driving by such a person should not be likely to cause a public danger.* If a licence holder/applicant can satisfy the above, a 3yr licence is normally issued. The 'till 70' licence may be restored if fit-free for 7yrs with drugs as needed (if no other disqualifying condition). *Single seizure:* OK to drive after 6 months if specialist says so and no abnormal tests (eg CT, MRI, EEG).

Epileptic drug withdrawal risks a 40% seizure rate in year 1. Those wishing to withdraw from medication should cease driving from the beginning of withdrawal and not recommence until 6 months after treatment has ceased.

Driving is prohibited in certain general categories

• Severe mental disorder (including severe mental impairment).
• Severe behavioural disorders—or drug abuse/dependency.
• Alcohol dependency[1] (including inability to refrain from drunken driving).
• Psychotic medication taken in quantities that impair driving ability.

Vision Acuity (±spectacles) must allow reading a 79.4mm-high number plate at 20.5 metres (~6/10 on Snellen chart). Monocular vision is allowed if visual field is full. Binocular field of vision must be >120°. Diplopia isn't allowed unless *mild* and *eye-patch correctable*. **Diabetic retinopathy** matters, but applicants/licence holders may not need DVLA visual field tests on a regular basis if vision meets required acuity and visual field standards, and a consultant confirms that it is stable, eg: • Visual field shows no deterioration during the last yr. • No further laser use in the last year or since their last licence renewal. • No change in retinal signs in the last year or since renewal.[250]

Drugs Driving or being in charge of a vehicle when under the influence (including side effect) of a drug is an offence under the Road Traffic Act 1988. Many drugs affect alertness and driving ability (check *Data-sheets*), and many are potentiated by alcohol, so warn patients not to drive until they are sure of side effects, not to drink and drive, not to drive if feeling unwell, and never to drive within 48h of a general anaesthetic.

Old age DVLA says: "progressive loss of memory, impairment in concentration and reaction time with possible loss of confidence, suggest consideration be given to cease driving." This is vague, as when reapplying for a licence (every 3yrs after 70) a driver simply signs to say 'no medical disability is present'.[251]

Fitness to fly: avoid hypobaric (high altitude) flights if...

• Climbing stairs causes troublesome dyspnoea (an easy screening test).
• Gas-filled dental caries (via putrifying bacteria): can cause severe toothache at altitude, and tooth damage may occur.
• Within 48h after diving below 50 feet (p814). Even at modest cabin altitudes death may occur. NB: barotrauma is worse on descent as the Eustachian tube is sucked flat by the low pressure in the middle ear, making the immediate equilibration of pressure more difficult.
• In uncontrolled cardiac failure, if O_2 supplements used at sea-level, wean off before air travel, to help see if air travel is OK. These patients must travel with enough supplementary O_2 to give intermittent use, eg at 2L/min.
• Confusional states and alcohol intoxication (synergistic with hypoxia).
• Pneumothorax; pneumomediastinum; or <10 days post-op to hollow organ.
• Neonates <3 days old, or women in the last 4 weeks of pregnancy (last 13 weeks if multiple pregnancy). See section on airlines, p8.
• Anaemia (Hb <7.5g/dL); GI bleeding; any recent tissue infarctions.

▶Encourage good hydration and mobility; use aspirin & compression stockings on long-haul flights—p16. NB: the list above is not exhaustive.

See International Air Transport Association advice.   medinet.co.uk/crit.htm

Fitness to do sporting activities and cardiac rehabilitation

GPs often have to advise on this. Ensure that those involved know you don't have a crystal ball. Common sense, and attention to warm-up exercise, is the key. If in an at-risk group, eg epilepsy + wanting to swim, or personal or family history of hypertrophic obstructive cardiomyopathy + wanting to do heavy exercise, get help. In epilepsy, swim with a friend, only in lifeguard supervised pools.[252] In CCF, mild work with hand weights need not be banned.[253]

Is this drug on the 'banned' list? See *Sports Medicine* in Mims Companion.

1 *Alcohol & driving:* anyone attempting to drive on a road, or public place (eg pub car park or a garage forecourt), may be required to give a breath test, to see if they are over the legal limit of alcohol: 35µg of alcohol/100mL of breath (or 80mg of alcohol/100mL of blood). The request must be made by a police officer.

Primary care

CFS entails severe, disabling fatigue for >6 months, affecting physical and mental functioning, present most of the time and feeling dreadful/relapse after mild exertion. ♀:♂≈3:1.[254] Myalgia, sleep and mood disturbance are common. *Predisposing factors:* Genetics; personality; anxiety/depression.[255] *Precipitating factors:* Infections ± psychosocial stress. *Perpetuating factors:*☀ Immunity↓, poor skeletal muscle, cognitive ability, endocrine & cardiovascular homeostasis.[256]

Physical correlates of CFS: Abnormal gene expression in 16 genes related to mitochondrial function (Epstein-Barr or parvoviruses could switch on this abnormal expression; this might form the basis for a diagnostic blood test).[257] Neutrophil apoptosis is ↑.[258] Electrodermal responses are somewhat characteristic.

Diagnostic criteria/work-up for 'query chronic fatigue syndrome' The Canadian criteria may be used for research purposes (>60 areas are investigated; some are controversial, eg ataxia).[259] In practice, exclude anaemia, TB, snoring, etc, with a history; physical exam; mental state (p324), urinalysis, FBC, U&E, TSH, ESR, LFT, glucose ± autoantibodies, creatine kinase, blood culture, and CXR.

THEN

Pursue abnormalities (eg ?TB/HIV if weight↓; ?depression if anhedonia, p336).

THEN ASK

Does the pattern fit CFS?—ie persistent or relapsing fatigue, not relieved by rest, and leading to substantial reduction in previous levels of activity.

THEN ASK

Are any exclusion criteria present?—psychosis (p316), bipolar depression (p354), dementia, anorexia (p348).
Are ≥4 of the following present for >6 months? • Unexplained muscle pain
• Impaired memory/concentration unrelated to drugs or alcohol use
• Polyarthralgia (but swelling suggests a joint diagnosis)
• Unrefreshing sleep
• Post-exertional malaise lasting over 24h
• Persisting sore throat not caused by glandular fever
• Unexplained tender cervical or axillary nodes.
If criteria met, call it CFS; if not fully met, call it 'idiopathic chronic fatigue'.
Co-morbid conditions are common, eg depression: consider diagnosing in a quantified way using formal diagnostic instruments (eg Beck inventory).

Treatment None is specific, and chronicity is common.[260] Aim for a therapeutic alliance with your patient. Some therapists aim to prevent somatic fixation: the strongest predictor of a poor prognosis is a fixed belief that symptoms are due only to physical causes. Allow non-threatening discussion about psychological issues, keeping an open mind. Make it clear that psychological symptoms are not the same as malingering: "Perhaps what starts as an illness may be not what keeps it going". Psychological factors affect outcome of many illnesses: why should this be different? *Proven interventions:* Graded exercise programmes (not the same as 'pacing[1]');[261,262] cognitive therapy (p374).
   Treating associated anxiety/depression (p340) may be the best way to improve quality of life.[263] Also address family and work problems, and other perpetuating factors (above). Talking with other patients sounds sensible, but this could prolong symptoms. Slow recovery is the norm (faster in adolescents).[261]

Trials of non-standard therapies Trials find modest benefit from methylphenidate (20mg/d)[264] and nicotinamide adenine dinucleotide (NADH).[265]

When to get help •Children with CFS •Unresponsive to the above measures •History of travel abroad •CNS signs •Walking difficulty •Fevers •Suicidal.

Prognosis Be optimistic. A key predictor of good outcome is emotional processing (expressing, acknowledging, and accepting of emotional distress).[266]

1 Pacing is setting a *realistic* exercise routine and sticking to it to avoid 'boom and bust' cycles. Proper rest between exercise (eg relaxation/meditation) is said to be vital.[267] Further reading: DoH CFS working party.

The prevalence of obesity (BMI >30kg/m²): USA 27%, UK 24%, Italy 10%.[268] Obesity is the commonest disorder of childhood and adolescence (see BMI charts, p227 and *preventing adult diseases in childhood*, p156).[269]

Obesity shortens life expectancy[270] (MI; stroke; hypertension; dyslipidaemia/ metabolic syndrome, thromboembolism, diabetes) and contributes to gout, sleep apnoea, cognitive diseases, and gallbladder disease.[268,272] In Framingham studies, obesity alone accounted for 11% of heart failure in men (14% in women).

Weight loss maintained for 2yrs, improves life expectancy and all the above complications.[273,274] (Less certainty with obesity-associated depression, cataracts, fatty liver disease, osteoarthritis, and benign intracranial hypertension.)

Obesity and cancer: Obesity is associated with ↑death rates from cancer of oesophagus, colon, rectum, gallbladder, pancreas, and kidney, independent of smoking. It also ↑ risk of death from stomach and prostate cancer in ♂and breast, cervical and ovarian cancer in ♀. This could be from increased inflammatory state in obesity. Risk of death correlates with BMI beyond 25kg/m².[272,275]

Mother/child: Obesity ↑ risk of pre-eclampsia (×2), diabetes (×4), thromboembolism, and maternal mortality. Rates of congenital deformities such as spinabifida and heart defects also increases.[276]

Hormonal changes in obesity Interactions between gut, brain, circulating metabolites and adipose tissue are all integrated to regulate food intake and attempt to maintain weight.[277] Cholecystokinin, GLP-1, ghrelin, and peptide YY, are examples of gut hormones with effects on brainstem, hypothalamus, or hippocampus, regulating hunger-satiety drive, food behaviour, and mood.[1,278]

Increased visceral fat enhances the degree of insulin resistance associated with obesity and hyperinsulinaemia. Together, hyperinsulinaemia and insulin resistance enhance the risk of the co-morbidities described above.[272]

Other endocrine changes include increased: leptin, TSH, insulin, IGF-1, androgens, progesterone, cytokines (IL-6), ACTH/cortisol, and decreased: GH, adiponectin[279] and parasympathetic activity.[280]

Typical needs Women: 2079Kcal/d (♂ ≈2605); most eat ≥10% more than needed. Once weight goes up, physical activity lessens, and weight increases further.

Measuring obesity BMI is still useful, but waist circumference (midway between lower ribs and iliac crest at the end of gentle expiration) correlates better with risk of complications even if BMI normal.[281] Reference intervals for obesity are lower in Asian people (obese=BMI >27.5) because their central fat is increased.[281]

Waist circumference for central obesity		
Europeans	♂≥94cm	♀≥80cm
South (s.) Asians	♂≥90cm	♀≥80cm
Chinese	♂≥90cm	♀≥80cm
Japanese	♂≥85cm	♀≥90cm♣♠
s.&central Americans: use s.asian data *pro tem*		
Africans + Middle East: use European *pro tem*		

Management The main problem is maintaining lost weight.

Non-pharmacological: There is strong evidence that combining a behavioural approach with more traditional dietary and activity advice leads to improved short-term weight loss and is currently the best lifestyle approach.[282,283]

Behavioural therapy: Setting goals, self-monitoring, family/friend/group (eg weight watchers), cognitive restructuring, problem solving, assertiveness.[284,NICE]

Diet/exercise example: 1000Kcal/day and 30min of moderate activity every day (≥5 days/wk)[285,286] adapted to maintain the weight loss.[283,286] 500kcal/day reduction without any change of activity leads to ~0.45kg of weight loss/wk. Easy! One may as well ask someone to hold their breath for a week.

---

1 Increasing ghrelin levels, through injections or calorie restriction in mice, gives anxiolytic- and antidepressant-like responses in forced swim tests. Ghrelin may defend against stress-induced depression.[287] Ghrelin ↑GH & cortisol secretion (and, in men, promotes restorative slow-wave sleep).[288]

"Doctor, I want to lose weight..."

- Is it you who wants to lose weight or have you been sent by someone else?
- Any plans? What have you tried? What is/was your maximum weight?
- Are you on anything that increases weight (pioglitazone; antipsychotics)?
- Your motivation is... eg to decrease BP medication or NSAIDs for OA (p689)?
- Would you accept a specific goal, eg 'lose 0.5kg/week eg with high-protein low-calorie, low carbohydrate diet?—or go to a weight-watchers group?'
- Can you change your obesogenic environment (eg less food stimuli)?[268,289]
- Can you commit to increase your exercise to maintain weight loss?
- Can you use a pedometer, join a gym, or do home-based exercise programs?
- Are you prepared to record food intake and energy expenditure?[290]
- Are you wanting a specific remedy (BELOW), if indicated (and no CI, eg BP↑)?

7 questions for weight-loss programmes to answer (*Mayo Clinic*)

1 Is there proof that it works (ask for evidence of long-term results)?
2 Any qualified dietician or specialist in behaviour modification employed?
3 Is the recommended intake nutritionally balanced?
4 Does the patient have to buy special products?
5 Will the patient receive advice on starting safe, moderate exercise?
6 How will the programme reward and monitor progress?
7 Is there support and follow-up for after the formal programme ends?

Specific therapies for obesity

Drug therapy Benefits are ↑weight loss (4-6kg added to diet alone), maintaining weight loss, improve vascular risks with weight reduction.[284]NICE Generally, stop if weight loss <5% at 12wks (less strict if diabetic).[284,291]NICE

Orlistat 120mg/8h PO. Intestinal lipase inhibitor; induces 5-10% weight loss in 50-60% which maintains for 4yrs. Explain to eat <60g fat/day otherwise steatorrhoea occurs. SE: oily spotting, flatus with discharge, faecal urgency[284,290]NICE CI: chronic malabsorption, cholestasis, breastfeeding (see BNF).

Bariatric surgery If all of these criteria are fulfilled: • BMI ≥40kg/m² or 35-40kg/m² and co-morbidities ↑risk. • All appropriate nonsurgical measures have been tried for >6 months • Involvement of a specialist obesity service. • No over-riding personality/behavioural problem.[284,292]NICE *Long term effects:* Iron, vitamin, and protein deficiencies; gallstones, weight regain.[292] Types of bariatric surgery: intragastric balloons, gastric banding (variable tightening); gastric bypass. NB: the morbidly obese are ghrelin and leptin hyporesponders with lesser intragastric balloon treatment efficiency.[293] Bariatric surgery in some cases can cure diseases caused by obesity such as type 2 diabetes.

Are we in a passive-dependent relationship with our obesity genes?
Exercise reduces the effect of FTO genes on obesity by 27%.(*Ruth Loos 2011 meta-analysis*)[294] So, at least to some extent, we can encourage our patients to take control.

1 **Websites for help with weight loss** www.weightlossresources.co.uk www.eating4health.co.uk www.toast-uk.org (Obesity Awareness Trust). www.whi.org.uk www.weightlossresources.co.uk
2 Genetic testing may be counter-productive: one study showed that people who were told they had ↑genetic susceptibility to obesity *increased* their dietary fat intake. We thank Dr Hamid Mani for his help with this topic.

What to do for the best?

Doctors are called on to make decisions about every patient they meet: few are curable at once, so making a plan for what to do for the best is the secret of success at the bedside. The aim here is to explain this secret, to enable you to flourish in the clinical world, and to keep you out of lawyers' offices.

Let us look at the steps of the history, physical, or mental examination, and investigations.

By the end of taking the **history**, you need to have acquired 3 things:

1 Rapport with the patient.
2 A diagnosis or differential diagnosis.
3 The placement of the diagnosis in the context of the patient's life.

Rapport: Consultations are shorter when rapport is good.[295 (N=116)] The patient is confident that he or she is getting the full attention of the doctor, and these patients are more understanding, and more forgiving when things go wrong. Doctors are far from infallible, so we need to have confidence that the patient will feel able to come back if things are not right, tell us what has happened, agree on an adjustment of the treatment, and, by giving feedback, improve our clinical acumen.

Diagnosis: Studies have shown that skilled physicians have made a provisional diagnosis soon after the consultation starts, and they spend the rest of the history in confirming or excluding it. What happens if you are not skilled, and you have no hint as to the diagnosis? You need to get more information.

• Pursue the main symptom: "tell me more about the headache..."
• Elicit other symptoms—eg change of weight or appetite, fevers, fatigue, unexplained lumps, itching, jaundice, or anything else odd?
• Get help from a colleague or even a diagnostic system—eg Mentor, p502.
• Check you still have rapport with the patient. Are you searching for a physical diagnosis when a psychological diagnosis would be more appropriate? Here you might ask questions such as "How is your mood?" "What would your wife or partner say is wrong?" "Would they say you are depressed?" "What would have to change for you to feel better?".

▶Do not proceed to the physical examination until you have a working diagnosis: the answer is rarely found there (<10%).

Placing the diagnosis in the context of the patient's life: If you do not do this, you will not know what will count as a cure, and, more specifically, different patients need different treatments—see p241. Some factors to focus on might be: the motivation of the patient to get better ("I've got to get my knee better so that I stay strong enough to lift my wife onto the commode"); their general health; social situation; drugs (not forgetting nicotine and alcohol); is help available at home; work (yes/no; type)?

At the end of the history, occasionally there is enough information to start treatment. Usually you may be only, say, 70% sure of the diagnosis, and more information is needed before treatment is commenced.

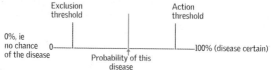

Fig 1.

It is time for the physical **examination**. This aims to gain evidence to confirm or exclude the hypothesis, to define the extent of some process, or to assess the progress of known disease. At each step, ask "What do I need to know?" Following the examination the diagram may look like this:

Primary care

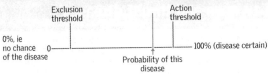

Fig 2.

Investigations If the action threshold has not been crossed, further information is need. Action thresholds vary from doctor to doctor, and from disease to disease. When the treatment is dangerous, the action threshold will be high (eg leukaemia). In self-limiting illnesses, eg pharyngitis, the action threshold will be lower. Note that 'action' may be that, in agreement with such a patient, only symptomatic treatment is needed, and future episodes could be managed without medical input.

Similarly, it may be important to move the probability of a serious but unlikely disease beyond the exclusion threshold.

Once the probability of a disease passes the action threshold, treatment can commence, if the patient wishes.

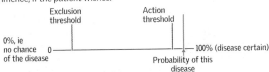

Fig 3.

Supposing neither the action threshold nor the exclusion threshold is exceeded, then more information is needed, eg from pathology, imaging, or the passage of time. Time itself is an investigation: it may reveal sinister causes or the benign nature of the disease. To use time this way, you need to be reasonably sure that immediate treatment is not required.

If there is still not enough certainty to initiate management, get further information, eg from books, computers, colleagues, further tests—or you may feel it appropriate to refer the patient at this stage. Or go round the process again, starting with the history—from a different viewpoint.

Once above the action threshold, it is time to decide what to do for the best. This is a decision shared by the doctor and the patient. It entails informed consent and consideration of:[296]

• The probability of the diagnosis.
• The likelihood of the different possible outcomes.
• The costs and side-effects of treatment.
• The hope and values of those affected, particularly the patient.
• What is possible, considering the skills, resources, and time available.

Finally, tell your patient how they will know if they are on the path to improvement or relapse, and if so, at what point to seek help (critical action threshold, below; record this in the notes)—eg if your peak flow falls by 40%, start this prescription for prednisolone, and come and see me.

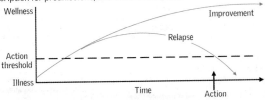

Fig 4.

7 Ear, nose and throat diseases

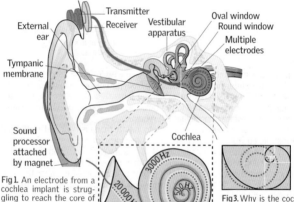

Fig 1. An electrode from a cochlea implant is struggling to reach the core of the cochlea's spiral, but unless it negotiates the ever tightening bends, lower tones (encoded near its core) are unheard, and speech will be distorted. [1-3]

Its spirals vary among mammals depending (perhaps!) on how much low-frequency sounds in their habitat most need amplification via the whispering chamber effect (**fig 3**, whereby sound travelling along a curved wall in a big room remains strong enough to be well-heard on its opposite side).

Cochlea (**fig 2**) is Latin for snail.

Fig 2. Our cochlea is a tapering spiral tube with 2.5 turns. Sometimes after an accident in the 7th embryonic week a child is born with only 1.5 turns (basal turn intact; Mondini's malformation). What is the result? No low-tone hearing. How is it diagnosed? Spiral CT, of course. [4]

Fig 3. Why is the cochlea's spiral (blue) different to simple spirals based on Fibonacci sequences (black)?
Low-tone hearing ranges from mice to whales in step with the pitch of the spiral; the tighter it is, the more sound energy in low-frequency waves is forced against the cochlea's outer wall. Trials show that this 'whispering chamber' effect augments low-frequency sound by ~20dB. [5-7]

Ideally, read this chapter with a good supply of ENT patients, ENT teachers and audiologists to hand. If unavailable, guides to ENT examination are found at www.ispub.com/ostia/index.php?xmlfilepath=journals/ijorl/current.xml. Free full text ENT journals/videos: www.entusa.com/qt_wmv1.htm. For those inspired to learn more, try www.bcm.edu/oto/othersa.html. *We thank Mr Chris Potter FRCS, our ENT Reader.*

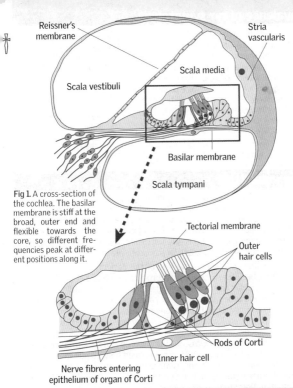

Reissner's membrane

Stria vascularis

Scala media

Scala vestibuli

Basilar membrane

Scala tympani

Fig 1. A cross-section of the cochlea. The basilar membrane is stiff at the broad, outer end and flexible towards the core, so different frequencies peak at different positions along it.

Tectorial membrane

Outer hair cells

Rods of Corti

Inner hair cell

Nerve fibres entering epithelium of organ of Corti

Fig 2. Inside the spiral: the organ of Corti. Hearing and balance rely on the ability of hair cells to sense tiny mechanical stimuli. Outer hair cells are actively motile structures that feed energy into the vibration of the inner ear and enhance sensitivity to sound and movement. The sounds they produce are called otoacoustic emissions (OAE). Detecting OAE is a good test of a healthy inner ear. OAE are detected in neonatal screening tests.[8] OAE and other hair cell functions are impaired by inner ear stressors, by various types of hereditary deafness, syndromic hearing loss,[9] and inner ear disease (eg Ménière's disease).   ©OUP

Active listening Within a few milliseconds of hearing sounds that might be meaningful speech (vs the same sounds played in reverse) we send impulses to the cochlear via medial olivocochlear efferents to improve perception of the speech-associated sounds. This effect it arises thanks in part to efferent effects on OAE. For other aspects of active listening, see fig 1, p371.[10]

From the index...ENT emergencies

▸▸Airway obstruction:
- •Complete (no breath sounds; aphonia; Heimlich manoeuvre[etc] p795
- •Incomplete (with, for example, wheeze or stridor) p566
- •Laryngeal oedema/anaphylaxis p237

▸▸Foreign body in the ear p538

▸▸Sudden sensorineural hearing loss p550

▸▸Perichondritis p536

▸▸Epiglottitis p566

▸▸Epistaxis p562

▸▸Nasal fractures p560

▸▸Nasal foreign body p560

▸▸Retropharyngeal abscess p564

▸▸Orbital cellulitis p420

▸▸Sudden parotid enlargement p578

▸▸Facial nerve palsy p574

▸▸Quinsy p564

▸▸Post-tonsillectomy bleeding p565

In one UK community study (n=15,788), ~20% reported current hearing troubles, eg difficulty with speech in background noise (few wore a hearing aid regularly). 20% reported tinnitus lasting >5 minutes. ~15% reported hayfever[et al] in the last year, 7% sneezing or voice problems, and 31% had severe sore throat/tonsillitis. ~21% reported ever having had dizziness in which things seemed to spin around the individual, 29% unsteadiness/light-headedness, and 13% reported dizziness in which the person seemed to move.[11] Nasal polyp symptoms (p567): 2%.[12]

ENT examination

Examination in ENT differs from some other specialties in that its regions are rather inaccessible. Illumination by a headlight (self-contained or with a separate light source and cable) has replaced the traditional head mirror with light source positioned behind the patient. Hands-free stereoscopic view of cavities is the aim. Patient positioning is also important. Rod lens and flexible fibreoptic scopes for nasendoscopy and laryngoscopy are now routine.

The ear (Position yourself to one side of the patient; begin on the better side, if applicable (otherwise you may forget to examine it at all). Inspect for *scars* (postauricular and endaural suggest mastoid and middle ear surgery respectively) and other abnormalities, eg *perichondritis*, which is a serious infection of the pinna, eg with pseudomonas after cosmetic piercing (vascular supply is impaired, leading to a *cauliflower ear*, ie neocartilage from disrupted perichondrium, unless urgent referral for abscess drainage is made). *To examine the auditory meatus*, pull the pinna up and back to straighten the bend. (In infants, the bony canal has not formed fully, so pull the pinna back and down.) Swab any discharge; remove wax carefully. Insert the largest comfortable aural speculum (don't probe too far—it's sensitive). Any infection/inflammation, stenosis, or exostoses (p538)?

Otoscopy: Practice is the key, (fig **3**, p539). Examine quadrants in turn. Identify the pars tensa, pars flaccida, the handle of the malleus and the cone of light (light reflex) that points to the toes (anteroinferior). Note colour, translucency, and any bulging or retraction of the drum—and *perforations* (size; position; site: marginal or central?). Perforation/retraction of the pars flaccida is serious (p544). Assess drum mobility using a pneumatic attachment for the otoscope or a special Siegle speculum. Lack of movement suggests perforation or middle ear effusion. On squeezing the balloon, the drum should move. Drum movement on a Valsalva manoeuvre means a patent Eustachian tube. Also: free field voice testing (whisper at 40cm); tuning fork test; VII nerve tests.

The nose (Testing smell is often omitted, but often fascinating.[1]) Sit face-to-face (knees together, to the patient's right). Inspect the external nose: size,

---

1 *Smell, sweat, darkness, dirt, and lust* Smells are as hard to name as emotions: when we are told by a novelist or a chef, we say "Yes: that's it!" Smells and emotions go hand in hand with memory. Engrams are the brain's map of memorable events; they include smells which can be the key to accessing the memory. Unrelated word pairs (eg *butter* and *church*) are recalled better if the smells at their encoding are re-presented when we try to recall them. MRI shows the olfactory cortex and anterior hippocampus mediate olfactory routes to hidden memory, and their attendant emotions.[13]

So when we test the sense of smell we are testing consciousness itself—which is no more or less than the interaction of emotion, memory, and sensation. When we re-smell the smells of youth, or re-smell a perfume from a distant *affaire de coeur*, we are transported, de-realized, and moved back to our former selves. For a moment we re-inhabit *lands of lost content* (p468) or torment. Olfaction plugs directly into the limbic system, enabling us to smell and interpret the dark. This expanding of the sense of smell to encompass all things struck Kipling on revisiting Lahore: '*the heat and smell of oil and spices, and puffs of temple incense, and sweat and darkness, and dirt and lust and cruelty.*'[14]

shape, deviations, or deformity. Lift the nose tip to inspect the vestibule. Check patency of each side either with a cold metal tongue depressor or by occluding each nostril in turn with the flat of your thumb: don't press the side in (distorts the other nostril). "Please sniff". *Thudicum speculum (anterior rhinoscopy):* Insert gently; assess mucosa, septum position, and the front of inferior and middle turbinates. Any polyps? Examine the rest of the nasal cavity with rigid endoscopy after spraying with xylometazoline & lidocaine. The middle meatus is a key nasal area as most of the sinuses ventilate via this cleft (between the middle and inferior conchae). The postnasal space (nasopharynx) contains the Eustachian tube orifices & the pharyngeal recess (of Rosenmuller), and may contain adenoids or naso-pharyngeal cancer. A postnasal mirror helps examine the nasopharynx via the oral cavity (these mirrors are usually only seen in clinical exams!). Examine the palate (it's the floor of the nose).

The throat •Position yourself as above; remove any dentures •Inspect lips and perioral region. Ask him to open his mouth without protruding the tongue. Then use a tongue depressor (with light) to retract each cheek: inspect the buccal mucosa, the parotid duct opening (opposite the upper 2nd molar), gums, teeth, floor of the mouth, and the retromolar trigone (mucosa behind the 3rd molar over the ramus of the mandible, a site of tumours that often involve periostium) •Depress the tongue; say "ah then aye" (checks palate movement and exposes more mucosa) •Examine the tonsils (prominent tonsils aren't always enlarged; deep crypts with debris can be normal) •Put on a glove for bimanual examination of the floor of the mouth; any submandibular gland stones or masses? •Palpate the tongue for early invisible tumours.

Free field voice testing NB: not so suitable in children.[15] Other tests: p540.
• Explain what you are about to do. Stand behind the patient.
• To test the right ear, use your left hand to rub the patient's left tragus to mask that ear, then 2ft (60cm), whisper a simple polysyllable, eg "41" or "chicken".
• The patient should be able to repeat what is said at least ½–⅔ of the time; failure represents hearing impairment. This is clarified by (a) coming closer (15cm) and (b) raising the voice to conversational levels—or a shout.

Indirect laryngoscopy (Now rarely done.) The posture is with head extended ("sniffing the morning air"). It is vital to explain what you are about to do.
• Anaesthetize the throat with a rather unpalatable topical 2% lidocaine spray; warn the patient not to eat anything hot for 1–2h after.
• Hold the protruded tongue with a swab with slight forward tension. With the other hand warm a mirror (not too hot!). Examine epiglottis and false cords (ventricular folds). On saying "hee", assess vocal cords and their movement.
• *Flexible nasendoscopy* (4mm) is now preferred to indirect laryngoscopy.

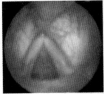

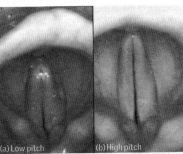

Fig 1. Vocal cords abducted for inspiration (above) and adducted for low (a), and high pitch phonation (b): NB elongation to raise pitch is done by the cricothyroid muscle.

(a) Low pitch

(b) High pitch

Courtesy of James Thomas.

The external ear (fig 1). The auricle is fibroelastic cartilage, covered by skin. The ear drum (figs 1, 3) is set obliquely, the external auditory canal is ~3cm anteriorly and ~2.5cm posteriorly. The canal's outer ⅓ is cartilage, having hairs and ceruminous (wax) glands in the skin; its inner ⅔ is bony and lined with sensitive skin.

Congenital anomalies The auricle develops from 6 hillocks derived from the 1st and 2nd branchial arches that appear at 4–6 wks with the intervening 1st branchial groove forming the external auditory canal. Any malfusion may give rise to accessory tags/auricles or a preauricular pit, sinus, or fistula. An infected sinus may be mistaken for an infected sebaceous cyst, but there is often a deep tract that lies close to the facial nerve. It must be removed to avoid further infection.
▶Auricular anomalies are frequently associated with middle ear anomalies.

Chondrodermatitis nodularis chronica helicis et antihelicis This Latin describes an exquisitely tender cartilaginous inflamed nodule dwelling on the upper helix♂ or antihelix♀ (fig 2). A more convenient name is Winkler's disease.[16] It is commoner in men who work outdoors. Causes: ?poor blood flow (avascular chondritis) from pressure (eg phone addicts)[17] or vasoconstriction from cold. A pressure-relieving prosthesis may help.[18] If not, excise skin and underlying cartilage (eg 'wide excision' or 'deep shave').[19]

Pinna haematoma Blunt trauma may cause bleeding in the subperichondrial plane elevating the perichondrium to form a haematoma. Arrange prompt evacuation. Aspiration is rarely adequate: firm packing conforming to the contours of the auricle may prevent reaccumulation.[20] Sometimes haematoma is found to be within the cartilage itself, which tends to be refractory.[21] Poor treatment leads to ischaemic necrosis, then fibrosis (a cauliflower ear). Secondary infection may cause major loss of cartilage.

Exostoses These are smooth multiple bilateral swellings of the bony canals and said to represent local bony hypertrophy from cold exposure, eg in aquatic sports. Symptoms: none, so long as the lumen is sufficient for sound conduction (so they are often picked up incidentally). When they hinder migration of wax or debris, or when they occlude the canal to cause conductive deafness, surgical removal is indicated. Osteomas (p699) are usually solitary.

Wax (cerumen) Wax is secreted in the outer ⅓ of the canal, to protect against maceration. Due to epithelial migration, the ear is self-cleaning; cotton buds are unnecessary and lead to deafness and discomfort if the wax impacts. Optimal treatment is suction under direct vision using a microscope—but syringing usually works too, using water at ~37°C; eg after softening with olive oil or bicarbonate drops daily for a week;[22] warn of post-op dizziness. Use of drops 30mins pre-syringing is just as good.[23] Or you can instil warm water 15min pre-op in un-oiled ears; this more than halves duration of syringing required.[24] But as 40% of the time oiling is all that is needed, the longer regimen has advantages. At syringing, direct the jet back and up. *Give up after 3 attempts.*[25] Dry the ear after.
▶Avoid syringing if the drum is perforated, if grommets (or within 1½yrs), cleft palate, or after mastoid surgery. *Complications:* Pain; otitis externa; vertigo (0.2%); perforated drum (≤0.2%).[25,26]

Ear FBs Foreign bodies are common if <5yrs old and in adults with learning difficulty. Organic FBs cause much inflammation. Many methods of removal described in the literature: **syringing** can be successful, eg with small objects; take care with objects that almost fill the canal as these may impact, and organic material may swell. **Suction** (± specially designed ends with soft flanges—may prevent FBs penetrating ever deeper), **glue**, **gum**, and **hooks** have their uses.
▶Batteries (eg from hearing aids) need urgent removal. Suction methods:
▶*Always use instrumentation under direct vision.* Difficult patients (eg young children; the anxious) are best referred directly, without inexpert attempts at removal to ↑chance of successful removal with few complications.

ENT diseases

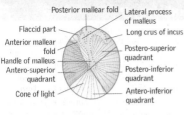

Fig 1. Left drum. The 4 arbitrary quadrants are indicated by solid lines and by the handle of the malleus. The light reflex points to the feet.

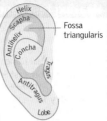

Fig 2. The pinna.

ENT diseases

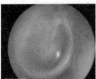

Fig 3. Normal right drum. If only patients could see how beautiful and delicate the drum is, amateur instrumentation of the ear would be far less common!

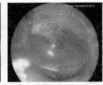

Fig 4. The left drum is retracted, along with the handle of the malleus (appears short). The lateral process will also become more prominent than normal.

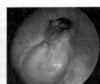

Fig 5. (Right drum) This crust in the attic represents a large underlying cholesteatoma.

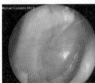

Fig 6. The (right) drum is opaque. There is prominence of blood vessels suggesting a middle ear effusion. This is one of several appearances of glue ear.

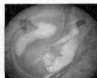

Fig 7. (Right drum) White patches are usually tympanosclerosis (calcium deposits), eg after infection or trauma. They are often of no significance; if severe can cause mild conductive hearing loss.

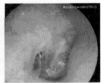

Fig 8. (Right drum) Posterior perforation. Posterior perforations may be serious, but this one is dry, and its posterior margin is defined. Traumatic perforations (eg barotrauma) are often posterior and linear, like a tear rather than a hole.

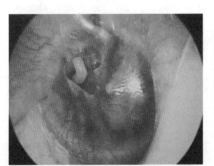

Fig 9. Posterior perforation exposing incudostapedial joint. The irregular shape suggests the cause is trauma. These images may look surprisingly clear: this is because they were taken through a Hopkins rod, rather than an otoscope.

Figs 3–8 courtesy of Michael Saunders FRCS. Fig 9 courtesy of Rory Herdman FRCS.

When assessing suspected hearing loss, determine its nature (conductive or sensorineural), its severity and its cause: is it treatable, and is it part of some other disease process—eg unilateral sensorineural hearing loss (SNHL) in acoustic neuroma? Remember also to assess the degree of disability.

Rinne tuning fork test See *OHCM* p468. If +ve in sudden sensori-neural deafness (air conduction > bone) ►refer same day (p550).● **Free field voice testing** p537.

Audiometry This quantifies loss and determines its nature. *Pure tone audiometry* is the standard measure—figs 1-7. Headphones deliver electronically generated tones at different strengths over frequencies of 250–8000Hz in a sound-proofed room. The patient says when he hears sounds 50% of the time at threshold. This intensity is recorded in decibels (dB) by the tester as the air conduction threshold. A bone conduction threshold is obtained by using a transducer over the mastoid process. Masking (→narrowband noise to the untested ear) prevents cross-stimulation of the non-test ear by raising its threshold. *Speech audiometry* examines speech discrimination above the threshold by asking patients to repeat words presented via headphones. It is assesses disability, and can predict whether a hearing aid would help.

Both pure tone and speech audiometry are subjective tests, *acoustic impedance audiometry (tympanometry)* is objective. A probe with an airtight seal is introduced into the meatus; it measures the proportion of an acoustic signal reflected back at varying pressures and generates a graph of compliance—see fig 3, p547. Tympanometry provides a useful measure of middle ear pressure. A normal ear shows a smooth bell-shaped compliance curve (type A). Fluid in the middle ear flattens the curve (type B). Negative middle ear pressure shifts the peak to the negative side or left (type C).

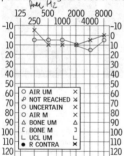

Fig 1. Normal hearing.

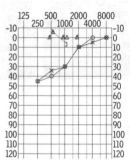

Fig 2. Bilateral middle ear congestion.

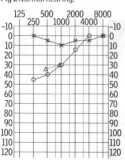

Fig 3. Right-sided Ménières.

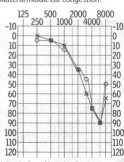

Fig 4. Noise-induced hearing loss.

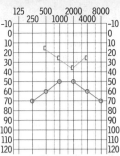

Fig 5. Right-sided otosclerosis, with Carhaarts notch at 2kHz on masked bone conduction.

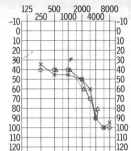

Fig 6. Typical presbyacusis—bilateral, symmetrical, high-frequency SNHL.

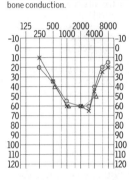

Fig 7. Cookie-bite loss (as if someone took a bite out of the top of the audiogram (isolated mid-range hearing loss). It is likely to be hereditary. Test siblings. Referral to a geneticist may be indicated. (In 'reverse cookie-bite' loss the bite is out of the lower edge.)

Abbreviations
m = masked
um = unmasked

Figs 1–7 ©C Potter

When to refer for speech therapy   Delay in talking: p215

0–1½ years old: Feeding difficulty eg from cleft lip/cerebral palsy.

2 years old: If vocabulary is <30 words or no phrases (but not if good communication skills without speech, and he or she seems on the edge of talking).

3 years old: Unintelligible speech, eg oromotor or verbal dyspraxia (with a quiet voice, poor lip control, with mouth always open and dribbling). Also consider if:
• Using sentences of 2 words only.
• No descriptive words or pronouns used.
• Comprehension↓, eg cannot identify ball or pen by 'which do we draw with?'
• Parental anxiety, if the child is going through a stage of non-fluency.

4 years old: Unclear speech/difficulty in carrying out simple commands.
• Sentences used are less than 3 words; vocabulary is limited.
• Stammering. The Lidcombe program is best started pre-school.[27] In this technique, parents provide verbal contingencies for periods of stutter-free conversation and moments of stuttering. Waiting for natural recovery is not acceptable because of negative social and cognitive consequences.

5 years old: Problems with 'r', 'th', and lisps or articulation difficulties. Also:
• Difficulty understanding simple sentences.
• Difficulty in giving direct answers to simple questions.
• Difficulty with sentence structure; immature sentences; word order.

6 years and older: Persisting articulation or comprehension problem. Also:
• Difficulty with verbal expression or other significant voice problems.

▶*Refer hoarseness and excessive nasality at whatever age they present.*

The cause is often non-otological (in 50%); look for sources of referred pain (OPPOSITE), eg throat and teeth: *does grinding/tapping hurt?*—see p580.

Otitis externa (OE) Minimal discharge, itch, pain and tragal tenderness due to an acute inflammation of the skin of the meatus, eg caused by moisture (swimming), trauma eg fingernails (a consequence from conditions causing itch, eg eczema/psoriasis), high humidity, an absence of wax, a narrow ear canal, and hearing aids.[28] *Pseudomonas* is the chief organism involved, though *Staphylococcus aureus* is another common offender. Hearing loss and canal stenosis (making hearing aids difficult to wear) can be sequelae. ΔΔ: Contact eczema (fig 1).

Aural toilet is the key to treatment. If severe, the meatus is narrowed. A thin Pope wick can be inserted and hydrated with eardrops, eg Sofradex® (framycetin + dexamethasone). An alternative is a strip of ribbon gauze soaked in ichthammol glycerine (very soothing) or aluminium acetate (astringent). After a few days, the meatus will open up enough for either microsuction or careful cleansing with cotton wool. Commercial Qtips® or cotton buds shouldn't be used: they are too large; instead thin out or make one yourself by wrapping a small piece of cotton wool gently around an orange stick. Use drops only short-term, as troublesome fungal infections can arise. Non-specialists should not syringe the ear.

►Beware persistent unilateral otitis externa in diabetics/immunosuppressed/ the elderly: the risk is malignant/necrotizing otitis externa (see BOX).

►OE which is resistant to treatment can be a sign of malignancy. Do biopsy.

Furunculosis This is a very painful staphylococcal abscess arising in a hair follicle. Pathologically it is identical to a boil anywhere else; if there is cellulitis consider flucloxacillin. Diabetes is an important predisposing factor.

Bullous myringitis These are very painful haemorrhagic blisters on deep meatal skin and on the drum (± serosanginous fluid behind it). Classically associated with influenza infection, but *Mycoplasma pneumoniae* has also been implicated as have a variety of other organisms. It may simply represent a variant of acute otitis media. Sensorineural hearing loss is much more frequent than previously thought. Treatment is generally supportive only, eg pain relief; oral antibiotics can be considered in cases with middle ear effusions.

Barotrauma (aerotitis) If the Eustachian tube is occluded, middle ear pressure cannot be equalized during descent in an aircraft or diving, so causing damage. *Risk factors:* Conditions inhibiting function of the Eustachian tube eg inflammation/infection. *Symptoms:* Severe pain as the drum becomes indrawn, eg from transudation or bleeding into middle ear. Barotrauma to the inner ear causes vertigo, tinnitus, and deafness. *Prevention:* Not flying with a URTI, decongestants into the nose (eg xylometazoline every 20min), repeated yawns, swallows/jaw movements. Inflating an Otovent® device is effective (it is recommended to air passengers with problems clearing the ears.)[29] Positive pressure (higher than Eustachian tube resistance) through mask to the nasopharynx can also help.[30] R: Supportive if simple barotrauma; effusions usually clear spontaneously, and most perforations heal.

Temporomandibular joint (TMJ) dysfunction *Symptoms:* Earache, facial pain, and joint clicking/popping related to malocclusion, teeth-grinding (bruxism) or joint derangement, and, importantly, stress, making this a biopsychosocial disorder which may become a chronic pain syndrome (p636).[31,32] *Signs:* Joint tenderness exacerbated by lateral movement of the open jaw, or trigger points in the pterygoids. *Imaging:* MRI. *Associations:* Depression;[33] Ehlers–Danlos, p642.[34] R: NSAIDs (PO or topical, eg diclofenac;[35] stabilizing orthodontic occlusal prostheses;[36] cognitive therapy (p374); physiotherapy; biofeedback; surgery (eg reconstruction);[37] acupuncture.[32]

Performing aural toilet (learn by watching an expert at work)

- Tools: otoscope, cotton wool, Jobson Horne probe, Crocodile forceps, which must be used under a direct headlight.
- Pull the pinna back and up to straighten the canal, and under direct vision, dry mop with Jobson Horne probe with a small piece of cotton wool on its serrated end.
- Clean the auditory meatus with a gentle rotary action; don't touch the drum.
- Replace the cotton wool as becomes soiled. Attend to the anterior-inferior recess, which often harbours debris.
- Intermittently re-examine the meatus, using the otoscope, during cleaning.
- Patients who have mastoid cavities (a surgical widened canal done to treat infection) should be followed up in the ENT department for irrigation and drying. Cavities repeatedly infected may need surgical repair of the posterior wall.
- Take swabs as needed and advise on ear care.

ENT diseases

Referred otalgia: when the cause is not in the ear

Referred (secondary) pain can arise from disease processes in the territories of the sensory nerves supplying the ear:

- *V:* The auriculotemporal nerve (a branch of the trigeminal nerve which supplies lateral upper half of pinna) may refer pain from dental disease and TMJ dysfunction (temporomandibular joint dysfunction, opposite).
- *VII:* A sensory branch of the facial nerve (supplies lateral surface of drum) refers pain in geniculate herpes (Ramsay Hunt syndrome, p652).
- *IX:* Primary glossopharyngeal neuralgia is a rare cause of pain often induced by talking or swallowing.
- *IX & X:* The tympanic branch of the glossopharyngeal nerve and the auricular branch of the vagus (supplies medial surface of drum) refer pain from the cancer of the posterior ⅓ of the tongue, pyriform fossa, or larynx, or from the throat to the ear, eg in tonsillitis or quinsy. Otalgia is common post-tonsillectomy (esp. in adults), so it is worth warning all patients.
- *C2,3:* The great auricular nerve (C2,3, supplying lower ½ of pinna) refers pain from soft tissue injury in the neck and from cervical spondylosis/arthritis.

Use of eardrops in otitis externa

▶Take a swab first, and do aural toilet. Is there chronic otitis externa that needs specialist attention? If not and no perforation, try local drops:

- Betamethasone 0.1% cheap and good for non-infected eczema.
- Framycetin + dexamethasone = Sofradex®.
- Polymyxin B + neomycin+hydrocortisone=Otosporin®.
- Gentamicin 0.3%+hydrocortisone 1% = Gentisone HC® drops; more costly than betamethasone but can be good: advised by some only as a 2nd-line agent, eg in *Pseudomonas* infections. To minimize risks of gentamicin ototoxicity, use for <2wks, and after baseline audiometry (if possible); explain risks and benefits of gentamicin esp. if tympanic perforation.
- Clioquinol 1% + flumetasone=Locorten-Vioform®, not if iodine sensitive).
- Sodium bicarbonate 5% drops are useful if wax is an additional problem.
- ▶Over-treating may lead to fungal infection: if suspected, try clotrimazole 1% solution/8–12h, continued for ≥2weeks after disappearance of infection.

Malignant/necrotizing otitis externa

This is aggressive, life-threatening infection of the external ear that can lead to temporal bone destruction and base-of-skull osteomyelitis. 90% are diabetic. Immunosuppression (and probably aural irrigation)[39] are other risk factors. The cause is usually *Pseudomonas aeruginosa* (also *Proteus* and *Klebsiella*). Treatment is by surgical debridement, systemic antibiotics, specific immunoglobulins, and, possibly, hyperbaric oxygen therapy.[40]

The character of the discharge provides clues to its source and cause:

Causes of discharge to consider
• Otitis externa/media.
• Cholesteatoma (rare but important). NB: crust in the attic/postero-superior quadrant often hides pathology, so remove it.

• *External ear:* Inflammation, ie otitis externa (OE) produces a scanty watery discharge, as there are no mucinous glands—see p542. Blood can result from trauma to the canal. Liquid wax can sometimes 'leak' out.

• *Middle ear:* Mucous discharges are almost always due to middle ear disease. Serosanguinous discharge suggests a granular mucosa of chronic otitis media (COM). An offensive discharge suggests cholesteatoma.

• *CSF otorrhoea:* CSF leaks may follow trauma: suspect if you see a halo sign on filter paper, or its glucose is ↑, or β_2 (tau) transferrin is present.

Acute otitis media (OM) entails middle ear inflammation; it presents with rapid onset of pain, fever±irritability, anorexia, or vomiting often after a viral upper respiratory infection. Chronic OM is inflammation with middle ear fluid of several months' duration. Common organisms: *Pneumococcus, Haemophilus, Moraxella*, other streps and staphs. In acute OM drum bulging causes pain, then purulent discharge if it perforates (often settles in 48h). R: Give analgesia. Amoxicillin (±clavulanate) for ≤7 days is 1st line.[41] Antibiotics are not always needed if well, *and follow-up is simple;*[42] but in one *NEJM* study $\binom{2011}{N=319}$[43] early use of co-amoxiclav did prevented significant morbidity.[44] SE: diarrhoea; resistance/'super-bugs'etc. Decongestants don't help much.[45]

Continuing discharge may indicate complications: mastoiditis which is rare (see below), and even rarer are petrositis; labyrinthitis; facial palsy; meningitis; intracranial abscesses. Mucopus may continue to drain when there is no mastoiditis, especially if grommets are in place. Treat with appropriate oral or topical antibiotics according to swab results. Do aural toilet to remove infected material from meatus. ▶*If discharge continues, get expert help.*

Chronic otitis media This is *mucosal* or *squamous*, and each may be *inactive* or with *active* inflammation.^Browning's classification There is discharge, ↓hearing, but little pain. For glue ear, see p546. Resolution is the rule (eg with antibiotic therapy, p543), but if secretions cannot drain, differentiation into squamous epithelium occurs ± more serious complications, eg a retraction pocket of the *pars tensa* or *flaccida* (fig1, p539).

Cholesteatoma (fig1; ie active squamous chronic otitis media) has serious rare complications (meningitis/cerebral abscess). Incidence: 1:10,000. Peak age: 5–15yrs. It is a misnomer as it is neither cholesterol nor a tumour (it *is* locally destructive around and beyond the *pars flaccida*). Δ: Foul discharge ± deafness; headache, pain, facial paralysis, and vertigo indicate impending CNS complications. R: Mastoid surgery is needed to make a safe dry ear by removing the disease; improving hearing is secondary.

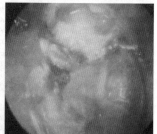
Fig1. Attic cholesteatoma; like cottage cheese with mucopus. ©Rory Herdman FRCS

Mastoiditis: Middle ear inflammation leads to destruction of air cells in the mastoid bone ± abscess formation. Beware intracranial extension. *Risk factors:* Withholding antibiotics in otitis media.[46] *Signs:* T°↑; tender mastoid; protruding auricle. *Imaging:* CT. R: Hospitalization, IV antibiotics, myringotomy ± definitive mastoidectomy.

ENT diseases

Hearing loss from middle ear causes: when to refer

Refer to community audiology service (if available) for:[47]
• Determination of severity and cause of hearing loss. Is it conductive?
• Is the hearing loss leading to a disability?

Refer direct to an ENT consultant if:
• Deaf for over 3 months—or difficulties with speech or learning—or
• Recurrent and persisting earache over a 3-month period—or
• Other disabilities making correction of deafness urgent.

Possibilities while the patient is waiting to be seen:
• Discourage passive smoking. What's it like at the childminder's?
• Encourage drinking from a cup, not a bottle (better Eustachian function).
• Encourage interlocutors to sit at the child's level, and to keep instructions short and simple. Explain the problem to all.
• Turn off the TV (less background noise, and this makes it more likely that the patient will look at the person speaking to him).
• Tell the teacher which side hears best (for class seating plan).
• Nasal steroids for 1 month—or
• **Co-amoxiclav** for 14 days (may be of little real benefit)—or
• Oral steroids for 5 days (eg **prednisolone** 1mg/kg/day PO).

ENT diseases

Tympanomastoid surgery for chronic otitis media

Canal wall down (CWD) and canal wall up (CWU) mastoidectomy are 2 surgical ways to address chronic middle ear cleft pathology. CWD probably results in worse hearing outcomes and a mastoid cavity which may require lifelong follow-up or later surgical obliteration. CWU surgery requires a second-look procedure at 1yr, but advances in MRI may obviate the need for this in the near future. NB: endoscopes are improving visualization in CWU techniques.[48]

Post-op complications include failure of the self-cleaning mechanism of the canal with either a skin-lined healed cavity (dry), or chronic (or URTI-associated) discharge ± blood and pain. Here, repeat visits are needed (eg ×3/yr) to the ENT ward for removal of wax and skin debris, debridement (see MINIBOX) and endoscopy to identify further infection or cholesteatoma.

Debriding an infected mastoid cavity
►Aim to remove all infected epithelium.
• Culture secretions
• Clean with hydrogen peroxide
• Remove debris/patches of granulation using suction and curette
• Silver nitrate cautery to polyps (avoid use anywhere near cranial nerve VII)
• Control bleeding with cotton balls (eg adrenaline-soaked).

Risk factors for otitis media

• URTI (and autumn/winter)
• Bottle-feeding
• Passive smoking
• Dummy/pacifier[49]
• Presence of adenoids
• Asthma
• Malformations (eg cleft palate)
• Gastro-oesophageal reflux/BMI↑ in adults

This is detected by otoscopy (fluid level or bubbles behind the drum) or indirectly, by tympanometry (fig 3). 50% of 3-yr-olds have ≥1 ear effusion/yr.[50] *In adults, exclude a postnasal space tumour as the cause of middle ear fluid.*

Glue ear/OME (otitis media with effusion; serous/secretory otitis media). ►*Hearing impairment noticed by parents is the mode of presentation in 80%.* The fundamental problem lies with dysfunction of the Eustachian tubes. The exact cause is unclear, but there are associations with upper respiratory tract infections, oversized adenoids and narrow nasopharyngeal dimensions. Bacterial biofilms present on the adenoids can be a source of infection, and are probably more important indicators of trouble than adenoid size. OME is commoner in boys, Down's syndrome, winter season, atopy, children of smokers and primary ciliary dyskinesia.[1] OME is the chief cause of hearing loss in young children, and can cause disastrous learning problems (rare). OME may cause no pain, so its presence may not be suspected.

History: Focus on poor listening, poor speech, language delay, inattention, poor behaviour, hearing fluctuation, ear infections/URTI, balance and, school work.

Signs: Variable, eg retracted or bulging drum. It can look dull, grey, or yellow. There may be bubbles or a fluid level, or superficial radial vessels and ↓drum mobility when tested with a Siegle speculum or with a pneumatic attachment.

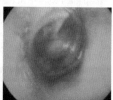

Fig 1. Glue ear with retracted drum & dull drumhead.
©R Herdman FRCS.

Tests: Audiograms: Look for conductive defects. *Impedance audiometry:* Look for flat tympanogram (fig 3; helps distinguish OME from Eustachian malfunction and otosclerosis).

R̩: It usually resolves over time. Explanation/reassurance + 3-monthly review may be enough.

Topical and systemic methods: NICE doesn't recommend antibiotics, diet change, antihistamines, decongestants, steroids—or acupuncture.[etc]

Hearing aids: Reserve for persistent bilateral OME and hearing loss if surgery is not accepted.

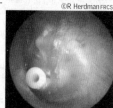

Fig 2. A grommet. ©R Herdman FRCS.

Surgery: If persistent bilateral OME + hearing level in better ear of <25–30dBHL($_{hearing\ loss}^{=decibel}$) confirmed over 3 months then myringotomy + suction of fluid, and insertion of air-conducting grommets ± adenoidectomy[2] (if hearing loss).[51] NICE also says surgery is an option if hearing loss is less severe but learning difficulties are to the fore. *Grommets* are preferred to T-tubes (tympanostomy tube), which cause too many complications[52] (eg residual perforation ≈50%). The main complications of grommets are infections and tympanosclerosis. Treat infections with aural toilet and antibiotic/steroid ear drops; grommet removal may be needed. Tonsillectomy doesn't help.[53]

Post-op: 90,000 operations/yr are done for OME in the UK (1 in 200 children). It is OK to swim with grommets, but avoid forcing water into the ear by diving. Some form of ear plug is wise, eg cotton wool and Vaseline® (esp. when shampooing as soap reduces the surface tension of water). Grommets extrude after ~3–12 months; recheck the hearing then; ~25% need re-insertion.

Prognosis: Language development sequelae, eg ↓reading skills, may persist.[54]

1 PCD/Kartagener's syndrome (p646) often causes otitis media and OEM throughout childhood (owing to loss of ciliary function in the Eustachian tube and middle ear), despite fairly continuous antibiotics. After 18yrs of age, the condition improves somewhat. Grommet placement do not improve ear function.[55]
2 Unless loss of hearing is a problem, adenoidectomy offers little benefit over watchful waiting in terms of URTI-associated stuffiness, mouth breathing and quality of life, as these symptoms get less with age.[51]

Grommets and hearing gain: what do meta-analyses say?

Use of grommets to ventilate the middle ear is common but controversial. In one careful review (Browning 2010) of research in children with OME the effect of grommets on hearing, as measured by standard tests, was small (~12dB) and diminished after 6 months (4dB) by which time natural resolution had led to improved hearing in non-surgically treated children[56] No effect was found on language or speech development or behaviour, or cognitive or quality-of-life outcomes. Tympanosclerosis (fig 7, p539) was seen in ~⅓ of ears receiving grommets. No effect was found on other child outcomes but data on these were sparse. No good study has been done in children with established speech, language, learning or developmental problems so no conclusions can be made regarding treatment of such children. Note that adenoidectomy added to grommets often gives the best results.[57] Target trial

ENT diseases

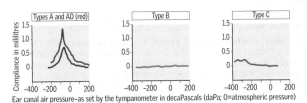

Ear canal air pressure–as set by the tympanometer in decaPascals (daPa; 0=atmospheric pressure)

Fig 3. Acoustic impedance audiometry (tympanometry).

Courtesy of Jane Jones, Oxford Radcliffe Hospitals NHS Trust.

Acoustic impedance audiometry (tympanometry) (fig 3) *Principles:* In normal ears, compliance of the drum (the amount of displacement in mL for a given sound—hence transmission of sound—peaks when middle ear pressure = ear canal pressure. So the peak of the tympanometry curve reflects middle ear pressure. *Operation:* The tympanometer has various sized probes that snugly fit most ears. As it continuously changes the pressure in the ear canal, a transmitter sends a sound to the drum. The wave that is reflected from the drum is then picked up by a microphone in the probe. The tympanometer measures the energy of the reflected sound. *Results:* If the middle ear space is filled with air, and the ossicles are intact, energy is absorbed by the drum, the ossicles, and inner ear structures, and the tracing will show a normal peak with normal compliance (TYPE A, PURPLE).

If there is disruption of the ossicles, or if part of the drum is flaccid, a large amount of energy will be absorbed into the drum which is free to move a lot—and it will move most when canal pressure=middle ear pressure (high compliance; type AD). Fluid in the middle ear makes the drum stiff, so most of the sound is reflected back to the probe—and changing the pressure in the canal has little effect—hence a low, flat result (low compliance, TYPE B). This finding must be related to ear canal volume (also measured by the tympanometer): if normal ≈ otitis media; if low ≈ wax occlusion; if high ≈ grommets or perforation. TYPE C: Shift in peak of the curve to the left found with negative middle ear pressure, eg as in developing or resolving otitis media.[58]

►*If you or a parent are worried, refer to a local community audiology unit.*

Congenital causes
Central (rare): Hyperbilirubinaemia/kernicterus, hypoxia, IVH.
Conductive: Anomalies of pinna, external ear canal, drum, or ossicles, congenital cholesteatoma, Treacher–Collins' (p655), Pierre Robin (p650).
Sensorineural hearing loss—SNHL (sometimes no cause is found):
- *Autosomal dominant:* Waardenburg (SNHL, heterochromia, fig1, p425 & telecanthus, ie ↑distance between medial canthi), Klippel–Feil, Alport (p648, 638).
- *Autosomal recessive:* Pendred (SNHL with goitre), Usher's syndrome (SNHL, retinitis pigmentosa), Jervell and Lange-Nielsen (JSNLL1—SNHL, long QT interval).
- *X-linked:* Alport's syndrome, Turner's syndrome.
- *Infections:* CMV, HSV, syphilis, rubella, toxoplasmosis, group B strep sepsis.
- *Ototoxic drugs.*

Perinatal and postnatal causes Anoxia, birth trauma, cerebral palsy, kernicterus, meningitis, ototoxic drugs, lead, skull fracture.

Universal newborn hearing screening (UNHS) Screening within hours of birth is the best way to ensure that deafness is diagnosed and managed **before 6 months old.** ►This does improve language.[59] Tests: *Otoacoustic emissions (OAE):* A microphone in the external meatus detects tiny cochlear sounds produced by movement in its basilar membrane in response to an auditory stimulus. OAE evaluates function of the peripheral auditory system, primarily the cochlea, the area most often involved in SNHL.[60] This is abnormal or equivocal in 3-8%.[61] Most of these 'failures' (84%) have external ear canal obstruction (collapsed ear canal or debris).[62] In these patients, ABR (see below) should be measured.[63,64] *Audiological brainstem responses (ABR):* The ears are covered with earphones that emit a series of soft clicks. Electrodes on the infant's forehead and neck measure brain wave activity in response to the clicks. ABR tests the auditory pathway from the external ear to the lower brainstem. *Prevalence of deafness found at UNHS:* 0.9-3.24 : 1000 for permanent bilateral hearing loss of >35dB; 5.95:1000 when unilateral and moderate hearing loss infants are counted.[65] No test performs perfectly![66]

Subjective hearing tests in the older child
- *7 months: Distraction testing* (suitable if aged 6-18 months, though not a very accurate technique): As the child sits on parent's lap, an assistant in front attracts the child's attention while a tester attempts to distract by making noises behind and beside child, eg with a rattle, conversational voice.
- *2-4 years: Conditioned response audiometry* (at 24-60 months): The child is trained to put pegs into holes or give toys to a parent on a particular auditory cue. This method can also obtain PTAs (pure tone audiograms) in an older child. *Speech discrimination:* (24-60 months): the child touches selected objects cued by acoustically similar phrases, eg *key/tree.*
- *5 years: Pure tone audiogram.*

Management Aim to provide as good hearing as possible to help language and education. Teachers of the deaf make arrangements for fitting hearing aids and help monitor progress. Children usually need higher gain from their aids than adults. Encourage parents to talk as much as possible to their deaf child. Children may be educated at ordinary schools with visits from teachers of the deaf, or, for the partially hearing, in special units in ordinary schools, or in schools for the deaf, depending on need. A *cochlear implant* may be suitable (BOX). NB: the shorter the duration of deafness, the better the outcome, so funding decisions must not be delayed. *Preventing post-implantation meningitis:* ►Give pneumococcal vaccine ≥2wks before implant (or vaccinate the unvaccinated if implant already *in situ*). ►Treat any otitis media promptly; if recurrent, insert grommets. ►Give IV antibiotics if mastoiditis suspected.[67]

ENT diseases

Cochlear implant issues[1]

Cochlear implant image: p534

They take ~2h to fit (under GA); an external device processes sound and transmits it across the skin to the subcutaneous receiver coil—to an electrode placed in the cochlea via the round window and directly stimulates the auditory nerve. The signal is not normal sound; rehabilitation is needed to understand the new sounds. Benefits: better lip-reading; recognition of environmental sounds, relief of isolation. Cost: ≤£35,000. Pre-op assessment is vital. Give pneumococcal vaccine. Selection criteria: best if language has been acquired. Age is no limit. Commitment is vital. Exclude central deafness.

Implants may be damaged by direct trauma, MRI, surgical diathermy, dental pulp testers and 'therapeutic' (short-wave and microwave) diathermy used in physiotherapy departments. www.bcig.org tel.: 0207 915 1301

Economic and ethical issues with cochlear implants These have been addressed by NICE. Guidance now states that they may be considered in profound sensorineural deafness whether a pre-language child or a deaf adult. Beware statements such as "after cochlear implant patients can lead normal lives" (this may only mean that *other* people don't notice the hearing problem). Post-op training is vital, and the user is by no means an inactive recipient. NB: quality is now sufficient for previously deaf people to be able to use mobile phones.

QALYs For multichannel cochlear implants, average cost per QALY (quality-adjusted life-year) for prelingually very deaf children is ~£13,413/QALY[68] which is in the middle of quoted estimates for costed NHS therapies (for a list, see *OHCM* p10). Implantation of those at least up to 70yrs old makes economic sense. NB: multiple disabilities are no bar to benefit from a device, but it is not clear that they merit extra consideration (they certainly merit full assessment).

Does deafness always count as a disability? Some deaf families particularly welcome the arrival of a deaf child, and some deaf couples selecting donors for artificial insemination choose a deaf father with a 'good' pedigree of deafness.[69] Such offspring will not grow up in a deaf world—so it is very debatable whether this is in the child's best interests, especially as in some areas sign language is dying out owing to the absence of congenital rubella.

BAHA: the bone-anchored hearing aid

This hearing aid augments bone conduction. It is best suited to conductive hearing loss, unilateral hearing loss, and children and adults with hearing loss who do not get on with 'in ear' or 'behind ear' aids. A trial of a bone conductor is traditionally used to determine whether BAHA will work well. They have a special benefits in some children with complex disorders because the children do not physically feel the presence of the hearing aid. On quality of life measures BAHA do very well. Complications are reported in 6% (eg skin regrowth around the titanium screw and non-osseointegration).[70-72]

Indications: Intolerance of conventional hearing aids (draining ear; mastoid cavity; topical sensitivity); congenital malformations (eg microtia; atresia); single-sided deafness. *Contraindications:* Average bone threshold worse than 45dB; non-compliance; poor hygiene; lack of bone volume.[73]

I t is not the actual sound itself that matters, but the reverberations that it makes as it travels through our mind. These are often to be found far away, strangely transformed; but it is only by gathering up and putting together these echoes and fragments that we arrive at the true nature of our experience. Virginia Woolf, 1926. Note that deepening the emotional content of music, for example, by association melody with concrete events in our lives depends on dealings in ancient sub-neocortical limbic regions such as the hippocampus, amygdala,[74] and anterior cingulate cortex, which form the hub of all our emotions, passions, and delights.

ENT diseases

Many cope well with mild hearing loss if given comprehensive rehabilitation.

Management Classify the deafness (BOX); find treatable causes. Exclude the dangerous (esp. if asymmetric): acoustic neuroma, cholesteatoma, effusion from nasopharyngeal cancer. *Palliative*: eg fitting a suitable aid. *Definitive*: eg surgery for perforations or otosclerosis. Severe sensorineural deafness (>100–120dB) may be helped by a *cochlear implant* (fig 1 p534 & 549 BOX 1) to stimulate residual neural tissue.

Is your hearing reduced?
• Do people 'mumble'?
• Do you keep saying "What?"
• Do you misunderstand names?
• Is your TV volume 'too loud'?
• Are noisy rooms a problem?

Sudden hearing loss • *If sensorineural:* ▶Immediate specialist referral, see BOX 3. *Definition:* Loss of ≥30dB in 3 contiguous pure tone frequencies over ≤72h. Incidence: 5–20 per 100,000/yr. ♂:♀≈1:1. Partial or complete spontaneous recovery occurs in 30–65%. Detailed evaluation reveals underlying diseases (eg noise exposure; gentamicin toxicity; mumps; acoustic neuroma; MS; vasculopathy; TB; rarities[1]) in 10%. *Tests:* BOX 3. Start rehabilitation early. *Prognosis:* Better if early presentation. Negative prognostic factors: Age <15yrs or >65yrs, ↑ESR, vertigo, hearing loss in the opposite ear, severe hearing loss.[75] There is evidence that idiopathic causes may respond to steroids ± hyperbaric O_2 therapy, if given promptly.[76] Anticoagulants, aciclovir, and carbamazepine are often given, but are of dubious efficacy.

• *Conductive:* A cause is 'always' found: infection, occlusion, trauma, fracture.

Otosclerosis Prevalence 0.5–2% clinically, 10% subclinically.[•] *Cause:* Autosomal dominant with incomplete penetrance; 50% have a family history. 85% are bilateral; ♀:♂≈2:1. *Pathology:* Vascular spongy bone replaces normal lamellar bone of otic capsule origin particularly around the oval window which fixes the stapes footplate. *Symptoms* usually appear in early adult life and are made worse by pregnancy, menstruation, and the menopause. There is conductive deafness (hearing is often better with background noise), 75% have tinnitus; mild, transient vertigo is common too. 10% have Schwartz's sign—a pink tinge to the drum; audiometry with masked bone conduction shows a dip at 2kHz (Cahart's notch). *Treatment:* Historically by fenestration. Fluoride may inhibit sclerotic progression.[77] Hearing aid or surgery to replace the adherent stapes with an implant[2] helps 90%. Microdrill and CO_2 laser stapedotomy give similar results.[78] Many prefer surgery to wearing an aid[79] (1–4% risk of a dead ear). **Cochlear implant** is another option (if severe).[80]

Presby(a)cusis (Age-related hearing loss from accumulated environmental noise toxicity.) Loss of high-frequency sounds starts before 30yrs; rate of loss is progressive thereafter. Deafness (loss of hair cells: see fig 3, p535) is gradual and we do not usually notice it until hearing of speech is affected with loss of high-frequency sounds (consonants at ~3–4kHz are needed for speech discrimination). Hearing is most affected in the presence of background noise. Hearing aids are the usual treatment. See pure tone audiograms on p541 (fig 2).

Tips on communicating with those who are hard of hearing
• Decrease background noise. Use of an induction loop system (eg a wire around the TV room) achieves this for those with suitably adapted aids (with a switch, ie the T setting; NB: some new aids are too small for these).
• Use short sentences. Be on the same level as the person you are addressing.
• Ensure that light falls on your face.

Unilateral sensorineural deafness Think of acoustic neuroma.

---

1 Stroke; sarcoidosis;[81] Takayasu's arteritis; *Chlamydia pneumoniae*; immune complexes; autoantibodies to inner ear proteins; anticardiolipin (ACL) antibodies; cellular immune defects.[82]
2 Middle ear implants: Surgical implantation of auditory devices is a rapidly growing area in the rehabilitation of deafness. They should be viewed as an alternative to conventional hearing aids for individuals who are either unable to wear hearing aids or reject them for any reason.[83]

ENT diseases

Classification of deafness

Conductive deafness There is impaired sound transmission via the external canal and middle ear ossicles to the foot of the stapes through a variety of causes. External canal obstruction (wax, pus, debris, foreign body, developmental anomalies); drum perforation (trauma, barotrauma, infection); problems with the ossicular chain (otosclerosis, infection, trauma); and inadequate Eustachian tube ventilation of the middle ear (eg with effusion secondary to nasopharyngeal carcinoma) all result in conductive deafness.

Sensorineural deafness results from defects central to the oval window in the cochlea (sensory), cochlear nerve (neural) or, rarely, more central pathways. Ototoxic drugs (eg streptomycin, vancomycin, gentamicin, chloroquine and hydroxychloroquine, vinca alkaloids), postinfective (meningitis, measles, mumps, flu, herpes, syphilis), cochlear vascular disease, Ménière's (p554), trauma, and presbyacusis are all sensorineural. *Rare causes:* Acoustic neuroma, B_{12} deficiency, multiple sclerosis, secondary carcinoma in the brain.

Choosing an aid: head-to-head speech *vs* cross-talk (amid noise)

Amplifying speech is a major factor to take into account when choosing an aid: get help from independent experts as digital technologies are constantly improving. We know that speech is best heard when listening binaurally. The benefits of directional microphones in hearing aids are also well documented in lab settings. If it is necessary to fit 2 aids, should they both be directional (symmetrical directional fitting)? Yes, if the speech comes from in front of the listener (head-to-head) and the noise sources are located to the side of or surround the listener. When speech is located to the side of the listener, use of directional processing on the ear adjacent to the speaker is likely to reduce speech audibility and thus degrade speech understanding.[84] NB: hearing aids with directional microphones cannot be fitted entirely within the ear canal, and so are more noticeable that smaller aids. Also, aids that fit in the canal may give better results with the telephone.

▶▶Managing sudden sensorineural deafness: a summary

▸▸Get expert ENT help.
▸▸Look for causes: WR; ANA; INR; TSH; blood glucose; cholesterol; ESR; FBC; LFT; viral titres; audiology; evoked response audiometry ± CXR; Mantoux; MRI; pANCA; lymph node and nasopharyngeal biopsy for malignancy/TB culture.
▸▸Imaging: gadolinium MRI; CT.
▸▸Audiometry and auditory brainstem evoked responses.
▸▸High-dose steroids are no more effective when combined with antivirals. One starting regimen is **prednisolone 80mg/24h PO** for 4 days tapered over 8 days.[85] Intratympanic dexamethasone may have a salvage role.

The bounds of 'normal' hearing

Both frequency (Hz) and sound pressure (decibels, dB) are important for the detection of sound by the human ear, though the relationship between the two is also important. Sound frequencies between 500 and 4000Hz are the most important for speech interpretation. Severe sensorineural deafness is defined as >100–120dB loss; significant hearing loss is considered as >35dB loss. Remember that decibels are a logarithmic scale, and that the range from 0 to 120dBs actually represents a million times relative increase in sound pressure. Another unit for the sound pressure (≈'volume' in common parlance) is the dyne/cm², which is not a logarithmic scale.

At high intensity (≥130dB), sound can also be a *painful* stimulus, showing an interesting (and variable) threshold relationship between useful information from special senses and painful stimuli (also present in the eye).

Tinnitus (Latin *tinnire,* meaning to ring) is a sensation of non-verbal sound not due to stimuli outside the body. Age of onset is 50-60yrs (peak). Ringing, hissing, or buzzing suggests an inner ear or central cause. Popping or clicking suggests problems in the external or middle ear, or the palate. Pulsatile sounds (*somatosounds*) may reflect anxiety, benign intracranial hypertension, vascular causes: glomus tumours (fig 1), carotid body tumours, carotid stenosis, arteriovenous malformations, aneurysms, hypertension,[86] and high-output cardiac states (Paget's, hyperthyroidism).[87]

Central tinnitus Most people get tinnitus, but automatically suppress it. If this suppression fails, tinnitus is intrusive and is perceived as a threat. Tinnitus training (below) reduces this threat. 4 areas of concern: *altered central processing; spontaneous otoacoustic emissions; crosstalk* between adjacent nerve fibres from myelin damage after trauma, and, very importantly *auditory–limbic interactions,* esp. the nucleus accumbens (mediates negative emotions, see functional MRI data).[88] It is likely that feedback connections from limbic regions block the tinnitus signal from reaching auditory cortex.[89] Diagnosing **subjective idiopathic tinnitus (SIT)** depends on excluding: 1 *Local causes,* eg hearing loss; presbyacusis; noise-induced; head injury; otosclerosis/post-stapedectomy; Ménière's. 2 *General: Cardiovascular:* BP↑, Hb↓, heart failure. 3 *Drugs:* Aspirin; loop diuretics; aminoglycosides, quinine, alcohol excess. Assess *psychological associations* (eg redundancy, divorce, retirement).

The patient *History:* Character (constant? pulsatile?); alleviating/exacerbating factors; otalgia; social surroundings (tinnitus is worse if isolated or depressed); drugs. *Impact:* does it disturbs sleep? *Associations:* deafness (prevalence rises to up to 100% in noise-induced trauma, 80% in severe deafness, and 70% in Schwannomas).[90] *Signs:* Otoscopy to detect drum mobility (patulous Eustachian tube or myoclonus of tensor tympani) and middle ear disease; hearing/tuning fork tests. BP & pulse. *Tests:* Audiometry (with masking), tympanogram (+stapedial reflex thresholds). ►In unilateral tinnitus do MRI to exclude acoustic neuroma (p553; 10% present this way). Hb; lipids; ?WR[et al]

R: Take time to explain tinnitus. Do tests to exclude acoustic neuroma (MRI) and transmitted noise (eg glomus tympanicum tumours, fig 1). Treat the treatable; support and reassure to help remodel symptoms. Positive attitudes help; avoid saying "it's untreatable; nothing can be done". Treat the whole person, not just a malfunctioning ear.

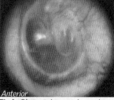

Anterior

Fig 1. Glomus tympanicum tumour: note red anterior mass and a small fluid meniscus around it.
©Rory Herdman FRCS.

- *Aids:* If hearing loss >35dB, a hearing aid that improves perception of background noise makes tinnitus less apparent. Masking with background white noise is no longer advised.
- *Psychological support* is vital; therapists use tinnitus retraining therapy (TRT makes tinnitus less intrusive, by sound therapy, and dispelling unfounded beliefs/fears). Cognitive therapy (p374) and patient groups help.
- *Music, massage* and other media may have a role.[91]
- *Drugs:* None are standard. Melatonin (~3mg at night, p404) *may* help, eg if sleep disturbance is bad; hypnotics are addictive. Betahistine only helps if Ménière's is the cause. Baclofen (10mg/12h PO up to 30mg/12h over 3wks) may also help. Anticonvulsants, eg carbamazepine, aren't much better than placebos but with side effects (in 18%). A meta-analysis of 'near or total eradication of tinnitus annoyance' showed no effect of anticonvulsants.[93]
- *Intratympanic dexamethasone* + oral alprazolam helped 76% (less for SIT of long duration) in one randomized study.[94][N=107]
- *Surgery:* Has little role. Destructive techniques are rarely justified.

Acoustic neuroma

These are typically indolent, histologically benign subarachnoid tumours that cause problems by local pressure, and then behave as space-occupying lesions. They are misnomers as they usually arise from the superior vestibular nerve schwann cell layer, hence the name *vestibular schwannoma*. *The patient:* Progressive ipsilateral tinnitus ± sensorineural deafness (cochlear nerve compression). Big tumours may give ipsilateral cerebellar signs or ICP↑ signs. Giddiness is common; vertigo rare. Trigeminal compression above the tumour may give a numb face. Nearby cranial nerves at risk: (V, VI, VII). *Tests:* MRI. ▶Do MRI in all those with unilateral tinnitus/deafness. ΔΔ: Meningioma. *Surgery:* (difficult, and often not needed, eg if elderly);[95] there are many methods with various ways of preserving hearing and the facial nerve (eg continuous intraoperative monitoring of evoked electromyograms).[96] Gamma knife surgery is one good way to ↓ neuroma volume. *Follow-up:* MRI detects expansion.

Noise and the dangers of excessive noise

Our waking and sleeping lives are bathed in seas of noise. Let's attend to our current soundscape: in my case, Sussex rain not quite drowned out by a string quartet and a phone ringing. For many it will be the unending roar of traffic, sirens, aircraft, urban strife, car alarms, and the shouts of the angry pursuing the drunk, maybe all occluded by MP3 earphones. What is the effect of all this noise?[97]

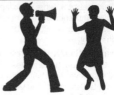

Fig 1. Noise causing helplessness.

- Pain (rape alarms hurt)
- Hearing fatigue ± tinnitus
- Presbyacusis/hearing loss
- Fatigue, somatization[103]
- Feelings of helplessness, fig 1
- Sleep disturbance and all its consequences[98,99]
- School problems (↓reading ability)[100]
- Cardiac output↓;[101] MI risk↑; hypertension[102]
- Neuroendocrine issues & CD4 cells & IgG↓[104]
- Poor memory, depression, even suicide[105]

Hyperacusis (auditory discomfort at 20-34dB) Peripheral causes: facial nerve palsy; myasthenia; tympanoplasty. Central: MS; AV malformations; work as a musician; migraine; pervasive refusal syndrome (unable to move/speak, closed eyes, tics, grimacing, hyperacusis ± hyperaesthesia). Management: earplugs.

Vibroacoustic disease (VAD) is a whole-body pathology (+loss of cilia) that develops in those exposed to ↑infrasound (0-20Hz) or deep noise (cabin crew, pilots, disc-jockeys). VAD causes abnormal growth of extracellular matrices (collagen & elastin) in blood vessels, pericardium,[106] trachea, and lung (fibrosis).

Avoiding noise-induced hearing loss Attend to sense, symbol, soma, and soundscape.[103] Turn the volume down. Avoid cities! Listen to nightingales; abide by health and safety rules; don't build houses near railways or runways;[107] wear ear muffs; support urban plans that address noise. Reframe auditory-somatic experience and address feelings of vulnerability, and defencelessness.[103]

Examining the nightingale's code:[1G] As a medical student, John Keats had a troubling time walking the noisy wards of Guy's Hospital, which were forever on the edge of chaos (p397): 'here, where men sit and hear each other groan' he reframed, for all time, the white noise and chaos of our lives into the sublime. Each midnight we must repeat this trick so that we can hear ourselves think, by trumping the groans of the sick by the nightingales of the mind.

Darkling I listen; and, for many a time,
I have been half in love with easeful Death,
Call'd him soft names in many a musèd rhyme,
To take into the air my quiet breath;

Now more than ever seems it rich to die,
To cease upon the midnight with no pain,
While thou art pouring forth thy soul abroad
In such an ecstasy!   *Ode to a Nightingale*

Vertigo can be *ghastly*. Find out if there other features: feeling unreal, panicky, loss of memory.

Vestibular (peripheral) vertigo is often severe, and may be accompanied by nausea, vomiting, hearing loss, tinnitus, and nystagmus (usually horizontal). Hearing loss and tinnitus are less common in central vertigo (it is usually less severe). Nystagmus may be horizontal or vertical with central vertigo, and may be different in each eye (eg the abducting eye in MS).

Is the symptom vestibular? "I'm dizzy" is ambiguous. Elicit the illusion! Ask "Did you or the world seem to spin (like getting off a playground roundabout?)" or "Which *way* are things going?" Those with vertigo often know without hesitation; if not, this is a cue to pursue other causes (lightheadedness ± a 'sense of collapse' can be vascular, ocular, musculoskeletal, metabolic, or claustrophobic). ▶Ask about duration of vertigo: seconds to minutes≈BPPV; 30mins to 30h≈Ménière's or migraine; 30h to a week≈acute vestibular failure.

Causes (often multifactorial)
Peripheral
● Ménière's disease
● Benign positional (postural) vertigo (BPV)
● Vestibular failure
● Labyrinthitis
● Cholesteatoma
Central
● Acoustic neuroma
● Multiple sclerosis
● Head injury
● Inner ear syphilis
● Vertebrobasilar insufficiency
Drugs (central/ototoxic)
● Gentamicin (neuronitis)
● Diuretics
● Co-trimoxazole
● Metronidazole

Examination/tests Assess CNS & ears (esp. middle ear). Test cranial nerves, cerebellar function & reflexes. Assess: nystagmus, gait, Romberg's test (+ve if balance is worse when eyes are shut, implying defective joint position sense or vestibular input) and Unterberger's (march up and down on the spot with arms stretched out in front and eyes closed; +ve if >45° turn in ≤50 steps).[108] Do provocation tests (*Hallpike test*, BOX). If equivocal, do audiometry ± electronystagmography; brainstem auditory evoked responses; calorimetry (the only way to test each labyrinth[1] separately; irrigate each canal with water 7°C above and below body T°: is nystagmus induced?); CT; MRI.

Ménière's disease Dilatation of the endolymphatic spaces[2] of the membranous labyrinth causes vertigo for ~12h with prostration, nausea/vomiting ± a feeling of fullness in the ear; uni- or bilateral tinnitus ± sensorineural deafness (eg fluctuating). Attacks occur in clusters (<20/month). *Cause:* A mystery! Δ: Electrocochleography; endolymphatic space MRI. R: Prochlorperazine as Buccastem® 3mg/8h PO (1st-line if vomiting) or betahistine 16mg/8h PO or chlortalidone may help.[109–111] Surgical approaches, eg endolymphatic shunts, seem logical, but robust evidence (using sham surgery for controls) is lacking. Labyrinthectomy may stop vertigo but causes total ipsilateral deafness; vestibular neurectomy spares hearing. Day-case installation of ototoxic drugs (gentamicin via a grommet) has been tried and can avoid deafness.

Acute vestibular failure follows a febrile illness in adults, eg in winter (eg herpes simplex virus type 1). Sudden vertigo, vomiting, and prostration are exacerbated by head movement. R: Try cyclizine 50mg/8h PO. Improvement occurs in days, though full recovery occurs within 2-3 weeks (longer if elderly). Methylprednisolone may also help, but valaciclovir does not.[112] It is impossible to distinguish from 'viral labyrinthitis' and so this term is best avoided.

Vertigo due to incomplete vestibular compensation After inner ear injury the brain adapts to the altered sensory input and the perception of vertigo fades over days to weeks—or never happens. Relapses in compensation (decompensation) in response to new physical or emotional stresses also occurs.

1 The cochlea (fig 1, p534) and the semicircular canals are called the **labyrinth** as its shape reminds us of the labyrinth built by Daedalus to imprison the Minotaur (½ bull, ½ man, who ate 7 virgins/yr). Like Daedalus, we are all prone to build structures such as books that seem designed for others to get lost in.
2 Also called *endolymphatic hydrops*. **Endolymph** is the fluid in the scala media (fig 3, p535) that is of a similar make-up to intracellular fluid. **Perilymph** is similar to CSF in composition, and is the fluid in the scala tympani and the scala vestibuli of the cochlea, that communicate at its apex via the helicotrema.

Benign positional vertigo

Attacks of sudden rotational vertigo lasting >30sec are provoked by head-turning. It is common after head injury. Other otological symptoms are rare.

Pathogenesis: Displacement of otoconia (=otoliths, ie calcium carbonate particles displaced from cells within in the endolymph) in semicircular canals.

Causes: Idiopathic, middle-ear disease, head injury, otosclerosis, spontaneous labyrinthine degeneration; postviral illness; stapes surgery (perilymph leak[113]).

Diagnosis: Establish important negatives: ►no *persistent* vertigo ►no speech, visual, motor, or sensory problems ►no tinnitus, headache, ataxia, facial numbness, or dysphagia ►no vertical nystagmus. *Hallpike test:*[1]

Treatment: Usually self-limiting in months; if persistent, try: • Vestibular habituation exercises (BOX 2). • *Reassurance* •↓Alcohol intake may help • *Drugs:* histamine analogues (betahistine); vestibular sedatives (prochlorperazine); antidepressants • Epley manoeuvres (fig 1) • *Last resort:* posterior semicircular canal denervation or obliteration (deafness may follow).

ENT diseases

Cawthorne Cooksey exercises for vestibular rehabilitation

1 *In bed:* Eye movements, slow, then quick; up and down; from side to side then focusing on finger moving from ~1 metre to 30cm away from the face. Then head movements at first slow, then quick, later with eyes closed bending forward and backward; turning from side to side.

2 *Sitting.* Eye movements and head movements as above, then:
• Shoulder shrugging and circling
• Bending forward and picking up objects from the ground

3 *Standing:* Eye, head and shoulder movements as before, then:
• Changing from sitting to standing position with eyes open and shut
• Throwing a small ball from hand to hand (above eye level)
• Throwing a ball from hand to hand under knee
• Changing from sitting to standing and turning around in between

4 *Moving about:* With eyes closed then open; ball games.

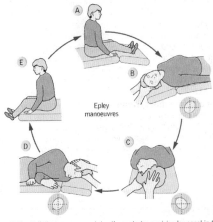

Epley manoeuvres

Fig 1. Otoconia repositioning with Epley head manoeuvres.[114] The ENT Dr/physiotherapist procures 4 sequential head movements with rest in each position for ~30sec. The aim is to reposition otoconia away from the sensitive posterior canals. This works in ~80% (a 2nd go may help).

1 The Hallpike manoeuvre rotates the posterior semicircular canal in the plane of gravity. Explain/reassure, and say "Keep your eyes open and look straight ahead". While supine, the head is held between the examiner's hands, turned 30-40° to one side and then rapidly lowered 30° below the couch's level. Ask the patient if they feel dizzy and look for nystagmus. If +ve, there is vertigo and rotary nystagmus towards the undermost ear, after a latent period of 5-10sec. This lasts <1min (adaptation). On sitting, there is more vertigo (±nystagmus). If any of these features are absent (no latency, no symptoms, and *persisting* nystagmus), seek a central cause.

The 2007 *European Position Statement* (EP3OS) defines rhinosinusitis (including nasal polyps, p557) as inflammation in the nose and paranasal sinuses with ≥2 symptoms, one of which must be nasal congestion or nasal discharge. Other symptoms of rhinosinusitis: facial pain or pressure, ↓ olfaction; endoscopic signs of nasal polyps or mucus ± pus discharged primarily from the sinuses, or CT showing mucosal changes within the sinuses. Rhinosinusitis symptoms are diagnosed as mild, moderate or severe—and as acute (ARS) or chronic (CRS, if lasting >12wks). **R:** Topical corticosteroids and oral antibiotics, are 1st line for adults with ARS. For adults with CRS with or without nasal polyps, EP3OS recommends that primary care physicians and non-ENT specialists prescribe topical steroids and nasal douching (p560) as 1st-line therapy.

Other causes of nasal congestion *Child:* Big adenoids, rhinitis, choanal atresia, postnasal space tumour (eg angiofibroma), foreign body (▸refer same day if *unilateral* obstruction ± foul/bloody discharge). *Adult:* Deflected nasal septum, granuloma (TB, syphilis, granulomatosis with polyangiitis, leprosy), topical vasoconstrictors, tricyclics. ▸*Refer urgently if:* •Numbness •Tooth loss •Bleeding •Unilateral obstructing mass •Tumour may be present. *Ask:* do symptoms vary? Is it both sides? Any effects on eating, speech, smell, or sleep (snoring)? Assess nasal deflection. Is either nostril **completely blocked** (does a mirror held under each nostril steam up)? Examine the postnasal space (scope or mirror).

Allergic rhinosinusitis may be seasonal (hay fever, prevalence ≈2%, high risk at 5–14yrs old) or perennial. *Cause:* IgE-mediatied inflammation from allergen exposure to nasal mucosa causing inflammatory mediator release from mast cells, eg from house dust mite (perennial) or pollen. *Symptoms:* Sneezing; pruritus; rhinorrhoea (bilateral & variable). *Signs:* Turbinates may be swollen and mucosae pale or mauve; nasal polyps. Skin tests may show allergens (avoid if prone to eczema, allergies, dermatographism, or on interfering antihistamines or steroids). Here, consider radio-allergosorbent (RAST) tests to find specific IgE. **R:** *Antihistamines:* Loratadine.[1] Systemic *decongestants* (pseudoephedrine 60mg/6h PO; CI: BP↑, hyperthyroidism, heart disease, MAOI use), *nasal sprays* (eg sodium cromoglicate 2%, 1 spray/4–6h), or *nasal steroids*, eg beclometasone 4–8×50µg puffs/24h. Steroid puffers may be used indefinitely, but steroid drops are systemically absorbed: use for <1 month at a time, <6 times/yr. *Oral steroids* or stat depot triamcinolone 40–100mg IM (buttock) may help the bad times. *Immunotherapy:*[2] ▸When rhinitis coexists with asthma (it does in up to 60%) a nasal steroid + an *anti-leukotriene agent* (zafirlukast 20mg/12h PO, adults only) may be better than loratadine/pseudoephedrine.[115,116] It may stop rhinitis triggering asthma.

Other causes of chronic rhinorrhoea/rhinitis Allergies, foreign body, CSF (eg after head injury; +ve for glucose), bacteria (eg TB), HIV, cystic fibrosis, Kartagener's syndrome, rheumatoid arthritis, atrophic, age (old man's drip[3]), pregnancy, the Pill, β-blockers, NSAIDs, decongestant overuse, antibody deficiency (p198), non-allergic rhinitis with eosinophilia (NARES).

---

1 Cetirizine, desloratadine, fexofenadine & mizolastine are all similar at a one-tablet-a-day dose and choice may be according to patient preference, availability, interactions, and price. Typically, antihistamines interact eg with erythromycin and other macrolides, grapefruit, fluoxetine, and systemic ketoconazole, but these effects are not seen with desloratadine (nor is antihistamine-associated ↑QT interval).[117]
2 Once-daily *sublingual immunotherapy* (SLIT) improves quality of life in grass-pollen-induced rhinosinusitis, eg once-daily grass allergen tablets (2,500; 25,000; or 75,000 SQ-T phleum pratense extract as Grazax®); start ≥4 months before the pollen season; continue for up to 3yrs.[118] *Injection immunotherapy* involves an induction course of the specific allergen. ▸SE: anaphylaxis (esp if asthma too), so administration should be under monitoring, with adrenaline and resus. equipment to hand. Beneficial effects can last for years![119]

The future for some patients may lie in **same-season ultra-short course allergy vaccine** (eg 4 injections of Pollinex Quattro® using natural allergens modified to enable higher doses).[120] N≈1028. SE: itch at injection site (risk of anaphylaxis not yet quantifiable, but there were no serious incidents in the above trial).
3 Old man's drip often occurs on eating, and ipratropium nasal spray (Rinatec®) may help.[121]

Typical patient: ♂ >40 years old.

Histology: Ciliated columnar epithelium with a thickened basement membrane and an avascular oedematous stroma. 90% are eosinophilic.[122]

Sites: Middle turbinates; middle meatus; ethmoids. Single, benign maxillary polyps may arise in the maxillary antrum, and prolapse to fill the nasopharynx (antrochoanal polyps). ►A polyp causing unilateral nasal obstruction may be sinister: refer promptly (esp. if pain or bleeding).

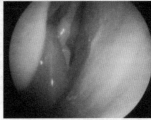

Fig 1. Polyp arising from right middle meatus. NB: the lower part of septum deviates to this side.
©R Herdman frcs

ENT diseases

Symptoms: Watery anterior rhinorrhoea, purulent postnasal drip, nasal obstruction, change in voice, anosmia/taste disturbance, sinusitis, headaches, mouth-breathing, snoring, mucocele (presents with a lump on the medial superior border of the orbit); pain (uncommon; eg over the dorsum of the nose).

Signs: It can be hard to distinguish hypertrophied inferior turbinates from polyps, but if a polyp, it is pale, mobile, and insensitive to gentle palpation.

Polyps associate with:
• Allergic rhinitis
• Non-allergic rhinitis
• Chronic ethmoid sinusitis
• Cystic fibrosis
• Aspirin hypersensitivity
• Asthma (eg non-atopic)

Drugs: 1% betamethasone, 1 drop/8h for 48h (longer courses may be safe). ►*Nose drop posture:* (fig 2) simply tilting the head back doesn't work![123] Bend double at hips, with nostrils pointing at the sky (Mygind position), or kneeling with the vertex/forehead on the floor (praying-to-Mecca). This may make polyps quickly diminish, and maintenance with beclometasone spray may then be tried, eg 8 puffs/24h (50µg/puff). 1–2wks of oral prednisolone may give short-term benefit, but the evidence is limited to poor trials,[124] eg at the high dose of 50mg/day for 2wks.[125] Balance benefit against risk (ohcm p361).[122] Anti-leukotrienes (p164) and continuous low-dose clarithromycin (250mg/24h for 2wks then 250mg/24h po) are also used.

Endoscopic polypectomy: If more than simple polypectomy is planned, do ct to show anatomical variations. Complications of endoscopic surgery are rare, but can include damage to

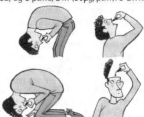

Fig 2. How to use nose drops—left two images; both the methods on the right are *equally* useless.

the optic nerve and csf leak (opposite). *Post-op:* • "Don't blow your nose until you are better" • Watch for bleeding • Abide by epistaxis advice (p562) • Topical steroids, eg beclometasone drops/12h (days 2 to 30) • 0.9% saline douched or sniffed from the palm to relieve crusting.

Children ►Nasal polyps are rare if <10yrs old; rule out neoplasms, cystic fibrosis, and meningocele/encephalocele (esp. if unilateral and <2yrs old).

A single unilateral 'polyp' ± epistaxis may turn out to be a sign of rare but serious intranasal pathology (eg nasopharyngeal cancer, glioma, lymphoma, neuroblastoma, or sarcoma).[138] Do prompt ct and get histology.

These are air-filled cavities in the bones around the nose, in continuity with the nasal cavity (fig 1). They are lined by ciliated mucosa; debris and mucus are swept towards and through ostia into the nostrils (fig 2). Viruses cause mucosal oedema and ↓cilia action, hence mucus retention and secondarily bacterial infection. Polyps/septal deviation→poor drainage→sinusitis. Current emphasis concentrates on recognizing and correcting these drainage problems. Sinusitis divides (imprecisely) into *acute* or *chronic* or *recurrent*: Symptoms:
• *Pain:* maxillary (cheek; teeth) or ethmoidal (between eyes), worse on bending.
• *Discharge* from nose, eg postnasal drip causing a foul taste in the mouth.
• *Nasal obstruction/congestion.*
• *Anosmia:* ↓smell; *cacosmia* (bad smell sensation without external source).
• *Systemic symptoms*, eg fever.

▶*Swelling is uncommon: exclude carcinoma or dental root infections.*

Differential diagnosis of sinusitis (non-sinus pain): migraine, TMJ dysfunction (p542), neuralgias, cervical spine disease, temporal arteritis, herpes zoster.

Causes of bacterial sinusitis (BS) Most follow viral infection. 4 others:
1 Direct spread (dental root infection or diving/swimming in infected water).
2 Odd anatomy: septal deviation, large ethmoidal bulla, polyps, large uncinate process (the part of ethmoid bone forming the maxillary sinus medial wall).
3 ITU causes: mechanical ventilation, recumbency, use of nasogastric tubes.[126]
4 Systemic causes: Kartagener's, immunodeficiency, or general debility.
5 Biofilms[1] denude mucosal cells of cilia and goblet cells.

Δ: A catheter attached to a syringe is as good as the 'suction trap' nasal collector.[127] Both may miss organisms growing within biofilms or in mucosal cells.[128] *Frequent bacteria: S. aureus, Pseudomonas aeruginosa, S. pneumoniae, H. influenzae,* and *Moraxella catarrhalis.* Fungi.[2]

Tests (None is usually needed.) ESR↑ & CRP↑ may be more reliable for BS than CT.[129] Endoscopy+CT is a sensitive method and helps plan surgery, identify underlying problems (anatomical pitfalls, eg low cribiform plates or vulnerable carotid arteries). Plain radiographs (occipitomental, occipitofrontal, and lateral views typically) and ultrasound are of little use. Normal radiographs cannot exclude sinus disease and 30% of normal sinuses show mucosal thickening.[130,131]

Treatment *Acute/single episode:* Most are self-limiting. After 5 days of symptoms, nasal douching (p560) and topical steroids/decongestants can be considered. Antihistamines are not routinely used as they may thicken secretions and complicate drainage. Antibiotics☞ (eg amoxicillin or co-amoxiclav).[132] N=214 may prevent complications. *Chronic/recurrent episodes:* (eg *S. aureus* or anaerobes.)[133] If antibiotics fail refer for *FESS* (functional endoscopic sinus surgery) tailored to the particular sinus affected.[134] High-volume, low-pressure rinsing of the surgical cavity can aid healing. Suction cleaning may be tried weekly starting 1wk post-op (continue until secretions, blood, and crusts disappear). **Fluticasone** nasal spray 200μg/12h starting 6 weeks post-op may have long-term advantages (fewer rescue courses of prednisolone & antibiotics needed at 5yrs).[135] Smoking cessation helps as tobacco irritates nasal mucosa and ↓cilia function.[136]

Complications Less common than previously (?from better health ± antibiotic use). *Mucocoeles* (esp. frontal sinus) may become infected pyoceoles. *Orbital cellulitis/abscess* (this is an emergency, p420). *Osteomyelitis* (classically staph, eg frontal bone). *Pott's puffy tumour* (subperiosteal abscess).[137] *Intracranial infection:* (Conscious level↓; cerebral irritability) Meningitis, encephalitis, cerebral abscess, cavernous sinus thrombosis.

---

1 A biofilm is an aggregate or micro-organisms on a living or inert surface.
2 Aspergillus (63%) candida, mucor.[138] 2 types: invasive or allergic, eg triggering asthma. Δ: culture; β-D-glucant; histology; ℞: (if invasive) antifungals+endonasal debridement;[139] HIV (may coexist; also diabetes or steroid use).

ENT diseases

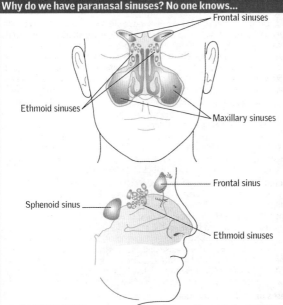

Fig 1. Sinus anatomy.   Redrawn with permission from Medtronic

Perhaps these pneumatic cavities are there to reduce the weight of our skull, Galen thought (but a pair of spectacles more than compensates) or maybe they moisten and warm the air as it goes to our lungs? Does their unique shape gives our voice its own timbre, so useful in recognizing each other when on different supermarket aisles? No!—according to studies of pitch, dynamic range, sound pressure, jitter, shimmer and noise-to-harmonics ratio![140] But they *do* make nitric oxide and aid immune defences![141]

Sinuses develop before (maxillary then ethmoid) and after birth (sphenoid then frontal) from invaginations in the nasal cavity that develop into the bones—another connection of sinus function with personal identity.

The maxillary sinus is particularly susceptible to congestion and subsequent infection, because its most dependent part lies below the level of the ostium (when standing), and so free drainage is impossible in this position.

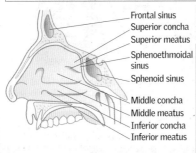

Frontal sinus
Superior concha
Superior meatus
Sphenoethmoidal sinus
Sphenoid sinus
Middle concha
Middle meatus
Inferior concha
Inferior meatus

Fig 2. The nasal conchae and meati. The table below shows the patterns of drainage of the sinuses & nasolacrimal duct.

Sinus	Meatus
Maxillary	Middle
Anterior ethmoidal	Middle
Middle ethmoidal	Middle
Posterior ethmoidal	Superior
Sphenoid	Spheno-ethmoidal recess
Frontal	Middle
Nasolacrimal duct	Inferior

ENT diseases

Undisplaced nasal fractures may need no treatment. If displaced, reduction (under GA) with post-op splintage is best within 2wks (complete setting occurs at 3wks). Advise to apply ice for the 1st 12h post-op; sleep with head elevated, sneeze through mouth, don't blow the nose or do vigorous exercise. Septal deviation may need septoplasty later. Post-traumatic nasal deformity is common (14–50%); this is reducible to 9% by complete nasal assessment (bony and septum), and primary septal reconstruction if severe septal fracture-dislocation.[142]

CSF rhinorrhoea Ethmoid fractures disrupting dura and arachnoid can result in CSF leaks. ►If not associated with trauma, ask: is it a tumour? Nasal discharge tests +ve for glucose (Clinistix® test—unreliable, so confirm with a lab glucose); CSF uniquely contains β_2 (tau) transferrin, tested for with immunoelectrophoresis (needs >0.5mL; the gold standard).[143] Conservative management: a lumbar drain and bedrest. Surgery is often not needed. Traumatic leaks should be covered with antibiotics and Pneumovax®.

Foreign bodies Most are self-inserted by children. Organic material presents early with purulent discharge; inorganic bodies may remain inert for ages. If a child is co-operative it may be possible to grab the object with forceps or a hooked instrument. An understanding parent/child team with good head immobilization (eg held between the parent's legs, wrapped in a blanket to stop wriggling) can make for successful removal. 2.5% **cocaine spray** (avoid in children) may shrink the mucosa and allow extraction with a sucker. Foley catheters can also be useful. Batteries need urgent removal. If GA needed, protect the airway.[144] A 'parental kiss' has been described with +ve pressure behind the object by blowing into the mouth whilst occluding the other nostril.

Causes of septal perforation After septal surgery (p561); trauma; nose picking; body piercings; nasal prongs (O_2 delivery); sniffing chrome salts or cocaine; malignancies (eg rodent ulcer); nasal steroid/decongestant sprays,[145] any chronic mucosal inflammation/granuloma—eg TB; syphilis; HIV, extra-GI Crohn's;[146] sarcoidosis; SLE; granulomatosis with polyangiitis; relapsing polychondritis (chondritis in auricles, nose and trachea ± non-erosive polyarthritis, eye inflammation, and vestibular or cochlear damage; it may be fatal).[147] Perforations irritate, whistle, crust, and bleed. *R:* Symptomatic. Closure is hard (may be done with rhinoplasty; a one-stage procedure).[148] Saline douche for crusts;[1] silastic buttons to occlude the hole.

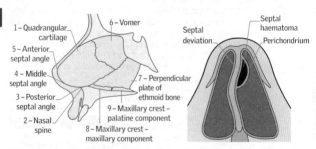

1 – Quadrangular cartilage
5 – Anterior septal angle
4 – Middle septal angle
3 – Posterior septal angle
2 – Nasal spine
6 – Vomer
7 – Perpendicular plate of ethmoid bone
9 – Maxillary crest – palatine component
8 – Maxillary crest – maxillary component
Septal deviation
Septal haematoma
Perichondrium

Fig 1. Is surgery needed for this case of septal deviation? Maybe, but you cannot rely on objective tests such as rhinomanometry.[149] Endoscopic repair may be superior to open procedures.[150] The main issues in nasal surgery are to stabilize the nose in the good position after surgery and preserve the cartilages and bones in the favourable situation and reduce the risk of deviation recurrence. Also it is necessary to avoid synechia formation, nasal valve narrowing, haematoma, and bleeding. Septoplasty can be safely performed without post-op nasal packing (may have complications such as pain, sleep problems and even toxic shock).[151]

ENT diseases

Septoplasty, septorhinoplasty

Septoplasty corrects a deviated nasal septum. Septorhinoplasty aims to straighten and or refashion the shape of the nose too for cosmesis and to help breathing by improving the airway. For an operative description of and pre-op assessment, see www.noseandsinus.com/BeckerSeptoplastyPaper.pdf

Complications: Bleeding (repacking may be needed); CSF leakage (nurse semi-upright; avoid blowing the nose; flap surgery may be needed); altered sensation of lips, gums and incisors. If a septal haematoma develops, drain and give IV antibiotics to prevent a septal abscess (formal drainage may be needed, and may not prevent septal perforation). Adhesions between the septum and the lateral nasal wall may need division.

1 Put 1 teaspoonful of salt in ≥500mL tap water (distilled if quality poor) and sniff the liquid from a cupped hand. A unilateral squirt from a 10mL syringe (or an old Beconase® container) is an alternative. Adding 1 teaspoonful of baking soda (sodium bicarbonate) improves the mucus-solvent properties of the irrigant.[152]

Respect all nosebleeds; they can be fatal. They are *anterior* or *posterior*; anterior bleeds that can be easily seen with rhinoscopy are simpler to treat and are usually less severe. Proceed as follows: G-up (gown, goggles, gloves), then:

▶▶Resuscitate as needed, eg if BP↓ or dizzy on sitting up. ABCs; IVI, SAO₂, etc. Monitor vital signs often.

▶▶History: Which side? Trauma? How much loss? On warfarin/aspirin? Note past medical history.

▶▶Ask him to apply pressure by pinching the *lower* part of nose for 15min while mouth-breathing and sitting forward so blood can be spat into a bowl.

▶▶Fully decongest (eg with ephedrine 0.5% drops).

▶▶Place ice pack on the dorsum of the nose (ice may also be sucked). If this doesn't stop the bleed...

▶▶Prepare silver nitrate cautery. Ask a nurse to help.

▶▶Encourage the patient to blow out nasal clots.

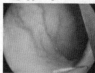

Fig 1. Vessels in Little's area (left side of septum; fig 2 for anatomy). These are the main cause of epistaxis in children. ©Rory Herdman

▶▶Look in side (headlamp+speculum); remove clots (gentle suction; spray on lidocaine and phenylephrine (vasoconstrictor); wait a few minutes.

▶▶Find bleeding points (eg indicated by prominent surface clot, often on the anterior septum. Apply cautery for ~10sec. Start from the edge of the bleeding point and move in on a radius. Remember: "silver nitrate cauterizes everything it touches." Keep it away from alae nasae. Get support to keep your hand steady. Never cauterize both sides of the septum (risks perforation)[153]

▶▶If you cannot see the bleeding point, refer to ENT.[154]

▶▶If bleeding continues, try an *anterior nasal pack* (paraffin gauze; Merocel®). Lubricate the pack (KY®); advance it all the way into the nose (direction is horizontal, *not* up). If all is well, remove after 24h. If bleeding continues, try a *postnasal pack* (Foley catheter, 16–18G filled with >10mL water);[1] get help from a colleague. Admit patients with packs and use the history to plan searches for a cause. If there is no more active bleeding, the patient may be discharged with an advice leaflet providing there are no other medical problems.

Causes/associations
- Trauma (local/facial)
- Local trauma or infection
- Hypertension
- Dyscrasia/haemophilia[et al]
- Alcohol intake↑
- Septal perforation
- Neoplasm

After the bleed...
- Don't pick your nose!
- Sit upright, out of the sun
- Avoid bending, lifting, or straining on the toilet
- If you sneeze, send it through your open mouth
- No hot food or drink
- Avoid alcohol/tobacco
- If it restarts, apply ice to the bridge of the nose, and hold the soft lower part *continuously* for 20 min; get help if this fails.

Anterior epistaxis is almost invariably septal; Little's area (Kiesselbach's plexus) is used to describe this area where anterior ethmoidal, sphenopalatine, and facial arteries anastomose to form an anterior anastomotic arcade (figs 1-2).

Serious posterior epistaxis More invasive procedures (see 2) may be best:

1 *Examination under anaesthesia:* If a discrete bleeding point is found it can be treated directly, eg with diathermy, otherwise repacking may be needed. Correction of septal deviation may improve access.

2 *Ligation:* The emerging gold standard is endoscopic ligation of the maxillary/sphenopalatine artery around the sphenopalatine foramen[156,157] This is preferred to transantral arterial ligation of maxillary artery or ligation of the anterior ethmoidal artery. Sometimes ligating 2 arteries is necessary (eg the contralateral one).[155] ▶▶Embolization can be lifesaving eg for bleeding not responding to surgical measures—but this can cause stroke.

1 An alternative is the Brighton device with anterior and posterior balloons: they are more expensive and inhalation of clot has been reported.[158]

ENT diseases

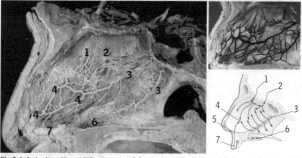

Fig 2. 1 Anterior ethmoidal artery (a.) **2** Posterior ethmoidal a. **3** Sphenopalatine a. (≥2 branches, as on the dissection). **4** Little's area (anterior ethmoidal, sphenopalatine, and facial arteries anastomose to form this anterior anastomotic arcade) **5** Septal branch **6** Greater palatine a. **7** Superior labial a. and branches (from facial artery).

Courtesy of Prof Tor Chiu who performed the dissection.

Tonsillitis (sore throat ± lymphadenopathy, especially jugulodigastric) often caused by Group A streps (eg *Streptococcus pyogenes*). Other pathogens include: staphs, *Moraxella catarrhalis*, mycoplasma, chlamydia, haemophilus. See fig 1.

Tests: Swabbing superficial bacteria in suspected cases is irrelevant and can lead to overdiagnosis.

R: Paracetamol ± Difflam® gargle if severe; antibiotics are unlikely to help (BOX 1) as most are viral, but if ill or (Centor criteria +ve):[1] penicillin, 250mg/6h usually PO (125mg/5mL, 5mL/6h PO if <6yrs); erythromycin if penicillin allergic) for 5 days; *not* amoxicillin (bad rash in almost all whose pharyngitis is from EBV). Consider alternating paracetamol/ibuprofen (both are antipyretic and analgesic).

<table>
<tr><td>Differential diagnosis:
• Epstein–Barr virus
• Agranulocytosis
• Leukaemia
• Scarlet fever; diphtheria</td></tr>
</table>

Complications of tonsillitis Ask yourself: is he immunosuppressed?

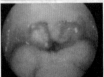

Fig 1. Tonsillitis in a child (erythema, follicle pus + narrow airway). Think of Kawasaki disease (p646) if peeling skin or platelets↓ ©Rory Herdman

• *Retropharyngeal abscess:* This is rare; typical patient: ill child with a stiff, extended neck/torticollis who fails to eat or drink. Lateral neck x-ray: soft tissue swelling. *R:* Incise and drain pus under GA (head-down, to prevent aspiration).

• *Peritonsillar abscess (quinsy)* presents with sore throat, dysphagia, peritonsillar bulge, uvular deviation, trismus, and muffled voice. Antibiotics[2] and aspiration (preferred to surgical drainage) are needed. Difficulties arise in examining the throat in an uncooperative child and escalate if needle aspiration rather than operative incision and drainage is tried.[159] Steroids reduce morbidity. There is a limited place for immediate tonsillectomy. **Technique for needle aspiration:** Learn from a colleague (the carotid artery is nearby). It is common to drain >10mL of pus with immediate benefit. Incision may be needed. For technique, see www.clinicaljunior.com/entoncallquinsy.html

• *Parapharyngeal and hypopharyngeal abscesses:* Medical therapy alone, especially in children, can resolve these.

• *Lemierre's syndrome:* Pharyngotonsillitis, internal jugular vein thrombophlebitis + septic emboli (to lungs, bone, muscle, kidney, liver etc). Cause: *Fusobacterium necrophorum.* *R:* High-dose IV benzylpenicillin,[2] clindamycin & metronidazole). Multiple debridments may be needed.[160-162]

Differential diagnosis of unilateral tonsillar enlargement
• True asymmetry. Do excision biopsy if malignancy possible.
• Apparent enlargement (shift ∴ peritonsillar abscess/parapharyngeal mass).
• Tumours: squamous cancer (70%). *Typical patient:* Elderly, with sore throat, dysphagia ± otalgia. *Treatment:* Radiotherapy; surgery; cytotoxics. In one study, survival for stage III and stage IV squamous cancer was 79% and 52%, respectively, over 2–15yrs.[163]

Scarlet fever If a rash develops on the chest, axillae or behind the ears, which is accentuated in skin folds, 12–48h after initial infection (±Pastia lines[3] and circumcoral pallor and a 'strawberry tongue') you are probably observing scarlet fever. *Start* penicillin as treatment. If after a week the child presents with odd movements, dizziness, walking difficulty or altered consciousness, you may be able to diagnose Sydenham's chorea or even a post-infectious demyelinating disorder, eg ADEM.[4]

---

1 Centor criteria: if T°↑, pus on tonsils, no cough but cervical adenopathy is present, +ve predictive value for strep throat is ~50%; if all 4 are –ve, the negative predictive value is 80%.
2 One IV regimen is penicillin 1.2g/6h + metronidazole up to 500mg/8h ± IV fluids ± stat steroid dose.
3 Confluent petechiae in skin creases (eg at elbow), that may persist as pigmented lines after acute phase.
4 Acute disseminated encephalomyelitis (ADEM) develops from antigenic mimicry with antibodies (eg to mycoplasma, streps or EBV) having crossreactivity to CNS epitopes.[164]

⊹ A holistic approach to the person with a sore throat

Don't focus on the throat, the swab, or the microbiology: home in on peo- ple's health beliefs and work to harmonize these beliefs with your own.

We often think patients expect antibiotics, and will be disappointed if they are not given. Often this is not the case. Does he attend with *every* sore throat? If not, why now? "My nephew is coming to stay, and my wife told me to come and get a prescription"—or symptoms may be worse than usual. If so, ibuprofen may help. But what may *really* help is dialogue. Strangely enough, there is evidence that rich dialogue reduces symptoms rather than merely making them more acceptable.[165]

But improving symptoms is not the only aim: dialogue may promote pa- tients' trust in their own body. It may be a stepping stone to active health rather than passive disease. It may stop your patient being a patient.

Don't do tonsillectomy unless you are sure that... ♦ 2009 SIGN

• Sore throats are in fact due to tonsillitis.
• 5 or more episodes of sore throat are occurring per year.
• Symptoms for at least a year.

NB: there is now a risk that too few tonsillectomies are being done. More and more adults and children are being hospitalized for throat infections. In 2000–1, there were 30,942 tonsil-related admissions for medical treatments. By 2008–09, this had risen to 43,641. entuk.org/position_papers/documents/tonsillectomy

Other indications: respiratory obstruction; suspicion of malignancy.

Methods The cold steel method uses good old-fashioned scissors, blades, snares and sutures. Cautery can be used ± a microscope; NICE recommends specific training in coblation[1] if used. Radiofrequency ablation can shrink tonsils.[166]

Complications of surgery (Mortality 1 in 16,000 to 1 in 35,000)[167] The worst (but rarely fatal) complication is bleeding.[168] Primary (<24h) often requires a return to theatre. Secondary (>24h, but typically after 5–10 days) is usually due to infection—here repeat surgery is rarely needed: try rest and antibi- otics. Use of the tonsillar gag may cause damage to teeth, the TMJ (p542), and posterior pharyngeal wall. Risk factors for haemorrhage: male; younger surgeon; older patient; heat (any kind) used for haemostasis. Use of single-use instruments (hated by some surgeons) need not cause more bleeding.[169]

Management of uncontrollable secondary bleeding post-tonsillectomy:
▸▸ Admit. High-flow O_2; IVI and resuscitate until urine flows at >30mL/min.
▸▸ Crossmatch blood and take to theatre as needed.
▸▸ IV antibiotic (co-amoxiclav is an option),[170] eg if T°↑, neutrophilia, or CRP↑.[171]

Most bleeding is not this severe and can be managed by hydrogen peroxide gargles, topical vasoconstrictors and admission for IV antibiotics.

See Royal College Audit 2003 www.rcseng.ac.uk/surgical_research_units/docs/National%20Prospec- tive%20Tonsillectomy%20Audit%20Final%20Report%202005.pdf

---

1 *Coblation* uses a plasma field of Na^+ created by passing a current through saline to vaporize and dis- sect adjacent tissue: surgical science at the cutting edge. It has less tissue-heating effect than diathermy.

Stridor is a musical noise heard in inspiration from partial obstruction at the larynx or large airways. **Sterto** is an inspiratory noise like snoring, coming from pharynx obstruction (its adjective is **stertorous**; commoner in the obese).

▶*Children's airways are narrower and more readily deformed than adult airways, so obstruction happens faster and more dramatically.*

▶*Look for other signs:* swallowing difficulty/drooling, pale/cyanosed, using accessory muscles of respiration; downward plunging of the trachea with respiration (tracheal tug); all are grave signs and mean impending obstruction.

Causes • *Congenital:* Laryngomalacia, web/stenosis, vascular rings.

• *Inflammation:* Laryngitis, epiglottitis, laryngotracheobronchitis, anaphylaxis.

• *Tumours:* Haemangiomas or papillomas (usually disappear with onset of immunity—but may require laser treatment before).

• *Trauma:* Thermal/chemical—or from intubation.

• *Miscellaneous:* Airway or oesophageal foreign body; vocal cord paralysis.

Laryngotracheobronchitis/croup is the leading cause of stridor with a barking cough (much commoner than epiglottitis). 95% are viral, eg parainfluenza (ribavirin can help, eg in immunodeficiency). Bacteria (*klebsiella*, diphtheria) & fungi are rare. If there is cough and no drooling, croup is almost always the diagnosis.[173] Usually self-limiting; treat at home (± antibiotics).

Severity grading of croup[172]
1 Inspiratory stridor ± barking cough
2 Grade 1 + expiratory stridor
3 Grade 2 + pulsus paradoxus
4 Grade 3 + cyanosis (± cognition↓)

Admit (eg to ITU) if severe. In children, CXR may show 'steeple sign' of a tapering trachea. Give **antibiotics**, humidified O_2, + nebulized **adrenaline** (5mL 1:1000, may buy time in severe disease needing ventilating), and **dexamethasone** 150µg/kg PO stat or **budesonide** 2mg nebulized. See also p158.

▶▶**Acute epiglottitis** is rarer than croup, eg $9/10^6$/yr, but mortality is high: 1% if respiratory distress. ♂:♀≈3:1. It's an emergency as respiratory arrest can occur. Often, history is short, septicaemia is rapid, and *cough is absent*. Also: sore throat (100%), fever (88%), dyspnoea (78%), voice change (75%), dysphagia (76%), tender anterior neck ±cellulitis (27%), hoarseness (21%), pharyngitis (20%), anterior neck nodes (9%),[174] drooling (head forward tongue out), prefers to sit, refusal to swallow, dysphagia. Typical cause: *Haemophilus* (vaccination has reduced prevalence); *Strep pyogenes*.

Managing epiglottitis
▶▶ Take to ITU; don't examine throat (causes resp. arrest)
▶▶ O_2 by mask till anaesthetist and ENT doctor arrive
▶▶ Give nebulized **adrenaline**, IV **dexamethasone**
▶▶ Visual diagnosis at nasopharyngeal intubation
▶▶ Blood/epiglottic culture
▶▶ Find cricothyrotomy kit
▶▶ IVI + penicillin G & ceftriaxone 2g/12h IV, p204
▶▶ Antipyretic, eg ibuprofen

Laryngomalacia This is the main congenital anomaly of the larynx (~60%) appearing within hours of birth (or up to a few months). Immature and floppy aryepiglottic folds and glottis ↑ laryngeal collapse in inspiration. Stridor may be most noticeable in certain positions, sleep, or if excited/upset. In 85%, no R_x is needed and symptoms usually improve by 2 yrs old. Problems may occur with concurrent laryngeal infections or with feeding.[175] Try surgery if severe. It can also develop in association with gastro-oesophageal reflux disease.[176]

Laryngeal paralysis accounts for 15-20% of all those with congenital laryngeal anomalies. *Cause:* Often unknown, but might be from vagal stretching at delivery. *Unilateral:* May manifest during the 1st few weeks of life with a hoarse, breathy cry that is aggravated by agitation, feeding difficulties ± aspiration. R_x: Supportive; most recover by 2-3 years. *Bilateral:* Inspiratory stridor at rest that worsens upon agitation ± significant respiratory distress. R_x: may need urgent airway intervention (intubation, tracheotomy)±surgery.[177,178]

⟶ Acute airway obstruction: management in adults

⟶ Let the patient sit/lie down in the position he is most comfortable.

⟶ Give O_2 or Heliox® (79% helium+21% O_2; it's less dense than air & O_2 ∴ more laminar flow in obstructed airways, and *may* reduce work of breathing, respiratory distress, and post-extubation stridor).[179]

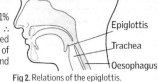

Fig 2. Relations of the epiglottis.

⟶ Nebulized racemic adrenaline.

⟶ Place an IV cannula, give **dexamethasone** or **hydrocortisone** IV.

⟶ Note O_2 saturation, respiratory rate, pulse and blood pressure.

⟶ Call the on-call ENT registrar and anaesthetist for help (eg via crash bleep).

⟶ Get the crash tracheostomy kit ready.

⟶ Brief history from relatives, keeping in view the common causes of stridor.

⟶ Do arterial blood gases if possible without causing delay or stress.

⟶ When the stridor improves, do a flexible nasendoscopy (ENT registrar) to visualize the airway, thereby giving an idea about the cause for stridor.

⟶ Get AP + lateral x-rays of neck & chest. www.clinicaljunior.com/entstridordoddi.html

Note on needle cricothyrotomy (*OHCM* p786) in children—jet O_2 at 15L/min through a wide-bore cannula (14G) placed in the cricothyroid membrane: allow O_2 in for 1 sec and exhalation (through partially obstructed upper airway) for 4sec. Useful in adults too.

If a surgical cricothyrotomy is used (not in children <12yrs; see *OHCM* p786) a tracheostomy in theatre is needed within 30min as jet insufflation oxygenates rather than ventilates, so CO_2 builds up.

Why is this child drooling?

Drooling is often normal if <3yrs old (eg associated with teething). So don't assume that drooling + stridor must mean epiglottitis if drooling predated the stridor (chronic causes below). Find out if oral incontinence is from ↓cerebral control of oral function, hypersalivation, or an obstruction to swallowing.

• ⟶Angioedema/anaphylaxis (p237) ⟶Rabies (*OHCM* p432) ⟶Epiglottitis

• Neurodisability, eg cerebral palsy, bulbar palsy (↓ oro-motor control).[180]

• Muscle problems (oesophageal dysmotility; cricopharyngeal achalasia)

• Ingestion of a foreign body, heavy metals, lithium, or caustic substances

• Head and neck trauma to swallowing structures

• Enlarged tonsils or adenoids ± nasal polyps/rhinosinusitis/severe tonsillitis

• Congenital lesions/nasal masses (eg an encephalocele or glioma).[1]

ENT diseases

---

1 Other causes in adults: ill-fitting dentures, reflux oesophagitis, Parkinson's, stroke, motor neurone disease. R: 'SPIT': **s**copolamine$^{et al}$ (anicholinergics ↓ salivary flow); **p**hysio/oral motor training (±palatal training appliances), attending to head **p**osition, education and training, suction aids, bio-feedback and support; **i**njections of botulinum toxin: gland excisions; **t**ransposition or excision of ducts.[181]

Hoarseness entails difficulty producing sound with change in voice pitch or quality ('breathy', 'scratchy', 'husky'). ►Investigate hoarseness (esp. in smokers) lasting >3wks, as it is the chief (and often the only) presentation of laryngeal carcinoma (p570). *Ask about:* Gastro–oesophageal reflux (GORD), dysphagia, smoking, stress, singing & shouting. Voice overuse is a common cause (prevalence >50% in eg teachers).[183]

Tests Laryngoscopy (to assess cord mobility, inspect the mucosa, exclude local causes); slow-motion videolaryngostroboscopy/acoustic analysis (causes have characteristic vibration patterns).

Specific causes *Reflux laryngitis (laryngopharyngeal reflux (LPR):* This is chronic laryngeal signs and symptoms associated with GORD. ~15% of all visits to the ENT clinics are because of LPR. *Treatment:* Twice daily proton-pump inhibitors for 2 to 4 months ± surgical fundoplication.[184]

Laryngitis: This is often viral and self-limiting, but there may be secondary infection with streps or staphs. It can also be secondary to GORD (see above) or autoimmune disease, eg rheumatoid arthritis. NB: in chronic laryngitis (lasting >3 wks), any bacteria found are likely to be colonizers only.[185] *Symptoms:* Pain (hypopharyngeal, dysphagia; pain on phonation), hoarseness; fever. ℞: Supportive. If necessary, give *penicillin v* 500mg/6h PO for 1 week. Steam inhalation may help. Chronic cord irritation from smoking ± chronic voice abuse may cause *Reinke's oedema* (a gelatinous fusiform enlargement of the cords, also associated with hypothyroidism—if conservative treatment fails, laser therapy may help).

Functional disorders of speech articulation: (ie cause unknown). *Aphonia:* Phonation yields no response (or a whisper) in seemingly normal cord adductors, eg in young women at times of stress (NB: there are many functional voice disorders which may result in laryngeal oedema ± nodules.) A good differentiating test is to ask patients to cough (needs functional adductors). It is a diagnosis by exclusion, eg allergic reactions may cause sudden aphonia, so don't assume a functional disorder without laryngoscopy. *Treatment:* Speech therapy is the best, with attention to emotional factors which may be present. *Spasmodic dysphonia:* Strained, effortful, hoarse voice + tremors, jerky voice onset, intermittent voice breaks, breathy spasms, hypernasality, failure to maintain voice.[186] *Children with functional speech disorders* have difficulty with specific speech sounds (eg /r/, /s/, /z/, /r/, /l/ and/or 'th'). Try to distinguish articulation disorders from phonological delay, consistent and varying ('inconsistent') phonological disorders and speech dyspraxia.

Differential: Before saying 'no cause can be found', consider generalized infiltrating entities of the larynx, such as hyperkeratosis (∵smoking, alcohol abuse, pollution), leukoplakia, also granulomata, papillomata, polyps, and cysts.

Less common causes

- *Intrinsic:* ↓Lubrication, eg sicca syn.; laryngocoeles; granulomas: eg Wegener's[*]; sarcoidosis; TB; syphilis.
- *Extrinsic pressure:* Goitre, carotid body tumour.[182]
- *Neoplasia:* Pancoast syndrome; larynx or thymus cancer; lymphoma; glomus tympanicum tumour (fig 1, p552).
- *Toxic:* Vomit; fumes[etc].
- *Injury* causing arytenoid subluxation; CVP lines.
- *Bacteria:* Epiglottitis; diphtheria; abscess; aortitis.
- *CNS causes:* Vagus lesion Guillain–Barré; myasthenia; other vocal cord pareses.
- *Endocrine:* Acromegaly, Addison's, myxoedema.

Rarer causes

- Mycotic aneurysm
- Subclavian aneurysm
- Malformations
- Mucormycosis/fungi in HIV
- Mucosal leishmaniasis
- Hamartoma/haemangioma
- Angioneurotic oedema
- Gouty cricoarytenoiditis
- Behçet's vasculitis of vasa nervorum of laryngeal nrv.
- Chondrosarcoma
- Relapsing polychondritis

Emergency presentations

- ►► Epiglottitis (p566)
- ►► Aortic dissection
- ►► Anaphylaxis
- ►► Acid/alkali ingestion
- ►► Trauma/foreign body

Get help to secure the airway.

ENT diseases (side margin)

Laryngeal nerve palsy

The recurrent laryngeal nerve supplies the intrinsic muscles of the larynx (apart from cricothyroideus, external branch of the superior laryngeal n.) and is responsible for both abduction and adduction of the vocal fold. It originates from the vagus, with a complex course: on the **left** under the ligamentum arteriosum, on the **right** under the subclavian artery, turning back in a cephalic direction to run in the tracheo-oesophageal groove. In its passage between the cricoid and thyroid cartilages it is vulnerable to compression from the cuff on an overinflated endotracheal tube. Symptoms of vocal cord paralysis are:
• Hoarseness with 'breathy' voice with a weak cough.
• Repeated coughing/aspiration (∵weak sphincter + supraglottic sensation↓).
• Exertional dyspnoea (glottis is too narrow to allow much air flow). NB: while at rest the contralateral cord can compensate by increased abduction.

In *partial* paralysis, cords are often fixed in the midline; in *complete* paralysis they are fixed mid-way ('paramedian'; *Semon's law:*◆❋ nerve fibres supplying the abductors are more susceptible to damage, and the median position is due to unopposed adduction).[187] NB: the Wagner–Grossman theory is discredited.

Causes: 30% are cancers (larynx in ~40%; thyroid, oesophagus, hypopharynx, bronchus, or malignant node). 25% are iatrogenic, ie after parathyroidectomy, oesophageal, or pharyngeal pouch surgery. Paralysis after thyroid surgery is seen in ≤5%, and is reversible in about 35%.[188] *Other causes:* CNS disease (polio; syringomyelia); TB; aortic aneurysm; 15% are idiopathic (≈'neurotropic virus').

Tests: CXR, barium swallow/meal, MRI, panendoscopy.

Treating non-malignant causes: Unilateral palsies can be compensated for by movement of the contralateral cord, but may need formal medialization in the form of bioplastique injections, or a thyroplasty, eg Isshiki-type.[189] *Reinnervation techniques:* ansa cervicalis-to-recurrent laryngeal nerve (RLN, eg after damage during thyroidectomy); primary RLN anastomosis, ansa-to-RLN+ cricothyroid muscle-nerve-muscle pedicle, ansa-to-thyroarytenoid implantation, ansa-to-thyroarytenoid neuromuscular pedicle, hypoglossal-to-RLN.[190]MET

Singer's nodules

Singer's nodules are caused by vocal abuse (untrained singers in smoky atmospheres). These are fibrous nodules (often bilateral) at the junction of the anterior ⅓ and posterior ⅔ of the cords. This is the middle of the membranous vocal folds (the posterior portion of the vocal fold is cartilage), and it may receive most contact injury during speech.

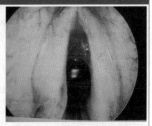

Fig 1. Singer's nodule (rt). ©R.Herdman FRCS

R: Speech therapy (if used early), or excision.

Vocal hygiene...Don't whisper! Don't shout!

• Drink plenty of fluids (8 cups/day, but not tea, coffee, alcohol, or cola).
• Get plenty of sleep: tiredness kills the voice.
• Avoid irritants (spicy foods, tobacco, smoke, dust, alcohol, aspirin gargles).
• Avoid eating late at night, as indigestion may affect the voice.
• Humidify your living and sleeping areas, eg damp towel on radiators, etc.
• Don't suck medicated lozenges; these numb the throat, and menthol is drying. You can keep your mouth moist by chewing pastilles or gum.
• Steam inhalations may help when you are ill (add nothing to them).

▶Use a multidisciplinary approach to investigation, diagnosis (imaging, histolotology, HPV virology[1]), staging (example below), and treatment (organ sparing or radical?). Have a low threshold for referral whenever symptoms in the MINIBOX occur (esp. in smokers).

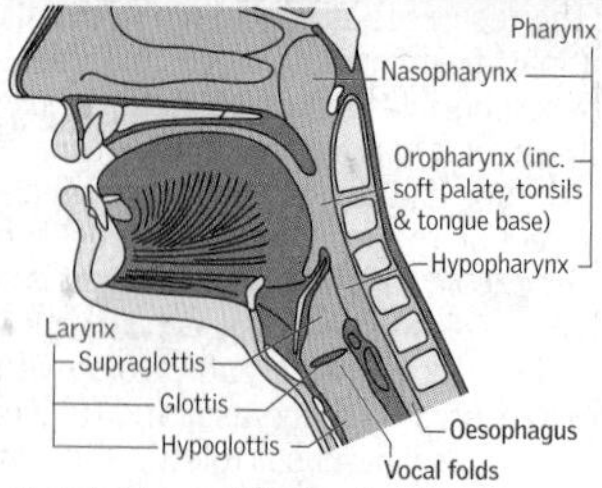

Nasopharyngeal cancer (fig 1) 25% of all cancers in China *vs* 1% in UK. *Associations:* •HLA A2 allele (↓survival with B17 & BW46) •HPV[1] •Epstein–Barr (EBV)[191] •Tobacco, formaldehyde, wood dust exposure[192]

Fig 1. Anatomy of the head and neck.

•Weaning on to salted fish (?N-nitroso carcinogens).
Staging: T1 Nasopharynx, oropharynx, or nasal cavity
T2 Parapharyngeal extension
T3 Bony structures of skull-base/paranasal sinuses
T4 Intracranial, cranial nerves, hypopharynx, orbit, infratemporal fossa/masticator space
N1 Unilateral cervical, unilateral or bilateral retropharyngeal nodes, above supraclavicular fossa, ≤6cm in the greatest dimension.
N2 Bilateral cervical above supraclavicular fossa ≤6cm
N3 >6cm. N3b Supraclavicular fossa.
Stage II=T1N1 to T2N0-1. Stage III=T1N2 to T3 N0-2.

Symptoms of HNSCC
•Neck pain/lump
•Hoarse voice >6wks
•Sore throat >6 weeks
•Mouth bleeding
•Mouth numbness
•Sinus congestion
•Sore tongue
•Painless ulcers
•Patches in the mouth
•Earache/effusion
•Lumps (lip, mouth, gum)
•Speech change
•Dysphagia; epistaxis

Lymph spread: Usually early to upper deep cervical nodes. Local spread may involve cranial nerves via the jugular foramen. *Signs:* Diplopia, conductive deafness (Eustachian tube affected), cranial nerve palsy (not I, VII, VIII), nasal obstruction, or neck lumps. Δ: Endoscopy/biopsy; PCR for EBV. NB: submucosal spread may mean the area *looks* normal. Stage by MRI, eg with STIR sequence (=short tau inversion recovery; better than CT).[193] R: Radiotherapy is mainstay (intensity-modulated/IMRT may cause fewer SE, eg xerostomia and dysphagia)[194] ± chemotherapy ± surgery (radical neck dissection). 3-yr survival for stage II: ~100% (93% for stage III; 69% for stage IV, in one study; worse if EBV +ve).[195,196]

Oropharyngeal carcinoma is often advanced at presentation. ♂:♀≈5:1. Histology: 85% are squamous. *Typical older patient:* Smoker with sore throat, sensation of a lump, referred otalgia, and local irritation by hot or cold foods, with risk factors: chewing or smoking tobacco (alcohol alone is not a risk factor but is synergistic with smoking). 30% of squamous pharyngeal tumours will have a 2nd primary within 10yrs. 20% are node +ve at presentation. *Imaging:* MRI with STIR (above) contrast-enhanced CT.[197] *Surgery,* eg with: jejunal flaps; tubed skin flaps (eg radial forearm or anterolateral thigh flaps); gastric pull-ups; transoral laser, robotic surgery and partial laryngeal surgery. *Radiotherapy* (eg intensity-modulated) may be 1st line if the tumour is T1 (<2cm) or T2 (>2cm but <4cm; NB: T3 is >4cm and T4 beyond oropharynx).

Hypopharyngeal tumours are rare and are usually a disease of the elderly. They can present as a lump in throat, dysphagia for solids then fluids, or as neck lumps. The anatomic limits of the hypopharynx are the hyoid bone to the lower edge of the cricoid cartilage: the 3 main sites are piriform fossa,

---

1 Note on human papilloma virus (HPV; oncogenic wart virus, one mode of transmission is sexual, p272). Head & neck cancers may be caused by HPV; they occur in younger people, and carry a better prognosis than those associated with smoking.[198] *Oral sex:* HPV16 cancer risk relates (partly) to number of partners.[199] *Kissing:* In those who had never had oral sex, risk of harbouring HPV increases if ≥10 lifetime or 5 recent open-mouthed kissing partners. HPV vaccination.♦ (p272) If this prevented *all* ENT HPV +ve cancers, this would increase its cost-effectiveness (and boys should get it too, esp. as HPV is overtaking smoking as the chief cause of these cancers).[200]

postcricoid region, and the posterior pharyngeal wall. Note premalignant conditions: leukoplakia and Patterson–Kelly–Brown syndrome (Plummer–Vinson)—in which a pharyngeal web is associated with iron deficiency, angular stomatitis, glossitis, and koilonychia: 2% risk postcricoid cancer. They are associated with previous irradiation, smoking and alcohol, but not as clearly as laryngeal carcinoma. Treatment options are radiotherapy and surgery in various combinations. The prognosis is poor with 60% mortality at 1 year.

Squamous cell laryngeal cancer (fig 1) *Incidence:* 2000/yr (UK). *Typical older patient:* Male smoker with progressive hoarseness, then stridor, difficulty or pain on swallowing ± haemoptysis ± ear pain (if pharynx involved). Regular cannabis users are at ↑risk.[201] *Typical younger patient:* HPV +ve.[1] *Sites:* Supraglottic, glottic, or subglottic. Glottic tumours have the best prognosis as they cause hoarseness earlier (spread to nodes is late). *Diagnosis:* Laryngoscopy+biopsy. HPV status; MRI staging.[202] *R̄:* Radical radiotherapy (eg IMRT above) or total laryngectomy ± block dissection of neck glands. There is debate about organ-sparing chemoradiotherapy *vs* laryngectomy, as well as laser *vs* radio-

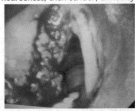

Fig 1. Laryngeal cancer along one vocal cord; it's just been biopsied, hence the bleeding. ©Rory Herdman FRCS

therapy for organ-sparing approaches. HPV +ve patients respond better to chemotherapy (2-yr survival 95% *vs* 62%), radiotherapy, and cetuximab. *Recurrence after radiotherapy:* Partial 'salvage' laryngectomy for *some* appears to be safe, effective, and gives reasonable preservation of laryngeal function.[203]

After total laryngectomy: Patients have a permanent tracheostomy, so must learn oesophageal speech. If a voice prosthesis is fitted at surgery, reasonable speech is possible within weeks. Give pre-op counselling. Discharge: eg <10d post-op, with a plastic stent or metal cannula to keep the tracheostomy open (discarded some weeks later). Excess secretions ± crusting around the stoma are common, needing meticulous attention—humidified stomal covers (eg Laryngofoam®) help here. Say to take care while having a bath, and to avoid fishing and deep water (unless expert training is to hand). *Complications:* Wound infection; pharyngocutaneous fistula; stenosis; pneumonias; post-radiation hypothyroidism (monitor TSH); pharyngeal stenosis; nodal metastasis.[204]

Rehabilitation/self-help: Suggest a laryngectomy club. (UK: 0207 381 9993)

Sinus squamous cell cancer (~1% of all tumours) *Typical patient:* Middle-aged or elderly. Suspect when chronic sinusitis presents for the first time in later life. *Early signs:* Blood-stained nasal discharge and nasal obstruction. *Later:* Cheek swelling, swelling or ulcers of the buccoalveolar plate or palate, epiphora due to a blocked nasolacrimal duct (fig 2, p419), ptosis and diplopia as the floor of the orbit is involved, and pain in maxillary division of the trigeminal nerve. Local spread may be to cheek, palate, nasal cavity, orbit, and pterygopalatine fossa. Patients present late because epistaxis, obstruction and headache only occur with large tumours. *Images:* MRI/CT ± endoscopy (with biopsy) is best. NB: coronal CT is needed to show bone erosion (esp. around the cribriform plate).[205] *Differential histology:* Squamous cell (50%), lymphoma (10%), adenocarcinoma, adenoid cystic carcinoma, olfactory neuroblastoma, or chondrosarcoma, benign tumours.[2] *Treatment:* Radiotherapy ± radical surgery. 5-yr and 10-yr overall survival rates are 77% and 66% respectively.[206]

---

2 Inverted papillomas (of Ringertz) are the most important benign tumours of the sinuses. They are exophytic masses that show distinctive epithelial invagination of the stroma without destroying the basal lamina. Total excision can therefore be difficult without taking wide margins. Most significantly, 2% show malignant change and 10% have a synchronous carcinoma.

ENT diseases

Dysphagia is difficulty in swallowing: unless it is associated with a transitory sore throat, it is a serious symptom: ▶*Endoscopy is essential.*

Painful swallowing is termed 'odynophagia'. *Globus pharyngeus* is a sensation of a lump in the throat, when not swallowing food, with no primary swallowing difficulty. Prevalence: 6%[9] Association: Hoarseness; mood↓.[207] *Tests:* Endoscopy (?hypopharyngeal cancer; pharyngeal pouch laryngeal cyst): Cause: Unclear. In a few there is cricopharyngeal overactivity[208] or ↑acid exposure at the laryngopharyngeal junction, with *normal* gastro-oesophageal pH.[209] *Treatment:* Reassure. NB: it is worsened by anxiety, and stress can form a vicious circle, but don't dismiss these patients as '*globus hystericus*'.[210]

The patient As examination is typically normal (unless anaemic), the history is central. Dyspepsia? Weight loss? Lumps?

1 Can fluid be drunk as fast as usual, except if food is stuck?
  Yes: Suspect a stricture (benign or malignant).
  No: Think of motility disorders (achalasia, neurological causes).
2 Is it difficult to make the swallowing movement?
  Yes: Suspect bulbar palsy, especially if he coughs on swallowing.
3 Is the dysphagia constant and painful?
  Yes (either feature): Suspect a malignant stricture.
4 Does the neck bulge or gurgle on drinking?
  Yes: Suspect a pharyngeal pouch (food may be regurgitated).

Tests FBC; ESR; barium swallow; rigid endoscopy with biopsy; oesophageal motility studies (this requires swallowing a catheter containing a pressure transducer). CXR. Ambulatory pH studies have no proven value.

Nutrition Dysphagia can cause malnutrition. Nutritional support may be needed pre- and post-treatment, eg via a percutaneous endoscopic gastrostomy (PEG) tube. Get expert (dietician's) help; see *OHCM* p586.[211]

Oesophageal carcinoma This is associated with achalasia, alcohol, smoking, Barrett's oesophagus (*OHCM* p708), tylosis (a hereditary condition causing hyperkeratosis of the palms), Patterson–Brown–Kelly (Plummer–Vinson) syndrome. Post-resection 5-yr survival is poor (*OHCM* p620).

Benign oesophageal stricture Causes: oesophageal reflux; swallowing corrosives; foreign body; trauma. *Treatment:* Dilatation (endoscopic or with bougies eg under GA). **Barrett's oesophagus** *OHCM* p686. **Achalasia** *OHCM* p240.

Pharyngeal pouch These are a common cause of dysphagia with gurgling. *Imaging:* Via the endoscope; barium radiology (fig 1) can help predict pouches that are unsuitable for stapling.[212] *Procedures:* Endoscopic stapling (NICE) involves stapling the bar of tissue that divides the pouch from the oesophagus. A specially designed endoscope gains access (under GA) to the bar and the openings of both the pouch and the oesophagus. In one study, other procedures included endoscopic laser surgery, external excision, cricopharyngeal myotomy; and pharyngoscopy with dilatation. Endoscopic stapling was abandoned in 15% (some declined further surgery).[213]

Malignant causes
• Oesophageal cancer
• Pharyngeal cancer
• Gastric cancer
• Extrinsic pressure, eg from lung cancer or node enlargement

Neurological causes
• Bulbar palsy (*OHCM* p510)
• Lateral medullary syn.
• Myasthenia gravis
• Syringomyelia (*OHCM* p520)

Other causes
• Benign strictures
• Pharyngeal pouch
• Achalasia*et al* (*OHCM* p240)
• Systemic sclerosis
• Oesophagitis
• Iron-deficient anaemia

ENT diseases

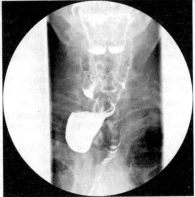

Fig 1. Pharyngeal pounch (called Zenker's diverticulum in the USA) "I've got this cough...seems to get worse watching the news on TV". When we hear this sort of absurdity, ask "What are you doing *before* the News comes on?". "Eating my dinner..." At this point ask about dysphagia, choking, chronic cough, regurgitation of undigested food, halitosis, weight loss, and aspiration. Listen to the neck after eating: any gurgles? Any lateral fullness/swelling?

Oesophageal mucosa is herniating backwards between cricopharyngeus and inferior pharyngeal constrictors. *Typical patient:* A man over 60. *Incidence:* 2/100 000/yr. *Treatment:* Surgery, eg day-case endoscopic stapling; note that flexible endoscopy can cause perforation when a pouch is unsuspected; hence the need for barium imaging.[214]

Reproduced from McGrath *et al*, *QJM* (2008) 101 (9): 747–748, with permission from Oxford University Press.

ENT diseases

Arising in the medulla, and emerging between pons and medulla, the facial nerve passes through the posterior fossa and runs through the middle ear before emerging from the stylomastoid foramen to pass into the parotid. Lesions may be at any part of its course. Branches in the temporal bone:

1 The greater superficial petrosal nerve (lacrimation).
2 Branch to stapedius (lesions above this cause hyperacusis).
3 The chorda tympani (supply taste to anterior ⅔ of the tongue) (fig 1).

Causes *Intracranial:* Brainstem tumours; strokes; polio; multiple sclerosis; cerebellopontine angle lesions (acoustic neuroma, meningitis).
Intratemporal: Otitis media; Ramsay Hunt syndrome; cholesteatoma.
Infratemporal: Parotid tumours; trauma.
Others: Lyme disease; sarcoid; Guillain–Barré; herpes; diabetes; Bell's palsy (fig 2).

Examination and tests Lower motor neuron lesions can paralyse all of one side of the face; but in upper motor neuron lesions, the forehead muscles may still work (they are bilaterally represented). Brainstem lesions produce only muscle weakness and may be accompanied by VI nerve palsies. Loss of lacrimation (Schirmer's test p418), stapedius reflex, taste (electrogustometry detects) and ↓submandibular saliva production (cannulate ducts) imply nerve lesions proximal to the origin of the relevant branches. Examine the parotid and the ears to exclude cholesteatoma and zoster (*Ramsay Hunt syndrome/herpes zoster oticus*, p652). Consider temporal bone radiography (CT). Electromyography reveals completeness of the lesion. In traumatic cases, examine the VII nerve. An incomplete palsy will probably recover; complete palsy demands surgical exploration in the presence of discontinuity of the nerve canal on CT.

Infection Otitis media causes a facial palsy in the presence of a dehiscent facial nerve and has an excellent prognosis. When cholesteatoma is present arrange emergency exploratory surgery. If rare acute necrotizing otitis externa is the cause, IV antibiotics (eg ticarcillin) and local toilet are needed.

Bell's palsy (20–30/100,000/yr). *Cause:* Inflammatory oedema from entrapment of VII in the narrow bony facial canal, eg as part of a viral polyneuropathy (herpes simplex or zoster, eg without vesicles) ± demyelination (V, X & C2 can be affected too). Onset is abrupt (eg after a nap; may be preceded by pain): the mouth sags, and dribbling, and watering (or dry) eyes occur + impaired brow-wrinkling, blowing, whistling, lid closure, cheek-pouting, taste, and speech.

Treatment: Protect the eye with glasses, and tape closed during sleep, ideally with well-fitting plastic cover over moistened gauze. If recovery is expected to take months, consider lateral tarsorrhaphy. Instil artificial tears regularly at slightest evidence of drying. There is good evidence that prednisolone helps, *if given early*[1] (eg in 1st 24h, eg 20mg/8h for 5 days, tail off over next 5 days). High-dose aciclovir or valaciclovir may also be indicated: see opposite.[215] Hooks & cheek plumpers improve appearance. Various facial reanimation procedures may be needed. Surgical exploration to check nerve continuity is controversial, but may be considered (graft with eg the lateral cutaneous nerve of the thigh).

Prognosis: ⅓ get full recovery. ⅓ have incomplete recovery of facial motor function (but don't have noticeable abnormalities.) The rest have permanent neurological and cosmetic abnormalities[216]

---

1 Many give steroids 'to reduce oedema' (esp. if <6 days since onset). Helpful studies: Hat & Shafshak[217] showing that benefit of steroids may be confined to those treated in 24h of onset. Spontaneous recovery is good-ish anyway. For every 3 people treated with steroids within 24h, 1 extra had a good recovery compared with no treatment; for ethical reasons, this study was not randomized. Older randomized studies were inconclusive, but did not look specifically at early treatment. Meta-analyses support steroids[218]

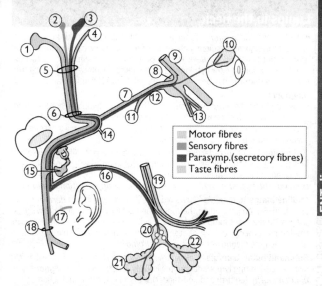

1 Facial nerve nucleus, deep in the reticular formation of lower pons
2 Spinal nucleus of V
3 Superior salivary nucleus
4 Solitary tract
5 Porus acusticus internus
6 Meatal foramen
7 Large petrosal nerve
8 Sphenopalatine ganglion
9 Superior maxillary nrv
10 Lacrimal gland
11 Large deep petrosal nrv
12 Vidian nerve
13 Nose & palate gland nrvs
14 Small petrosal nerve at geniculate ganglion
15 Stapedial nerve
16 Chorda tympani
17 Auricular branch
18 Stylomastoid foramen
19 Lingual nerve—visceral motor VII & taste VII & general sensory to tongue (V₃)
20 Submandibular ganglion
21 Submandibular gland
22 Sublingual gland

Fig 1. Facial nerve branches.

Reproduced from *Oxford Handbook of Clinical Medicine*, with permission

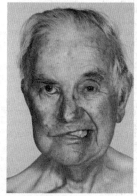

Fig 2. Bell's palsy: the patient is trying to smile, but his right lower lid is drooping, the naso-labial fold is slack, and the lips do not move. ©OUP data bank

▶Whenever you see someone with Bell's palsy within 3 days of its starting, ask about preceding pain in the ear, stiff neck, or a reddish auricle: if these are associated with severe paralysis, the cause is likely to be zoster (without vesicles: *zoster sine herpete*)—and high-dose antivirals are indicated,•※ eg valaciclovir 1g/8h PO for 7 days[219] (+prednisolone).

If there are no prodromal features, zoster is less likely and lower doses of antivirals may be used (eg valaciclovir 500mg/12h PO for 5 days).

▶*Don't biopsy neck lumps!* Refer any possibly malignant neck lump to ENT, where thorough assessment and search for a primary can be done, eg in a dedicated fast-track '2-week rule' neck lump clinic[220] with access to fine-needle aspiration (FNA for cytology—beware pulsatile lumps!) and CT/MRI (MRI is better). ▶Culture any specimens for TB: don't put it all in formalin.

Diagnosis

• *How long has the lump been present?* If <3 weeks, lymphadenopathy from a self-limiting infection is likely, and extensive investigation is unwise.

• *Which tissue layer is the lump?* Is it intradermal? (eg from sebaceous cyst with a central punctum, or a lipoma.)

If the lump is not intradermal, and not of recent onset, allow yourself to feel the intoxicating pleasure of a hunt beginning over complex terrain. But remember—you are vastly outnumbered by a pack of diseases, so be cunning. *The first step in this process is a proper appreciation of anatomy.*

Midline lumps In patients <20yrs old, the likely diagnosis is a *dermoid cyst,* or, if it moves on protruding the tongue and is below the hyoid, a *thyroglossal cyst* (a fluctuant lump developing in cell rests in thyroid's migration path; treated by surgery). If over 20, it's probably a thyroid mass, unless it is bony hard, when the diagnosis may be a *chondroma.*[221]

Submandibular triangle (Below jaw; above anterior belly of digastric.) If <20yrs, self-limiting lymphadenopathy is likely. If >20, exclude *malignant lymphadenopathy* (eg firm and non-tender). ▶Is TB likely? If it's not a node, think of *submandibular salivary stone, tumour,* or *sialadenitis.*[222]

Anterior triangle (Below digastric and in front of sternomastoid.) Nodes are common (see above): remember to examine the areas which they drain (is the spleen enlarged?—this may indicate lymphoma). *Branchial cysts* emerge under the anterior border of sternomastoid where the upper ⅓ meets the middle ⅓; age <20. The popular theory is that they are due to non-disappearance of the cervical sinus (where the 2nd branchial arch grows down over 3rd and 4th) but this is not universally accepted. Lined by squamous epithelium, their fluid contains cholesterol crystals. Treat by excision. *Cystic hygromas* (macrocystic lymphatic malformations) arise from the jugular lymph sac and transilluminate brightly. Treat by surgery or hypertonic saline sclerosant. *Carotid body paragangliomas* are very rare, move from side-to-side, but not up and down, and splay out the carotid bifurcation. They are firm (softness is rare) and pulsatile, and do not usually cause bruits. They may be bilateral, familial, and malignant (5%). This tumour should be suspected in tumours just anterior to the upper third of sternomastoid. Diagnose by MRI. Treatment: extirpation by vascular surgeon. If the lump is in the superoposterior area of the anterior triangle, is it a *parotid tumour?* (more likely if >40yrs). A *laryngocele* is an uncommon cause of a lump in the anterior triangle: it is painless, more common in males, and is made worse by blowing.[223]

Posterior triangle (Behind sternomastoid, in front of trapezius, and above the clavicle.) If there are many small lumps, think of *nodes*—TB or viruses, eg HIV or EBV (infectious mononucleosis) or, if over 20yrs, consider lymphoma or metastases. The primary may be head and neck (eg tongue base, posterior nasal space, tonsils, etc) or bronchus, gut, breast, or gonad (in that order of likelihood). *Cervical ribs* may intrude here.[224]

Tests Ultrasound shows lump consistency. CT defines masses in relation to their anatomical neighbours. Do virology and Mantoux test. CXR may show malignancy or reveal bilateral hilar lymphadenopathy, when you should consider sarcoidosis. Fine-needle aspiration (FNA, fig 7).

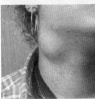
Fig 1. Branchial cyst.

Fig 2. Goitre.

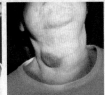
Fig 3. Infected cyst.

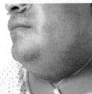
Fig 4. Deep cervical abscess.
Figs 1–6 ©Bechara Ghorayeb.

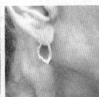
Fig 5. Lymph node metastases.

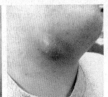
Fig 6. Submandibular abscess.

Fig 7. Pivotal role of fine needle aspiration cytology (FNAC).[225]

Fig 8. Procedure for suspicious node if FNAC +ve.

- EGA: examination under GA
- LCUC: large cell undifferentiated ca
- MDT: multidisciplinary team
- SCC: squamous cell ca
- US: ultrasound

Reproduced from Balm et al Int J Surg Oncol, 2010.

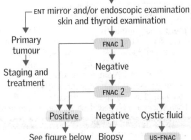

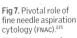

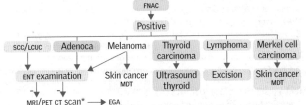

▶Refer all patients with unexplained salivary gland masses.

The 3 major pairs of salivary glands are: *parotid*, *submandibular*, and *sublingual*. ~800 smaller glands are distributed through the upper aerodigestive tract.

History and examination Dry mouth/eyes; lumps; swelling related to food; pain. Look for external swellings, secretions (in mouth first), do bimanual palpation for stones, test VII nerve, any regional nodes?

Inflammation is usually due to infection or an obstructing calculus (calcium phosphates and carbonates form around a nidus of cells and organisms).

Classification Are symptoms unilateral, or bilateral? Acute or chronic?

Acute bilateral symptoms are usually due to mumps (eg if young/unvaccinated, p142). ΔΔ: staphs, TB, HIV, ALL, Heerfordt's syndrome (acute sarcoidosis, with uveitis, fever and salivary/lacrimal gland swelling, ie uveoparotid fever).

Acute unilateral symptoms are also likely to be due to mumps but acute parotitis may occur by ascending oral infection. This occurs post-op but is now rare, unless dehydrated or poor oral hygiene; it is managed by oral hygiene, heat, massage, hydration, antibiotics (depends on culture and sensitivities). If the duct stops draining pus, or there is increasing pain and pyrexia, think of abscess formation which needs draining through the skin, in theatre.

Recurrent unilateral symptoms are often from stones (submandibular in 80%. Pain/swelling is worse on eating). The gland may be red, swollen, and tender (not always infected). Δ: plain radiography; sialography. *Treatment:* Remove distal stones via the mouth; excise the gland if it contains the stone.

Chronic bilateral symptoms may be associated with dry eyes and mouth ± Sjögren's or Mikulicz's syndromes (*OHCM* p698). *Treatment* is hard. If chronic infection is the cause, simple antibiotics will fail: what is needed is prolonged treatment with **oxytetracycline** 250mg/12h 1h ac PO.

Fixed swellings may be malignant, idiopathic or due to sarcoidosis.

Tumours '80% are in the parotid, 80% of these are benign pleomorphic adenomas, 80% of these are in the superficial lobe'. 10% are submandibular (50% are malignant here). ▶Remove any salivary gland tumour if present for >1 month (or examine cells by fine-needle aspiration: this does not lead to seeding along its track; exception: proven pleomorphic adenoma if elderly: safe to observe for years). VIIth nerve paresis suggests malignancy. As tumours grow by budding and have no capsule, lumpectomy leads to seedling deposits, so partial parotidectomy is needed. NB: sialograms (*OHCM* p597) + CT are useful pre-op.

Classification *Benign:*	*Intermediate:*	*Malignant:*
Pleomorphic (mixed parotid) adenoma	Mucoepidermoid tumour	Adenoid cystic cancer
Adenolymphoma (Warthin's tumour)	Acinic cell cancer	Adenocarcinoma
Haemangioma/lymphangioma (child)	Oncocytoma	Squamous cell cancer

Pleomorphic adenoma: Middle age; slow growth; removed by superficial parotidectomy or enucleation.◆* Radiotherapy has a role if there was intraoperative spillage, or in residual disease, or recurrences (seen in ~1–2% at 12-yr follow-up).

Adenolymphoma: Usually elderly men; soft. *Surgery:* Partial parotidectomy.

Carcinoma: Rapid growth; hard fixed mass; pain & VIIth nerve palsy. R: Surgery + radiotherapy. PET scan is better than CT and MRI for staging, detecting local recurrence and regional lymph node and distant metastases.[226]

Adenoid cystic ca: Rare tumour of exocrine mucous glands (salivary, lacrimal, lid). Painful slow growing mass + late recurrences + perineural infiltration + distant mets. Survival: 88%, 69% and 52% at 5, 10 and 15yrs[227] Follow-up: ▶for life.

Complications of surgery: VIIth palsy; salivary fistula; Frey's syndrome (BOX 3).

Assessing salivary lumps

- Note size, mobility, and extent of the mass, as well as fixity to surroundings. Any tenderness? Bimanually palpate the lateral pharyngeal wall for deep parotid tumours (any parapharyngeal space extension?).
- Also bimanually examine submandibular and sublingual masses.
- Assess surrounding skin as regional metastases from skin or mucosal malignancies may present as salivary gland masses.
- Cranial nerve examination may show neural infiltration.[228]

The dry mouth (xerostomia)

Signs Dry, atrophic, fissured oral mucosa; also:

- Discomfort, causing difficulty eating, speaking, and wearing dentures.
- No saliva pooling in floor of mouth.
- Difficulty in expressing saliva from major ducts.

Complications Dental caries; candida infection.

Management[229]

- Increase oral fluids; take frequent sips.
- Good dental hygiene; no acidic drinks and foods that demineralize teeth.
- Try a saliva substitute, eg sst® tablets (contain polyethylene and cottonseed oil). 'Allow a tablet to dissolve in the mouth—while moving it around with your tongue.' Up to 16 tablets per day may be needed.

Typical causes
• Hypnotics & tricyclics
• Antipsychotics
• β-blockers; diuretics
• Mouth breathing
• Dehydration
• ENT radiotherapy
• Sjögren's syndrome
• SLE and scleroderma
• Sarcoidosis
• HIV/AIDS
• Parotid sialoliths; 40% are radio-opaque *vs* >80% if submandibular

- Chewing sugar-free gum or sweets may ↑salivary flow.[230]
- Pilocarpine (Salagen®) is rarely satisfactory.[231,232] Cholinergic SE: sweating, lacrimation, rhinitis, amblyopia, diarrhoea, urinary frequency. Pilocarpine mouth washes may obviate these (difficult to obtain, but may be made by diluting pilocarpine eye-drops in water).[233] $N=40$
- *Irradiation xerostomia:* Acupuncture may help, eg as an 8-needle regimen of 3 weekly sessions followed by monthly sessions.[234] $n=50$

ENT diseases

Łucja Frey and her misconnection syndrome (fig 1)

"Doctor...when I eat, or even just *think* of food, a sweaty rash crops up on my cheek." Duphenix first described gustatory sweating in 1757. Its cause was mysterious until 1923, when a soldier presented to Łucja Frey, a pioneering Polish neurologist (the first female neurologist we know of, and the most tragic). Her soldier had a bullet in his parotid, and gustatory sweating. Frey's brilliant dissections showed how the auriculo-temporal branch of the trigeminal nerve sends parasympathetic fibres to the parotid and sympathetic fibres to facial sweat glands. During resprouting after injury, fibres switch course to cause gustatory sweating. How misguided...

You don't have to be shot to get Frey's syndrome. Other causes: birth trauma; parotid surgery (in 23%, so pre-op counselling is vital but only understood fully by neuroanatomists; NB: +ve Minor's iodine starch tests that detect subclinical cases are seen post-op in 62%). Management is hard, but not always needed. Botulinum toxin has been tried.

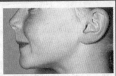
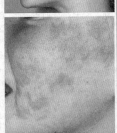

Fig 1. Frey's syndrome before and after eating.

Reproduced from *Frey's syndrome: a masquerader of food allegy*, Nahin Hussain, Muthu Dhanarass, William Whitehouse, *Postgrad Med J* 86 (1011), with permission (BMJ Publishing Group Ltd).

Frey was murdered by Nazis with all her patients in the Lwow ghetto in 1942.

▶Any oral ulcer which has not healed in 3 weeks should receive specialist assessment for biopsy to exclude malignancy (*OHCM* p238).

Causes of facial pain Tooth pathology, sinusitis, temporomandibular joint (TMJ) dysfunction, salivary pathology, migraine, trigeminal neuralgia, atypical facial pain (no clear cause), trauma, cluster headache (*OHCM* p461), angina, frontal bone osteomyelitis (post sinusitis), ENT tumours.

▶When helping a patient with a dental infection pay attention to these features—before consulting a maxillofacial surgeon, or a dentist (GDP).

1 *Is it the teeth?* History: *Is the pain...*
- Worse with sugar and heat? } Tooth is alive
- Worse or better with cold? } (pulpitis)
- Intermittent?

Is the pain...
- Worse with percussion? } Tooth dead
- Constant/uninterrupted? } (osteitis/abscess)

Is the pain...
- Exacerbated by movement } Abscess
  between finger and thumb }

Radiography (usually helpful): Orthopantogram (OPT) is useful for imaging molars and pre-molars. If incisors are suspected, request periapical radiographs of the tooth in question. Interpretation of radiograph...

• **Abscess**
(Tooth tender to percussion)

• **Periodontal disease**
(Tooth mobile)

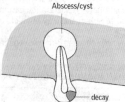
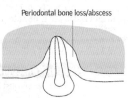

Fig 1. Distinguishing between (a) absess of the tooth and (b) periodontal disease.

2 *Trismus:* (Opening mouth is difficult because of spasm or pain.) This is a sign of severe infection. Ask the patient to open mouth wide and measure how many fingers breadth between the incisor teeth. Trismus always requires maxillofacial advice. Other causes: tetanus; neoplasia.

3 *Facial swellings due to dental infection:* Usually subside with oral antibiotics. ▶If swelling is related to the lower jaw, assess for airways obstruction; if spreading to the eye, assess the second cranial nerve. If in any doubt, refer to a maxillofacial surgeon.

4 *Bedside observations:* Temperature (very important), pulse and blood pressure. This information must be to hand *prior* to referral. Systemically unwell patients require maxillofacial advice/admission.

5 *Systemic disease complicating dental infection:* Any immunocompromise (eg HIV, leukaemia, diabetics, those on steroids); patients at risk of endocarditis; coagulopathy (eg haemophilia or warfarin). Seek specialist advice. In one HIV study, lesions included: candidiasis (29%), ulcers (15%), salivary gland disease (9%), necrotizing ulcerative gingivitis/periodontitis (5%), linear gingival erythema (4%), labial molluscum contagiosum (3%), oral warts (2%), hairy leukoplakia (2%), and herpes zoster (1%).[235]

Dental caries Although on the decline in the West due primarily to fluoride,

ENT diseases

this condition is increasing exponentially in developing countries. Causes: bacteria (esp. *S. mutans*), substrate (sugars) and susceptible tooth surface. In otherwise healthy individuals it is an entirely preventable disease.

Rampant caries is a variant found in children exposed to excessive sucrose in the forms of coated dummies, 'health' drinks, and prescribed medicines.

Radiation caries (eg post head & neck radiotherapy, eg with jaw osteoradionecrosis). *Treatment and complications:* Pain ± infection. Toothache pain responds best to NSAIDs, eg **ibuprofen** 200–400mg/8h PO after food (can buy it from pharmacists), and dental infection to **penicillin** and **metronidazole**, but drug treatment is never definitive, and a dental referral is required.

Periodontal disease Virtually all dentate adults have gingivitis, caused by bacterial and polysaccharide complexes at the tooth–gingival interface (=plaque). Toothbrushing is the only answer. Pathogens: herpes; streps.*et al*

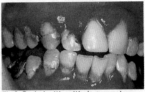

Fig 2. Periodontitis with damange to supporting tissue including bone. © BMJ.

Vincent's angina is a smoking or HIV associated, painful, foul-smelling, ulcerative gingivitis, caused by anaerobes (*Fusobacteria*) ± spirochetes (*Borellia vincentii*). ℞: penicillin 250mg/6h PO + metronidazole 200mg/8h PO.

Causes of gingival swelling: Fibrous hyperplasia (congenital or from phenytoin, ciclosporin, nifedipine); pregnancy, HIV, scurvy, leukaemic deposits.

Periodontitis (pyorrhoea) is a progression of localized inflammation from the gums into the ligament supporting a tooth. Associations: anaerobes; calcified bacterial deposits (calculi, tartar); poor oral hygiene. It needs a dentist.

HIV and periodontal disease: HIV causes linear gingival erythema, necrotizing ulcerative gingivitis and necrotizing ulcerative periodontitis.

Causes of juvenile periodontitis: Poor nutrition; immunosuppression; wcc↓; neutrophil dysfunction (leucocyte adhesion deficiency, Chediak–Higashi or Papillon–Lefevre syndrome, with palmar keratosis), granulomatous disease.[236]

Malocclusion Inappropriate positioning of the teeth in the jaws or between the jaws themselves is common. Those with prominent upper teeth are particularly prone to trauma, and those children at risk (eg in epilepsy) or those involved in contact sports should be referred to an orthodontist. Those with severe facial or jaw disharmony who may be unable to chew or have psychological difficulty with their appearance may be amenable to surgical correction by an oral or maxillofacial surgeon.

Wisdom teeth These declare themselves in early adult life. Like the appendix, they are something of a vestigial organ. Impaction can cause pain (fig 3). They account for an enormous number of inpatient operations. If asymptomatic and not exposed to contamination by the mouth, they don't usually need removal. Complications are pain and infection and they may be involved in

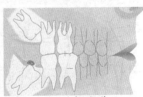

Fig 3. Impacting wisdom teeth.

fractures of the mandible. Post-op recovery is often complicated by pain and swelling; pain responds well to NSAIDs and poorly to opiates (eg dihydrocodeine. Infection complicates up to 30% not receiving antibiotics. Penicillin and metronidazole (as above) are standbys.

Teething An acute sore mouth during tooth eruption is often caused by viral infections (eg herpetic). The onset of eruption of first deciduous teeth (fig 1, p221) correlates with the fall-off in transferred maternal antibody.

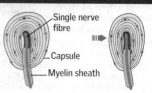

Fig 1. Under pressure: the right Pacinian corpuscle is feeling the strain. Filippo Pacini, the Italian anatomist, born in 1812, saw the corpuscles that now bear his name in a hand he was dissecting as a medical student in an anatomy class in Pistoia hospital in 1831, when he was 19.[1]

These corpuscles (~1mm in diameter) transmit pressure sensations. We can feel our clothes as soon as we put them on—whereupon we stop feeling them, as these corpuscles only respond to *changes* in pressure.

No one took his observations seriously, and Pacini heads our list of brilliant medical students ignored by their narrow-mined professors. For example, he discovered the cause of cholera in 1854, 30 years before Koch's 'first' description.[2]

Pacini was the first medical student to understand what it is to feel pressure, without buckling. In his case, his chief pressure was the need to look after his two sick sisters. These duties eventually bankrupted him, and he died in a poorhouse in Florence in 1883.[2]

We dedicate this chapter to him, and everyone else feeling the strain.

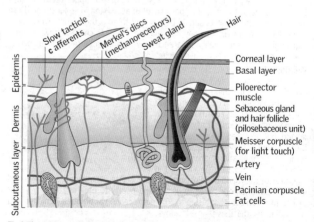

Fig 2. The anatomy of pleasure. All pleasure is sensory, and as our skin is our largest organ, let us rejoice in our unmyelinated tactile c afferents which mediate all tactile pleasure by sending impulses to our insular cortex rather than to mundane somatosensory areas.[3]

Holistic approaches to dermatology

Because our skin is our most superficial organ, dermatology is never given due weight; but the skin is also our heaviest organ, and although its wounds only ever seem skin deep, their effects cast long shadows over the psyche because people judge our health and beauty by the condition of our skin.[4,5]

Our skin displays a more varied range of signs and reaction patterns than any other organ. Recognizing these may allow diagnosis of unsuspected systemic diseases (see p588). Primarily skin conditions such as eczema and psoriasis (p594) are not only the domain of dermatologists but are likely to be encountered by us all, regardless of our field of practice. A practical knowledge and clinical confidence in diagnosing skin disease is thus a most valuable asset—and we all need to know how the dermatological aspects of our patients' lives interact to form those complex social and biological matrices that are the lives of our patient with chronic skin conditions.

Dermatologists do not confine themselves to the skin. Skin symptoms are features of many medical (p588) and psychiatric illnesses, eg body image problems, dermatitis artefacta, neurotic excoriations, and trichotillomania (neurotic pulling out of one's hair).[6]

Psychocutaneous events There is an association between depression/social phobia and psoriasis, and between obsessive–compulsive disorder, stress, and acne. If you doubt the relevance of psychocutaneous phenomena, look no further than Dennis Potter's *Singing Detective*, Philip Marlow.[7]

The psycho-physiology of acne is instructive. Sebaceous glands and their secretions are involved in a pathway like the hypothalamic–pituitary–adrenal axis, mediating a direct link between oily skin and the stress hormone CRH (corticotrophin releasing hormone) which acts on sebaceous glands. So think of CRH as an autocrine hormone for human sebocytes that exerts homeostatic lipogenic activity, with testosterone and growth hormone inducing CRH negative feedback. These findings implicate CRH (hence stress) in mediating acne, seborrhoea, androgenic alopecia, skin ageing, and xerosis. Substance P is another route connecting stress, seborrhoea, and acne.[8,9]

Telemedicine, virtual outreach, and dermatology delivery

Traditionally, dermatologists see patients on wards and in central clinics: convenient for them, but less convenient for patients who live far away, and this paradigm does not allow for useful interaction between the referring doctor and the specialist. Also, urgency cannot be assessed until the patient presents (unless a photograph is sent with the referral letter; this simple idea requires e-mail, digital cameras, and technical commitment). Telemedicine uses high-quality video links and computer equipment to form a virtual consultation. Is the expense entailed worth it? Are there problems—even for this, the most visual of specialties?

Advantages	*Disadvantages*[10,11] N=3170
Travel times are less	Expense is not outweighed by ↓travel time
Fewer tests ordered	No proper sharing of patients' problems
Teaching referring GPs	Technical problems can waste whole sessions
Patient satisfaction	Extra time needed from GPs and consultants
Fewer follow-ups	Important clinical cues are lost in telemedicine

We thank our Specialist Reader, Dr Jonathan Bowling, and our Junior Reader, William Hunt, for their help with this chapter.

History Duration of rash/lesions; site of onset, spread, and distribution of lesions; symptoms (itch, pain); aggravating factors (sunlight, heat); previous treatments; medical conditions and medications; family history (psoriasis, atopy); occupation (industrial chemicals); pets. Family and personal history of allergy/atopy (eg to animal danders), migraine.

Examination Examine all the skin, the hair, and nails. To communicate with a dermatologist, it is customary to translate your findings into rather garbled Latin or Greek (see below—but English will usually do just as well).

Distribution Symmetrical flexural (atopic eczema, fig 1 on p596); contact with jewellery or cosmetics (allergic contact dermatitis); areas exposed to sun, eg backs of hands, face, neck (photosensitivity); grouped lesions (herpes virus); symmetrical extensor surfaces (psoriasis, p594). Are there crops of lesions? Monomorphic (Greek for all taking one form or shape) or polymorphic?

Pattern Ring (fungal—active edge with healing centre, p598); linear (Köbner phenomenon, below), targetoid (erythema multiforme).

Terms used to describe lesions and processes in dermatology	
Alopecia	Hair loss
Atopy/atopic	Prone to allergic eczema, asthma, or rhinitis; *typical patient:* city-based child in a 1-child family of high socio-economic class.[1,2]
Atrophy	Thinning and loss of skin substance
Autosensitization	General lowering of the irritation threshold triggered by intense local inflammation, eg a fungal foot infection or a local area of contact dermatitis may produce a generalized itchy rash (=autoeczematization='id reaction')
Bulla	Blister larger than a vesicle (see below, ie >0.5cm diameter)
Crust	Dried brownish exudate
Erosion	Superficial break in epidermal surface; heals without scarring
Erythema	Reddening of the skin which blanches on pressure
Excoriation	A scratch which has broken the surface of the skin
Filiform	Long, irregular projections, which may be threadlike, or broader, like close-packed tombstones on a mound (seen in warts)
Fissure	Crack, often through keratin
Induration	An area of cutaneous or subcutaneous hardening or thickening
Köbner phenomena	Skin lesions which develop at sites of injury—seen in psoriasis (p594), lichen planus, plane warts, and vitiligo
Lichenification	Skin thickening with exaggerated skin markings, as a result of repeated trauma (eg in response to itch). See fig 1, p585
Macule	Defined, flat area of altered pigmentation; big macules are *patches*
Nodule	Solid lump >0.5cm in diameter; subcutaneous or intradermal
Papule	Raised well-defined lesion, usually less than 0.5cm in diameter
Plaque	Raised flat-topped lesion, usually over 2cm in diameter
Purpura	Purplish lesion resulting from free red blood cells in the skin; it doesn't blanch on pressure, and may be nodular (vasculitis)
Pustule	Well-defined, pus-filled lesion
Scale	Fragment of dry skin
Scar	Permanent replacement of skin area with connective tissue
Ulcer	Loss of epidermis and dermis resulting in a scar (unlike erosions)
Vesicle	Blister less than 0.5cm in diameter
Weals/urticaria	Transient pale papules with pink margins, eg 'nettle rash' (=hives)

Let's stop excoriating our pustules and admit that jargon inflates our self-importance.

---

1 Allergic conjunctivitis and urticaria are other features.

Ointments, creams, lotions: 3 ends of a spectrum

▶Ointments are for dry skin, and creams are for moist areas. Any topical compound is more or less like an idealized *ointment* (greasy as has no added water), *cream* (oil-in-water or water-in-oil emulsions) or *lotion* (water-based; typically made from powders). Lotions are less common (used as a coolant, eg calamine lotion). If a large area of skin is involved, a large volume of cream or ointment is needed, eg 500g. Use clean procedures when getting creams out of pots, eg remove cream with a clean spoon first. Close tubs of ointment after use. Pump dispensers are a good way around bacterial contamination. Regimens may be complex, and you may get annoyed at the patient's 'poor compliance'—until you reframe this as loss of *concordance* (compliance is when the doctor and the patient share the same view as to what is important[13]). Then you may get annoyed with yourself (just as bad). Avoid both by getting a nurse to help plan treatment through dialogue, and understanding lifestyle constraints. ▶Dermatology/practice nurses are invaluable in teaching topical therapies, and in optimizing concordance. ▶Topical treatment is not enough: take steps to improve coping behaviour and quality of life.[14]

Concordance: harmony + singing the same song.

Dermatology

Latin[L] & Greek[G] for dermatologists

Alba[L]=white (as in albino).

Cutis[L]=skin (sub[L]=under, eg subcutaneous).

Derma[G] δεμα=skin (intra[L]=within, hence intradermal=within the skin).

Eczema[G], from ekzein, to break out, boil over: ek, out; (zein=to boil).

Erythema[G]= redness (eg of the skin).

Impetere[L]=to attack (as in impetigo).

Indurare[L]=to harden (as in induration).

Lichen[L]=tree moss; lichenification to dermatologist means like Morocco leather, a condition caused by scratching (fig 1).

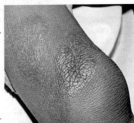
Fig 1. Lichenification.

Livedo[L] livid (furious, red/blue); *reticulum*[L]=net[L]. Livedo reticularis, p588.

Lupus[L]=wolf.

Macula[L]=stain/spot (immaculate; without stain; macula peccati=the stain of original sin).

Mens/mentem[L]=mind; nature; temper; mentum=chin (submental=below the jaw).

Muto (mutat)[L]=I (he) change(s)/mutate(s).

Papilla[L]=nipple or teat (so papule; papilloma).

Pilus/pili[L]=hair (hence fur coat; pelt)/hairs.

Pityriasis[G]=grain husk, scale; pityuron=bran.

Psoriasis[G]=to have the itch (psora=itch; NB: psoriasis often does not itch).

Purpura[L]=purple (imperial) colour; porphyra.[G]

Rosea[L]=pink; akme[G]=acne (summit; acme; pimple);[15] acne rosacea=pink pimples, p600.

Seborrhoeic=making *sebum*[L] (suet, grease).

Senex[L]=old man.

Tel[G]...telos=end+angeion=+vessel+ekstasis =extension, hence telangiectasia.

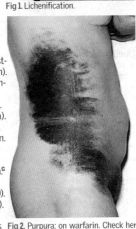
Fig 2. Purpura: on warfarin. Check her INR *now*! Is vitamin K needed?

Topicos[G]=surface (hence *top*ography; creams are *top*ical).

Vesica[L]=purse, bladder (fluid-filled blister). *Vitellus*[L]=spotted calf (vitiligo).

So...try translating *lupus pilum mutat, non mentem* (the wolf can change his coat but not his nature); but it is unkind to think of dermatologists as wolves: think of them as leopards who *can* change their (and our) spots.

Possible causes of patterns of skin disease

White lesions
- Pityriasis versicolor: superficial slightly scaly infection with the yeast *Malassezia furfur*; appears depigmented on darker skins; ℞: p598.
- Pityriasis alba: post-eczema hypopigmentation, often on children's faces.
- Vitiligo (*vitellus* is Latin for *spotted calf*): white patches ± hyperpigmented borders. Sunlight causes itch. *Associations*: Autoimmunity: pernicious anaemia, thyroid or Addison's, DM, alopecia areata. ℞: (unsatisfactory): try cosmetic camouflage, narrowband UVB PUVA (p595)[16] ± potent topical steroids.

Ring-shaped lesions • Basal cell cancer (rodent ulcer; p590): pearly papule + central ulcer.
- Tinea: active red scaly edge + central healing.
- Granuloma annulare (fig 1; ~1cm ring on hand).
- Erythema multiforme: target-like lesions, eg on extensor limb surfaces (fig 2 p588).
- Rarely, leprosy.

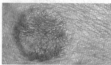

Fig 1. Granuloma annulare.
©Dr Jonathan Bowling.

Brown pigmented lesions Apart from sun-related freckles there are:
- Lentigos: persistent brown macules, often larger than freckles (fig 2).
- Café-au-lait spots: faint brown macules; if >5, consider neurofibromatosis.[17,18]
- Seborrhoeic keratoses/warts: benign greasy-brown warty lesions usually on the back, chest, and face; very common in the elderly.
- Chloasma (melasma) are brown patches especially on the face, related to pregnancy or Pill use. The condition may respond to topical azelaic acid.
- Systemic diseases: Addison's (palmar creases, oral mucosa, scars); haemochromatosis; porphyria cutanea tarda (+ skin fragility and blisters).

Round, oval, or coin-shaped (discoid) lesions • Bowen's disease (fig 7).
- Discoid eczema (fig 5 & p602): itchy, crusted/scaly eczema, worsened by heat.
- Psoriasis: well-defined scaly red/pink plaques (p594). Distribution on extensor surfaces, scalp and natal cleft distinguishes it from discoid eczema (also, scales are thicker, get silvery on rubbing, and bleed on lifting).
- Pityriasis rosea: herald patch; oval red lesions with scaly edge, eg on trunk.
- Erythema chronicum migrans (fig 3). See p588.
- Impetigo: well-defined red patches, covered with honey-coloured crust, fig 6.

Linear lesions • Köbner phenomenon: psoriasis, lichen planus.
- Dermatitis artefacta: linear or bizarre-shaped lesions, induced by patient.
- Herpes zoster: polymorphous vesicles/pustules in dermatomal distribution.
- Scabies burrows (fig 8, the mite is visible as a speck just above the red area).
- Cutaneous larva migrans (fig 4), eg from strongyloidiasis (OHCM p442).

Subcutaneous nodules Rheumatoid nodules, rheumatic fever, PAN, xanthelasma, tuberous sclerosis, neurofibroma, sarcoidosis, granuloma annulare.

Itch (pruritus) ▶ *Itch can be very distressing.* Skin will usually be scratched or rubbed and a number of secondary skin signs are seen: excoriations (scratch marks); lichenification (skin thickening, fig 1 on p585); papules or nodules (local skin thickening). *Causes*: Dry (and older) skin tends to itch. Determine if there is a primary skin disease or is itch due to systemic disease.
- Itchy lesions: *scabies* (burrows in finger-webs, wrists, groin, buttock; *urticaria* (transient wheals, dermatographism); *atopic eczema* (flexural eruption, lichenification, fig 1 on p596); dermatitis herpetiformis (very itchy blisters on elbows, shoulders); lichen planus (flat violet wrist papules).
- In ~22%, itch is caused by a systemic disease:[19] *Fe↓* (koilonychia, pale); *lymphoma* (nodes, hepatosplenomegaly); *hypo/hyperthyroidism; liver disease* (jaundice, spider naevi); *chronic renal failure* (dry sallow skin); *malignancy* (clubbing, masses); *drugs.* Do FBC, ESR, ferritin, LFT, U&E, glucose, TSH, CXR.

Treatment: Treat any primary disease; bland emollients (eg Diprobase®) to soothe dry skin; emollient bath oils; sedative antihistamines at night.

Lentigos are brown macules/patches. Some are premalignant. Fig 2: lentigo maligna (melanoma *in situ*)—precursor to invasive lentigo maligna melanoma. Typical patient: Caucasian >40yrs. It develops in sun-damaged skin. It is flat, irregular, and variably pigmented (darker areas may be invasive). Not all show ABCDE signs of malignancy.[1] Use dermoscopes[2] ± biopsy in equivocal lesions.[20] Excision is best (>5mm margins); if impossible, try radiotherapy or topical 5% **imiquimod** × 5/wk (*typical time to clear:* 9 wks; do repeated biopsy over the next years[21] to spot dangerously common occult recurrence).[22]

Dermatology

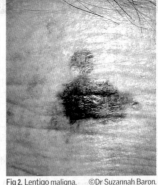

Fig 2. Lentigo maligna.   ©Dr Suzannah Baron.

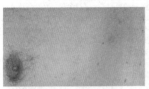

Fig 3. Erythema chronicum migrans.
Courtesy of Dr Jonathan Bowling.

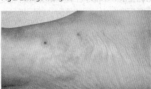

Fig 4. Cutaneous larval migrans.
Courtesy of Dr Jonathan Bowling.

Fig 5. Discoid/nummular eczema (p602).
Dr Jonathan Bowling (& figs 7 & 8).

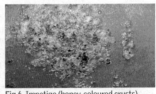

Fig 6. Impetigo (honey-coloured crusts).
Courtesy of Dr Samuel Da Silva.

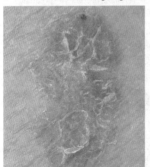

Fig 7. Bowen's disease.

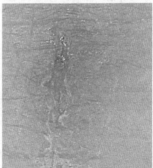

Fig 8. Scabies burrow (and mite, top).

1 A for asymmetry; B for border irregularity; C for colour (non-uniform browns, blacks, reds, whites, or blues); D for diameter >6mm; E for evolving over time.[23]
2 The dermoscope is a battery-operated handheld microscope-like instrument using epiluminescence for evaluating pigmented skin lesions. It allows vision through the stratum corneum.[24]

Dermatology

Diabetes *Flexural candidiasis; necrobiosis lipoidica* (waxy, shiny red/brown plaques, then atrophic/yellow, on shins. ♀:♂≈3:1); *folliculitis; skin infections.*

Coeliac disease *Dermatitis herpetiformis* (very itchy/"burning" blisters on elbows, scalp, shoulders, ankles). *Treatment:* long-term gluten-free diet.[25,26] It responds quickly to **dapsone** (50-200mg/day PO). *SE:* haemolysis, LFT↑, agranulocytosis. *CI:* G6PD deficiency. Small risk of lymphoma in chronic disease.[27]

Inflammatory bowel disease •*Erythema nodosum* (tender ill-defined subcutaneous nodules, eg on shins; other causes: sarcoidosis, drugs, TB, streps) •*Pyoderma gangrenosum:* recurring nodulo-pustular ulcers, ~10cm wide, with tender red/blue overhanging necrotic edge, healing with cribriform (pitted) scars. *Site:* eg leg; abdomen; face. Other causes: autoimmune hepatitis; neoplasia; Wegener's•; myeloma. ♀:♂ >1:1.

Rheumatoid arthritis (RA) Rheumatoid nodules; vasculitis (nodular purpura, with ulcers).

Systemic lupus erythematosus (SLE) *OHCM* p556. *Facial butterfly rash; photosensitivity* (face, dorsum of hands, V of neck); *red scaly rash; diffuse alopecia.* Δ: Autoantibodies; skin biopsy with immunofluorescence.

Erythema multiforme (fig2) *Minor form:* Target lesions, usually on extensor surfaces esp. of peripheries, palms, and soles. *Major form:* (Stevens-Johnson syndrome/toxic epidermal necrolysis, p601) associated with systemic upset, fever, severe mucosal involvement, including conjunctivae. *Cause:* Herpes simplex (70%);[1] mycoplasma; viruses (minor form); drugs esp. sulfonamides, penicillins (major form). *R:* Treat the cause; supportive care, steroids (controversial; may ↑mortality), other immunomodulators.[28] *Major complications:* Strictures of mucous membranes, eg with severe eye problems.[29]

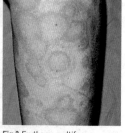
Fig 2. Erythema multiforme.

Erythema migrans (fig 3 p587) We all need to be good at this rash as it's the best way to diagnosis Lyme disease, as serology is difficult. ►<50% give history of a tick bite. City and rural people have similar risk. A papule becomes a spreading red ring, lasting weeks to months. *R:* 3wks PO doxycycline 100mg/12h, amoxicillin 500mg/8h, or cefuroxime.[30]

Cutaneous vasculitis (capillaritis/venulitis/arteriolitis) Signs: Variable, eg palpable purpura, eg on legs; nodules; ulcers; livedo reticularis. Causes: idiopathic (often); thiazides; neoplasia; systemic vasculitis, eg polyarteritis nodosa (PAN), Henoch-Schönlein purpura (vasculitic rash on legs/buttocks ± arthralgia, abdominal pain and glomerulonephritis); Wegener's• granulomatosis.

Livedo reticularis (fig3) Non-blanching vague persisting, red/blue zig-zags enclosing more normal skin, like diamond-shaped holes in a net, eg on legs (*reticulum* is latin for net). Causes/triggers: cold, pregnancy; RA; SLE; lymphoma; PAN; TB; polymyositis; Raynaud's; Sneddon's cerebral infarction; (cryoglobulins; sticky platelets; Ca²⁺↑; intra-arterial injection; cholesterol emboli; homocystinuria; ♀:♂ >1:1. *R:* Treat cause±bath PUVA.[31]

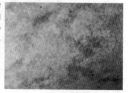
Fig 3. Livedo reticularis.

1 Erythema multiforme may be precipitated by orolabial and genital herpes recurrences and by recurrences on buttocks and other sites. Episodes of erythema multiforme are not always associated with clinical herpetic recurrences. Herpes-associated erythema multiforme can be controlled by continuous oral aciclovir; it is not prevented by aciclovir if a herpes simplex recurrence is present or just passed.[32]

Lupus erythematosus (LE): 5 types of skin change: 1) *Chilblain LE:* Cryoglobulin/cold agglutinin -ve; ℞: antimalarials, steroids, pentoxifylline, or dapsone.[33]

2) *Chronic cutaneous (discoid) LE:* Inflamed plaques + scarring ± atrophy; may respond to: ↓sun exposure, topical steroids, antimalarials (hydroxychloroquine).

3) *Subacute cutaneous LE:* Widespread, non-scarring round or psoriasis-like plaques in photodistribution. ANA or Ro/La +ve.

4) *Acute systemic lupus erythematosus (SLE):* Specific malar induration forming butterfly rash or widespread indurated erythema on upper trunk.

5) *Non-specific cutaneous LE phenomenon:* Vasculitis, alopecia, oral ulcers, palmar erythema, periungual erythema, Raynaud's phenomenon.

CREST: Scleroderma[1]/morphea with: calcinosis cutis; Raynaud's; œsophageal dysmotility; sclerodactyly; ↑telangiectasia. Typically anti-centromere +ve.

Sarcoidosis (Hypopigmented areas, waxy deposits; biopsy shows non-caseating granulomata). Plaques are red/violet, indurated, and shiny, eg on face and extremities. They may become annular in shape and the centre of the plaque may atrophy. If seen with telangiectasia, use the term angiolupoid.

Lupus pernio (fig 1) (diagnostic of sarcoidosis): chronic sarcoid plaques eg on nose, ears, lips, and cheeks ± permanent scarring. Granulomatous infiltration of nasal mucosa and respiratory tract may precede nasal septum destruction. Bulbous, sausage-shaped fingers signify underlying bone cysts. ℞: Alefacept (T-cell inhibitor) may be effective.[34]

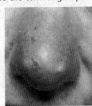

Fig 1. Lupus pernio of the nose. © OTM/OUP.

Darier–Roussy subcutaneous nodules may be seen on arms and legs (typically non-tender). Fish-like ichthyosiform sarcoid presents as dark polygonal scaly patches on the legs.[35] It may respond to steroids.[36] Verruciform (warty) lesions, erythroderma, oral lesions, nail dystrophy, and scarring alopecia also occur.[37]

Paraneoplastic skin phenomena[38]

If a tumour makes transforming growth factor (similar to epidermal growth factor and binds the same receptors) distant keratinocytes flourish excessively, and a range of proliferative paraneoplastic signs erupt, eg sudden flocks of seborrheic keratoses (*Leser-Trélat sign*), *tripe palms* (ridged velvety lesions), and *florid cutaneous papillomatosis* and *acanthosis nigricans*—symmetrical darkening and velvety skin thickening, most often of axillae, sides of the neck, and groin, seen with gastric cancer and lymphoma (also: obesity; acromegaly, Cushing's, DM, and thyroid disorders).[39] *Pruritus* (p586) may be paraneoplastic; others (all 6 are rare):[2]

1 *Amyloidosis:* Purpura ('raccoon eyes' if periorbital, fig1 *OHCM* p364), macroglossia; low-voltage ECG, nephrosis, carpal tunnel syndrome, neuropathy. Malignant associations: myeloma, lymphoma, and endometrial cancer.[40]

2 *Paraneoplastic pemphigus:* An autoimmune mucocutaneous disease associated with lymphoproliferative disorders (eg leukaemia); also melanoma; mesenchymal sarcomas; BCC; bronchogenic carcinoma.[41] Signs: severe oral and conjunctival ulceration resembling Stevens-Johnson's syndrome.[42]

3 *Dermatomyositis:* Heliotrope (red/purple) lids; periungual redness; Gottron's papules (flat violet knuckle papules) from lung, breast, ovary, or colon ca.

4 *Erythroderma* (>50% of skin is too red) eg from lymphoreticular neoplasia.

5 *Acquired ichthyosis:* Dry scaly skin; recent onset points to lymphoma or cancer; as one lost soul in denial said: "Pay no attention to the dry scales that discolour my skin, nor to the way my flesh wastes away." *Dante Purgatorio*

6 *Hypertrichosis lanuginosa* (An increase in downy lanugo hair); associated with lung, bladder, gallbladder, rectum, colon, uterus, and breast cancer.

---

1 Connective tissue disease with chemokine-mediated ✒️ ↑deposition of extracellular matrix in skin.[43]

2 Ask the lab to characterize paraneoplastic antibodies (eg anti-Hu) from lung cancer (*OHCM* p539).

Actinic (solar) keratoses (AK) (fig 3) Pre-malignant crumbly yellow-white scaly crusts occur on sun-exposed skin from dysplastic intra-epidermal proliferation of atypical keratinocytes. *UK prevalence:* If 40yrs old, 21%; if 70yrs old, 52%. *Natural history:* May regress/recur. *ΔΔ:* Bowen's, psoriasis, seborrhoeic wart, BCC; if in doubt, biopsy. *Treatment:* See BOX. *Prevention:* Education; hats; sunscreens ± ↓dietary fat—but enough vitamin A. [44-46]

Basal cell carcinoma (BCC = rodent ulcer) Typically, a pearly nodule with rolled telangiectatic edge on the face. Metastases are very rare. It is locally destructive (esp. if multinodular). Lesions on the trunk can appear as red scaly plaques with raised smooth edge. *Cause:* UV exposure may induce mutations in TP53 tumour-suppressor gene. [47] *R̄:* Excision; radiotherapy if a big lesion, eg in the elderly. Cryo ± curettage can be used if non-critical site; [48] consider imiquimod if superficial. [49]

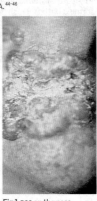

Bowen's disease (fig 4) Slow-growing red scaly plaque, eg on shin. *Histology:* Full-thickness dysplasia/carcinoma *in situ*. May progress to squamous cell cancer (esp. if hyperkeratotic). *R̄:* Cryo (≤5sec if on face); topical fluorouracil (BOX); photodynamic therapy. [50]

Leprosy (fig 5) Rare; suspect in any hypopigmented anaesthetic skin lesion.

Fig 1. BCC on the nose.

Leukoplakia (p607). **Lentigos** (p587) **Melanoma** (p592).

Metastatic cancer Skin metastases are uncommon but well recognized in association with carcinomas of breast (fig 6), kidney, and lung. Non-Hodgkin's lymphoma and leukaemia can also metastasize to the skin. Metastases are usually firm, rather inflammatory lesions; often on the scalp or trunk.

Mycosis fungoides The chief skin lymphoma (CD4 helper T-cell). [51] Well-defined red scaly patches or plaques on trunk/limbs. *Δ:* Biopsy *R̄:* Topical steroids, PUVA (p595; if early [52]), electron-beam radiation. Leukaemic phase (Sezary syndrome) is associated with erythroderma and circulating Sezary cells, [53] and deletions on chromosome 10q. [54] 5yr survival: 90%; most deaths are from sepsis. [55]

Paget's disease of the nipple (fig7) An itchy, red, scaly, or crusted nipple, from intraductal breast cancer (with a mass in 50%). *Δ:* Biopsy. *ΔΔ:* Eczema (but eczema is bilateral, non-deforming, and waxes and wanes), so... ►*always consider a biopsy in "nipple eczema"*. Also consider ultrasound, mammography and sentinel node biopsy. *Surgery:* Mastectomy or lesser surgery ± radiotherapy. [56-58]

Squamous cell cancer (fig 2, the commonest skin cancer after BCC) A persistently ulcerated or crusted firm irregular lesion often on sun-exposed sites, eg ear; hand dorsum; bald scalp (here it may develop in a pre-existing AK, above). Also related to smoking (on lower lip), chronic inflammation, eg venous leg ulcers, and HPV (eg genital area or periungual, like verrucas, p570). [59] *R̄:* Excision. Topical imiquimod or 5FU if superficial. [60] Metastases are rare, frequent at some sites, eg the ears.

Syphilis Isolated painless genital ulcers (1° chancre [fig 8]). Pityriasis rosea-like copper-coloured scaly rashes affecting trunk, limbs, palms, and soles (2° syphilis). See *OHCM* p431. Are other sexually transmitted infections present?

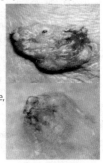

Fig 2. Squamous cell ca.

Dermatology

Options in actinic keratoses (AK)

- *Surgical excision and curettage:* Excision of AKs is used only if invasive SCC is suspected or recurrent lesions are present. Curettage (±electro-surgery or cryotherapy) has very good cure rates.[61]
- *Cryotherapy:* Warn that blisters may form afterwards; they may be burst, repeatedly, with a sterile needle; advise antiseptic cream to prevent infection ± aspirin for pain (adults).
- *Chemical peeling:* It can be an alternative for treatment of extensive facial actinic keratoses. Recurrence rate is 25-35%.[61]
- *Photodynamic therapy:* Application of a topical photosensitizer followed by activation by a light source can give long-term prophylaxis for AKs and may ↓ incidence of AK-related SCC.[61]
- *Fluorouracil (5FU)* 5% cream once-daily, with this sequence of events: erythema→vesiculation→erosion→red, sore ulcers→necrosis→healing epithelialization. This inflammatory response is in pre-actinic lesions: healthy skin is less harmed. Using pulsed therapy (eg with gaps of a week or more) reduces this problem (if severe, 8-hourly Fucibet® may help).
- *Diclofenac gel (3%)* is effective (mechanism unknown); used twice daily for 2 months, it is well tolerated.[63,64] N=96 It may be tried on AK intruding on mucosa (eg from the lip's vermilion). SE: dry skin; rash.[65] Expect ≥75% near or complete clearance within 90 days in ≥75% of patients.[66]
- *Imiquimod* 5% (3×weekly for 4wks to lesions; assess after a 4wk treatment-free gap; repeat once if persisting; allow to stay on site for 8h, then wash (soap & water). It augments cell mediated immunity by inducing interferon-α.[67,68] SE: itch, 'burning', erythema, erosion, oedema, scabs, 'flu-like symptoms.

Dermatology

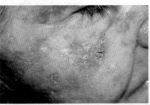

Fig 3. Solar keratosis.

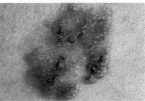

Fig 4. Bowen's disease.

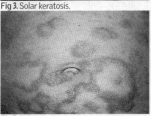

Fig 5. Leprosy.

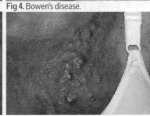

Fig 6. Breast cancer metastasis.

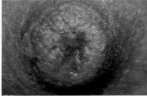

Fig 7. Paget's disease of nipple.

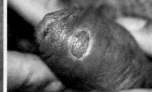

Fig 8. Primary syphilis chancre.

Figs 3-8 courtesy of Dr Samuel da Silva: *www.atlasdermatologico.com.br*

Malignant melanoma (fig 1) ♀:♂≈1.3:1. *UK incidence:* ≥10:100,000/yr (↑in the last 20yrs by ~300% in ♂ and ~200% in ♀). 5-yr survival is rising (now >80%). ~4% have a family history of melanoma. *Mortality:* 1.9:100,000/yr in UK.[69]

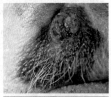

Risk: UV exposure†; sunburn, fair complexion, many common/dysplastic moles, +ve family history, old age. 66% are related to BRAF mutations.[70] *Early diagnosis:* ►Everyone should know what early melanomas look like, and know how to get help.

Signs: Most arise in normal skin, a few in dysplastic naevi. All changing moles are suspect (esp. if edges irregular or colour varies). Use a magnifying glass. ►Excise all new irregular black lesions *however small*[71] and all ABCDE lesions (opposite).

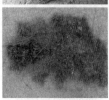

ΔΔ: Benign melanocytic lesions; non-melanocytic pigmented lesions, eg seborrhoeic keratoses, common if >50yrs; they feel greasy, and look as if they are stuck on. Benign moles tend to be <5mm across, with uniform colour/shape, but melanomas are often different shades of brown, black, or blue. If melanomas incite inflammation, pink-reds may appear. If immune response is active, areas of regression with dermal scarring appear as grey-white.[72,73] They may be nodular or flat. *Unusual sites:* Sole, eye, anus, vagina, palate.*etc*

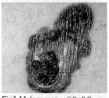

Treatment: For *any* unusual, growing, or changing pigmented lesion, excision biopsy must be considered (with a 1cm *margin of normal skin* around the lesion for every mm of depth, up to 3cm (there is no evidence for wider excision, so Fig 1. Melanomas. ©Dr S Baron. don't do incisional biopsies for '?melanoma'. Prognosis depends on excision completeness and tumour depth ('Breslow thickness' is a major prognostic sign). If <1mm thick, disease-free 5-yr survival is >75% (if >4mm it's 50%).[1]

Metastatic melanoma: Sentinel node mets ≈ poorer prognosis.[74] Ask an oncologist to match molecular analysis of the tumour with the most appropriate agent,[2,75] eg pegylated interferon alfa-2b, interleukin 2 ± cytotoxics[78] (10–30% respond) or ipilimumab (targets CTLA-4) ± dacarbazine.[77,78]

Slip-slop-slap-seek-slide 'Slip on a shirt, slop on sunscreen,[3] slap on a hat, seek shade, and slide on sunglasses'—see BOX.

Pigmented naevi/moles 3% of us have ≥2 pigmented naevi at birth and 20–50 small naevi as teenagers. Numbers peak before ~50yrs. By old age, they are relatively rare. Most naevi are not pre-malignant. *Lesions <5mm across with uniform colour and outline don't need histology unless they've grown or changed.* The benign *halo naevus* occurs most often on the back of young adults. The 'white' halo is not sinister and results from loss of melanocytes by lymphocyte action.[79] When a prepubertal child 'has an obvious melanoma', the diagnosis may well be a benign *Spitz (compound) naevus* with nests of spindle-shaped melanocytes.[80]   See also *SCC* (p590) and *MCC*.[4]

---

1 TNM staging is complex; note that melanoma thickness and ulceration not level of invasion are used in the *T* category (except for *T1*); the number of metastatic nodes rather than gross dimensions is used in the N category; site of distant metastases and LDH† are used in the M category. Stage IIb is thickness ≥4mm, node -ve for example; stage III is any primary tumour node +ve.[81]

2 Various inhibitors of v-Raf murine sarcoma viral oncogene homologue B1 (BRAF) yield high response rates in those harbouring BRAF-V600E mutations. Mutations in c-kit respond to imatinib.[82]

3 Sunsense® products are good, eg Sunsensitive SPF50+® (said to be water-resistant for 4h).

4 Compared with melanoma, Merkel cell cancer occurs in an older people, more often on head & neck, and in a higher %age of men (62 *vs* 57%). MCC metastasizes more. 10-yr survival is less (18 *vs* 61%).[83]

We all have a genetic skin type which determines sensitivity to UV.

Skin type	Do you burn or tan?	Those affected
I	"I always burn easily, but I never tan"	Caucasians (many Celts)
II	"I always burn, but tan minimally"	Caucasians
III	"Sometimes I burn; I always tan"	Caucasians
IV	"I rarely burn, and always tan well"	Caucasians
V	"I rarely burn, and always tan deeply"	Dark-skinned eg Latin, Indian
VI	"I never burn, but tan if very exposed"	Black Africans

This helps predict individual susceptibility for development of skin cancers and manifestations of photo-ageing. While persons in groups I-II are at highest risk, most skin cancers cluster in type II & III people: type I people know from experience to stay out of the sun. How to determine type:[84]

• When you first go out in the sun each summer do you sunburn?
• If so, do you always burn? Easily? Do you ever blister when you burn?
• Can you tan? Does it take a long time or do you tan easily?
• Do you develop a deep tan or just a shade beyond your normal colour?

Ask about freckles and melanomas (self + family), and past sunbed and sunburn (esp. blistering). "Do you use sun-screens and do skin selfexamination (use mirrors or a friend for hard-to-see areas)? Are your jobs/hobbies outdoor? Are you pregnant?" (expect mole darkening). Is hair red/blond? Are the eyes blue? Note number and type of all moles (examine all over).

▶Don't just diagnose today's melanoma: prevent tomorrow's by educating all the family.[85] ▶Avoid sunbeds and over-exposure (esp. around noon). ▶Use protective clothing/sunscreens[3] (may be less good).[86] We often ignore advice as sunlight feels good, and tans look good. This is why the fashion industry turns out to be a key co-educator.[87] *Tailor advice to individual risk.* ▶Those at most risk benefit from professional skin exam every 6-9 months. "Would you like information about harmful effects of sunlight?"

When to refer ABCDE: Asymmetric lesions, Border irregular, Colour irregularity, Diameter >6mm, or Evolving over time. Refer if ≥3—or if there is a clear spontaneous change in any of A, B, C, or D—or itching, pain, or bleeding.

Sunscreens[3] and melanoma prevention The SPF (sun protection factor) indicates how long an individual can be exposed to sunshine without burning, eg SPF8 means that an individual can stay out in the sun 8 times longer than the time it would normally take them to burn. Protection varies depending on skin type (and thickness of application, so SPF50 ≈ SPF15 unless plastered on thickly). SPF refers UVB. Many sunscreens contain UVA-block too, graded on a 'star-rating', which as yet, is not internationally standardized.

Sunscreens protect by blocking light (eg titanium dioxide) or by absorbing light by photochemical reaction (eg benzophenones; cinnamates).

3 melanoma paradoxes: 1 Sunnier European countries have lower melanoma mortality.[88] **2** Occupational sun exposure is unrelated to melanoma risk.[89] **3** Sun exposure ↑survival from melanoma.[90] Why? One of sunshine's best effects, apart from banishing British gloom, is to ↑vitamin D, which has antineoplastic effects (↑cell differentiation & apoptosis, and ↓angiogenesis & metastases).[91] Early deaths from lack of UVB ≈ 22,000/yr for white Americans:[92] *much* more than the 8000 deaths from melanoma.[93] This is due to fewer deaths from bladder and lung cancer.[et al] Survival from cancers reflects vitamin D synthesis which in the UK is ~⅓ that at the equator.[94] What does this mean? Not "Let's all go down to the beach for noon-time orgies of photosynthesis". Ask instead: "How do we get the benefit without the risk?" Diet? Slip-slop-slap-supplements?◆☀ So...serum vitamin D levels of 70-100nmol/L might be a reasonable target for melanoma patients (and for everyone else).[89]

Tans are sexy and sun protection products are expensive and a pain to use...so our advice to young people is almost guaranteed to fail: peer-advocacy is a better bet.

Dermatology

Psoriasis is a chronic inflammatory skin condition affecting ~2% of Caucasians of any age, peaking in the 20s (type 1) and 50s (type 2). ♀:♂ ≈ 1:1. There are 2 pathologies: *epidermal proliferation* (with abnormal differentiation) and T-cell driven *inflammatory infiltration* of the dermis and epidermis. TNF-α (tumour necrosis factor), activated T cells, macrophages, and dendritic cells play a central role in the pathogenesis of psoriasis.[95] In many, psoriasis is preceded by a strep infection activating T cells (vaccination might be possible).[96]

30% have a family member with psoriasis. HLA associations: HLA-CW6, HLA-B13, B17, DR7. If both parents have psoriasis, risk to offspring is ~50%. *Triggers:* Stress, infections (esp. streps), skin trauma (Köbner phenomenon), drugs (lithium, NSAIDs, β-blockers, antimalarials), alcohol, obesity, smoking, and climate.

Signs (figs 1-4) Symmetrical well-defined red plaques with silvery scale on extensor aspects of the elbows, knees, scalp, and sacrum. Flexures (axillae, groins, submammary areas, and umbilicus) also frequently affected but lesions are non-scaly. *Nail changes* (in 50%): pitting, onycholysis (separation from nail-bed), thickening and subungual hyperkeratosis. *Small plaques* (guttate psoriasis) are seen in the young (especially if associated with concurrent streptococcal infection). *Pustular variants* (sterile) can affect the palms & soles.[97,98] *Generalized (erythrodermic) psoriasis* (and generalized pustular psoriasis) may cause severe systemic upset (fever, ↑WCC, dehydration)—also triggered by rapid withdrawal of systemic steroids. *Other signs:* Köbner phenomenon (p584); Auspitz sign: pinpoint bleeding on scale removal; 'pepper pot nail pitting; 'grease-spots'.

Systemic signs 7% develop a seronegative arthropathy—5 types: 1 Monoarthritis or oligomonoarthritis 2 Psoriatic spondylitis 3 Asymmetrical polyarthritis 4 Arthritis mutilans (destructive) 5 Rheumatoid-like polyarthritis.

Tests None is routine; histology: epidermal keratinocyte hyperproliferation, parakeratosis ± intra-epidermal neutrophil microabscesses (of Munro).[99]

ΔΔ Eczema; tinea (solitary or few lesions; asymmetrical; expanding); mycosis fungoides (asymmetric, less scaling, do biopsy); seborrhoeic dermatitis.

Management Education is vital; control, not cure, is realistic. Assess severity and proportion of skin affected. Find out what he/she finds most distressing. Encourage a support group (Psoriasis Association) **Remove triggers** (above). *If mild:* Creams are mostly used, eg the vitamin D analogue calcipotriol + betamethasone 0.05% (once daily Dovobet®;[1] it ↑quality of life).[100] Others: Tar: Messy (esp. ointments—reserve for inpatient use); Alphosyl HC®, twice daily, is cleaner. **Dithranol:** Available in creams for use in short-contact regimens (apply carefully to affected skin; wash off after ½h): start at low concentrations (0.1%); increase as tolerated (eg 0.25%, 0.5%, 1%). SE: burning (avoid flexures); staining (avoid on face). **Tacalcitol** may be applied once daily before going to bed (max 5g/day, and only up to two 12-week courses/yr). For flexural disease, topical steroid/antibiotic/antifungal preparations can be useful (Trimovate®). *Psoriatic arthropathy:*[2] Consider etanercept, infliximab,[101] or methotrexate.[102] *Moderate to severe psoriasis:* Risk:benefit ratio seems most favourable for Goeckerman PUVA (see BOX), followed by etanercept or adalimumab (BOX).[103]

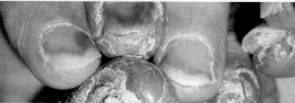

Fig 1. Psoriasis affecting the nails.   Courtesy of Dr J Bowling.

Dermatology

Recalcitrant psoriasis[1]

Be holistic! This is a biological as well as a social injunction. 60% of patients with psoriasis are depressed. Cytokine levels correlate with depression and TNF antagonists (below) directly reduce depressive symptoms in psoriasis.[104]

Tazarotene (once daily topical retinoid): for mild/moderate psoriasis affecting <10% skin surface. Avoid in pregnancy. Wash hands after use. Avoid contact with eyes, face, intertriginous areas, hair-covered scalp, inflamed skin; avoid exposure to uv light/PUVA etc. Don't use emollients or cosmetics within 1h of use. NB: **clobetasol 0.05% cream** was better in one trial.[105]

Phototherapy with a selective broadband ultraviolet (uv) source with little emission <290 nanometres is less photocarcinogenic than narrowband UVB;[106] avoid if history of photosensitivity; most suitable for guttate/small plaque psoriasis. PUVA: UVA + oral/topical psoralen; suitable for extensive large plaque disease (oral psoralen) and localized psoriasis (topical psoralen); limit total dose to 1000J/150 treatments to avoid undue skin ageing and risk of skin cancer (esp. squamous cell carcinoma); can be combined with oral retinoids (re-PUVA) to ↓light dose needed to clear lesions. Goeckerman regimen: hospital day-based ℞ for 3 weeks with coal tar applied once or twice daily then washed off before total body UVB (then shower to wash off scales).

Non-biologic oral drugs
Severe psoriasis often needs oral drugs (get help).
• **Methotrexate** 10-20mg/week PO; most useful in elderly patients; avoid if young in view of long-term risk of hepatic fibrosis. Monitor FBC & LFT.
• **Ciclosporin:** 2.5-5mg/kg/day PO; good, but SE bad (BP↑; renal dysfunction).
• **Acitretin:** Oral retinoid; useful for moderate/severe disease; SE: teratogenic; dry skin and mucosae; ↑lipids; glucose↑; ↑LFT (reversible). Check lipids, glucose, LFT at start, then every 2wks for 8wks, then every 12wks. In the UK, use is limited to hospitals. Starting at 25-30mg/24h PO; typical maintenance: 25-50mg/day; adjust according to response. Exclude pregnancy, and avoid donating blood for >1yr and pregnancy until >2yrs after the last dose.
• **Hydroxycarbamide:** 0.5-1.5g/24h PO. SE: marrow suppression.[107]

Biological drugs
inhibit T-cell activation and function, or neutralize cytokines. They also can potentially ↓ adverse systemic side effects because of their high specificity for pathogenic cells without affecting cells of other organs.[95] If psoriasis hasn't improved eg with ciclosporin, methotrexate and PUVA or these have had side effects, consider **ustekinumab** or **etanercept** (eg 25mg SC, twice weekly for ≤24wks).[108] This tumour necrosis factor (TNF-α) inhibitor can also help joints in psoriatic arthropathy (and ↓radiographic progression).[109] It is usually well tolerated. SE: vomiting, oesophagitis, cholecystitis, pancreatitis, GI bleeds, ischaemia, emboli, BP↑↓, dyspnoea, demyelination, seizures. Specialist use only. Alternatives: **infliximab, adalimumab.**NICE[110]

Dermatology

"I feel stigmatized: He keeps staring at me...I expect he thinks I'm contagious."

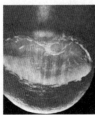

Fig 2. Onycholysis. Nail pitting may also be present.

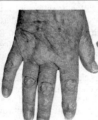

Fig 3. Plaques on hand.

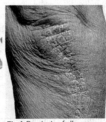

Fig 4. Psoriasis of elbow.
Figs 2, 3, & 4 © Dr S Baron.

1 In stable plaque psoriasis, apply Dovobet® to <30% of body surface for ≤4wks; max 15g/day or 100gwk; repeat if needed after ≥4wks. Avoid face, genitals and scalp. **Dermovate shampoo®** can help the scalp.
2 Psoriatic arthropathy may signify endothelial dysfunction and impaired coronary microcirculation, so consider a vigorous approach to controlling cardiovascular risk factors.[111]

Acute eczema causes a rash with less scale and less demarcated than psoriasis. Eczema may be atopic, hypersensitive (type VI), or be caused by irritants or venous stasis. See also discoid eczema (p602 & fig 5, p586). Different types may co-exist. Ask about work, hobbies, and other exposures to allergens.

Atopic eczema (fig1) *Causes:* Multifactorial: *Genetic:* A family history of atopy is common (70%); Overactive TH2 lymphocytes produce IL4 & IL5, stimulating IgE production. *Infection:* Staphs colonize lesions and toxins act as a superantigen. *Allergens:* ↑IgE is common. *RAST* (radioallergosorbent ↑testing) identifies specific antigens, eg house dust mite or animal dander. Altered microbial exposure may have a role (probiotics improve this, see BOX). *Diet:* Some atopic children have food allergies, eg dairy products ± egg which exacerbate eczema. Although infantile eczema is common (~2% of UK infants), most grow out of it before 13yrs old. *R̶:*

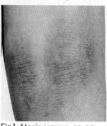

Fig 1. Atopic eczema. ©Dr S Baron

• Management involves control, not cure. Dry skin itches and is susceptible to irritants, so use emollients liberally, even when eczema is less active. They treat dryness and act as a barrier. Ditto for bath emollients, eg Oilatum® or Aveeno® (oat oils). Use soap substitutes as emulsifying ointment.

• Emollients (use at least twice a day). In severe eczema, greasy emollients are best, eg 50/50 emulsifying ointment and liquid paraffin (~£3/week); Epaderm® costs ~£7/week. In less severe eczema, less greasy preparations are more acceptable, eg Diprobase® (~£7/week).

• Daily[112] steroid ointment for active sites. Strength depends on severity, site, and age. *Face, flexures, groins:* 1% hydrocortisone. Potency of clobetasone 0.05% is one step above hydrocortisone (use on face for <1wk, under supervision).[113] *Elsewhere:* Get control in ≤1wk with higher-potency betamethasone 0.1% ointment; ↓strength soon (betamethasone 0.025%). Clobetasol is jolly potent; use briefly only on thick skin (∵ skin thinning, telangiectasia, adrenal suppression). Haelan tape® (fludroxycortide) is good at healing fissured digits. Oral anti-staph antibiotics (topical fusidic acid helps little compared to fluticasone or tacrolimus).[114] If systemic R̶ needed, ciclosporin may be best (get help).

Irritant dermatitis We are all susceptible to irritants. Hands are often affected; redness ± weeping precedes dry fissuring. *Common irritants:* detergents, soaps, oils, solvents, alkalis; water (if repeated). It often affects bar staff and cleaners. *R̶:* Avoid all irritants; hand care (soap substitutes; regular emollients; careful drying; cotton or cotton-lined rubber gloves for dry and wet work respectively; as-needed use of topical steroids for acute flare-ups).

Allergic contact dermatitis (Type IV reaction) Common allergens: nickel (jewellery, watches, coins, keys); chromates (cements, leather); lanolin (creams, cosmetics); rubber (foam in furniture); plants (primulas); topical neomycin, framycetin, antihistamines, or anaesthetics (haemorrhoid creams). The pattern of contact gives clues to the allergen. There is often a sharp cut-off where contact ends. Secondary spread elsewhere is frequent (auto-sensitization). *R̶:* Consider patch testing and avoidance of implicated allergens; topical steroid appropriate for severity (↓ strength and stop as it settles).

Adult seborrhoeic dermatitis This common red, scaly rash affects scalp (dandruff), eyebrows, nasolabial folds, cheeks, and flexures. Cause: eg overgrowth of skin yeasts (*Malassezia*). It can be severe if HIV+ve. *R̶:* Mild topical steroid/antifungal preparations, eg Daktacort® or ketoconazole 2% cream or shampoo (or metronidazole 0.75% gel). Treat intermittently, as needed.[115]

Holistic care of children with atopic eczema

Identify triggers (irritants, infections, inhalants, ingest substances/foods). Find out how family life works to harmonize regimens with daily lifestyles. Say to report any severe weeping rash eg around the mouth: this may be *eczema herpeticum* (Kaposi's varicelliform eruption):[1] ►► IV aciclovir may be needed.

►Also get help if: nightly loss of sleep; ↓social functioning; incessant itch; bleeding; oozing; extensive skin thickening/redness/excoriation. Tacrolimus, bandages, phototherapy ± systemic therapy may be needed. Dermatology nurses play a big role in giving practical support for parents. They can show how to apply creams and occlusive dressings, eg stockinet suits, which aid emollient absorption, and prevent drying and scratching. If less severe...

• Dry skin is itchy, so scratching is a big problem; it may become a habit (distraction therapies/star charts can help). Use leave-on emollients over the whole body often (500g/week). Turn down the heating (avoids drying).

• Sedating antihistamines help, eg hydroxyzine or alimemazine. High doses may be needed in breaking the itch-scratch cycle, and in enabling sleep.

• Encourage joining a national eczema association (in UK, 020 7388 4097).

• Discourage elimination diets. Only occasionally is there a clear trigger (eg confirm a dairy allergy with a RAST test; if +ve, get a dietician's help).

• Reducing exposure to house dust mite may help (high filtration vacuuming of mattresses, limiting of carpet use; Gore-tex® mattress covers).

Use *mild potency topical steroids*; for severe flares moderate potency steroids (for ≤5 days if on face; for <2wks for axillae/groins) *may* be needed.[116] NICE

Non-steroidal immunomodulation: Pimecrolimus 1% cream and tacrolimus 0.03% ointment have a role if >2yrs old; use sparingly twice daily on any skin, including face & flexures, for ≤3wks (usually by a dermatologist, if topical steroids have failed or skin thinning would be a problem). Stop if no effect after 2wks. SE: pruritus, burning, acne (*not* skin atrophy).[117] One advantage is that benefits keep developing even after treatment stops.[117] It does help itch.[118] *Cautions:* Infection at treatment site; uv exposure. CI: Erythroderma; pregnancy/lactation. SE: Tingling, pruritus, folliculitis, acne, herpes simplex, ↑sensitivity to hot and cold, alcohol intolerance. NB: tacrolimus ointment is said to be better, with faster onset of action than pimecrolimus in atopy.[119]

Preventing infantile eczema

Exclusive breastfeeding for the 1st 3 months associates with less atopic eczema in children with a 1st degree relative with atopy.[120] Antigen avoidance diets in high-risk women in pregnancy has little effect[121] but during lactation this *might* ↓ infant atopic eczema. If a mother wants to try antigen avoidance, point out that it may not work. Prenatal diets rich in fish oil (n-3PUF) may help.[122] If breastfeeding is impossible, many try soya milk, but this doesn't work; milk with hydrolysed casein (Nutramigen®; Pregestimil®) does.[123] N=595

Probiotics are dietary supplements containing potentially beneficial bacteria to assist developing body's gut flora. The idea is that altered microbial exposure may underlie the rise of allergic diseases in affluent areas. Probiotics have been found to ↓ incidence of IgE-associated eczema in infancy.[124]

Reducing exposure to house dust mite: High-filtration vacuuming of mattresses; acaricidal sprays, eg benzyltannate; Gore-tex® mattress covering; washing bedding at 55°C. NB: meta-analyses doubt the efficacy of these.[125]

Abbreviated Williams diagnostic criteria for atopic eczema[126]

A child must have an itchy skin (or parents report scratching) + ≥3 of: 1 Onset before 2yrs. 2 Past skin crease involvement. 3 History of generally dry skin. 3 Personal history of other atopy or history of atopy in 1st degree relative. 5 Flexural dermatitis or on cheeks/forehead and outer side of limbs if <4yrs.

Dermatology

---

1 This is a primary herpes infection in skin traumatized by eczema; it may be fatal.

Fungi Superficial mycoses are the commonest of human fungal infections—and are limited to skin, hair, nails, and mucous membranes. They include dermatophytes (ringworm), superficial candidosis, and Pityrosporum infections. 3 genera of dermatophytes affect humans: Epidermophyton, Trichophyton and Microsporum. Spread is from man to man (anthropophilic, eg *T. rubrum*, fig 2), animal to man (zoophilic, eg *M. canis*) or soil to man (geophilic, eg *M. gypseum*). A ringworm infection is a round, scaly, itchy lesion whose edge is more inflamed than its centre. It is called tinea followed, in Latin, by the part affected, eg tinea pedis (foot); cruris (groins); capitis (scalp); unguium (nail); corporis (body, fig 1). Infection caused by yeasts of Candida genus (eg *C. albicans*) are common (esp. in immunocompromised онсм p441), and mainly affect mouth, vagina, glans, skin folds/ toe web; nail areas. They are often pink and moist ± satellite lesions. Other yeasts causing infection: *Malassezia* species (eg *M. furfur*; 11 species are recognized and are tricky to distinguish):[127] Pityriasis versicolor (multiple hypo- or hyperpigmented scaly macules on the upper trunk and back). Pityrosporum folliculitis and seborrhoeic dermatitis (*R*: once-daily **ketoconazole** cream). **Δ**: Skin scrapings from the edge (active margin) of lesion. Collect specimens from hair-pulls and nail clippings in folds of black paper (to contrast with white scrapings). Wood's light causes fluorescence in some fungi and can help diagnosis, and suggest areas for scrapings. Microscopy (added кон dissolves keratin) and culture (takes 6 wks) also help. Take skin swabs if candidosis is suspected. *R*: **Dermatophytes:** Skin: **terbinafine** or **imidazole** creams (eg clotrimazole) twice daily for 2wks. Scalp: **griseofulvin** or **terbinafine** PO for children for 2 weeks. Nails: **terbinafine** PO for 3 months if deemed essential. Explain about SE (headache; dizziness; taste disturbance; arthralgia; LFT↑; psychiatric illness; vertigo) and interactions (β-blockers; antidepressants). *Candida:* Mouth: **nystatin** (eg oral suspension, 1mL/6h for 1 week). Vagina: **imidazole** cream ± pessary (eg Canesten Combi®). *Pityriasis versicolor:* **Selenium sulphide** shampoo daily for 1 week; wash off after 10mins or twice-daily imidazole creams.

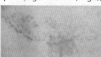

Fig 1. Tinea corporis.
Courtesy of Dr Susannah Baron.

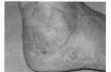

Fig 2. *Trichophyton rubrum.*
Courtesy of Dr Jonathan Bowling.

Bacteria *Impetigo:* Contagious superficial infection caused by *Staph aureus* (±*Strep pyogenes*). *Peak:* 2-5yrs. Lesions (often well-defined) usually start around the nose & face with honey-coloured crusts on erythematous base (±superficial flaccid blisters). *R*: Try topical antibiotics first (**fusidic acid, mupirocin**). Give oral antibiotics (eg **flucloxacillin** 125mg/6h PO, in a child) if more severe.[128]

Erysipelas: Sharply defined superficial infection caused by *Strep pyogenes*. Often affects the face (unilateral) with fever and ↑wcc. *R*: Systemic **penicillin** (see below). Recurrent cases may need prophylactic antibiotics.[129]

Cellulitis: Acute infection of skin and soft tissues (eg legs). *Cause:* β-haemolytic streps ± staphs. It is deeper and less well-defined than erysipelas. *Signs:* pain, swelling, erythema, warmth, systemic upset and lymphadenopathy. *R*: ▶Elevate the legs. **Benzylpenicillin** 600mg/6h IV (or **penicillin v** 500mg/4-6h PO) + **flucloxacillin** 500mg/6h PO. If penicillin-allergic, try **erythromycin** 500mg/12h PO.

Skin TB: *Lupus vulgaris*—55%; a patch of red-brown 'apple jelly nodules' (on white skins) eg on face/leg, which forms a scar in which new nodules may grow; ♀:♂ ≥2:1. *Scrofuloderma* (27%; suppurating nodules over TB foci), TB verrucosa cutis (6%; indolent warty plaques); *TB gumma* (5%); *tuberculids* (7%, symmetric generalized exanthems, eg Bazin's erythema induratum/lichen scrofulosorum).[130]

Warts (fig 1) Cause: human papillomavirus (HPV) in keratino-
cytes. Large numbers can occur if immunosuppressed. *Com-* Fig 1. Wart. OUP
mon warts: Most common in children/young adults; often
resolve spontaneously (some are stubborn). Complications: scc, p590. Treat-
ment: "wait and see" or salicylic acid (keratolytic, eg **Salatac®**gel); cryother-
apy (if ≥7yrs) or once-daily topical **5-fluorouracil** (for 6wks; adults & chil-
dren; unlicensed).$^{Glasjo}_{regimen}$ [131] Oral zinc sulfate (≤600mg/d) appears to help.[132]

Plantar warts: Large confluent lesions (mosaic warts) often resist treat-
ment. T½≈2yrs. They are infectious. Avoid excision. After abrading it, try
salicylic acid under an occlusive plaster, eg as Occlusal®. Combination
therapy eg topical **cantharidin 1% + podophyllotoxin 5% + salicylic acid 30%**
(CPS) is often better than cryo (double freeze-thaw cycles are better than
single ones, but not for hand warts).[133] Recalcitrant warts may respond to
photodynamic therapy; use is non-standard.[134] NB: schools expect children
to wear **verruca socks** for swimming. One uncontrolled study showed pub-
lic shower users got more plantar warts than locker room users who didn't
use such showers.[135] *Plane warts:* Flat skin-coloured or brown lesions; tend
to Köbnerize (p584) in scratch marks; they often resist treatment.

Genital warts (condylomata acuminata): R: Cryo ± podophyllin: terato-
genic) or imiquimod cream. Screen for other STI. Women with genital warts
(or whose partners have them) may need yearly cervical cytology (HPV16 & 18/
cervical cancer, p273). Prevention: p272. If a child, suspect abuse.

Other wart treatments: Radiofrequency ablation, infrared coagulation, anti-
virals (cidofovir), bleomycin, interferon intralesional injection, topical 5FU.[136]

Molluscum contagiosum *(pox virus)* These pink papules have an umbili-
cated (depressed) central punctum. White material can be expressed and
microscoped to confirm the diagnosis (molluscum bodies). Common in chil-
dren. They resolve spontaneously (may take months). Gentle cryo may be
tried. It is more common in atopic eczema. If florid, suspect HIV.

Herpes simplex (gingivostomatitis or recurrent genital or perioral infec-
tion) Infection can be triggered by fevers, sunlight, immunosuppression.
Eruption often preceded by symptoms of burning/itching. *Signs:* Grouped
painful vesicles on erythematous base which heal without scarring. *Treat-*
ment: Often none needed. Topical aciclovir may prevent or reduce severity
of recurrences. Systemic treatment is indicated in certain circumstances
(immunosuppressed; frequent recurrent genital herpes). There is evidence
that Bell's palsy may be related to recurrent herpes infection.

Herpes zoster Varicella-zoster
virus becomes dormant in dorsal
root ganglia. Recurrent infection
affects one or more dermatomes
(p762, esp. if immunosuppressed).
Pain and malaise may precedes the
rash *Signs:* Polymorphic red pap-
ules, vesicles, pustules (fig 3). Post-
herpetic neuralgia: see OHCM p400. R:
If mild, none. If severe (or immuno-
suppressed) try aciclovir 800mg 5×/
day PO for 1wk (SE: confusion; LFT↑;
GFR↓) or famciclovir 250mg/8h PO
for 1wk (SE: headache, confusion).
Varicella-zoster vaccine (if >60yrs)
and immune globulin (postexpo-
sure) are preventives.[137]

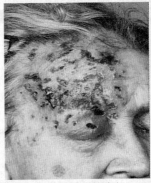

Fig 3. Ophthalmic zoster (shingles).

Dermatology

The 5 pillars of acne (1) Basal keratinocyte proliferation in pilosebaceous follicles (androgen- and CRH- driven, p583), (2) ↑sebum production, (3) *Propionibacterium acnes* colonization, (4) inflammation, (5) comedones (white- & black-head) blocking secretions, hence papules, nodules, cysts, and scars (face, neck, upper torso). It is almost universal in teenagers: it causes much angst (nature in one of her darkly ironic moods picks the fairest skin at its vainest moment for her fiercest pustules). Most with acne don't have ↑androgens but their sebaceous glands are more sensitive to androgens (p583).

Differential diagnosis Acne rosacea—no comedones; diffusely red nose, cheeks, chin, and forehead; telangiectasia; flushing, especially after alcohol.

R℞ Be holistic; subtle doctors use acne consultations to promote mental health by giving patients a vocabulary to describe their misery, and so to control it. Dispel myths: it is NOT due to filth, lack of washing, etc. But diet may be important (↑glycaemic loads *may* have a role).[138] Ask about mood, fears of social rejection (not always unfounded). Suicidal ideation is a red flag. Stress reduction is important (modulates sebaceous gland hormones & cytokines).

Mild acne Mainly facial comedones; if to be manually removed♀, do at ovulation, before sebaceous orifices narrow.[139] Topical R℞: (singly or combined): **benzoyl peroxide** (as low a strength as works, eg 2.5%, or 10% as a twice-weekly wash; more may irritate); **azelaic acid** (15% gel, twice daily for <6 months); roll-on antibiotics (**clindamycin**, as Dalacin T®); with azelaic acid it is synergistic.[140]

Moderate acne (inflammatory lesions, face ± torso): **Doxycycline** or **minocycline**[141] (erythromycin if pregnant or <12yrs old) for ≥4-6 months with topical **benzoyl peroxide** (start at 2.5%, not 5 or 10% to avoid irritation).[142] Make topical antibiotics the same as the oral drug to ↓drug resistance. Topical retinoids (creams/gels): **adapalene** or **isotretinoin** used either alone or with benzoyl peroxide (Epiduo® gel) or erythromycin (Isotrexin® gel).[142]

Severe acne (nodules, cysts, scars): **Isotretinoin** is 1st choice eg 0.5-1mg/kg/day for 20wks (to ↓sebum production and pituitary hormones).[141,143] Marked benefit occurs in virtually all patients (permanent ~65%). SE: teratogenic (good contraception must be used during and for 1 month after treatment); dry skin, lips, mucosae; myalgia; headache (benign intracranial hypertension reported); depression;[1] hepatitis; ↑lipids.[144] Monitor triglycerides, AST, ALT, cholesterol, and FBC often.[141] Alternative (if ♀ and wanting contraception): co-cyprindiol (Dianette®)—see combined oral contraception, p300. Other putative indications for isotretinoin: moderate acne not responding to antibiotics; presence of scarring and severe psychological problems.

Acne rosacea

This is a chronic relapsing/remitting disorder of blood vessels and pilosebaceous units in convex central facial areas typically in fair-skinned people. Prevalence: 10%. Pre-rosacea features: flushing[2] triggered by stress/blushing, alcohol & spices. Grade I to III signs: erythemato-teleangiectasies, papulopustules, and inflammatory nodules. Severe subtypes: rosacea conglobata; rosacea fulminans; rosacea with lymphoedema ± blepharitis/conjunctivitis. In men, rhinophyma (swelling + soft tissue overgrowth of the nose) may occur. *Cause:* Unknown. *Chlamydia pneumoniae* may have a role.[145] *Plan/R℞:* Avoid irritants & sun overexposure. Help with avoiding blushing (CBT, p374) may help social functioning.[146] Topical **azelaic acid** ± **metronidazole** (0.75% gel/12h for 8wks) for mild/moderate disease,[147] or **doxycycline** eg 40mg[148] PO for 16wks. **Azithromycin** 500mg/day PO for 2wks helps (it's anti-inflammatory *and* kills *C. pneumoniae*).[149] Isotretinoin (above) and lasers (eg 532nm) are rarely needed.

---

1 Don't deny R℞ if depressed: those with pre-existing depression have most to gain (eg ↑quality of life).
2 *Flushing* ΔΔ: Menopause; alcohol; food intolerances; toxins; drugs (nicotinic acid, bromocriptine, tamoxifen, cyproterone acetate, ciclosporin); mastocytosis (p602); carcinoid; pheochromocytoma.

10% of hospital patients develop a drug eruption during their admission, so... know the main culprits, and how to classify and treat them.

Types of reaction *Maculopapular* or *ex-anthematous:* (fig 1) This is the commonest type, presenting with generalized erythematous macules and papules eg on the trunk ± fever and eosinophilia—eg within 2wks after onset of therapy. *Drugs:* Penicillins; cephalosporins; anti-epileptics.

Urticaria:[1] *Signs:* wheals (fig 2 on p584); rapid onset after taking drug ± association with angio-oedema/anaphylaxis. It can result from both immunological and non-immunological mechanisms. *Drugs:*

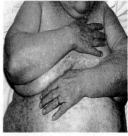
Fig 1. Penicillin rash.

morphine & codeine cause direct mast cell degranulation; penicillins & cefalosporins trigger IgE responses; NSAIDs; ACEi.

Exfoliative dermatitis: Signs: Widespread erythema and dermatitis; erythroderma. *Causative drugs:* Sulfonamides; allopurinol; carbamazepine; gold.

Erythema multiforme major (Stevens-Johnson syndrome): The more severe variants of erythema multiforme are usually due to drugs. *Signs:* Target lesions and polymorphic erythema, eg with blistering mucosae (conjunctivae, oral, labial, genital) if severe. *Drugs:* Sulfonamides; anticonvulsants.

Toxic epidermal necrolysis (TEN): the bad bad end of the erythema multiforme/ Stevens-Johnson syndrome (SJS) spectrum. *Signs:* Widespread erythema, then necrosis of large sheets of epidermis. Mucosae severely affected. Risk of TEN in HIV patients is 1000-fold higher.[150] Mortality: ~30%. *Drug causes:* Sulfonamides; anticonvulsants; penicillins; allopurinol; NSAIDs. Manage in a dermatology or burns unit. Short-term dexamethasone pulse therapy,[151] IV Ig.

Lichenoid: This is similar to lichen planus but it rarely shows typical signs of idiopathic lichen planus. It can be very itchy. *Drugs:* β-blockers; thiazides; gold; antimalarials.

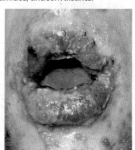
Fig 2. TEN/Stevens-Johnson syndrome
© Dr Susannah Baron.

Fixed drug eruption: Lesions recur in the same area each time a particular drug is taken. *Drugs:* paracetamol, tetracyclines, sulfonamides, aspirin.[152]

Management A clear history of the onset and duration of the rash is essential. Record *all* drugs taken (herbal remedies, etc). Stop the likely offender. If the clinical diagnosis is in doubt, a prick test or skin biopsy may be helpful but is not always so. In order to confirm the suspicion of drug sensitivity, some advocate rechallenge with the suspected drug once the patient has recovered. While this may be the ideal, re-challenge may be dangerous (beware erythroderma and anaphylaxis). Not unreasonably, patients may also object to this.[153] Many drug rashes need no intervention. Give regular emollients for dryness or itch. Very itchy rashes, eg lichenoid or dermatitic, may need short courses of topical steroids. Urticaria: prompt antihistamine with IV **hydrocortisone**/IM **adrenaline** (=epinephrine, p237) if anaphylaxis. More severe eruptions, eg erythema multiforme are best managed by specialists.

1 Other triggers of *acute urticaria*: Animals; rubber; shellfish; nuts; dairy products; stings; viruses.[134] *Chronic urticaria*: Food additives; autoantibodies which attack mast cells, which release histamine

Lichen planus Lesions (eg on flexor aspects of wrists, forearms, ankles and legs) are purple, pruritic, poly-angular, planar(flat-topped) papules, seen at any age + white lacy markings (known as Wickham's striae). Lesions elsewhere: scalp (scarring alopecia), nails (longitudinal ridges), tongue, mouth (lacy white areas on inner cheeks), and genital lesions. Lesions often arise at sites of trauma. Usually persists for 6-18 months. ℞: Topical steroids (± topical antifungals) are 1st-line (esp. in oral disease, eg fluticasone spray). Moderate to potent topical steroids help itch. Use systemic steroids only if severe. [155]

Haemangiomas *Strawberry naevae* occur in neonates as a rapidly enlarging red spot. Most go by the age of 5-7 years. No treatment is required unless a vital function is impaired, eg obscuring vision. [156]

Pyogenic granuloma/lobular haemangioma (fig 1) is a lesion thought to arise as a result of minor trauma, typically occurring on fingers. It is not infectious or granulomatous. It appears as a moist red lesion which grows rapidly and often bleeds easily. *Treatment:* Curettage.

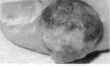

Fig 1. Pyogenic granuloma.
Courtesy of Dr Jonathan Bowling.

Pityriasis rosea This is common, often affecting young adults, and may have a viral cause (eg herpes hominis HHV-6 & HHV-7). [157] A rash is preceded by a herald patch (ovoid red scaly patch with a scaly edge, similar to but larger than later lesions). Tends to affect the neck, trunk, and proximal limbs. There is no treatment. It is self-limiting (recovers in 2-12wks). Oral erythromycin may help treat the rash and decrease the itch. [158]

Alopecia Hair loss is *scarring* or *non-scarring*. Non-scarring causes may be reversible, but scarring alopecia implies irreversible loss. Scalp disorders may be signs of skin elsewhere: (look for signs of lichen planus, and *SLE*).

Non-scarring alopecia: nutritional (Fe or Zn deficiency); *androgenetic* (♀ & ♂) *autoimmune* (alopecia areata: smooth round patches of hair loss on scalp; hairs like exclamation marks are a typical feature; often spontaneously regrows; total scalp hair loss=alopecia totalis; total body hair loss = alopecia universalis—its treatment is difficult: consider topical or intralesional steroids, or *minoxidil*, or dinitrochlorobenzene); *telogen effluvium* (shedding of telogen phase hairs after period of stress, eg childbirth, surgery, severe illness).

Scarring alopecia: lichen planus; discoid lupus erythematosus; trauma.

Blistering disorders *Infection* (eg herpes); *insect bites* (eg on legs); *drugs* (ACEi; furosemide); *dermatitis herpetiformis*, (p588); *friction*; *discoid eczema*;[1] *Zn↓*; *autoimmune blistering disorders (ABD)*, eg *pemphigoid*—the chief ABD in the elderly—due to IgG autoantibodies to basement membrane (bullous pemphigoid antigens 1 & 2). *Signs:* Tense blisters on an urticated base. *Skin biopsy:* (+ve immunofluorescence; linear IgG and C3 along the basement membrane). ℞: clobetasol cream up to 40g/day is better than oral steroids. [159]

Pemphigus affects younger people (<40yrs) than pemphigoid and is due to IgG autoantibodies against desmosomal components (desmoglein 1 & 3). This leads to acantholysis (keratinocytes separate from each other). Drugs may cause it, eg ACEi, NSAID, phenobarbital, L-dopa. *Signs:* Flaccid blisters which rupture easily to leave widespread erosions. The oral mucosa is often affected early. *Skin biopsy:* +ve immunofluorescence (intercellular IgG giving a crazy-paving effect). ℞: prednisolone (60-80mg/day PO, eg life-long in low doses). IVIs of *rituximab* and *immune globulin* may have a dramatic effect. [160]

1 Discoid (=nummular, ie coin-shaped) eczema may begin with vesicles. [161] Typical patient: ♂ 50-70yrs or ♀ 20-30, with somewhat symmetrical round/oval very itchy vesicles, or papular plaques often on legs (or trunk/arm, *not* face) with well-defined irregular margins (p587 fig 5). They may crust and get infected by staphs before flattening into hyperpigmented macules. It recurs at the same sites. Sunlight may improve it. Cause: unknown; patch test +ve in ~50% (if +ve, avoid culprits). [162] ℞: lukewarm baths + moisturizers + steroid ointment (eg high-potency, preceded by a 20min water-soak [163]) + oral antihistamine.

Photosensitivity For classification of susceptibility to ultraviolet, see p593.
Photosensitivity denotes conditions triggered by light (eg solar urticaria; polymorphic light eruption). Photoaggravation describes disorders worsened by light but not due to abnormal sensitivity to light (eg recurrent herpes labialis; rosacea). Photosensitivity can occur to visible light, UVA (320-400nm) or UVB (290-320nm). ►Usually a *careful history* allows accurate diagnosis.

• A rash every summer, for example, suggests that uv has a role.
• How long does the rash take to appear? Within 30min suggests solar urticaria; polymorphic light eruption may take days to appear.
• Itching suggests polymorphic light eruption or solar urticaria.
• Face rashes, including the V of the neck, but sparing periorbital skin.
• The dorsum of the hands and the arms are other typical sites.
• As hands are usually relaxed in the semi-flexed position, skin around DIP joins is less affected than that around the knuckles and PIP joints.
• Is there a family history? If so, refer to genophotodermatologist. Is it xeroderma pigmentosum, Bloom's syndrome, or Cockayne's syndrome?
• Pain (± family history) suggests erythropoietic protoporphyria (sun may hurt so much that a child quickly avoids it, so there is pain but no rash).
• Was the rash related to starting a drug (eg nalidixic acid)? See below.
• Are there papules: this suggests polymorphic light eruption.
• Any blisters or linear marks where plants have scratched the skin (phytophotodermatitis from furocoumarins)? Ask about hobbies/work.

Polymorphic light eruption: This is a common idiopathic disorder typically affecting young women in spring. After light exposure, itchy red papules, vesicles, and plaques develop on exposed sites, often improving over the summer due to a phenomenon called 'hardening'. Smoking and alcohol may trigger it.[184] ℞: Sun-avoidance; sun-protection (high factor UVA + UVB sunscreen). Acute attack: potent topical steroids ± a short course of systemic steroids. Severe cases: desensitization (UVB phototherapy or PUVA therapy).[165]

Porphyria cutanea tarda: (The commonest porphyria) The 1° abnormality is ↓uroporphyrinogen decarboxylase in liver. *Causes/triggers:* some alleles of haemochromatosis gene; HIV; hepatitis C; alcohol; oestrogen,↑iron,↓ascorbic acid. *Signs:* Vesicles/bullae in sun-exposed sites, hypertrichosis, hyperpigmentation, skin fragility, and scarring (milia). *Tests:* ↑LFT; ↑ferritin; ↑plasma, faecal & urinary porphyrins (protect urine from the light and ensure it gets analysed promptly; phone lab). ℞: Remove precipitants; sun-avoidance/protection; regular venesection until ferritin in normal range; chloroquine, ascorbic acid.[166,167]

Systemic lupus erythematosus: (OHCM p556) Light exposure often triggers erythematous rashes, with systemic flare. A variant of lupus, subacute LE, is associated with marked photosensitivity and anti-Ro antibodies.

Drugs often cause of photosensitivity, so ►*look up details of all drugs taken*. Frequent offenders: thiazides (sunburn-like or lichenoid rash); tetracyclines/sulfonamides (sunburn-like); tricyclics; phenothiazines; NSAIDs; amiodarone (sunburn-like eruptions). It may take months to settle, after drug withdrawal.

Ordinary urticaria *Acute:* Rash (eg to latex) lasts <6wks. Skin prick or blood RAST tests (p596) may help. *Chronic:* Idiopathic, but can be autoimmune in ~45% of patients (IgG against IgE receptor,[188] causing degranulation, p610) or seen with collagen, thyroid or sinus disease. **Physical urticaria** is caused within minutes by an external trigger, eg heat, cold, exercise, or trauma (dermatographism). **Contact urticaria** arises eg on contact with food, insect bites, or pet saliva. **Urticaria pigmentosa** (fig 1, p610) May be caused by *H. pylori*. **Urticarial vasculitis** Cutaneous lesions resemble urticaria, but histologically show features of a vasculitis. Also: flitting arthralgia, GI symptoms obstructive lung disease especially in smokers. If complements are low, it may be associated with SLE, Sjögren's syndrome, or cryoglobulinaemia. ℞: Antihistamine, NSAIDs, but some patients may need immunosuppressive therapy.[169]

Venous leg ulcers (fig 2) *Risk factors:* Varicose veins, DVT, venous insufficiency, poor calf muscle function, arterio-venous fistulae, obesity, leg fracture. Venous hypertension from damaged valves of the deep venous system causes superficial varicosities and skin changes (lipodermatosclerosis, fig 2). Minimal trauma typically over the medial malleolus causes ulcers.

Typical causes
• Gravity/stasis
• Neuropathy
• Vascular: venous 75%; arterial 10%; mixed 15%
• Trauma

Rarer causes
• Pyoderma gangrenosum (eg with Crohn's; UC)
• Sickle-cell disease
• Vasculitis (SLE, rheumatoid)
• Vasculitis (eg SLE)
• Cryoglobulinaemia
• Malignancy
• Leishmaniasis

Management: Graded compression is the mainstay. Do Dopplers first to exclude arterial disease (ensure the ankle–brachial pressure index is >0.8, OHCM p658). 4-layer compression bandaging is applied with ~40mmHg pressure at the ankle, tapering off to ~18mmHg below the knee. This reduces superficial venous pressure. Ulcers heal more quickly with occlusive dressings which absorb exudate and improve comfort. Treat varicose eczema (fig 3) with emollients and topical steroids. Infection is most chiefly caused by *Staph aureus, Pseudomonas*, and β-*haemolytic strep*. These should be treated empirically (broad-spectrum penicillin: macrolide or quinolone) until definitive sensitivities are available. Avoid topical antibiotics as they ↑ the risk of resistance and contact dermatitis. Ulcers which don't heal on adequate treatment for 3 months must be investigated further (eg biopsy for malignancy). Once an ulcer is healed, patients should follow advice aimed at preventing recurrence: wearing compression stockings, skin care, leg elevation, calf exercises, and suitable diet. Annual recurrence rate: ~20%.[170]

Asteatotic eczema (eczema craquelé) Commoner in the elderly, this particularly affects the lower legs with a dry eczema which polygonally fissures into a crazy-paving pattern (fig 1). Emollients and soap substitutes help.[171] 1% pimecrolimus cream may help itch. Rare (paraneoplastic) association: lymphoma (suspect if the eczema is difficult to treat).

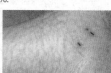
Fig 1. Eczema craquelé. ©Dr Baron.

Pruritus is a common complaint in the elderly. *Skin causes: Eczema; scabies* (appearance can be in the elderly); *pemphigoid/pre-pemphigoid eruptions; asteatotic eczema; generalized xerosis. Medical causes: Anaemia; polycythaemia; lymphoma; solid neoplasms; hepatic* and *renal failure; hypo-* and *hyperthyroidism; diabetes (candidiasis)*. Excluded by blood tests.

Pressure sores If made immobile by age, stroke, or cord lesions, uninterrupted pressure on skin leads to ulcers and extensive, painful, subcutaneous destruction, eg on the sacrum, heel, or greater trochanter. Protein malnutrition and arteriopathy make this more likely, particularly if nursing is poor. They are a big problem. Cost: >£800 million/yr.[172,173] A full-thickness sacral sore causes much misery and extends hospital stay by months. ►This should make prevention a central preoccupation, not just on long-stay geriatric wards, but in *all* acute wards, where most pressure sores start. Nurse education, ↑staff numbers, and nursing comatose patients prone (with a prone-head support system) may help.[174] Don't rely on special mattresses![175]

Staging	Stage	
	Stage	I: Non-blanching erythema over intact skin
	Stage	II: Partial thickness skin loss, eg shallow crater
	Stage	III: Full thickness skin loss, extending into fat
	Stage	IV: Destruction of muscle, bone, or tendons

Prevalence: ~7% of inpatients have pressure sores; >70% are over 70yrs. Up to 85% of paraplegic patients have pressure sores. *Complications:* Osteomyelitis.

Treatment and prevention of pressure sores

- Prevent the condition getting worse (see below).
- Optimize nutrition (get systematic help).[176] Insulin if hyperglycaemic.
- Treat systemic infection with antibiotics (evidence is lacking on whether antimicrobials are effective in the treatment of pressure ulcers.)[177 NICE]
- Dress the area. There is no convincing evidence from randomized trials which favours any one type of dressing.
- Elevation may increase perfusion around heel pressure sores.[178]
- Debridement of dead or necrotic tissue, or other debris, from the wound.
- Topical negative pressure treatment.
- Vascular reconstruction, if needed, and if practicable.
- Split thickness skin grafts.
- Neurosensory myocutaneous flap surgery.

Prevention
- Find an interested, knowledgeable nurse to educate the patient.
- Proper positioning, with regular turning (eg every 2h, p768-p776, alternating between supine, and right or left lateral position). Use pillows to separate the legs.
- On ITU, anatomical foam supports do prevent heel pressure ulcers.[179]
- Functional electrical stimulation can prevent sores in paraplegics, by inducing the buttocks to change shape, and by improving blood flow. A good randomized trial (N=44 patients aged ~85yrs with hip fracture) showed that a DeCube® mattress with removable cubes for provision of rest for pressure points can halve the incidence of pressure sores.[180]

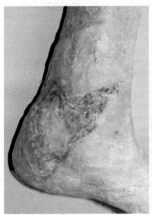

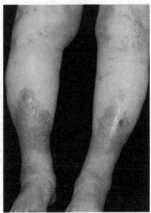

Fig 2. Venous leg ulcer (with eczema). Is there healthy granulation tissue on the ulcer floor? Remove all that over-ripe camembert pus to find out. Pain is frequent in these patients (who are often obese, so compounding immobility).   ©Dr S Baron.

Fig 3. Varicose eczema with hyperpigmentation and lipodermatosclerosis (an ill-defined band causing leg tapering, as if a bottle with a tightish neck were pouring liquid rhubarb down towards the ankle).
©Dr J Bowling..

Skin disease is a burdensome stigma for HIV patients and a challenge to us all due to severity and recalcitrance.[181] Skin problems are markers of HIV progression, so understanding them is vital.[182] They are classified as *primary* (eg seroconversion illness) or *secondary* (eg opportunistic infections that correlating with ↓CD4 levels). The full scope of primary HIV skin disease has yet to be elucidated.

▶*Any new lesion in HIV patients must prompt a hunt for unusual organisms.* With highly active antiretrovirals (HAART, OHCM p415), some are becoming less common. HIV skin pathologies may co-exist with conditions reflecting the same risk exposure (eg secondary syphilis rash or condylomata lata, or sometimes rare complications, eg chronic annular plaques of nodular tertiary syphilis).[183]

Infections HIV +ve people are at ↑risk from common pathogens (in their nastier guises, eg MRSA) and commensal organisms that don't normally cause disease.

- *HIV seroconversion* causes an acute mononucleosis-type illness, usually accompanied by a non-specific maculopapular eruption affecting the upper trunk, associated with lymphadenopathy, malaise, headache, and fever.
- *Thrush* may be severe, disseminated, and treatment-resistant, involving the posterior pharynx and oesophagus. ℞: Topical **nystatin**; systemic **imidazoles**.
- *Tinea* (eg on head) is a common and early HIV-related mycosis.[184]
- *Warts* are common; oral warts cause cancers (p570); *verrucas*: Risk↑ ×4.
- *Molluscum contagiosum:* (eg face; genitals). ℞ (difficult): cryotherapy, topical **retinoids**, cautery, or curettage. ∆∆: Disseminated cryptococcosis.
- *Malignant syphilis:* Multiple cutaneous ulcers and leonine features.[185]
- *Cryptococcosis:* Looks like facial molluscum contagiosum. ℞: **Fluconazole**.
- *Helminths:* Non-blanchable macules; examine sputum, faeces, etc for eggs.[186]
- *Scabies:* Severe variants, eg crusted are more common in advanced HIV disease. Paradoxically, patients may not complain of severe itch. A widespread scaly, crusted eruption occurs (highly infectious p608). ℞: **Permethrin** lotion. **Ivermectin** may also be of benefit (but side effects may be serious).

Inflammatory disorders *Seborrhoeic dermatitis:* (31%) Red scaly patches on hairy areas and naso-labial folds & flexures. ℞: **Ketoconazole** cream. Others:

- *Oral pigmentation* (29%), *xerosis/ichthyosis* (23%), *pyodermas* (22%).
- *Psoriasis:* Treating HIV will often improve response to standard ℞ (p594).
- *Eosinophilic folliculitis:* The cause of this intensely itchy rash is unknown ∆: Biopsy. ℞: 0.1% **tacrolimus**, topical **steroids**, UVB therapy, PUVA therapy.[187]
- *Drug reactions* are common in HIV (esp. co-trimoxazole's maculopapular eruptions or erythema multiforme; toxic epidermal necrolysis; fig 2 p601).
- *Pityriasis rubra pilaris* is rarely the presenting feature of HIV, eg with palmo-plantar keratoderma, long horny keratotic spiny follicular papules coalescing to form orange plaques, eg over ears, limbs, and trunk.[188] Cause: unknown.
- *Darier's disease:* (= keratosis follicularis; rare) reflects Ca^{2+} dysregulation of synthesis, folding, and trafficking of desmosomal proteins, eg from mutations in ATP2A2).[189] Signs: many follicular keratotic red-brown papules on scalp, face, retroauricular area, ears, sternum, upper trunk, hands, axillae & groins.[190]

HIV & nail changes: Onychomycosis (30%; eg *Trichophyton rubrum*; multiple fungi are often cultured in a single patient); melanonychia (15%); leukonychia (14%); transverse lines (7%), onychoschizia (7%), clubbing (6%).[191]

HIV & skin neoplasia Kaposi (BOX), BCC, skin lymphoma, MCC,[1] leukoplakia (fig 2).

IR(I)S (Immune reconstitution (inflammatory) syndrome) With antiretrovirals, immunity begins to recover, but then responds to previously acquired opportunistic infection with a powerful inflammatory response, paradoxically worsening symptoms, often involving the skin. You may confuse this with serious HIV progression. IRS is hardly ever fatal.[192,193]

Dermatology

Herpes simplex virus infection: This can be increasingly troublesome as HIV progresses. Painful ulcers and erosions develop, eg around mouth and genitals. Any ulcerated or eroded area is HSV until proven otherwise. ℞: High-dose **aciclovir** (oral or IV). Aciclovir resistance may develop and **foscarnet** is an alternative. Start a more highly active antiretroviral therapy (HAART).[194]

Varicella zoster: This may occur with atypical signs. Ulceration and post-herpetic neuralgia may be more frequent and severe. In advanced disease, disseminated infection occurs. ℞: High-dose **aciclovir** (IV if systemic disease).

Kaposi's sarcoma (KS): Cause: HHV-8 (herpes hominis virus). There is proliferation of vascular endothelial & lymphoreticular cells ± multicentric skin nodules/plaques (fig 1). 4 types: classic KS (typically on legs), endemic (African) KS, iatrogenic KS, and epidemic AIDS-related KS, often multi-organ (skin is not always involved);[195] incidence is falling thanks to HAART (*OHCM* p415). HHV-8 seroprevalence is higher in men who have sex with men (NB: *no* heterosexual spread).[196] Kiss transmission (if much saliva exchanged) may be important in HIV+ve & -ve men.[197]

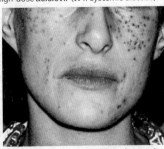

Fig 1. Kaposi's sarcoma. Purple macules, papules, nodules, and plaques affecting limbs, and face ± periorbital purpura/raccoon eyes (ΔΔ: skull fracture, myeloma, amyloidosis, *OHCM* p355, fig 1), and neuroblastoma).[198] Also seen in mucosae, eg oral, tongue, appendix, prepuce.   ©Dr S Baron.

ΔΔ: Bacillary angiomatosis (*Bartonella* species); pyogenic granuloma.

℞: *(if HIV +ve)* HAART; radiotherapy can palliate symptomatic disease (esp. if unable to tolerate chemotherapy, eg liver failure). Local ℞: intralesional chemotherapy, cryo, laser, photodynamic treatment, and excision.[199] Systemic **interferon-α** or chemotherapy (eg pegylated-liposomal **anthracyclines & paclitaxel**). In resource-limited settings, consider IV **vincristine**, oral **etoposide** or IM **bleomycin**.[200] HAART does not greatly influence other HIV malignancies.[201]

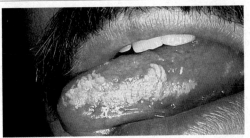

Fig 2. Oral hairy leukoplakia (adherent white plaques) is caused by Epstein-Barr virus in oral mucosa. 'Corrugated' would be a better term than 'hairy' as there are no hairs. Associations: HIV (esp. if CD4 <200/mm³);[202] immunosuppressives (steroids), eg in transplant patients; lamotrigine. ℞ (if needed): Topical **podophyllum** 25% resin + **aciclovir** 5% may work[203] ± systemic **aciclovir** or **valaciclovir**.[204] *Other oral signs of HIV:* KS, candida, linear gingival erythema, and necrotizing ulcerative periodontitis/gingivitis.   ©Prof D. Rosenstein

1 MCC (Merkel cell cancer) is a rare, aggressive neuroendocrine skin malignancy, and positively correlates with UV exposure and immunosuppression; see p502.

Dermatology

Dermatology

Scabies (*Sarcoptes scabei*; fig 1) A highly contagious, common disorder particularly affecting children and young adults. Spread: direct person to person, eg by holding hands or *prolonged* hugs. The ♀ mite digs a burrow (pathognomonic sign—a short, wavy, grey or red line on the skin surface) and lays eggs which hatch as larvae. The itch and subsequent red rash is probably due to allergic sensitivity to the mite or its products. *Signs:* It presents as very itchy papules, vesicles, pustules, and nodules affecting finger-webs (esp. first), wrist flexures, axillae, abdomen (esp. around umbilicus and waistband area), buttocks, and groins (itchy red penile or scrotal papules are virtually diagnostic). In young infants, palms and soles are characteristically involved. The eruption is usually excoriated and becomes eczematized. Mites can sometimes be extracted from burrows and visualized microscopically; eggs can be seen in skin scrapings. Crusted or Norwegian scabies is seen in the elderly or immunocompromized. They harbour up to 2 million mites and are highly contagious. If it occurs on your ward, get help. Simultaneous mass prophylaxis may reduce the need for ward closures.[205]

Management: A good explanation (verbal + written) will aid concordance between the patient's and the doctor's requirements, and will promote the chances of successful cure.[206] Permethrin 5% dermal cream is probably the most effective topical agent. It is also drug of choice for pregnant women. Preparations are applied to all areas of the skin, from the neck down, for 24h. Areas which are washed during this period (eg hands) should have treatment re-applied. **Malathion** is a good second choice. Oral **ivermectin** is also effective (200µg/kg stat (may need repeating).[207] All members of a household should be treated at the same time, even if asymptomatic. The rash and symptom of itch will take a few weeks to settle, occasionally longer. A suitable anti-pruritic such as **crotamiton** cream (Eurax®) (which also has anti-scabetic activity) can be useful during this period. *Example of written advice:*

• Take a warm bath and soap the skin all over.
• Scrub the fingers and nails with a firm brush. Dry your body.
• Apply **permethrin** or **malathion** 0.5% liquid (not if pregnant or <6 months old). Remember to paint *all* parts, including soles (+head if <2yrs old).
• Wash off after 24h. If you wash your hands before 24h is up, reapply the liquid to the parts you have washed. Avoid the eyes!
• Use fresh pillow cases and sheets, if you have any.
• Treatment may worsen itch for 2 weeks—so use calamine lotion or Eurax®.

Headlice (*Pediculus capitis*; fig 2) are common in children; but spread is only by head to head contact. Lice are 3mm long and have legs adapted to cling to hair shafts. Eggs (nits) are bound firmly to the scalp hairs and when empty appear white. *Signs:* Itch ± papular rash on the nape. *Neurotoxic agents:* (work in ~70%—alcohol based: take great care not to ignite): **Malathion, carbaryl, phenothrin** (repeat after 1 week). Resistance is a problem so many health boards operate treatment by rotation. *Non-irritant options:* **Dimeticone** (4%; repeat at 1wk).[208] Hot air at temperatures lower than blow-dryers can be effective.[209] Meticulous combing (see box). Only treat head-to-head contacts (over the past 5wks) if they have lice (say to have a careful look).

Crab lice (*Phthiriasis pubis*) Often sexually transmitted and affect pubic hairs. Eyebrows, eyelashes, and axillae may also be involved. *Management:* Topical **malathion** to all affected (or potentially affected) areas. Look for evidence of other sexually transmitted diseases. Treat all sexual contacts.

Flea bites (*Pulicidae*) spread plague, typhus, and cat-scratch disease. The animal (eg cat or dog) which spreads the flea may not itch or scratch itself. Flea bites cause a papular urticaria in a sensitized individual. Treatment: de-flea pets; de-flea household carpets and soft-furnishings.

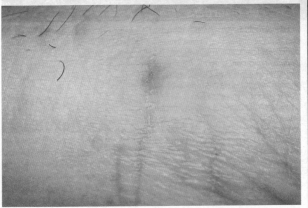

Fig 1. "Doctor, have I caught scabies?" "Do you recall sharing bedding, clothing, or towels with anyone, 4–6 weeks ago? Have you cuddled a pet? Or been to an institution? Is the itching worse at night?" Look for rows of irregular or s-shaped red furrows in web spaces, axillae, ventral skin on wrist, knee or penis (also palms & soles in children). Here is a scabies burrow with a mite just visible (with the eye of faith) beyond the red area. ©Dr J Bowling.

Advice on detection combing for head lice

Seeing lice is hard; using a special fine comb (prescribable, or bought at chemist) is 3-4-fold better than simple measures.[210] Here's how to do it.

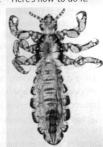

- Wash hair with ordinary shampoo, rinse, and apply lots of ordinary conditioner.
- Comb the hair with a normal comb to untangle it; then use the fine-toothed comb. Slot its teeth into the hair roots so they touch the scalp; draw it through to the hair tips.
- Ensure all hair is combed; check comb for lice after each stroke (use a magnifying glass). If lice seen, clean comb by wiping it on tissue, or rinse it before the next stroke. Combing takes ~1h. NB: nits (empty eggshells) don't mean live lice, as they can stick to hair even if lice have gone.
- After all hair combed, rinse out conditioner.
- Repeat combing every 4 days; only stop when no more lice have been seen for 12 days.[211]

Fig 2. *Pediculus humanus.*
©Prof S. Upton, Kansas Univ.

The flea (as lovers' go-between)

Mark but this flea, and mark in this
How little that which thou deny'st me is;
Me it suck'd first, and now sucks thee,
And in this flea our two bloods mingled be;
Confess it; this cannot be said
A sin, or shame, or loss of maidenhead,
Yet this enjoys before it woo,
And pamper'd swells with one blood made two,
And this, alas, is more than we can do.
Oh stay, three lives in one flea spare,
Where we almost, nay more than married are:
This flea is you and I, and this
Our marriage bed, and marriage temple is.

John Donne, to his lover, circa 1600.

Mastocytosis (urticaria pigmentosa) There are too many mast cells in the skin (± other organs), eg in nests or as a single mastocytoma. These release histamine, leukotrienes, and heparin (with systemic effects) and proteases (local effects). Adults have mutations of the stem cell factor receptor (kit D816V).[212]

Signs: red-brown itchy macules/papules (fig 1) which urticate, ie become more itchy, swollen, red (± weals) if scratched—Darier's sign. Also: head-

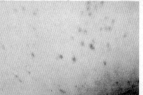
Fig 1. Mastocytosis. *Courtesy of Dr Sue Burge.*

ache, palpitations, syncope, flushing, wheeze, D&V, hepatosplenomegaly, osteoporosis, osteosclerosis, anaemia, eosinophilia, mast cell leukaemia (rare).[213]

ΔΔ: Multiorgan multifocal infiltrates of mast cells, plus one of: **a)** >25% of mast cells have abnormal morphology **b)** C-kit mutation at codon 816 **c)** Mast cells in marrow express CD2 or CD25 **d)** Serum tryptase↑.[214] *ΔΔ:* Sarcoid; histiocytosis.

R̃: Avoid triggers (eg aspirin, heat, cold). Try antihistamines + disodium cromoglicate. UVB phototherapy,[215] Nd:YAG lasers, interferon, and cladribine may help. D816V kit mutation predicts resistance to imatinib, while the FIP1L1-PDGFRA mutation suggests a good response to low-dose imatinib.[216]

Lasers in dermatology

Lasers (light amplification by stimulated emission of radiation) have an increasing role. The destructive energy of lasers can be concentrated in time and space, and the light's wavelength can be adjusted to match the target lesion. Energy can be selectively taken up by targets as long as the volume delivered is less than the target's capacity to absorb it. If this limit is exceeded, unnecessary destruction is caused. Variables to specify—an example from treating keloid scars: wavelength 585nm, pulse duration 0.45msec, spot size 5mm, mean fluence per pulse 7Joules/cm², treatment interval: 6 weeks. NB: melanin in dark skins may be a problematic competing chromophore.

Photoacoustic damage by shock waves (intense energy over picoseconds).

Photocoagulation implies less rapid, and less intense treatment.

Selective photothermolysis is somewhere between the above 2 categories. It may produce minimum scarring.

Examples of laser-treatable skin disorders *Tuberous sclerosis:* (p638) Angiofibromata (misnamed adenoma sebaceum) can cover much of the face.

Port wine stain: (OHCM p703) Best treated when young (small, smooth lesions).

Strawberry naevi: (p602 & fig 1 p121) These do *not* need treatment, unless they fail to resolve spontaneously. If they ulcerate, get expert advice.

Flat, pigmented lesions: Problematic unless known to be benign.

Tattoos: If multicoloured, multiple wavelengths must be used.

Scars: Raised, red, nodular *keloid scars* may appear ugly (and itchy); lasers can help somewhat. *Acne scars* (atrophic or 'ice-pick').

UV phototherapy UVA315-400nm & UVB290-315nm stabilizes many skin conditions when topical or systemic agents disappoint. In the neonatal nursery blue light (459–460nm) reduces bilirubin levels and prevents kernicterus. Psoralens and UVA (PUVA): see p595. Narrowband UVB (311nm) can help atopic dermatitis, psoriasis, vitiligo, morphea, mastocytosis, and lymphocytic infiltrative diseases (mycosis fungoides, alopecia areata and pityriasis lichenoides).[217] Protect the eyes. Local delivery of narrowband UVB can be given by excimer laser (308nm).

To construct a coherent identity, we must distinguish what belongs to the external, perceived world from what belongs to our inner world. The skin marks this boundary and can become the battle-field where different identities fight for dominance (see case report[1]). In a famous thought-experiment, Arthur Rimbaud spells out the advantages of connecting with universal monstrosities by receiving grafts of warts to his face, for gleeful cultivation[218]—in order to free himself from not just from his past selves, but from the stability of identity in general and so to become strong, aware, and visionary. Dermatologists rarely recommend his methods, but unless we develop the flexibility to understand this and related points of view,[1] our patients with self-mutilation and dermatitis artefacta will never be understood by us.

The range of self-destructive skin phenomena: *neurosis/obsessiveness*, neurotic excoriations (compulsive picking at the skin), and *trichotillomania*— and *psychosis* ("I make holes in my skin to let the demons out") and *dermatitis artefacta* reflecting difficulties with the solidity of these patients mental and physical limits. For these men and women (not necessarily patients) their real skin is metaphorically linked to the fantasized mental structure that delimits individual mental space. They are said (according to the *Anzieu moi-peau hypothesis*) to show a **pathology of action** and attack their own skin, paradoxically, to test the solidity and reliability of their own limits.[219]

Dermatitis artefacta 3 key signs differentiate dermatitis artefacta from other psychodermatoses: **1** Lack of direct suicide ideation. **2** Denial of responsibility for the lesions. **3** Resistance to the idea that the lesions are important unconscious non-verbal messages (eg dealing with emotional deprivation).

Associations: Any chronic medical or skin condition, eg acne, alopecia, leg ulcer (which they may encourage); also psychosocial problems, eg borderline personality, p366; stress; unemployment; depression; anorexia nervosa (in 33%); chronic pain syndrome; sexual conflicts. There is overlap with Münchhausen's and other pathomimicry, factious or somatizing syndromes.

Epidemiology: Typical age: any, eg as young as 3yrs.[220,221] ♀:♂≈6:1. In conscript armies sex ratios may reverse (there is usually obvious secondary gain).

Signs: Variable (simply showing images can be very misleading). Look for unusual/inexplicable features.

Diagnostic work-up: **Background:** Is there borderline personality disorder or anorexia nervosa? Any secondary gain? What does the family think? Is there a spouse? If not, why? (Could the rash be protecting your patient from an unfortunate marriage?) But don't ask too many questions: you risk only getting answers in reply, when what you need is **insight**. **Histology:** non-specific. Self-injection of foreign matter eg causing abscesses is provable by spectrometry.

Treatment: Supportive care will only gain traction once issues surrounding emotional deprivation, isolation, insecurity and other psychological states are addressed. Don't just prescribe antidepressants or antipsychotics and move on. Spend time with your patient and develop a rich therapeutic alliance. Include the family. Avoid addictive drugs. Find a specialist (GP, dermatologist, or psychiatrist) who enjoys a nice juicy holistic challenge of epic ectodermal proportions and who can roll skin and brain into a single unified management plan. Don't lapse into idle confrontations. If this method is to be tried it must be carefully planned. Acceptance may be a better approach.

---

1 14-yr-old girl presented with many large, deep ulcers with unnatural shapes on her left forearm, leading to a provisional diagnosis of dermatitis artefacta. Psychiatric examination revealed that she had dissociative identity disorder and that mutilations only occurred when one of her identities was assumed.[224]

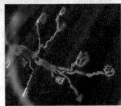

Fig 1. Immunofluorescent labelled image of the motor unit including the neuromuscular junction (NMJ). Axons and nerve terminals (in green) are marked with antibodies against neurofilament and synaptophysin respectively. Acetylcholine receptors (in red) are labelled with rhodamine-α-bungarotoxin. Blockade at the NMJ is just one arm in the triad of:

Muscle relaxation
Hypnosis and
Analgesia

that is required for effective anaesthesia. See p622 for how we can interpose at this junction in the safest possible manner.

Image courtesy of Prof. Mendel Rimer, School of Biological Sciences, University of Texas, Austin.

Other relevant pages Pain relief in labour (p66); resuscitation after delivery (p107); neonatal ITU (p108); ventilating neonates (p110); major injury (p724); choosing the correct dose of lidocaine according to body weight (p729); pain relief in children (p719); Bier's block (p744). **Online resources** www.frca.co.uk

Introduction

Anaesthesia evolved from humble origins in 1842 when CW Long gave ether, but he failed to report this landmark in pain relief. Then, in 1844, Horace Wells used nitrous oxide for tooth extraction (p617), and in 1846 WTG Morton gave the first surgical anaesthetic with ether. It is now a highly sophisticated specialty in its own right. While the triad of anaesthesia (hypnosis, analgesia, and muscle relaxation) remains the fundamental principle behind general anaesthesia for surgery, the role of the anaesthetist has expanded to encompass not only the provision of ideal operating conditions for surgery, but also intensive care, resuscitation, alleviation of acute and chronic pain, obstetric anaesthesia and anaesthesia for diagnostic procedures. A detailed knowledge of general medicine, physiology, pharmacology, the physical properties of gases and the workings of the vast array of anaesthetic equipment are essential in order to practise well.

▶We emphasize that this short chapter is no substitute for a specialist text or for experience on the ward and in theatre or clinic. The main aim is to enable understanding of the issues anaesthetists face, and to prepare one's mind for intelligent discussions on anaesthetic issues.

We thank Dr Mike Nathanson—our Specialist Reader for this chapter.

Aims To ensure that patients: • Get the right surgery • Are happy and pain free • Are as fit as possible • Have individualized decisions on type of anaesthesia/analgesia taking into account risks, benefits, and wishes.

Past history screen:
• MI or IHD
• Asthma/COPD
• Hypertension
• Rheumatic fever
• Epilepsy
• Liver/renal disease
• Dental problems
• Neck problems
• GI reflux or vomiting (needing rapid sequence induction—see p626)
• Past anaesthesia/ problems (eg intubation difficulty/PONV)
• Recent GA?

The pre-operative visit Have the symptoms, signs or patient's wishes changed? If so, inform the surgeon. Assess cardiovascular and respiratory systems, exercise tolerance, existing illnesses, drug therapy, and allergies.

Assess past history—see MINIBOX.

Family history Ask about malignant hyperthermia (p628); dystrophia myotonica (OHCM p514); porphyria; cholinesterase problems; sickle-cell disease (test if needed). Does the patient have any specific worries?

Drugs Ask about allergy to any drug, antiseptic, adhesive bandage, & latex.
• *ACE inhibitors:* No special action is required if BP & U&E are OK.
• *Antibiotics:* Aminoglycosides, colistin, and tetracycline prolong neuromuscular blockade, even *depolarizing* neuromuscular blockers.
• *Anticoagulants:* Know the indication. Check the INR and switch warfarin to heparin pre-operatively, leaving sufficient time for the INR to drop to <1.5 before surgery. Admit early, and discuss the plan of action so that all goes smoothly. Avoid epidural/spinal blocks. Beware regional anaesthesia.
• *Anticonvulsants:* Give the usual dose up to 1h before surgery. Give drugs IV (or by NGT) post-op, until able to take oral drugs. *Sodium valproate:* an IV form is available (give the patient's usual dose). *Phenytoin:* give IV slowly (<50mg/min). IM phenytoin absorption is unreliable.
• *Beta-blockers:* Continue up to and including the day of surgery as this reduces the likelihood of a labile cardiovascular response.
• *Bronchodilators:* Continue and consider supplementing with nebulizers.
• *Contraceptive Pill:* See BNF. Stop 4 weeks before major (or leg) surgery, restarting at 2wks post-op if mobile.
• *Digoxin:* Continue up to and *including* morning of surgery. Check for toxicity and check plasma K⁺. Suxamethonium ↑serum K⁺ by ~1mmol/L, and can lead to ventricular arrhythmias in the fully digitalized.
• *Diuretics:* Beware hypokalaemia. Check U&E.
• *HRT:* Stop before hip surgery; use heparin thromboprophylaxis + stockings.
• *Insulin:* Stop insulin on day of surgery and start a GKI infusion (glucose, potassium, and insulin). See OHCM p591.
• *Levodopa:* Possible arrhythmias when the patient is under GA.
• *Lithium:* Check for a recent serum level; non-depolarizing muscle relaxants may be potentiated. Beware post-op toxicity ± U&Es imbalance: p354.
• *Monoamine oxidase inhibitors:* Get expert help as interaction with narcotics and anaesthetics may lead to hypotensive/hypertensive crisis. Newer selective MAOIs are safer.
• *Ophthalmic drugs:* Anticholinesterases used to treat glaucoma may cause sensitivity to, and prolong duration of, drugs metabolized by cholinesterases, eg suxamethonium. Beta-blocker eye drops may cause systemic symptoms of bronchospasm/hypotension.
• *Steroids:* If the patient is on or has recently taken steroids at an equivalent of >10mg prednisolone per day give extra cover for the peri-operative period (p616). See BNF section 6.3.2 for steroid equivalence doses.
• *Tricyclic antidepressants:* These enhance the effects of adrenaline in addition to exerting anticholinergic effects causing ↑HR, arrhythmias and ↓BP.

It is the anaesthetist's duty to assess suitability for anaesthesia. It requires an appreciation of the patient's wishes and desires, as well as their pre-morbid state. It requires an understanding of the proposed surgery and the particular anaesthetic techniques to suit both the patient and the surgeon. It requires this to be done for a range of situations within a range of surgery, eg dedicated pre-operative assessment clinics by day, trauma theatres by night. Planning and preparation with the patient are invaluable (see BOX), though when necessary, the ability to bring a patient safely into theatre for life-saving surgery as soon as possible comes with the confidence gained through experience. The *ward doctor* assists with a good history and examination, but should not be responsible for consent (*OHCM* p570), though can discuss post-operative complications—both general (*OHCM* p578) and specific (*OHCM* p582). DoH guidelines are that the consenting doctor must be capable of performing the procedure or have been specially trained in taking consent.[1] ►Be alert to risk factors (see BOX). Communicate your concerns to the anaesthetist. Other issues:

- DVT prophylaxis (eg p706)
- Frozen section (tell pathology)
- Perioperative antibiotics (*OHCM* p572)
- Bowel prep (*OHCM* p572)
- Post-op physio
- On-table x-rays.

Tests Be guided by age, history, examination and proposed surgery, finding the safe balance between too many investigations and too few. Be guided by NICE, which takes into account the grade of surgery, from grade 1 (minor) to grade 4 (complex+) and beyond: cardiovascular and neurosurgery.ₙᵢcₑ NB: tests may not be needed for young fit adults having intermediate surgery, eg knee arthroscopy.

- *FBC*, ward test for *blood glucose*, and *U&E*—see MINIBOX for when to check . If Hb <10g/dL tell anaesthetist. Investigate/treat as appropriate.
- *Group & save* for all major surgery; *crossmatch* according to local transfusion guidelines, depending on pre-op Hb and type of surgery. Consider using autotransfusion devices, such as specialized suction and drains.
- *LFTs* in jaundice, malignancy, or alcohol abuse. *Amylase* if needed (eg trauma).
- *Blood glucose* in diabetic patients (*OHCM* p576).
- *Drug levels* as appropriate (eg digoxin, lithium).
- *Clotting studies* in liver disease, DIC, massive blood loss, already on warfarin or heparin.
- *Virology:* HIV, HBsAg in high-risk patients—after appropriate counselling.
- *Sickle-cell test* in those from Africa, West Indies, or Mediterranean area—and others whose origins are in malarial areas (including most of India). Take consent before performing the test, and offer genetic counselling.
- *Thyroid function tests* in those with thyroid disease.
- *CXR:* If known cardiorespiratory disease, pathology or symptoms.
- *ECG:* In those with cardiorespiratory disease—ie poor exercise tolerance, angina etc, BP↑, past rheumatic fever/Kawasaki's (p646)—and age >60 (high incidence of 'silent' ischaemia).
- *Lateral c-spine x-ray:* Consider in rheumatoid arthritis/anklyosing spondylitis/Down's syndrome to check for atlanto-axial instability.
- *Urinalysis* is not specifically indicated, though may be useful.

Check U&Es if:
• On diuretics
• Diabetes
• Burns victim
• Major trauma
• Hepatic/renal disease
• Intestinal obstruction/ ileus
• Parenteral nutrition.

If the patient needs referral to another medical team for optimization or investigation, ensure that both the patient and surgeon are involved and aware.

---

1 Use only words the patient understands. Ensure he believes your facts and can retain pros and cons long enough to inform his decision. Make sure his choice is free from pressure from others. A patient may complain if: • He is unaware of what will happen • He has not been offered all options • He was sedated at the time of consent • He changed his mind • He was not told a treatment was experimental • A 2ⁿᵈ opinion has been denied • Details of prognosis were glossed over.

Risk factors in the perioperative period[2]

• *Age:* The risk of dying doubles every 7 years from the age of 10. Such that the mortality risk at 90 is 5000× greater than the risk at age 10.
• *Sex:* Men are 1.7× more likely to die than women of the same age.
• *Socioeconomic status:* The impoverished are 2× as likely to die as the rich.
• *Aerobic fitness:* Ask about a patient's functional capacity—this can be measured in metabolic equivalents (METs), where 1 MET equals the basal metabolic rate. Ask the patient if they can walk indoors or 100m on level ground (2-3 METs), or climb 2 flights of stairs (4 METs) or participate in strenuous sport (eg singles tennis; skiing ~10METs). When functional capacity is high, the prognosis is excellent, even in the presence of other risk factors. A low functional capacity has been associated with poorer outcomes in thoracic surgery, although it has less predictive power with non-cardiac surgery.[3] In the pre-assessment clinic aerobic fitness can be assessed by a shuttle walk, or cardio-pulmonary exercise testing.
• *Diagnosed myocardial infarction (MI), heart failure, stroke, kidney failure* (creatinine >150μmol/L), *peripheral arterial disease:* Multiply long-term mortality risk by 1.5. Angina (without MI) and transient ischaemic attacks increase risk to a lesser degree.
• *Other:* Ask about COPD/asthma, smoking, diabetes, hypertension and hypercholesterolaemia as these may contribute to perioperative risk. ►Post-op chest infections are ×6 more likely in smokers. Stopping smoking 6-8 weeks pre-op is best but stopping smoking even 1 day pre-op is of benefit.[4]

Pre-op fasting Assoc. of Anaesthetists of Great Britain & Ireland 2010[5]

• *Fast the patient:* For elective surgery, if there is no GI co-morbidity, allow clear fluids (including black tea or coffee) ≥2h pre-op; all other intake (ie food/solids) up to 6h beforehand. In emergency surgery, it may be best to restrict all oral intake to ≥6h pre-op. Involve the anaesthetist in any decisions if the situation is unclear. Children undergoing elective surgery are allowed formula/cows' milk/solids upto 6h pre-op; breast milk up to 4h pre-op and clear fluids up to 2h pre-op. Chewing gum may be allowed up to 2h pre-op.

ASA score   ASA = American Society of Anesthesiologists

1	Normally healthy
2	Mild systemic disease, but with no limitation of activity
3	Severe systemic disease that limits activity; not incapacitating
4	Incapacitating systemic disease which poses a threat to life
5	Moribund. Not expected to survive 24h even with operation
6	Brain dead patient whose organs are being removed for donor purposes

This should reflect the health of the patient at the time of surgery. There is a slot for ASA numbers on most anaesthetic charts; the prefix 'E' denotes emergencies. NB: in most (but not all) studies ASA correlates with morbidity.[6]

Patient safety: use of checklists

►*Follow local procedures.* Safety must be a leading concern.[7] Checklists help achieve safety by reducing complex tasks to component parts, and by ensuring that nothing is omitted, eg:[8] • Identity • Procedure • Consent • Equipment check • Site marked • Allergies? • Aspiration risk? • Anticipated blood loss >500mL (7mL/kg if a child)? • Have team members introduced themselves by name & role? • Any patient-specific concerns? • Post-op: have equipment failures been addressed? • Have surgeon & anaesthetist liaised over recovery? *Full checklist:* www.who.int/patientsafety/safesurgery

Anaesthesia

Historically most patients would have received some sort of premedication to allay anxiety and contribute to a smooth induction of anaesthesia by decreasing secretions (more important when ether was used), promoting amnesia and analgesia, and decreasing vagal reflexes. With increasing amounts of day-surgery and greater awareness of "hangover" effects from premedication routine use of anxiolytics is far less common. However, there are a variety of reasons patients may receive certain pre-operative medications which may improve patient outcome and satisfaction (see MINIBOX.)

Premedication: 7As
• Analgesia
• Anxiolysis
• Amnesia
• Antacid
• Anti-emesis (see BOX)
• Antibiotics
• Anti-autonomic.

Timing ~2h pre-op for oral drugs.

Anxiolysis and amnesia Bear in mind that amnesia may add to the unpleasantness of the experience, though it can be useful in those not wanting to know, and children. The most common agents used are benzodiazepines. These should be prescribed by the anaesthetist.

Examples for the 70kg man:
• Lorazepam 2mg PO.
• Diazepam 5mg PO.
• Midazolam 0.05–0.1mg/kg PO. NB: relaxing music may be as effective as midazolam in reducing anxiety.[9]

Examples for children: (Always use oral premeds in children as first choice.)
•Midazolam 0.5mg/kg (tastes bitter so often put in paracetamol suspension).
•Local anaesthetic creams: Tetracaine 4% (Ametop®; apply 45min before inserting IVI) is more popular than EMLA®, as it does not vasoconstrict.
►NB: *The presence of a parent at induction is more powerful than any premedication in reducing anxiety.*[10]

Specific premedications *Analgesia:* Pre-emptive analgesia in elective patients aims to dampen the pain pathways before the signals start to arrive, thus modulating longer term pain response.[11,12] Patients admitted for acute procedures, who have pain pre-operatively should be given adequate pain relief. *Antacids:* For reflux either ranitidine 150mg PO or omeprazole 40mg PO/IV the night before and then 2h pre-op can be given—ranitidine reduces both gastric pH and volume. Emergency caesareans: see p78. ►Aspiration is a much greater risk in emergency surgery, pregnancy, diabetes, and with a hiatus hernia, causing fatality in ~1 in 70,000 of all anaesthetics. *Antibiotic prophylaxis:* See OHCM p572. *Beta-blockers* can be used to reduce the risk of peri-operative ischaemia. *Bronchodilators:* eg salbutamol nebulizer. *Nitrates:* Can be applied as a patch or IVI as in cardiac surgery. *Steroids: Minor operations:* eg 25–50mg hydrocortisone IV at induction. *Major operations:* 50mg hydrocortisone IV at induction, then repeat 3 times (8-hourly before restarting oral); ditto if adrenal insufficiency or adrenal surgery, or steroid therapy within last 3 months with over 10mg of prednisolone per day.

Common reasons for cancellation
• Current or still symptomatic respiratory tract infection.
• Patient not in optimum condition, eg poor control of drug therapy (insulin for diabetic patients, digoxin, thyroxine, phenytoin); exacerbation of illness.
• Recent myocardial infarction (eg within last 3 months).●✷
• U&E imbalance (particularly K⁺); anaemia.
• Inadequate preparation (results not available, not crossmatched/fasted).
• Undiagnosed or untreated hypertension or uncontrolled atrial fibrillation (heart rate > 100/min).
• Insufficient ITU beds, staff, or theatre time or other logistical problems.

Post-operative nausea and vomiting (PONV)

This remains one of the more unpleasant side effects imposed by anaesthesia, and is experienced by at least 25% of patients. Control is desirable not least for comfort, but also for minimization of post-op complications such as:

- Dehydration
- Electrolyte imbalance
- Metabolic imbalance (metabolic alkalosis)
- Pulmonary aspiration
- Hernia formation
- Damage to site of surgery (direct, eg ENT, or indirect, eg neurosurgery)
- Inability to take oral medication
- Delayed discharge

The exact mechanisms of action for all the factors involved (see MINIBOX) are unknown, though the central mechanisms behind the vomiting reflex are somewhat better understood.

It is initiated in the vomiting centre of the medulla (see fig 1), which itself receives input from higher centres, the chemoreceptor trigger zone (CTZ), afferent somatic and visceral fibres, and the vestibular apparatus of the middle & inner ear. Of these, the CTZ in the *area postrema* (located in the floor of the fourth ventricle) is probably the most important.

PONV risk factors:
- *Patient factors:*
  - Female
  - Previous history
  - Obesity
  - Motion sickness
  - Pre-operative anxiety
  - NB: smoking is protective
- *Anaesthetic agents:*
  - Opioids
  - Nitrous oxide (N₂O)
  - Etomidate/ketamine
  - Volatile agents
  - NB: TIVA total IV anaesthesia with propofol ↓PONV
- *Surgery type:*
  - GI
  - GU/Gynae
  - Neurosurgery
  - Middle ear
  - Ophthalmic
- *Post-op factors:*
  - Dehydration
  - Hypotension
  - Hypoxia
  - Early oral intake[13]

For specific anti-emetics and their mode of action see *OHCM* p241, and in this book on p630. Neurokinin 1 (NK₁) receptor antagonists, eg aprepitant (80mg PO, given 3h prior to anaesthesia), are a new class of antiemetics which appear more effective than 5-HT₃ antagonists (e.g. ondansetron).[14] Non-pharmacological approaches such as P6 acupuncture point stimulation are effective.[15]

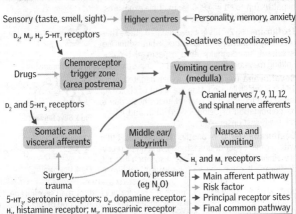

Fig 1. The neural pathways, receptor sites and triggers for PONV.

5-HT₃, serotonin receptors; D₂, dopamine receptor; H₁, histamine receptor; M₁, muscarinic receptor

Reproduced from Postoperative nausea and vomiting: Barry Miller, Anaesthesia and Intensive Care Medicine: 7:12; 453–455. 2006, with permission from Elsevier

Careful checking of equipment is vital before any anaesthetic or sedative procedure. Check anaesthetic machine (*plugged in* and *on*) plus:
- Tilting bed or trolley (in case of vomiting).
- High-volume suction with rigid Yankauer/long suction catheters.
- Reliable oxygen supply, capable of delivering 15L/min.
- Self-inflating bag with oxygen reservoir, non-rebreathing valve, and compatible mask (a 'bag-valve-mask' system).
- Oropharyngeal, nasopharyngeal, and laryngeal mask airways.
- A range of anatomical facemask sizes.
- Anaesthetic circuit: make sure that there are no obstructions to the flow. Check the vaporizers, flowmeters, and ventilator.
- Laryngoscope with range of blade sizes, spare bulbs, and batteries.
- Tracheal tubes (range) and catheter mount.
- Intravenous infusion cannulae and fluids (warmed if necessary).
- Anaesthetic and resuscitation drugs and anaesthetic gases.
- Defibrillator.
- Monitoring equipment (eg pulse oximeter ± end-tidal CO_2 monitor, p628).

Inhalational agents

These are volatile liquids which readily vaporize, permitting administration by inhalation in O_2-enriched air or an O_2/N_2O mix. They help maintain anaesthesia and decrease awareness (by an unclear mechanism).

Halothane (fig 1) This is a colourless, pleasant-smelling gas (which, unlike the other agents, is **not** an ether) first used as an anaesthetic agent in the 1950s. It has little analgesic effect, but decreases cardiac output (vagal tone ↑, leading to bradycardia, vasodilation, and hypotension). It sensitizes the myocardium to catecholamines (beware in patients with

Fig 1. Halothane.

arrhythmias; surgical infiltration with local anaesthetic and adrenaline). Halothane is no longer used in the UK—it has been replaced by safer inhalational agents (below), due to the rare but serious complication of postoperative hepatitis (up to ~1 in 4,000 for multiple exposures; less frequently in children).[18]

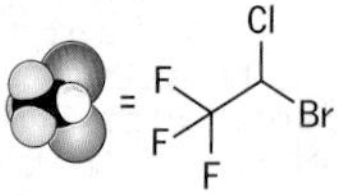

Isoflurane (fig 2) This is a halogenated ether. Theoretically induction should be quick, but isoflurane is irritant, so coughing, laryngospasm, or breath-holding may complicate the onset of anaesthesia.

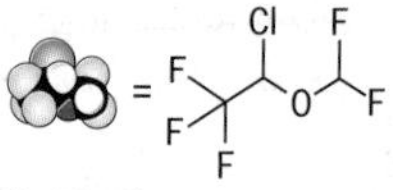

Fig 2. Isoflurane.

Sevoflurane (fig 3) This is a halogenated ether which is well tolerated. It is the agent of choice for inhalation induction of general anaesthesia due to its combination of being low irritant, and having relatively fast onset—offset.

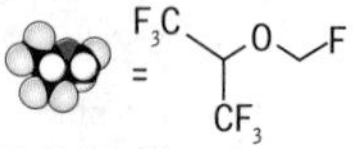

Fig 3. Sevoflurane.

Desflurane (fig 4) is another halogenated ether with a rapid onset of anaesthesia, and quick recovery. Having perhaps the lowest absorption into fat, desflurane is often chosen for surgery in the morbidly obese as it provides for the quickest recovery

Fig 4. Desflurane.

post surgery.[19] However, it is more of a respiratory irritant than sevoflurane, so is sometimes only used for maintenance rather than induction of anaesthesia. It may also have greater depressant effects of the cardiovascular system than sevoflurane. Stopping inhalation reverses all the above effects—except for hepatitis resulting from drug metabolism. ►All can cause malignant hyperthermia (p628).

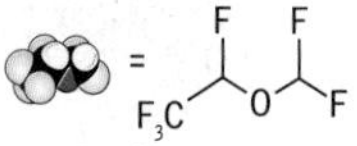

Anaesthesia

The ease with which the agent vaporizes in the chamber (=*volatility*) is a function of its *saturation vapour pressure* (svp) and the temperature of the liquid. Agents with a higher svp (eg isoflurane) need less gas to flow over them to reach a given concentration.

A vaporizer should ideally deliver a predictable and controllable concentration of anaesthetic agent to the patient for inhalation. There are 2 main types of device that can be used to create the inhaled vapour:

• **High-resistance devices:** eg the plenum vaporizer. Inhalational agents are added to the fresh gas flow by passing a fraction of the carrier gas (N_2O/O_2 or O_2–enriched air) through a chamber—the plenum ($\approx$ 'full space').

Anaesthesia

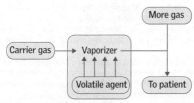

Fig 1. Schematic diagram of a high-resistance device.

This requires a positive pressure to drive it and it is therefore a high-resistance device. It works as a *precision* vaporizer, which delivers more accurate concentrations by overcoming the effect of temperature variation with a heat sink or a valve to vary gas flow. The plenum cannot be used inside the patient circuit as its internal resistance is so high.

• **Low-resistance draw-over devices:** eg Oxford miniature vaporizer, Goldman vaporizer. The patient's breathing generates enough flow to drive the gas flow. With the increase in the use of low-flow anaesthesia, low-resistance vaporizers have been developed that fit directly into the breathing circuit.[20] Accuracy/efficiency depends on the exact device used.

▶Cross-contamination and overdose in multiple devices can be a problem, though precautions are taken against this.[21]

• **Potency** The potency of an inhaled agent can be given by its **minimum alveolar concentration (MAC)**, which is the concentration that will produce no movement response to incision of the skin in 50% of unpremedicated patients. It is not a useful clinical measurement, but it can be used to compare potency of the different inhalational agents. It is affected by a number of factors, eg age, thyroid status and anxiety state of the patient.

Footnotes in History

Inevitably, not all stories along the trail of discovery and development in medicine are joyous ones. In 1844, the dentist Horace Wells was subject to the first tooth extraction under anaesthesia with the *'Exhilirating or Laughing Gas'*, nitrous oxide. Taking up the technique, he subsequently went on to spectacularly fail to anaesthetize a patient in a demonstration of tooth extraction at the Massachusetts General Hospital, leaving the patient in agony as he performed the procedure. For Wells, this was the start of a downward spiral into chloroform addiction, and ultimately suicide in jail after being arrested for throwing sulphuric acid at two prostitutes. Let's allow it to be a sombre testament to us all to make sure that we look after ourselves and our colleagues.[22,23]

This tale was sourced from The Greatest Benefit to Mankind, *by Roy Porter, Fontana Press, 1999*

Anaesthesia

Propofol (2,6-diisopropylphenol; $t_{\frac{1}{2}}$=30–600min)[1] This lipophilic phenol derivative is produced commercially as an emulsion in soybean oil and has become the most commonly used IV anaesthetic agent in the developed world. Its good recovery characteristics and anti-emetic effect make it popular, especially in day-case surgery.[24] It is fast-acting and its offset of action is due to rapid redistribution, and not metabolism.

- *Dose examples:* Induction = 2mg/kg IVI at 2–4mg/sec. Maintenance = 4–12mg/kg/h IVI. NB: ▸Rapid injection can cause cardiovascular depression (↓BP), and respiratory depression can occur when combined with IV narcotics. For procedural sedation: 0.5–1mg/kg IVI over 1–5min. Dose needs to be reduced in the elderly, debilitated and shocked. Dose also depends partly on premed use: with midazolam induction dose requirements for propofol are reduced by 20–50%. This effect seems to be more pronounced in the elderly.[26,27]

▸**Contraindications:**
- Extremes of age
- <17yr for sedation
- Egg or soy allergy[25]
- Compromised airway[2]

- *Uses:* It is used in induction and maintenance of GA, and for sedation during regional anaesthesia, short procedures, and as a sedative in ITU (though contraindicated in children for this last use). Once opened, use ampoules or discard, because of the risk of bacterial growth.
- *Problems:* Pain on injection occurs in up to 40% of patients. This can be minimized by either adding a small amount of lidocaine (eg 2mL of 1%) to the propofol, or by pre-injection of local anaesthetic.[28]

Thiopental sodium ($t_{\frac{1}{2}}$=11h) a barbiturate that is typically mixed with water to give a 2.5% solution (ie 25mg/mL). It has a rapid onset of action (arm–brain circulation time about 30sec). Effects last 3–8min, and awakening is due largely to redistribution, not metabolism. Some 30% of the injected dose is still present in the body after 24h, giving rise to a hangover effect. It has been replaced by propofol as the most popular induction agent.

- *Dose examples:* 100–150mg (less if elderly/debilitated) IV over 10–15sec (longer if elderly/debilitated), followed by further quantity if needed according to response after 30–60sec (or up to 4mg/kg; max 500mg).
- *Uses:* Induction of GA; it is also a potent anticonvulsant—used in status epilepticus management when other measures have failed (p208).
- *Problems:* Anaphylaxis is rare (1 in 20,000). Is a negative inotrope so can drop cardiac output by 20%. May also lead to bronchoconstriction. ▸*Intra-arterial injection* produces pain and blanching of the hand/limb below the level of injection due to arterial spasm, followed by ischaemic damage and gangrene—following inadvertent brachial artery puncture in the antecubital fossa. This is less of a problem now that an indwelling cannula is obligatory (compared with the historical use of a needle).

▸**Contraindications:**
- Airway obstruction
- Barbiturate allergy
- Fixed cardiac output states
- Hypovolaemia/↓BP
- Porphyria
- Compromised airway[2]

- *Treatment:*
  1 Leave the needle in the artery and inject a vasodilator, eg papaverine.
  2 Ask an experienced colleague to perform, brachial plexus or stellate ganglion block. (This should dilate vessels and ↓ischaemia.)
  3 Heparin IV to stop thrombus forming.
  4 Give pain relief—postpone surgery unless desperate.

Extravascular injection causes severe pain and local necrosis. ▸Get expert help. Infiltrate with hyaluronidase 1500IU dissolved in 1mL water through the cannula.

1 The pharmacokinetics are best modelled by a three-compartment model.
2 A compromised airway is a relative contraindication to any IV induction, regardless of the agent used.

Other IV anaesthetic agents

Etomidate (t½=3.5h) This is a carboxylated imidazole and is used as an induction agent. *Dose:* 0.15–0.3mg/kg. *Uses:* Histamine release is not a feature, but rapidity of recovery and cardiovascular stability are; therefore it is often used in emergent patients with trauma/head injuries for whom avoidance of even a brief episode of hypotension is important. *Problems:* Be aware it can induce involuntary muscle movements, nausea, and adrenal suppression.[29,30] Local thrombophlebitis can occur after injection.

Ketamine (a phencyclidine derivative, produced as a racemic mixture; N-methyl-d-aspartate receptor antagonist; t½=2.2h) *Dose example:* 2mg/kg usually gives 5–10min of surgical anaesthesia (for long procedures—see *BNF* 15.1.1). *Uses:* Mainly for paediatric anaesthesia and procedural sedation. Cardiac output is unchanged or increased, and so it is a good 'on site' or 'in the field' agent, as it can be given IM, producing profound analgesia without compounding shock. Ketamine has potent bronchodilatory properties, so can be considered during intubation in status asthmaticus.[31] *Problems:* Hypertonus and salivation, but there is some maintenance of laryngeal reflexes (but do not rely on this). Recovery is slow. Emergence phenomena are troublesome (delirium, hallucinations, nightmares; all made worse if the patient is disturbed during recovery). ►Avoid in the hypertensive patient, those with a history of stroke or raised intracranial pressure (further ↑ produced), patients with a recent penetrating eye injury (risk of ↑ intra-ocular pressure), and psychiatric patients. Avoid adrenaline infiltrations. In the UK, the Home Office classifies it as a class C drug as it is prone to misuse ('Special-κ').

Ideal weight and drug dosages To avoid excessive dosage in obese patients it may be best to calculate the dose on the basis of ideal body weight (IBW).

> Ideal body weight in kg:
> ♂ = 50kg + 2.3kg for each inch over 5 feet tall.
> ♀ = 45.5kg+2.3kg for each inch over 5 feet tall.

See www.globalrph.com

The ideal (but imaginary) IV anaesthetic agent

The ideal IV agent would be stable in solution and in the presence of light, be water-soluble and have a long shelf-life. It would be painless when given IV; non-irritant if injected extravascularly (with a low incidence of thrombosis) with some pain (as a warning) if given intra-arterially. Furthermore:
• It should act rapidly within one arm–brain circulation.
• Recovery should be quick and complete with no hangover effect.
• It should provoke no excitatory phenomena.
• Analgesic properties are advantageous.
• Respiratory and cardiovascular effects should be minimal.
• It should not interact with other anaesthetic agents.
• There should be no hypersensitivity reactions.
• There should be no post-op phenomena, eg nausea or hallucinations.

The ideal (but imaginary) inhaled anaesthetic agent[32]

Inhaled agents have advantages (eg no IV access required, more precise control) and disadvantages (eg claustrophobic) over IV agents. The ideal inhaled agent should:
• Have low solubility in blood and tissues (to allow rapid recovery).
• Be resistant to any degradation.
• Have no injurious effects on vital tissues.
• Be administrable in a reliable and known concentration.

These act on the post-synaptic receptors at the NMJ. There are two main types:

Depolarizing agents Suxamethonium (=succinylcholine) is the only one commonly used. It is a partial agonist for acetylcholine receptors and causes initial fasciculation through depolarization of the post-synaptic membrane, then paralysis by inhibiting the restoration of normal membrane polarity. Suxamethonium is rapidly inactivated by plasma cholinesterases. *Dose:* 1–1.5mg/kg *IV uses:* It has been the most popular paralytic agent in rapid sequence inductions (RSI) for several decades due to its rapid onset (30–60sec), and short duration (3–5min). Both these aspects are important in rapid sequence induction. The rapid onset lessens the time between induction and intubation—decreasing the risk of aspiration and potential hypoxia. The short duration means that if intubation is impossible, the patient regains muscle tone, and starts protecting their own airway again. Its popularity may start to wane with the increasing use of rocuronium (below). *Side effects:* ↑K⁺ (enough to raise the plasma K⁺ by ∼0.5–1.0mmol/L—avoid in paraplegia and burns!). Beware that K⁺ liberation is increased with multiple sclerosis, Guillain–Barré, stroke, and crush injury. Suxamethonium increases intra-ocular pressure (eg increases risk of vitreous extrusion). 30% of patients get post-operative muscle pains. Repeated doses of suxamethonium may lead to bradycardia—more common in children—treat with atropine. ►Beware suxamethonium apnoea (p628).

Non-depolarizing agents These drugs are competitive antagonists of acetylcholine (ACh)—that is they compete with ACh at the NMJ—but without producing initial depolarization (so no fasiculations). Their action can be reversed by anticholinesterases (eg neostigmine) which lead to an increase in the amount of ACh available at the NMJ. They are used during balanced anaesthesia to facilitate IPPV and surgery. Examples include: *Rocuronium:* Lasts 10–15min. Typically given at dose of 0.6mg/kg IBW (ideal body weight p621)—although in RSI has been used at doses of 0.9–1.2mg/kg to produce intubating conditions within 60 sec. Rocuronium has few side effects—although has been known to cause anaphylaxis. Excretion is via the liver. Historically, rocuronium has not been used for RSI due to its duration of action. The availability of *Sugammadex* (a reversal agent for rocuronium) is allowing this to change. At doses of 16mg/kg (given 3–5min post rocuronium) sugammadex is able to reverse rocuronium faster than the time taken for suxamethonium to wear off.[33] Given its lower side effect profile, RSI with rocuronium could be considered an attractive alternative to RSI with suxamethonium. *Vecuronium:* Lasting 20–30min, it is used if cardiovascular stability is important. **Adult dose:** 0.1mg/kg IV then 20–30µg/kg IV as needed. *Sugammadex* also reverses vecuronium. *Atracurium:* Lasting ∼20min. Metabolism is by *Hoffman elimination* (spontaneous molecular breakdown), so it is the drug of choice in renal and liver failure. **Dose:** 0.5mg/kg IBW IV then 100–200µg/kg IBW IV as needed.

Other non-depolarizing agents include cisatracurium and mivacurium.

Note on neuromuscular blockers in those with myasthenia In general, these patients are resistant to suxamethonium and very sensitive to non-depolarizing relaxants (action may be prolonged: lower doses may be needed). Warn patients that mechanical ventilation may be needed post-op. Liaise closely with a senior anaesthetist. A small dose of atracurium is most commonly used.

Action at the NMJ: mayhem, mischief or medication?

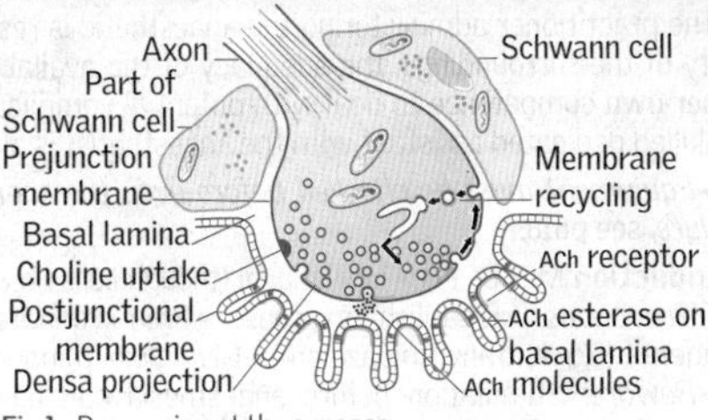

Procession at the synapse (fig 1) With the arrival of an action potential at the nerve terminal comes the release of acetylcholine (ACh) by exocytosis of vesicles at the presynaptic membrane. ACh then diffuses across the synaptic cleft (~75nm wide), its fate then being one of:

Fig 1. Procession at the synapse

Labels: Axon · Part of Schwann cell · Prejunction membrane · Basal lamina · Choline uptake · Postjunctional membrane · Densa projection · Schwann cell · Membrane recycling · ACh receptor · ACh esterase on basal lamina · ACh molecules

1 Hydrolysis in the synaptic cleft by acetylcholinesterase (AChE) to choline and acetate.
2 Diffusion into circulation (to be broken down by pseudocholinesterase).
3 Binding to post-synaptic nicotinic ACh receptors (NAChRs).
4 It is the last of these that continues the signal procession at the post-synaptic membrane by opening an ionophore channel linked to the receptor, allowing the influx of Na^+ cations. Membrane depolarization ensues, creating an endplate potential that results in muscle contraction. Hydrolysis of ACh whilst bound to the receptor causes termination of the endplate potential, bringing the trigger to contraction to an end.

Although there is a degree of receptor redundancy in the system for safety, the skeletal neuromuscular junction is nonetheless a site where lethal paralysis can take place. But agents that meddle here are not all bad.

Mayhem...

- *Curare:* eg tubocurarine, reversible NAChR blocker; poison used in South America extracted from plants (eg *Chondrodendrum tomentosum*, *Strychnos toxifera*) and used to tip darts for hunting.
- *α-Neurotoxoins:* eg α-bungarotoxin, irreversible NAChR blockers found in snake venom (eg Taiwanese banded krait, *Bungarus multicinctus*); multiple research uses, including immunostaining techniques (see fig 1, p612).
- *Botulinum toxin:* produced by *Clostridium botulinum*; blocks exocytosis.
- *Organophosphates:* insecticides which irreversibly inhibit AChE, causing prolonged binding of ACh at the post-synaptic membrane and depolarization.
- *Sarin:* odourless and colourless high SVP agent (see p619), infamous as a nerve gas; related to organophosphates.

...mischief...

- *Nicotine:* mimics the effect of acetylcholine at the receptor.
- *Myasthenia gravis:* autoimmune depletion of NAChRs on the post-synaptic membrane (OHCM p516).
- *Eaton–Lambert syndrome:* defective ACh release at the pre-synaptic membrane; paraneoplastic or autoimmune syndrome, with antibodies *vs* the pre-synaptic voltage-gated Ca^{2+} channels—OHCM p516.

...or medication?

- *Suxamethonium:* depolarizing NAChR blocker (see OPPOSITE).
- *Vecuronium:* non-depolarizing NAChR blocker (see OPPOSITE).
- *Neostigmine:* anticholinesterase that prevents breakdown of ACh in the synaptic cleft, increasing the efficacy of ACh.
- *Edrophonium:* another anticholinesterase, which was used diagnostically in myasthenia gravis (Tensilon® test); also used to reverse effects of non-depolarizing blockers, though worsens effect of depolarizing blockers.
- *Botulinum toxin:* used to relieve disability from focal spasticity, and in blepharospasm, spasmodic torticollis and severe hyperhidrosis.

Anaesthesia

The practitioner administering the anaesthetic is responsible for the suitability of the surroundings, the adequacy of the available equipment, and his or her own competence to deal with potential complications. The presence of a skilled dedicated assistant with the anaesthetist is also vital.

▶*Equipment must be checked before even the shortest anaesthetic procedure,* see p618.

Induction May be IV OR inhalational (though IM is possible with ketamine, p621). *Intravenous:* •Establish IV access. •Pre-oxygenate, and give co-induction agents (e.g. fentanyl/midazolam) •Give a sleep-inducing dose of eg propofol. ▶*Beware:* Stimulation before anaesthesia can have drastic consequences (coughing, breath-holding, laryngospasm). Remember: noise is a stimulus too. *Gaseous:* •*Either* start with sevoflurane in oxygen according to age and clinical state. •*Or* give nitrous oxide: oxygen 60%:40% mixture with a volatile agent, eg sevoflurane. In children, it is less frightening to start with a hand cupped from the end of the circuit onto the face than to apply the mask direct to the face. •Establish IV access as soon as asleep.

Indications for gaseous induction
• At the patient's request. • Difficult IV access • Children
• Some patients with partial airway obstruction (actual or potential, eg foreign body, tumour, or abscess), though awake fibre-optic intubation is an

Airway control This is maintained by holding a mask onto the face, by inserting a laryngeal mask airway, or by intubation (p627). To prevent airway obstruction, standard chin lift and/or jaw thrust manoeuvres are used. It may be facilitated by the use of an airway adjunct (eg oropharyngeal or nasopharyngeal), ▶*but this may produce vomiting or laryngospasm* at light levels of anaesthesia.

Ensure the patient is adequately anaesthetized (see p626), as laryngoscopy and tracheal intubation can produce a harmful *adrenergic stress response* with adverse increases in pulse and BP. Concurrent short-acting opiates or esmolol IVI can attenuate this in a dose-dependent way.[34]

Aspiration

Aspiration of foreign material into the respiratory tract can occur at any time around anaesthesia. It is unlikely to occur if a tracheal tube is *in situ*. It may occur with a LMA (p627). It can be the result of passive regurgitation, or of active vomiting. If suspected (direct visualization at laryngoscopy, coughing, vomiting, laryngospasm, bronchospasm, $S_AO_2\downarrow$, tachypnoea, wheeze and crepitations on auscultation), then immediately do the following:
➡ Apply cricoid pressure, unless actively vomiting (risks oesophageal rupture).
➡ Use suction to clear the mouth of debris.
➡ Intubate with an ET tube, use soft catheters to suction out the upper airway.
➡ Refrain from ventilating whilst undertaking these procedures, providing oxygenation levels are acceptable (to prevent dispersion of aspirate).
➡ Empty the stomach with an NGT at the first available opportunity.
➡ Put the patient head down and in the left lateral position.
➡ Cancel surgery, unless it is for an emergency.
➡ Consider ongoing ventilatory support to ensure adequate oxygenation.
➡ Arrange a CXR. Further investigation may be needed, eg bronchoscopy.
➡ In the absence of faecal contamination of the airway, consider withholding antibiotics until sensitivities are known (eg from bronchial lavage).

Mechanical ventilation

Indications Ventilators are used in anaesthesia when there is an operative need for muscle paralysis, or when muscle paralysis is part of a balanced GA for a long operation. (Ventilators are used in intensive care for

Overview of ventilator modes:
• Pressure controlled
• Volume controlled

ventilatory support in reversible acute respiratory failure—this is a different topic: see eg p110.)

Modes[1]

• Whenever the patient is paralysed and intubated, *intermittent positive pressure ventilation* (IPPV) is mostly used. These ventilators have controls to alter:

   • Tidal volume—which provides precise control of volume and P_aCO_2 (ie volume controlled)
   • Pressure necessary to inflate the lungs (ie pressure controlled)—which reduces risk of barotrauma.

   Other controls may be available to adjust:

   • Respiratory rate
   • Inspiratory time
   • Inspiratory flow waveform
   • End-tidal pause
   • I:E ratio (I:E = the ratio of inspiratory to expiratory time).

• Another form is *controlled mandatory ventilation* (CMV), which controls the drive and rate of ventilation in the presence of paralysed spontaneous breathing, and is in practice the same as IPPV.

• Some ventilators deliver *synchronized intermittent mandatory ventilation* (SIMV) which allows the patient to start breathing spontaneously when paralysis wears off, providing assistance if these breaths are inadequate. These are less common in theatre, and more often used in intensive care units.

▶It is mandatory for ventilators to have disconnect, high-pressure, and oxygen failure alarms.

Whichever mode is used, *positive end expiratory pressure (PEEP)* is often a useful adjunct. PEEP allows a pressure to be exerted at the end of expiration, which help splint open alveoli, increasing the surface area available for gas exchange, thereby reducing the amount of "shunt" (areas of lung which are perfused but not ventilated). A typical PEEP value would be ~5cm H_2O. High levels of PEEP may lead to reduced venous return due to a rise in intrathoracic pressure.

Familiarity with ventilators and ventilation is best gained from direct observation of their use. If you are interested in finding out more, then pursue the opportunity of a placement in the intensive care unit.

Lung compliance
Compliance =
$$\dfrac{\text{change in volume}}{\text{change in pressure}}$$
This is a useful concept in ventilation, as it relates to the behaviour of various parts of the respiratory tract. Poor compliance means only a small change in volume for a big change in pressure.

---

1 High-frequency oscillatory ventilation (HFOV) is used in preterm infants and neonates (p110).[38]

Intubation Passing an ET tube through the cords into the trachea protects the airway and ensures that ventilation can take place. Most commonly needed in:

- Risk of vomiting/aspiration (▶▶p 624) of gastric contents: eg reflux oesophagitis, abdominal disease, major trauma, non-fasted, hiatus hernia, pregnant >15wks.
- Management of difficult airways. If difficulty is suspected, ensure senior help is available and consider fibre-optic or awake intubation.
- An inaccessible or shared airway (eg as in head and neck surgery).
- Conditions when muscle paralysis facilitates surgery, eg abdominal surgery.

▶*Paralysed patients cannot breathe—and so require ventilation.*

Muscle relaxation increases the ease of intubation—the norm is a short- or long-acting muscle relaxant, as appropriate: *Short-acting:* Suxamethonium, typically 1-1.5mg/kg IV. Use if risk of vomiting ↑ or when difficulty with intubation is anticipated. *Long-acting:* Many are available, eg rocuronium/vecuronium (see p622), but they take longer to provide suitable conditions for intubation. Rocuronium provides suitable intubating conditions in 60-90s, but vecuronium may take >2min.

Rapid sequence induction (RSI) Used where the risk of aspiration is high.
- Pre-oxygenate with 100% O_2 for 3min to provide an O_2 reservoir in the lungs for use during the period of induced apnoea.
- *Sellick's manoeuvre* on induction: firm backward pressure (aim for force of 10N ≈ 1kg) on cricoid cartilage occluding oesophagus may stop gastric reflux to the larynx.[36,37]
- Give induction agent (eg propofol) then immediately give muscle relaxant (eg suxamethonium).[38] Wait 60sec for muscle relaxant to work. The trachea is then intubated, and the cuff of the ET tube inflated.
- Once the ET tube is positioned and cuff inflated, cricoid pressure may be released, and a volatile agent added to maintain anaesthesia.
- Give a longer-acting muscle relaxant (ie non-depolarizing) when suxamethonium wears off.

RSI: a quick overview
• NGT and IV access
• Pre-oxygenate
• IV induction
• Fast muscle relaxant
• Cricoid pressure
• ET intubation.

Maintaining anaesthesia (see BOX 'Gauging depth of anaesthesia', p631)
1 Volatile agent added to N_2O/O_2 mixture as before. Either spontaneously breathing or ventilation, with or without opiates. If the patient is ventilated, muscle relaxants are generally used.
2 IV infusion anaesthesia, eg propofol ± opiates. Maintenance dose, p620.
3 High-dose opiates with mechanical ventilation. ▶NB: There is a considerable risk of awareness with this, and it is only used in exceptional circumstances.

Whatever the technique, the dose and concentration of each drug is adjusted according to the level of anaesthesia achieved *vs* the desired level (determined by monitoring vital signs—eg HR, BP, signs of sympathetic stimulation, p631).

End of anaesthesia Change inspired gases to 100% oxygen only, then:
- Discontinue any infusions of anaesthetic drugs.
- After ascertaining that some spontaneous reversal has occurred (use a peripheral nerve stimulator), reverse any residual muscle paralysis with neostigmine (~2.5mg in adults) + an anticholinergic to prevent muscarinic side effects (↓HR, salivation), eg atropine/glycopyrronium.
- Once spontaneously breathing, inspect mouth and oropharynx under direct vision. Remove ET tube then administer oxygen by facemask.
- If no problems, transfer to recovery, but be prepared to reassess at any time.

Anaesthesia

Intubation technique

Preparation is the key. Assess the neck pre-op. Prediction of difficult intubation may be possible with assessment of the Mallampati classification (how much of the soft palate is obscured on looking into the open mouth), thyromental and sternomental distances.[39] Know your PLAN A (e.g tracheal tube); PLAN

Difficult intubation:
• Obese
• Short neck
• Receding chin/mandible
• Protruding teeth

B (ILMA/LMA—both below); PLAN C (bag-mask ventilation/wake pt if able) and PLAN D (needle/surgical crycothyroidectomy) before you start.[40]

ET tube sizes: (mm internal diameter, ID):

> *Adult ID:* ♂ = 8.5mm, ♀ = 7.5mm
> *Children ID* = [age in years/4] + 4.0mm
> *Neonate ID* = 3–3.5mm
> *Length (oral)* = [age of child/2] + 12.5cm
> *Length (nasal)* = [age of child/2] + 14.5cm

NB: Broselow tape-measures are said to be more accurate.

• Lubricate the tube, and check that its cuff and the laryngoscope work.
• Position the patient with neck flexed and head extended using a pillow ('sniffing the morning air').
• Hold the laryngoscope in the left hand; open the mouth with the right.
• Slide the laryngoscope blade down the right side of the tongue into the vallecula (area between tongue and epiglottis), guarding the lip and teeth with the fingers of your right hand.
• Lift the laryngoscope blade upwards and away from yourself. ►*Do not lever on the teeth or you may damage them.*
• Lift the epiglottis from view: the cords should become visible. When they are, insert the tube with your right hand (anatomy—p 567).
• Once the cuff of the ET tube is beyond the cords, remove the laryngoscope; ask the assistant to inflate the cuff to prevent air leak.
• Attach to the circuit. Gently inflate lungs. Watch the chest move. Do both sides move equally? Is the abdomen moving and not the chest?
• Auscultate both sides of chest. Is air entry equal? Fix the tube with a tie.
• Confirm correct placement with capnography (detects CO_2, p628).

►*Remember: if in doubt, take it out.* It is safer to re-intubate than to risk leaving a tube in the oesophagus. Tubes may slip down a main bronchus (usually right). If so, withdraw until both sides of the chest move equally and air entry is equal (so avoiding collapse in the unventilated lung, or pneumothorax on the overventilated side). If you are having problems intubating:
►Adequate oxygenation is top priority: • Get senior help • Employ the local or national failed intubation guidelines • Do not repeat the dose of suxamethonium: allow the relaxant to wear off whilst maintaining oxygenation • Consider a LMA (below).

Laryngeal mask airway (LMA) is used in 50% of elective UK surgery, and in cardiac arrests where a skilled intubator is not present. It consists of a tube with a cuff designed to sit over the larynx. A cuff takes ~30mL of air (depends on size). It is more efficient than masks. Advantages are that **no laryngoscope is needed** (no damage to teeth or cord stimulation), and **ease of insertion**. Lubricate the cuff, and slide over the palate so the device sits over the larynx. Learn the method on a mannequin; practise with an anaesthetist. It is available in a range of sizes from 1.0 to 5.0. It is safe and effective.[41] Specialized LMAs can assist with difficult intubation (eg an Intubating Laryngeal Mask Airway, ILMA),[42] and may allow air and fluid to be aspirated from the stomach (eg Proseal®).[43]
If unable to intubate? Employ failed intubation guidelines.[40]

The continuous presence of the anaesthetist is by far the most important monitor. Clinical monitoring of the patient supplemented by (not substituted by) a range of monitors of the patient and the anaesthetic delivery apparatus is mandatory. The process begins prior to induction of anaesthesia and continues throughout. ►*A warm, pink, and well-perfused patient is the aim.* Sweating and lacrimation invariably indicate something is wrong: *Respiration:* Rate, depth. *BP:* Intra-arterial in long/tricky cases (also allows ABG analysis). *T°:* Particularly important in infants, as the large surface area to body mass may lead to hypothermia. A warm environment, warming blankets, and warm IV fluids, are important in long cases. *Pulse oximetry:* Computes HR and arterial O_2 saturation. *ECG:* Reveals rate, arrhythmias, and ischaemia. *CVP:* Helps differentiate hypovolaemia from ↓cardiac function. Insert when large blood loss is anticipated, or in unstable patients. *Capnography* is essential: a low end-tidal CO_2 warns of a displaced ET tube, emboli, and more. Inspired oxygen concentration and end-tidal volatile agent concentration should also be monitored. Also monitor urine output, neuromuscular status, and ventilator pressures. Alarms should be set to appropriate levels prior to the case.

Some complications of anaesthesia

►*The commonest respiratory complication is airway obstruction from loss of muscle tone in the soft palate ('swallowing the tongue').*

►►**Anaphylaxis** See p237 and *OHCM* p780. ►►**Aspiration** See p624.

Atelectasis and pneumonia Atelectasis is best seen on CT (not CXR). It starts within minutes of induction, and is partly caused by using 100% O_2. ℞: Good pain relief aids coughing. Arrange physiotherapy + antibiotics (*OHCM* p161).

Awareness This is most distressing for patients. Paralysis makes its diagnosis difficult; the BIS monitor (p631) may ↓incidence. *Prevalence:* Much less than 1% even in emergency/obstetric anaesthesia (here doses are minimized, to avoid shock). It is still rarer in other contexts (eg 0.2%). See p631 for assessment.

Bronchospasm If intubated, check tube position (carina stimulation may be the cause: withdraw tube slightly). Check for pneumothorax. Ventilate with 100% O_2. Increase concentration of volatile agent if he is 'light'—most volatiles (especially sevoflurane) are good bronchodilators. Salbutamol ± aminophylline 250mg IV. $MgSO_4$ 2g IV may help Give hydrocortisone 100mg IV.

►►**Laryngospasm** The cords are firmly shut. Treat with 100% oxygen. Deepen anaesthesia—attempt to ventilate. It may be necessary to paralyse and intubate.

►►**Malignant hyperthermia:** Rare, autosomal dominant, life-threatening condition triggered by exposure to suxamethonium or volatile anaesthetics. Suspect when there is unexpected ↑oxygen consumption, hypercapnia and tachycardia. Rapid temperature rise (>2°C/h) may be a late sign. *Treatment:* Stop trigger agents (install a clean breathing circuit); ►► *Get help.* Hyperventilate with 100% O_2; maintain anaesthesia with IV agent (eg propofol); abandon surgery; muscle relaxant with *non-depolarizing muscle relaxant.* Give *dantrolene 2.5mg/ kg IV* as initial bolus, then 1mg/kg as needed to a maximum of 10mg/kg. Check for and treat hyperkalaemia; arrhythmias; acidosis; myoglobinaemia (mannitol/ furosemide/sodium bicarbonate/renal replacement therapy); coagulopathy; raised creatinine kinase. Take to ICU; counsel family, refer for follow up.[44]

Suxamethonium apnoea Abnormal cholinesterase leads to prolonged receptor inactivity. Ventilate until relaxant effect has worn off.

Shivering ± hypothermia May be treated by radiant heat/warming blankets. Shivering can be treated with clonidine, pethidine, tramadol or nefopam[40,2] Be aware that shivering increases O_2 consumption 5-fold.

Autonomic learning...

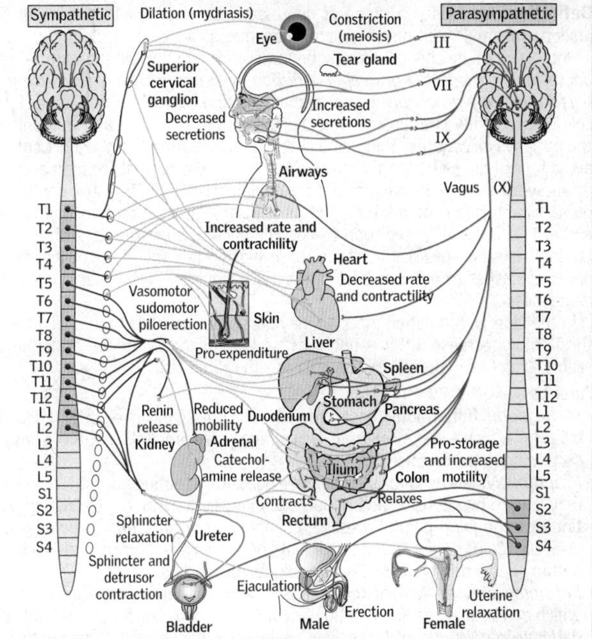

Fig 1. The autonomic nervous system may be primitive, but it is anything but simple. Many of the drugs used in anaesthesia (eg atropine, β-blockers) have an effect on this system, and at more than one place at once. This means that it is useful to remind yourself of exactly where each arm of the autonomic nervous system spreads its tendrils, and how it mediates effects:

Sympathetic			
Site		**Neurotransmitter**	**Receptor type**
Pre-ganglionic	All	ACh	NAChR
	Adrenal gland[1]	ACh	NAChR
Post-ganglionic	Sweat glands	ACh[2]	MAChR[2]
	All other	NA	NAR

Parasympathetic			
Site		**Neurotransmitter**	**Receptor type**
Pre-ganglionic	All	ACh	NAChR
Post-ganglionic	All	ACh	MAChR

Key: ACh = acetylcholine, NAChR = nicotinic acetylcholine receptor, MAChR = muscarinic acetylcholine receptor; NA = noradrenaline; NAR = noradrenaline receptor
1 The sympathetic fibres that innervate the adrenal gland are pre-ganglionic
2 This is the main oddity: sweat glands have MAChRs in the sympathetic system

NB: there are a number of other (co-)transmitters in the autonomic system (such as ATP to adenosine receptors). The gut also has a large independent neuronal network.

If only we could let our minds learn with the same autonomy that it has to control the function of individual organs and homeostasis. Perhaps it is best that we are able to switch off our higher functions from time to time, leaving the autonomic nervous system to its usual business!

Definition Sedation is a range of depressed conscious levels from relief of anxiety (minimal sedation) to general anaesthesia (see BOX).

Doctors in many specialties may be required to administer sedation. ►*The doctor giving moderate or deeper sedation must not also be responsible for performing any procedure* (such as manipulation of a dislocated joint). Her sole responsibility is to ensure that the sedation is adequate, and to monitor the patient's airway, breathing, and circulation. Sedation is not a short cut to avoid formal anaesthesia, and it does not excuse the patient from an appropriate work-up or reasonable fasting (►risking aspiration of gastric contents, p624). Monitoring is mandatory, and must include at least pulse oximetry, HR and BP.[45] It is easy for sedation to become general anaesthesia, with its attendant risks (see p628). The loss of the 'eyelash reflex' (gentle stroking of the upper eyelashes to produce blinking) is a good guide to the onset of general anaesthesia.

In the elderly, ↓cognition after GA may persist for months;[46] regional anaesthesia may decrease it,[47] it is unclear if sedation can obviate it—although it seems reduction in duration of anaesthesia may limit risk.[48]

Agents

• *Midazolam:* Initial adult dose 2mg IV over 1min (1mg if elderly). Further 0.5–1mg IV as needed after 2min. Usual range 3.5–7.5mg (elderly max 3.5mg). SE: psychomotor function↓.[49]

• *Propofol:* Widely used for sedation, see p620. Rapid acting anaesthetic—but may lead to hypotension and apnoea. In many circumstances (eg manipulation of large joint; painful dressing changes) a *narcotic analgesic* may be used too (eg morphine in 1–2mg aliquots IV, or shorter-acting opioids such as fentanyl) as propofol doesn't have analgesic properties.

• *Ketamine* may be administered. This is a dissociative anaesthetic agent which can be used as an induction agent (1.5–2mg/kg), or for procedural sedation (~1mg/kg). It produces deep analgesia with superficial sleep without loss of airway reflexes or hypotension. Side-effects include nausea, vomiting, emergency delirium and hallucinations. Ketamine and propofol can be combined in a single syringe to produce a sedative agent with less hypotensive effects than propofol alone, and less nausea/emergence problems than ketamine.[50,51] This is sometimes referred to as a *ketofol* sedation.

►Remember the need for oxygen and equipment to support ventilation as well as appropriate monitoring when undertaking any form of sedation.

Recovery from anaesthesia

• Oxygen supplementation via facemask: as much and for as long as necessary to counteract hypoxia due to diffusion hypoxia, respiratory depression, or ventilation/perfusion mismatch.[1]

• Monitor pulse and BP; keep the patient warm.

• Look for hypoventilation (?inadequate reversal—check with nerve stimulator; narcosis—reverse opiates with naloxone—*cautiously* to minimize pain; check for airway obstruction). Ensure adequate analgesia.

• Return the patient to the ward when you are satisfied with his cardiovascular and respiratory status and pain relief.

• Give clear instructions on post-operative fluid regimens, blood transfusions, oxygen therapy, pain relief, and physiotherapy.

• Post-operative nausea and vomiting (PONV, p617) is partly preventable by a 5-HT₃ receptor antagonist, eg granisetron or dexamethasone.[52] Metoclopramide is less effective.[53,54]

---

1 For a short duration (<5min) while very soluble nitrous oxide is diffusing out of the circulation into the alveoli, the concentration of O_2 in alveolar gas will be falling (diffusion hypoxia).[55]

Anaesthesia

Level of sedation

Minimal sedation (anxiolysis): is a drug-induced state where the pa[t]
is still able to respond to speech. Cognitive function and coordination ar[e]
impaired but airway, breathing and cardiovascular systems are unaffected.

Moderate sedation (conscious sedation): is drug-induced reduction
of consciousness during which the patient is able to make a purposeful response to voice or *light touch*. Response to pain only indicates deeper sedation. At this level of sedation no airway adjuncts are required, breathing and
cardiovascular function should be adequate.

Deep sedation: drug-induced reduction in consciousness to a point where
the patient cannot be easily roused but does respond *purposefully* to painful stimuli (withdrawal is *not* purposeful). At this level airway intervention
may be required (jaw thrust/ chin lift). Spontaneous ventilation may become
inadequate.

General anaesthesia: drug-induced loss of consciousness during which
patients are not able to be roused, even with repeated painful stimulation.
Airway typically requires intervention, spontaneous ventilation is frequently
inadequate and cardiovascular function may be impaired.

(Based on American Society of Anesthesiologists Guidelines, 2009)[56]

▶*Typically procedural sedation of patients outside of the operating theatre
or ICU for is confined to ASA 1 or 2 category patients* (see p615).

Gauging depth of general anaesthesia

Lack of inappropriate levels of general anaesthesia in a patient should be
suspected in the presence of:
• ↑HR[s]
• ↑BP[s]
• Lacrimation[s]
• Dilated pupils[s]
• Movement
• Laryngospasm
• Note that many of these responses are mediated by autonomic sympathetic
  drive (=[s], see p629), and all should be picked up with appropriate and con-
  tinual monitoring (p628).

Other measures: Bispectral index (BIS) EEG monitoring can help assess the
depth of GA—and can also reduce PONV and anaesthetic consumption, but not
cost or time to discharge.[57] Evoked potentials (auditory and somatosensory)
have also been used.[58]

▶*No single method is reliably accurate, and these cannot replace the vigilance and clinical suspicion of the anaesthetist.*

Local anaesthetic agents

Local anaesthesia is used either alone or to supplement general anaesthesia, by reducing nerve conduction of painful impulses to higher centres (via the thalamus), where the perception of pain occurs. Local anaesthetics act by impairing membrane permeability to sodium, resulting in a membrane-stabilizing effect, thereby blocking impulse propagation. ►Regional techniques (i.e. to whole limb/lower half of body) may lead to loss of consciousness or loss of airway, and so require the same facilities, expertise, and precautions as for general anaesthesia (eg full resuscitation facilities)

Types of local anaesthetic agents (LA):

1 **Lidocaine (lignocaine)** ($t_{\frac{1}{2}}$=2h) Max dose in typical healthy adult=3mg/kg IBW up to 200mg. Max dose of lidocaine + adrenaline = 7mg/kg IBW up to 500mg.

2 **Prilocaine** ($t_{\frac{1}{2}}$=2h) Moderate onset. The dose is 3–5mg/kg IBW. 400mg is the maximum dose in adults. Very low toxicity, so it is the drug of choice for Bier's block (IV regional anaesthesia). If <6 months old, then particularly susceptible to methaemoglobinaemia.

3 **Bupivacaine** ($t_{\frac{1}{2}}$=3h) Slow onset and prolonged duration. More cardiotoxic than other local anaesthetics. Contraindicated in IV regional anaesthesia (Bier's block). Dose for local infiltration is 2mg/kg IBW to a max of 150mg.

4 **Levobupivacaine** (isomer of bupivacaine[1]) is less cardiotoxic. Dose for local infiltration or peripheral nerve block: 2mg/kg (max 150mg). Use <150mg (use 5–7.5mg/ml solution) for epidural; <15mg for intrathecal.

5 **Ropivacaine** ($t_{\frac{1}{2}}$=1.8h) Dose: 3mg/kg IBW. Less cardiotoxic than bupivacaine. Less motor block when used epidurally. Contraindicated for IV regional anaesthesia and paracervical block in obstetrics.

6 **Tetracaine** ($t_{\frac{1}{2}}$=1h) Slow onset. High toxicity. *Drops* for topical anaesthesia to eye (the eye must be covered with a patch following use), and now *topically* (AMETOP®) as an alternative to EMLA®. Also available as a gel (combined with adrenaline and lidocaine) which can be used on open wounds

7 **Cocaine:** very high toxicity. Short duration of action. Used in ENT surgery

NB: 0.5% solution=5mg/mL. 1% solution=10mg/mL. So for a 70kg man, the maximum dose of lidocaine is 20mL of 1% or 10mL of 2% solution. NB: systemic absorption is increased from areas of increased vascularity (eg intercostal blocks, scalp wounds); certain commercially available preparations contain *adrenaline* which slows systemic absorption of LA. However, systemic effects from the adrenaline may arise and prove hazardous, especially in CVS disease or ↑BP. *►Adrenaline is contraindicated in digital or penile blocks, and around the nose or ears (due to concerns of causing local ischaemia/necrosis).*

Toxicity From excess dose, too rapid absorption, or direct IV injection. *Features:* Peri-oral tingling; numb tongue; anxiety; lightheadedness; tinnitus; seizures; apnoea; collapse; direct myocardial depression; coma. *Treatment:*[59] ↠Stop injection of LA; ►Call for help; Ensure ABC; Give 100% O_2. *CVS collapse:* Try standard therapies first; then consider lipid emulsion (Intralipid®). This may work by binding to the LA and thus reducing the amount of free LA in the circulation.[60] Initial dose of 1.5ml/kg of 20% Intralipid® over 1 min (can repeat twice more after 5min) plus infusion (15mL/kg/hr;max combined dose of 12ml/kg). If in circulatory arrest manage with standard ALS protocols plus Intralipid®. Recovery from LA-induced cardiac arrest may take >1h. *Seizures:* Benzodiazepines/propofol/thiopental in small incremental doses.

Anaphylaxis Occurs more commonly with the esters (eg tetracaine/cocaine), but can occur with the amides (1–5 in above list) (↠p237 and OHCM p806).

---

1 Racemic mixtures contain D & L isomers; the D isomer may cause cardiac problems.[61] NB: stereo-isomerism describes molecules having the same formula but there are 2 possible mirror-image structures (enantiomers). R (rectus)/D (dexter) enantiomers rotate light to the right; S (sinister)/L (levo) enantiomers to the left.

▶*Explain the procedure, as co-operation helps. Get informed consent* (OHCM p554).

Infiltration Use a small gauge needle. **Lidocaine** 1% is the most common agent. Frequent aspiration is important. Remember that after initial injection, subsequent injections through infiltrated areas hurt less. Likewise, infiltration through the cut edges of a laceration is less painful than through the skin. **Levobupivacaine** 0.25% can be infiltrated around and into the operative wound prior to waking from GA.

Topical Tetracaine to eye. **Lidocaine** 4% spray to cords prior to intubation (nil by mouth for 4h afterwards avoids aspiration).

Nerve blocks Lidocaine 1%, prilocaine 1% (3% or 4% is available for dental use), or **levobupivacaine** 0.25%. Nerve stimulation increases success rate. Accurate placement (eg aided by ultrasound-guided nerve location) of an appropriate concentration of agent is the most effective method of inducing anaesthesia.

A practical example *Femoral nerve block:* Direct injection or catheter placement into the femoral sheath.
1 Mark out the inguinal ligament (pubic tubercle to the anterior superior iliac spine). Palpate, and mark, the femoral artery.
2 Insert short-bevel needle (insulated if nerve stimulator is used) 1cm lateral to the artery, just below the ligament. A 'click' is felt on traversing the skin, and again on traversing the fascia lata. Find the position either by eliciting paraesthesia or with a nerve stimulator.
3 Aspiration test, then inject eg 0.25% **levobupivacaine** 20–30mL.

Specific peripheral blocks and their uses	
Block type	**Examples of use**
Bier's block (p744)	Hand/forearm manipulation or surgery
Cervical plexus	Carotid endarterectomy[62]
Interscalene (brachial plexus)	Shoulder surgery (good prolonged post-op pain relief)
Axillary block	Hand/forearm surgery
Lumbosacral plexus (psoas compartment block)	Hip surgery (combined with a sciatic nerve block)
Ilioinguinal–iliohypogastric nerve	Inguinal hernia repair
Femoral nerve (see above)	Femoral fracture, knee surgery (when combined with a sciatic block)
Sciatic nerve	Surgery below the knee
Popliteal & saphenous nerves	Ankle or foot surgery

▶Ensure that the anaesthetized area is positioned and protected sufficiently both intra- and post-operatively to avoid injury.

▶Complications from nerve blocks include:
- Nerve damage
- Overdose
- Inadvertent IV injection
- Damage to adjacent structures
- Haemorrhage
- Infection
- Incorrect nerve block (eg accidental phrenic nerve block with brachial plexus block)
- Skin injury (from accidental pressure/heat).

Anaesthesia

▶*Explain the procedure: co-operation helps. Get informed consent (OHCM p570).*

▶*If unfamiliar or learning, these techniques are only to be practised under the direct supervision of an anaesthetist.*

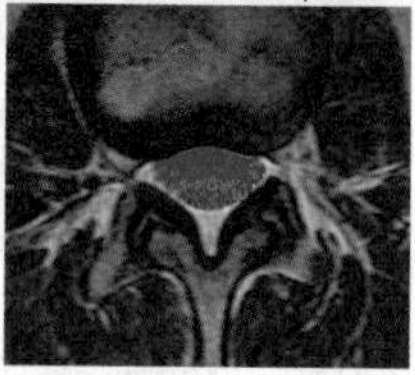

Spinal anaesthesia Anaesthetic into the *subarachnoid space*. The aim is to anaesthetize the spinal nerve roots passing through here.

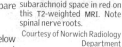

- Insert IV cannula and start IV crystalloid—eg 500mL.
- Check BP; position patient—sitting or left lateral
- Surgical scrub; mask, gown & gloves. Prepare back.

Fig 1. Approximation of the subarachnoid space in red on this T2-weighted MRI. Note spinal nerve roots.
Courtesy of Norwich Radiology Department

- Infiltrate skin with 1-2mL 1% lidocaine.
- Insert a 25G spinal needle at L3/4 space (ie below spinal cord). Free flow of CSF confirms correct placement. Rotate the needle through 180° to ensure that all the needle aperture is in (avoids patchy blocks).
- Inject 1-3mL 0.5% Marcain Heavy® (bupivacaine + dextrose, a hyperbaric solution that falls by gravity). NB: much less LA is needed in pregnancy. Consider adding a small amount of opioid to prolong the analgesic effect.
- Achieving a low, high, or unilateral block is only possible if the patient is left in position for a protracted period prior to surgery (usually unrealistic).
- Monitor BP—may ↓; if so, give crystalloid ± vasopressors (eg **ephedrine** 3–6mg IV repeated as needed (p632), or **phenylephrine** 50–100μg).

A small total drug concentration is required—producing sympathetic blockade (vasodilation, ↓BP), sensory blockade (numbness) and finally motor blockade (↓ or absence of lower limb power).

Complications of spinal anaesthesia: • Total spinal block (↓BP, ↓HR, anxiety, apnoea, LOC)—see below • Headache—see below • Urinary retention • Permanent neurological damage (very rare).

Extradural (epidural) anaesthesia[63]

This is anaesthetic into the **extradural space**. Insertion of indwelling catheter allows prolonged instillation of LA and/or opiates. Larger volumes of LA are required than with spinal anaesthesia. Opioids enhance sensory and not motor block. Lumbar most common site, but cervical/thoracic possible (needs great skill).

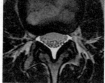

- Use aseptic technique, with patient sitting, or in the left lateral position.
- Check BP. Start IV crystalloid—eg 500mL.

Fig 2. Approximation of the extradural space in yellow on this T2-weighted MRI.
Courtesy of Norwich Radiology Department

- L3/4 commonest site. Infiltrate 1–2mL 0.5% lidocaine.
- Insert 16G Touhy needle until held firm in ligamentum flavum (~2–3cm)
- 'Loss of resistance' technique finds epidural space: 10mL 0.9% saline via Touhy needle is difficult to inject while in ligaments, but once in the epidural space, sudden loss of resistance enables easy injection.
- Fine-bore epidural catheter threaded, needle withdrawn, and catheter placed to needle depth plus 3–5cm. Check you can't aspirate fluid from catheter.
- Administer 2mL test dose of anaesthetic and wait 3min. If there has been inadvertent intrathecal placement this will result in spinal anaesthesia.
- Inject needed dose, eg 10mL 0.25% plain bupivacaine in 5mL aliquots.
- Secure catheter in place.
- Monitor BP every 5min for 15min (slower onset than spinal; therefore hypotension takes longer to be revealed).

Complications of epidural anaesthesia *Dural puncture:* <1%. CSF leak may not be obvious; hence the importance of test dose. Push oral fluids, with caffeine. Nurse flat. Give analgesics for headache, laxatives to prevent constipation/straining. Blood patch is usually necessary if headache lasts >24–48h. Inform a consultant. *Vessel puncture and inadvertent injection:* Treat with ABC remembering: O_2, IVI, pressor drugs, atropine if bradycardia (due to block of sympathetic outflow to heart T2–4). *Hypoventilation:* Motor block of intercostals; may need control of ventilation. *'Total spinal'*—ie injection of a large epidural dose into the CSF. Marked hypotension. Apnoea. Loss of consciousness. Treatment: ABC resuscitation and 100% O_2. Treat ↓BP. ➤➤*Death will occur from asphyxia if treatment is not prompt. Epidural haematoma or abscess:* Aim for early diagnosis to prevent permanent CNS damage. ➤➤Get emergency neurological review and MRI.[64] *Other:* Patchy or unilateral block. Nerve root damage.

Benefits of epidural anaesthesia In obstetric practice (p66) there is no excess risk of caesarean section,[65] though superior outcome with regional anaesthesia compared with GA has not been confirmed.[66] Epidural local anaesthetics cause less GI paralysis compared with systemic or epidural opioids, with comparable pain relief.[67] Epidurals may also ↓post-op risk of respiratory failure.[63]

Caudal (sacral epidural) Left lateral; prone or semi-prone positions; aseptic technique. Palpate sacral hiatus (4–5cm above coccyx tip). This is often not easy. Another method is to palpate the posterior superior iliac spines: the line joining them forms the base of an equilateral triangle with the sacral hiatus at the apex. Insert 21G block needle perpendicular to skin through the sacrococcygeal membrane into the sacral canal. A 23G needle may be useful for infants. Aspirate, and inject up to 20mL 0.5% bupivacaine in the adult. If injecting is difficult (there should be no resistance), or swelling occurs, the needle is in the wrong place—so **stop**! Withdraw the needle and start again. *Indications* Provides anaesthesia for the sacral region—commonly used in children. Useful, eg in scrotal surgery, low cavity forceps (needs experience because of risk of injecting into baby's head), hernias or haemorrhoids.

GA or LA? Abdominal, pelvic and lower limb surgery are ideal for regional neuraxial techniques (eg hernia repair, THR). However, in day-case surgery neuraxial techniques may be associated with a prolonged stay.[68] For some operations, outcome may be better with neuraxial techniques—one study found marginal benefits of fewer deaths and DVTs in hip fracture surgery.[MET][69] Remember that they can also be used as an adjunct to GA, reducing the stress response and postoperative pain.[70]

Absolute contraindications to **all** *neuraxial anaesthesia:*
1 Anticoagulant states (risk pressure damage to cord from bleed—there is an extensive local vertebral venous plexus).
2 Local sepsis (risk of introducing infection to CSF).
3 Shock or hypovolaemic states (effective reduction in circulating volume due to vasodilatation).
4 Raised intracranial pressure (➔coning).
5 Unwilling or uncooperative patient.
6 Fixed output states (eg mitral and aortic stenosis).

Relative contraindications to **all** *neuraxial anaesthesia:*
• Neurological disease—procedure may be blamed for change in state.
• Ischaemic heart disease.
• Spinal deformity or previous surgery.
• Bowel perforation (theoretical risk of ↑parasympathetic activity, peristalsis and peritoneal soiling).

♱ John Keats, the best known medical student to die of unrequited love, showed that the life of the spirit entails the capacity to feel pain, but, as usual, Nature has been over-generous in endowing us with this capacity—so making the treatment of pain paramount: analgesia promotes wellbeing, sleep, and the honeyed indolence preceding recovery or the easeful passage into oblivion. We tend to think simplistically about

That some stream of lightning
From the old man in the skies
Can burn out that suffering
No right-taught man denies.
But a coarse old man am I,
I choose the second best,
I forget it all awhile
Upon a woman's breast. WB Yeats
Daybreak and a candle-end

pain, assuming that when pain is submitted to us we must respond with something analgesic or anaesthetic—but there are other approaches...see quote.

Remember also that pain relief aids physiotherapy (allowing coughing and mobility), preventing pneumonia. Pain also exacerbates hypo/hyperventilation, hypertension, and tachycardia, and can lead to urinary retention.

Methods of analgesia (See *OHCM* p576 and *OHCM* p534)[1]

1 *Oral:* Try paracetamol: 1g/6h—then:
- *NSAIDs:* Diclofenac 50mg/8h (remember danger of GI bleed; cover with ranitidine or misoprostol; caution in asthma). Effects on renal function are minimal if pre-op U&E is normal[71] but be cautious if hypovolaemic.
- *Tramadol* 50–100mg/4–6h PO/IV. Fewer SEs than morphine, but less potent.
- *Opioids,* eg morphine sulphate solution. NB: most are poorly absorbed from the gut.
- *Neuropathic agents:* eg gabapentin for neuropathic pain associated with chronic regional pain syndrome (CRPS, p739) or diabetic/vascular neuralgia. See *BNF* section 4.8.1.

2 *Sublingual:* Buprenorphine (an uncommonly used synthetic opiate; 'controlled' drug): 0.4mg/6h sublingually, or buccal fentanyl drops/lozenges.

3 *Inhalational:* Nitrous oxide/oxygen (Entonox®), useful for labour pains, changing dressings, and physiotherapy.

4 *Intramuscular:* Rarely used—eg morphine 10mg IM; Pethidine 100mg IM

5 *Subcutaneous:* Used in palliative care e.g diamorphine

6 *Intravenous:* Boluses or continuous infusion. Patient-controlled analgesia (PCA). The patient can give himself boluses, avoiding the risks of continuous infusion. Remember to program maximum dose limit.

7 *Regional anaesthesia (RA):* p634. Epidurals (opiates, or LA, boluses or continuous infusion). Many techniques used (intercostal nerve, brachial plexus, femoral nerve blocks).

8 *Transcutaneous fentanyl patches.*

9 *Transcutaneous electrical nerve stimulation:* (TENS).

Chronic pain No single treatment will be effective for every patient. Treatment may be broadly categorized into three categories—pharmacological, physical and psychological. The British Pain Society recommends individualized pain management programmes based on the principles of cognitive behavioural therapy for those with chronic pain which cannot be remedied with drug and physical treatments alone. These consist of education on pain physiology, psychology and self management of pain problems.[72] Pharmacological treatments include simple analgesia, opioids tricyclic antidepressants, neuropathic pain medicines (e.g gabapentin) and epidurals for low back pain. Interventions which may help certain patients include acupuncture and hypnosis.

Pain in children See p719 for narcotic and other analgesia in painful conditions such as sickle-cell disease. For post-op relief, see p172.

Anaesthesia

Deming's definition: Quality is meeting customer requirements at a price they are willing to pay. On this view, anaesthesia has various 'customers' rating its quality: surgeons, hospitals, tax-payers, and patients, and these groups may have conflicting requirements.[73]

The most important customer is the patient, and their chief requirement is pain relief—but don't focus on this narrowly. Patients are also very keen to have a friendly anaesthetist explaining what to expect. This is the chief area of disparity between what anaesthetists think patients should want and what they actually want. The best approach to anaesthesia does not regard these tasks as separate: they are complementary.[1]

EBM in anaesthesia: possible limitations

In anaesthesia research, surrogate or intermediate outcomes predominate as the end-points, which is a weakness when the results serve as the evidence on which to base clinical decisions. More importantly, in interventions requiring skill, dexterity, and dynamic decision-making, do not assume that equally good outcomes are achievable by all, by the simple application of the results of EBM.[74] That said, section 1 of *Bandolier's Little Book of Pain*[75] [2] offers valuable insight on the approach to the evidence base for the treatment of pain.

Patient-centred anaesthesia   ☺

Anaesthetists must form brief but intimate relationship with their patients, often under difficult circumstances. As well as doing a good technical job, they need to be aware of subjective areas that are of particular importance to patients. These are centred around physical comfort and respect. In one study, ratings for information provision, involvement, and emotional support were rated significantly less important than physical comfort and respect. Ratings did not differ very much *vis à vis* inpatient *vs* day surgery, surgical service, type of anaesthetic, or anaesthetist.[76] Comfort may centre around needleless induction of anaesthesia and good peri-operative care in non-frightening surroundings.[77] Also, avoiding nausea/vomiting (p617) are top priorities.[78] NB: information booklets can improve satisfaction.[79]

Patient-centred anaesthesia cannot flourish in a vacuum: if the whole context of care is patient-centred the need for anaesthetic care itself may be less. For example, in obstetrics where there is a one-to-one relationship between the midwife and the mother, the need for epidurals is ~50% less (and the 2nd stage of labour is shorter) than when less personal methods are used.[80]

One way to improve patient-centred anaesthesia is to control distractions in the anaesthetic work place: time and motion studies show that it is relatively easy for anaesthetists to be distracted by extraneous interruptions.[81] Exactly how to limit this in busy NHS practice is a challenge.

Patients can be confused by an uncertain locus of responsibility. In some cultures (eg in Japan) chief responsibility for peri-operative care lies with the surgeon. In other cultures, responsibility is shared—with confusing results unless the surgeon and the anaesthetist co-operate closely.[82]

1 See the Bandolier website for the 2007 Oxford league table of analgesia efficiency, which outlines the NNT for different analgesics in acute pain.[83]
2 The authors would like to thank Mr Christopher Constant for bringing this resource to their attention.

Anaesthesia

See also *OHCM* p708–731.

To have *any* disease is unfortunate, but to have a rare disease is doubly so: the patient must often wait for ages for a diagnosis, and then he must contend with his physician's lifelong morbid interest in him. Having a rare disease is common! (~30 million in Europe): 5000 diseases have prevalences of <1:2000.[1] See rare.diseases.org & geneticalliance.org for assistance with rare diseases.

Alport's syndrome x-linked or auto-somal recessive sensorineural deafness, pyelonephritis, haematuria, and renal failure (glomerulonephritis+ basket weaving of GBM). x-linked forms are caused by mutations in COL4A5 genes that encode the α5-chain of type-IV collagen. *R:* No effective treatment is available, but they may do well on dialysis or after kidney transplant. Bone marrow transplant might be an option in future. Typical age at death (♂): 20–30yrs.[2,3]

Asperger's syndrome Autistic features (p394) *without* autistic aloneness or linguistic difficulty. It is less severe than autism.[4] It is possible to teach better recognition of emotions and how to predict emotional responses.[5]

Bardet–Biedl syndrome Autosomal recessive A key cause of chronic renal failure in children.[6] *Signs:* Renal calyceal clubbing/blunting, calyceal cysts ± fetal lobulation; retinal dystrophy; IQ↓; hypogonadism; obesity; anosmia; polydactyly. Lack of paraparesis distinguishes it from Laurence–Moon–Biedl synd., p648. ♂:♀≈1.3:1.[7]

Batten's syndrome (juvenile neuronal ceroid lipofuscinoses)[8] Apoptosis of photoreceptors & neurons from defects in the CLN3 gene causes vision↓, childhood dementia, fits, ataxia, spasticity, athetosis, dystonia, and early death (in teens). *Tests:* Skin biopsy;[8] lipopigments in lymphocytes and urine.[9]

Becker's muscular dystrophy x-linked recessive There are mutations in the dystrophin gene (xp21), but unlike Duchenne (p642) (where there is near-total loss of dystrophin) there is 'semifunctional' dystrophin, and milder symptoms and later onset, slower progression but more calf enlargement in adolescence. *R:* Symptomatic. Steroids may help (monitor creatine kinase).[10] Genetic counselling[11,12] (p154).

Beckwith–Wiedemann syndrome is the chief cause of macroglossia;[13] other signs: macrosomia, visceromegaly, omphalocoele, hemihypertrophy, microcephaly, hypoglycaemia, feeding difficulty. Overexpression of IGF2 gene at locus 11p15 causes embryonal tumours (esp. Wilms, p133) in ~8%.[14]

Bourneville's disease (tuberous sclerosis; epiloia=EPIlepsy, LOW Intelligence + Adenoma sebaceum, see fig 1) Autosomal dominant (AD) multi-organ calcified hamartomatous tubers. Loci on 9q34 (TSC1, making *harmatin*) & 16p13 (TSC2 makes *tuberin*; mutations here are worst). *Prognosis:* often benign.

Diagnosis: Try to get 2 major features (*), or 1 major and 2 minor.[15]
- *Eye/CNS:* Fits (at presentation in 90%),[16] autism,[17] subependymal astrocytoma*, hydrocephalus, periventricular calcification, ↓IQ, phacomata (white or yellow retinal tumours in ~50%), retinal nodules* & achromatic patches.
- *Skin and hair:* Hypomelanic macules ('ashleaf' macules, which are Wood's lamp +ve)*, adenoma sebaceum (warty nasolabial angiofibromas*; fig 1), *café-au-lait* spots, butterfly rash, periungual fibromas* (fig 2), skin tags, sacral plaques (shagreen patches, like shark skin), white lock.
- *Mouth and teeth:* Pitted tooth enamel, gingival fibromas.
- *Bone:* Sclerotic lesions, phalangeal cysts, hypertelorism.
- *Kidney:* Angiomyolipomas*, multiple cysts, haematuria.
- *Lungs:* Honeycomb lung, pneumothorax, 'muscular hyperplasia of lung'.
- *Heart:* Rhabdomyomas*, BP↑, cardiomyopathy, haemopericardium.
- *Lymph nodes:* Lymphangiomyomatosis*, Castleman tumour.
- *Bowel:* Polyps ± Peutz–Jeghers, *OHCM* p700.
- *Liver and peritoneum:* Carney's complex (p699). *Also:* Precocious puberty.

The hidden faces of Jack, some gunpowder—and a spark

We are surrounded by eponyms commemorating the Great and the Good, from the Reith Lectures and the Booker Prize, to the 100° proof of Jack Daniels and Johnnie Walker. Medical eponyms are pickled in something almost as intoxicating: the hidden recesses of our own minds. We store away the bizarre, the fearsome, and the mundane—and then, years later, as if playing some dreadful game of snap, we match these features with the person sitting in front of us, and say: "Dandy–Walker!" or "Prader–Willi!" Here we deal a pack and a half (84 cards) to play with, plus a few jokers, and fascinating and frightening games they can be. But as the years go by we wonder more and more about the people behind the eponyms. We read about these quacks and geniuses—but it is always rather unsatisfying: history shows us everything except the one thing we want to see: the spark that made these eponymous characters truly original. We resign ourselves to the fact that we can only ever see one face of the jack. More years pass and inexplicable events teach us that we all have hidden faces we never directly see or know (p325). *So the possibility arises that these hidden faces are regarding each other.* That is the sensation we have on conjuring with the names of Dandy and Walker and the rest: a sensation that we are not alone—that we are *accompanied*.

Whether we are connoisseurs of Johnnie Walker or Dandy–Walker and its diagnosis, we are relying on hidden processes going on in the dark over many years, to give us the spirit that burns with a steady flame when we are mixed with gunpowder—and that spark. This 'steady flame' is the old definition of alcoholic proof above 100°.[1] It is also our reward for having transformed raw knowledge into something illuminating, by the hidden processes of fermentation and distillation.

This special learning sometimes goes to our heads, and, drunk on knowledge, we career up and down the wards causing havoc until we learn to apply judgment as well as knowledge (as Benjamin Disraeli observed: in order to be successful as a the Queen's First Minister, it is unpardonable to have a good memory: it is vital to be able to forget).

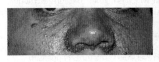

Fig 1. Adenoma sebaceum.

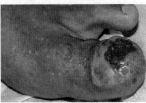

Fig 2. Periungual fibroma.
Both figures courtesy of Dr Samuel da Silva.

1 Spirits were once graded by the ***gunpowder test:*** a mixture of water and alcohol 'proved' itself if one could pour it on gunpowder and a spark could induce it to burn with a steady flame. If it did not, the liquor was too weak. A 'proven' liquor was defined as 100 degrees proof (100°).[18]

Unusual eponymous syndromes

Who cares about history? Medical history is worse than bunk: it's an unaffordable distraction.

Briquet's syndrome (fat-folder syndrome) Hypochondria (p334) with somatization with >13 medically unexplained symptoms in various organs (see BOX).

Bruton sex-linked♂ agammaglobulinaemia See p199.

Buchanan's syndrome (truncus arteriosus) A single artery arises out of the base of the heart, supplying pulmonary *and* systemic vasculature. The aorta may be divided. There is cyanosis from birth. Surgical correction is possible.

Capgras syndrome (clonal pluralization of the self)[19] A 'delusion of doubles' that oneself or a friend has been replaced by an exact clone, who is an impostor. *Cause:* Psychosis; head injury; B₁₂↓; pituitary or right occipitotemporal lesion; multiple sclerosis.[20] Quetiapine may help. *Myself am ever mine own counterfeit* [21] Michelangelo; Sonnet XLI

Castleman's disease Angiofollicular lymph node hyperplasia + benign vascular mediastinal tumour. *2 types:* Hyaline vascular and plasma cell type (T°↑), anaemia, weight↓). Frank lymphoma is rare. POEMS syndrome may be present (BOX).[22]

Chediak–Higashi syndrome Immunodeficiency, hypopigmentation, photophobia, nystagmus, weakness, tremor, fever, platelets↓, liver↑, ± lymphoma. WBCs contain big peroxidase granules. *Cause:* 1q43 mutation (CHS1/LYST gene).[23] Fatal in 90% by 10yrs of age without marrow transplantation.[24]

Conradi–Hünermann syndrome (chondrodysplasia punctata) Saddle nose, nasal hypoplasia, frontal bossing, short stature, stippled epiphyses, optic atrophy, cataracts, IQ↓, flexural contractures. *Cause:* Genetic or effects of warfarin given during the 1st trimester of pregnancy.[25]

Cornelia de Lange syndrome Autosomal dominant mutation in NIPBL gene on 5p13 causes short stature + abnormal head shape (brows meet in midline) ± hirsutism, low-set ears, wide-spaced teeth, single palmar crease, IQ↓, fits, self-harm, abnormal temporal lobes, recurrent otitis media.[26] Sporadic in 99%.[27]

Corrigan's syndrome This is congenital aortic regurgitation.

Cotard's syndrome (nihilistic delusions) We deny our existence, or believe we are rotting, or we demand burial, thinking we are a corpse. *Nihil* is Latin for nothing; a good nihilist will *annihilate* all trace of himself, *leaving only such trace upon earth as smoke leaves in air, or foam in water.* Dante Alighieri Inferno XXIV 50
Cause: Depression, alcohol, syphilis, parietal lobe lesion, or just being born, "for there is in everyone a deep instinct which is neither that for destruction, nor for creation. It is simply the longing to resemble nothing." Albert Camus

Crigler–Najjar syndrome ↓Gluconyl transferase activity causes nonhaemolytic unconjugated hyperbilirubinaemia (jaundice ± CNS signs) in the 1st days of life. Autosomal dominant form is mild but autosomal recessive form is severe and may need liver transplant before irreversible kernicterus happens.[28]

Dandy–Walker syndrome Congenital obstruction of the foramina of Luschka and Magendi leads to progressive enlargement of the head, congested scalp veins, bulging fontanelle, separation of the cranial sutures, papilloedema, bradycardia (fig 1). R: Drain the CSF into a body cavity.

De Clerambault's syndrome (erotomania) The patient is persistently deluded that a celebrity, a politician, or someone of a higher social status is in love with her.[29] She derives satisfaction from having been 'chosen', and may make trouble by publicizing her view of his feelings. ►*Always have a chaperone!* Homoerotomania may be complicated by Fregoli delusions (eg the love object of a teenage boy was a neighbour believed by him to be his father). Stalking is one manifestation. *Also:* IQ↓; schizophrenia; mania; left frontal lobe lesion.[30]

Diamond–Blackfan syndrome (erythrogenesis imperfecta) ↓Erythroid production (Hb↓, platelets↑, MCV↑) causes pallor ± limb anomalies. *Cause:* 25% due to mutations in RPS19 gene on 19q13.[31,32] R: Steroids ± marrow transplant are tried—or stem-cell transplant from a donor embryo created by IVF (preimplantation genetic diagnosis confirms HLA matching).[33] See BOX 4.

Helping people with Briquet's syndrome (see p334)

- Give time—don't dismiss these patients as just the 'worried well'.[34]
- Explore with the patient the factors perpetuating the illness (disordered physiology, misinformation, unfounded fears, misinterpretation of sensations, unhelpful 'coping' behaviour, social stressors).
- Agree a management plan which focuses on each issue and makes sense to the patient's holistic view of him or herself.
- Treat any depression (p340, eg **escitalopram**[35]); consider cognitive therapy; make the patient feel understood; broaden the agenda, negotiating a new understanding of symptoms including psychosocial factors.[36]

Cloning our wives

In idle moments, we might think that it would be useful to clone our wives. This is what men with Capgras syndrome have accomplished. But could we really cope with this? Men with Capgras syndrome get very destabilized by not knowing who they are talking to—the genuine or the fake wife.[37] It is an example of a delusion called the 'clonal pluralization of identities'.[38] As such, it is the best example we have of a purely metaphysical disease. When a man with Capgras syndrome asks his wife with all solicitude: "*How are we today?*"—he means *every word* he utters. And he never knows the answer.

Castleman's lymph node hyperplasia with POEMS syndrome

POEMS syndrome entails: peripheral neuropathy, organomegaly/hyperplasia, endocrinopathy, a monoclonal paraprotein, and skin lesions. Interleukin-6 excess is also a feature. Children with unexplained chronic inflammatory symptoms ± PUO ± failure to thrive may need detailed soft tissue tests to reveal associated vascular tumours.

Creating donor embryos to donate stem cells: good idea?

Bishops, authors, bigots and philosophers like to sound off about the morals of creating embryo brothers and sisters for the purpose of providing spare parts—in this case, an umbilical cord for harvesting stem cells—eg to populate the failing marrow of a 6-year-old with Diamond–Blackfan syndrome. To create a new human in this way is thought to be using people as means, not ends. Proponents of this argument ignore the need to state what *would* be a 'good enough' reason to create an embryo. Behind the oft-used expression 'a much hoped-for baby' lies a raft of reasons most parents would rather not look at in too much detail: the hope is often unconsciously selfish (who will look after me in my old age?). Yet when parents have a very specific and altruistic motive—they are questioned remorselessly. What patient-centred ethics teaches is that special circumstances require special sensitivity. Anyone witnessing parents taking these sorts of decisions will be well aware that concepts such as 'designer babies' are unhelpful (and in any case guarded against by the Human Fertilisation and Embryology Authority, p293).

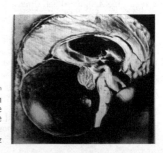

Fig 1. Dandy-Walker dilatation of the 4th ventricle. The large cyst is actually an enlarged 4th ventricle and not separate from it. The 3rd and lateral ventricles are much enlarged, secondarily.

Courtesy of Professor Ralph Józefowicz

DiGeorge's syndrome A deletion of chromosome 22q11.2 causes absent thymus, fits, small parathyroids (∴Ca²⁺↓), anaemia, lymphopenia, growth hormone↓, ↓T-cell-immunity. It is related to velo-cardio-facial syndrome: characteristic face, multiple anomalies, eg cleft palate, heart defects, cognitive defects. [39,40]

Di Guglielmo's disease (erythromyelosis) Dysplastic RBCs infiltrate liver, spleen & heart. Hb↓; MCV↔; WCC↓, platelets↓; LDH↑; B₁₂↑. Immunoperoxidase stain shows antihaemoglobin antibody. Steroids, splenectomy±transfusions may be tried. [41]

Duchenne's muscular dystrophy [X-linked recessive] Mutations in dystrophin gene (xp21) result in near-total loss of dystrophin (so muscles get replaced by fibroadipose tissue and ↑cytotoxic c cells). Presents in boys of 1–6yrs, with a waddling, clumsy gait. No abnormality is noted at birth. Gower's manoeuvre: on standing, he uses his hands to climb up his legs. Distal girdle muscles are affected late; selective wasting causes calf pseudohypertrophy. Wheelchairs are needed at 9–12yrs. *Prevalence:* 1:3500 births. *Creatine kinase* is ↑; ►measure in all boys not walking by 1½yrs, so that genetic advice may be given. Scoliosis and many chest infections occur. *Muscle biopsy:* Abnormal fibres surrounded by fat and fibrous tissue. *R:* Aim to maintain walking (eg using knee–ankle–foot orthoses). Gene therapy may be an option. [42] **Prednisolone ± creatine** supplements can help, but don't allow wheelchair abandoning. [43] A disease-modifying agent (AVI-4658) is under development. [44] *Prognosis:* Vital capacity <700mL is a bad sign. Ventilation improves longevity (median age at death is now 31yrs). [45] *Carrier ♀:* 80% of have abnormal chemistry. *Prenatal screening* is available.

Ebstein's anomaly A congenital defect with downward displacement of the tricuspid valve (±deformed leaflets) atrializing the right ventricle causing right-sided heart failure. There may be no symptoms, or cyanosis, clubbing, triple rhythm, systolic, and diastolic murmurs. It can be associated with other cardiac malformations. *Tests:* ECG: tall P waves, ↑P–R interval; right bundle branch block. *Survival:* ~67% at 1 year and ~59% at 10 years. [46,47]

Edwards syndrome During meiosis chromosomes undergo condensation, pairing, crossing-over, and disjunction. Stringent regulation of the distribution and quantity of meiotic crossovers is critical for proper chromosome segregation. Failure to faithfully segregate meiotic chromosomes often results in severe genetic disorders, eg Edwards syndrome/trisomy 18 (fig 3), [48] our 2ⁿᵈ commonest trisomy (Down's is 1ˢᵗ p152). ♀:♂ ≈ 2:1 (girls live longer; mean ≈10 months). [49]

Ehlers-Danlos syndrome [Autosomal dominant] is a collagen disease (figs 1 & 2) with hyperelasticity. *6 types:* Type II, for example, is caused by COL52A mutations; in type IV COL381 mutations upset encoding of type III collagen. *Δ:* Urine pyridinolines.

Eisenmenger's syndrome A congenital heart defect which is at first associated with a left-to-right shunt may lead to pulmonary hypertension and hence shunt reversal. If so, cyanosis develops (± heart failure and chest infections), and Eisenmenger's syndrome is said to exist. Monitor S_AO₂, PCV & BMI. [50,51]

Erb's scapulohumeral dystrophy ♀:♂ ≈ 1:1. *Onset:* 10–60yrs. *Early sign:* cannot raise hands above head, then (in order): deltoid→erector spinae→trunk muscles→pelvic girdle→thigh. Often mild & asymmetric; lifespan is shortened.

Fallot's tetrad (OHCM p151 fig 1) Pulmonary stenosis, overriding aorta, interventricular defect, and RVH. It is the commonest cyanotic congenital heart disorder (10%; 3–6/10,000). *Signs:* Cyanosis as ductus closes, dyspnoea, faints, squatting at play (this ↑peripheral vascular resistance, so reduces right-to-left shunt), clubbing, thrills, absent pulmonary part of S₂, harsh systolic murmur at left sternal base. *Tests:* Hb↑. CXR: wooden shoe heart contour + RVH. ECG: RVH. Echo shows anatomy & degree of stenosis. Cardiac CT/MRI helps plan surgery. *R:* O₂. Place in knee-chest position. Morphine to sedate and to relax pulmonary outflow. Long-term β-blockers. 'Total repair' entails VSD closure and correcting pulmonary stenosis, eg before 1yr, and may result in normal life, with driving possible if no syncopal attacks. *Prognosis:* Without surgery, mortality rate is ~95% by age 20. 20-yr survival is ~90–95% after repair.

x-linked muscular dystrophies

1. Duchenne's muscular dystrophy (severe)
2. Becker muscular dystrophy (benign)
3. Emery–Dreifuss muscular dystrophy (benign; early contractures)
4. McLeod syndrome (benign with acanthocytes)
5. Scapuloperoneal (rare).

Myotonic dystrophy and other autosomal muscular dystrophies

1. Myotonic dystrophy (autosomal dominant; Steinert disease)
2. Congenital myotonic dystrophy
3. Facioscapulohumeral muscular dystrophy (Landouzy–Dejerine p468)
4. Early childhood autosomal recessive Duchenne-like limb-girdle dystrophy
5. Late-onset (Erb-type) autosomal recessive limb-girdle dystrophy (usually scapulohumeral; rarely pelvifemoral)
6. Autosomal dominant limb-girdle dystrophy
7. Oculopharyngeal muscular dystrophy
8. Distal myopathies
9. Non-progressive myopathies.   homepages.hetnet.nl/~b1beukema/ziekspieren.html

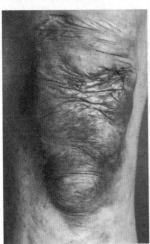

Fig 1. In Ehlers–Danlos syndrome, skin is poor-healing, fragile, and easily bruised or torn, with wide scars as thin as cigarette paper. Look for piezogenic papules (easily compressible outpouchings of fat through defects in the dermis on the sides of the feet). Also: hypotonic, hypermobile joints; flat feet; GI bleeds/perforation; mitral valve prolapse;[52] dissecting aneurysms.[53]

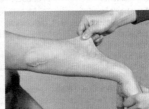

Fig 2. Elastic skin in Ehlers–Danlos (EDS). Bennett's paradox: the woman at a drag ball is the true impostor for, unlike everyone else, she is what she seems. So with EDS, which doesn't behave like a connective tissue disease *because it really is one* (a true disease of collagen). Other 'connective tissue diseases' are really diseases of something else.

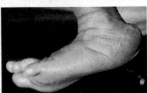

Fig 3. Rockerbottom feet, as seen in Edwards syndrome. Other signs: rigidity with limb flexion, odd low-set ears, receding chin, proptosis, cleft lip/palate ± umbilical/inguinal herniae; short sternum (makes nipples look widely separated). The fingers cannot be extended (index finger overlaps 3rd digit).

Reproduced from eMedicine.com, 2007.
Available at: http://www.emedicine.com/ped/
topic652.htm with permission

Post-op problems: • Residual VSD + pulmonary hypertension, if big • Ventricular tachycardia • Complete heart block • Right ventricular aneurysm • SBE (risk is lowish) • Dilated cardiomyopathy • Pulmonary or aortic regurgitation. NB: when pregnant (may be unproblematic), do careful fetal echo.[54]

Fanconi anaemia x-linked or auto-somal recessive Progressive marrow failure + absence of radii, thumb hypoplasia, syndactyly, missing carpal bones, skin pigmentation, microsomy, microcephaly, strabismus, cryptorchidism, IQ↓, deafness, short stature, and ↑risk of leukaemias and solid tumours. *Survival:* 70% at 5yrs post-marrow transplant (umbilical cord blood stem cells are also tried, p641). There are 12 groups and subtype A is the commonest.[55,56] *R:* Gene therapy is planned.[57]

Galeazzi fracture Radius shaft fracture with dislocation of the distal radio-ulnar joint.

Ganser syndrome Disorientation + pseudodementia + 'approximate answering',[58] eg the answer to "How many legs has the chair in that corner got?" might be: "What corner? I don't know what a corner is. I don't see a chair... five." Absurd remarks only occur as answers to questions. Intellectual deficit is inconstant (hence the 'pseudo'). Hysteria, hallucinations, and fluctuating consciousness are common. *Causes:* Temporoparietal lesion;[59] head injury.[60]

Gaucher's syndrome Autosomal recessive Mutations in glucocerebrosidase gene on chromosome 1q21 cause Gaucher's, the commonest lysosomal storage disease. ⅔ present before the age of 20. Three forms are defined based on the presence of CNS signs. 1 Presents at <5yrs old with splenomegaly.[61] 2 Acute neuropathic form (3–6 months old). 3 Chronic neuropathic form appears like a type 1 with progressive horizontal saccade-initiation failure and developmental delay. Other CNS signs: rigid neck, dysphagia, catatonia, reflexes↑, IQ↓. *Δ:* Measure acid β-glucosidase activity in peripheral WBCs. Death may be from pneumonia or bleeding. *R:* IVI of imiglucerase (specialist use only) helps haematology and organomegaly, but not bone indices, in type 1 & 3.[62] Miglustat is an oral inhibitor of glucosylceramide synthase (for type I). *Prognosis:* Worse if early onset.

Hand–Schüller–Christian syndrome (HSC; Langerhans' cell histiocytosis; histiocytosis x, Letterer-Siwe eosinophilic granuloma of bone) Monoclonal Langerhans-like cells are pathognomonic of this 'neoplastic', destructive, infiltrative disease in which bone, liver, skin, and spleen show lytic foci of eosinophils, plasma cells, and histiocytes. Lesions may show on a ⁹⁹technetium-labelled bone scan. It occurs in children and adults, eg starting with a polyp at the external auditory meatus. Other signs: see MINIBOX. A lethal 'leukaemia' picture is seen in infants. *R:* Bone surgery, steroids, cytotoxics, and radiotherapy may induce remissions.[63,64]

Signs of HSC
• Diabetes insipidus*
• Exophthalmos*
• Lytic bone lesions*
• Failure to thrive; dyspnoea
• Scalp lumps/skin erosions
• Eczema-like rash/pustules
• Cord compression ± fits
• Ear discharge, stomatitis
• Honeycomb lung
• Hepatosplenomegaly
• Lymphadenopathy
• T°↑; anaemia; ↓platelets
*Classic triad; seen in 10%

Hartnup's disease Autosomal recessive Increased ↑GI & urinary loss of neutral amino acids involving a transporter for monoamino-monocarboxylic acids.[65] Look for niacin deficiency: diarrhoea, dementia, and dermatitis (skin is thick, scaly, and hyperpigmented where light-exposed). Also: nystagmus, ataxia, bruxism (teeth grinding), diplopia, reflexes↑. Gene: SLC6A19. *R:* Nicotinamide & B vitamins.[66,67]

Hunter's syndrome (mucopolysaccharidosis II) x-linked recessive (33% are due to a new mutation). Iduronate sulfatase (IDS) deficiency results in deafness, IQ↓, short stature, chronic diarrhoea, unusual face, hepatosplenomegaly (like Hurler's disease, p646 but it is milder and almost always without corneal clouding). Also look for joint contractures including ankylosis of the temporomandibular joint; spinal stenosis; and carpal tunnel syndrome. Death: late childhood (but may be at >30yrs). *Δ:* Definitive diagnosis is made by enzyme analysis for iduronate sulfatase in leucocytes or cultured skin fibroblasts. *Prenatal Δ:* Ultrasound.[68] *R:* Human recombinant idursulfase.[69]

Huntington's chorea ^{Autosomal dominant} A triad of progressive motor, cognitive, and emotional symptoms + spiny neuron loss in the neostriatum, due to excessive repeats of 'CAG' in the huntingtin gene. Normally, there are <28 repeats. Symptoms usually do not appear until adulthood (~30-50yrs). *Penetrance:* A large number of repeats means the disease is more likely. 29-35 CAG repeats means no signs but they may pass Huntington's to their children. 36-39 CAG repeats means ↓penetrance. If >40 CAG repeats, 100% get Huntington's disease if they live long enough. *Early findings:* ↓Auditory & visual reaction times (needs special equipment) then mild chorea (flitting, jerky movements, odd extraocular movements, ↑reflexes, ↓rapid alternating movements. Unpredictable motor impairment is found until chorea starts. Abnormal ocular saccades may indicate imminent manifest signs. *Late signs:* Personality change, self-neglect, apathy, clumsiness, fidgeting, fleeting grimaces (may be mistaken for mannerisms), chorea, and dementia. Ethical dilemmas surround testing, as symptoms may only start after procreation has finished. Careful pre-test counselling is vital.[70]

Hunt's syndrome (pyridoxine cerebral deficiency) Intractable neonatal fits cause death unless given **pyridoxine** (50mg IV under EEG control).

Hurler's syndrome (mucopolysaccharidosis 1h; MPS1h) After briefly normal growth, there is physical and mental decline, hydrocephalus, thick skin, hirsutism, coxa valga, nodules over scapulae, and CCF. Cause: ↓α-L-iduronidase, hence blocking degradation of dermatan sulfate & heparan sulfate and ↑mucopolysaccharides in urine, cartilage, periosteum, tendons, valves, meninges & eye. *Skull x-ray:* Thick bone; absent frontal sinuses; deformed pituitary fossa. *Marrow:* Metachromatic Reilly bodies in lymphocytes. *R̥:* ►Laronidase must start *promptly*[71] ± stem cell transplantation. Death is often at ≤10yrs.

Hutchinson's triad (congenital syphilis) Deafness + keratitis + pointed teeth.

Ivemark's syndrome This is the association of congenital asplenia with ostium primum atrial septal defects (± pulmonary valve atresia or stenosis).

Kartagener's syndrome Primary ciliary dyskinesia (inflexible, poorly beating cilia) is called Kartagener's syndrome if associated with situs inversus (dextrocardia).[73] Clearance of mucus & bacteria is poor, hence chronic sinusitis and bronchiectasis. ♂ infertility, otitis media, and salpingitis are common. *R̥:* Antibiotics, continuous or intermittent, are used to treat airway infections. Children are good candidates for long-term low-dose preventive antibiotics.

Kawasaki disease A vasculitis inflames small to medium arteries causing aneurysms to form. *Cause:* Unknown (? reaction to infection). *Median age:* 10 months.[74] 3 phases: 1 *Acute:* Lasts 1-2wks; the child has T°↑+ major signs (see BOX 1), also diarrhoea ± jaundice. 2 *Subacute:* Lasts ~2wks: ►coronary arteritis—like PAN; ie non-atheromatous coronary artery disease ± *infarction* in ~24% (♂:♀≈5:1; commoner than rheumatic fever as a cause of acquired heart disease).[74] 3 *Convalescent:* Takes ~7wks. *Tests:* ESR & c-reactive protein↑; bilirubin↑, AST↑, α₂-globulin↑, platelets↑. *ΔΔ:* Stevens-Johnson syndrome, measles, streps, infectious mononucleosis. *R̥:* Aspirin (30-50mg/kg/day until fever resolves, then 3-5mg/kg/day). Immunoglobulin 2g/kg as a single IVI dose *usually* causes rapid (diagnostic) improvement.[75] If not, a 2nd dose may help. *Follow-up:* Echo; 3D coronary magnetic resonance angiography accurately defines aneurysms (it is a non-invasive alternative when transthoracic echo quality is insufficient, and angiography is too invasive).[76,77]

Klinefelter's syndrome (XXY or XXYY polysomy + variable Leydig cell defect) The chief genetic cause of ♂ hypogonadism; 1:2000 births manifests in adolescence with psychopathy, ↓cognition, ↓libido, ↓sexual maturation. *Associations:* T₄↓, DM, asthma, ?oncogenesis. Androgens and surgery for gynaecomastia may help. Lifespan is normal, but arm span may exceed the body length by 10cm.

Kugelberg–Welander spinal muscular atrophy ↓Anterior horn cell (BOX 2).

Diagnostic criteria for Kawasaki disease

Fever for ≥5 days + at least 4 of the following:*
1 Bilateral non-purulent conjunctivitis
2 Neck lymphadenopathy (>1.5cm across)
3 Pharyngeal injection, dry fissured lips, strawberry tongue
4 Polymorphous rash (especially on the trunk)
5 Changes in extremities: arthralgia, palmar erythema or later, ►fingertip desquamation + swelling of hands/feet.

*Kawasaki disease may be diagnosed with <4 of these features if coronary artery aneurysms (CAA) are present.

►Incomplete forms exist, so get expert help *today* while wresting with this difficult, important diagnosis.[78] IVIG given ≥10 days after illness onset resolves inflammation but can be too late to prevent coronary artery lesions.[79]

There is paradoxical data that incomplete or atypical forms are *more* likely to have complications such as CAA: the reason is that Kawasaki thought his disease was always benign and self-limiting, so over-optimism may be built into the definition of the syndrome.[80]

Kugelberg–Welander spinal muscular atrophy (type 3 SMA) Autosomal recessive

SMA entails loss of anterior horn cells and all the dignity they engender. Starting after 18 months old, there is lack of mobility, then wheelchair dependence—and often need for help with toileting and, in its later stages, with ventilation. But as symptoms start during the most adaptive years, people with this syndrome often don't think they are ill, and are resentful when we decide for them when symptoms are pronounced that they should not be resuscitated. Here are two contrasting views from patients with SMA.

Life is a millstone...Let me die now	Message from a militant dynamo...
"Let me die at the moment of my choosing, with dignity". In some jurisdictions (eg Montana, USA) assisted suicide is justified in terminal conditions. Note that *terminal* doesn't imply *now in its end-stage*: it is 'an incurable and irreversible condition, for the end stage of which there is no known treatment which will alter its course to death, and which...will result in a premature death.'	"My first big demo...I took hundreds of [us] wheelchair users onto Westminster Bridge and stopped the traffic...*Not dead yet!* placards round our necks...*rights not charity!* To my partner: "If I should ever seek death—there are several times when my [progressive spinal muscular atrophy] challenges me—I want to guarantee that you are there supporting my continued life and its value. The last thing I want is for you to give up on me, especially when I need you most."
Is physician (or carer) assisted suicide for those with SMA valid? Some with SMA want this—but not Jane Campbell (see OPPOSITE), SMA's most vocal victim/non-victim.	And for those with no partner? "It's our role as a caring society to be that someone..."[81] Jane Campbell House of Lords 2009

Klippel-Feil syndrome ^{Autosomal recessive or dominant} Congenital fusion of cervical vertebrae, nystagmus, deafness and CNS signs. The clinical triad seen in 50% is: short neck, low posterior hairline, and limited neck movement. *Mirror movements* are said to occur if *voluntary* movements in one limb are *involuntarily* mimicked by the other. Possible cause: KFS gene on chromosome 8.

Landouzy-Dejerine (fascioscapulohumeral) muscular dystrophy ^{Autosomal dominant} Deletion on 4q35 results in weakness of the shoulder muscles, eg on combing the hair, appears at 12-14yrs of age. There is difficulty in closing the eyes, sucking, blowing, and whistling. Scapulae wing and the lips pout, and the facial expression is 'ironed out'. Adult myoglobin is reduced and fetal myoglobin and sarcolemma nuclei are increased.[82,83] Surgical scapulopexy may help.[84]

Laurence-Moon syndrome ^{Autosomal recessive} Retinitis pigmentosa, obesity, polydactyly, hypogenitalism, ↓IQ, ↓body hair, azoospermia, CNS[85] and renal abnormalities (calyceal clubbing, cysts, or diverticula; fetal lobulation; end-stage renal failure in 15%). It is distinct from Bardet–Biedl syndrome p638 (no polydactyly).

Leber's hereditary optic atrophy is the commonest mitochondrial DNA disorder and causes irreversible blindness/scotomas in young adults, and ↑risk of neoplasia. A mutation (G→A) in mitochondrial DNA coding for a dehydrogenase enzyme is proposed (a type of cytoplasmic inheritance). Idebenone may help.[86]

Lesch–Nyhan syndrome x-linked (only fully expressed if ♂) deficiency of hypoxanthine-guanine phosphoribosyl transferase (HPRT) causes 3 problems: *Uric acid overproduction:* Hyperuricaemia (orange crystals in the nappy) causing renal stones ± renal failure, and gout. *CNS:* Motor delay, IQ↓ (eg <65), clonus, choreoathetosis, hypotonia, and fits. *Behavioural problems:* Cognitive dysfunction, compulsive, agitated, self-mutilation (lip/foot biting, head banging, face scratching—may be unilateral). Smiling aggression to others may occur. *Δ:* Measurement of HPRT enzyme activity in blood. Diagnosis is confirmed by identifying a mutation in the HPRT gene. *Prognosis:* Death is usually before 25yrs, from renal failure or infection. *R:* Good hydration (urine flow↑); allopurinol prevents urate stones, but not CNS signs. Deep brain stimulation can stop automutilation,[87] as can (less subtle!) removal of teeth.[88]

Lewy body dementia A common type of dementia with intracytoplasmic neuronal inclusion bodies (fig 1) in brainstem/cortex + fluctuating cognitive impairment, parkinsonism, hallucinations, and visuoperceptual deficits. *R:* Cholinesterase inhibitors (eg rivastigmine). Overlap with Alzheimer's and Parkinson's diseases makes treatment hard as antiparkinsonian agents can precipitate delusions, and antipsychotics worsen parkinsonism.[89]

Li-Fraumeni syndrome Families suffer high rates of cancer in their young. As well as devastating families, it fascinates geneticists as families inherit a germline nonsense or oncogene-like missense mutation in one *p53* allele; see BOX.

Martin-Bell (fragile x) syndrome (semi-dominant; prevalence: 1:5700) is the main form of inherited cognitive impairment, and is a leading single-gene disorder. *Cause:* A stretch of CGG-repeats in FMR-1 gene (fragile x mental retardation-1) on xq27, that lengthens as it is transmitted from generation to generation. Once the repeat exceeds a threshold length, no fragile x protein is made, and disease results. *Signs:* ↓Flexibility in adapting to the changing demands that life brings (↓attentional set-shifting),[90] big testes, big jaw, high forehead, ↓IQ (not always);[91] poor learning, facial asymmetry, long ears, short temper. Also: hyperactivity, emotional and behavioural problems, anxiety, mood swings, autism, tactile defensiveness (little eye contact; no hugging; hypersensitive to touch & sound, ?from slowed mid-trimester maturation of the sensory cortex). *Tests:* Prenatal tests are possible. Screening could be general or of high-risk groups (eg families with >1 retarded ♂). Screening for carrier status leads to labelling and stigmatization, and is rejected by some families.[92]

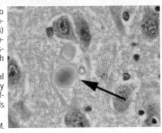

Fig 1. Lewy body (arrow). NB: there are no generally accepted biomarkers to distinguish dementia with Lewy bodies (DLB) from other dementias. Think of DLB whenever there is progressive anxiety, depression, apathy, agitation, sleep disorder with psychosis and memory disorders.

The best imaging candidate may be striatal dopamine transporter system scintigraphy using FP-CIT SPECT.[93] EEG is helpful—but difficult and the application of criteria needs an expert.[94]

Courtesy of Kondi Wong / NLM.

Li–Fraumeni syndrome, p53, and the guardian of the genome

p53 is a tumour-suppressor gene (chromosome 17p13.1; encoding nuclear phosphoprotein, a transcription factor allowing passage through the cell cycle). In this syndrome, as only one allele is affected, development is normal until a spontaneous mutation affects the other allele. Somatic mutation of p53 occurs at both alleles in 50–80% of spontaneous human cancers. Cells with a p53 mutation do not pause in G1 (a phase in which DNA repair takes place, and faulty DNA purged), but proceed straight to S1 (DNA replication), which is why p53 protein is known as the 'guardian of the genome'. Examples of cancers caused this way: early-onset breast cancer; brain tumours; sarcomas; leukaemia; lymphoma; melanoma; adrenal cortex carcinoma.[95]

Note that tumours are associated with more than one syndrome, eg adrenal cortex tumours are associated with familial cancer syndromes such as the Beckwith–Wiedemann and Li–Fraumeni syndromes, the Carney complex (p699), multiple endocrine neoplasia type 1, congenital adrenal hyperplasia, and the McCune–Albright syndrome (p650).[96]

In a retrospective study of 200 cancer-affected carriers of TP53 germline mutations, 15% developed a 2nd cancer, 4% a 3rd cancer, and 2% a 4th cancer.[97] In some populations (eg in South Brazil) there is a high prevalence of otherwise rare mutations in p53, partly explaining high rates of colon and other cancers (eg fatal stomach cancers in children as young as 12).[98]

McCune–Albright syndrome Polyosteotic fibrous dysplasia of bone, irregular areas of skin pigmentation and facial asymmetry ± precocious puberty.

Monteggia fracture # of the proximal ⅓ of ulna, with angulation + radial head subluxation, caused forced pronation. Open reduction/plating aids good alignment (5wks in plaster). Wait for full union (~12wks) before normal arm use.[99]

Morquio's syndrome (mucopolysaccharidosis IV $^{Autosomal}_{recessive}$) Lysosomal storage disease caused by ↓N-acetylgalactosamine-6-sulfate sulfatase. *Signs:* Stature↓; deaf; weakness; broad mouth; widely-spaced teeth; aortic regurgitation.[100] IQ↔.

Moyamoya disease Vascular disease at the circle of Willis causes strokes/TIAs (alternating hemiplegia, dyspraxia, fits, involuntary movements, headache).[101] *Typical patient:* Japanese girl, with triggering infection (eg tonsillitis) or hyperventilation (CO_2↓ causes vasoconstriction). *Digital subtraction angiography:* Collateral vessel formation 'like a puff of smoke'. *MRI/CT:* Multiple infarctions in watershed areas. ℞: Bypass surgery may be possible.[101]

Niemann–Pick disease $^{Autosomal}_{recessive}$ A neurovisceral lysosomal lipid storage disorder.[102] After years of normal growth, there is physical and mental decline, psychosis, wasting, and hepatosplenomegaly from abnormal metabolism of sphingomyelin. Other signs: brown skin patches; a cherry red spot on the macula; AST↑. Δ: Sphingomyelinase activity in peripheral blood white cells.[103]

Noonan syndrome Hypertrophic cardiomyopathy, VSD/ASDs, bruising (APTT↑; ↓factors VIII, XI, XII), ptosis, down-slanting eyes, low-set ears, webbed neck. Height, IQ, social functioning & hearing are ↓,[104] but not severely. ~50% have germ-line PTPN11 mutations (± associated neuroblastoma$^{et\,al}$).[105] *ECG:* Left axis deviation⁴⁵%, small R wave in v6²⁴%; abnormal Q wave⁶%.[106] *Prevalence:* 1:5000.

Ondine's curse Failure of migration neural crest cells→autonomic dysfunction →central alveolar hypoventilation→apnoea during sleep.[107] Ondine was a nymph who sacrificed her immortality by falling in love with a prince who promised to honour her with every waking breath. As she began to age, the prince lost interest. Ondine was furious, uttering her curse: "for as long as you are awake, you shall breathe. But should you ever fall asleep, that breath will desert you".

Othello syndrome (morbid jealousy) A lover believes, against all reason, that his beloved is being sexually unfaithful, thinking that she is plotting against him, or deliberately making him impotent. He may engage a spy, and obsessively examine her underwear for signs of sexual activity. Associations: alcohol, schizophrenia, depression, right frontal lobe problems.[108] ►Get psychiatric help: jealousy is the most deadly of all the passions, and outlasts all others.[109] "Without my having seen Albertine...there would flash from my memory some vision of her with Gisèle in an attitude which had seemed innocent to me at the time; it was enough now to destroy the peace of mind I had managed to recover, I had no longer any need to go and breath dangerous germs outside, I had, as Cottard [p640] would have said, supplied my own toxin."$^{Marcel\,Proust:\,ch2\,of}_{Sodome\,\&\,Gomorre}$

Patau's syndrome (trisomy 13) Cleft lip & palate, microcephaly, omphalocele, hernias, patent ductus arteriosus, VSD ± dextrocardia, capillary haemangiomata, and polycystic kidneys. Hands show flexion contractures ± polydactyly/narrow fingernails. *Antenatal management:* See BOX 3. *Typical survival:* A few days; 5% survive >6 months. *Prevalence:* 1 in 7500 births.[110]

Pick's dementia *Prevalence:* 15:100,000 aged 45-64yrs. *Signs:* Before cognitive loss, look for:[111] character change, frontal lobe signs, eg tactless disinhibition ± stealing, practical jokes, callousness, sexual (mis)adventures, fatuous euphoria/depression, odd eating habits/impaired satiety,[112] jargon dysphasia. Delusions (rare).[113] *Tests:* MRI. ℞: Drugs, eg memantine$^{et\,al}$, often fail.[114] See BOX.

Pierre Robin syndrome Poor neonatal feeding & breathing due to micrognathia (short chin) ± cleft palate or eye abnormality. Prevent the tongue slipping back by nursing on the belly (chest elevated on pillow) or by surgery.[115]

Distinguishing Pick's dementia from Alzheimer's disease (AD)

Histology: Instead of the neurofibrillary tangles of AD, look for severe atrophy, neuronal loss, gliosis, ballooned neurons (Pick cells), and argentophilic neuronal inclusions (Pick bodies) especially in frontal and temporal cortical regions. (Pick's is a type of frontotemporal dementia and all types tend to show disinhibition, character change, increased appetite, sexual misconduct and language problems.)[116]

Epidemiology: Pick's runs a shorter course, starting earlier than AD. ♂:♀ >1:1

A good history from carers is quite good at distinguishing the conditions. *Sensitivity:* 79%. *Specificity:* 90%.[117] See OPPOSITE for discriminating signs. NB: memory and visuospatial dysfunction may less affected than in AD.

On examination: Reflexes such as grasp, suck, and snout; plastic rigidity.

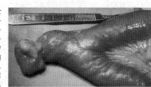

Fig 1. Meckel's diverticulum *Prevalence:* ≤2%. ≤2 inches long, and >2 feet from the ileocaecal valve (antemesenteric aspect of ileum); it contains gastric and pancreatic tissue. Δ: Radioisotope scan; laparotomy may be the cause of occult GI pain and bleeding (brick red stools, or dark becoming bright). It is a leading cause of rectal bleeding (± GI obstruction) in children.   ©Dr Thomas Tracy.

Hyper-endocrinopathies, McCune–Albright syndrome, and the Taiwanese giant

In the McCune–Albright syndrome, precocious puberty is not the only endocrinopathy: hyperthyroidism and Cushing's also occur. In the case of the 'Taiwanese giant' (an unfortunate name) excess growth hormone production has also been found.[118] Deformities, fractures, and pain further complicate the picture (sometimes ameliorated by IV pamidronate). The craniofacial fibrous dysplasia may encroach on the optic nerve, causing visual problems. GNRH analogues have been used (experimentally) to treat the precocious puberty.[119]

The cause may be a mutation of the GNAS 1 gene coding for the α subunit of the stimulatory guanine-nucleotide binding protein, G-protein, which activates adenylate cyclase (∴ ↑intracellular cyclic AMP).[120]

Ethical considerations...severe trisomy conditions

If the patient's views are known, comply with them. This excellent principle only gets us so far in obstetrics, where there are 2 potential patients whose needs may be in conflict eg during antenatal diagnosis of a uniformly lethal condition (L+) or a uniformly severe commonly lethal condition (L±, eg trisomy 13 or 18). What do doctors actually do with these uncomfortably nested bombs? Not every doctor will discuss termination even for L+ conditions, but most do. If the mother decides to continue her pregnancy and is requesting obstetric non-intervention, 99% of us comply with her views for both L+ and L± conditions.[121] Most of us try to be encouraging for such management, but some of us are non-directive or discourage this management. In continuing pregnancies where the mother changes her mind and wants a late termination, most of us are willing to comply for both L+ (71%) and L± (82%) conditions. What do we make of these discrepancies? Patients may be offered different options based on doctors' ethical or religious backgrounds. If the doctor does *not* comply with patient wishes he or she may be wise to get a second opinion, and should be prepared to be challenged through the Courts, where opposing ethics are decided one way or another, for better or worse, by judges who may never have heard of trisomy—that, of course, is their great strength: their superb ignorance immunizes them against bias.

Captain Pollard syndrome A state of mind (known to all doctors) caused by destroying the very person we had hoped to protect due to over-indulging views of colleagues. In 1821 he found himself eating his 17-yr-old cousin (whom he had promised to protect) while adrift without food on the Pacific after a series of giving way to the other's views on how to conduct his fatal whaling expedition.

Pompe's glycogen storage disease (GSD-II) ↓Lysosomal $α_{1,4}$-glucosidase activity leads to progressive weakness and failure to thrive. 2 forms: infantile and late-onset.[122] IQ↓ & sepsis occur. Glycogen accumulates in heart (do echo); muscle; liver; CNS; kidney; adrenals. ℞: Alglucosidase alfa prolongs life and can reverse cardiomyopathy. Gene therapy might be curative in future.[123]

Prader–Willi syndrome (PWS) *Cause:* Loss of paternal contribution of the proximal part of the long arm of chromosome 15. *Prevalence:* 1:25,000. Δ: See BOX. *Signs:* Blue eyes and blond hair ± hypersomnolence,[124] hyperphagia/pica (eg for dog biscuits, or shop-lifting food). Toddlers may be passive, autistic, or introverted or develop unstable moods. Those who are extrovert may develop psychosis. *Tests:* Chromosome analysis. EEG: slow spike & wave activity.[125]

Ramsay Hunt syndrome (herpes zoster oticus) Severe otalgia, often in the elderly, precedes VII & other cranial nerve palsies. Zoster vesicles appear around the ear, in the deep meatus (± soft palate & tonsillar fossa). There may be vertigo ± sensorineural deafness.[126] ℞: Valaciclovir 1g/8h PO[127] + prednisolone (p574).[128]

Rett disorder x-linked. Development: Normal at first. Diagnosis (according to DSM IV-TR): *A: All of the following:* • Normal prenatal and perinatal development • Normal psychomotor development for ~5 months after birth • Normal head circumference at birth. *B: Onset of all of the following after a period of normal development:* • ↓Head growth between 5 and 48 months old • Loss of previously acquired purposeful hand skills between 5 and 30 months (development of stereotyped movements, eg hand wringing or hand washing) • ↓Interest in social activities early in the course • Ataxic gait or trunk movements • Impaired expressive & receptive language + psychomotor retardation. Δ: Sequencing of MECP2 gene mutations (the cause in 70%).[129,130]

Reye's syndrome Encephalopathy occurs days after a febrile viral illness (varicella, influenza). Aspirin intake is a risk factor[131] (and maybe antiemetics/antihistamines). Median age:[UK] 14 months. *Tests:* Transaminases↑; glucose↓; blood ammonium↑ (correlate with survival); INR↑. Liver biopsy: swollen, pleomorphic mitochondria (ATP↓, gluconeogenesis & ureagenesis↓). CNS MRI: cerebral oedema; white matter changes.[132] ΔΔ: Inherited metabolic disorders (IMD). See BOX.

Russell Silver syndrome A heterogeneous congenital disorder, characterized by severe intrauterine and post-natal growth retardation, dysmorphic facial features, asymmetrical growth, small stature and precocious puberty. The cause usually unknown. *Association:* Wilms'. Aberrant genomic imprinting (eg involving chromosome 11p15.5) may be to blame.[133] In imprinting, DNA sequences have conditional behaviour depending on if they are maternally or paternally inherited. The idea is that there is some imprint put on the DNA in the mother's ovary or in the father's testes which marks that DNA as being maternal or paternal, and influences expression in their progeny.[134,135]

Shakhonovich's syndrome (hypokalaemic periodic paralysis) Attacks (1-24h) of flaccid paralysis, spreading up from the legs triggered by: stress, menses, cold, carbohydrate loads, rest after exercise, or liquorice. Speech, eye movements & swallowing are OK. *Age:* ~7-21yrs. *Signs:* During attacks, muscles feel firmer than usual. Reflexes: diminished. *Genes:* Mis-sense mutations of CACNA1S (type 1) & SCN4A genes (type 2) affecting the voltage sensor of the transmembrane segment of Ca^{2+} channels (type 1) and Na^+ channels (type 2).[136] *Tests during attacks:* ➤K^+↓; PO_4^{3-}↓; urate↑; WCC↑; glycosuria.[137] ℞: IV/oral K^+ can help; acetazolamide prevents some attacks, depending on genetic diagnosis. *Genetic counselling.*[138] ΔΔ: Hypokalaemic thyrotoxic periodic paralysis.[139]

Diagnosing Prader–Willi if <3yrs old

Likely if > 5 points if 3 from major criteria

Major criteria (1 point each)
- Feeding problems ± failure to thrive
- Hypogonadism
- Developmental delay ± ↓IQ
- Rapid weight gain (1-6yrs of age; NB: wt normal in 26%, if aged 6–17)[140]
- Central hypotonia
- Characteristic facial features

Minor criteria (½ point each)
- ↓Fetal movement/infantile lethargy
- Short stature ± small hands and feet
- Esotropia/myopia
- Speech articulation defects
- Sleep disturbance ± sleep apnoea
- Hypopigmentation
- Thick viscous saliva
- Skin picking

Prader-Willi syndrome (PWS) and epigenetic proof of existentialism

Chromosome 15q11-q13 is a critical region for PWS and Angelman syndrome (AS, a totally different syndrome of frequent laughter, ataxia & hypotonia giving a puppet-like gait—*happy puppet syndrome*).[141] PWS results from loss of expression of paternally expressed genes and AS of maternally expressed genes from the same locus. How do the genes know where they come from? They bear an imprint of their origin. This is genetic imprinting—an example of epigenetics—ie transgenerationally-transmissible functional changes in the genome that can be altered by environmental events and don't involve an alteration of DNA sequences. What we expose our genes to today may be influencing the lives our grandchildren can lead. Mouse models show that this can be inherited down unlimited generations.

In humans we know that permanent reactions to stress (eg increased glucocorticoid receptor sensitivity, eg after a terrorist outrage) can be inherited down at least one generation.[142] Another example of the environment controlling genomic events is the association of Beckwith-Wiedemann syndrome (p638) with embryos that have been stored and treated in unusual ways during IVF. Furthermore, changes in our diet may activate certain pathways leaving an imprint that is passed to the next generation (Kaati's hypothesis is supported by data on harvest yields in Overkalix in northern Sweden: a propensity to diabetes is inherited only if there is a surfeit of food during the time leading up to one's grandfather's puberty).[143,144]

A cardinal precept of genetics has always been that we cannot choose what we pass on to the next generation. But epigenetics opens up an unlimited dialogue between genes and our environment. It is likely that we can be responsible by *free choice* whether a gene is turned on or off (eg by exposing ourselves to pesticides or smoke)—and this turning-off may be inherited in an unchanging way. ►*We need to nurture our own genome carefully for future generations*. Does this mean that we have a duty to be happy and lead a stress-free life? We don't know. What we do know is that the existentialists have a point—it is as if we are all now responsible for everything forever. And this knowledge may itself be stressful. By confronting this stress and making free choices we can authenticate our dialogue with our genes.

Staging and treatment of Reye's syndrome

Stage 2 (or worse) should prompt rapid referral to a tertiary centre able to monitor ICP and intra-arterial pressure. Stage 2 criteria: inappropriate verbalizing, combative or stuporose, purposeful or non-purposeful response to pain, sluggish pupillary responses, intact eye reflex. *Management:* ►Correct hypoglycaemia with a *continuous* IVI of 10–15% glucose. Restrict fluids; do blood glucose every 2h; give **vitamin K** 0.25mg/kg slowly IV (monitor prothrombin time); lower ICP (p200). Aim for 40mmHg cerebral perfusion pressure (=systolic BP minus ICP). Control T° and seizures. *Mortality:* <20%, from brainstem dysfunction. Since abandoning aspirin in children, incidence has fallen to ≤1-6 patients/yr/10⁶ children <16yrs.[145]

Still's disease (systemic-onset juvenile idiopathic arthritis/JIA) presents with systemic upset eg in a prepubertal girl with synovitis, cartilage erosion ± fever, pericarditis, iridocyclitis, pneumonitis (lung biopsy specific), lymphadenopathy, splenomegaly. It is a cause of walking on tip-toes (ΔΔ: short Achilles tendon; habit; muscle contractures; cerebral palsy).[146] 88% get arthritis (8% mono-, 45% oligo-, 47% polyarticular)—eg of knee (68% of patients with arthritis), wrist (68%), and ankle (57%).[147] Latex is –ve.[148] *Other subgroups:* juvenile ankylosing spondylitis; psoriatic arthritis; ulcerative colitis-associated arthritis; juvenile-onset rheumatoid arthritis: here Rh factor is +ve, and systemic upset is rarer (eg DIC, liver/renal failure; amyloid; cardiac tamponade; sterile endocarditis; peritonitis; macrophage activation/cytokine storm).[149]

Adult-onset Still's disease (AOSD) diagnostic criteria—all of: daily fever >39°C; arthralgia/arthritis; Rh factor *and* antinuclear factor –ve *plus any* 2 of: WCC >15 × 10⁹/L; rash; serositis (pleural/pericardial); hepatosplenomegaly; adenopathy—*provided* that SBE, leukaemia & sarcoid are excluded.

Tests: WCC↑; ESR↑; CRP↑ (≈poor response); Hb↓; ferritin↑; LFT↑; albumin↓; echo.[150] *R:* ▶The chief challenge for the child is to negotiate between their protected status as a 'sick child', their own responsibility in illness management, and the need to achieve a normal lifestyle.[151] Try mild exercise; then rest for 1h each day. If hips are affected, physio to prevent contractures by encouraging extension (eg lying prone on the floor to watch TV). Splinting, traction, and non-weight-bearing exercises help. Hot baths help morning stiffness. Consider **tocilizumab** (may halt radiographic progression by blocking interleukin-6 receptors; SE dyslipidaemia), **methotrexate** (may help uveitis too), **penicillamine**, **gold**, and **hydroxychloroquine**.[152] Intra-articular **triamcinolone** may be tried.[153] Synovectomy[154] may conserve joint function.[155]

Sydenham's chorea (St Vitus dance) This is still the chief cause of chorea in children, and is a major manifestation of acute rheumatic fever (p166). It may be the *only* feature, appearing up to 6 months after clinical and lab signs of strep infection have abated. This may start with emotional lability and a preference for being alone (± attention span↓). Other non-motor features: include obsessions, compulsions, attention deficit, ↓verbal fluency, ↓executive function.[156] Motor signs: purposeless movement, worsened by stress and disappearing on sleep, with clumsiness, grimacing, a darting lizard's tongue and unclear speech. The term PANDAS (paediatric autoimmune neuropsychiatric disorder associated with streptococcus) denotes a putative subset of obsessive-compulsive disorder and Tourette's syndrome (OHCM p714) that bears some resemblance to Sydenham's chorea.[157] ΔΔ: Wilson's disease, juvenile Huntington's, thyrotoxicosis, SLE, polycythaemia, Na⁺↓, hypoparathyroidism, kernicterus, encephalitis lethargica, subdural haematoma, alcohol, phenytoin, neuroleptics, hereditary chorea, neuroacanthosis. *R:* Often self-limiting, but treat if chorea interferes with life. **Sodium valproate** (15-20mg/kg/day) or **carbamazepine** can control chorea within 1 week.[158] Despite treating active and recurrent strep infections vigorously, chorea may persist.[156]

Syme's amputation An amputation immediately proximal to the ankle.

Tay–Sachs disease Autosomal recessive Type I gangliosidosis affecting ~1:4000 Ashkenazi Jewish births. It is a disease of grey matter. There is ↓lysosomal hexosaminidase A. Low levels of enzyme are detectable in carriers. Children are normal until ~6 months old, when developmental delay, photophobia, myoclonic fits, hyperacusis and irritability occur. Ophthalmoscopy: cherry-red spot at macula. Death at ~3-5yrs of age. Prenatal diagnosis may be made by amniocentesis.

Tolosa–Hunt syndrome Painful ophthalmoplegia + ipsilateral ocular motor nerve palsies, from non-specific granulomatous inflammation in the cavernous sinus, superior orbital fissure, or orbit. Maxillary sinusitis may trigger it. MRI may show enhancement of one cavernous sinus. Corticosteroids may cure.[159,160]

Treacher–Collins syndrome $^{\text{Autosomal}}_{\text{dominant}}$ Lower lid notching, oblique palpebral fissures, flattening of malar bones ± hypoplastic zygoma. If these are associated with mandibular defects, ear defects, and deafness, it is called Franceschetti's synd. *Cause:* TCOF1 gene mutations. *Reconstructive surgery* is an option.[161]

Turner's syndrome (XO monosomy or mosaic, eg 45,X/46,XX or 45,X/47,XXX; uncorrelated with ↑maternal age). *Prevalence:* 1:2500 girls. *Signs:* Short stature (eg ≤130cm, but depends on mother's height);[162] hyperconvex nails; wide carrying angle (cubitus valgus); broad, shield-shaped chest; hypoplastic breasts/lack of secondary sexual features (but pregnancy *is* possible);[163] inverted (not always widely spaced)[164] nipples; ptosis; nystagmus; webbed neck; low posterior hairline;[165] coarctation of the aorta; left heart defects; leg lymphoedema. Gonad dysgenesis (streak ovary)/absent and puberty may not occur. *Typical mode of death:* Heart disease. R: **Somatropin** (human GH; eg 0.6–2u/kg/wk SC, or in divided nightly doses) adds a median of 5.1cm to final stature (6.4cm if GH + **oxandrolone** ≤0.1mg/kg/day); don't give if epiphyses are fused. NB: GH prolongs the normal state of insulin resistance seen in puberty (resultant hyperinsulinaemia may ↑anabolic effects of insulin on protein metabolism in puberty).[166] If hypogonadic, HRT, eg 2mg **estradiol valerate** + **levonorgestrel** 75µg at night, can start at 13yrs.◆ *Association:* Crohn's disease.[167]

Ulysses syndrome After the Trojan war, Ulysses (the Latin name for Odysseus), King of Ithaca, had many perilous and perhaps pointless adventures before he returned to his starting place. Similarly, many of our incurable patients start out with a problem, and end with the same problem, after many risky and futile tests have advanced their case not one jot, as we have not had the courage to say: "Let's not *do* anything". It is always easier to do new scans or daring operations, and Ulysses syndrome describes this superfluity. But there is an ambiguity here: "Ithaca has given you the beautiful voyage...If you find her poor, Ithaca has not cheated you..." Why not? Because the journey teaches patients the one thing that has eluded us: namely wisdom. _{Konstantinos Kavafis; *Ithaca*}

Von Gierke's syndrome (type 1a glycogen storage disease; GSD 1a) $^{\text{Autosomal}}_{\text{recessive}}$ Glucose-6-phosphatase is low. GSD1a is the severest glycogenosis. Δ: Mutation analysis of G6PC gene. GSD1a accounts for 20% of glycogenoses in some centres.[168] *Signs:* Hepatomegaly/renomegaly, growth retardation, hypoglycaemia, lactic acidaemia, hyperuricaemia, failure to thrive, lumbar lordosis, dyslipidaemia, adiposity, xanthomata over joints and buttocks, bleeding tendency, and delayed tooth eruption.[169] *Complication:* Hepatic adenoma; hepatocellular cancer.[170]

Werner's syndrome (WS; progeria) $^{\text{Autosomal}}_{\text{recessive}}$ WS is characterized by precocious ageing after a shallow puberty (no growth spurt), with bird-like pinched nose, loss or greying of hair, cataracts, skin atrophy/ulcers, ↑peripheral fat, dyslipidaemia, and diabetes.[171] The complex molecular and cellular phenotypes of WS involve features of genomic instability and accelerated replicative senescence. The gene involved (WRN) has been cloned, and its gene product (WRNP) is a helicase. Helicases play important roles in a variety of DNA transactions, including DNA replication, transcription, repair, and recombination, and in WS unwinding of DNA pairs is disordered.[172] R: **Pioglitazone** may reduce insulin resistance.[173]

Winkler's disease p538.

Wiskott–Aldrich syndrome (WAS) is a severe x-linked primary immunodeficiency (p198) with eczema, recurrent infections, autoimmune disorders, IgA nephropathy ± haematopoietic neoplasia. Platelets are too few and too small. Without marrow transplant, most die before adulthood. WAS protein gene mutations also cause x-linked thrombocytopenia, intermittent thrombocytopenia, and neutropenia.[164] *Prenatal diagnosis:* Direct gene analysis with single-strand conformation polymorphism (SSCP), and hetero-duplex formation (HD).[165] R: *Antibiotics* ± IV immunoglobulin for infections. Hematopoietic stem cell transplant is 1st choice therapy. Gene therapy is awaited.

Orthopaedics

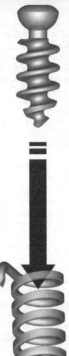

Fig 1. *When the spi-
ral meets the helix,
the orthopod gets
his fix.*

A&E* and associated topics

Relevant pages in other chapters *Paediatrics*: ch 2; *rheumatology OHCM* p540.

Sources/further reading *Internet:*   www.worldortho.com;   www.wheelessonline.com[1]
secure.facs.org/trauma/atls/information.html;   www.anatomy.tv;   www.e-anatomy.org;
the image bank at: www.trauma.org

Books: Practical Fracture Treatment, 4th ed, McRae and Esser, ISBN 0443070385;
Advanced Trauma Life Support® (ATLS®) *Manual*, 7th ed; ISBN 1880696142.

1 ►Many detailed treatments are described in this chapter, and it is not envisaged that the inexperienced doctor will try them out except under appropriate supervision. The importance of
enlisting early expert help (either at once or, if appropriate, by calling the patient back to the
next morning's clinic) cannot be overemphasized.

We thank James Hopkinson-Woolley and Winnie Chen and James Sewell our Specialist Readers for
this chapter, and Fabio Conteduca for permission to use the image in figure 1—and Dr Tom Turmezei
for his masterful commentaries on the many images he supplied.

Remain in light...

▶It's better to ask than to remain in the dark; see p701 for bone & joint types.

ankylosis	Stiffening of a joint with fibrous or bony union across it
arthro-	Relating to a joint (prefix)
arthrodesis	The surgical fusion of a joint
arthropathy	A pathological process occurring within a joint
arthroplasty	Creation of an artificial joint (eg total hip replacement)
arthroscopy	Minimally invasive ('keyhole') joint inspection/surgery
articular	Relating to a joint surface or capsule; extra-articular = outside the joint capsule; intra-articular = within the joint capsule
closed	Of a fracture, contained totally inside the body (not open)
comminuted	Of a fracture, having more than 2 parts
multifragmentary	Of a fracture, having several discernible (and countable) parts; may be preferred to 'comminuted' by some
nerve injuries	For axonotmesis, neurotmesis and neurapraxia, see p760
open	Of fractures: having any communication with the outside world
osteotomy	Surgical cutting, wedging, and then realignment of a bone
palmar	The anterior aspect of the wrist and hand (preferred to volar)
-physis	For physis, epiphysis, etc., see p683
pseudarthrosis	A false joint across which movement can occur in a bone
radicle (radiculo-)	Nerve fibres that come together to form a spinal nerve root
reaming	Surgical widening of the medullary cavity of a bone
spondylo-	Relating to a vertebra (prefix; from Greek)
spondylolisthesis	Slippage (Greek olisthos = slippery) of one vertebra forward on top of the other
spondylolysis	A defect in the pars interarticularis of a vertebra
spondylosis	Term used for generalized degenerative disease of the spine
subluxation	Partial dislocation of a joint—as opposed to full dislocation
torticollis	Means 'twisted neck' (from Latin)—see p660
valgus	Deformity of part of a limb laterally from the normal axis
varus	Deformity of part of a limb medially from the normal axis

*A&E nomenclatures

A&E stands for Accident & Emergency; the word 'accident' is often dropped, and emergency medicine has emerged as a speciality in its own right—which centres on the 'knowledge and skills required for the prevention, diagnosis, and management of the acute and urgent aspects of illness and injury affecting patients of all age groups with a full spectrum of physical and behavioural disorders. It is a specialty in which time is critical'.[1]

Principles of orthopaedic examination

Going through clinical examination with an expert is the best way to learn, but this experience can be reinforced by taking principles and background reading with you into the arena. Most orthopaedic examinations can be developed on the following structure, whether for hip, elbow, ankle...

1 For each of:	2 Do the following:	3 Then remember to test:

• Skin
• Soft tissues
• Bone
	• Look
	• Feel
	• Then, move the limb:
	  • actively
	  • passively (the Dr does the work)
	  • versus resistance.
		• Ligaments
		• Neurovascular status
		• Any special tests, eg:
		  • knee meniscal tests
		  • hip fixed flexion deformity.

▶Remember to examine one joint above and one joint below the joint in question, ie for the hip, examine the knee and lumbar spine. This will uncover any referring pathology. When thinking of movement limitation: active loss = neuromuscular deficit; passive loss = bony or soft tissue impediment.

▶▶If you suspect a cervical spine injury, immobilize the neck with hard collar, sandbags,[1] and tape. NB: if very restless, use hard collar only, as otherwise the neck is vulnerable when the body moves on an immobilized head.

Examination The posture of the neck and any bone tenderness (midline and over the spinous processes) are noted. If safe to remove collar, check the range of movements: flexion & extension (mainly atlanto-occipital joint); rotation (mainly atlanto-axial joint); lateral flexion (whole of cervical spine). Rotation is the movement most commonly affected. Examine arms: test for root

For root lesions, test:
• c5: shoulder abduction
• c6: elbow flexion
• c7: elbow extension
• c8: finger flexion (grip)
• t1: finger abduction

lesions (see MINIBOX); test the reflexes (biceps c5; brachioradialis c6; triceps c7). Motor nerve roots and dermatomes are given on p716 and p762. If cord compression is suspected examine the lower limbs for signs of this (p770), eg upgoing plantars, hyperreflexia. The main sites of injury are c6 & 7, followed by c2. ~10% of c-spine fractures will have another spine fracture elsewhere, so always examine the whole spine. ▶Take neurological signs very seriously.

Imaging In minor trauma use the NEXUS or Canadian C-spine rule to decide if an x-ray is required.[2] Major trauma may need CT as first-line imaging (p779).[3]
When examining the image, follow 4 simple steps (ABCs):
1 *Alignment:* Check alignment of the following: •Anterior vertebral bodies; •Posterior vertebral bodies •Posterior spinal canal •Spinous processes (fig 1).
  • A step >3mm is abnormal (<25%=unifacet; >50%=bifacet dislocation).
  • Atlas–dens interval (ADI)—normal if <3mm (adults) or <5mm (children).
  • 40% of <7-yr-olds have anterior displacement c2 on c3 (in this pseudo-subluxation the posterior spinal line is maintained).
2 *Bone contour:* Trace around each vertebra individually.
  • Anterior/posterior height difference of >3mm (implies *wedge fracture*). In general <25% difference is stable and >25% difference is unstable.
  • Pedicles (*hangman's #*, fig 4) & spinous processes (*clayshoveller's #*).
  • Avulsion fractures of the vertebral body (*teardrop #*).
3 *Cartilages:* The disc space margins should be parallel (>11° is abnormal).
4 *Soft tissues:* Check the soft tissue shadows:
  • Retropharyngeal—c1–c3 <7mm; c4–c7 <22mm/1 vertebral body (fig 2).
  • Spinous process separation (interspinous ligament rupture). Spiral CT can help diagnose fractures here.[4]

▶All 7 cervical vertebrae must be seen, along with the c7–t1 junction: do not accept an incomplete image—a 'swimmers' view of c7–t1 may be needed.

▶A cross-table lateral in the best hands will still miss at least 15% of injuries.

Other views and investigations
• Open mouth 'peg' view (OMV, fig 3) for suspected odontoid peg fractures and c1 fractures (total lateral mass overhang of c1 on c2 should be <8mm).
• CT is used to image areas not adequately assessed on plain films (p779).
• MRI is vital for assessing ligamentous disruption, disc prolapse, and the neural elements (spinal cord and nerve roots), all of which can only be inferred from CT and plain radiography. Whole spine assessment is best.

Spinal cord injury without radiological abnormality (SCIWORA) is a condition in which there is a neurological deficit (ie spinal cord injury) in the absence of a lesion on plain radiographs (pathology may be visible on MRI). It most commonly occurs in paediatric cervical spine injuries and is treated in the same manner as a spinal fracture with appropriate immobilization and referral. Clinical evidence of the injury in children may be delayed in up to 50%, so always consider the injury if the mechanism is appropriate.[5]

---

1 If there is marked kyphosis, avoid hard collars to stabilize the spine, as the extension produced may be more than is natural for the patient: so collars may *cause* spinal injury.[6]

Orthopaedics and trauma

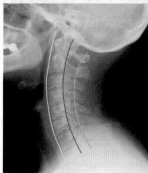

Fig 1. The lines to check for discontinuity on a lateral c-spine radiograph:
Yellow = anterior spinal line
Red   = posterior spinal line
Green   = spinolaminar line
Blue   = tips of spinous processes.
Note that we can see all the way to c7–T1.

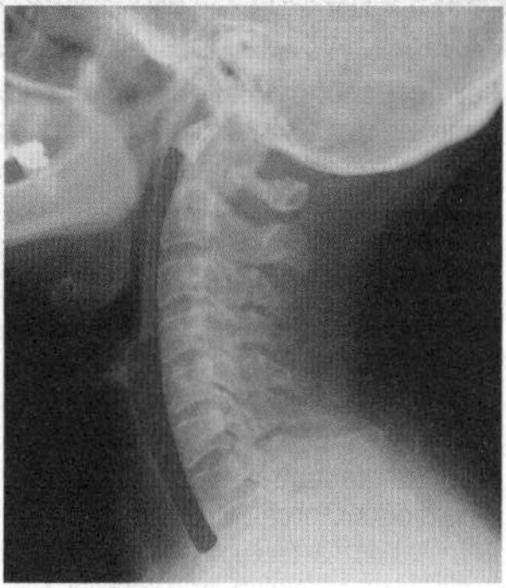

Fig 2. More important areas to look at on the lateral c-spine radiograph:
Yellow = ADI should be <3mm in adults
Red   = before c1–c3 should be <7mm
Blue   = before c4–c7 should be <22m.
ADI is the distance between the anterior aspect of the odontoid peg and the posterior of the anterior arch of C1.

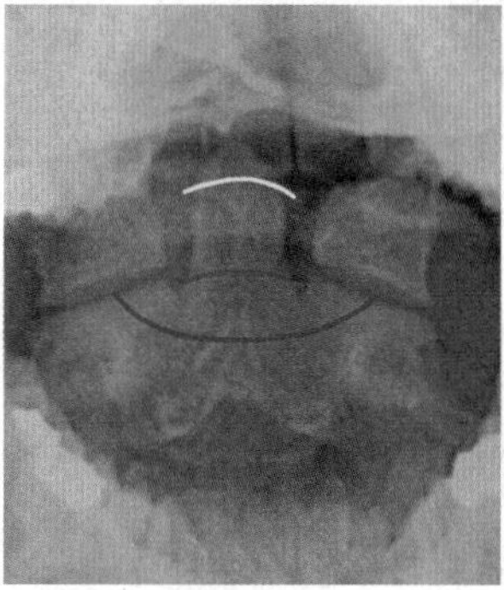

Fig 3. Odontoid peg fractures are best seen on the omv. There are 3 types:
Type I   = through the tip
Type II = through the base
Type III = into the body of c2.
Remember to check for the overhang of c1 on c2 (<8mm in total).

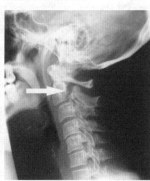

Fig 4. Lateral radiograph of the c-spine showing a fracture through the pedicles of the c2 vertebra—the hangman's fracture, which is traumatic spondylolisthesis of c2.

Courtesy of Professor Peter Scally.

Figures 1–3 Courtesy of The Norfolk and Norwich University Hospitals (NNUH) Radiology Department.

The paediatric cervical spine

Below the age of ~9yrs, the cervical spine needs to be assessed as an entirely different entity, as it creates very different patterns of normality and abnormality. The most important point to make here is that is best to ask a specialist's opinion—ie ask a Paediatric Radiologist. Nonetheless, remember:
▸▸ Injury is commonest in the upper spine.
▸▸ SCIWORA (see OPPOSITE).
▸▸ Growth plates (physes) and synchondroses can be mistaken for fractures.
▸▸ c2-3 and c3–4 can demonstrate pseudosubluxation.
▸▸ c7–T1 does not need to be visualized unless ≥8yrs old.

Cervical spondylosis (See *OHCM* p512) Degenerative changes of the cervical spine; eg featuring degeneration of the annulus fibrosus and bony spurs narrow the spinal canal and intervertebral foramina. Very common: ~90% of men >60yrs and women >50yrs. Usually asymptomatic, but can cause neck and arm pain with paraesthesiae—sometimes with myelopathy (spastic weakness and, later, incontinence). Images and treatment: see *OHCM*.

Cervical spondylolisthesis This is displacement of one vertebra upon the one below. *Causes:*

1 Congenital failure of fusion of the odontoid process with the axis, or fracture of the odontoid process (skull, atlas & odontoid process slip forward on axis).
2 Inflammation softens the transverse ligament (fig 1) of the atlas (eg rheumatoid or complicating throat infections), so the atlas slips forward on the axis.
3 Instability after injuries. The most important consequence of spondylolisthesis is the possibility of spinal cord compression. Treatments used include traction, immobilization in plaster jackets, and spinal fusion.

Prolapsed cervical disc Central protrusions (typically of c5/6 & c6/7) may give symptoms of spinal cord compression (p770; refer to neurosurgeon). Posterolateral protrusions may cause a stiff neck, pain radiating to the arm, weakness of muscles affected by the nerve root, and depressed reflexes. *Tests:* MRI is the preferred image (fig 2). *Treatment* is with NSAIDs, and a collar. As pain subsides, physiotherapy may help to restore mobility. Surgery is occasionally indicated, in the light of CT/MRI findings.

Cervical rib Congenital development of the costal process of the c7 vertebra is often asymptomatic but may cause thoracic outlet compression (figs 3–4). Similar symptoms with no radiological abnormality is called a scalenus or 1st rib syndrome. Thoracic outlet compression involves the lowest trunk of the brachial plexus (fig 3 & p765) ± the subclavian artery. Pain or numbness may be felt in hand or forearm (often on the ulnar side); there may be hand weakness and muscle wasting (thenar or hypothenar). *Diagnosis:* Weak radial pulse ± forearm cyanosis. Specific manoeuvres (eg Adson's test) are not reliable. Radiographs may not reveal cervical ribs, as symptoms may be caused by fibrous bands. Arteriography may show subclavian compression. *Treatment:* Physiotherapy to strengthen the shoulder elevators may improve symptoms, but rib removal or band division may be needed.

Spasmodic torticollis (cervical dystonia) The commonest adult focal dystonia. Episodes of a sudden stiff painful neck with torticollis are due to trapezius and sternocleidomastoid spasm. *Social withdrawal can be a problem. Causes:* Genetic; trauma. *Treatment:* If not self-limiting, heat, manipulation, relaxants, and analgesia may help. If severe, wearing a collar may help initial discomfort but may prolong symptoms. Botulinum toxin (p460) is a safe and effective option.[7,8] *Adjuncts:* Anticholinergics, benzodiazepines, baclofen.[9]

Infantile torticollis This may result from birth damage to sternocleidomastoid. *Typical age:* 1–36 months. *Signs:* Tilted head (ear nearer shoulder on affected side). ♂:♀≈3:2. Retarded facial growth on the affected side, hence facial asymmetry. Early, there is a tumour-like thickening in the muscle (may be palpable). *ΔΔ:* Spasmus nutans or 'nodding spasm' (head-nodding; torticollis; nystagmus); acquired late-infancy torticollis from rare CNS disorders (eg gangliocytoma). If there is an associated muscle mass, biopsy may be reassuring by showing a benign fibrous lesion.[10] *Treatment:* Self-limiting in 97%. If persistent, physiotherapy helps by lengthening the muscle; division at its lower end is more drastic.[11]

Acute whiplash Acceleration–deceleration injury (eg from RTA/sport) with no radiographic abnormality or neurological signs. May benefit from early mobilization and an early return to activity.[12] See also p758.

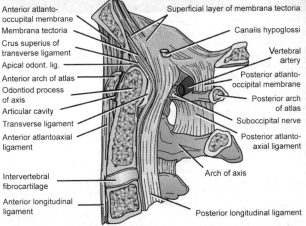

Anterior atlanto-occipital membrane
Membrana tectoria
Crus superius of transverse ligament
Apical odont. lig.
Anterior arch of atlas
Odontiod process of axis
Articular cavity
Transverse ligament
Anterior atlantoaxial ligament
Intervertebral fibrocartilage
Anterior longitudinal ligament

Superficial layer of membrana tectoria
Canalis hypoglossi
Vertebral artery
Posterior atlanto-occipital membrane
Posterior arch of atlas
Suboccipital nerve
Posterior atlanto-axial ligament
Arch of axis
Posterior longitudinal ligament

Fig 1. Cut-away sagittal view of the atlas and the axis cervical vertebrae, showing the ligaments around the odontoid peg.

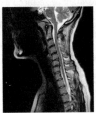

Fig 2. T2-weighted sagittal MRI of the cervical spine showing intervertebral disc protrusion at the C5/6 level.

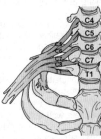

C4
C5
C6
C7
T1

Fig 3. Cervical rib causing compression of the inferior trunk of the brachial plexus (p765). The distal part of the rib can also cause stenosis in the subclavian artery, with post-stenotic dilatation (visible on arteriography).

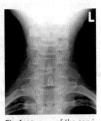

L

Fig 4. AP x-ray of the cervical spine showing bilateral rudimentary cervical ribs in the form of prominent transverse processes (the condition is a spectrum). They are usually a unilateral radiographic finding, though the contralateral side may still have a ligamentous band present. The presence of a cervical rib increases the likelihood of the brachial plexus being *prefixed*—ie arise from C4–C8 rather than C5–T1.

Figures 2 & 4 courtesy of the Norfolk and Norwich University Hospitals (NNUH) radiology department.

Anatomically, the glenohumeral joint is lax, depending far more on surrounding rotator cuff muscles than bony structures for stability—ie the tendons of supraspinatus (abduction), subscapularis (internal rotation), infraspinatus (external rotation), and teres minor (external rotation + extension). Biceps' long head traverses the cuff, attaching to the top of the glenoid cavity (figs 1–3).

History Occupation? Any previous trauma? *Where* is the pain: shoulder or neck? Does shoulder movement make it worse? If all movements worsen pain, suspect arthritis or capsulitis; if only some movements, suspect impingement. General health ok: if aches and pains all over, is it fibromyalgia or polymyalgia?

Examination Strip to waist. To assess glenohumeral movement, feel the lower half of the scapula to estimate degrees of scapular rotation over the thorax. Half the range of normal abduction is by scapular movement. Test *abduction* by raising hands from the sides sideways to above the head; *flexion* by raising hands forwards and up; *extension* by backward movement of elbows; *external rotation* by holding elbows against sides flexed at 90° and moving the hands outwards (normal 80°); and *internal rotation* by placing the back of the hand against the lumbar spine and moving the elbows forward; an easier test is to assess how far behind her back she can reach: 'imagine you are doing up a bra'. This is the last movement to recover after shoulder soft-tissue surgery.

The muscles used for movement at the shoulder joint
- *Flexion:* (forward movement) pectoralis major, deltoid (ant. ⅓), coracobrachialis.
- *Extension:* Deltoid (posterior ⅓); latissimus dorsi, pectoralis major, and teres major begin the extension if the shoulder starts out flexed.
- *Abduction:* Supraspinatus for first 15°, then deltoid.
- *Adduction:* Pectoralis major, latissimus dorsi, teres major, subscapularis.
- *Medial rotation:* Pectoralis major, deltoid (middle ⅓), latissimus dorsi, teres major, subscapularis.
- *Lateral rotation:* Teres minor, infraspinatus.

Rotator cuff muscles
• Subscapularis
• Teres minor
• Infraspinatus
• Supraspinatus

Scapula movement on the chest wall NB: serratus anterior prevents 'winging' of the scapula as pressure is placed on the outstretched hand.
- *Elevation:* (shrug shoulders) Levator scapulae, trapezius
- *Depression:* Serratus anterior, pectoralis minor
- *Forward action:* (=protraction, eg punch) Serratus anterior; pectoralis major
- *Retraction:* (brace shoulders) Trapezius, rhomboid.

Recurrent shoulder dislocation (For initial dislocation, see p740.) 2 types: *Atraumatic:* (5%) The patient is often a teenager with no history of trauma, but having general joint laxity. Remember AMBRI: atraumatic (ie 'born loose'); multidirectional; bilateral; treat by: rehabilitation; inferior capsular shift surgery only if rehab fails. *Traumatic:* Dislocation is anterior (sometimes inferior, rarely posterior) and secondary to trauma (may be mild). Remember TUBS: traumatic; unilateral; Bankart lesion (see below); surgical treatment. Abduction + lateral rotation of the arm (eg donning a coat) may cause dislocation. The capsule is attached to the neck of scapula but detached from the glenoid labrum (Bankart lesion). There may be a posterolateral 'dent' in the humeral head, called a Hill–Sachs lesion (seen on radiographs with arm medially rotated). *Treatment:* Open repair may yield better results than arthroscopic repair,[13] though latest arthroscopic techniques (eg suture anchor fixation + capsule plication) merit further study.[14] With the rarer recurrent posterior dislocation, the capsule is torn from the back of the neck of scapula, the humeral dent is superomedial, and it is abduction & medial rotation which causes dislocation (eg seizure). *Treatment:* Surgery—if prompt closed reduction fails.[15] Recurrent *subluxation* is also recognized (disabling and difficult to treat).

Orthopaedics and trauma

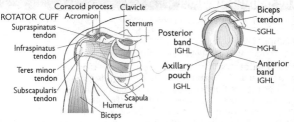

Fig 1. Shoulder anatomy (without deltoid): anterior view.

Fig 2. The glenoid surface of the gleno-humeral joint, and the glenohumeral ligaments (GHLs)—superior (SGHL), medial (MGHL), and inferior (IGHL).

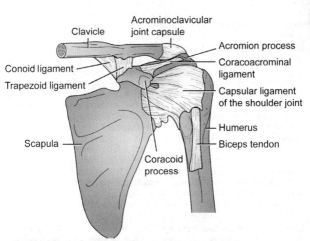

Fig 3. Shoulder and acromioclavicular (AC) joint ligaments: anterior view.

Some specific specialist shoulder examination tests

There are many specific shoulder examination tests that can be performed:
- *Neer's test:* Passive flexion of shoulder with a pronated arm, whilst scapula is stabilized. A painful arc between 60° and 120° = impingement.
- *Drop arm sign:* Patient lowers arm slowly from 160° abduction. If patient can't control the arm, and it drops quickly to the side = rotator cuff tear.
- *Jobe test:* Patient internally rotates arm whilst in 90°abduction and 30° forward flexion with an extended elbow. Attempt to further abduct against resistance which result in pain = supraspinatus weakness or injury.
- *Speed's test:* Patient starts with arm flexed forward 60°, elbow extended and forearm in supination, and attempts to flex shoulder forward against resistance. Pain on palpation of long head of biceps tendon during this manoeuvre = biceps tendonitis.
- *Apprehension test:* With elbow flexed at 90°, the forearm supine, abduct and externally rotate arm to 90°: apprehension=anterior joint instability.
- *Scarf test:* Forced adduction of arm across the neck: pain=AC joint disease.

There are a further host of tests, but the above represent a useful quotient for the budding upper limb orthopod.[16]

'*There is little evidence to support or refute the efficacy of common interventions for shoulder pain...*',[17] so it is vital to clarify expectations before any course of treatment. Remember that the neck may refer pain via C5 to the deltoid region and via C6, C7, and C8 to the superior border of the scapula.

Rotator cuff tears Tears in supraspinatus tendon (fig 1)—or adjacent sub-scapularis and infraspinatus—may be from degeneration, or less commonly, a sudden jolt or fall. Patients complain of shoulder *weakness* and pain. Night pain may affect sleep as patient is unable to keep the arm in a comfortable position (adducted without rotation). Partial tears cause a painful arc (below); complete tears limit shoulder abduction to the 45–60° given by scapular rotation. If the arm is passively abducted beyond 90° deltoid's contribution to abduction comes into play, which is then possible from this point. Full-range passive movement is present. Typical age: >40yrs.[18] *Imaging:* US (good for tendon imaging), MRI (better for imaging of labral tears,[19] or MRI-arthrography (reveals communication between joint capsule and subacromial bursa). *Treatment:* Incomplete: expectant. Complete: prompt referral for assessment for open or arthroscopic repair.

Painful arc syndrome (on abducting 45°–160°) *Causes of pain on abduction*:

1 *Supraspinatus tendinopathy* or partial rupture of supraspinatus tendon gives pain reproduced by adducting pressure on the partially abducted arm. Typical age: 35–60. Only a proportion will have a painful arc (others have increasing pain up to full abduction), which is why the term *impingement syndrome* (as the tendon catches under the acromion during abduction between, eg 70° and 140°) is preferred. NB: tendon rupture can also be asymptomatic.[20] *Treatment:* Active shoulder movement with physiotherapy and pain relief; subacromial bursa injection of steroid, eg triamcinolone acetonide 40mg with local anaesthetic may help;[21] arthroscopic acromioplasty.

2 *Calcifying tendinopathy:* One of the acute calcific arthropathies. Typical age about 40yrs. There is acute inflammation of supraspinatus. Pain is maximal during the phase of resorption. *Treatment:* Physiotherapy; NSAIDs; steroid injection; rarely, excision of calcium. See fig 2.

3 *Acromioclavicular joint osteoarthritis:* This is common. Try steroid injections or excision of the lateral end of the clavicle.

Long head of biceps tendinopathy Pain is in the anterior shoulder and characteristically ↑ on forced contraction of biceps. ℞: Pain relief; hydrocortisone injection to the tendon may help, but risks tendon rupture. Technique: p710.

Rupture of long head of biceps Discomfort occurs after 'something has gone' when lifting or pulling. A 'ball' appears in the muscle on elbow flexion, like a 'Popeye' muscle. *Treatment:* Repair is rarely indicated as function remains.[1]

Frozen shoulder (adhesive capsulitis) may follow modest injury in older people. Pain may be severe and worse at night (eg unable to lie on one side). Active and passive movement range is reduced. Abduction↓ (<90°) ± external rotation↓ (<30°). It may be associated with cervical spondylosis (more global restriction of movement). *Treatment:* NSAIDs, intra-articular steroid (see p710 for technique), physiotherapy, manipulation under anaesthetic. Local nerve block may provide short-term pain relief.[22] Meta-analyses of randomized trials are said not to support any one option, but they did not include Der Windt's trial which strongly favoured injections. Resolution may take years.

Shoulder osteoarthritis (fig 3) This is not so common as hip or knee OA. Good success rates (especially for pain relief) are being achieved by joint replacement—complications: infection, dislocation, loosening, periprosthetic humeral/glenoid fractures, nerve injury, prosthetic fracture; ectopic ossification. Timing of surgery is important, so that the rotator cuff and glenoid are not too worn for good stability.[23]

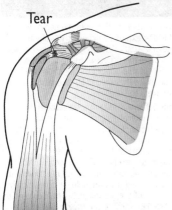

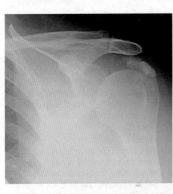

Fig 1. Rotator cuff tear in the supraspinatus tendon. See p663 for muscle names.

Fig 2. AP radiograph of the left shoulder showing calcifying tendinopathy in the left supraspinatus. The gleno–humeral joint also appears subluxed, though this is most likely 'deltoid inhibition' caused by pain.

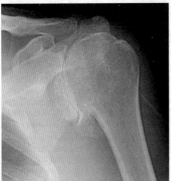

Fig 3. AP radiograph of the left shoulder showing osteoarthritis: loss of joint space, subchondral sclerosis, osteophytes, glenoid erosion and humeral head deformity are all present.

Figs 2 & 3 Courtesy of The Norfolk And Norwich University Hospitals (NNUH) Radiolology Department.

1 Conversely, if it is the biceps *insertion* that is avulsed, surgical repair will be required.

The elbow joint is formed by an articulation of the distal humerus with the proximal radius and ulna (fig 1). Flexion/extension occur at the ulnohumeral joint and is possible through a range of 0°–150°. With the elbow flexed, supination/pronation of 90° should be possible—this occurs at the radiohumeral and proximal radioulnar articulations. Acceptable upper limb function requires a 100° arc in each plane, ie 30°–130° extension/flexion and 50° pronation/supination.[24] Pain at the elbow may radiate from the shoulder.

Lateral epicondylitis (tennis elbow) There is inflammation where the common extensor tendon arises from the lateral epicondyle of the humerus ± rupture of aponeurosis fibres. *Presentation:* Pain is worst when the tendon is most stretched (wrist and finger flexion with hand pronated). Pain is felt at the front of the lateral condyle. Ask the patient to extend the wrist, and then to resist extension of the middle finger: is pain elicited? *Radiography:* Nonspecific. *Treatment:* Pain often subsides in time, but some favour injection of the tendon origin (p710).[25] If this fails, physiotherapy may help, or an epicondylitis brace; with severe disability, excision of the diseased part of the common extensor origin and repair of the extensor mechanism gives relief in 80% of recalcitrant disease, but there is a lack of RCTs for surgery.[26] Meta-analyses are equivocal on the best form of treatment.

Medial epicondylitis (golfer's elbow) This is less common than tennis elbow. Steroid injection may help, but be wary of the ulnar nerve that runs behind the epicondyle and the brachial artery that runs anteromedially.[27]

Olecranon bursitis (student's elbow) This is a traumatic bursitis following pressure on the elbows, eg while engrossed in a long book. There is pain and swelling behind the olecranon. Other causes are septic and gouty bursitis (look for tophi). The bursa should be aspirated—send fluid for Gram stain and microscopy for crystals. Traumatic bursitis may then be injected with hydrocortisone. Septic bursitis should be formally drained and will need a course of antibiotics.[28]

Ulnar neuritis (also 'cubital tunnel syndrome') Osteoarthritic or rheumatoid narrowing of the ulnar groove and constriction of the ulnar nerve as it passes behind the medial epicondyle, or friction of the ulnar nerve due to cubitus valgus (a possible sequel to childhood supracondylar fractures) can cause fibrosis of the ulnar nerve and ulnar neuropathy. *Presentation:* Sensory symptoms usually occur first, eg ↓ sensation over the little finger and medial half of ring finger. Patients may experience clumsiness of the hand and weakness of the small muscles of the hand innervated by the ulnar nerve (adductor pollicis, interossei, abductor digiti minimi and opponens digiti minimi). *Tests:* Nerve conduction studies may confirm the site of the lesion. *Treatment:* Surgical decompression ± transposition of the nerve to in front of the elbow (often only required if the nerve subluxes over the medial epicondyle after decompression).

Deformities *Cubitus valgus:* The normal degree of valgus ('carrying angle') at the elbow is 10° in ♂, and 15° in ♀. Fractures at the lower end of the humerus or interference with the lateral epiphyseal growth plate (ie causing arrest) may lead to the angle being greater. As a result, ulnar neuritis and osteoarthritis may occur. Treat if necessary. Association: Turner's syndrome. *Cubitus varus:* This may occur after poorly reduced supracondylar fractures.

Osteoarthritis of the elbow (fig 2). Osteochondritis dissecans and fractures involving the joint are risk factors. *Tests:* Flexion, extension and forearm rotation may be impaired. Loose bodies may cause restriction of movement, eg loss of full extension. *Treatment:* Surgery is rarely needed (procedures include: removal of loose bodies, debridement, radial head excision, joint replacement). Joint replacement may also be performed for rheumatoid arthritis of the elbow.

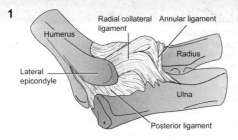

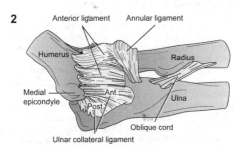

Fig 1. The ligaments around the elbow joint—posterolateral view of the right elbow (1) and anteromedial view of the left elbow (2). Stability of this joint is mainly from bony factors, though ligaments do play an important part—eg the annular ligament wraps around the head of the radius (which can pop out in a 'pulled elbow'), and also allows smooth pronation/supination. Remember that the joint is made up from 3 articulations: radio-humeral, proximal radioulnar, and humeroulnar.

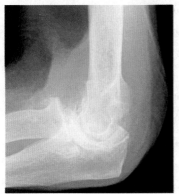

Fig 2. Lateral x-ray of the elbow showing degenerative changes of osteo-arthritis. There is loss of joint space, osteophyte formation, bony deformity, and subchondral sclerosis. Movement is painful and severely restricted.

© Norfolk and Norwich University Hospitals (**NNUH**) Radiology Department.

Orthopaedics and trauma

Dupuytren's contracture Progressive, painless fibrotic thickening of the palmar fascia with skin puckering and tethering. Ring and little fingers are chiefly affected. It is often bilateral and symmetrical. As thickening occurs there may be MCP joint flexion. If interphalangeal joints are affected the hand may be quite disabled. Surgery (eg fasciectomy) aims to remove affected palmar fascia and release contractures. As a guide, if he cannot place his palm flat on a flat surface (*Hueston's table-top test*), refer for surgery. There is tendency for recurrence.[29]

Causes/associations
Often multifactorial:
• Genetic (AD)
• Smoking
• Diabetes
• Antiepileptics
• Peyronie's disease
(OHCM p722)

Ganglia These smooth, multilocular swellings are cysts containing jelly-like fluid in communication with joint capsules or tendon sheaths. Treatment is not needed unless they cause pain or pressure (eg on median or ulnar nerve at the wrist, or lateral popliteal nerve at the knee). They may disappear spontaneously. Local pressure may disperse them (traditionally a blow from a Bible!) Aspiration via a wide-bore needle may work, or they may be surgically dissected out, which may give less recurrence;[30] problems include painful scars, neurovascular damage (esp. in palmar wrist ganglia), and recurrence.[31]

De Quervain's disease This refers to stenosing tenosynovitis (thickening and tightening) of the abductor pollicis longus and extensor pollicis brevis tendons (at the anterior border of the anatomical snuff box) as they cross the distal radial styloid. Pain is worst when these tendons are stretched (eg lifting a teapot), and is more proximal than that from osteoarthritis of the 1st carpometacarpal joint. *Finkelstein's sign* is pain elicited by sharply pulling on the relaxed thumb to cause ulnar deviation.[32] *Cause:* Unknown but symptoms can be exacerbated by over use of the tendons (eg wringing clothes). *Treatment:* First try rest (thumb spica splint), ice, and NSAIDs. Hydrocortisone injection at tendon site during the 1st 6 months of symptoms is effective in 90% of patients. If injection (p710) and rest fail to relieve, decompression of the tendons is provided by splitting the tendon sheaths. >80% do well post-op.[33,34]

Trigger finger (tendon nodules) Probably caused by a swelling of the flexor tendon or tightening of the flexor tendon sheath. Ring and middle fingers are most commonly affected, and the thumb especially in babies and children. Swelling of the tendon sheath, along with nodule formation on the tendon, proximal to the A1 pulley (fig 3) prevents the smooth gliding of the tendon. As a result the tendon 'catches' causing the finger to lock in flexion. As extension occurs, the nodule moves with the flexor tendon, but then becomes jammed on the proximal side of the pulley, and has to be flicked straight, so producing triggering. *R:* Simple immobilization is initial treatment of choice: if severe, steroid injection into the region of the nodule may be tried (not if the patient is a child, has renal failure or diabetes). Risk of recurrence is high, so surgery may be needed.[35,36]

Volkmann's ischaemic contracture follows compartment syndrome or interruption of the brachial artery near the elbow (eg after supracondylar fracture of humerus, p740). Muscle necrosis (especially flexor pollicis longus and flexor digitorum profundus) results in contraction and fibrosis causing a flexion deformity at wrist and elbow, with forearm pronation, wrist flexion, thumb flexion & adduction, digital metacarpophalangeal joint extension, and interphalangeal joint flexion. ▶Suspect compartment syndrome if a damaged arm has no radial pulse, and passive finger extension is painful (a crucial sign, p736). *Treatment:* Remove constricting splints, warm other limbs (promote vasodilatation). If pulse doesn't return within 30min, explore the artery. Treating contractures: release of compressed nerves ± tendon lengthening and transfers to restore lost function.[37]

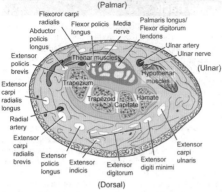

Fig 1. Cross-sectional view of the wrist showing the contents of the carpal tunnel and the extensor tendons of the hand. When trying to describe local anatomy of the hand, it is easier to use the terms *ulnar* and *radial*, rather than medial and lateral, which can cause confusion. *Dorsal* refers to the posterior surface, while *palmar* refers to the anterior surface.[1]

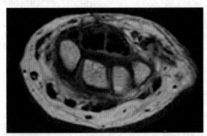

Fig 2. Axial T1-weighted wrist MRI; note labels on fig 1.
© Norfolk and Norwich University Hospitals (NNUH) Radiology Dept.

Flexor tendons pulley mechanisms (fig 3)

In order to stop the long flexor tendons of the hand bowing when the fingers are flexed, the fingers have a number of pulleys (that are well-placed thickenings in the flexor sheath) attached to the bones and volar plates beneath. Named morphologically as either 'A' for annular, or 'c' for cruciate, there are 5 A-pulleys and 3 c-pulleys. The most important are A2 (which is at the proximal end of the proximal phalanx) and A4 (at the middle of the middle phalanx), both of which need to be preserved during any surgery to prevent bowing of the flexor tendons. Sometimes mountaineers, and others hanging on by their fingertips, partially damage the A2 pulley (typically). Stop climbing! Apply ice and buddy-taping/splinting. Then do only light exercises (rubber doughnut squeezes; mild stretches) until 2wks after pain and swelling subside. Visible bowing of the tendon may indicate that surgery is needed; get help ± MRI.

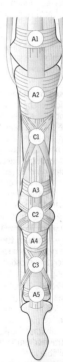

Fig 3 Pulley system.

1 The International Federation for Societies for Surgery of the Hand recommends the term 'palmar' over 'volar'.

History The commonest musculoskeletal complaint is back pain. Attention should be paid to the nature of the pain, exacerbating and relieving factors, and the history of onset. ► It is important to know if bowel or bladder function is affected (signifying cord or cauda equina compression and should set alarm bells ringing: refer at once (MRI in <4h). See MINIBOX, p676, for other sinister symptoms). With low back pain, it is not uncommon for pain to radiate down the leg (sciatica), and may be accompanied by nerve root signs (see below).

Examination With the patient standing and wearing only underwear, inspect the back for abnormality and palpate for local tenderness and deformity. Movements assessed are *forward flexion* (stretch forward to touch toes with knees straight)—look to see how much movement is due to back flexion and how much by flexion at the hips—with back flexion the back has a gently rounded contour. On bending fully forwards, expansion of a line drawn from 10cm above L5 to 5cm below it by <5cm is firm and quantifiable evidence of movement restriction. Look for a rib hump—a sign of scoliosis; *extension* (arch spine backwards); *lateral flexion* (lean sideways so hand moves down corresponding thigh) and *rotation* (keep pelvis fixed but move shoulders round to each side in turn—mostly from the thoracic spine). Movement at the costovertebral joints is assessed by the difference in chest expansion between maximal inspiration and expiration (normal=5cm). Iliac crests are grasped by the examiner and compressed to move sacroiliac joints and see if this reproduces the pain. Compare leg length; quantify discrepancy and muscle wasting (measure thigh and calf circumference). If there are leg symptoms ensure *neurologic assessment* of L4 (knee reflex), L5 (weakness of ankle and great toe dorsiflexion, sensory loss in medial foot and 1st/2nd toe web space) and S1 (ankle reflex, weakness of plantar flexion) roots.

Straight leg raising *Why?* To test for an underlying herniated disc (98% of which will be at the L4–S1 levels) *How?* Keeping the knee extended, lift the patient's leg off the couch and note the angle to which the leg can be raised before eliciting pain. If 30-70°, Lasègue's sign is said to be positive. *Mechanism?* This stretches the sciatic nerve and causes root pain (a characteristic lancinating pain distributed in the relevant dermatome, and made worse by coughing or sneezing). The crossed straight leg raise involves lifting the unaffected leg. If this reproduces pain in the affected side it is said to be positive. It is less sensitive but more specific for an underlying herniated disc. **Alternatively:** sit the patient up in bed with legs out in front. This can be done while examining another system, and may prove pain-free if the patient is not genuine. All these tests may still give false positives and negatives, hence the importance of a good history combined with the examination.[38]

Other parts of the body to examine ► Remember to examine hip joints (p680) and gait. Other relevant areas are the iliac fossae (important in days when tuberculous psoas abscesses were common), abdomen, pelvis, rectum, and major arteries. The commonest tumours to metastasize to bone are: breast, bronchus, kidney, thyroid, and prostate so it may be relevant to examine these.

Tests For acute low back pain seen in primary care, tests are not usually needed in the first 4 weeks. FBC, CRP (infection), ESR (if high, think of metastases or myeloma, and do electrophoresis ± bone marrow aspirate), alkaline phosphatase (high in Paget's disease and tumours), calcium. In the absence of trauma, MRI is the gold-standard imaging investigation and is sometimes available in the primary care setting. Radioisotope scanning is a non-specific investigation, but may reveal 'hot spots' of tumour or pyogenic infection.

On the following pages you can find: • Kyphosis/scoliosis • Causes of back pain • Management of back pain • Specific and sometimes sinister back pain.

Laid flat by a wealth of evidence

Entering the search term 'back pain' in Pubmed delivers 42,099 entries (at the time of writing), with 392 meta-analyses! Holding back throes of exasperation: where do you start, what do you look for, and how can you filter? (See also p636.) Does this wealth of evidence exist because back pain is such a common condition, because there are so many different treatment options, or because we are not yet to be able to offer definitive therapy to our patients? Before embarking on a more targeted search, an answer dawns that it is most likely a combination of all these factors, unfairly pitted against a complex mix of anatomy (just think of the number of structures in the back that can be injured), individuality, susceptibility, cause, tolerability, and treatment efficacy.

As we stand up to the challenge laid down by evolution (and search engines alike), those without back pain can count themselves lucky, while those struck horizontal by our primitive postural problems try not to think of the irony that we are lying in the plane in which our vertebral column originally worked!

Orthopaedics and trauma

Kyphosis is a spinal thoracocervical flexion, sometimes with a lordosis of the lumbar spine. Treat the underlying cause if indicated. NB: congenital kyphosis is much less common than congenital scoliosis, but is more serious, as cord compression and paraplegia sometimes develop rapidly, eg during adolescence.[39]

Causes of kyphosis
• Osteoporosis
• Spina bifida
• Calvé's and Scheuermann's osteochondritis (p702)
• Cancer; wedge fractures
• Tuberculosis; polio
• Paget's disease
• Ankylosing spondylitis

Scoliosis This is lateral spinal curvature with secondary vertebral rotation. The chief cause is idiopathic, and normally involves muscle spasm. Classification:
• Idiopathic (may be infantile, juvenile or adolescent).
• Congenital (failure of formation or segmentation—see BOX, opposite).
• Neuromuscular (neuropathic, eg UMN/LMN lesion or myopathic, eg cerebral palsy or muscular dystrophy).
• Syndromic (eg Marfan's, OHCM p720, or neurofibromatosis, OHCM p518).
• Other (eg tumour, infection, trauma).

Remain in light...
• *Kyphosis:* anterior curvature of the spine (kyphos = hump-backed)
• *Lordosis:* posterior curvature of the spine (lordos = bent back)
• *Scoliosis:* lateral curvature of the spine (skolios = curved)

Idiopathic scoliosis There is lateral curvature (a Cobb angle) of the thoracic or lumbar spine of >10°. It is usually accompanied by a degree of rotation of the spinal column. Adolescent idiopathic scoliosis (AIS) is the most common spinal deformity; girls are more often and more severely affected than boys and the convexity is more commonly to the right. Complications in later life revolve around pain, cosmesis, and impaired lung function. Thoracic problems tend to give more severe deformity than lumbar. Rib deformity causes a characteristic hump on the convex side of the curve which becomes manifest on asking the patient to bend forwards. Curvature increases while the affected person continues to grow, so usually the earlier the onset the worse the deformity.

Since the advent of screening, scoliosis has been detected in 1.5–3%; of these only ~6% progress. The younger the child, and the greater the Cobb angle at presentation, the more the risk of progression—double curves progress more than single curves, and a scoliosis in girls is more likely to progress than one in boys. Thoracolumbar or lumbar curves progress the least. Treatment is needed in 2.75:1000 screened. Where curvatures are >30° and growth is completed, or >20° if growth is in progress, orthopaedic referral is recommended. When curvatures are progressing, attempts to halt it may be made using a Boston or Milwaukee distraction-derotation brace (particularly for double curves, or if the apex of the curve is higher than the 8th thoracic vertebra[1]) until the child is old enough for any spinal surgery that may be indicated. NB: it can be hard to persuade a child to wear a brace for the ≥20h/day that is optimal!—bracing will not correct the deformity but has a role in slowing/preventing curve progression. Surgery involves deformity correction with spinal fusion and stabilization (pedicle screws and longitudinal rods). Intra-operative spinal cord monitoring reduces the most feared post-op complication—paralysis (it now occurs in 0.2%). ►When scoliosis in youth gives pain (especially at night), exclude osteoid osteoma (p699), osteoblastoma, spondylolisthesis (p674), and spinal tumours.

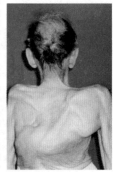
Fig 1. Kyphoscoliosis.

Atlas
Axis

7th cervical
1st thoracic

12th thoracic

1st lumbar

5th lumbar

Coccyx

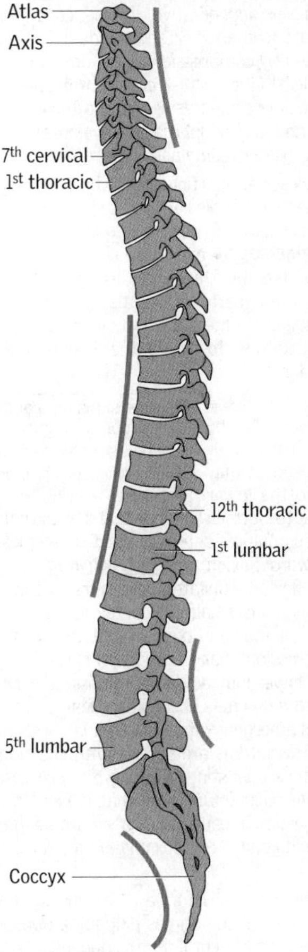

Fig 2. The vertebral column.

During development, the vertebral column initially has a *primary curvature* (anteriorly concave, as for the thoracic and sacral curvatures in red), then goes on to develop *secondary curvatures* in the cervical and lumbar regions (in blue). The normal vertebral body count is 7 cervical, 12 thoracic, 5 lumbar, 5 sacral, and then some coccygeal (3–5). There is some variation, eg L5 can be fused to the sacrum (sacralization) or S1 can be distinct from the sacrum (lumbarization), though total numbers remain constant (even across some mammalian species, especially in the cervical region—eg the giraffe also has 7 cervical vertebrae).[40]

Remember that there are 8 cervical spinal nerve roots, with the C1 root arising from above the C1 vertebra, the C8 root from above the T1 vertebra, and from T1 onwards the root exiting below the corresponding vertebra. This occurs because during development the incipient spinal nerves develop through the embryonic sclerotomes, with the upper part of the C1 sclerotome joining with the last occipital sclerotome to form the base of the occipital bone, and the lower part of the C1 sclerotome forming the C1 vertebra with the upper C2 sclerotome—and so on. Defective induction of vertebral body formation on one side of the body (=hemivertebra) may cause a severe *scoliosis*, and incorrect or absent induction of vertebral arch closure by the neural tube causes the degrees of *spina bifida* (p140).

---

1 Boston braces worn for >18h/day do prevent progression of large curves at a mean of 9.8 years after bracing is discontinued.[41]

Backache is often from low back strain or degenerative disease. *Local pain* is typically deep and aching (from soft tissue and vertebral body irritation). *Radicular pain* is stabbing, and is caused by compression of the dorsal nerve roots, and projects in a dermatomal distribution. *Other causes:* Retroperitoneal (duodenal ulcer, pancreatic cancer, aortic aneurysm; pain is often lumbodorsal and spine movements pain-free and full); neoplasia (eg myeloma); local infection; disc lesions; arthritis; osteoporosis/osteomalacia; renal colic.

Mechanical pain The spine is a complex series of articulations (fig 2, and fig 1 on p673), with spongy discs between vertebral bodies acting as shock absorbers, and a multitude of articulating facet joints. Problems in one part affect function of the whole. Spasm of vertebral muscles can cause significant pain. Upright posture provokes big forces on the spine, eg when lifting, and discs may rupture (if young), vertebrae fracture (elderly) or soft tissues tear (low back strain). NB: with low back strain the exact mechanism may be elusive; if there are no sinister features (▶p676) take time to explain the diagnosis and management; see p676 for imaging guidance.

Disc prolapse (fig 1). Lumbar discs are those most likely to rupture (esp. L4/5 & L5/S1). Typically, one is seized by severe pain on coughing, sneezing, or twisting a few days after back strain (onset may be insidious). Pain may be confined to the lower lumbar area (lumbago), or may radiate to buttock or leg (sciatica) if the herniated nucleus pulposus compresses a nerve root. *Signs:* Forward flexion

Danger signs of cauda equina compression
▸▸Saddle-area sensation↓
▸▸Incontinence/retention of faeces or urine
▸▸Poor anal tone (do PR)
▸▸Paralysis ± sensory loss
▸▸*Do MRI within 4h*

(p670) and extension limited, ± lateral flexion—unilaterally and inconstantly. With L5/S1 prolapse, S1 root compression causes calf pain, weak foot plantar flexion, ↓sensation (pinprick) over sole of foot and back of calf, and ↓ankle jerk. With L4/5 prolapse (L5 root compression), hallux extension is weak and sensation↓ on outer dorsum of foot. If lower lumbar discs prolapse centrally, cauda equina compression (p770, and MINIBOX) may occur. *Tests:* MRI (or CT) if intervention is contemplated—▸▸as an emergency if cauda equina compression is suspected—or if rest fails and symptoms are severe, with CNS signs such as reflex or sensory changes, or muscle wasting. *Treating disc prolapse:* Brief rest and early mobilization + pain relief (p676) is all that is needed in 90% (±physiotherapy). Discectomy is needed in cauda equina syndrome, progressive muscular weakness, or continuing pain.[42] See BOX on p677 for surgical options.

Spondylolisthesis There is displacement (usually forward) of one lumbar vertebra upon the one below (usually L5 on S1, sometimes palpable). *Causes:* Spondylolysis (defect in pars interarticularis of neural arch); congenital malformation of articular processes, osteoarthritis of posterior facet joints (older people). Onset of pain with or without sciatica is often in adolescence ± hamstring tightness and abnormal gait. *Diagnosis* is by plain radiographs. *Treatment* may involve wearing a corset, or nerve release and spinal fusion.

Lumbar spinal stenosis (LSS) and lateral recess stenosis (figs 2 & 3). Facet joint osteoarthritis (the only synovial joints in the back) may produce generalized narrowing of the lumbar spinal canal or simply of its lateral recesses. Unlike the pain of lumbar disc prolapse, this causes: • Pain worse on walking with aching and heaviness in one or both legs causing the person to stop walking (= 'spinal claudication') • Pain on extension. • Negative straight leg raising test. • Few CNS signs. *Tests:* MRI (CT and myelography are less good options). *Treatment:* Canal decompression (removing its posterior wall) gives good results if NSAIDs, epidural steroid injections, and corsets (to prevent exaggerating the lumbar lordosis of standing) fail to help.[43]

Notes on the *cauda equina* (=horse's tail)

The cord tapers to its end, the *conus medullaris*, at L1 in adults. Lumbar and sacral nerve roots arising from the *conus medullaris* form the *cauda equina*. These spinal nerve roots separate in pairs, exiting laterally through the nerve root foramina, providing motor and sensory innervation of the legs and pelvic organs. Compression may be from extrinsic tumours, primary cord tumours, spondylosis, spinal stenosis, achondroplasia, fluorosis, central disc herniation, trauma, spinal subarachnoid haemorrhage, abscess, tuberculoma, or vertebral collapse secondary to malignancy.[44]

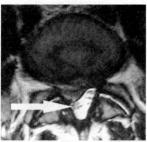
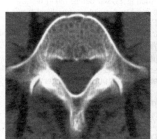

Fig 1. Axial MRI image at the L5/S1 level showing a right-sided paracentral disc prolapse. Observe the displaced nerve roots within the CSF-filled dural sac (arrow). Remember that CSF is white on T2-weighted MRI.

Picture courtesy of Mr Mark Brinsden, FRCS.

Normal lateral recess (3–5mm) · Stenosed lateral recess (<2mm) · Pedicle of L5 · Inferior articular facet of L4 · Superior articular facet L5 · L4 lamina · L4 spinous process

Fig 2. L5 cross-section showing lateral recess stenosis. This is usually caused by degenerative disease of the facet joint, but rarely can be from congenitally shortened pedicles.

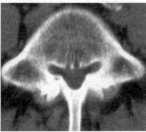

Fig 3. Cross-section CT images at L5, one with spinal stenosis (right). Observe the difference in spinal canal shape and dimensions caused by osteoarthritis of the facet joints posterolaterally. Factors contributing to spinal stenosis: disc prolapse, spondylolisthesis, hypertrophy of the ligamentum flavum. Identify the spinal canal contents at this level, including the thecal sac and the two L5 nerve root sheaths that occupy the lateral recesses.

Images courtesy of Mr Mark Brinsden FRCS.

Orthopaedics and trauma

Back pain is common. 80% of Western people get it at some stage in their lives. 50 per 1000 industrial workers have time off work because of it each year. In the UK it accounts for 11 million lost working days/yr (£3.8 billion/yr in lost production). A GP expects 20 people per 1000 on her list to consult with it each year (only ~10% are referred to hospital). Fewer than 10% of those referred to a specialist need surgery. Physiotherapy may be carried out in hospital or general practice. Most back pain is self-limiting: of those attending GPs, 70% are better after 3 weeks, 90% by 6 weeks, irrespective of treatment. But remember: the cause of back pain can be sinister—cancer, infection, or cord or cauda equina compression—and an approach is needed that detects these promptly. Age is important: only 3% of those aged between 20 and 55 have 'spinal pathology' (eg tumour, infection, inflammatory disease) compared with 11% of those <20yrs, and 19% >55yrs. ▶Pain brought on by activity and relieved by rest is *rarely* sinister. See MINIBOX. Refer those with any suggestion of cord or cauda equina compression (p770), or with deteriorating unilateral signs *at once*. If cancer or infection is suspected, refer promptly. ▶Do FBC, ESR, LFT etc (p670) whenever pain lasts >4weeks, whatever the age.

Backache is sinister if
• ≤20 or ≥55 years old
• Violent trauma
• Alternating sciatica (both legs involved)
• Bilateral sciatica
• Weak legs
• Weight loss
• Fever or unwell
• ESR↑ (>25mm/h)
• Taking oral steroids
• Progressive, continuous, non-mechanical pain
• Systemically unwell
• Drug abuse or HIV +ve
• Spine movement in all directions painful
• Pain unrelated to mechanical events
• Local bony tenderness
• CNS deficit at more than one root level
• Pain or tenderness of thoracic spine
• Bilateral signs of nerve root tension
• Previous neoplasia

Imaging In general, don't do imaging such as CT/MRI before blood tests, and reserve for when symptoms are chronic (ie >4 weeks, unless significant trauma or there are alarm features, see BOX). Plain radiographs correlate poorly with symptoms, and irradiate gonads. ~25% of asymptomatic adults show lumbar degenerative changes on plain films; 50% have coincidental bulging discs.[45]

Treating biomechanical back pain Often hard! 'Get on with your life within the limits of the pain' gives better results than physiotherapy with lateral bending exercises. Avoid bed-rest after the 1st 48h (a board under the mattress helps). Avoid slouching. Advise on how to rise from lying, avoid stooping, bending, lifting, and low chairs.[46,47] *Analgesia* breaks the pain–muscle spasm cycle (paracetamol ≤4g/24h PO, ± NSAID, eg ibuprofen 400mg/8h PO pc or naproxen.[1] Opioids may be needed early. *Warmth* helps, as does swimming in a warm pool. If acute spasm persists, try a *muscle relaxant* such as diazepam 2mg/8h PO for a short while, but warn about side effects (eg drowsiness).[48] *Cognitive therapy in groups* (p372–6) helps tackle unhelpful beliefs about backache and fears about retarting activity. *Antidepressants* can help refractory pain, but not level of functioning.[49] *Physiotherapy* in the acute phase can ↓pain and spasm. In convalesence, use *education* on lifting and exercises to strengthen the back muscles. Many consult osteopaths or physiotherapists or chiropractors for *manipulation*, but studies show that it is unlikely to provide relief beyond that attained from other standard therapies.[50] Referral for epidural anaesthesia, and corsets may help + orthopaedic referral; but note that spinal fusion is no better than intensive rehabilitation.[51]

---

1 cox-2 inhibitors have an uncertain role; heart SE are problematic so don't use in arteriopaths. Naproxen with misoprostol, eg Napratec® is one choice as gastric protection from of misoprostol translates into ↓mortality. ▶Avoid in fertile women. Alternative: nabumetone 1g PO at night; in severe pain 0.5–1g in morning as well; elderly 0.5–1g daily. In one study, the adjusted odds of death for Arthrotec® was 1.4 and 3 for naproxen.[52] Naproxen may be associated with fewer thrombotic events. If current peptic ulcer and NSAID unavoidable, try omeprazole + celecoxib.

Surgery for lumbar disc prolapse

There are a number of procedures that can be performed for the treatment of lumbar disc prolapse:

- **Lumbar microdiscectomy** (fig 1) is the most common procedure, and involves microscopic resection of the protruding disc (nucleus pulposus) from a posterior approach, with the patient anaesthetized in the prone position with lumbar spine flexion. Occasionally the overlying medial facet is partially removed. Complication rate is 2–4% (infection, bleeding, nerve damage).
- **Endoscopic discectomy** (fig 2) is similar in principle to lumbar microdiscectomy, though is less invasive.
- **Laser discectomy** involves radiographically assisted placement of a delivery device into the disc, through which a laser can be introduced to remove disc material.
- **Lumbar disc arthoplasty** (replacement with an artificial disc) is a concept that has been around since the late 1980s, and is becoming more common.[53]
- **Interspinous spacers** relieve pressure that cause the disc to protrude by causing distraction of the spinous processes (= 'dynamic stabilization').[54] Longterm effectiveness is unknown.
- **Chemonucleolysis**, which used to be more common, involves injection of chymopapain (a proteolytic derived from papaya) into the nucleus pulposus—it has been part of practice since the 1960s. There has been controversy surrounding the procedure, with shadows hanging over the efficacy of the techniques and side effects of the agent (eg possible anaphylaxis). It is less invasive than other techniques though is probably less effective than surgical discectomy.[55]

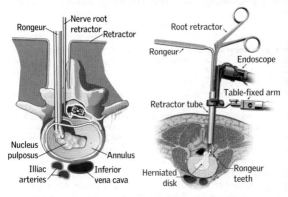

Fig 1. Lumbar microdiscectomy.
Reproduced with kind permission of Dr Aaron Filler; *Do You Really Need Back Surgery?* OUP, 2004.

Fig 2. Endoscopic discectomy.
Kindly provided by Medtronic Sofamor Danek, Inc. METRx® System incorporates technology developed by Gary K. Michelson, MD.[54]

Typical causes of back pain according to age:	
15–30yrs	Prolapsed disc, trauma, fractures, ankylosing spondylitis (*онсм*, p552), spondylolisthesis, pregnancy
>30yrs	Prolapsed disc, cancer (lung, breast, prostate, thyroid, kidney)
>50yrs	Degenerative, osteoporosis, Paget's disease (*онсм* p699), malignancy, myeloma (*онсм* p362); lumbar artery atheroma (which may itself cause disc degeneration)

Rarer causes Spinal stenosis; cauda equina tumours; spinal infection (usually staphylococcal, also *Proteus, E. coli, Salmonella typhi*, TB). Often there are no systemic signs of infection.

Spinal tumours These may be of spinal cord, meninges, nerves, or bone. They may be primary, secondary, lymphoma, or myeloma. They may compress the cord, causing pain, lower motor neurone signs at the level of the lesion, upper motor neuron signs and sensory loss below—or bowel and bladder dysfunction. Peripheral nerve function may be impaired resulting in pain along the course of the nerve, weakness, hyporeflexia & ↓sensation (p762). With cauda equina involvement there is often urinary retention ± saddle anaesthesia (p770). When the deposit is in the spinal canal and there is no bone involvement, there may be no pain, just long tract signs. When bones of the back are involved there is progressive, constant pain and local destruction of bone. Metastases tend to affect cancellous bone, but focal lesions cannot be seen on radiographs until 50% of bone mass is lost. There may be muscle spasm and local tenderness to percussion. Bone collapse may result in deformity, or cause cord or nerve compression. *Tests*: ESR; PSA; electrophoresis (for myeloma); LFT. Plain radiographs; CT; MRI; isotope bone scans; bone biopsy.

In those with past cancer and current back pain, it is best to do a bone scan first (fig 1), with plain radiographs of any hot spots suggesting metastases.

Pyogenic spine infections This is a notoriously difficult diagnosis as all signs of infection may be absent (eg no fever, tenderness, or WCC↑, but the ESR is often↑). It may be secondary to other septic foci. Pain occurs, and movement is restricted by spasm. It is usually an infection of the disc space (discitis). *Risk factors:* Diabetes mellitus, immunosuppression, urinary surgery, or catheterization. Half of infections are staphylococcal; *Streptococcal, Proteus, E. coli, Salmonella typhi* and TB also occur. *Tests:* ESR↑; WCC↑; radiographs shows bone rarefaction or erosion, joint space narrowing ± subligamentous new bone formation. Technetium bone scans and MRI (fig 2) are better. *Treatment:* As for osteomyelitis (p696), resting the back with bed rest, brace, or plaster jacket. Surgery may be needed.

Spinal TB Rare in those born in the West, this tends to affect young adults, giving pain, and stiffness of all back movements. ESR↑. Abscesses and cord compression may occur (Pott's paraplegia). Radiographs show narrow disc spaces and local osteoporosis early, with bone destruction leading to wedging of vertebrae later. In the thoracic spine, paraspinal abscesses may be seen on radiographs, and kyphosis on examination; with lower thoracic or lumbar involvement abscess formation may be related to psoas muscle in the flank, or in the iliac fossa. MRI (not CT) is the ideal way to delineate cord compression. Treatment is anti-TB drugs (eg for 1yr; p160) + abscess drainage. Fixation + bone grafting, or metal rods, plates, or wires needs highly specialized services. If a syrinx (tubular cavity) develops, complete CNS recovery is not expected.[56]

Central disc protrusion This neurosurgical emergency is suggested by bilateral sciatica, perineal or 'saddle' anaesthesia and disturbance of gut or bladder function. ►Prompt decompression may prevent permanent incontinence.

Diagnostic triage: which group encompasses your patient?

Simple lumbar pain:
- Aged 20–55 with 'mechanical' backache, eg caused by twisting and worse on moving
- Patient well in himself; no fevers; no weight loss

Nerve root pain:
- One leg hurting more than the back
- Radiation to foot/toes
- Hip flexion reproduces the pain in leg;
- Localized neurological signs

►For features of potentially sinister back pain, see MINIBOX, on p676.

►Signs demanding immediate (same-day) referral: gait or sphincter disturbance; saddle anaesthesia—these suggest cauda equina compression.

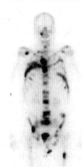

R   L

Fig 1. Bone scan showing multiple metastases from prostatic cancer, including infiltration of the pelvis, ribs, left femur and spinal column.

© University Hospital NNUH NHS Trust.

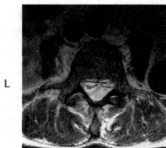

Fig 2. Axial T2-weighted MRI of the lumbar spine showing an epidural abscess in the posterior portion of the spinal canal causing mild stenosis.

© Norfolk & Norwich University Hospital (NNUH) NHS Trust.

Why do some people get intractable back pain?

39% of adults have, or have had, an intermittent chronic back problem, and much energy is expended on frequently fruitless searches for the causes listed opposite. Imaging may be non-specific (subclinical disc protrusion, facet joint arthritis, or minor spondylosis). Risk factors for chronicity:
- Smoking
- Coexisting cardio-respiratory disease
- Psychological morbidity
- Poor work conditions
- Low income/social class
- Number of children (for women *and* men).

Be cautious of blaming sitting at work for chronic back pain. Meta-analyses do not find in favour of this popular association.[57]

Vascular problems may underlie chronicity (hence associations with smoking and heart disease), and pain may be maintained by involvement of the sympathetic chain, which may mediate hyperaesthesia, hyperpathia (excess pain from minor noxious stimuli), allodynia (pain from minor skin stimulation)—but surgical sympathectomy often only provides temporary relief. This implies central neuromodulation of stimuli producing a complex regional pain syndrome. Dorsal horn receptor fields may expand and have their thresholds changed by peripheral injury, so pain is more intense, and appreciated over a wider area than simple anatomy would predict.[58]

The movements examined at the hip are described in fig 1.[59] Internal rotation is often the first movement to be restricted by hip disease.

Questions Are activities of daily living affected?—walking distance, ability to climb stairs (only one at a time possible?), difficulty getting out of low chairs. Remember that pain in the knee may be referred from the hip.

Examination Follow the routine for joint examination (p657); then also perform the following tests.

Measurements Apparent leg length disparity (with the lower limbs parallel and in line with the trunk) is called either 'apparent shortening' (eg due to pelvic tilt or fixed adduction deformity—which gives the apparent shortening on that side) or 'apparent lengthening' (eg due to fixed hip abduction). In these cases, there is no true disparity, as detected by measuring between the anterior superior iliac spine and medial malleolus on each side with the pelvis held square (fig 2) and the lower limbs held equally adducted or abducted or by comparing leg length by positioning the lower limbs perpendicular to a line joining the anterior superior iliac spines.

Fixed deformity Joint or muscle contractures prevent limbs from being put in the neutral position. With fixed adduction deformity, the angle between the limb and the transverse axis of the pelvis (line between both anterior superior iliac spines) is <90° but with fixed abduction deformity it is >90°. Fixed flexion deformity is detected by the *Thomas test:* With the patient supine on an examination couch, flex the good hip up towards the chest until the lumbar lordosis is obliterated (check by finding it impossible to pass a hand between the patient and the couch in the small of the back). If there is a fixed flexion deformity the thigh on the affected side will lift off the couch as the lumbar lordosis is obliterated. NB: to assess the full range of extension, have the patient prone on the table and then extend the hip.

The Trendelenburg test is a test of the function of hip abduction and the ability to support the pelvis when standing on one leg. In this state, it is normal for the pelvis to rise on the side of the lifted leg. A +ve test is when the pelvis falls on the side of the lifted leg. *Causes:* 1 Abductor muscle paralysis (gluteus medius and minimus) 2 Upward displacement of the greater trochanter (severe coxa vara, below, or dislocated hip) 3 Absence of a stable fulcrum (eg un-united fractures of the neck of the femur).

Gait If a hip is unstable or painful, a stick is used on the opposite side (the reverse is true for knees) so as to off-load the hip abductors on the affected side. *Antalgic gait:* Shortening of the stance phase[1] on the painful leg occurs, with quick and short steps. *Short-leg gait:* Discrepancy in length is compensated for by adduction of the long leg at the hip and abduction of the short leg creating pelvic drop, or an *equinus* deformity. *Trendelenburg gait:* A waddling gait caused by weak hip abductors, in which the trunk tilts over the weakened side (can be bilateral) in the stance phase. See *OHCM* p459.

Other joints to examine Spine, knee, sacroiliac joints/pelvis.

Coxa vara (fig 3) This term is used to describe a *hip* in which the angle between the neck and the shaft of femur is less than the normal 125°.

Causes: Congenital; slipped upper femoral epiphysis; fracture (trochanteric with malunion, un-united fractures of neck of femur); due to softening of bones (rickets, osteomalacia, Paget's disease). *Consequences:* True shortening of limb; Trendelenburg 'dip' on walking makes the affected person limp.

---

1 The *stance phase* of gait starts when the forward foot foot makes contact with the ground. Then there is loading, mid- and terminal stance (+preswing)—before the shorter *swing phase* starts.

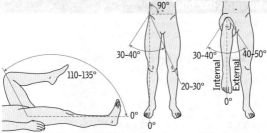

Fig 1. Ball and socket (eg the hip) joints have 3 axes of movement: flexion–extension (left); ab- & adduction (middle); and external & internal rotation. External rotation of the ball in the socket is achieved by movement of the shin across the midline, as in the diagram (40°–50°). After trauma, a hip at rest in external rotation is likely to be fractured; if internally rotated dislocation is more likely. These abnormal positions occur because of the change in the fulcrum of the force across the hip joint from the iliopsoas muscle (which inserts on to the lesser trochanter of the femur).

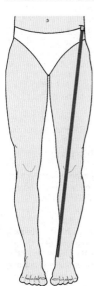

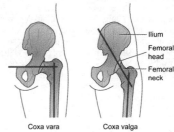

Fig 3. Coxa vara (L) and coxa valga (R).

Fig 2. Measuring leg length: from the anterior superior iliac spine to the medial malleolus.

▶When a child complains of pain in the knee, always examine the hip. ▶Is T°↑? If so, do urgent blood culture ± ultrasound-guided aspiration.

Differential diagnosis
You must rule out:
• Septic arthritis
Then consider:
• Tubercular arthritis²⁻⁵ʸʳ
• Perthes' disease⁴⁻⁷ʸʳ
• SUFE¹⁰⁻¹⁶ʸʳ
• Inflammatory arthritis
And by exclusion:
• TSOH

Transient synovitis of the hip (TSOH; irritable hip) is the chief cause of hip pain in children. It is a diagnosis of exclusion (exclude: septic arthritis; Perthes' disease; and slipped upper femoral epiphysis). Examine the hip clinically and investigate with plain films (figs 1 & 2), FBC, ESR/CRP. Ultrasound is helpful (fig 3), and can guide needle aspiration when pus is suspected, so obviating need for arthrotomy.⁶⁰ Admission for observation, rest and analgesia (eg ibuprofen) may be needed.⁶¹ If other joints are involved, consider juvenile idiopathic arthritis (p654).

Perthes' disease (Legg–Calvé–Perthes' disease: fig 5) This is osteochondritis of the femoral head and affects those aged 3–11yrs (typically 4–7). It is bilateral in 10–15%. ♂:♀≈4:1.⁶² The disease process is likely secondary to avascular necrosis of the developing femoral head.⁶³ It presents with pain in hip or knee and causes a limp. On examination all movements at the hip are limited, especially internal rotation and abduction. Early radiographs ± MRI show joint space widening. Later there is a decrease in size of the femoral head with patchy density. Later still, there may be collapse and deformity of the femoral head with new bone formation. Severe deformity of the femoral head risks early arthritis—40yrs post diagnosis, ~40% will have a joint replacement. The younger the patient the better the prognosis (due to increased ability to remodel). For those with less severe disease (<½ the femoral head affected on lateral radiographs, and joint space depth well preserved) treatment is bed rest and NSAIDs until pain-free, followed by radiographic surveillance. If prognosis poorer (>½ femoral head affected, narrowing of total joint space) surgery may be indicated.⁶⁴

Slipped upper femoral epiphysis (SUFE)¹ Affects those aged 10–16yrs. 20% are bilateral. ♂:♀≈3:1. About 50% of patients are obese. There is displacement through the growth plate with the epiphysis always slipping down and back. The exact cause is unknown, though it is likely to be a combination of hormonal and bio mechanical factors. It usually presents with limping and pain in the groin, anterior thigh, or knee. Can the patient weightbear (stable) or not (unstable)? This is important in predicting the risk of complications.⁶⁵ Flexion, abduction, and medial rotation are limited (eg lying with foot externally rotated). Δ: anteroposterior (fig 1) + frog-leg lateral radiographs of both hips. Treatment, regardless of severity, is stabilization across the physis. Reduction first may improve function and reduce likelihood of further surgery, but may increase the risk of avascular necrosis (AVN).⁶⁶ If untreated, consequences may be avascular necrosis of the femoral head or malunion predisposing to arthritis.⁶⁷ ▶Symptoms may be mild so have a high index of suspicion if in correct age group. If occurring in those <10 or >16yrs, then consider an endocrinopathy, eg hypothyroidism, hypogonadism or growth hormone imbalance.

Tubercular arthritis This is rare in the UK, but worldwide there is a resurgence of TB. Children aged 2–5yrs and the elderly are most commonly affected. The symptoms are pain and a limp. All hip movements cause pain and muscle spasm. *Tests:* An early radiographic sign is rarefaction (↓ bone density). Later there is fuzziness of joint margins and narrowing of the joint space. Later, bony erosion may be seen. Ask about contacts. Check ESR, CXR, and Mantoux test (*OHCM* p398). Synovial membrane biopsy confirms the diagnosis of TB arthritis. *Treatment (eg of hip):* Rest + anti-TB drugs (p160), given by experienced personnel. Arthrodesis may be needed if much joint destruction has occurred.

1 It may be that unrecognized SUFE can cause later osteoarthritis of the hip.

Orthopaedics and trauma

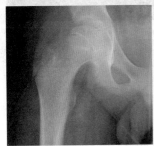

Fig 1. AP radiograph of the right hip showing a SUFE. The changes are subtle, but note that a line (the line of Klein) drawn along the upper edge of the femoral neck in **fig 2** would intersect the femoral head, but would not in **fig 1**. More reliable, though even harder to appreciate, is the widening of the physis—most prominent at the lateral edge.

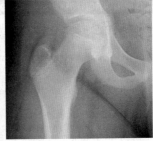

Fig 2. Normal AP radiograph of the right hip. Practice your saccadic eye movements between the two to appreciate the slip downwards and medially.

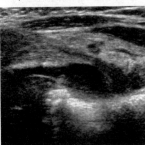

Fig 3. Hip US, showing joint effusion—the low reflectivity (black) area superficial to the femoral neck and head.

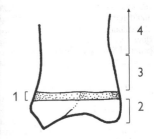

Fig 4. Bones such as the femur grow from a cartilaginous growth plate called a *physis* (1); the end of a bone beyond the growth plate is called the *epiphysis* (2); the shaft of a long bone is called the *diaphysis* (4); the ossified portion of bone in a transitional zone between the epiphysis and diaphysis is called the *metaphysis* (3) and it should always have a smoothly curved cortex. The diaphysis continues (arrow) to the metaphysis at the other end of the bone. The stem, *-physis*, comes from the Greek for 'growth'. An *apophysis* is a bony outgrowth independent of a centre of ossification. Epiphyseal injuries are covered on p737.

Image by Tom Turmezei.

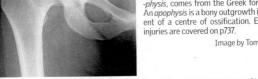

Fig 5. Right hip radiograph showing modelling deformity of the femoral head, consistent with prior Perthes' disease.

Figures 1, 2, 3 and 5 Courtesy of Norfolk and Norwich University Hospital (NNUH) Radiology Department.

DDH refers to a spectrum of pathology from stable acetabular dysplasia to established hip dislocation. It has replaced the term congenital dislocation of the hip (CDH). A world-wide systematic review (in unscreened populations) estimated prevalence of diagnosed DDH at 1.3 per 1000.[68] UK incidence: 2 per 1000 live births. ♀:♂≈6:1; left/right hip incidence≈4:1; bilateral in ⅓.

At-risk babies:
• Breech birth
• Caesar for breech
• Other malformations
• Positive family history
• Birth weight↑
• Oligohydramnios
• Primip/older mother
• Postmaturity

Diagnosis Identify all those infants at risk (see MINI-BOX). If high risk, infant should have ultrasound at 2–4 weeks, with treatment instigated by 6 weeks if required. All babies should have their hips examined in the 1st days of life and at 6 weeks.[1] Detection of DDH is user dependent, but improves with training and guidance.[69] The Ortolani and Barlow manoeuvres (fig 1) detect unstable hips, but will both be negative in an irreducible dislocated hip, so use other tests as well (see BOX p685). ►Be alert to DDH throughout child surveillance (p150) as a hip may be normal at birth, and become abnormal later. Early diagnosis is important as if appropriately aligned in the first few months of life, a dysplastic hip may normalize.

Ultrasound is the imaging of choice, up to 4.5 months, as it is non-invasive and dynamic. In a large series (Nottingham, UK) 40:1000 babies had evidence of instability on routine ultrasound screening; only 3:1000 required treatment. However, routine ultrasound screening for DDH remains controversial, on account of the high rate of spontaneous resolution of dysplasia and instability combined with the lack of definitive data on functional outcome of interventions.[70,71]

Treatment If neonatal examination suggests instability arrange ultrasonography. Hips that remain unstable at 6 weeks require prompt treatment. Typically treatment involves splinting in flexion-abduction in an orthosis known as the Pavlik harness.[72] Excess abduction (in splint) may cause **avascular necrosis** of the head of femur—the worst possible outcome of treatment. *From 6–18 months* examination-under-anaesthetic, arthrography and closed reduction are performed followed by a period of immobilization in a *spica* hip bandage (*spica* refers to the pattern of bandaging, from the Latin for an 'ear of corn'), as the harness is less than 50% successful beyond 6 months of age. Open reduction is sometimes required if closed techniques fail. *After 18 months* (delayed presentation) open reduction is required with corrective femoral/pelvic osteotomies to maintain joint stability.[73]

Club foot

Neonatal club foot is also known as *talipes equinovarus*. ♂:♀ >1:1; bilateral in 50%. The foot deformity consists of: 1 Inversion; 2 Adduction of forefoot relative to hindfoot (which is in varus); 3 Equinus (plantarflexion) deformity. The foot cannot be passively everted and dorsiflexed through the normal range. The preferred treatment, starting as early as possible, is now the **Ponseti method**,[74] in which the foot is manipulated and placed in a long leg plaster cast (which aims to correct the forefoot adduction and hindfoot varus deformity) on repeated occasions. It is important that deformity correction is *gradual*. If this does not work, operations on soft tissues and/or bones of the foot may be carried out later (from 2 years). Associated with myelomeningocoele, arthrogryposis and prune belly syndrome.

---

1 The importance behind picking up DDH is that for a hip to develop normally the femoral head must articulate with the acetabulum. Failure to identify the problem early means that there is no development of the acetabulofemoral joint, posing real problems for any prospect of surgical correction.

Orthopaedics and trauma

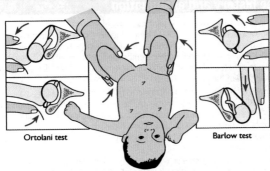

Fig 1. Hip tests: the Ortolani test and the Barlow manoeuvre.

Hip tests for DDH

Ortolani manoeuvre This test relocates a subluxed or partially dislocated hip. With the child's hips flexed and abducted, place your fingers on the greater trochanter and try to lift up the femoral head and relocate it into the acetabulum. The test is positive when there is a palpable 'clunk' as the hip relocates. The test will be negative if there is an *irreducible* dislocation.

Barlow manoeuvre This test aims to sublux or dislocate an unstable hip. Start with hip flexed and adducted slightly. Gently apply axial load to the femur and try to dislocate the femoral head with the thumb. The test is positive when the femoral head is felt to dislocate; this action may be accompanied by a 'clunk'. Beware repeated Ortolani and Barlow manoeuvres which may induce instability.

Galeazzi test Looks for apparent shortening of femur caused by dislocation of femoral head. The child lies supine on an examination table with the hips flexed, the feet flat on the table, and the ankles touching the buttocks. The test is positive when the knees are at different heights. This test will be negative if both hips are dislocated as there will be no apparent discrepancy.

Other signs Unequal leg length and asymmetrical groin creases may also suggest DDH (although not present in bilateral cases). Other signs include a widened perineum and buttock flattening on the affected side. If child is >3 months old, limited abduction (<60°) of hip whilst in flexion may be the most sensitive test for DDH.[75] In older children signs may be: delay in walking and abnormal waddling gait (affected leg is shorter). With bilateral involvement the lumbar lordosis is increased.

The knee is the largest human joint in terms of volume and surface area of cartilage and is most susceptible to injury, age related wear, inflammatory arthritis and septic arthritis. It consists of a hinge joint between the femur and tibia. The patella is a sesamoid bone embedded in the quadriceps tendon. It articulates with the trochlear groove of the femur and increases the mechanical advantage of the quadriceps.

History Is non-traumatic pain intrinsic to the knee (localized knee pain/with weakness/limited range of movement/effusion) or referred (vague pain ± radiation from hip or back). If traumatic ask about mechanism of injury, noises (clicks/pops/crunching), swelling (and how rapidly it developed), direct impact to the knee, inability to weight bear, locking (meniscal injury), and giving way (cruciate injury).

Examination Examine supine with legs fully exposed. Look for alignment, quadriceps wasting and for swelling. Even 5-10mL of fluid will 'fill in' the medial and lateral peripatellar dimples giving the knee a general fullness. Confirm by placing the palm of one hand above the patella over the suprapatellar pouch, and thumb and forefinger of the other hand below the patella. Fluid can be moved between the two by squeezing one hand, then the other. If >15mL fluid is present it may be possible to feel a *patellar tap* (milk fluid towards centre of knee then ballott patella against the anterior surface of the femur). Palpate the medial and lateral joint lines (for osteoarthritis/meniscal/plateau injuries), the patella, the popliteal fossa and femoral condyles.

Check active and passive movement. Flexion should be enough for the heel to touch the buttock. Compare extension with the 'good' side. Check to see no evidence of crepitus or 'locking'. Ensure patella tendon is intact by examining active knee extension/straight leg raise.

Examine the *medial* and *lateral collateral ligaments* with the knee flexed 20°-30° (to relax the posterior capsule and the cruciate ligaments); one hand lifts the ankle, the other stabilizes the knee. Stress the knee by abducting the ankle while pushing the knee medially with the hand behind the knee (tests the *medial* ligament with a *valgus* stress force). Reverse the pressures to give adducting force to test *lateral* ligament (ie *varus* stress). If these ligaments are torn the knee joint opens more widely when the relevant ligament is tested (compare knees against each other, as general laxity may be present).

Test the *cruciate ligaments* (figs 1 & 3) with the knee 90° flexed (anterior/posterior drawer tests) and at 20° of flexion (Lachman's test). The *anterior* cruciate ligament prevents *anterior* glide; the *posterior* prevents *posterior* glide. Excessive glide in one direction (compare knees again) suggests damage to the relevant ligament. A more sensitive test to determine if symptoms are really due to cruciate ligament damage (which can be asymptomatic) is the 'pivot shift test'.[1]

McMurray's rotation test is an unreliable way of detecting pedunculated *meniscal tears*. With the knee flexed, the tibia is laterally rotated, then the knee is extended. This is repeated with varying degrees of knee flexion, and then again with the tibia medially rotated on the femur. The test is designed to jam the free end of a pedunculated meniscus in the joint—a click being felt and heard and pain experienced by the patient as the jammed tag is released as the knee straightens. This test may not detect bucket-handle tears (p754). NB: normal knees often produce patellar clicks. Simply eliciting joint-line tenderness may be a more valid test when combined with a history of mechanical locking.

Arthroscopy enables internal structures of the knee to be seen and a definite diagnosis may be made. It also enables a wide range of operations to be done as day-case surgery. This is routinely preceded by MRI.

1 This is so-called because it was found to be positive in patients (eg American Football players) who reported to their surgeon that "When I pivot (on my leg) something shifts".

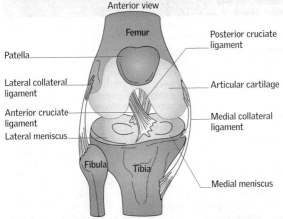

Anterior view

Femur

Patella

Posterior cruciate ligament

Lateral collateral ligament

Articular cartilage

Anterior cruciate ligament

Medial collateral ligament

Lateral meniscus

Fibula Tibia

Medial meniscus

Fig 1. The anatomy of the right knee—as seen from in front. The medial collateral ligament is much broader than the lateral ligament, and its deep fibres are firmly attached to the medial meniscus. The lateral ligament and the lateral meniscus are interposed by the popliteal tendon (see **fig 2**), and hence are not connected.

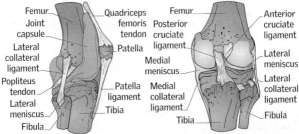

Femur

Joint capsule

Quadriceps femoris tendon

Femur

Anterior cruciate ligament

Posterior cruciate ligament

Lateral collateral ligament

Patella

Medial meniscus

Lateral meniscus

Popliteus tendon

Patella ligament

Medial collateral ligament

Lateral collateral ligament

Lateral meniscus

Tibia

Fibula

Fibula

Tibia

Fig 2. The synovium of the right knee joint: lateral (left) and posterior views. Note that the synovium extends up behind the patella (remember for joint aspiration, p708), and that both cruciate ligaments are extrasynovial (but are intracapsular). NB: the joint capsule is distended in these images by infusion of fluid.

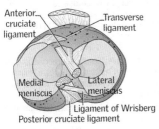

Anterior cruciate ligament

Transverse ligament

Medial meniscus

Lateral meniscus

Ligament of Wrisberg

Posterior cruciate ligament

Fig 3. Tibial plateau and ligaments. Note that on the tibial plateau the attachments in the midline from anterior to posterior are:
• Tranverse ligament
• Anterior horn of medial meniscus
• Anterior cruciate ligament
• Anterior horn of lateral meniscus
• Posterior horn of lateral meniscus
• Posterior horn of medial meniscus
• Posterior cruciate ligament.

The common symptoms are anterior knee pain or pain and swelling. Anterior knee pain can be due to many causes (see below).

Patellofemoral pain syndrome (PFPS) Is common in young athletes—especially runners—and may be associated with overuse as well as lower limb malalignment and patella tracking abnormalities. Patella aching is felt after prolonged sitting or on climbing stairs. There may have been a recent increase in sporting activity or trauma—especially history of patella subluxation/dislocation. Effusion is rare. Medial retropatellar tenderness and pain on patellofemoral compression occur: +ve Clarke's test = pain on patellofemoral compression with tensed quadriceps muscles. There may be either decreased or increased patella mobility. *Diagnosis* is clinical. *Treat* by relative rest—if due to increased training, with structured rehabilitation. Quadriceps strengthening exercises are the mainstay of treatment, but many will benefit from hip strengthening exercises as well.[76] Reasonable results are also reported with electrical stimulators.[77] NSAIDs may only be effective in reducing pain for a few months.[78] If symptoms last >1yr, arthroscopic lateral retinacular release may be tried. Shaving the posterior surface of the patella gives uncertain results.

Bipartite patella (figs 1 & 2) is a congenital fragmentation of the patella, found in ~1%. This is usually an incidental radiographic finding (not to be interpreted as a fracture pattern), but may give pain if the superolateral fragment is mobile with tenderness over the junction. Extra fragment excision may relieve pain.[79]

Recurrent patella subluxation A tight lateral retinaculum causes the patella to sublux laterally, giving medial pain. The knee may give way. It is commoner in girls and with valgus knees. It may be familial, or associated with joint laxity, a high-riding patella (*patella alta*), or a hypotrophic lateral femoral condyle. *Signs:* Increased lateral patellar movement, accompanied by pain and the reflex contraction of quadriceps (ie a +ve patellar apprehension test). Contralateral instability and young age at time of initial subluxation are risk factors for chronic recurrence.[80] Treatments vary (RCTs are needed). If vastus medialis exercises fail to help, lateral retinacular release with medial soft tissue realignment may be of benefit.[81] Patellar tendon transfer is rarely needed.[82]

Patella tendinopathy (jumper's knee) is usually initiated by micro- or macro patella tendon tears, eg associated with sudden sporting loads. It can occur anywhere in the patellar tendon, and settles with rest ± NSAIDs. If unable to rest, steroid injection around (not into) the tendon may help. Eccentric contraction exercises (tension whilst lengthening the muscle) may also help.[83]

Iliotibial tract syndrome Typically presents with lateral knee pain and tenderness over lateral femoral epicondyle. Thought to be due to overuse and associated with movement of the iliotibial tract (thickened lateral edge of the tensor fascia lata) and the lateral femoral epicondyle. Common in runners, it usually settles with sport modification, rest, ice, and NSAIDs, but may need steroid injection[84] and hip adductor strengthening.[85]

Medial shelf syndrome The synovial fold above the medial meniscus is inflamed. Pain is superomedial. There may be brief locking of the knee (mimicking a torn meniscus). *Diagnosis:* Arthroscopy. *Treatment:* Rest, NSAIDs, local steroid injection, or division of the synovial fold arthroscopically.

Hoffa's fat pad syndrome This is impingement of the infrapatella fat pad. Think of it in those with meniscus or ligament-type symptoms when imaging shows they are intact. MRI may show a hypertrophic Hoffa pad impinging between articular surfaces (which causes pain under the patella). There may be hydrarthrosis or haemarthrosis (from arteriole rupture). Extending a bent knee while putting pressure on the patellar tendon margins elicits pain and a defensive behaviour.[86]

'All these hags'

Once, after a stay in hospital with a fracture, a patient who was not quite as deaf as she was supposed to be, told one of us (JML) how she had overheard a newly arrived orthopaedic surgeon say to the ward nurse "What are we going to do with all these hags?". As he progressed down the ward, turning first to the left and then to the beds on the right, his mood became morose, then black—as if he was getting angry that all these 'hags' were clogging up his beds, preventing his scientific endeavours. But what was really happening, my patient suspected, was that, as he turned to left and right, he was really nodding goodbye to his humanity, and, dimly aware of this, he was angry to see it go. On this view, these rows of hags were like buoys in the night, marking his passage out of our world. We all make this trip. Is there any way back? The process of becoming a doctor takes us away from the very people we first wanted to serve (Captain Pollard syndrome, p652). Must medicine take the brightest and the best and turn us into quasi-monsters?

The answer to these questions came unexpectedly in the months that followed: sheer pressure of work drove this patient's observations out of my mind. It was winter, and there was 'flu. In the unnatural twilight of a snowy day I drifted from bed to bed in a stupor of exhaustion with a deepening sense of a collapse that could not be put off...It was all I could do to climb into bed: but when I awoke, I found I had somehow climbed into a patient's bed, who had kindly moved over to make space for me, and was now looking at me with concern in her eyes. Herein lay the answer: the hag must make room for the doctor, and the doctor must make room for the hag: *we are all in the same bed*.

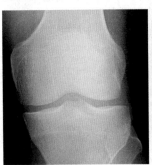

Fig 1. Bipartite patella at the usual position of the superolateral edge.

Figs 1 & 2 courtesy of Norfolk and Norwich University Hospital (NNUH) Radiology Department.

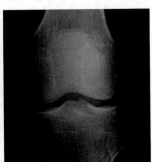

Fig 2. The same image as fig 1, but 'windowed' to make the lesion more obvious (the bean-sized fragment is between 1 and 2 o'clock). This has been one of the major advantages of digitized image viewing.

Other causes of anterior knee pain

Chrondromalacia patellae, where there is softening of the articular cartilage of the patella.

Loose bodies Variable symptoms, may have locking, effusion, intermittent sudden pain associated with movement.

Osgood–Schatter disease Adolescent patients with tenderness at tibial tubercle (see p704).

Prepatella bursitis *(housemaid's knee)* Swelling anterior to patella, typically occurs following trauma or overuse (see p690).

Orthopaedics and trauma

Arthritis Knee swelling may occur with any arthritic process. *Primary osteoarthritis (OA)* can be defined as degeneration of the articular cartilage and surfaces of a joint with no predisposing factors—in this sense, the disease is idiopathic, though current research is suggesting many of these cases have subtle underlying congenital/developmental defects. In *Secondary OA* there is an underlying precipitant to the degenerative process (see MINIBOX). OA is associated with ↑BMI, genetic factors, age and occupation. Patients complain of pain on initiating movement. Stiffness follows inactivity, but often resolves in <30mins. In the knee, OA particularly affects the posterior patella and the medial compartment, so tending to varus deformity. *Treatment:* NSAIDs, knee support (Tubigrip®), weight loss, local steroid injections, knee replacement (p706), or osteotomy (to correct varus deformity). Some may benefit from augmentation of the synovial fluid within the joint with hyaluronan (see BOX).[1] ▸Remember that a unilaterally swollen knee may be a septic arthritis. Diagnosis is made on the basis of aspiration, so avoid steroid injections prior to this (p708). ▸*Aspiration of a replaced joint must be done under sterile conditions in theatre.*

Secondary OA causes
• Post traumatic
• Post-operative
• Post-infective
• Malposition
• Mechanical instability
• Osteochondritis dissecans (below)

Meniscal cysts *Typical patient:* A young man, with past trauma, then insidious development of cyst. *Pain:* Over the joint line. Lateral cysts are 5–10× more common than medial. Swelling may disappear with full flexion. The meniscus is often torn radially (an otherwise unusual direction) so there may be knee clicking and giving way. Δ: MRI. *Treatment:* Arthroscopic decompression.[87]

Ligament tears, meniscus lesions, patellar dislocation See p754.

Osteochondritis dissecans Subchondral bone becomes avascular, and may progress to fragments of bone and overlying cartilage (osteochondral fragments) breaking away from the bone to form loose bodies. *Cause:* Unknown. *Typical site:* Lateral side of the medial femoral condyle. *Typical patient:* 13–21-year-olds.[88] *Symptoms:* Pain after exercise with intermittent knee swelling. Locking may occur. *Imaging:* MRI reveals articular surface defects/loose bodies *Treatment:* Stable lesions are treated conservatively, as spontaneous healing can occur. Unstable fragments may be pinned in place. Loose bodies may be removed and the defect drilled to promote fibrocartilage formation.[89]

Loose bodies cause knee locking (all movements may be jammed unlike locking from torn menisci when only extension is limited). Also, there is effusion/swelling. *Diagnosis:* Plain films ± US (helps show if fragments are intra-articular).[90] ΔΔ: Tophi (gout).[91] *Causes:* Osteochondritis dissecans (≤3 loose bodies), osteoarthritis (≤10 loose bodies), chip fractures of joint surfaces (≤3 loose bodies) or synovial chondromatosis (>50 loose bodies). When locking is a problem, loose bodies are best removed—eg arthroscopically.

Bursitis ~16 bursae surround the knee. Most commonly affected are: the *prepatellar bursa* ('housemaid's knee') where swelling over the anterior inferior patella is due to inflammation and fluid in the bursa due to friction (kneeling); the *infrapatellar bursa* ('clergyman's knee'—they kneel more upright); and the *semimembranous bursa* in the popliteal fossa (a popliteal cyst which differs from the 'Baker's cyst' which is a herniation from the joint synovium). Prepatellar bursae may be aspirated, have hydrocortisone injected to decrease recurrence. If very persistent it may need excision. Pain may be relieved by topical NSAIDs. Aspiration distinguishes friction bursitis from suppurative bursitis, which needs drainage and antibiotics, eg flucloxacillin 250mg/6h PO (adults).

---

1 This technique involves a 5-week course (2mL/wk) of high molecular weight intra-articular hyaluronan derivatives (eg Synvisc®). Any effusion is drained to dryness. A 5-week course may be repeated at 6 months. See BOX OPPOSITE for efficacy.

NB: knee OA is the commonest joint disease in Europe (fig 1).
• Women (especially if >55yrs old) are at greater risk.[92]
• Weight loss in women reduces risk of getting OA symptoms.[93 n=796]
• *Paracetamol* (±tramadol) & *quadriceps-strengthening* exercises can help.[94]
• Trials comparing *NSAIDs* are often flawed because the drugs compared tend not to be used in comparable doses, as expressed as a fraction of the maximum daily dose.[95 16 trials] *Topical ibuprofen* may be as good as oral in older patients, and has fewer SE.[96]
• There seems to be benefit from *intra-articular steroid injections* in the short term, but long-term results are unclear.[97] Some trials report benefits which only last a week or so.[98 N=98]
• *Hyaluronan* is a physiological substance found in synovial fluid that gives lubrication and protection to articulating surfaces. Cochrane meta-analyses suggest that intra-articular injection of hyaluronan (visco-supplementation) has a role in the therapy of knee osteoarthritis, providing pain relief and improved functionality for periods longer than steroid injection. There are a number of available formulations, though analysis limitations meant that no singular one could be recommended above the others.[99 % trials]

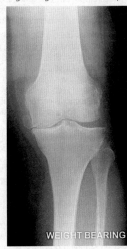

WEIGHT BEARING

Fig 1. Degenerative change of OA in the left knee. Note *genu varus* deformity, and how the medial compartment is most affected.
Courtesy of Norfolk & Norwich University Hospital (NNUH) Radiology Dept.

• *Transcutaneous electrical nerve stimulation (TENS)* for knee osteoarthritis is a noninvasive modality in physiotherapy. Different modes of TENS setting (high rate and strong burst mode) show significant benefit in relief of pain and stiffness over placebo.[100]
• While *exercise* is known to have beneficial effects in knee osteoarthritis, improving both functionality and pain, the appropriate intensity level of exercise regime remains unclear and open to further investigation.[101]
• *Knee replacement* (p706) is often the treatment of choice. However, 21% of patients are still getting knee pain one or more years post-op. Significant complications include preventable thromboembolism. Intermittent pneumatic compression devices and low molecular weight heparin are significantly better than warfarin and aspirin in preventing DVT. Incidence of asymptomatic PE: 11.7% for aspirin, 8.2% for warfarin, and 6.3% for pneumatic compression group. (Numbers of symptomatic PEs are too small to produce reliable statistics.)[102 23 trials]
• Post-operative aseptic loosening and other problems requiring revision are a problem in 9% over 5yrs for unicompartmental prostheses (7% over 4yrs for bicompartmental prostheses). Serious infections may be less in those centres doing many procedures.[103]

Ankle and foot examination 25° of extension (dorsiflexion) and 30° of flexion (plantarflexion) are the norm at the tibiotalar joint. Inversion and eversion are from the subtalar and midtarsal joints. Toes should have between 60° and 90° extension. Note any callosities. Examine the arches (fig 1). Watch as the toes are lifted off the ground, and on standing on tiptoe. Examine gait and shoes (normal wear pattern is medially under ball of foot, posterolaterally at heel).

Hallux valgus The big toe deviates laterally at the metatarsophalangeal joint (fig 2). Associated with genetic predisposition, female gender, age, type of footwear and BMI. Pressure of the metatarsophalangeal joint against the shoe leads to bunion formation. Secondary arthritis in the joint is common. Bunion pads and plastic wedges between great and second toes may relieve pain, but severe deformity requires surgery. Many different operations are used. Generally, the deformity is corrected with a metatarsal osteotomy—up to ⅓ are unsatisfied with the result.[104] End-stage MTP joint OA (*Hallux rigidus*) is treated with arthrodesis (joint fusion).

Pes planus (flat feet) The medial longitudinal arch (fig 1) collapses—leading to the whole sole (or near to it) coming in contact with the ground. Flat feet are normal when a child is learning to walk. The medial arch develops over the next few years. In adults flat feet are associated with dysfunction of the posterior tibialis tendon (PPT) (a dynamic stabilizer of the medial arch). In most, it is asymptomatic and may not need intervention if the arch restores itself on standing on tiptoe (ie a 'mobile' flat foot). Pain may develop medially over the PPT

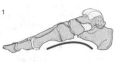
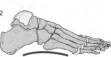

Fig 1. The medial (1) and lateral (2) longitudinal arches of the foot.

and there may be progressive forefoot abduction and hindfoot valgus deformity with loss of ability to heel rise, as the condition progresses. Weight loss, supportive shoes (with insoles), orthosis may help in mild cases.[105] Prevention: studies of feet in India show that going barefoot until 6 years old keeps feet healthy. Pain and limitations in sport tend to be post-op complications (eg after the Viladot procedure), so don't advise surgery lightly.[106]

Pes cavus Accentuated longitudinal foot arches which do not flatten with weight-bearing. May be idiopathic, or associated with an underlying neurological condition (see MINIBOX). Claw toes may occur, as weight is taken on metatarsal heads when walking (hence causing pain). *Other symptoms:* Difficulty with shoes; foot fatigue; mobility↓; ankle instability/sprains; callosities. **If foot used to be normal, refer to a neurologist.**

Pes cavus associations
• Spina bifida
• Cerebral palsy
• Polio
• Muscular dystrophy
• Charcot–Marie–Tooth dis.
• Syringomyelia
• Friedreich's ataxia
• Spinal tumour

MRI may help establish any underlying disease. If orthoses and custom footwear fail, surgical procedures include (if vascular supply is good) soft-tissue releases, tendon transfers, arthrodesis.[107]

Lesser toe deformities
1 *Hammer toes:* These are extended at the MTP joint, hyperflexed at the PIP joint and extended at the DIP joint. Second toes are most commonly affected.
2 *Claw toes:* Extended at the MTP joint but flexed at both PIP and DIP joints. The operative treatment for both hammer and claw toes is metatarsal shortening (flexible deformity) or PIP joint arthrodesis (fixed deformity).
3 *Mallet toes:* Flexion deformity of the DIP joint in isolation treated with flexor tenotomy (flexible deformity) or DIP joint arthrodesis (fixed deformity).

Classification of severity of hallux valgus deformity

	Hallux valgus angle (HVA)	Intermetatarsal angle (IMA)
Normal	<15	<9
Mild	15–20	9–11
Moderate	20–40	11–18
Severe	>40	>18

NB: sources vary in definitions.

Surgery may be problematic. Mild and moderate deformities may be corrected with a distal metatarsal osteotomy (eg Mitchell's or Chevron osteotomy). Severe deformities also require correction of the intermetatarsal angle (eg Scarf osteotomy).[104,108]

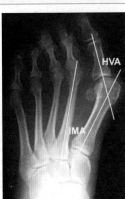

Fig 2. Weightbearing AP image showing a hallux valgus deformity and the hallux valgus angle (HVA) and intermetatarsal angle (IMA).

Courtesy of Professor Peter Scally.

Footnotes in History

By the time we get down to the foot, our anatomical interest is flagging, but on close inspection '*we would never have believed, my dear José, that so much glory could fit into a shoe*'.[Gabriel García Marquez 1989, The General in His Labyrinth] Feet made for walking are really quite old—some 4–7 million years, according to Sterkfontein Man's remains.[1] The significant thing about these old feet is that they can and did take us anywhere. We started off swinging from tree to tree in an African forest, and began quite a journey on foot that has taken us not only to the furthest reaches of our own world, but also to another—with some extra help. And how long will those historical footprints last on the moon? Perhaps another few million years.[109]

▸Look at a wet footprint and wear on the shoe sole to assess functional anatomy of the loaded foot. Many of the conditions mentioned in 'the foot' (p692) can be painful. Other causes of pain are mentioned here.

Young children rarely complain of foot pain: if in the sole think of a foreign body. Shoe pressure on a prominent navicular bone, or sometimes an accessory bone, or a prominent posterosuperior *os calcis* may need surgical trimming. Osteochondritis (p702) of foot bones may be the cause (do radiography).

Metatarsus primus varus 1st metatarsal midline angulation. Typical patients: teenagers. It may be familial. If deformity is great, a metatarsal or wedge osteotomy may be tried.[110] Tarsal bone coalitions can also cause pain.

Ingrowing toenails Typically the big toe. Incorrect nail cutting ± pressure of shoes predispose to the lateral nail digging into its fleshy bed, which reacts to becoming heaped up infection-prone 'proudflesh'. *Conservative treatment* involves tucking cotton-wool soaked in surgical spirit under the proudflesh and awaiting nail growth (then cut it straight with edges protruding beyond flesh margins). Antibiotics may help the young.[111] Recurrent infections may need surgery. *Nail avulsion* plus *chemical matrixectomy* (with phenol or sodium bicarbonate) to the nail bed is better than simple avulsion[112] (but there may be more post-op infection.[113]

Adult forefoot pain (metatarsalgia) Increased pressure on the metatarsal heads causes pain. *Treatment:* insole supports, surgery other than for rheumatoid arthritis is unpredictable. Other causes include synovitis, sesamoid fracture, and traumatic injury.

Morton's metatarsalgia Pain is from pressure on an interdigital neuroma between the metatarsals (eg from fashion shoes). Pain usually radiates to the lateral side of one toe, and the medial side of its neighbour (eg toes 3 & 4). A compression test of the affected web space is quite specific. MRI helps, and ultrasound if by an experienced worker.[114] Neuroma excision may be needed.[115]

March (stress) fractures occur in the shaft of the 2nd or 3rd metatarsals and may follow excess walking. Radiographs may be normal, or have subtle periosteal changes: the history should raise suspicion and prompt a scouring search of the metatarsi. Radionuclide bone scans are more discriminating. Treatment is rest and analgesia. If pain is severe, try a plaster cast while awaiting healing.

Pain in the heel *Causes:* (✓ means *may* respond to steroid injection)
- Diseases of the calcaneum
- Rupture of calcaneal tendon (p712)
- Postcalcaneal bursitis (back of heel)
- Plantar fasciitis ✓ [1]
- Lymphoma (in children)
- Arthritis of the subtalar joint
- Calcaneal paratendinopathy ✓
- Tender heel pad ✓
- Infection.

MRI may have a role in undiagnosed heel pain (eg from occult stress fractures).[116] Apart from calcaneal diseases and tendon rupture, conservative treatment (eg shoe alteration to prevent rubbing) may help. If not, with postcalcaneal bursitis the bursa may be surgically removed.

Corns Focal friction-dependent hyperkeratotic intradermal nodules develop bony pressure points (eg the top of hammer toes, fig 1), which stop keratinized skin cells coming to the surface. A bursa-like structure may form around these islands. Likelihood↑ if neuropathy eg diabetes. Unlike calluses they have a core of keratin, occur only on the foot, and cause pain.[117] *Management:* Optimize footwear (not too tight or loose, ± an instep); chiropody (± softening with salicylic acid) or excise the corn (try to remove its core without causing bleeding). More radically, remove the culprit bone too (eg hammer toe condylectomy).[118]

---

1 If proximal planar fasciitis doesn't respond to injections, extracorporeal shockwave therapy is a reasonable alternative to surgery.[119]

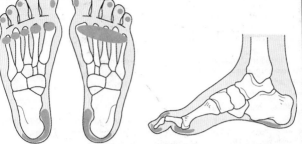

Fig 1. Pressure points in a foot with hammer toe.

Talus and Talos—a better grasp of what we are looking at

It can be difficult to identify and orientate a bone (or indeed any anatomical structure) in isolation—a flashback for some to an old-style anatomy viva. Building up a picture of what you are looking at using context can make the task easier. This context can be provided by a number of means, for example by using a combination of imaging, anatomy prosection and dissection, and functional techniques.

The aim is to bring anatomy to life in our own minds as close to that which we see in our patients before us, almost as if constructing a mental animation. In the 1963 film, *Jason & the Argonauts*, Ray Harryhausen famously animated articulated skeleton warriors (grown from the teeth of the Hydra by King Aeëtes of Colchis) in a feat of which most students of anatomy would be jealous. In the same film, Harryhausen also animated the bronze automaton Talos (not to be confused with the talus, fig 2), forged by Hephaestus as a gift from Zeus to Europa, queen of Crete. Although there are many permutations to classical myth, in the film version Jason slays Talos by dislodging a bolt in his heel that caused exsanguination of the ichor from the single vein that ran from his neck to his heel—perhaps reflective of the understanding of anatomy and physiology in those ancient times.

The Left Talus

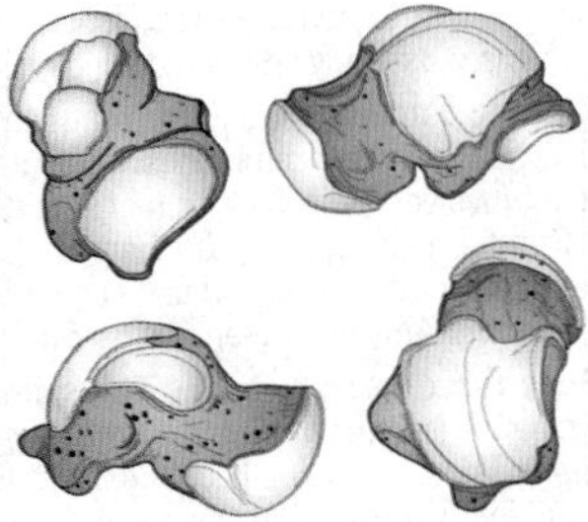

Fig 2. The talus bone of the foot—not easy to identify or orientate in isolation. Which view is which?[1]

So, although every student will have their own methods of learning anatomy, the process of study may be helped by thinking of animation—or even *'anatimation'*—and not just the stationary. Technology has come a long way from 1963, with the development of excellent aids, tools and resources that can enhance the learning of anatomy, eg at www.anatomy.tv and www.e-anatomy.org.

[1] Top left = inferior view; top right = lateral view; bottom left = medial view; bottom right = superior view.

This is an infection of bone. Its incidence reduces as living standards rise. It can be categorized as acute haematogenous, secondary to contiguous local infection (with or without the presence of vascular disease), or vertebral (see below). All forms can progress to chronic osteomyelitis.[120] Infection may spread from boils, abscesses, pneumonia, or genitourinary instrumentation, though often no primary site is found.

Common organisms
• *Staphylococcus aureus*
• *Pseudomonas*
• *E. coli*
• Streptococci
Other organisms
• *Salmonella* (esp. with sickle cell disease)[121]
• *Brucella*[122]
• *Proteus/Klebsiella*[123,124]
• Mycobacteria
• Fungi[125]

Clinical features See BOX, opposite.

Tests ESR/CRP↑, WCC↑. Blood culture (+ve in 60%). Bone biopsy and culture is gold standard—but rarely required for acute osteomyelitis. Swabs from discharging sinuses may give misleading results.[126] Radiographic changes are not apparent for 10–14 days but then show haziness ± loss of density of affected bone, then subperiosteal reaction, and later, sequestrum and involucrum (see BOX, OPPOSITE & figs 1–3). NB: infected cancellous bone shows less change. MRI is sensitive and specific (88% and 93%, vs 61% and 33% for isotope scans)—and avoids ionizing radiation, but isotope scans are still sometimes required (eg in presence of prostheses causing imaging artefact).[127]

Treatment Drain abscesses and remove sequestra by open surgery. Culture all sequestra. Antibiotic: vancomycin 1g/12h and cefotaxime 1g/12h IVI until the organism and its sensitivities are known. Continue for 6 weeks. Alternative treatments for

Complications
• Septic arthritis
• Fractures
• Deformity
• Chronic osteomyelitis

adults are fusidic acid or clindamycin. Ciprofloxacin 500mg/8–12h PO is suitable for *Pseudomonas* osteomyelitis, but be guided by sensitivities and a microbiologist. In children, prevalence of *Haemophilus influenzae* osteomyelitis is reducing due to the HIB vaccination.[128]

Chronic osteomyelitis Poor treatment results in pain, fever, and sinus suppuration with long remissions. Radiographs show thick irregular bone. Treatment involves radical excision of sequestra (infected dead bone), skeletal stabilization, 'dead-space' management (often needs plastic surgical input) and antibiotics (as above, modified according to sensitivities) for ≥12 weeks. *Complications:* Amyloid, squamous carcinoma development in sinus track.

Bone TB (eg vertebral body = Pott's disease).[129] This represents 1–3% of all TB; incidence is rising, rare in UK. Spread is haematogenous or via nearby nodes. *Signs:* Local pain, swelling, and 'cold abscess' formation ± joint effusion are common. With joint involvement there is pain, swelling, pain on movement and muscle wasting. Also: weight↓; malaise; fever; lethargy. *Differential diagnoses:* Malignancy; other infections; gout; rheumatoid. *Imaging:* Radiographic changes: bone rarefaction (=reduction in density/solidity), periostitis changes, cyst formation. Later there is loss of joint space, erosions and bony ankylosis. Also look for soft tissue swellings (abscess; tenosynovitis/bursitis). MRI is especially useful in analysing soft tissue changes. Bone scans may be useful in diagnosing dactylitis (a feature of childhood TB). One recent meta-analysis showed PET to be superior to all other forms of imaging, with a sensitivity of 96% and a specificity of 91%.[130] *Other tests:* Aspirated pus is creamy and may be positive on culture or ZN stain; ESR↑; Mantoux +ve; CXR; HIV tests. *Treatment:* Drain abscesses, immobilize affected large joints. Standard 6-month courses (OHCM p386) of eg isoniazid (300mg/day), rifampicin (600mg/day) and pyrazinamide (1.5g/day) may not be long enough. Late arthroplasty or arthrodesis is needed for gross joint destruction.[131]

Orthopaedics and trauma

Patterns of infection Cancellous bone is typically affected in adults—commonly in vertebrae (IV drug use) and feet (diabetics); in children, vascular bone is most affected (eg in long-bone metaphyses—esp. distal femur, upper tibia). Infection leads to cortex erosion, with holes (*cloacae*). Exudation of pus lifts up the periosteum interrupting blood supply to underlying bone and necrotic fragments of bone may form

Risk factors
• Diabetes
• Vascular disease
• Impaired immunity
• Sickle cell disease
• Surgical prostheses
• Open fractures
• Impaired immunity

(*sequestrum*). The presence of sequestra is typical of chronic infection. New bone formation created by the elevated periosteum forms an *involucrum*. Pus may discharge into joint spaces or via sinuses to the skin.

The patient Pain of gradual onset over the course of a few days—with tenderness, warmth, and erythema at the affected part; unwillingness to move; slight effusion in neighbouring joints; signs of systemic infection. All signs are less marked in adults.

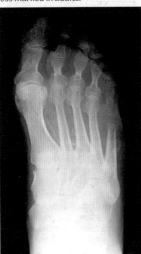

Fig 1. Osteomyelitis causing destruction of the 5th metatarsal head and the base of the 5th proximal phalanx. Note also the vascular calcification in this patient, who had diabetes.

Images courtesy of Norfolk and Norwich University Hospital (NNUH) Radiology Department.

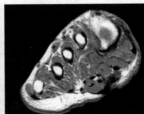

Fig 2. Axial T1-weighted MRI of the foot through the metatarsals, showing reduced signal within the first metatarsal (from replacement of the marrow fat with pus) consistent with osteomyelitis.

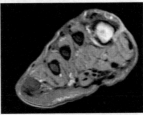

Fig 3. Axial T1-weighted MRI of the same patient as fig 2, this time with FAT SAT (fat saturation) and IV gadolinium contrast. The effect of this technique is to suppress the marrow fat and enhance the infection.

Orthopaedics and trauma

Tumours present with pain, swelling or pathological fracture. Bone is a common site for secondaries (eg from breast, bronchus, prostate, kidney). Primary bone neoplasia is rare: incidence of 9 per million population/year.[132] Delays in diagnosis are common. Metastases are blood-borne and usually arise in the lungs or other

Radiological features
• Bone destruction
• New bone formation
• Soft tissue swelling
• Periosteal elevation

bones. Staging is done with MRI or combination techniques such as PET-CT.[133] Treatment of these rare and highly aggressive primary tumours is best carried out in multidisciplinary specialist treatment centres.

Osteosarcoma is the most common malignant primary bone tumour.[1] Primary osteosarcoma typically affects adolescents and arises in the metaphyses of long bone, especially around the knee. Secondary osteosarcoma may arise in bone affected by Paget's disease or after irradiation. *Radiography:* Bone destruction and new bone formation, often with marked periosteal elevation (sunray spiculation and Codman's triangle, respectively). *Treatment:* Resection + chemotherapy, eg doxorubicin, cisplatin and methotrexate.[134] A cure rate of ~60-70% is achievable.[134]

Giant cell tumour Rare tumour—characterized by multinucleated giant (osteoclast like) cells—hence also called osteoclastoma. This histologically 'benign', primary skeletal neoplasm, with unpredictable biological aggressiveness, is commonest in 20-44-yr-olds.[135] It occurs around epiphyses (esp. knee). The tumour is osteolytic and often slowly progressive, sometimes resulting in pathological fracture. *Treatment* is by detailed and thorough curettage resulting in 75% cure. Recurrences are usually treated by wide excision.

Ewing's sarcoma This malignant round-cell tumour of long bones (typically diaphysis) and limb girdles, usually presents in adolescents. Radiographs show bone destruction, concentric layers of new bone formation ('onion-ring' sign) and a soft tissue mass. MRI is helpful. Typically those with Ewing's sarcoma have a t11:22 chromosomal translocation. *Treatment:* Chemotherapy, surgery and radiotherapy are required. The key adverse prognostic factor is metastases at diagnosis (5-year recurrence-free survival is 22%—vs 55% if no metastases at diagnosis).[136]975

Chondrosarcoma may arise *de novo* or from malignant transformation of chondromas. It is usually associated with pain or a lump and presents in the axial skeleton of the middle-aged. 'Popcorn calcification' is typical on radiography. MRI/CT will better define tumour extent. *Treatment:* It doesn't respond to chemotherapy or radiotherapy, so treatment is by excision. Inadequate surgery is accompanied by local recurrence, often of a higher grade of malignancy. The cure rate depends on the type and grade of chondrosarcoma at diagnosis.

Malignant fibrous histiocytoma is the rarest primary bone tumour. It arises in middle age, often at the site of a previous bone abnormality (eg bone infarcts). Treatment is as for osteosarcoma.

Chordomas arise from notochord remnants in the spine and are typically sacral, and quite big before a diagnosis is made. Bladder & bowel sphincter problems may occur. Radical surgery + pre-op radiotherapy cure <20%. The others may have a slow and difficult death.[137]

Surgical reconstruction (after excising a bone tumour) may involve replacing affected bone with a metal and polyethylene endoprosthesis—as an alternative to amputation. Excellent and durable reconstruction is possible using massive endoprostheses or bone allografts. 85% of patients now have limb salvage following chemotherapy for primary bone tumours.

---

1 There are many different subtypes, including intramedullary, periosteal, parosteal & telangiectatic.

Osteochondroma is the commonest benign bone tumour, usually occurring about the knee, proximal femur, or proximal humerus. Presents as a painful mass associated with trauma. Seen on x-ray as a bony spur arising from the cortex and usually pointing away from the joint. *Treatment:* Remove if causing symptoms, eg pressure on adjacent structures. Any osteochondroma continuing to grow after skeletal maturity must be removed because of risk of malignancy (arises rarely in solitary osteochondromas but in up to 10% of patients with hereditary multiple exostoses—an autosomal dominant inherited condition).

Osteoid osteoma is a painful benign bone lesion that occurs most commonly in long bones of males 10–25yrs old (and also often in the spine). It appears as local cortical sclerosis on radiographs with a central radiolucent nidus. Within the nidus there may be a small nucleus of calcification The nidus produces prostaglandins leading to pain unrelated to activity, and relieved by aspirin (and other prostaglandin inhibitors) *Treatment:* CT guided biopsy and radiofrequency ablation.[138] NB: in young adults, any bone pain responding to aspirin within 15min could be caused by an osteoid osteoma. Plain radiographs may miss these tumours. CT is the best imaging modality.[139]

Chondroma These benign cartilaginous tumours may arise from bone surfaces or within the medulla (=enchondromata). They may cause local swelling or fracture. *Treatment* is rarely needed, except to exclude malignancy (chondrosarcoma—see OPPOSITE). NB: Carney's syndrome is gastric leiomyosarcoma, plus pulmonary chondroma plus a non-adrenal paraganglioma.[140]

Fibrous dysplasia of bone is a developmental abnormality where bone is not properly formed. May lead to pain and increased risk of fracture. Surgical stabilization is sometimes needed. In the polyostotic form bisphosphonates may help relieve symptoms.

Soft tissue sarcomas (STS)[1]

STS are uncommon (~1500/yr in UK) but can arise in any mesenchymal tissue, originating from fat, muscle etc, presenting as a painless enlarging mass. Risk factors include neurofibromatosis type 1 (*OHCM*, p518) and previous radiotherapy. *Diagnosis:* Any lump that has any feature from

Consider STS malignant if
• Bigger than 5cm
• Increasing in size
• Deep to the deep fascia
• Painful

the MINIBOX is to be considered malignant until proved otherwise. *Imaging* with MRI followed by needle biopsy at a specialist sarcoma unit is recommended. Pathological diagnoses include rhabdo-myosarcoma (most common in children), liposarcoma, leiomyosarcoma, fibrosarcoma etc. Gene expression profiling is helping to improve diagnosis and indicate tumours which may respond to chemotherapy. *Treatment* is by excision with wide margins followed by radiotherapy for most. Alkalylating agents: trabectedin has a role.[1] Most adult STS are not sensitive to other chemotherapy but it may be used for metastatic disease. *Prognosis* is related to histological grade, size and depth of the tumour. High-grade, large, deep tumours have <50% 5yr survival. STS in children often respond well to chemotherapy; survival is better.

Gastrointestinal stromal tumours (GIST)

GIST is an easy-to-misdiagnose submucosal sarcoma arising chiefly in the upper GI tract. It is the commonest GI mesenchymal neoplasm. *Treatment:* Surgery. ~50% recur and spread to liver. Imatinib can help.[141]

---

1 NICE have advised on care of soft tissue sarcoma: www.nice.org.uk/page.aspx?o=csgsarcoma.[142]

Osteogenesis imperfecta (OI) is an inherited disorder of type I collagen that results in fragile, low density bones. It affects 1 in 20,000. OI has historically been classified into four forms (although type IV, the most diverse, has recently been expanded into types IV–VII).

I	The mildest and most common form. It is autosomal dominant. Associated with blue sclerae (due to increased corneal translucency) and 50% have hearing loss. Fractures typically occur before puberty. There is a normal life expectancy.
II	Lethal perinatal form with many fractures and dwarfism; it is recessive.
III	Severe form—occurs in about 20%. Recessive. Fractures at birth + progressive spinal and limb deformity, with resultant short stature; blue or white sclera; dentinogenesis imperfecta common (enamel separates from defective dentine, leaving teeth transparent or discoloured); Life expectancy is decreased.
IV	Moderate form, autosomal dominant. Fragile bones, white sclerae after infancy.

Radiographs: Many fractures, osteoporotic bones with thin cortex, and bowing deformity of long bones. *Histology:* Immature unorganized bone with abnormal cortex. *Treatment:* Prevent injury. Physio, rehab and occupational therapy are key. Osteotomies may correct deformity. Intramedullary rods are sometimes used in long bones. Medical treatments include bisphosphonates Current research is looking at the possibility of gene therapy.[143]

Achondroplasia is the most common form of *dis*proportionate short stature. It occurs due to reduced growth of cartilaginous bone It is autosomal dominant, but ~80% are from spontaneous mutation. 95% are caused by mutation in the gene encoding fibroblast growth factor receptor type 3 (FGFR3).[144] Affected babies have large heads (>97th centile) with ventriculomegaly and frontal bossing, normal trunk length, short limbs, and fingers all the same length. Gross motor skills develop later—only 50% sit unsupported at 9 months, and only 50% walk alone at 18 months.[144] Condition specific growth charts are available to monitor development.[145,146] Adults are short with ↑lumbar lordosis, bow legs, and short proximal arms & legs. Lifespan, mental & sexual development are normal. Complications include tibial bowing, joint hypermobility, hydrocephalus, foramen magnum compression (5–10%), recurrent otitis media and hearing loss, sleep apnoea (75%) and ↑BMI *Radiographs:* Short proximal long bones (rhizomelic shortening) & wide epiphyses. *Treatment:* Involves monitoring for potential complications. Growth hormone has been tried.[147]

Hereditary multiple exostoses (HME ≈ diaphyseal aclasia) is an autosomal dominant disorder in which certain proteins accumulate in the Golgi apparatus leading to cartilage-capped tumours (exostoses/osteochondromata) developing from affected cartilage at the end of long bones. These point away from the nearby joint. If severe, bones are broad and badly modelled, causing short stature as well as forearm, knee, and ankle deformity. Beware of malignant transformation to chondrosarcomas[2] or osteosarcomas. HME is usually caused by defects in various EXT genes which encode enzymes catalysing synthesis of heparan sulfate, an important component of the extracellular matrix. *Treatment:* Removal of symptom-producing exostoses.[148]

Osteopetrosis Lack of differentiation between cortex and medulla of bone (from underlying failure of osteoclastic bone resorption) results in very hard dense 'marble' bones that are brittle. Anaemia and thrombocytopenia may result from decreased marrow space. Deafness and optic atrophy can result from compression of cranial nerves. Lack of remodelling preserves variations of ossific density causing the characteristic 'bone within a bone' appearance.

---

1 See Neurofibromatosis (OHCM p518), Marfan's (OHCM p720), Ehlers–Danlos & Morquio's, p143.
2 *Cartilage tumour classification:* Is the lesion benign or malignant? Is the lesion a pure or impure cartilaginous tumour? Is the epicentre of the lesion intraosseous, juxtacortical, or in the soft tissues? The most common benign tumours are enchondroma, osteochondroma, chondroblastoma, and chondromyxoid fibroma. Chondrosarcoma is malignant.[149]

Developmental bone biology

Because bone is ossified, we tend to think of it as the architectural rock around which our living tissues are constructed. But bone maintenance and development is a highly dynamic and regulated process sensitive to a wide variety of hormones, inflammatory mediators, growth factors, and genetic influences which become aberrant whenever there are deletions, insertions, and missense mutations.[150] The concept of a *master gene* is useful to indicate how genes relate and interact. Master genes encode proteins that can control other genes by directly binding to their DNA, for example, transcription factor OSF2 (osteoblast specific transcription factor 2) gene is thought to serve as a master gene regulating expression of other genes, allowing mesenchymal stem cells to differentiate into osteoblasts. OSF 2 maps close to a chromosomal locus on chromosome 6P21 (thought to be important eg in craniocleidodystosis). NB: master genes make a mockery of genes *vs* environment questions. One gene is an environment for another, and the effects of each may be catastrophic in some environments or negligible in others.

Remain in light...the different types of bone

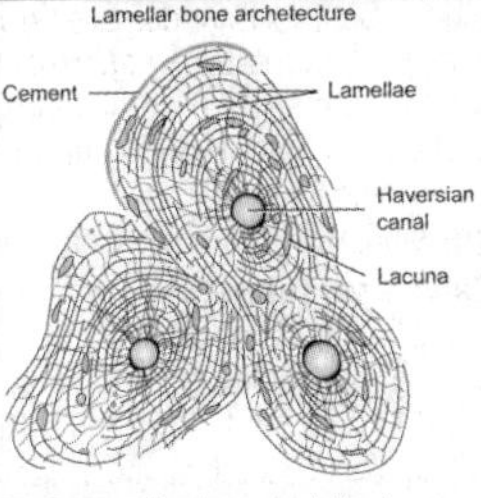

- *Cancellous* Trabeculations form a network of parallel lamellae, the spaces being filled with connective tissue or bone. This type of bone does not make callus when healing; also called 'spongy' bone.
- *Cartilagenous* Formed from growth plates (p683).
- *Compact* Non-cancellous bone that is formed from Haversian canals and concentric lamellae.
- *Cortical* The superficial thin layer of compact bone.

Fig 1. Lamellar bone architecture.

- *Endochondral* Develops in cartilage that has been destroyed by calcification and subsequent resorption.
- *Heterotopic* Forms outside the normal skeleton either from a pathological process (eg in the heart) or as a reaction to local trauma/surgery.
- *Lamellar* The overall normal type of adult bone (subdivided into cancellous and compact), characterized by repeating architectural patterns—fig 1.
- *Membranous* Formed from intramembranous ossification (eg clavicle).
- *Sesamoid* Bone formed in a tendon where it passes over a joint (eg the pisiform bone in flexor carpi ulnaris, and the patella).
- *Woven* Embryonic bone in which the connective tissue fibres are arranged and interlaced irregularly.

Remain in light...The different types of joint

- *Cartilagenous, primary* Hyaline cartilage between the bone ends. Only types are the costochondral and sternochondral (1st rib) joints.
- *Cartilagenous, secondary* As above, but with a layer of fibrocartilage between the layers of hyaline cartilage. Only types (that all lie in the midline) are the manubriosternal, intervertebral, pubic symphysis, xiphisternal and sacrococcygeal joints.
- *Fibrous* Fibrous tissue between bones; eg radio-ulnar interosseous membrane.
- *Synovial* Joint cavity containing synovial fluid, with hyaline cartilage on the bone surface; eg acetabulofemoral, glenohumeral.
- *Synovial, atypical* Joint cavity containing synovial fluid, with fibrocartilage on the bone surface ± a fibrocartilage disc; eg acromioclavicular and sternoclavicular joints (with discs). NB: fibrocartilage is found on the articulating surface of any bone that undergoes intramembranous ossification.

The osteochondroses are a group of conditions characterized by the abnormal endochondral ossification of epiphyseal growth during childhood. Osteochondrosis (also called osteochondritis) occurs in the wrist, elbow, hip, knee, ankle, fingers, toes and spine. The underlying cause of most osteochondroses is unknown, although inheritance, overuse/trauma, rapid growth and anatomic configuration may be predisposing factors. All osteochondroses undergo an interuption of blood supply to the epiphysis, followed by bone and cartilage necrosis, revascularization and regrowth of bone

Scheuermann's disease The commonest cause of kyphosis in 13–16-yr-olds. It is an autosomal dominant. The normal ossification of ring epiphyses of several thoracic vertebrae are affected. Deforming forces are greatest at their anterior border, so vertebrae are narrower here, causing kyphosis. During the active phase, vertebrae may be tender. Patients appear round shouldered and 'hunched'—they tend to present for deformity rather than pain. *Radiographs:* Irregular vertebral endplates, Schmorl's nodes ± disc space ± anterior wedging. 3 adjacent vertebral bodies of at least 5° of wedging is pathognomonic. Schmorl's nodes are herniations of the intervertebral disc through the vertebral endplate. *Treatment:* If posture control (eg standing during lessons rather than sitting) and exercise (eg swimming) fails, physiotherapy ± spinal braces can help, though curvature may recur over time after discontinuation of bracing. Surgery may be tried for severe kyphosis (>75°) with curve progression, refractory pain, or neurological deficit.[151]

Calvé's vertebra Presents with symptoms similar to Scheuermann's disease but in a younger age group (typical age is 2–10yrs). Unlike Scheuermann's disease is not due to ischaemic necrosis but to eosinophilic granulomata (detected via CT guided biopsy)—thus it is not a true osteochondrosis. Typical site is a thoracic vertebra; if cervical/atlas, torticollis may result. *Symptoms:* Pain ± tenderness over the affected vertebra; slight kyphosis. *Imaging:* Radiographs/CT/MRI can show dense, flattened vertebral body with disc space preserved; bone scans can show a hyperactive spot. *ΔΔ:* Sarcoma; osteomyelitis. *Treatment:* Bed rest ± plaster cast immobilization.

Kienböck's disease Affects male adults 20–40 years. Pain is felt over the lunate (esp. during active wrist movement). Grip is impaired due to pain. Associated with negative ulnar variance. *Radiographs:* Dense lunate with a little depth reduction early; more marked flattening later, leading later to osteoarthritis. *Treatment:* Early: manage symptomatically with splinting and analgesia; early + sufficiently symptomatic: ulnar lengthening or radial shortening, capitates shortening; late + symptomatic: proximal row carpectomy, intercarpal arthrodesis, total wrist arthrodesis.[1] Once arthritis is established, lunate excision does not help. Wrist arthrodesis is the last resort.

Panner's disease/Osteochondritis dissecans (OCD) of the elbow represent a continuum of disease of the capitellum. Panner's disease is the avascular necrosis of the ossific nucleus of the capitellum. Mostly presents in boys under 10yrs, causing lateral elbow pain and swelling. Conservative managment is usually all that is required. OCD of the elbow affects the surface below the cartilage of the anterior capitellum. A loose body is formed (1–3cm across) from a convex joint surface when a segment of subchondral bone and cartilage becomes avascular and separates from underlying bone. Adolescents experience early aching and effusions after use, and sudden painful locking of joints once pieces have separated to make loose bodies. *Radiographs:* Lucent areas in a piece *about* to separate, the defect from which the piece *has* separated, and loose bodies *after* separation. *Treatment:* Stable lesions are managed conservatively in a hinged brace. Unstable lesions may need fixation ± removal of loose bodies. Closed wedge resection may lead to revascularization.[152]

The navicula is the bone at the top of the foot and is separated from the metatarsals by the 3 cuneiform bones with which it articulates. Moving proximally, it articulates with the talus. Navicula is Latin for a small ship.

Köhler's disease Children affected are 3–5-yr-olds. Pain is felt in the mid-tarsal region and they limp. There may be navicular tenderness. *Radiographs:* Dense, deformed bone (fig 1). *Treatment:* Symptomatic: resting the foot or wearing a walking plaster. *Prognosis:* Excellent, with very few longterm problems.[138]

Freiberg's disease (infraction) This may be classed as an osteochondritis dissecans of the lesser metatarsal heads, most commonly the 2nd. It presents as forefoot pain, that worsens with pressure, usually starting around the time of puberty. There may be microfractures at the junction of the metaphysis and the growth plate—precise aetiology is unknown. *Radiographs:* Epiphysis of a metatarsal head becomes granular, fragmented and flattened. *Treatment:* Good shoes ± metatarsal pad. Limit activity for 4–6 weeks. If severe, consider removal of affected bone with bone grafting or interpositional arthroplasty and use of a walking plaster.

Eponyms of osteochondroses

Eponym	Site affected
Friedrich disease	Clavicle
Froelich disease	Humeral condyles
Panner's disease (p702)	Capitellum of humerus
Kienböck's disease (p702)	Lunate bone (in adults)
Scheuermann's disease (p702)	Vertebral ring epiphyses
Perthes' disease (p682)	Hip
Blount disease	Proximal tibial epiphysis
Osgood–Schlatter disease (p704)	Tuberosity of the tibia
Sinding–Larsen disease (p704)	Secondary patellar centre
Köhler's disease (above)	Navicular bone
Sever's disease (p704)	Calcaneal apophysis
Freiberg's disease (above)	Head of 2nd or 3rd metatarsal

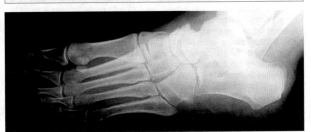

Fig 1. Oblique radiograph of the left foot, showing sclerosis and deformity of the navicula, secondary to Köhler's disease.[1]

Images courtesy of Norfolk and Norwich University Hospital (NNUH) Radiology Department.

1 Patients with Kienbök's disease who avoid surgery tend to change profession, whereas surgery often results in being unable to return to the previous occupation.

Osgood–Schlatter's syndrome (OSS) is tibial tuberosity apophysitis that affects children 10–15yrs old. ♂:♀≈3:1. The 'accepted theory' suggests that repeated traction causes inflammation and chronic avulsion of the secondary ossification centre of the tibial tuberosity, leading to inflammation, hence its association with physical overuse. The pain below the knee is worse on strenuous activity and quadriceps contraction (lift straight leg against resistance). The tuberosity looks enlarged and is tender. OSS is self-limiting in >90% of cases. *Radiographs:* Tibial tuberosity enlargement (± fragmentation). Note the appearance of a normal immature tibial tuberosity, fig 1. MRI shows the tendonitis. NB: diagnosis is clinical, not simply radiological. *Treatment:* Standard treatment is limitation of activity, ice, oral anti-inflammatories, knee padding and physiotherapy. Plaster cast immobilization is now uncommonly used as it leads to quadriceps wasting—short-term immobilization in a brace is occasionally used.[153] Tibial tubercle excision may be recommended if the above fail.[154]

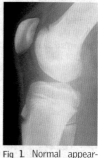

Fig 1. Normal appearance of an immature tibial tuberosity on x-ray.
Courtesy of Norfolk and Norwich University Hospital (NNUH) Radiology Department.

Sinding Larsen's disease (jumper's knee) Traction tendinopathy with calcification in the proximal attachment of the patellar tendon, which may be partially avulsed. Symptoms, treatment are similar to Osgood–Schlatter's disease (above), but the onset tends to be 1–2yrs earlier.[155]

Sever's disease This common calcaneal apophysitis is probably from strained attachment of the Achilles tendon. It is usually self-limiting. Typical age: 8–13yrs. There is pain behind the heel (bilateral in 60%) ± limping, and tenderness over the lower posterior calcaneal tuberosity. *Radiographs:* Often normal. *Treatment:* Physiotherapy and heel raise. If needed, a below-knee walking plaster may give pain relief. Most are well after 5 weeks.[156]

Avascular necrosis (osteonecrosis) *Sites of infarction:* Hip (commonest), knee, shoulder. *Imaging:* MRI is best; sclerotic or porotic bone due to infarction; joint surface odd, osteochondral fragments.[157] *Local causes:* Trauma (eg fractured neck of femur); secondary to rheumatoid, severe osteoarthritis, psoriatic arthropathy, or neuropathic joints. *Systemic:* Thalassaemia, sickle-cell (+ any cause of microthrombi, eg platelets↑ in leukaemia), NSAIDs/steroids (eg post-transplant), SLE, scleroderma, SBE, dyslipidaemia, alcoholism, pancreatitis, diabetes, big burns, radiation, divers (p813), Cushing's & Gaucher's diseases. *Treatment:* Immobilization; analgesia; for hips, arthroplasty.[158]

Sport and exercise medicine

Sport and exercise medicine is a relatively new medical specialty that, in its broadest sense, encompasses performance in sport and the care of injury.

The ever-increasing standards and demands in professional sport have driven competitors to new heights and lengths (the consequences of which for some are justifiably punishing), but by far the largest group of those undertaking sport do so for pure enjoyment. The importance of health and exercise running in partnership cannot be understated, and helping all those who enjoy sport to be healthy and safe has become a multidisciplinary field with substantial breadth of expertise (see MINIBOX). There are also other facets to this specialty, including performance in extreme environments and supporting those with medical illness in sporting activity.

Specialties involved:
• Clinical medicine
• General practice
• Orthopaedics
• Radiology
• Physiology
• Anatomy
• Biomechanics
• Kinetics
• Physiotherapy
• Podiatry
• Nutrition
• Pharmacology
• Epidemiology
• Psychology

Overuse injuries are a major cause of morbidity—see p715 for overuse phenomena outside sport.[159,160] Repetitive activity, a mainstay of sport (eg as in baseball pitching, cycling, golf, running), causes tissue damage over time, with rate of injury exceeding rate of recovery. There are many theories on the role of stress, mechanical fatigue, and inflammatory factors in causation. Symptoms depend on the site and type of tissue involved (eg nerve, muscle, bone, tendon, ligament) but usually equate to local pain exacerbated by use. Problems commonly seen include *shin splints* (shin soreness, common in unfit runners on hard surfaces and due to muscle tears, mild anterior compartment syndrome or stress fracture) and *tennis elbow*, p666.[1 84]

Treatment This usually involves rest, physiotherapy, technique evaluation, NSAIDs, local corticosteroid injection (►beware the complication of tendon rupture), or surgery on specialist advice. The threshold for treatment (especially surgery) may be different for professional sports players. For *soft tissue injuries*, the treatment in the first 24h is 'RICE':

Rest:	A splint or plaster cast may help
Ice:	Cold is anaesthetic and a vasoconstrictor. Apply ice packs (eg a packet of frozen peas wrapped in a cloth) or cold compresses intermittently for <10min at a time, to avoid cold injury
Compression:	Strapping restricts swelling and further bleeding
Elevation:	Ideally elevate the affected part above the heart to improve drainage from the affected part and to reduce pain

►Correct management reduces pain, recovery time and later disability.

Rehabilitation Passive stretching to maintain joint mobility and muscle length, then progressive active exercise until the full range and strength of movement is restored, eg wobbleboards for ankles. Sportsmen must then retrain to full fitness. Also consider NSAIDs, rubefacients, and ultrasound.

Prevention and safety are a vital part of good training and performance.
• Is the patient preparing the body for activity with a proper warm-up? Inadequate warm-up increases the risk of injury.
• Cooling-down is also important in reducing muscle soreness.
• Is (correct) protective equipment being worn?
• Many acute and chronic injuries are caused by unsuitable equipment, faulty technique, or unwise training schedules. ►Get advice from a coach.

---

1 Other relevant pages: Golfer's elbow, p666; tennis elbow, p666; iliotibial tract syndrome, p688; march fracture, p694; plantar fasciitis, p694; soft tissue injuries, p715; fractures in general, p734; injuries to the hand, p746; knee ligament injury, p754; ankle strain, p756; head injury, p758; heat exhaustion/injury, p788.

Joint replacement has been used for at least 70yrs.[1] Each year ~80,000 hips and >80,000 knees are replaced in England and Wales.[161]

Hip replacement This is carried out to relieve pain and disability caused by arthropathies of the hip—85% are to replace osteoarthritic hips. Other conditions which may result in replacement are: rheumatoid arthritis, avascular necrosis of head of femur; congenitally dislocated hip; fractured neck of femur. Women outnumber men by ~2:1; and the over 65-yr-olds account for 2 in every 3 procedures.[163] Many prostheses are available; most consist of a metal femoral component with an intramedullary stem sometimes held in place by bone cement, and a plastic acetabular component—fig 2. Early success of operation occurs in 90%.

Early complications
• VTE 4%
• Dislocation 3%
• Deep infection 2%
• Fracture 1%
• Nerve palsy 1%
• Limb-length discrepancy 1%
• Death 0.4–0.7%[164]

Later problems of loosening or infection are heralded by return of pain. If plain radiographs are inconclusive in the case of loosening, strontium or technecium scans may reveal increased bone activity. Suspected sepsis should be investigated by WCC, ESR, and ultrasound-guided aspiration. Revision arthroplasty is more successful for loosening than for infection. *Joint survival:* By 9–10yrs post-op 11% of implants have been revised. Be cautious in recommending replacement to those in their 60s who are likely to cause excessive wear of the prosthesis. Earlier replacement is used for rheumatoid arthritis as joints tend to be grossly affected younger—and excessive delay may result in surgery upon very rarefied osteoporotic bone. Central migration of the prosthesis via perforation of the medial acetabular wall is a rare cause of external iliac artery and bladder injury.[165] *Hip resurfacing* is an evolving method to consider for active people ≤65yrs with endstage arthropathy (fig 3). It is experimental as long-term data are sparse.[166] [NICE] In a 2008 trial, 93% had good/excellent results at 2–8yrs, and no loosening; revision rate: 4%.[167]

Knee replacement consists of resection of articular surfaces of the knee, then resurfacing with metal and polyethylene components. Replacement may be total or partial (unicompartmental). Indications for knee replacement: pain at rest, or disturbing sleep, or making housebound. Pain correlates poorly with radiological signs. Success rate: 95%. *Joint survival:* 90% last 15yrs (better than hips). Revision rates are similar. Quality of life can be transformed, even if >80yrs old.

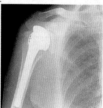

Fig 1. AP image shoulder hemi-arthroplasty.
Courtesy of Norfolk and Norwich University Hospital (NNUH) Radiology Department.

Other joints Joint spacers are used in finger joints for rheumatoid, with success. Elbow replacements are beginning to show some success. Shoulder replacement (fig 1) success rates are approaching those of knees.

Preventing pulmonary emboli (PE) Follow local evidence-based protocols. DVT occurs in ~⅔ of major orthopaedic events, but fatal PE in only 0.1–0.2%.[168] [n=130,000] Low-molecular weight heparin (LMWH) halves DVT rate and lowers risk of fatal PE by ~75%.[169] In major orthopaedic surgery, low-molecular weight heparin (LMWH) is preferable to ordinary heparin. CI: uncontrolled bleeding/risk of bleeding (eg peptic ulcer); endocarditis; children. *Dose example:* **Dalteparin** 2500U 2h pre-op and at 12h post-op, then 5000U once/day for 1 week. In knees, **fondaparinux** 2.5mg/day may be better than enoxaparin.[170] [n=1049] The oral agents **dabigatran** and **rivaroxaban** may be easier to take. DVT/PE prophylaxis may need continuing for 28–25 days post-hip surgery and 10–14 days post-knee surgery.[2] NB: if rate of fatal PE is always ≪0.1%,◆ in some centres prophylaxis *may* not be warranted.[171]

Infected hip and knee prostheses

This may be a disastrous complication of joint replacement—presenting with pain, loss of function, fever, or wound inflammation. Perioperative wound complications, obesity, increased age, diabetes mellitus, steroid use and rheumatoid arthritis increase risk. Staphyloccal skin commensals are the most common infective organisms *Investigations:* CRP/ESR, blood culture and aspiration of joint. Plain radiographs may show peri-prosthetic loosening. CT/MRI may be of limited use due to artefact. Gallium/labelled leukocyte imaging may be useful in hard to diagnose cases *Treatment:* Early on, debridement + antibiotics may be enough. Later, with loosening of components, radical debridement must include removal of all prosthetic material, as well as any involved bone and soft tissue. Sometimes reconstruction by exchange arthroplasty works, eg for less virulent infections. Antibiotics may be needed for months. Patient selection is vital, eg those without draining sinuses, without immunocompromise, and with adequate bone quality after debridement.[172] The Mayo Clinic reports a 13% failure rate with a 2-stage reconstruction.

Another alternative may be the removal of all foreign material and allowing ankylosis to occur, ie a Girdlestone pseudarthrosis, for the hip.

SBE–style antibiotic prophylaxis ± antibiotic-impregnated cement?

• *Dentistry-associated prosthesis infection* with oral bacteria is very rare and risks of antibiotics are palpable (>500 penicillin-caused deaths/yr, in the USA), and SBE-style prophylaxis is not recommended.
• *Colonoscopy + polypectomy* may be more risky than dentistry; some recommend prophylaxis, if <6 months since replacement.

The best prophylaxis might be achieved with a combination of gentamicin-impregnated cement, systemic antibiotics for >24h, and surgery performed in ultra-clean environments (laminar air flow theatres/surgeons in 'space suits', although the additional cost of this may be prohibitive or prove to be ineffective). Reimplantation need not require use of cement: hydroxyapatite coated total prostheses are an alternative.[173] See fig 2 for the usual constituents found in bone cement.

Other systemic long-term complications of joint replacements[174] Fine fragmentation may lead to metal poisoning (eg cobalt) targeting mitochondria: suspect if visual/hearing loss and 24h urine cobalt excretion >1.5µg/L.

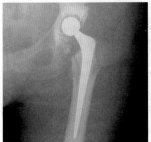

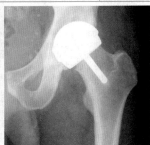

Fig 2. AP radiograph of a cemented total hip arthroplasty. *Bone cement* usually contains: methylmethacrylate (forms the polymer); a starter, initiator + inhibitor chemicals; an antibiotic (eg gentamicin ± clindamycin); a colouring agent (eg chlorophyll, hence green colour); and a radiopacifier (eg ZrO_2 or $BaSO_4$).[1]

Fig 3. AP radiograph of the left hip after Birmingham hip resurfacing.[2]

Images courtesy of Norfolk and Norwich University Hospital (NNUH) Radiology Department.

1 The first hip replacement was done by Philip Wiles at the Middlesex Hospital in 1938. The Charnley low friction arthroplasty was first used in the 1960s.
2 For DVT/PE prophylaxis, NICE recommends using either LMWH, fondaparinux, dabigatran or rivaroxaban for 10–35 days post-op depending on the type of surgery, and agent chosen.

Joint aspirations *Diagnostic role:* Any blood, crystals, or pus?[175] *Therapeutic role:* For tense effusions, septic effusions, and haemarthroses. Approaches for specific joints are given below and on p710. ►Remember that aspiration of a joint with a prosthesis should only be done under the strictest sterile conditions (ie in the operating theatre) to minimize risk of introducing infection.

Steroid injections to inflamed joints, bursae, or tendon sheaths aim to ↓inflammation and relieve pain, perhaps by ↓prostaglandin synthesis, stabilizing mast cells, or ↓tissue calcification, or increasing vascularization and permeability of synovium. *Side effects:* Skin atrophy (hydrocortisone acetate is safer than triamcinolone), haemarthrosis, facial flushing, urticaria, Charcot's arthropathy, post-injection flare syndrome (synovitis with fever), paresis, and septic arthritis (≤1 in 14,000 injections). ►*It is essential that steroids are not used in septic conditions* and, if any doubt at all exists, results of synovial fluid culture should be awaited. Remember the possibility of tuberculous synovitis—especially in immigrant populations. Repeated injections are more dangerous: beware ligamentous laxity, joint instability, calcification, or tendon rupture.

Preparations are available: **hydrocortisone acetate** (cheapest, shortest acting), **methylprednisolone**, and **triamcinolone**. They may be mixed with 1% lidocaine. When triamcinolone is used for injecting near short tendons, 10mg strength is preferred to 40mg as tendon rupture has been reported after the latter. Despite our best intentions 'joint' injections often fail to meet their target (50% in one study in which contrast material was also injected); those off-target are less likely to relieve symptoms.[176]

Conditions responding reasonably well to steroid injection Localized subdeltoid bursitis; supraspinatus, infraspinatus, and subscapular tendinopathy; shoulder arthritis; tennis and golfer's elbow, arthritis of elbow, radioulnar, acromioclavicular, and sternoclavicular joints; ganglia; trigger fingers; de Quervain's disease; strains of collateral and cruciate ligaments of knee; suprapatellar, infrapatellar, and Achilles tendinopathy; plantar fasciitis; traumatic arthritis of metatarsophalangeal joints; and sesamo-first-metatarsal joint.

Preparation Check you have swabs, needles, and sterile bottles. For aspiration of viscid fluid (eg haemarthrosis) use a 19G needle. For the larger joints use a 21G needle, and for fingers and toes a 23G needle. Locate joint margins carefully before cleaning with chlorhexidine in 5% spirit or surgical spirit; once the skin is clean use scrupulous aseptic no-touch technique. Remember that antiseptics and local anaesthetics take 3min to work; even then, the skin is clean but not sterile. Samples for microbiology should be sent in sterile containers, those for cytology or crystal examination in heparinized or FBC containers.

Knee joint The patient lies with knee supported slightly flexed and muscles relaxed. Palpate the joint space behind patella either medially or laterally—the lateral approach may be less reliable.[177] Insert a needle horizontally between the patella and femur. Slight resistance is felt on traversing the synovial membrane; it should be possible to aspirate fluid, and injection fluid should flow easily. *Usual doses:* 25–50mg **hydrocortisone acetate**, 40mg **methylprednisolone**, 20mg **triamcinolone**. Repeat injections should be longer than 3 months apart. If injection is used for prepatellar bursitis, give 25mg hydrocortisone acetate into the most tender spot.

The ankle Plantar flex foot slightly, palpate joint margin between tibialis anterior (the most medial) and extensor hallucis longus (lateral to tibialis anterior) tendons just above tip of medial malleolus. Inject 25mg **hydrocortisone** acetate into the joint.

Orthopaedics and trauma

Synovial fluid in health and disease

Blood, crystals or pus? Aspiration of synovial fluid is used diagnose haemarthroses, or infectious or crystal (gout and pseudogout) arthropathies.

	Appearance	Viscosity	wbc/mm³	Neutrophils
Normal	Clear, colourless	High	<200	<25%
Non-inflammatory, eg OA	Clear, straw	High	<5000	<25%
Haemorrhagic, eg tumour haemophilia, trauma	Bloody, xanthochromic	Variable	<10,000	<50%
Acute inflammatory[1]	Turbid, yellow	Decreased		
• Acute gout			~14,000	~80%
• Rheumatic fever			~18,000	~50%
• Rheumatoid arthritis			~16,000	~65%
Septic	Turbid, yellow	Decreased		
• TB			~24,000	~70%
• Gonorrhoeal			~14,000	~60%
• Septic (non-gonococcal)[2]			~16,000	~95%

For inflammatory causes of arthritis: Synovial fluid wbc >2000/mm³ is 84% sensitive (84% specific); synovial fluid neutrophil count >75% is 75% sensitive (92% specific). ►NB: not all labs are equally skilful.[178]

Pathological fractures

Definition A fracture that occurs in diseased or abnormal bone. Disruption of bony structural integrity means that even trivial forces can produce a fracture, so suspect a pathological fracture if the energy of the trauma is abnormally low for the resulting injury. Common sites include the subtrochanteric femur and the proximal humeral shaft.

Causes The commonest causes are osteoporosis (so-called 'fragility' fractures) and bony metastases (eg from breast or prostate primaries). Rarer causes include osteomalacia, osteitis (bone infection), primary bone tumour and osteogenesis imperfecta.

Management If the underlying diagnosis is unclear, then do rigorous directed investigation, eg in a search for a primary cancer. Without treating the bone metastases, the chances of healing are nearly zero. Chemo- and

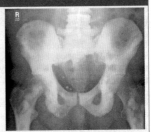

Fig 1. Diffuse bony sclerotic lesions, putting the patient at risk from pathological fracture.

ΔΔ: Metastasis from prostate and breast, and rarely GI carcinoma; primary lymphoma; multiple myeloma.

►Remember to image the whole femur if a proximal pathological fracture is identified—the forces through any fixation device could snap any other surrounding infiltrated bone.

Courtesy of Norfolk and Norwich University Hospital (NNUH) Radiology Department.

radiotherapy with fixation (eg intramedullary nail insertion ± bone cement) may allow slow healing.

Prevention Prevention of fracture from metastatic deposits may include external beam irradiation and prophylactic intramedullary nail insertion.[179] Osteoporosis prevention is also a major issue, covered by NICE.[180]

►Remember pathological fractures, as prevention is important and treatment may be different.

1 Includes eg Reiter's syndrome, pseudogout, SLE etc.
2 Includes Staphs, Streps, Lyme, and *Pseudomonas* (eg post-op).

Orthopaedics and trauma

Shoulder injection As shoulder pain from soft tissue causes is common (lifetime incidence ~10%), and pain can be chronic (≤23% resolve within 4wks), this is one of the most commonly injected joints. But we do not know *who* to inject or *when* in their illness, as trials are few, and the best ones cast doubt on the benefit of *any* injection.[21] *Anterior approach:* (aspiration, synovitis, frozen shoulder) seat the patient with arm relaxed by side of chest. Feel the space between head of humerus and glenoid cap ~1cm below coracoid process. Insert 21G green needle into the joint space (enters joint space when almost up to hilt) and inject 25–50mg hydrocortisone acetate. ▶Do not go medial to the coracoid process *(neurovascular structures, p765 fig 2).* *Lateral approach:* (subacromial bursitis, painful arc syndrome) inject 25–50mg hydrocortisone acetate with lidocaine just below the lateral tip of the acromion, pointing downwards and advancing medially. If the needle is withdrawn from touching the head of humerus with slight pressure on the plunger, a drop in pressure is felt as the bursa is entered. Painful arc pain may be reproduced. A 2nd injection may be given after >48h.

Tennis elbow (see also p666) 25mg hydrocortisone acetate with 1mL lidocaine is injected with force to area of maximal tenderness over lateral humeral condyle moving to and fro down to bone several times. A second injection may be needed, eg after 2 weeks. Warn the patient that symptoms may worsen briefly after the injection has been given, and that long-term (>6 weeks) relief of symptoms may not be provided—better results may be obtained with physiotherapy and elbow manipulation.[181,182] Avoid triamcinolone and Depo-Medrone®—because injections are superficial, fat necrosis may occur.

Elbow joint injection With elbow flexed at 90°, inject 25mg *hydrocortisone acetate* between proximal head of radius (locate by rotating patient's forearm and feeling the radial head rotate) and lateral epicondyle by lateral approach (needle 90° to skin), or posteriorly between olecranon and lateral epicondyle. ▶Avoid the posteromedial aspect, as the ulnar nerve lies behind the epicondyle.

Biceps tendinopathy is worsened by externally rotating the arm. Insert needle parallel to tendon (if resistance, it is in the tendon: withdraw a bit); inject 25mg hydrocortisone acetate into tendon sheath and 25mg into joint. Ultrasound guidance for this injection increases accuracy.[183]

Wrist injection Inject 25mg hydrocortisone acetate 1-1.5cm deep between extensor tendons of ring and little fingers between ulnar head and lunate.

De Quervain's tenosynovitis Extensor pollicis brevis and abductor pollicis longus tendons—on traversing the extensor retinaculum on the dorsal wrist—may cause a tender swelling (p668). With needle almost parallel to skin pointing proximally, inject 25mg hydrocortisone acetate slowly just distal or proximal to the radial styloid, at the site of maximum tenderness. If needle in tendon, injection is difficult so withdraw until easy flow occurs.

Carpal tunnel Introduce the needle just proximal to the distal wrist crease, to the ulnar side of palmaris longus (locate before starting by resisting active flexion of the wrist), angled at ~45°in a *distal to proximal* direction. ▶Do not use local anaesthetic. If the patient jumps or reports an 'electric shock' then you are probably in, or touching, the nerve. Redirect the needle towards the ulnar side and then inject 25mg hydrocortisone acetate. The intention is to deliver steroid around the flexor tendons and not into the carpal tunnel itself. If the first injection fails, consider repeating with 10–20mg triamcinolone. A splint worn for the next few days may mitigate symptoms which can occur at the time of injection.

Trigger finger Insert needle at MCP skin crease parallel to flexor tendon, pointing to palm. Palpate tendon thickening in palm; proceed as for de Quervain's.

First carpometacarpal joint of thumb Avoiding radial artery, inject 25mg hydrocortisone acetate at base of first metacarpal at 1cm depth in anatomical snuffbox (aim at base of little finger). ▶In all areas, learn from an expert.

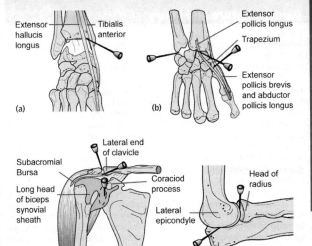

Fig. 1.
(a) Dorsal aspect of the right ankle indicating anatomical landmarks—shown here is the anterior ankle approach.
(b) Dorsal aspect of the right wrist indicating anatomical landmarks—shown here from left to right are the injection sites for the wrist joint, de Quervain's tenosynovitis & the 1st carpometacarpal joint.
(c) Diagrammatic representation of the anterior aspect of the right shoulder region. The blue areas indicate synovial membranes of the subacromial bursa and the glenohumeral joints—shown here are the anterior shoulder approach (below) and the acromioclavicular joint approach (above).
(d) The right elbow, flexed—shown from left to right the posterior and lateral approaches.[184]

The main tendons to rupture are the extensor tendons of the fingers, the Achilles tendon (fig 2), the long head of biceps (p664), supraspinatus (p664), and the quadriceps expansion (fig 1). The cause may be sharp or blunt trauma (anything from sporting injuries to rubber bullets). Ultrasound aids diagnosis, but its usefulness is largely operator-dependent.

Mallet finger Often caused by a sudden blow to an extended finger—e.g. hit by basketball on outstretched finger—which leads to rupture of the extensor tendon at the distal phalanx. *Treatment:* Splint the affected digit for 6 weeks (in slight hyper-extension) using a Stack splint or a moulded aluminium splint. If untreated the mallet finger may develop into a swan-neck deformity. If conservative treatment fails, or the mallet finger is associated with a large avulsion fracture (>30%) refer to a hand surgeon for consideration of surgical fixation.[185]

Boutonnière deformity Rupture of the central slip of the extensor tendon (at the base of the middle phalanx) allows the lateral bands of the extensor mechanism to slip towards the palm, turning them into flexors of the PIP joint. The result is flexion at the PIP joint and hyperextension of the DIP joint. It can occur following injury (forced flexion of extended PIP joint or volar dislocation of distal finger at PIP joint) or secondary to rheumatoid arthritis. Acute injuries are typically treated by splinting PIP in complete and constant extension, allowing movement at DIP and MCP joints. Referral to hand therapy is recommended.

Achilles (calcaneal) tendon rupture Typified by sudden pain at the back of the ankle during running or jumping as the tendon ruptures. Pain may be perceived as a 'kick' rather than actual pain. It is possible to walk (with a limp), and some plantar flexion of the foot remains, but it is impossible to raise the heel from the floor when standing on the affected leg. A gap may be palpated in the tendon course (particularly within 24h of injury). *The squeeze test* (Simmonds' test) is sensitive: ask the patient to kneel on a chair, while you squeeze both calves—if the Achilles is ruptured, there is less plantar flexion on the affected side. *Treatment:* Tendon repair (percutaneous or open) is often preferred by young, athletic patients. Late-presenting ruptures usually need reconstructing.[186] Surgery has a lower re-rupture rate, but risks potentially devastating infection. Conservative treatment may be most suitable for smokers, diabetics and those >50yrs old. Conservative management usually requires initial casting in equinus position. Typically there is no weight bearing for 6–8 weeks.

Quadriceps expansion rupture Injury may be direct (eg blow) or indirect (stumbling causing sudden contraction of the apparatus). The quadriceps expansion (fig 1) encloses the patella and inserts into the tibial tuberosity as the patellar tendon. *Non-traumatic causes:* Pseudogout; Wilson's disease; renal failure with hyperparathyroidism.[187] *Treatment:* Rupture can occur at the site of quadriceps insertion to the patella, through the patella by fracture, or by avulsion of the patellar tendon from the tibial tuberosity. In all with extensor mechanism disruption (no straight leg raising) surgery is mandatory. After repair, the knee is immobilized for >4 weeks; then intensive physiotherapy helps regain knee function. Many have persistent weakness.[188]

Tenosynovitis Tendons and surrounding synovium may become locally inflamed (?from strain) so causing pain, eg supraspinatus tendinopathy and bicipital tendinopathy (p664) and de Quervain's (p668). Acute frictional synovitis at the wrist is another example, with swelling over wrist and thumb extensors. If palpation doesn't detect crepitus, at some sites, stethoscope auscultation reveals sounds like bronchial breathing.[1] *Treatment:* In wrist tenosynovitis, a splint for 3 weeks (leaving the fingers free) may be needed to allow inflammation to subside.

1 'Breathing' on the painful right arch on great toe flexion with 'vesicular'-type breathing on the unaffected left side.[189]

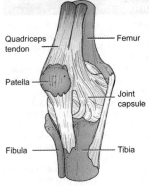

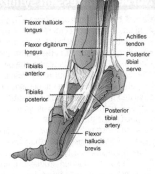

Fig 1. The extensor expansion of the knee.

Fig 2. The medial aspect of the ankle, showing the extensor and flexor tendons of the foot. The Achilles tendon tends to rupture ~5cm proximal to its insertion into the calcaneus. Also note the ordering of the flexor tendons posterior to the medial malleolus, from anterior to posterior—this can be remembered with the mnemonic Tom, Dick and, Harry:

- Tibialis posterior
- Flexor digitorum longus
- Posterior tibial artery
- Posterior tibial nerve
- Flexor hallucis longus.

Carpal tunnel syndrome (CTS) ▶This is the commonest cause of hand pain at night. It is due to compression of the median nerve as it passes under the flexor retinaculum. ♀:♂>1:1. *Signs* are in the median nerve distribution:
- Tingling or pain is felt in the thumb, index, and middle fingers.
- When the pain is at its worse, the patient characteristically flicks or shakes the wrist to bring about relief. Pain is especially common at night and after repetitive actions. Affected persons may experience clumsiness.
- Wasted thenar eminence & ↓sensation over the lateral 3½ digits (*not* 5ᵗʰ).
- Lateral palmar sensation is spared as its supply (the palmar cutaneous branch of the median nerve) does not pass through the tunnel.
- *Phalen's test:* holding the wrist hyperflexed for 1min reproduces the symptoms. (This is more reliable than *Tinel's test*—tapping over the tunnel to produce paraesthesiae. Note: Phalen's flexing, Tinel's tapping.)
Tests: Nerve conduction studies are unnecessary if history and examination are conclusive. US may be useful, MRI is less diagnostically accurate; neither are routine.[190,191]

Posterior interosseous nerve (PIN) compression The branch is compressed on passing through the proximal supinator muscle, eg after forearm fracture or excessive exercise. Patients experience weakness of thumb and finger extension. Electromyographic studies are typically positive **Radial tunnel syndrome** involves compression of the same nerve, but presents with lateral forearm pain rather than weakness. Electrodiagnostic studies tend to be negative *Examination* may show weakness of long finger extensors, and short and long thumb extensors, but no sensory loss. *Treatment* Rest, splints, NSAIDs. are first line. Steroids injections may help. In resistant cases surgical decompression of areas of potential compression of the PIN (eg the arcade of Fröhse, ie the free edge of supinator).[192]

Anterior interosseous nerve compression This median nerve branch may be compressed under the fibrous origin of flexor digitorum profundus, causing weakness of pinch and pain along the forearm's radial border. Examination shows weakness of the long thumb flexor and flexor profundus to the index finger—the patient will be unable to flex the DIP joint of the index finger and PIP joint of the thumb to make a rounded 'O' shape *Treatment* Initial conservative managment with surgical decompression if required.

Ulnar nerve compression at the wrist Uncommon. Compression occurs at Guyon's Canal. Loss may be motor or sensory. Compression can be due to a mass or external compression (in cyclists). *Diagnose* clinically, US may help.

Meralgia paraesthetica is a symptom complex of numbness, paraesthesiae, and pain (eg burning/shooting) in the anterolateral thigh, caused by lateral femoral cutaneous nerve entrapment, eg under the lateral part of the inguinal ligament (or neuroma, or other mononeuropathy). *Causes:* Tight jeans; body armour; seatbelts; patient-positioning devices (eg for hip surgery); ↑intra-abdominal pressure (eg pregnancy, obesity, ascites); ★diabetes mellitus, ★tumours,[193] repetitive contraction of inguinal muscles during sports training,[194] herniorrhaphy, pregnancy, pelvic osteotomy (eg for grafts).[195] ∆∆: Lumbar disc hernia. ℞: (often self-limiting but may recur[196]). Lose weight if needed, rest, NSAID ± carbamazepine[197] ± cortisone and local anaesthetic injection at the anterior superior iliac spine gives unpredictable results.

Common peroneal compression Nerve compression against the head of fibula (eg plaster casts, thin patients lying unconscious, proximal fibula fracture, squatting, obstructed labour)[198] causes inability to dorsiflex the foot. Sensation may be ↓ over the dorsum of the foot. *Treatment:* Most recover spontaneously but surgical decompression may be needed (eg if >3 months without improvement). Physiotherapy and splint until foot-drop recovers.

---

1 Ulnar nerve compression at elbow, p666; brachial plexus injury, p764; peripheral nerve injury, p760 & p716.

Managing carpal tunnel syndrome

Treat any treatable association (see MINIBOX) Rest, weight reduction and wrist splints are first line treatment.[199] 20% of cases will spontaneously resolve. For carpal injection, see p710. (Symptom relief beyond 1 month compared to placebo is unproven.)[200]

More permanent results are obtained from decompression by flexor retinaculum division.[201] Although a certain proportion (~7%) have worse symptoms post surgery. Full implications of endoscopic techniques are uncertain.[202]

CTS associations
- Myxoedema
- Pregnancy; the Pill
- Gout & pseudogout
- Diabetes; obesity
- Cardiac failure
- Acromegaly
- Rheumatoid arthritis
- Premenstrual state
- Amyloidosis

Overuse phenomena at work

Activity requiring repetitive actions, particularly those associated with prolonged muscle contraction, may lead to chronic symptoms. Employers have a duty to provide a safe working environment and well-designed chairs and tools, and frequent short breaks. Chang-

Synonyms
- Non-specific arm pain
= Work-related upper limb injury
= Occupational overuse syndrome
= Isometric contraction myopathy
= RSI (although, see fig 1)

es of posture and activity help to reduce work-related 'non-specific arm pain'. If no diagnosis has been made, this term is preferred to the fallacious *repetitive strain injury (RSI)*—see fig 1. The cost of these injuries in suffering, and hours lost from work, is considerable as treatment of established symptoms is often difficult and may necessitate change in employment—if one is available.

Compensation is a vexed issue, and recent court judgments have gone in favour of employers in some instances, and in favour of patients in others. Some people argue that the condition does not exist as a separate medical entity, emphasizing lack of histopathology. It should be noted that this is not a prerequisite for a disease (see *Sudden infant death*, p148)—and in any case histopathology is sometimes demonstrable. Treatments tried include splinting (may prolong the problem), physiotherapy, β-blockers for relaxation, and the Alexander technique for posture re-education.

Those who use vacuum cleaners, assemble cars, or play stringed instruments may all develop overuse phenomena, as can sports players (p705).

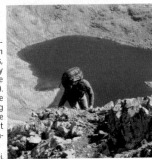

Fig 1. Why is the term repetitive strain injury a fallacy? Just because chest pain from angina can be provoked by walking up hills, walking up hills does not cause coronary artery stenosis (although the idea for some may be enough to cause a little heart flutter). And so, because use of the arm may provoke the symptoms of an underlying condition (eg carpal tunnel syndrome, osteoarthritis at the base of the thumb, de Quervain's disease), it does not mean that it is the cause of the underlying condition.

Courtesy of Dr Tom Turmezei.

Orthopaedics and trauma

Upper limb[203]		
Nerve root	**Muscle**	**Test by asking the patient to:**
C3,4	Trapezius	Shrug shoulder (via accessory nerve).[204]
C4,5	Rhomboids	Brace shoulder back.
C5,6,7	Serratus anterior	Push arm forward against resistance.
C5,6	Pectoralis major (clavicular head)	Adduct arm from above horizontal, and push it forward.
C6,7,8	Pectoralis major (sternocostal head)	Adduct arm below horizontal.
C5,6	Supraspinatus	Abduct arm the first 15°.
C5,6	Infraspinatus	Externally rotate arm, elbow at side.
C6,7,8	Latissimus dorsi	Adduct arm from horizontal position.
C5,6	Biceps	Flex supinated forearm.
C5,6	Deltoid	Abduct arm between 15° and 90°.
Radial nerve (C5–8)		
C6,7,8	Triceps	Extend elbow against resistance.
C5,6	Brachioradialis	Flex elbow with forearm half way between pronation and supination.
C5,6	Extensor carpi radialis longus	Extend wrist radially with fingers extended.
C6,7	Supinator	Arm by side, resist hand pronation.
C7,8	Extensor digitorum	Keep fingers extended at MCP joint.
C7,8	Extensor carpi ulnaris	Extend wrist to ulnar side.
C7,8	Abductor pollicis longus	Abduct thumb at 90° to palm.
C7,8	Extensor pollicis brevis	Extend thumb at MCP joint.
C7,8	Extensor pollicis longus	Resist thumb flexion at IP joint.
Median nerve (C6–T1)		
C6,7	Pronator teres	Keep arm pronated against resistance.
C6,7	Flexor carpi radialis	Flex wrist towards radial side.
C7,8,T1	Flexor digitorum superficialis	Resist extension at PIP joint (while you fix his proximal phalanx).
C8,T1	Flexor digitorum profundus I & II	Flex the DIP of the index finger, with the PIP held in extension.
C8,T1	Flexor pollicis longus	Resist thumb extension at interphalangeal joint (fix proximal phalanx).
C8,T1	Abductor pollicis brevis	Abduct thumb (nail at 90° to palm).
C8,T1	Opponens pollicis	Thumb touches base of 5th finger-tip (nail parallel to palm).
C8,T1	1st and 2nd lumbricals	Extend PIP joint against resistance with MCP joint held in flexion.
Ulnar nerve (C7–T1)		
C7,8,T1	Flexor carpi ulnaris	Flex wrist towards ulnar side.
C7,C8	Flexor digitorum profundus III & IV	Flex the DIP of the little finger, with the PIP held in extension.
C8,T1	Dorsal interossei	Abduct fingers (use index finger).
C8,T1	Palmar interossei	Adduct fingers (use index finger).
C8,T1	Adductor pollicis	Adduct thumb (nail at 90° to palm).
C8,T1	Abductor digiti minimi	Abduct little finger.
C8,T1	Flexor digiti minimi	Flex the little finger at MCP joint.
The musculocutaneous nerve (C5–6)		
C5,6	This may be injured at the brachial plexus, causing weakness of biceps, coracobrachialis, and brachialis. Forearm flexion is weak, ± some loss of sensation.[1]	

Sources: MRC Handbook; www.rad.washington.edu/atlas; www.medmedia.com/05/324.htm

See p762 for dermatomes and peripheral nerve distributions.

NB: root numbers in **bold** indicate that that root is more important than its neighbour. ►Sources vary in ascribing particular nerve roots to muscles—and there is some biological variation in individuals. The above is a reasonable compromise, and is based on the MRC guidelines.

Lower limb[205]

Nerve root	Muscle	Test by asking the patient to:
L**4,5**, S1	Gluteus medius & minimus	Internal rotation at hip, hip abduction.
L5, S1,2	Gluteus maximus	Extension at hip (lie prone).
L**2,3,4**	Adductors (obturator nerve)	Adduct leg against resistance.
Femoral nerve (L2–4, posterior division)		
L1,2,3	Iliopsoas	Flex hip with knee flexed and lower leg supported: patient lies on back.
L2,3	Sartorius	Flex knee with hip external rotated.
L2,3,4	Quadriceps femoris	Extend knee against resistance.
Obturator nerve (L2–4, anterior division)		
L2,3,4	Hip adductors	Adduct the leg.
Inferior gluteal nerve		
L5,S1,S2	Gluteus maximus	Hip extension.
Superior gluteal nerve		
L4,5,S1	Gluteus medius & minimus	Abduction and internal rotation of hip.
Sciatic nerve (including the common peroneal nerve[CP] & tibial nerve)		
L**4**,5[CP]	Tibialis anterior	Dorsiflex ankle.
L**5**,S1[CP]	Extensor digitorum longus	Dorsiflex toes against resistance.
L**5**,S1[CP]	Extensor hallucis longus	Dorsiflex hallux against resistance.
L**5**,S1[CP]	Peroneus longus & brevis	Evert foot against resistance.
L5,S1[CP]	Extensor digitorum brevis	Dorsiflex 2nd–4th toes (muscle of foot).
L5,**S1**,2[T]	Hamstrings	Flex knee against resistance.
L4,5[T]	Tibialis posterior	Invert plantarflexed foot.
S1,2[T]	Gastrocnemius	Plantarflex ankle joint.
L5,**S1**,2[T]	Flexor digitorum longus	Flex terminal joints of toes.
S1,2[T]	Small muscles of foot	Make sole of foot into a cup.

Quick screening test for muscle power

Shoulder	Abduction	C5	Hip	Flexion	L1,2
	Adduction	C5, 7		Extension	L5,S1
Elbow	Flexion	C5, 6	Knee	Flexion	S1
	Extension	C7		Extension	L3,4
Wrist	Flexion	C7,8	Ankle	Dorsiflexion	L4
	Extension	C7		Plantarflexion	S1,2
Fingers	Flexion	C7–8			
	Extension	C7			
	Abduction	T1 (ulnar)			

Quantifying strength

The UK MRC scale objectifies strength (reasonably well):

Grade 0 No muscle contraction	**Grade 3** Active movement, with gravity eliminated
Grade 1 Flicker of contraction	**Grade 4** Active movement against resistance
Grade 2 Some active movement	**Grade 5** Normal power

Grades 4–, 4, and 4+ describe movement against slight, moderate, and strong resistance. Dynamometers help quantify strength.[206][n=30] Remember to test proximal muscle power: ask the patient to sit from lying, to pull you towards himself, and to rise from squatting. **Gower's sign** (observed in a child with muscular dystrophy and proximal muscle weakness) shows the patient standing from a squatting position by 'climbing' sequentially up his own legs. ►Also, observe walking (easy to forget, even if the complaint is of walking difficulty!). See p680 and *OHCM* p471 for gait disorders.

▶All patients should be asked specifically if they require pain relief. Clinical assessment is expedited by relieving pain. There is some evidence to show that nurse initiated analgesia in Emergency Departments reduces time to relief of pain.[207,208] No acute pain is uncontrollable. If systemic analgesia is required, select the analgesic most appropriate to the type of pain. In pleuritic or musculoskeletal pain, NSAIDs are often more efficacious than a narcotic. NB: there are NO contraindications to narcotic analgesia (other than well-defined allergy which is very rare). If in doubt, TREAT!

Adjuncts Splint and elevate fractures and dislocations; RICE (p705).

Local anaesthesia Local infiltration of wounds with 1% lidocaine; digital nerve block in finger injuries; femoral nerve block for fractured shaft of femur. NB: use plain lidocaine (no added adrenaline) for finger blocks.

Non-opioid systemic analgesia Paracetamol 1g/4–6h; aspirin 600mg ± codeine 15–60mg/6h. NSAIDs: see below. **Ketamine** is a dissociative agent which can be used in subanaesthetic doses to provide analgesia. It should be used under the authority of a consultant.

NSAIDs Ibuprofen 400–800mg/8h PO. Diclofenac 75mg PR/IM STAT (max dose 150mg in 24h) is useful in management of renal colic. Indometacin 100mg PR stat can also be used in acute pain, eg from renal colic or gout. Ketorolac is an injectable NSAID. Dose if >16yrs old: ~10mg IM/IV over >15sec, every 2–6h, up to 90mg/day (60mg if old or <50kg). ▶NSAIDs ought to be avoided if there is a history of renal impairment, peptic ulceration or inducing acute asthma.

Gas Entonox® is a 50% mixture of nitrous oxide in O_2. It is self-administered using a demand valve system and can provide a good level of analgesia for short procedures (eg finger relocation) or when awaiting other forms of analgesia. Nitrous oxide is now increasingly available in variable concentrations upto 70%—and is no more likely to result in adverse effects than Entonox®.[209]

Opioid analgesia should be given IV as a bolus or infusion (IM is too slow and unpredictable). **Morphine** dose: 50–100µg/kg, eg 2.5–7.5mg IV slowly. Further increments should be titrated to the patient's response, initially at 5min intervals. Respiratory depression is unlikely with careful titration. ▶*There is no defined maximum dose*; a typical total dose is 10–20mg. Antiemetics are not always required routinely, but may be helpful in alleviating symptoms of nausea and vomiting (avoid metoclopramide in children: risk of oculogyric crisis). Naloxone (0.1–0.2mg stat IV, then 0.1mg every 2mins until responsive) can be used to reverse effects of overdose. Fentanyl (1–2µg/kg IBW, eg 50–100µg IV) is useful for short procedures requiring conscious sedation (cardioversion, reduction of dislocated shoulder). Meptazinol is an opioid option, and can be given as 200mg every 3–6h PO—effects are only partially reversed by naloxone. Tramadol is a synthetic opioid analgesic that has weak agonist activity at mu opiate receptors and inhibits serotonin and noradrenaline reuptake in the spinal cord; dose: 50–100mg/6h PO.

Sedation Sometimes IV sedation is required for the sake of comfort *and* cooperation—eg joint relocation, fracture reduction (p734) or cardioversion (*OHCM*, p784). It is important that, if possible, one person is in charge of drug administration and monitoring (HR, BP, O_2 sats, GCS) and one person is in charge of the procedure. NB: this is not always possible, eg in remote locations, where single physician procedural sedation will be required.[210] Midazolam is an effective sedative and should be titrated to response, starting with 2.5mg IV by slow injection (1mg in elderly) and given in further 0.5–1mg increments. It is unusual for more than 5mg to be required. It can be given with morphine, though remember that morphine also has sedative effects. The use of propofol and/or ketamine is useful in experienced hands. ▶Monitor the patient throughout and after the procedure until GCS normal.

Children with trauma needing pain relief

Hospitals can be frightening. Toys, friendliness, a quiet room and a simple explanation of what is going to happen go a long way to avoid creating distress.

- Introduce yourself to the child (and their parents), get down to their eye level, and reassure them (and their parents).
- Be positive and relaxed, let them know they are brave, and that you are going to make them feel better and want to "fix" what ails them.
- Be aware that children who experience pain and discomfort with medical procedures are more likely to be anxious and experience greater pain in the future with similar procedures.
- Consider intranasal fentanyl (1.5µg/kg initial dose—via an atomiser, in divided doses between the nostrils—a second dose eg 0.75µg/kg can be given after 5 min) for burns and fractures—there is usually time to give this before examination.
- For IV cannulation and venepuncture use topical local anaesthetic (eg EMLA —needs 60mins to work or LMX-4—needs 30min to work)—unless access is needed emergently.
- Do you need to suture a wound? Consider the alternatives (p730).
- Do you need to inject local anaesthetic? Consider needle-free alternatives —for example 70% nitrous oxide +/– topical wound anaesthetic. It is rarely worth an injection for a single suture.
- Use oral sucrose in neonates.
- If local anaesthetic is necessary, use the smallest needle possible to infiltrate the wound (an insulin syringe needle (30G) or dental syringe needle (27–30G) is ideal).
- Buffering local anaesthetic with 8.4% sodium bicarbonate (9 parts anaesthetic to 1 part sodium bicarbonate) and using anaesthetic that is warmed to body temperature may reduce the pain associated with infiltration.
- Use some sort of distraction as you are doing your procedure—play music or a DVD, ask the parents or a nurse to blow bubbles for the child, engage them in conversation about their brothers/sisters/pets or other interests. If there is a play therapist available—they may prove as effective in reducing pain as local anaesthetic!
- Infiltrate wounds through the open wound edge rather than puncturing intact skin—inject slowly, and use the minimal volume of anaesthetic.
- If suturing or other painful procedures are unavoidable, consider sedation (see OPPOSITE): **morphine**, **fentanyl**, or **ketamine** (p802) are the agents of choice. Oral ketamine is a potent, short-acting analgesic at 3–10mg/kg. The injectable form can be used PO in a flavoured drink. It is a class C drug^UK.

Explain to the child and the parents what you are going to do. Take your time, don't rush the child or the parents. Wrap the child in a blanket. Enlist enough nurses to hold the child and immobilize the part you are suturing. Warn the parents of possible distress. If they prefer not to be present, try to sit them out of earshot. Showing the child the result in a mirror, offering a big bandage, and giving an 'I was brave' badge can help. GA is rarely justified; if it is, the wound should probably be sutured by a plastic surgeon.

This is a subjective way of quantifying the conscious state of a person. It can be used by medical and nursing staff for initial and continuing assessment. It has value in predicting ultimate outcome. 3 types of response are assessed:

- **Best motor response** This has 6 grades:

  6 *Carrying out request ('obeying command'):* The patient does simple things you ask (beware of accepting a grasp reflex in this category).

  5 *Localizing response to pain:* Put pressure on the patient's finger nail bed with a pencil then try supraorbital and sternal pressure: purposeful movements towards changing painful stimuli is a 'localizing' response.

  4 *Withdraws to pain:* Pulls limb away from painful stimulus.

  3 *Flexor response to pain:* Pressure on the nail bed causes abnormal flexion of limbs: decorticate posture.

  2 *Extensor posturing to pain:* The stimulus causes limb extension (adduction, internal rotation of shoulder, forearm pronation): decerebrate posture.

  1 *No response to pain.* ▸NB: record the best response of any limb.

- **Best verbal response** This has 5 grades.

  5 *Oriented:* The patient knows who he is, where he is and why, the year, season, and month.

  4 *Confused conversation:* The patient responds to questions in a conversational manner but there is some disorientation and confusion.

  3 *Inappropriate speech:* Random or exclamatory articulated speech, but no conversational exchange.

  2 *Incomprehensible speech:* Moaning but no words.

  1 *None.* ▸NB: record the best level of speech.

- **Eye opening** This has 4 grades.

  4 *Spontaneous eye opening.*

  3 *Eye opening in response to speech:* Any speech, or shout, not necessarily request to open eyes.

  2 *Eye opening to response to pain:* Pain to limbs as above.

  1 *No eye opening.*

An overall score is made by summing the score in the 3 areas assessed, eg: no response to pain + no verbalization + no eye opening = 3.

- *Severe injury:* GCS ≤ 8 (airway needs protection with endotracheal intubation).
- *Moderate injury:* GCS 9–12.
- *Minor injury:* GCS 13–15.

Dramatic changes in GCS level can be seen in substance overdose, eg gamma-hydroxybutyrate. It is not unknown for patients to walk out just hours after presenting with a GCS of 3.[211]

AVPU An abbreviated coma scale, AVPU, is sometimes used in the initial assessment ('primary survey') of the critically ill:

  A = alert
  V = responds to vocal stimuli
  P = responds to pain
  U = unresponsive

Paediatric GCS See p201.

Orthopaedics and trauma

This algorithm (fig. 1) assumes that only one rescuer is present, with no equipment. (If a defibrillator is to hand, get a rhythm readout, and defibrillate, as needed, as soon as possible.) First, remove yourself, bystanders and the casualty from obvious dangers. Then shake and shout to the casualty to check responsiveness. If unresponsive:

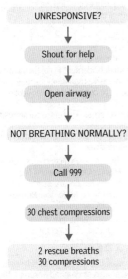

UNRESPONSIVE?

↓

Shout for help

↓

Open airway — (head tilt; chin lift; if non-responsive turn on back)

↓

NOT BREATHING NORMALLY? — (look, listen, feel; if breathing place in recovery position and go for help)

↓

Call 999 — (if alone, go at this stage for help/ call emergency services, eg **999** or **112**)

↓

30 chest compressions — (give **30** at a rate of ~**100** per min)

↓

2 rescue breaths
30 compressions — (each breath over **1** second) (chest compressions to rescue breaths at **30:2**)

Fig. 1. Adult basic life-support algorithm.
© Resuscitation Council, UK, 2010.

▶Continue resuscitation until help arrives/takes over, until normal breathing resumes or until you become exhausted (change every ~2min if there is more than one of you).

▶Do not interrupt resuscitation; only stop and reassess if the victim starts breathing normally.

Managing the airway
• Open the airway by chin-lift/head tilt or by jaw thrust (if trained and there is a possibility of spinal injury).
• Use a close-fitting mask if available, held in place by thumbs pressing downwards either side of the mouthpiece; palms against cheeks.

Chest compressions
• Cardiopulmonary resuscitation (CPR) involves compressive force over the lower sternum with the heel of the hands placed one on top of the other, directing the weight of your body through your vertical, straight arms.
• Depth of compression: 5–6cm.
• Rate of compressions: 100–120/min.

Orthopaedics and trauma

Murders by firearms Australia 59; UK 14; New Zealand 10; USA 9300 (+17,000 suicides). Historically gunshot wounds (GSWs) have been divided into low velocity (<1000ft/sec eg most handguns) and high velocity (>1000ft/sec—eg military rifles). Low velocity wounds lacerate and crush tissues. High velocity weapons are more destructive due to cavitation and the shock wave produced. When faced with a GSW or other penetrating injury consider the following:

▶ Initial management is in accordance with ATLS protocols.
▶ Minimal surface injury may hide much deeper injury, depending on the weapon used, the mechanism of injury, bullet speed. Factors such as tumble, yaw and trajectory can exacerbate internal injury.
▶ Some low velocity wounds (eg in limbs with no vascular/bone involvement) can be treated with irrigation and minimal debridement in ED, then with oral antibiotics and outpatient review. Non-operative management may also be suitable for some abdominal GSWs—(use CT to confirm no peritoneal breach or solid organ injury).
▶ Most victims are young and fit with good reserves. Therefore cardiorespiratory decompensation indicates severe injury.
▶ If the weapon (eg knife) is still *in situ*, do not remove it until the patient is on the operating table—the danger is exsanguination.

Define and record each injury. *Low-velocity* bullets leave dirty tracks, requiring exploration, excision, and *delayed* closure. *High-velocity* weapons (eg military rifles) are extraordinarily destructive due to the temporary cavity caused by the missile and likely fatal if to the head, thorax or abdomen. Ruthless and massive debridement is essential. Tetanus prophylaxis: p730.

Penetrating chest injuries may damage pleura, lung, great vessels, heart, mediastinum, diaphragm, and abdominal contents. The commonest injury is haemopneumothorax from damage to lung and chest wall. This requires a large (adult: 32G) chest drain: if drainage is initially >1500mL (='massive'), or >300mL/h, thoracotomy is needed. If available, attach an autotransfusion device to the drain. Deterioration or cardiac arrest demands prompt thoracotomy. Wounds of intercostal vessels, great vessels, or heart can cause massive haemorrhage. ▶Anterior wounds medial to the nipple line and posterior wounds medial to the scapulae must also prompt thoughts of thoracotomy.

Sucking chest wounds must be closed at once, eg by Vaseline® gauze pads sealed on 3 sides only (acts as flutter valve)—complete the seal on chest drain insertion. ▶▶Relieve tension pneumothorax by needling the chest on the side of the suspected lesion *before* inserting a 32G chest drain (OHCM p780) or doing radiographs (delay may be fatal). Prophylactic antibiotics may be indicated.[212]

Respiratory embarrassment due to pain, flail chest, or diaphragmatic injury requires intubation and ventilation. Insert a chest drain if there is any chance of a tear to lung, bronchus, or chest wall.

Cardiac tamponade 15% of deep chest injuries involve the heart. *Diagnosis:* Clinical diagnosis using Beck's triad = rising JVP, falling BP, and a small, quiet heart (± pulsus paradoxus) is difficult in the trauma situation. Portable ultrasound is more reliable)—a black stripe seen around the heart indicates fluid. ▶▶Pericardial aspiration may buy time before thoracotomy. *Procedure:* (OHCM p787) Insert an 18G needle to the left of the xiphoid. Aim at the left shoulder, but with the needle angled downwards at 45° to the horizontal. *All these patients need:* Crossmatching of ≥6 units of blood, then: •2 large-bore IV cannulae for vigorous fluid replacement. • Monitoring: vital signs; blood gases; CXR; ECG monitoring. • ITU care with a chest drain immediately to hand, and facilities for immediate thoracotomy (eg if any deterioration, or a cardiac arrest).

Abdominal injuries All but the most superficial injuries need admission and exploration, never just observation. Suspect abdominal injury with all penetrating chest trauma: the liver is up to the 4th rib (right). ▸▸See p726.

Limb injury Nerves, tendons, and vessels are endangered, so examine limbs in good light, testing *pulses* (their presence doesn't exclude arterial injury), *sensation* and *sweating*. Direct pressure will staunch bleeding. ▸Do not use a tourniquet: it may augment ischaemic damage, and you may forget to take it off (exception: extremity amputation—or where blood loss is a mortal threat).

Saving lives in trauma

Trauma is a ruthless killer. Every day 16,000 people worldwide are estimated to die from trauma. 1000 times as many are thought suffer a significant injury, with long-term morbidity having a significant impact on populations.[213] Road traffic accidents (RTAs)—or motor vehicle accidents (MVAs)—are the highest risk activity, causing 45,000 deaths (2% of all causes) in the USA in 2002.[214]

It was in the US that the approach to caring for trauma patients began to change. In 1976 (after a light aircraft crash in which he lost his wife) the reflections of the pilot, Nebraskan orthopaedic surgeon Dr James K. Styner, drove him to create the means of disseminating education of the optimum care of trauma patients to those for whom trauma did not play a major part in everyday medical practice. By 1978, the American College of Surgeons (ACS) had taken on the *Advanced Trauma Life Support* (ATLS®) course as a means to maintain this standard of care for all those subject to trauma.

It was broadly based on vital, yet novel concepts such as the 'golden hour',[1] treating the most life-threatening injury first,[2] and direct action when signs for action are identified. Now in its 7th edition, the course (and its handbook, ISBN 1880696142) cover the basic and advanced aspects of life-saving trauma care from chest injury, to the biomechanics of injury, to frostbite.

The programme also promotes the value of leadership and teamwork, skills that come to the fore in the heat of the moment, sometimes from the most unexpected quarters.

---

1 The first hour after injury is vital for the short- and long-term prognosis of patients who survive the initial trauma, and this timeframe is called the 'golden hour'. The actions of a carer during this period have profound effects on subsequent mortality and morbidity.

2 ABCDE: **a**irway, **b**reathing, **c**irculation, **d**isability, **e**xposure—see p725.

On news of major trauma, summon experienced help (eg senior traumatologist). ▶▶Remember ABCDE (see OPPOSITE for the generic approach).

Blunt chest injury If breathing spontaneously, give ALL patients O_2 at 15L/min through tight-fitting mask with reservoir.

- *Quality of breathing:* Stridor (± voice change) ≈? sternoclavicular fracture/posterior dislocation: get expert help at once as intubation may be difficult owing to tracheal compression, until the dislocation is reduced—by extending the shoulders, and grasping the clavicle with a clamp (eg towel clip) and manually reducing the fracture. Cover & seal open chest wounds on 3 sides.

- *Assume spinal instability:* Keep neck immobile with sandbags, collar, tape.

- ▶▶*Is there tension pneumothorax?* Needs urgent treatment: Relieve by inserting a large (14–16G) cannula (2ⁿᵈ ICS, midclavicular line) then a chest drain. *Signs:* breath sounds, respiratory distress; pulse; BP; tracheal deviation (away from tension); cyanosis; neck veins distended, asymmetrical appearance of chest.

- *Haemorrhage control and fluid resuscitation:* Apply pressure and elevation to any actively bleeding part. Crossmatch (▶ask for group-compatible blood—only takes 5–10min); glucose stix; 2 wide-bore saline IVIs (femoral catheter or saphenous cutdown anterior to medial malleolus if no IV access).[215] Take systolic BP. If <90mmHg and blood loss is the probable cause; give 2L of warmed crystalloid stat IV until BP↑; urine flows (>30mL/h; catheterize as soon as feasible) and crossmatched blood arrives. NB: colloid is no longer the resuscitation fluid of choice.[216] If intraperitoneal bleeding is suspected, see p726. ▶Have a low threshold for suspicion of abdominal injury

- ↓BP + ↑JVP + *quiet heart sounds:* = *cardiac tamponade:* ▶▶see p722.

- *Level-of-consciousness:* (GCS/AVPU, p720). If fits occur give ≤8mg lorazepam ~4mg as a slow bolus (~2min) into a large vein—or buccal midazolam (p208); beware apnoea. Check pupil size every few mins. If pupils unequal, summon neurological help; give 20% mannitol 1g/kg (5mL/kg) IV (↑cerebral blood flow). See p728 for head injury.

- *Injury extent:* Remove clothes (large scissors). Do *circumferential burns* need escharotomy to ↓laryngeal pressure? Any *surgical emphysema* (chest drain needed?). Is there a *flail chest* (a segment has no bony continuity with thorax, with paradoxical respiration)? The main problem is the underlying injured lung (sensitive to *over & under* resuscitation; intubate & ventilate).

- Chart ALL obs every few minutes and make sure someone is time-keeping.

- *ECG:* ST & conduction problems ≈ myocardial damage: extent is revealed via direct inspection by thoracic surgeon.

- *Imaging:* CXR, cervical spine (p658) and pelvis x-rays. *CXR implications:*
  - If free air, do thoracocentesis (or formal chest drain) for pneumothorax.
  - If persistent large pneumothorax after chest drain suspect bronchial tear.
  - # of ribs 1–3 ≈ ?airway/big vessel[1]
  - # of >2 ribs in 2 places ≈ ?flail chest
  - Bowel gas in chest≈?diaphragm injury
  - Coils of NGT in chest≈?diaphragm injury
  - # of sternum ≈ ?myocardial contusion
  - Respiratory distress+CXR OK≈?aspiration
  - Wide mediastinum ≈ ?aortic rupture[1]
  - Deviation of oesophagus≈?aortic rupture[1]
  - Ribs 9–12# ≈ ?abdominal trauma
  - CXR fluid level ≈ haemothorax
  - Diaphragm contour↓ ≈ ?rupture
  - Liver raised ≈ ?diaphragm injury
  - Mediastinal air ≈ lung barotrauma
  - # of scapula ≈?airway injury
  - Tracheal deviation ≈ ?aortic injury[1]
  - No aortic knob ≈ ?ruptured aorta.[1]

FAST (focused assessment with sonography for trauma) and emergency echocardiography are other useful tools in the evaluation of trauma patients. (see p727)

- *Secondary survey:* Head-to-toe exam. Examine all peripheral pulses. 30% of fractures are missed in resus rooms; target further imaging appropriately.

- In lung contusion (ventilate if S_AO_2 <90%).

- Give *tetanus toxoid* booster ± *human anti-tetanus immunoglobulin* (p730).

1 Have a low threshold for contrast-enhanced aorta CTs, especially if deceleration injury.

Orthopaedics and trauma

The ATLS® programme uses the ABCDE mantra to inculcate the care methodology for the trauma situation (see also BOX 'Saving lives in trauma', p723). It prioritizes direct treatment according to the most life-threatening injury identified and avoids delay. ▸▸Remember to act immediately...

Primary survey

▸▸A=airway + O_2 + cervical spine. Approach the patient with arms ready to immobilize the neck from the caudal end; CT is the best method of assessment if high/moderate risk for cervical fracture.[217] Assess the airway; jaw thrust can be used to help maintain patency. Give 100% O_2 to all patients. Talk to the patient—if they are able to talk back, then significant airway or breathing compromise is unlikely. Trauma to: ▸▸airway obstruction/head and neck trauma: see p758; ▸▸spine, p766.

▸▸B=breathing + ventilation. Check air entry with auscultation; also auscultate the heart; inspect, palpate and percuss the chest wall for further evidence of injury. Check RR. ▸▸Chest trauma, p722-4.

▸▸c=circulation + haemorrhage control. Check GCS/AVPU, skin perfusion, BP & pulse. Note that the pulse pressure narrows before the BP drops. Estimate the volume of any blood loss (OHCM p609). Control any visible haemorrhage with local pressure, and consider possible sources of occult haemorrhage if no source identified but the patient is shocked, ie examine abdo, pelvis, femora (MINIBOX). NB: blood loss estimates from the scene of injury are unreliable.

Get 2L of *warmed* Ringer's lactate solution/Hartmann's solution/0.9% saline running stat via 2 separate points of venous access (take bloods first from one—including pregnancy test for ♀).[216] Crossmatch an overestimate of the amount of blood loss. RBC replacement will be needed

Occult blood loss sites
• Tibial/humeral # [(0.75L)]
• Femoral # [(1.5L)]
• Pelvic # [(several L)]
• Chest/abdomen [(all)]

with >1.5L blood loss. Remember the possibility of cardiac or neurogenic shock with a low BP *and* HR or if unresponsive to fluid resuscitation. Young, fit patients have excellent reserves, and so haemodynamic instability may represent extreme compromise. ▸▸Abdo trauma, p726. ▸▸Pelvic trauma, p750. ▸▸Limb trauma, p738-57.

▸▸D=disability. Check GCS (if not already done), pupillary reflexes, gross evidence of a lateralizing injury or spinal cord level. Also check BM. ▸▸Head injury, p728. ▸▸Spinal trauma, p766.

▸▸E=exposure. Check and maintain body temperature using rewarming methods. Totally undress the patient, cutting all clothes off if necessary. ▸▸Hypothermia, OHCM p860.

Adjuncts to the primary survey can add life-saving information: CXR, lateral c-spine x-ray and pelvic x-ray (and *no* other x-ray until after the secondary survey); urinary catheter to accurately assess urine output (▸exclude urethral injury first); NGT insertion (▸not in presence of facial #); O_2 sats and then ABG to accurately assess oxygenation.

▸▸NB: if there is any change in the state of the patient or if there has been a problem identified and treated during the primary survey, begin the primary survey over again—eg laparotomy may even precede 'D'.

Secondary survey Now the patient is stabilized, *every inch must be scrutinized* for another injury, working from scalp to toe. More focused imaging can take place. Includes more focused examination (eg PR exam, otoscopy) and tests (eg limb x-ray, full c-spine series). ▸Remember tetanus—p730.

PRINCIPAL SOURCE: ADVANCED TRAUMA LIFE SUPPORT, 7/e, AMERICAN COLLEGE OF SURGEONS

Orthopaedics and trauma

▶▶After any trauma, the abdomen and chest may be sites of occult blood loss (see MINIBOX, p725). *Always* consider intra-abdominal bleeding or pelvic fracture (p750) if BP↓ and no source of loss is found.

Penetrating injuries mostly require prompt laparotomy/laparoscopy. ▶*Remember that all but the most superficial injuries will require exploration*—laparotomy is indicated if the posterior rectus sheath is breached. Remember that the diaphragm rises up to the 4th ICS on the right and up to the 5th ICS on the left; diaphragmatic rupture may also expose abdominal contents to injury in the chest. Assess degree of penetration (if uncertain) under local anaesthetic, by extending the wound, if necessary. Ask for expert assistance with this. The most commonly injured abdominal organ in penetrating trauma is the liver (MINIBOX).

Stab involvement:
Liver (40%)
Small bowel (30%)
Diaphragm (20%)
Colon (15%)

Blunt trauma Deceleration forces may tear bowel from mesentery, liver from vena cava, bladder from bladder neck, pancreas from retroperitoneum, and aorta from itself.[1] The spleen is the most commonly injured abdominal organ in blunt trauma (MINIBOX). ▶A ruptured spleen is suggested by shock, abdominal tenderness and distension, left shoulder-tip pain, and an overlying rib fracture.

Blunt involvement:
Spleen (~50%)
Liver (~40%)
Small bowel (~10%)
Retroperitoneal (15%)

Key questions: *Are vital signs stable? Is laparotomy needed?* (BP↓; GI, GU, or PR bleeding; evisceration; +ve ultrasound or peritoneal lavage). *Tests* CVP measurements, CT, and ultrasound may all mislead. There is no substitute for monitoring vital signs and examining the abdomen *often*. Systolic BP doesn't fall consistently until ≥30% of blood volume is lost. ▶NB: any visceral injury may cause bruising in the flanks, absent bowel sounds, and muscular spasm.

Management Maintain airway; ensure adequate ventilation. Give high-flow O₂ (15L/min). Treat shock (p725). Crossmatch blood. Then:

1 If the patient does not respond quickly, take straight to theatre for an exploratory laparotomy (after urgent CXR to rule out pneumothorax and after passing of a nasogastric tube).

2 Baseline observations: HR, BP, respirations, temperature, urine output.

3 Look for signs of GU injury (suggested by haematuria):
   • Blood at the urethral tip, signifying ruptured urethra.
   • Test the urine. Is there frank or microscopic haematuria?
   • Do a rectal exam to assess bowel integrity, presence of blood, or high-riding prostate (this suggests bladder neck injury).
   • If any suspicious signs, seek urological help to plan urethral repair. Rarely, GU trauma needs ureteroureterostomy, ureteroneocystostomy, or even kidney autotransplantation.

4 Consider peritoneal lavage or FAST scanning (BOX 1).

5 Arrange a prompt exploratory laparotomy if there is:
   ▶▶Shock (eg ruptured spleen)   ▶▶Penetration to unknown extent
   ▶▶Peritonism (ruptured viscus)   ▶▶Pneumoperitoneum (OHCM p609, fig 1)
   A non-functioning kidney on IVU is a *relative* indication. Don't deny analgesia on finishing your assessment, simply for fear of masking signs.

6 *Blood tests* FBC (raised WCC may occur in ruptured spleen), U&E, amylase.

7 *Radiology* Primary survey adjuncts as for p725. Abdominal images are part of the secondary assessment: consider these along with IVU, thoracolumbar spine, and other injured sites. See BOX OPPOSITE for the implications of radiology investigations.

---

1 ▶Thinking of mechanisms in trauma is essential, as it will trigger thought of injuries that may remain occult until too late (such as the above).

Emergency ultrasound

Investigations are often required in abdominal trauma because physical examination alone may yield equivocal results. **Focused Assessment with Sonography for Trauma (FAST)** has all but replaced diagnostic peritoneal lavage (DPL) as the bedside investigation of choice in abdominal trauma. as it is a rapid, repeatable and non-invasive test. It is used to evaluate the evaluate the patient for free peritoneal or pericardic fluid—which in the context of trauma is assumed to be blood. The FAST consists of four windows—the peri-hepatic, perisplenic, pelvic and pericardic It is considered positive when intra-abdominal or pericardial fluid is seen, and negative in the absence of this. FAST scanning can detect more than 100-250mL of fluid in the abdomen.[218] However its sensitivity is user dependent and it is not sensitive at detecting liver and spleen tears[219] or hollow viscus injuries.

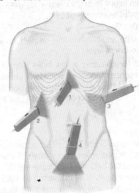

Fig. 1. Shown are four transducer positions in the FAST: (1) pericardial area, (2) right upper quadrant, (3) left upper quadrant, and (4) pelvis.
Reproduced from ACS Surgery: Principles and Practice, American College of Surgeons. © Decker Intellectual Properties, 2012

It has been found to decrease the time to recognition of intraabdominal trauma, the time to theatre, and reduce the number of CT scans performed.[220–222] However it has not been shown to reduce mortality.[223] The role of FAST is therefore best confined to use with haemodynamically unstable patients—who can't be transferred to CT for more definitive imaging. In such patients FAST can be used to identify whether the cause for haemodynamic instability is intraabdominal or intra-thoracic. Sonography at the bedside can also be used to evaluate the chest for a haemothorax or pneumothorax. It has greater sensitivity for small pneumothoraces than CXR, especially in the supine trauma patient.

Radiographic implications in abdominal trauma

- *Lower rib fracture* = ?liver/spleen trauma
- *Pelvic fracture* = ?rectal/urethral injury
- *Spine fracture* = ?renal/pancreatic/aortic/caval trauma
- *Free gas* = bowel rupture
- *Bowel displaced* = ?haemoperitoneum.

In the UK, manage according to NICE guidelines. This is a summary.[224]

Definition Any trauma to the head other than superficial injury to the face.

Emergency care As always, treat ABCDE—Airway, Breathing, and Circulation, Disability, Exposure (p725).

▸▸Give O₂ and treat shock.

▸▸Protect the cervical spine.

▸▸Note pupil sizes and reactivity.

▸▸*Do not neglect other injuries.* Primary brain damage occurs with the initial trauma. The clinical imperative is to prevent or ameliorate secondary brain injury, ie further neuronal death: successful management of A, B & C is the first step.

Cranial injuries:
• Skull fracture
Intracranial injuries:
• Diffuse axonal injury
• Extradural bleed*
• Subdural bleed*
• Subarachnoid bleed#
• Intracerebral bleed
• Cerebral contusion
OHCM images on: *p487; #p483.

Ask about: • Injury time and mechanism—impact or acceleration/deceleration. • Trend in consciousness level.

Check *ears and nose* for bleeding or CSF leaks (oto- & rhinorrhoea respectively—p560). The presence of these or blood behind the tympanic membrane may indicate a fractured base of skull. Bruising over the mastoid (**Battle's sign**) and periorbital bruising ('**raccoon eyes**') are late and unreliable signs of fractured base of skull.

Neurological assessment

• Write full notes; record times.

• Assess the *Glasgow Coma Score* (GCS, p720) *accurately* and *repeatedly*. Record all 3 parameters (motor, eyes, and verbal). If there is a difference between the sides, record the better result. If there is the possibility of a spinal injury, check for a response such as grimacing to a painful stimulus applied above the clavicles. Assess and record any contribution to mental status from alcohol or other drugs.

• *Pupils*—check size and reactivity every few minutes until stable. Unequal pupils are less important if conscious, but a grave sign in coma.

• *Spinal cord*—look for localizing neurological long tract signs ie: assess power, tone, reflexes, and all sensory modalities, comparing right side *vs* left, upper body *vs* lower. Check for priapism and anal tone.

• *Low BP* together with an inappropriately *low pulse* rate indicates sympathetic disruption in cervical spinal cord injury.

Medical management of head injury There are a number of specialist intensive care measures that can prevent secondary injury and optimize recovery:

• *Avoidance of hypotension:* Keep systolic BP >90. Even a single episode of low BP is associated with worse outcomes in severe traumatic brain injury.[225]

• *Avoidance of hypoxia:* Keep P_aO_2 >60mmHg or sats >90%.

• *Careful IV fluid therapy:* ▸Treat hypovolaemia (∴ cerebral hypoperfusion); ▸do not overload (preventing cerebral oedema); do not use glucose preparations (which damage brain tissue).

• *Hyperventilation:* Avoid in the first 24h post injury. After this use only as a temporizing measure for reduction of acute elevations of ICP. Hyperventilation reduces P_aCO_2, which causes cerebral vasoconstriction, thus reducing the effects of ↑ICP.[1] However, vasoconstriction may lead to increased ischaemia thereby worsening neurological injury.[226]

• *Mannitol:* 0.25–1g/kg of 20% mannitol solution causes osmotic diuresis, aiming to reduce ICP; useful in acute deterioration. Avoid systemic hypotension.

• If fits occur (in any situation), see p724.

---

1 Cerebral perfusion pressure (CPP) = mean arterial blood pressure (MABP) – intracranial pressure (ICP).

Orthopaedics and trauma

Investigating and managing head injury patients

Imaging	Urgent CT head if:	Cervical spine (x-ray/CT) if:
	• GCS <13 at initial assessment • GCS <15 at 2h post injury • Open or depressed skull or basal skull fracture • Post-traumatic fit • Focal CNS deficit • >1 episode of vomiting • Retrograde amnesia >½h	*Patients with neck pain or tenderness + one of:* • Age >65 • Dangerous mechanism • Unsafe to assess range of movement • Inability to rotate neck 45 degrees to the left and right • Extremity paraesthesiae • Focal CNS deficit
	CT head if any LOC/amnesia & • Age >65 years • Dangerous mechanism of injury • Coagulopathy	CT cervical spine if: • GCS <13 at initial assessment • Intubated • Patient is has multi-region trauma requiring CT scanning • Abnormal plain films • Ongoing clinical suspicion

▶▶If CT abnormal, GCS <15, or significant symptoms or signs, you must admit 'under a consultant with specialist training in managing head injured patients'. Those not fulfilling the admission criteria may be discharged with a *head injury information sheet*. Tertiary referral to a neurosurgical service should be according to agreed local guidelines/policy.

See also 'The neck', p658 and 'Does he need a radiograph?', p778.

Imaging diffuse axonal injury (DAI)

This important and historically underestimated type of brain injury is usually the result of rotational acceleration/deceleration forces to the unrestrained head, causing microscopic shearing of axons, though not necessarily at the precise moment of injury.

Brain areas at risk
• Hemispheric white matter • Corpus callosum • Brainstem.[227]

Delay can be in the order of hours to days (ie as part of secondary injury).

Imaging with CT may show the typical patterns of intraventricular haemorrhage, hemispheric intra-parenchymal haemorrhage, haemorrhage in the brainstem and corpus callosum, though often no abnormality is visualized (in 50–80%).[228] MRI is the superior modality, as it is more sensitive at revealing the presence of injury.[229]

Outcome of injury is often a persistent vegetative state (p776): likelihood correlates with the site and number of lesions present on imaging.

NB: see p758 for **Injuries to the face and neck**.

Orthopaedics and trauma

Principles of management Where possible, convert dirty ragged wounds into clean wounds that can be reconstructed simply eg by waiting for healing by secondary intention (may be suitable for small wounds in inconspicuous places or concave areas) or perform primary closure by suturing or other means. Other more complex options in the reconstructive ladder include skin grafts, flaps, tissue expansion and tissue engineering, and require specialist care.

Important points in the management of wounds

1 Irrigation, irrigation, and more irrigation with 0.9% saline or clean tap water. It is vital to clean the wound well as soon as possible particularly if the patient is referred to specialist care that could incur further delay.

2 Infiltrate with **lidocaine** (blocks voltage-gated Na⁺ channels to prevent depolarization) 4mg/kg plain or 7mg/kg with adrenaline. See opposite. Lidocaine is a vasodilator (∴ increases its own systemic clearance). **Adrenaline** is used where vasoconstriction to reduce bleeding is useful and if the predicted dose of lidocaine needed would exceed 4mg/kg. 1 in 200,000 adrenaline is most suitable for daily use (1:1000 is 1mg/mL). Use the minimum strength for job. Local anaesthesia (LA) will still work at dilute concentrations but you will need to wait for longer; for suturing 0.5% provides a good effect with less toxicity. Infiltrate through devitalized tissue of the wound using a small volume to avoid distorting the tissues. Local blocks are also an option. Use a fine needle (eg insulin syringe or dental syringe), warm the local anaesthetic and inject slowly to reduce pain. Topical anaesthetic—eg LET (lidocaine 4%, epinephrine 0.1% & tetracaine 0.5%) may help. Wait for anaesthetic (3min) and vasoconstrictor effect (7min).

3 Remove debris, foreign bodies and necrotic tissue; ragged or shelved skin edges may need trimming. Avoid excessive tissue resection on the face where reconstruction may be difficult. Abrasions need to be scrubbed thoroughly otherwise permanent tattooing will occur after re-epithelialization.

4 Use absorbable subcutaneous sutures (Vicryl®/PDS®) to bring skin edges together and avoid skin tension. Use interrupted monofilament (nylon/Prolene®) on the skin in most cases for optimal apposition 6'0 for the face, 5'0 or thicker for other areas. Very thick sutures are not needed as the strength of repair lies in the deeper layer. Avoid skin tension and wound inversion. Vicryl Rapide® or other absorbables may be considered as skin sutures in non-cosmetic areas: brush suture knots away after a week. (Sutures: OHCM p572.)

5 Remove sutures at the correct time to minimize risk of unsightly permanent stitch marks: face 5 days, upper limb/body 7–10 days, lower limb 14 days.

Suture alternatives avoid sharps and the need for removal. *Steristrips*: Good for non-hairy skin that is unlikely to get wet. Avoid too much traction (may cause fragile skin to blister). They may be combined with buried dermal absorbable sutures. *Glues:* (eg Dermabond®) After haemostasis, place directly on top of accurately apposed and dried skin edges. Avoid thick layers as the exothermic reaction may hurt. Allow to dry for 30sec, then apply another thin layer. Avoid getting the glue inside the wound as it is cytotoxic. Post-op: 'you can shower, but don't soak or scrub'. *NEJM 2008 video* tinyurl.com/57k3vf

Antibiotics Often not needed,[230] unless human/animal bite, hand wound.[231]

Tetanus Prophylaxis is vital. A full course (p151) provides good immunity. Vaccinate those who have not completed their schedule and where there is uncertainty.[1] Human immunoglobulin is for wounds that are prone to cause tetanus eg involving manure, extensive necrosis (give vaccine and Ig in different arms).

---

1 A full adult course if unimmunized would be 0.5mL of 'combined tetanus & low-dose diphtheria and inactivated polio vaccine' IM repeated × 2 at monthly intervals with boosters at 10 & 20yrs.

We thank Prof Tor Chiu for this page.

Calculating lidocaine (= lignocaine) doses[232]

For more information on local anaesthetic doses, toxicity, and onset and duration times. For lidocaine doses (*without adrenaline*):

Percentage	Concentration (mg/mL)	Approx. allowable volume (mL/kg)
0.25%	2.5	1.12
0.5%	5	0.56
1%	10	0.28
2%	20	0.14

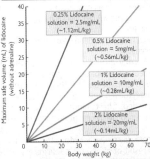

Fig 1. Maximum safe volume of plain lidocaine by body weight.

0.25% Lidocaine solution = 2.5mg/mL (~1.12mL/kg)

0.5% Lidocaine solution = 5mg/mL (~0.56mL/kg)

1% Lidocaine solution = 10mg/mL (~0.28mL/kg)

2% Lidocaine solution = 20mg/mL (~0.14mL/kg)

Max. safe dose of lidocaine *without adrenaline*: 3mg/kg; *with adrenaline*: 7mg/kg. Use different strengths for different jobs: 0.25-0.5% for infiltration & IV regional anaesthesia; 1% for nerve blocks, epidural anaesthesia, and IV regional anaesthesia; 2% for nerve blocks.

NB: 1%=10mg/mL.

Wound healing and associated problems

Wound healing is a fascinating but complex web of physiology: to attempt to explain it in detail would be unflattering to such a remarkable process.[233]

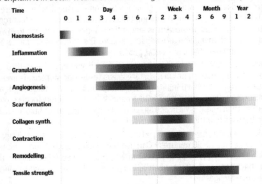

Fig 2. The above diagram outlines the important and overlapping stages during the wound healing process—NB: milestones are variable. Courtesy of Dr Tom Turmezei.

Wound healing problems Wound healing capability ↓ with ↑age, malnutrition, DM, steroid therapy, smoking (p737), peripheral vascular disease and irradiation. Wound infection worsens scarring and so topical **chloramphenicol** can be used to reduce the risk of cosmetic insult (eg on face). *Keloid scarring* is exaggerated scarring (from excess collagen production, especially type III) to beyond the confines of the initial wound and can appear progressively and after a delay. *Hypertrophic scarring* is exaggerated scarring within the confines of the initial wound, is often associated with a wound across a joint surface, and tends to regress. Both are more common in dark-skinned individuals.

Orthopaedics and trauma

The majority of burns are minor; non-specialist staff will see very few major burns. Their task should be to ensure the rapid and safe transfer to Burns units (with ITU resources and access to burn surgery) experienced in their care. Staff should be familiar with ATLS and EMSB protocols (Early Management of Severe Burns).[234]

Airway and breathing Inhalational injury can occur by many mechanisms: thermal, chemical/acids, irritant or systemic effects. Direct damage to lung parenchyma is rare. Risk of inhalational injury is best judged by clinical assessment—have a high index of suspicion (there is no single diagnostic sign). Thermal damage to the upper airway may cause airway obstruction through oedema which may be exacerbated by concomitant cutaneous injury.

• *History* Fire in enclosed space eg house fire.
• *Signs* Burns of oropharynx, burnt nasal hairs, change in voice, soot in upper airway or sputum or bronchoscopic evidence.
• *Management* ▸▸Give high-flow O_2. Formal airway assessment by an ICU anaesthetist is advisable. ▸Early expectant intubation is preferable. Difficulty with ventilation may be related to thoracic burns if they are deep and circumferential and so restrict breathing movements—an escharotomy (see Decompression, opposite) may be needed. Chest injuries such as tension pneumothorax or flail chest may be caused by the event eg force of explosion, running/jumping to safety.
• *Carboxyhaemoglobin (COHb)* Check COHb particularly within the first hour, as levels can drop quickly; blood gas result of >10% COHb confirms exposure (oximetry is unreliable). 100% O_2 will reduce the half life of COHb from 250 to 40min (there are very few indications for using hyperbaric oxygen except for deteriorating neurological signs—COHb blood levels are not a good indicator).
• *Cyanide (CN)* Comes from burning foam and disrupts cellular metabolism. It is not readily measured in the clinical situation—suspect where there is persistent evidence of tissue poisoning (mechanism of toxicity is cytochrome inhibition). The safest treatment is single-dose sodium thiosulfate followed by hydroxocobalamin given as early as possible. The effects of CO and CN are often overestimated. (Also see OHCM, p854.)

Circulation Insert 2 large-bore IV cannulae even if you have to go through burnt skin. The estimation of burn surface areas (BSA—see MINIBOX) is important as the size of the burn injury reflects magnitude of inflammatory reaction; subsequent fluid shifts may lead to shock if uncorrected (occurs over hours rather than minutes as in actual haemorrhage). The aim of fluid 'resuscitation' in burns is to anticipate and prevent shock.

First Aid •Remove burnt clothing •Cool burns and warm patient: irrigate with cool water for 10–20 minutes •Can use clingfilm in thermal burns (do not wrap circumferentially) •Cooling gels/masks simple to use especially for the face, but have the most effect when left exposed to the air •Chemical burns need continued irrigation.

Burn surface area (BSA) Use rule of 9s (MINIBOX) or a burn chart—eg Lund and Browder (OHCM, p859).

Fluids There are several commonly used formulae for fluid administration—the **Parklands formula** (below) is often preferred to formulae using colloids (Muir & Barclay) but the actual dangers of the latter are probably overestimated, particularly in uncomplicated patients. The administration of colloid is generally regarded as being safe after the 1st day (when capillary permeability recovers) but is not always given; similarly blood is advocated by some but rarely given.

Wallace rule of nines
• Arm (all over) 9%
• Leg (all over) 18%
• Front 18%
• Back 18%
• Head (all over) 9%
• Genitals/perineum 1%

Orthopaedics and trauma

We thank Prof Tor Chiu for help with this page.

Parklands formula Time of injury is taken as the start time and with any delay, the deficit needs to be calculated and given:

> Volume of Hartmann's (mL)[1] = 4 × body weight (kg) × BSA (%).
> • ½ is given in the 1st 8h • The other ½ in the next 16h.

▶NB: do not confuse the formulae: Muir & Barclay use half the volume but in the form of colloid. Use the appropriate fluid with the formula. All formulae represent starting points: tailor continuing fluids to the response. The patient should be catheterized as the best single measure is the urine output—aim for more than 0.5mL/kg/h.[235] The temperature gradient (core and periphery) is used in some units to measure peripheral perfusion.

Burn depth This has implications for healing/scarring but assessment can be hard, particularly for intermediate-thickness burns. Many burns, especially scalds in children, are mixed depth. Also, burns can evolve for up to 48h. In A&E, the most important aspect of assessing burn depth is *erythema*; to avoid over-estimating burns, don't count mild redness, blisters or oedema. Laser Doppler imaging (LDI) can provide reliable objective measures of burn depth but machines are costly.

• *Full-thickness burns* are white/grey/black, thick and insensate and can cause constriction if circumferential
• *Superficial burns* are painful, red and have blisters.

Decompression Full thickness burns are tough and inflexible; if circumferential, they can have a tourniquet-like effect and hinder breathing or limb circulation. Also, big volumes of crystalloid may lead to marked soft tissue swelling. In such cases *decompression* may be needed, which may involve escharotomy (incising inflexible burn eschar along prescribed lines) and fasciotomy. It is rarely needed at once and, contrary to some advice, it is best performed under controlled conditions ie in the operating theatre and under GA.

Transfer and dressings There is no need for anything fancy. Simple cleaning of the wound with sterile 0.9% saline is adequate. Blisters should be left alone unless tense and causing pain.

• Apply cool wet dressings for pain relief.
• Using Clingfilm® covered with blankets to keep warm is adequate.
• Hands (and feet) can be put into clean plastic bags, and should be elevated.
• Analgesia should be adequate; use IV opiates if necessary, titrated to comfort. Tetanus prophylaxis is given as necessary (p730).

Paediatric burns Standard estimation of area cannot be applied: Wallace's rule of 9s must be modified but is then rather unwieldy, and specific burn charts are more reliable. For small burns you can use the patient's palm and fingers—equivalent to ~1% BSA—to estimate burn size. There is a lower threshold to begin resuscitation (10% BSA).

• Maintenance fluids in the form of dextrose-saline are given, and a higher urine output is needed: >1mL/kg/h.
• Keep warm as there is a greater tendency to hypothermia.
• Be alert to possibility of non-accidental injury.

Because of advances in wound management in specialized burns centres (eg autologous split-thickness skin grafts ± cultured fetal skin fibroblasts) even 95% burns are survivable by 50% of children.[236]

Mortality risk prediction The percentage of burnt surface area + age gives a very rough prediction of mortality (though it's usefulness has been reduced by improvements in burns care.) For example:
• 10% burn in a 20-yr-old ≈ 30% risk of mortality
• 10% burn in a 90-yr-old ≈ 100% risk of mortality.

In general, burns mortality is related to surface area involved, inhalational injury, age and comorbid illnesses.

---

1 In electric shock injuries, higher volumes of fluid may be needed; see p789.

Orthopaedics and trauma

Description
- *Site:* Bone(s) fractured; part of bone (proximal, shaft, distal etc)
- *Obliquity:* Transverse; short oblique; spiral; multi-fragmentary
- *Displacement:* Angulation; translation; rotation; impaction, foreshortening
- *Soft tissues:* Open/closed; neurovascular status; compartment syndrome.

NB: when giving a displacement description, this refers to the **distal** fragment. For angulated fractures, eg in the hand, the terms 'apex dorsal' and 'apex palmar' can also be used.

Seven key questions
• How many fractures?
• Can I see all the bone?
• What is broken?
• Are the bones normal?
• Any trapped air?
• Any foreign body?
• More plain films needed (IVU, CT, arteriogram)?

Clinical features Pain; loss of function; tenderness; deformity; swelling; crepitus; abnormal movement or positioning of a limb; soft tissues.

Fracture healing (see also p738) A rule-of-thumb for fracture healing is given by the 'rule-of-3s'. A *closed, paediatric, metaphyseal, upper limb* fracture is the simplest and will heal in 3 weeks. Any 'complicating factor' doubles the healing time, ie adult; diaphyseal; lower limb; open injury. For example an *adult (6), diaphyseal (12) forearm* fracture may take 12 weeks to heal. Likewise an *open (6), adult (12), diaphyseal (24), tibia (48)* may be expected to heal in 48 weeks (almost a year!) to heal. Metaphysis and epiphysis are defined on p683.

Methods of managing fractures Immobilize and reduce the part (if needed, p736), eg using a plaster of Paris cast. The problem with this method is that 'fracture disease' follows immobilization—muscle atrophy, stiff joints, and osteoporosis—so anything speeding return of function may be beneficial.[1] If possible, fractures involving joint articulations should be treated by open reduction, accurate reconstruction of the joint surfaces, and fixation, such that immediate movement can occur—see MINIBOX for the other indications for open reduction internal fixation (ORIF). Otherwise, secondary osteoarthritis is inevitable. Prompt internal fixation, eg with plates and screws, nails or wires (Kirschner), of all fractures in those with polytrauma leads to large reductions in serious complications (fat embolism, acute respiratory distress syndrome), as well as lessening the time during which mechanical ventilation is needed.[237]

External fixation uses wires into bone, a bar, and a means (clamps) of attaching the bar to the screws to align and engage the fractured cortices. The wires may be driven through the bone and out of the far side of the limb, so that a second bar can add stability. Further rigidity is afforded by another set of screws at 90° to the first set. Because the intervention is away from the field of injury, this method is very useful when there are burns, loss of skin and bone, or an open fracture.

Indications for ORIF
• Failed conservative Rx
• 2 #s in 1 limb
• Bilateral identical #s
• Intra-articular #s
• Open #.

Pathological fractures See p709.

---

1 Healing may be speeded by ~64 days with pulsed ultrasound (it's non-standard).[217]

Fixation

Screw insertion to unite the fragments typically begins with temporary wire or bone clamp fixation. A pilot hole is then drilled into bone, which must be substantial enough to support the screw head. Both near and far cortices are drilled with the pilot drill. Countersinking decreases incidence of stress risers and microfractures of the bone as the head of the screw compresses into the near cortex. The pilot hole

Fixation options
• Kirschner wires (K-wires)
• Cannulated screws
• Staples
• Self-tapping screws
• Osteosynthesis lag screws
• Herbert headless screws[238]
• Absorbable pins

is measured to aid selection of the best length of screw. Distal threads have a smaller diameter than proximal threads to give thread cutting action for self-tapping screws. Have eg 2 threads of the screw exiting the far cortex to assure that the largest threads of the screw purchase the far cortex. (Add eg 2mm to the pilot measurement.)

Lag screw technique An oversized countersunk hole is drilled through the near cortex. The distal portion of the hole is drilled with a diameter corresponding to the core diameter of the screw. As the screw tightens, its distal end engages the threaded hole of the distal fragment. The undersurface of the screw head contacts the countersink hole and pulls the distal fragment against the proximal fragment causing compression. A lag effect can only occur if the screw can pass freely through the gliding hole. Lag screws are most appropriate for oblique fractures.[239]

Gustilo classification of open fractures[240]

Type I	*Low-energy* wounds <1cm long, eg caused by bone piercing skin
Type II	*Low-energy* wounds >1cm, causing moderate soft tissue damage
Type III	All *high-energy* injuries irrespective of wound size:
	• IIIA fractures have *adequate* local soft tissue coverage
	• IIIB fractures have *inadequate* local soft tissue coverage
	• IIIC implies arterial injury needing repair

▸▸Emergency management of open fractures: the 7 'As'

1 *ATLS:* As with all emergencies manage in an ABC fashion. In the multi-trauma patient be careful not to be distracted by the open fracture, but complete a primary survey assessing Airway, Breathing, Circulation and Disability - treating life threatening injuries as they are discovered. Correct shock (p725); give blood if >1.5L lost or continued bleeding. Control of bleeding may require open surgery.

2 *Assessment:* Neurovascular status, soft tissues and *photograph* wound (reduces number of wound inspections).

3 *Antisepsis:* Take a swab from the wound, use copious irrigation with sterile 0.9% saline (eg 3L), then cover with a large antiseptic-soaked dressing.

4 *Alignment:* Align fracture and splint (also provides pain relief).

5 *Anti-tetanus:* Check status and immunize appropriately (p730).

6 *Antibiotics:* 3rd generation cephalosporin, eg **ceftriaxone** 1g/24h IV[241] ± **metronidazole** if grossly contaminated; antibiotics prevent early infection.[242]

7 *Analgesia:* Intravenous opiate analgesia titrated to effect.

A displaced fracture needs realignment (reduction) unless function and appearance of the limb are satisfactory. For example, a small displacement acceptable in a fracture of the femoral shaft might not be acceptable in the radius, where it could interrupt supination. Reduction also allows freeing of any structures trapped between bone ends. Accurate reduction aids revascularization (vital in subcapital fractures of the femur) and prevents later degeneration if fractures involve joints. Internal and external fixation has removed the need for much traction in adults, but it is still used for children.

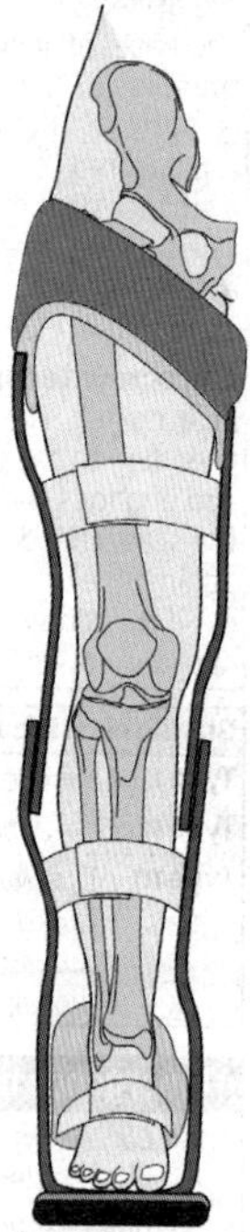

Fig 1. Thomas' splint.

Methods of reduction

- *Manipulation* under anaesthesia (for analgesia and muscle relaxation) and radiographic screening. NB: if under GA, consent for ± ORIF (open reduction + internal fixation, p134) in case closed reduction is unsuccessful. ▶▶Occasionally reduction will be required immediately, ie in A&E before an x-ray is even taken (eg for fracture-dislocation of the ankle or knee).
- *Traction* (see below & fig **2**) may be used for eg femoral shaft fractures or spinal injury.
- *Open reduction* aids accuracy, eg before internal fixation.

Methods of traction The next problem is to hold the reduction in place by using traction or fixation during healing, which takes from 2 weeks (babies) to >12 weeks (p734).

- *Skin traction* uses adhesive strapping to attach the load to the limb. The problems are that the load cannot be very great, and that sensitivity to the adhesive may develop.
- *Fixed traction* The Thomas' splint (fig **1**). Weight can be added over a pulley (at the foot end) to relieve pressure on ischial tuberosity.
- *Skeletal traction* Using a pin through bone, bigger forces can be employed (eg Steinmann or Denham pin in the distal femur/proximal tibia for femoral shaft fractures, Gardner–Wells tongs or Crutchfield skull callipers for cervical spine traction).
- *Balanced traction* (fig **2**) The weight of the limb balanced against the load. This can enable to patient to easily lift the leg off the bed, eg for a bed pan.
- *Gallows traction* (fig **2**) is suitable for children up to 2yrs of age. The buttocks rise just above the bed.

The ward nurses will be experts at setting up and adjusting traction devices, so ask if you can watch and help. See BOX, p735 for methods of fixation.

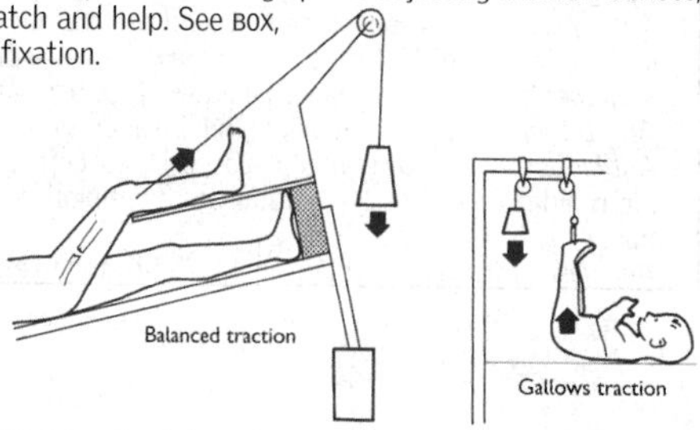

Fig 2. Traction: balanced traction, and gallows traction.

Smoking and tissue healing—the consequences of a cigarette break

Trauma patients need to knit back together well, and they face a number of complications without adding tobacco into the physiological equation. Not only do smokers increase risk of perioperative complication—such as venous thromboembolism, respiratory tract infection & cardiac ischaemia—they also reduce their chances of healing well, potentially undoing all the hard graft of the surgical team in theatre (eg plastics, orthopaedics, general surgery).

What damage are smokers doing? Nicotine increases the time it takes for a fracture to unite **and** reduces quality of bone healing. Tobacco smoking also reduces tissue oxygenation and wound healing. This is particularly pertinent for operations on the lower extremities—eg Achilles tendon repair (p712) or calcaneal fracture ORIF (p756)—because of the precarious local blood supply combined with a propensity for compartment syndrome, ▸p738.

Is it justifiable to withhold surgery from smokers?[1] Perhaps 'yes', if a given problem has a non-operative alternative with similar outcome yet potentially disastrous complications exacerbated by smoking: eg a calcaneal ORIF spiralling out of control into an amputation. Also perhaps 'yes', if resources must be distributed across a population in whom smokers are shown to fare much worse with a given operative management. The ethical counterpoise would be from a discriminatory angle, both in terms of costs and the concept of self-inflicted harm—eg in comparison to dangerous sporting activity.

How to approach the issue? Careful informed consent will be vital, though whether scare tactics are allowed is another matter altogether. Abstaining for 6 to 8 weeks prior to elective surgery will reduce many of the side-effects of smoking, but this is not a luxury afforded to trauma patients, and for some the stresses of what has happened may be too much to place on top of stopping smoking.[2] Do smokers mobilize more keenly in the post-op period in response to their craving to get off the ward for a cigarette? There appear to be no studies to answer this yet! For giving *advice on stopping smoking*, see p512.

Salter and Harris classification of epiphyseal injury

I   Seen in babies or pathological conditions (eg scurvy)

II   The commonest injury, with the fracture line **above** the growth plate

III There is a displaced fragment, with the fracture line **through** the growth plate

IV   Union across the growth plate may interfere with bone growth

V   Compression of the epiphysis causes deformity and stunting

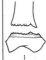

Fig 3. Salter and Harris classification of epiphyseal injury.

Injuries to and around the growth plate can be very difficult to distinguish from normal appearances, especially when they are viewed obliquely. Most physes are in plane that makes it relatively easy to diagnose the injury (eg distal radius, and to a lesser extent proximal femur), whereas some cross the plane of the x-ray at multiple angles (eg proximal humerus). With these trickier physes, it is wise to liaise with someone with experience. Also consider comparison with the contralateral side.

---

1 With pressure to provide a cost-effective and fair service in the NHS, there are strong arguments from both parties. The debate certainly does not allow for smoke without fire...[244]

2 Though even stopping one day before surgery has been shown to improve outcome.

Orthopaedics and trauma

Complications Synopsis: see MINIBOX. *Fat embolism:* Typically arises on day 3–10. Signs: confusion, dyspnoea, pulse↑, P_aO_2↓, fits, coma, T°↑, petechial rash. CXR/CT: small subpleural nodular opacities.[245] ►►Take to ITU ►►Get expert help ►►Correct shock ►►Monitor CVP & urine output ►►Treat respiratory failure (OHCM p180). Aim for early mobilization. Early fixation of fractures is preventive. Mortality: 10–20%.

Crush and compartment syndromes are a cause of ischaemia. Fluid loss, DIC, and myoglobin release cause renal tubular necrosis: dialysis may be needed. Correct hypovolaemia vigorously. Watch urine output & plasma K$^+$. A limb's dead weight when immobile or in coma may cause crush injury/compartment syndrome in a vicious cycle of pressure→vascular occlusion→hypoxia→necrosis →pressure↑. Look for tell-tale signs of redness, mottling, blisters, swelling, and *pain on passive muscle stretching.*
►►Compartment syndrome is limb- and life-threatening. Avoiding problems caused by delay requires vigilance and perhaps intracompartmental pressure measurement (NB: diagnosis is clinical; normal values for intervention are controversial). *Prompt fasciotomy is life-/limb-saving.[246]*

Late complications
- *Wound sepsis:* Early wound cleaning is vital. Infection arises in ~8% of closed fractures if internal fixation is used. Ceftriaxone 2g IVI at induction halves risk.[247]
- *Failure of fixation:* eg plates or nails break, or dislodge.
- *Joint stiffness, contractures, malalignment* (=malunion).
- *CRPS:* Joint stiffness and patchy osteopenia—see OPPOSITE.
- *Psychological problems in mobilizing:* eg 'compensation neurosis'.
- *Non-union (atrophic or hypertrophic)* This is said to have occurred when there is no evidence of progression towards healing, clinically or radiologically.
- *Delayed union* is when the fracture has not healed within the time reasonably expected for *that* fracture (p734). *Causes of delay:*
  - A fracture in a bone which has finished growing.
  - Poor blood supply (eg lower tibia) or avascular fragment (eg scaphoid).
  - Comminuted/infected fractures, eg after open reduction/internal fixation.
  - Generalized disease such as malignancy or infection.
  - Distraction of bone ends by muscle; open reduction ± internal fixation prevents this. NB: osteoporosis ± old age don't necessarily delay union.

Managing non-union Broadly, a non-union occurs from inadequate or abnormal biology or mechanics. Management is aimed at optimizing biology (infection, blood supply, bone graft) or the mechanics (skeletal stabilization).

Complications
Immediate:
• Internal bleeding
• External bleeding
• Organ injury, eg brain
• Nerve or skin injury
• Vessel injury (limb ischaemia: OHCM p658)
Later—local:
• Skin necrosis/gangrene
• Pressure sores
• Infection
• Non- or delayed union
Later—general:
• Venous or fat embolism
• Pulmonary embolism
• Pneumonia
• Renal stones

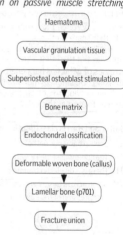

Haematoma
↓
Vascular granulation tissue
↓
Subperiosteal osteoblast stimulation
↓
Bone matrix
↓
Endochondral ossification
↓
Deformable woven bone (callus)
↓
Lamellar bone (p701)
↓
Fracture union

Fig 1. Bone healing.

Complex regional pain syndromes (CRPS)

CRPS type I is a deranged sequel to limb trauma *without* nerve injury (CRPS I≈ algodystrophy ≈ reflex sympathetic dystrophy, RSD). If nerve lesions are present, the term CRPS II (causalgia) is used. Here it is helpful to bear in mind that after a partial nerve lesion there is ↑activity in undamaged afferent c fibres with neuropeptide release (∴ vasodilatation within their innervation territory). But CNS phenomena are important too. Animal studies show ↑expression of the N-methyl-D-aspartate (NMDA) receptors in models of neuropathic pain (and NMDA receptor blockers such as memantine can improve symptoms).[248] Another proof of central effects is the finding of substantial reorganization of somatotopic CNS maps—leading to mislocalization of tactile stimuli.[249]

CRPS type I is a 'complex disorder of pain, sensory abnormalities, abnormal blood flow, sweating, and trophic changes in superficial or deep tissues'. The central event may be loss of vascular tone or supersensitivity to sympathetic neurotransmitters. Pathogenesis is obscure, the idea of exaggerated regional inflammatory responses is supported by the fact that IgG labelled with indium (^{111}In) is concentrated in the affected extremity.[250]

Causes Injury esp distal and esp upper limb—eg fractures, carpal tunnel release, ops for Dupuytren's, tendon release procedures, mastectomy, transradial cardiac catheterization,[251] knee surgery, crush injury, ankle arthrodesis, amputation, hip arthroplasty, rotator cuff injury, zoster, myocardial infarction, stroke, cancer, spontaneous/idiopathic.

Presentation Typically patients have initial trauma—commonly in a hand or foot—which may be trivial or severe. This is followed weeks or months later by pain, allodynia/hyperalgesia, vasomotor instability and abnormal sweating. Pain is often burning in nature and may extend to the whole limb. The limb may be cold and cyanosed, or hot and sweating (locally). T° sensitivity may be heightened. The skin of the affected part may be oedematous, or, later, shiny and atrophic. Hyperreflexia, dystonic movements, and contractures may occur. Symptoms are often worse after exercise, and may include weakness, hyperalgesia, clumsiness, inability to initiate movements, spasms, dystonias, and allodynia (a stimulus not usually painful now hurts). There are no systemic signs (no fever, tachycardia, or lymphadenopathy).

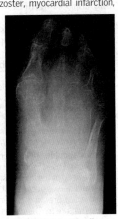

Fig 2. CRPS type I, with diffuse osteopenia and destruction of the 2nd and 3rd metatarsals.

Image Courtesy of Norfolk and Norwich University Hospital (NNUH) Radiology Department.

Imaging *Radiographs:* Patchy osteopenia greater than expected from disuse; joint space not narrowed (*no* thinned cartilage)—see fig 2. *Bone scintigraphy:* Characteristic uniform uptake, with increased limb perfusion on the dynamic phase.

• **Treatment** ►Refer to pain clinic/multidisciplinary team (physio + OT).
• Encourage optimism and pleasurable things. Ultimately, with appropriate care, CRPS is self-limiting.
• Avoid bad habits of trying to protect the affected by keeping it immobile, (leads to stiffness). Educate on using the limb in activities of daily living.
• Effective painkillers often have amitriptyline eg 25mg/d PO ± NSAIDs.

Other treatments include: tricyclics; gabapentin; ketamine; clonidine (α₂-adrenoceptor agonist with anaesthetic and analgesic sparing effects); calcitonin; postganglionic sympathetic blocks (guanethidine; bretylium).[252]

Fracture of the clavicle Historically thought to be caused by a fall onto an outstretched hand, most seem to occur after a direct blow to the shoulder. Fractures are most common in the middle third. Management is typically a broad arm sling with follow up x-rays at 6 weeks to ensure union. Fractures at the lateral end may need internal fixation if there is non-union (figs **1 & 2**). ►Remember the possibility of neurovascular injury (brachial plexus; subclavian vessels) + pneumothorax as complications.

Scapula and acromion fractures These represent high-energy transfer injuries, so assess carefully to exclude other injuries.

Acromioclavicular (AC) joint dislocation The patient has a tender prominence over the AC joint. Adduction of the arm across the body will cause increased pain. Subluxation can be confirmed by supporting the elbow and gently pushing down on the clavicle to improve the contour of the shoulder. On x-ray check for congruity of the underside of the acromion with the distal clavicle. Radiography may be normal, so if suspicious, request bilateral weight-carrying views. These injuries rarely require anything more than sling support and early mobilization. A small number (<5%) have persistent symptoms and require surgery.

Fracture of the proximal humerus may result in 2–4 fragments (eg Neer classification).[253] Most are stable osteoporotic fractures in the elderly.[254] Minimally displaced fractures may be managed conservatively. Open fractures, pathological fractures, 3 or 4 part fracture-dislocations or those with neurovascular injury (brachial plexus/axillary artery) will need operative management.[254] Prognosis and complications (eg avascular necrosis) worsen with ↑ number of fragments.

Fracture of the humeral shaft Often caused by a fall on an outstretched arm. Marked displacement may make the diagnosis easy. Non-operative management is adequate for >90% of these fractures.[255] Splinting with a humeral brace and gravity traction by means of a no. 1 'collar and cuff' sling usually gives satisfactory reduction. Immobilize for 8–12 weeks. Surgical options include intramedullary nailing and compression plating. ►Radial nerve injury may cause wrist-drop, but damage can also be a complication of surgery, so *document function pre-operatively.*

Anterior shoulder dislocation may follow a fall on an arm or shoulder (figs **4 & 5**). *Signs:* Loss of shoulder contour (flattening of deltoid), an anterior bulge from the head of the humerus, which may also be palpated in the axilla. ►Check pulses and nerves (including the axillary nerve supplying sensation over lower deltoid area) pre- and post-reduction. Before reduction, do radiography (*is there a fracture too?*)—unless this is a case of recurrent dislocation, when just a post-reduction image may be needed. Relieve pain (eg intra-articular local anaesthetic, parenteral opioid, Entonox® through the procedure). Treatment: *Simple reduction:* Apply longitudinal traction to the arm in abduction, and replace the head of the humerus by gentle pressure. *Kocher's method:* Flex the elbow to 90°, abduct the shoulder, externally rotate the shoulder/humerus and then abduct the upper arm back across the front of the body before internally rotating the shoulder. Risk: humeral #. Remember to obtain a radiograph post-reduction. Support the arm in internal rotation with a broad arm sling. Surgery may be needed eg if young/athletic, or recurrent dislocation (eg Bankart repair + capsular shift). *Is there an underlying connective tissue disorder?*

Posterior dislocation of the shoulder is rare and presents with a limitation of external rotation. It may be hard to diagnose from an anteroposterior radiograph ('light-bulb' appearance of humeral head); lateral radiographs are essential. Refer to an orthopaedic surgeon. www.ncemi.org/cse/cse0905.htm

Inferior shoulder dislocation Rarer; from hyperabduction; high incidence of complication: neurovascular injury, tuberosity avulsion, rotator cuff tear.

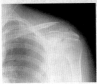
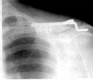
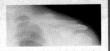

Fig 1. Comminuted distal clavicular fracture—an injury requiring ORIF...

Fig 2. ...Hook plate repair of fig 1-type injury. Remember nearby vessels!

Fig 3. Healed mid-clavicular fracture in a different patient—note deformity. Often, surgical repair is not needed for clavicle fractures, as healing and long-term function are good.

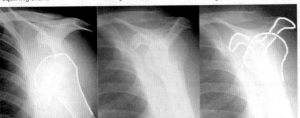

Fig 4–6. Anterior dislocation of the shoulder (fig 4)[1] and a post-reduction image (fig 5—copied and highlighted, fig 6). The dislocation can be painful, so positioning is difficult for the radiographer. These are attempted lateral views of the scapula. After reduction, the head of the humerus lies in the centre of the 'Y' with the coracoid process anterior and the acromion posterior.

Figs 1–3 courtesy of Norfolk and Norwich University Hospital (NNUH) Radiology Department; Figs 4–6 courtesy of Professor Peter Scally.

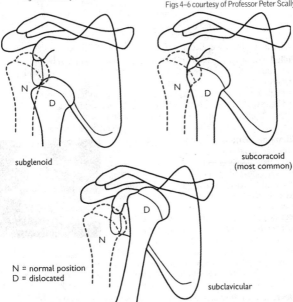

subglenoid

subcoracoid (most common)

N = normal position
D = dislocated

subclavicular

Fig 7. Types of anterior shoulder dislocation.

1 The humeral head can sometimes lie low in the glenoid fossa with surgical neck fractures, from 'deltoid inhibition'—relaxation of the muscle from pain, causing subluxation; it is **not** a fracture-dislocation.

Orthopaedics and trauma

The humerus • *Supracondylar fracture:* is the most common fracture of childhood, with a peak incidence between the ages of 5 and 7 years.[256] These fractures may compromise brachial artery, median (typically anterior interosseous branch), radial or ulnar nerve function so check neurovascular status. Keeping the elbow in extension after injury prevents exacerbating brachial artery damage from the time of injury. *Management:* Avoid flexing the elbow by >90°. Type I fractures (see box) can be managed with and above elbow back slab and sling. Type II fractures may require reduction under sedation/GA. Type III fractures generally require ORIF (eg with K-wires).[256]

• *Fracture of the medial condyle:* These may require surgery if a fragment is in the joint or if there are ulnar nerve compression symptoms.

• *Fracture of the lateral condyle:* Surgical fixation may be required. Complications include cubitus valgus and ulnar nerve palsy.

• *T-shaped intercondylar humerus fracture:* This is a supracondylar fracture with a break between the condyles.

The elbow *Imaging:* Presence of an elbow fracture is suggested by an 'anterior sail sign' or 'posterior fat pad sign'.[1] *Management:* If no # obvious, but an effusion is present, treat initially with a broad arm sling. Re-x-ray after 10d (# more easily seen): if clear, start mobilization. For fractures, internal fixation may be needed. Physiotherapy and early mobilization are vital in preventing stiffness.[257]

Fractures of the radial head The elbow is swollen and tender over the radial head; flexion/extension may be possible but pronation & supination hurt. Radiography often shows an effusion, but minor fractures are often missed. Undisplaced fractures can be treated in a collar and cuff sling—if displaced or fragment prevents supination/pronation: if clear, internal fixation or excision of the radial head may be needed.[258] *Complications:* 3–14% are associated with the 'terrible triad' of radial head fracture, elbow dislocation and coronoid process fracture—resulting in joint instability and post traumatic complications.[259] Radial nerve injury may occur with severe anterior displacement but is rare.

Pulled elbow Typical patient: 1–4-yr-old who has been lifted by the arms in play, causing the radial head to slip out of the annular ligament (fig 1; p667) The arm is held slightly flexed and twisted inwards. Reduction can be achieved through the examiner cradling the elbow, with thumb/forefingers over the radial head and either hyperpronating or supinating and flexing the elbow. Hyperpronation may be more successful.[260] Imaging is not needed. Caution parents not to pull arm of child, as this condition recurs in up to 25%.

Elbow dislocation A fall on a not yet fully outstretched hand, with elbow flexed, causes posterior ulna displacement on the humerus, and a swollen elbow, fixed in flexion. Brachial artery and median nerve damage are rare. *Reduction (±GA):* Stand behind the patient; flex the elbow to relax biceps brachii. With your fingers around the epicondyles, push forwards on the olecranon with your thumbs, and down on the forearm. Hearing a clunk heralds success. This may be aided by traction at the wrist. A post-reduction image is needed to exclude fractures. Immobilize in a backslab for 10 days. *Complications:* Stiffness, instability, ectopic ossification, radio-ulnar joint disruption.[261]

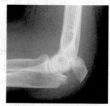

Fig 1. Displaced olecranon fracture needing fixation.
Courtesy of Norfolk and Norwich University Hospital (NNUH) Radiology Department;

Olecranon fracture ORIF, eg tension band wiring, if displaced fracture.

Elbow arthroplasty In comminuted distal humerus fractures, ORIF may be difficult, eg in osteoporotic bones. Hence the occasional use of total arthroplasty as a primary procedure.[262]

Gartland classification of supracondylar fractures

There are 2 chief categories: *extension* (95%) and *flexion* types.

Type I	Non-displaced fractures
Type II	Angulated with an intact posterior cortex
Type III	Posterior displacement—which is unstable[263]
	• **IIIA** is *posteromedial* and threatens the radial nerve
	• **IIIB** is *posterolateral* and threatens the median nerve, esp. the anterior interosseous branch, which innervates deep flexors to the index finger as well as flexor pollicis longus (pincer grip); it is an entirely motor nerve—so injury is easily missed

Falling children often get a buckle (ie **torus**) forearm fracture when the dorsal cortex crumples on pressure through an outstretched arm. The volar cortex is intact (check carefully to make sure). The distal fragment is angulated dorsally. There is usually local tenderness and swelling (torus is Latin for mound). As they are stable, a splint or short-arm cast for 3 weeks may be sufficient.[264] In greenstick fractures, one cortex fails in compression and the other fails in bending or rotation. The deformation can continue to angulate with growth.[265]

NB: **Monteggia/Galeazzi fractures** See p650 & p644.

Reduction of a fracture of the distal radius (Colles' type)

- Ensure that there is adequate local or regional anaesthesia (p744). Traction should be applied to the hand with an assistant to provide counter-traction at the elbow. The fracture can often be felt to disimpact with 'clunk'.

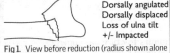

Dorsally angulated
Dorsally displaced
Loss of ulna tilt
+/- Impacted

Fig 1. View before reduction (radius shown alone in lateral view only).

- **Exaggerate** dorsal angulation while maintaining distal traction to stop the inelastic dorsal periosteum from preventing reduction by longitudinal traction.
- Correct dorsal and radial angulation, again maintaining distal traction. Aim for anatomical alignment:

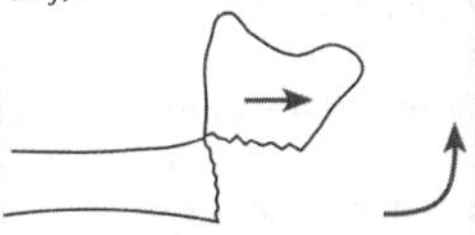

Fig 2.

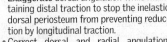

- Apply plaster of Paris (POP), moulded to provide 3-point pressure—this should maintain the reduction in ulnar deviation and with some wrist flexion.

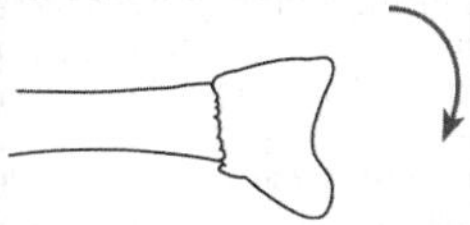

Fig 3.

- Maintain traction while the POP is applied (get all the kit ready beforehand). This is most easily done by pulling on the thumb and 1st finger against counter-traction. This applies both palmar and ulnar deviation.
- Support in a sling, once a radiograph has shown a good position (dorsal tilt <10°; radial shortening <2mm; radial inclination >15°; articular step <2mm and distal radio-ulnar joint congruence).
- Split cast to allow for swelling
- Check x-ray in 5d, when swelling has reduced; the plaster is then completed.
- ▶ Inability to get a good position may indicate soft tissue interpositioning.
- ▶ Finding good staff with experience saves remanipulating in theatre.

1 The *anterior fat pad* can be seen on lateral elbow x-ray as a radiolucent triangle in front of the distal humerus. It can be present in a normal elbow, and is only abnormal when raised off the bone by an effusion. A visible *posterior fat pad* is always abnormal. Absence of either of these signs makes a fracture very unlikely. Other things to check on the lateral x-ray: *anterior humeral line* (which should cross the anterior third of the capitellum) and *alignment of the radial shaft* with the capitellum (which it should bisect).

Distal radial fractures—eg Colles' type (common in osteoporotic post-menopausal women who fall on an outstretched hand). There is dorsal angulation and displacement producing a 'dinner-fork' wrist deformity (the fingers are the prongs). Avulsion of the ulna styloid process may also occur. *Treatment:* For reduction, Bier's block method (= IV regional anaesthesia) is best—but the young (<12) and elderly may not tolerate the prolonged time of cuff inflation. The use of a double cuff is controversial—a properly applied and checked tourniquet should suffice.

1 Place a loose tourniquet around the upper arm.
2 Place a small cannula on the back of the hand on the injured side, and a larger one in the antecubital fossa of the uninjured arm (in case you need to give rescue drugs).
3 Empty the arm of blood either by raising above the heart for 1min or by the use of an Esmarch bandage.[266]
4 Inflate the cuff to 100mmHg above systolic BP.
5 Inject 30–40mL 0.5% prilocaine[1] into the injured limb. ►*Never use bupivacaine for a Bier's block* (cardiotoxic if cuff is accidentally deflated).
6 Allow anaesthetic to develop (5–10min), then manipulate the fracture (p743).
7 30min after the injection deflate the tourniquet, at which point the anaesthesia will wear off.[1]
8 Other methods such as direct infiltration of the haematoma (haematoma block) are less effective.[267,268] The alternative is GA. *Complications:* Median nerve symptoms (should resolve after good reduction); ruptured tendons (esp. extensor pollicis longus); malunion & nonunion; CRPS type I (p739).

Smith's fracture Sometimes called a 'reverse Colles' fracture', in this injury the distal radius fractures with the fragment angled and displaced *forward/palmarly*. Fixation is needed in these fracture more commonly than in Colles' fractures, as the fracture fragment tends to migrate palmarly.

Bennett's fracture Carpometacarpal fracture/dislocation of thumb. ℞: Percutaneous wire fixation. Good reduction reduces risk of future OA.[269]

Scaphoid fracture Common and easily missed on radiography; results from falls on the hand. *Signs:* Tender in anatomical snuff box and over scaphoid tubercle, pain on axial compression of the thumb, and on ulnar deviation of the pronated wrist, or supination against resistance. *Imaging:* Request a dedicated 'scaphoid' series. If –ve, and fracture is suspected MRI has been shown to be sensitive and cost-effective.[270] CT is an alternative. If neither is available, cast and re-x-ray in 2 weeks. Nondisplaced fractures involving the waist may be immobilized in a neutral forearm cast for several weeks until union. Percutaneous cannulated screw fixation allows the patient to return to work earlier but does not affect the long-term outcome.[271] *Complications:* Avascular necrosis: the proximal pole relies on interosseous supply from the distal part.

Wrist dislocation (eg scapholunate or lunotriquetral) May be anterior or posterior. Manipulation and often open reduction, and plaster immobilization eg for 6 weeks. Median nerve compression may occur.[272]

►Beware eponymy: See BOX, 'Today we have naming of parts...'

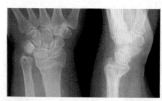

Fig 1. AP and lateral views of the left wrist. What type of wrist fracture is this: Colles', Smith's or Barton's?
Courtesy of Norfolk and Norwich University Hospital (NNUH) Radiology Department.

A-P views

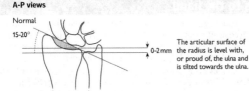

Normal
15-20°

The articular surface of the radius is level with, or proud of, the ulna and is tilted towards the ulna.

0-2mm

Unacceptable reductions

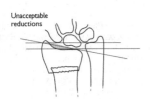

Note loss of radial length and reduction in ulnar tilt of the radius.

Lateral views

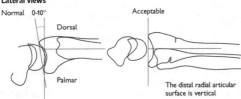

Normal 0-10°

Dorsal

Palmar

Acceptable

The distal radial articular surface is vertical

Unacceptable

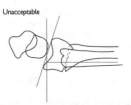

The distal radius surface is dorsally angulated. If allowed to heal in this position it will cause a marked restriction in function.

Fig 2.

'Today we have naming of parts...'

Be careful in immediately labelling a distal radial fracture as a *Colles' fracture*; a *Smith's fracture* has volar displacement and angulation, while a

*Today we have naming of parts. Yesterday,
We had daily cleaning. And tomorrow morning,
We shall have what to do after firing. But today,
We have naming of parts...* Henry Reed
From the *Dragon Book of Verse*, OUP

Barton's fracture is an intra-articular fracture involving the dorsal aspect of the distal radius (fig 1 is a reverse Barton's, involving the palmar surface). Have a quick think before firing off '*Colles' fracture*' and be better off for simply describing the fracture pattern that you see.

---

1 To get 0.5% prilocaine, dilute the 1% solution with an equal volume of 0.9% saline. ► NB: sudden early release of prilocaine into the circulation may cause seizures.

✠ ▶*There are no minor injuries to the hand.* Any breach of the integument may be the start of a chain of events that leads to loss of our most useful appendage. Contrary to beliefs of poets, our fingers are *not* protected from accidents by an invisible ring of shining:* *they are very frequently injured.*

Infections *Staph aureus* is the most common bacteria associated with hand infection (80%). Others include Streps and Gram -ves. *Paronychia:* infection under the eponychial fold. In the early stages, antibiotics may cure this, but once a collection forms, drainage is required. Occasionally part of the nail needs to be removed. *Felon:* an infection in the pulp of the distal finger. x-ray to look for a foreign body as the source of infection. Incise either into area of maximal fluctuance or a high lateral incision.[273] Blunt dissection is needed to break up septae, and a drain left in place. *Pyogenic flexor tenosynovitis* Bacterial infection of flexor tendon sheath—which can spread via the carpal tunnel to the forearm. Signs include swollen fingers, with tenderness over flexor sheath, and pain on extension of fingers. Treat urgently with IV antibiotics and surgery (see **fig 2**). A chronic 'cold' abscess of the tendon sheath suggests tuberculosis.[274] *Osteomyelitis:* Infection in the bone occurs through direct spread from an open fracture or contiguous spread following trauma. Haematogenous spread may occur in children, but is rare in adults. X-rays may show osteolysis, periosteal reactions and sequestrum or involucrum (p697). Treatment requires IV antibiotics, and surgical debridement. *Septic arthritis:* Infection occurs within a joint space. Pain is severe with movement of the joint. Delay in treatment leads to destruction of cartilage. If possible obtain joint aspirates to help identify the responsible organism. Treat with IV antibiotics and washout of the joint. *Bite wounds:* Bites from pets typically occur to children 5–10 and are often found on hands, feet and faces. Adults may get 'fight bites'—these occur when a fist strikes the teeth of an opponent. They may appear to be unassuming lacerations found over the 4th and 5th metacarpals which can overlie fractures, deep fascia or tendon injuries. Rigorous cleaning and irrigation is required. Give tetanus prophylaxis if needed. Most are allowed to heal be secondary intention. Antibiotic treatment (eg amoxicillin + clavulinic acid) is generally advocated.[275]

Nerve injury (p716 & p764) Examine sensory and motor function. Nerves smaller than the digital nerve at the level of the DIP joint are rarely reparable. Function is better if the injured nerve serves a single modality (motor or sensory). Let an expert decide the method of repair: primary, secondary, or nerve graft.[276]

Tendon injuries
- Failure to extend the MCP joint ≈ extensor tendon division. 75% are closed injuries.[277]
- Failure to flex the DIP joint against resistance ≈ flexor digitorum profundus division. If this is intact but flexion of the PIP joint is affected, there is division of superficialis. Flexor pollicis longus section leads to inability to flex the interphalangeal joint of the thumb. In general, flexor tendon injuries are best treated by primary repair (most are open injuries). If there is loss of tendon substance or delayed presentation, a staged repair with a silastic implant to keep the tendon sheath open, followed by a tendon graft, may be needed. Intensive hand physiotherapy with supervision is essential.

---

* *B*right clasp of her whole hand around my finger
My daughter, as we walk together now.
All my life I'll feel a ring invisibly
*Circle this bone with shining...*Stephen Spender
To My Daughter

Limb surgery in bloodless fields

This can be achieved with pneumatic tourniquets, which must have adequate width and curve, and be applied for as brief a time as possible.[278]

'Bruner's rules': These minimize risk of ischaemic limb changes.
• Width of tourniquet: 10cm for the arm; 15cm for legs.
• Apply to the upper arm, or mid/upper thigh.
• Use ≥2 layers of orthopaedic wool to provide adequate padding (make sure it does not get wet with the skin preparation fluid, which should be aqueous, so that if wetting happens inadvertently, 'chemical burns' do not occur).
• Inflation—arm: 50–100mmHg above systolic BP; leg: double systolic BP.
• Deflation—must be within 2h.
• Re-application after only brief reperfusion is inadvisable.[279]
• Avoid heating the limb (cooling is better, if feasible).[280]
• Apply only with the utmost caution to an unhealthy limb.
• Ensure the apparatus is calibrated weekly, and is well maintained.
• Document duration and pressure of tourniquet use.

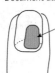

Sub-ungual haematoma
Release with needle by 'drilling' down—twiddling it between finger and thumbs; *or* by heating a paper clip to white heat and burning a hole through the nail.

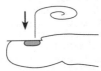

If left, the blood does not clot for up to 24hrs, therefore there is a throbbing pain due to pressure. This sometimes works (relieving the pressure) up to 2 days after the original injury.

Beware: subungual lacerations to the nail bed

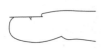   Nail removed

Remove the nail first—then stitch.
Also remove nail if there is nail avulsion.

Fig 1. Procedure for the evacuation of a subungual haematoma.

Hand incisions—fig 2
A: pulp space drainage;
B & B¹: lavage of flexor tendons;
C: drainage of radial bursa;
D: drainage of the ulnar bursa;
E & E¹: for the mid-palmar space;
F: drainage of the thenar space.

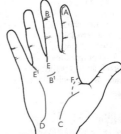

Fig 2.

Orthopaedics and trauma

Metacarpal fractures The base of the 2nd and 3rd metacarpals (MCs) form the functional centre of the hand around which the movement of the hand is centred. Thus, whilst malalignment and imperfect reduction may be tolerated in the 5th MC (<40° volar angulation), far less is permitted in the 2nd MC (<10°). The 5th metacarpal is most commonly involved, often from a punching injury. Managment may vary depending on whether the fracture is in the head/neck/ shaft or base of the MC, however, stable closed fractures can be managed in a splint/cast for ~2 weeks, with the wrist in partial extension (20°–30°), MCP joints in 70-90° flexion with fingers in extension. Unstable fractures may require K-wires/ORIF.[281] Longer periods of splinting in plaster or 'boxing glove' bandage can cause a stiff hand, eg from joint adhesions/contracture, flexor tendon fibrosis and collateral ligament shortening.

Refer any fractures with obvious rotational deformity (a clinical, not a radiological decision), as this can be disabling. Rotational fractures disclose themselves by producing a rotation of the fingers—see BOX; they usually require operative fixation (plate & screws), as do fractures of ≥2 metacarpals.

►Beware wounds overlying metacarpophalangeal joints (often from the teeth of the punched victim, as they are contaminated, and may communicate with the joint).

Fractures of the proximal phalanx Spiral or oblique fractures occurring at this site are likely to be associated with a rotation deformity—and this must be corrected (see BOX). Often, the only way to do this accurately is by open reduction and fixation, eg with a single compression screw.[282]

Middle phalanx fractures Manipulate these; splint in flexion over a malleable metal splint, strapping the finger to its neighbour ('neighbour strapping'). The aim is to control rotation, which interferes with later finger flexion.

Distal phalanx fractures may be caused by crush injuries and are often open. If closed, symptoms may be relieved by trephining the nail to reduce swelling. Rarely, split skin grafts from the thenar eminence may be needed for partial amputations of the finger tip.[1 283]

Mallet finger The tip of the finger droops because of avulsion of the extensor tendon's attachment to the terminal phalanx or rupture of the terminal part of the tendon. If the avulsed tendon includes a piece of bone, union is made easier—using a special splint, eg with 0° of extension. Use for 6 weeks.[284] Surgical intervention may be indicated if the fracture fragment is >30% of the joint surface.[285] Poorer outcome is associated with delay in splinting.

Gamekeeper's thumb This is so-called because of the laxity of the ulnar collateral ligament of the metacarpophalangeal joint of the thumb during the forced thumb abduction that occurs when wringing a pheasant's neck. The same injury is described in dry ski slope participants who fall and catch their thumb in the matting ('skier's thumb'). Diagnosis can be difficult as the thumb is so painful to examine, but to miss this injury may condemn the patient to a weak pincer grip—inject 1–2mL 1% plain lidocaine around the ligament to facilitate examination. Differentiation of complete *vs* partial tears of the ligament is crucial because the treatment for complete tears is surgical. Radiographic evaluation will detect a bony avulsion fragment.

Partial tears (clinically stable), or those associated with undisplaced avulsion fractures of the proximal phalanx, can be adequately treated using simple short-arm thumb spica casting.

---

1 For fingertip injuries in general, loss of <1cm² finger pulp skin should be able to heal by secondary intention.

Fig 1. Nail avulsion.

• If the nail margins are all intact, this is usually not needed. Look carefully at the dorsal nail fold, the nail root may have been avulsed then slipped back.
• Warn the patient the nail may not re-grow (or may regrow improperly). Get consent.
• Ring block the finger and test it is numb.
• Push one jaw of a small straight clamp down one side of the nail at its edge.
• Close clamp firmly. Warn the patient to look away.
• Turn the clamp on its long axis as if opening a sardine can. The nail will wrap round the clamp and peel off its nail bed.
• Having repaired the nailbed, replace the nail to serve as a splint. Ensure the nail fits into the nail fold, to minimize scarring along it. The old nail will drop out as the new one grows.

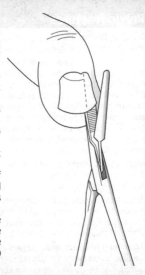

Assessing rotational deformity

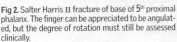

Assessing for rotational deformity in finger and metacarpal fractures is essential, as lasting deformity can be disabling. It cannot be accurately assessed with the fingers extended, so ask the patient to flex their fingers: they should all point to the scaphoid. Alternatively, look at and assess the nails end on in this position. Refer to a specialist if rotation is detected, as manipulation may be required; function and perhaps livelihood are at stake.

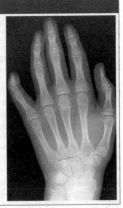

Fig 2. Salter Harris II fracture of base of 5th proximal phalanx. The finger can be appreciated to be angulated, but the degree of rotation must still be assessed clinically.

Image courtesy of Norfolk and Norwich University Hospital (NNUH) Radiology Department.

Rang's aphorism: *The pelvis is like a suit of armour: after damage there is much more concern about its contents than about the structure itself.*

Owing to the ring structure of the pelvis, single fractures are often stable (see BOX) and just need a few weeks' rest. In contrast, ≥2 fractures in the pelvis (with one above the level of the hip) renders the ring unstable and is a serious injury, with internal injuries in 25%. The force producing the fracture may be anteroposterior (AP), lateral compression (LC), vertical shear or a combination and is correlated with the pattern of organ injury and overall outcome.[286] Signs to look for include leg length discrepancy, abdominal distention, bruising, perineal or scrotal haematoma, and blood at the urethral meatus. For some examples of pelvic fractures, see the BOX 'Stability of pelvic fractures' and figs 1 to 3.

Malgaigne's fracture (20% of all pelvic fractures, 60% of unstable ones) There is disruption of the pelvis anteriorly and posteriorly with displacement of a fragment containing the hip joint.

Acetabular fractures *Common sites:* posterior lip or transverse. CT scans are needed to define injuries exactly[287] (easy to miss on x-ray as the acetabular columns are difficult to trace). *Treatment:* open reduction and reconstruction of the articular surface—to delay the onset of secondary osteoarthritis.[1]

Examining patients with suspected pelvic fracture ►Gentle palpation of the iliac crests, pubic symphysis, sacrum/coccyx and posterior SI joints is required. The pelvis may be gently compressed (once) to assess stability but 'rocking the pelvis' is no longer recommended, as it is painful and may disturb the retroperitoneal haematoma, so exacerbating haemorrhage. The diagnosis is principally made from the pelvis radiograph/CT scan.

Complications
- ►*Haemorrhage* (see BOX 'Shock with pelvic fracture', eg internal iliac artery). Check foot pulses, BP, CVP, and urine output often. Transfusion often needed.
- ►*Bladder rupture*—may be intraperitoneal or extraperitoneal (more common).
- ►*Urethral rupture*—often at the junction of the prostatic and membranous parts in males. The appearance of a drop of blood at the end of the urethra is suggestive. He may be unable to pass urine (avoid repeated tries). On rectal examination, the prostate may be 'high riding' i.e. elevated out of reach. NB: CT is the image of choice in trauma patients with haematuria.
- ►*Vaginal and rectal perforation*—look for bleeding. Both are rare.
- ►*Paralytic ileus*—this may occur with or without operative fixation.
- ►*Trapping of the sciatic nerve*—there is persistent pain.

Treatment Relieve pain and replace blood (BOX 1). If urethral rupture is suspected, ATLS guidelines suggest performing a retrograde cystourethrogram (RUG) before catheterizing; a suprapubic catheter may be needed. However, be aware that this may interfere with interpretation of pelvic angiograms. One study suggests a single, blind, gentle attempt at urethral catheterization will not worsen urethral injuries.[288] Get urological help. A small volume of urine suggests bladder rupture. A cystogram or CT is needed. If no pelvic fluid is seen on CT, bladder rupture is unlikely.[289,290]

Reassuring signs on a pelvis radiograph:
- Symphysis pubis separation <1cm
- Integrity of superior & inferior rami
- Integrity of the acetabula & femoral necks
- Symmetry of ilium & sacroiliac joints
- Symmetry of the sacral foramina, eg by evaluating the arcuate lines
- No fracture of transverse process of L5.

1 See fig 4, *OHCM* p719, for a surface rendered 3D reconstruction of a superior acetabular fracture.

Orthopaedics and trauma

Shock with pelvic fracture

This carries a mortality of 14–55% (towards the higher end if base excess on arterial blood gas analysis is ≤ –5).[291,292]

►► *Is the patient pregnant?* This poses big problems, eg ↑pelvic blood flow. Maternal haemorrhage is probably more important than direct uterine trauma in determining fetal outcome.[293]

►► *Resuscitate* vigorously and meticulously: see p725.

►► *Ways to reduce blood loss:* Avoid manipulations of the pelvis. Internally rotate both lower legs to close an 'open-book' fracture. Apply a pelvic binder. Compression may help reduce blood loss in AP fractures, but excessive compression, especially in lateral compression fractures may exacerbate it. Traction applied to the legs may help. Surgical reconstruction may then be undertaken. NB: pneumatic antishock garments (PASGs) are not designed for specifically for the stabilization of pelvic fractures.

►► *Alternatives:* External fixation frame.[294]

►► *Is there associated abdominal and pelvic injury?* Look and think hard. In one series of pelvic fractures there were splenic lesions (37%), diaphragm (21%) and bladder ruptures (24%), liver lacerations (19%), urethral lesions (17%), intestinal lesions (17%), and kidney rupture (9%).[295]

►► *Imaging:* Sometimes diagnosis is hard. Prompt spiral CT identifies those needing a special procedure, such as angiographic embolization.[296]

►► *Ordering of interventions matters*—eg laparotomy with surgical packing of retroperitoneum and mechanical stabilization of fracture will control venous bleeing. Angiography with embolization will target arterial bleeding. In practice it can be hard to decide if bleeding is arterial or venous in origin. The majority of patients will have venous bleeding—however, hypotensive, fluid unresponsive patients may be more likely to have arterial bleeding.[297]

►► Inter-disciplinary co-operation is vital—and must be practised.

The stability of pelvic fractures

When assessing the stability of a pelvic ring fracture, two important vectors need to be considered: vertical stability and rotational stability. The presence of vertical stability may mean that operative fixation is not required, depending on factors such as concomitant visceral injury, haemodynamic instability or inadequate mobilization. Pelvic ring fractures can therefore be categorized as one of the following:

1 *Vertically stable, rotationally stable:* eg isolated pubic rami (fig 1) or iliac wing fractures
2 *Vertically stable, rotationally unstable:* eg ispi- or contralateral ('bucket handle' type—fig 2) lateral compression fractures; 'open book' fracture (look for widening at the SI joints from rupture of the otherwise strong SI ligaments and diastasis (=separation) of the pubic symphysis).
3 *Vertically unstable, rotationally unstable:* eg fracture through the ipsilateral SI joint and pubic rami (fig 3). NB: a clue to the presence of vertical instability is superior migration of the pelvic fragment.

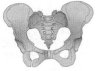
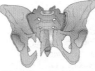
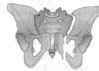

Fig 1. A vertically and rotationally stable pelvic fracture.

Fig 2. A vertically stable, rotationally unstable pelvic fracture—contralateral lateral compression type.

Fig 3. A vertically and rotationally unstable pelvic fracture. ►►Expert help is needed here.

Orthopaedics and trauma

►Currently there are ~75,000 patients with hip fractures annually in the uk. This number is set to rise to >100,000 by 2020. 10% will die within 1 month of this fracture; >30% will die within 1 year.[298]

Intracapsular fractures occur just below the femoral head (see figs **1** & **2**). This often causes *external rotation*, *adduction* and *shortening*.[1] The injuring force can be trivial and the patient may be able to walk (but with difficulty). As the medial femoral circumflex artery supplies the head via the neck, ischaemic necrosis of the head may occur, particularly if there is much displacement. *Treatment:*

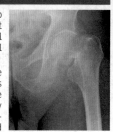

Fig 1. AP radiograph of the left hip showing a sub-capital fracture of the femoral neck. This may be easily appreciated on this view, but a lateral is vital for less obvious injuries.
Courtesy of Norfolk and Norwich University Hospital (NNUH) Radiology Department.

- Assess vital signs. Treat shock with crystalloid, but beware incipient heart failure. If central venous access is present, monitor CVP.
- Relieve pain (eg morphine 0.1mg/kg IV + femoral nerve block + an antiemetic).
- Images: a good quality lateral is essential (see fig 1). 5% of fractures can be missed unless CT is used.
- Prepare for theatre: FBC, U&E, CXR, ECG, crossmatch 2U, consent.
- Sort out medical problems pre-op: ►get help from an ortho-geriatrician.
- If displacement is minimal, multiple screw fixation *in situ* is appropriate, as the risk of avascular necrosis is much less. In displaced fractures the head is excised and a prosthesis inserted.[299]

Intertrochanteric-extracapsular fractures (between greater & lesser trochanters—see fig 2). They occur in an older age group and, as blood supply is adequate, non-union is rarer. ℞: Dynamic hip screw (DHS) fixation. The principle of the DHS is to stabilize the fracture but allow compression by sliding. Surgery is associated with ↓length of hospital stay and improved rehab.[300,301]

Femoral shaft fracture ►Require considerable force—think of injuries elsewhere and manage ABCs. 500–1500mL of blood may be lost in a simple fracture—look for swelling and check distal pulses (possible femoral artery injury). Sciatic nerve injury may also occur. The proximal bone fragment is flexed by iliopsoas, abducted by gluteus medius, and laterally rotated by gluteus maximus. The lower fragment is pulled up by the hamstrings and adducted (with external rotation) by the adductors. *Treatment:* Stabilize patient in ED with resuscitation and traction. Definitive treatment is typically with a locked intramedullary nail introduced proximally over a guide wire that is manipulated across the fracture under fluoroscopic control. This allows early mobilization.

Condylar fractures and tibial plateau fractures Being intra-articular, these demand accurate joint reconstruction to minimize later OA. Hinged cast braces can be used for tibial plateau fractures.

Posterior hip dislocation (eg to front-seat passengers if the knee strikes the dashboard). Feel for the femoral head in the buttock. The leg is *flexed*, *internally* rotated, *adducted*, and *shortened*. ►The sciatic nerve may be lacerated, stretched, or compressed; early MRI diagnosis may prevent later equinus foot deformity. *Treatment:* Reduction under GA, by lifting the femoral head back into the joint. Traction for 3 weeks promotes joint capsule healing.[302]

---

1 This is opposed to the **internal rotation** found in hip dislocation. These positionings are explained by the changes in the fulcrum for the force applied by iliopsoas to the proximal femur in either condition. ►NB: **pathological fractures** are discussed on p709.

Types of proximal femoral fractures

The same principles apply for describing proximal femoral fractures as for any other (p734). Here are pattern-specific descriptive terms that are useful to remember (fig 2):

- *Intra-*[itn] *and extra-*[ext]*capsular fractures:*[304]
  1 Subcapital [itn]
  2 Transcervical [itn]
  3 Basicervical [itn]
  4 Intertrochanteric/pertrochanteric [ext]
  5 Reverse oblique/transtrochanteric [ext]
  6 Subtrochanteric [ext]

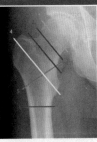

Fig 2. The fracture pattern in the proximal femur will determine the treatment.

Courtesy of Norfolk and Norwich University Hospital (NNUH) Radiology Department.

Determining the type and site of fracture is important, to determine management. Eg:

- Undisplaced intracapsular (1 or 2) → AO screw fixation/conservative (AO = Arbeitsgemeinschaft (Osteosynthesefragen).
- Displaced intracapsular (1 or 2) → (hemi)arthroplasty.[305]
- Basicervical (3)/intertrochanteric (4) → DHS fixation (p752).
- Transtrochanteric (5)/subtrochanteric (6) → DHS fixation can be used, but an intramedullary hip screw (IMHS) is usually preferred.

NB: different surgeons may favour one fixation method over another.

Garden classification (not commonly used, as it is based purely on the AP radiograph findings) This classifies intracapsular femoral neck fractures—it correlates with prognosis, IV being the worst.

I	Incomplete undisplaced fracture with the inferior cortex intact; look for trabecular disruption
II	Complete undisplaced fracture through the neck
III	Complete neck fracture with displacement; there is abduction and internal rotation of the proximal fragment in the acetabulum
IV	Fully displaced fracture with the proximal fragment in the neutral position

Preventing hip fractures

- Prevent falls: eg good lighting, less sedation, & keep-fit programmes.[1]
- Teach exercise and balance training, eg with tai chi[1] classes for the elderly. This lessens fear of falling, and can halve rates of multiple falls.[306]
- Prevent osteoporosis: eg exercise, bisphosphonates (see p709).
- Ensure good vitamin D intake (plasma levels ≥30nmol/L; esp. in northern climes). A lack of vitamin D and calcium is associated with hip fracture whether or not patients are osteoporotic.
- Follow-up meta-analyses have cast doubt over whether hip protectors decrease risk of hip fracture in the elderly. Acceptability by users remains a problem, because of discomfort and practicality.[307]

The following may prevent complications after hip injury

- Early mobilization to prevent thromboembolism.
- Co-ordinated multidisciplinary inpatient rehabilitation.
- Good nutrition—but meta-analyses do not provide much support for specific multi-nutritional commercial food supplements.

---

1 The Chinese characters for tai chi chuan can be translated as the 'supreme ultimate force'—an odd concept, one might think, to find in village halls—until one combines this with the Chinese concept of yin-yang —the dynamic duality (male/female, active/passive, dark/light, forceful/yielding, etc.) seen in *all* things. Think of tai chi as meditation combined with mobile yoga sequenced into sets of movements inspired by the animal kingdom and martial arts traditions. In Chinese philosophy and medicine there exists the concept of 'chi', a vital force that animates the body. One aim of tai chi is to circulate 'chi' through the body to promote health and vitality. Another aim of tai chi is to foster a calm and tranquil mind, focused on the precise execution of movements.

The patella *Dislocation:* Is typically lateral—often as the result of a twisting motion of the lower leg, combined with contraction of the quadriceps. The knee is flexed with a lateral deformity. Reduction is achieved with gentle medial pressure, combined with extension of the knee. Radiographs should be obtained post reduction to ensure no fracture to the patella. Check the extensor mechanism of the knee post reduction. Ensure a period of immobilization in cast/posterior splint or brace. Rehabilitation will require quadriceps strengthening exercises. *Recurrent dislocation* may be related to developmental abnormalities around the knee and may warrant surgery to strengthen the medial expansion. *Patella fracture* usually results from a fall onto a flexed knee or due to dashboard injury in motor vehicle collision. Non-displaced fractures with an intact extensor mechanism may be managed conservatively. Displaced fractures are likely to require operative fixation.

The knee *Injury to a collateral ligament* is common in sport. *Mechanism:* The medial ligament is most commonly injured by a blow to the lateral aspect of the knee whilst the foot is fixed (putting valgus stress on the knee); vice versa for the lateral ligament. *Signs:* Effusion ± tenderness over affected ligaments. Rest is needed, then firm support. See p686 for examination techniques. NB: surgery is rarely needed for isolated medial collateral ligament injury.[308] In lateral injury, surgery is required if there is instability; also look for associated common peroneal nerve injury. *Anterior cruciate ligament (ACL) tear:* Typically follows a twisting injury to the knee with the foot fixed to the ground. *Signs:* Effusion; haemarthrosis; +ve 'draw' sign (immobilize the patient's leg by sitting on his foot, and then with the knee in 90° flexion, grip the upper tibia and try to draw it towards you, away from the femur; the reverse 'set back' suggests a **posterior cruciate tear**—eg in car crashes as the knee strikes the dashboard). Do a 'pivot shift test' (p686). Examination under GA may be needed. *Treatment:* This is problematic. 3 weeks' rest and physio may help. In the young, or ↑knee instability, consider ligament reconstruction (autograft).[309,310]

Meniscal (semilunar cartilage) tears: Medial meniscus tears (eg 'bucket-hadle') follow twists to a flexed knee (eg in football). Adduction + internal rotation causes *lateral meniscus* tears. Extension is limited (knee locking) as the displaced segment lodges between femoral and tibial condyles. The patient must stop what he is doing, and can only walk on tiptoe, if at all. The joint line is tender, and McMurray's test is +ve (p686). If the 'handle' of the 'bucket' becomes free at one end ('parrot beak' tear), the knee suddenly gives way, rather than locking. MRI gives tear location, morphology, length, depth, and stability, and helps predict tears requiring repair.[311] Look for avulsions on x-ray. Management is conservative when possible, though arthroscopy is usually needed for locked knees, cysts, or persisting symptoms after injury.

Typical injury triad: ACL + medial collateral ligament + medial meniscus.

Occult bone injury: If MRI/x-rays are -ve, don't put everything down to '*minor problems with the meniscus*'. Detailed MRI (STIR[1] + dynamic contrast to show periosteal oedema)[312] may show: •Subchondral fracture eg of the posterior margin of the medial tibial condyle.[313] •Stress fracture (intramedullary and periosteal oedema with high signal intensity)[314] •Tibial plateau oedema.

Tibia fracture *Avulsion fractures* of the intercondylar region often occur with anterior cruciate injury. Arthroscopic reduction may be tried.[315] Sliding traction, or surgery with open elevation of the joint surface may be needed. Open shaft fractures are common as there is little anterior covering tissue. Soft tissue stripping may devascularize the bone leading to poor union in tibia fractures. With *closed fractures*, operative or non-operative management can depend on patient variables (eg kneeling occupation), fracture (eg stability) factor, and surgeon's preference. *Open fractures:* See *managing open fractures* (p735).

Pretibial lacerations

The shin (esp. if elderly) has poor blood supply. It is vulnerable to flap wounds (fig 1). *Treatment:* Try hard to iron out **all** the flap, repositioning it carefully: an ideal tool is the wrong end of a Vacutainer® needle, sheathed in rubber. The important thing is to evacuate the haematoma to prevent tension (tension→breakdown→plastic surgery)—so skin closure with adhesive strips (eg Steristrip®) is better than sutures, as they can be loosened if the tissues swell. Wound glue may be better still.[316] Dress, and advise a support bandage, and leg elevation. Review to check for infection, wound tension, and necrosis.

Before
Flap retracts back

Good
No tension in flap.
Held with adhesive sutures.

Bad
Flap stretched tight and likely to necrose.

Fig 1. Flap wounds.

Bone marrow contusions reveal the mechanism of injury

Bone marrow contusions are often seen on knee trauma MRIs. These osseous injuries result from a direct blow, from compression impact from adjacent bones, or from traction from avulsion injury. The distribution of oedema gives valuable clues to associated soft-tissue injuries.

5 contusion patterns are associated with soft-tissue knee injuries:
1 *Pivot shift injury:* Oedema involves the posterolateral tibial plateau and the midportion of the lateral femoral condyle.
2 *Dashboard injury:* Oedema is in the anterior aspect of the proximal tibia.
3 *Hyperextension:* Results in the 'kissing' contusion pattern involving the anterior aspect of the proximal tibia and distal femur.
4 *Clip injury:* Results in a big area of oedema in the lateral femoral condyle and a small area of oedema involving the medial femoral condyle.
5 *Lateral patellar dislocation:* Causes oedema involving the inferomedial patella and the lateral femoral condyle (anteriorly).

So you can infer the mechanism of injury by patterns of oedema, and hence predict which specific soft-tissue abnormalities are present.[317]

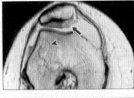

Fig 2. Axial view fat-suppressed fast-spin echo MRI in patella dislocation injury. Full-thickness chondral fracture (arrow) of the medial patella facet is seen as an area of increased signal intensity. Bone contusion oedema of the subjacent marrow (arrowhead) involving the lateral femoral condyle was caused by impaction of the patella against the epicondyle.[1]

Courtesy of Hollis M. Fritss, MD.

Some other leg fractures

- **Isolated fibular fracture:** A supportive dressing may be sufficient.
- **Toddler's fracture:** This is a spiral fracture of the distal tibial shaft seen in toddlers. Treatment is supportive, eg analgesia and crêpe bandaging. ►►These should **never** occur in a child who is not yet walking, so you must think of NAI in such cases and alert the paediatric team (p146).

1 STIR = Short T1 Inversion Recovery MRI (has specific timing to suppress the signal from fat).

Orthopaedics and trauma

Ankle ligament strains Twisting inversion accounts for the common strain to the anterior talofibular part of the lateral ligament (fig 2). *Signs:* Stiffness, tenderness over the lateral ligament, pain on inversion. If there is tenderness at either malleolus or inability to walk (eg 4 steps) do radiographs to rule out fracture (see p778). *Treatment:* Consists of RICE (rest, ice, compression, elevation). Medial deltoid ligament strains (fig 2), due to eversion, are rare. Supervized walking exercises and diapulse therapy relieve pain. NB: minor sprains may respond to rest and simple analgesia ± topical NSAID (ibuprofen, ketoprofen, piroxicam). *Prevention:* Good footwear may be more important than shoe-heel height. Proprioceptive training can ↓incidence of ankle sprains in athletes,[318] but this may only hold for recurrence.[319] For athletes, consider trade-off between prevention of injury and performance restriction.[320]

Malleolar and metatarsal fractures

• Either malleolus may be fractured by the above injuries. Rotation causes oblique lateral malleolar fracture (hard to see except on lateral radiographs), or a proximal fracture of the 5th metatarsal (avulsion by peroneus brevis). *R:* In general stable fractures only involve one side of the ankle (AO/Weber A1/B1 fractures—see fig 1). Stable or minimally displaced fractures maybe treated non-operatively in a cast. Unstable or displaced fractures require surgery.

• *Maisonneuve's fracture* Proximal fibular fracture + syndesmosis rupture, and medial malleolus fracture or deltoid ligament rupture. If 2 bones dislocate where no true joint exists, the term *diastasis* ('standing apart') is used. ►Always examine the proximal fibula with 'ankle sprains'. *R* is surgical, with restoration of the ankle mortise and placement of 1–2 suprasyndesmotic screws.[321]

• *Lisfranc fracture-dislocation at the 1st tarsometatarsal joint* ►This is a commonly missed fracture in multitrauma patients, but it can also occur by stepping awkwardly off a kerb. It may cause compartment syndrome of the medial foot (± later arthritis and persistent pain).[322] *Images:* On plain x-ray look for widening of the gap between the medial cuneiform and the base of the 2nd metatarsal. Because of the overlapping bones, subluxations can be hard to see. CT helps.[323] *R:* Achieve precise anatomic reduction. Open reduction and temporary screw or K-wire fixation may be best.[324]

Other fractures *Fractured neck of talus* can occur after forced dorsiflexion, and is a serious injury because interruption of vessels may lead to avascular necrosis of the body of the talus. *R:* Displaced fractures require ORIF.

Os calcis fractures Often bilateral, after serious falls (which is associated with worse outcome).[325] ►Always look for associated spinal fracture. *Signs:* Swelling; bruising; inability to weight bear. Check Bohler's angle on lateral x-ray: the angle between lines from the anterior process to the peak of the posterior articulating surface and from the same to the posterior calcaneal process: <20° is abnormal. *R:* ►*Does the fracture enter the subtalar joint?* Some only opt for conservative treatment in extra-articular fractures, or minor displaced intra-articular fractures in nonambulatory patients. Others opt for surgery, but it is not clear that operative management has better outcomes, even for intra-articular fractures.[326]

Mid-tarsal (eg calcaneocuboid) dislocation produces a painful, swollen foot. The navicula proximal articular surface may not articulate with the talus. *R:* Early manipulation + plaster cast for, eg 7 weeks.[327]

2nd metatarsal march fracture: Shaft # may simply require rest. Several weeks of crutches may be useful. Severe pain may be better managed with a cast.

Fractures of the toes: Simple protective dressings usually suffice.

NB: consider dedicated bone algorithm CT for all complex fractures in this region.

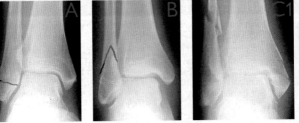

Fig 1. A simplification of the *AO WEBER classification* of malleolar fractures.[328]

Images courtesy of Professor Peter Scally.

a1	Transverse fibula fracture at or below the joint line with no medial injury
a2/3	Transverse fibula fracture below joint line + medial injury (ligament / fracture)
b1-3	Fibula fracture at the joint line (B1) + medial injury (B2) + posterior injury (B3)
c1/2	Oblique fibula fracture above a ruptured tibiofibular ligament + medial injury
c3	Maisonneuve's fracture, i.e. proximal fibular fracture + medial injury

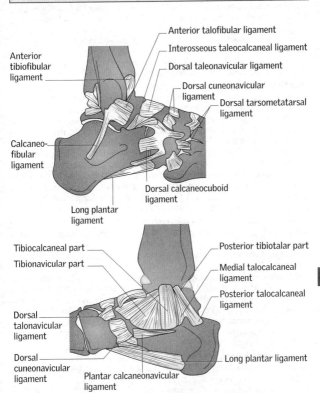

Fig 2. Ligaments of the ankle and hind/midfoot: *(top)* lateral and *(bottom)* medial views. The medial view is dominated by the various parts of the deltoid ligament.

Assault is the commonest cause of facial trauma, with young men the most affected. Facial laceration and mandible fracture are the commonest injuries.[329]

▶*If there is airway obstruction, summon expert help promptly.* Remove blood, loose/false teeth, and vomit from the mouth. Lie in the semi-prone position to prevent obstruction (p799) from a swollen injured tongue, but always beware of cervical spine trauma with injuries above the clavicle. If the pharynx is swelling or there is fracture of the larynx, try gentle intubation. If impossible, do cricothyrotomy (OHCM p786), then tracheostomy. Blood aspiration is prevented by direct pressure to the bleeding site.

Precautions with possible neck trauma Injury to the cervical spine should be considered in any trauma situation, especially if: high energy; patient complaining of neck pain; patient unconscious. CT is the best method if high/moderate risk for cervical fracture.[217] See p658 for assessing neck injuries.

Lacerations of the face Clean meticulously. Alignment of the tissues and antisepsis must be exact to produce a good cosmetic result.
• *Simple lacerations:* Consider glue or steristrip closure (p730).
• *Complex lacerations:* Is there a plastic surgeon available?
• *Mammal bites:* Give antibiotic cover: p782, eg **co-amoxiclav** 1 tab/8h PO.[231]
• *Rugby player's ('cauliflower') ear:* Aspirate/drain haematoma (repeat every few days) and then strap pressure dressing against the head.
• *Ruptured ear drum:* NSAIDs for analgesia, and advise to keep ear dry.
• *Avulsed teeth* may be replaced (p784). If inhaled, do expiratory CXR. Bleeding socket: bite on adrenaline-soaked pads, or use sutures.
• *Eye injury, nose fractures, and nose bleeds:* See p452, p560, & p562.

Mandible injury *Signs:* Local tenderness and swelling; jaw malocclusion; a mobile fragment; bone may protrude into the mouth in open fractures; if comminuted, the tongue may make airway management extremely difficult, so get expert help. *Diagnosis:* Orthopantogram (OPG) radiographs. Enlist expert dental help. *Treating TMJ dislocations:* Place (gloved) thumbs over the back teeth and press downwards, while at the same time levering the chin upwards with your fingers (both hands). Consider midazolam sedation: see p718.

Blows to the chin may cause fracture at the impact site, or indirect fractures near the temporomandibular joint. *Fractures:* Open reduction + internal fixation with miniplates is better than wiring teeth together for 6 weeks. Try to get onto a daytime consultant list, rather than at night. Complicated fractures may benefit from lag osteosynthesis. Complications: infection; non-union.[330]

'Whiplash' injury (a source of some controversy) is cervical strain caused by sudden neck extension with rebound flexion. It is common, often in rear-end crashes. Hyperextension causes damage to the anterior musculoligamentous structures. Subsequent protective muscle spasm causes pain and stiffness, which may be severe. *Treatment:*[331] Reassure physical injury is rare. Emphasize positive attitudes to prognosis and recovery are important. Encourage prompt return to usual activity and occupation. Suggest active mobilization (if tolerated), eg with gentle stretching and posture control, as exercise enhances recovery. Aim to prevent chronicity and 'disuse syndrome' through advocating self-management with analgesia. Collars, rest and negative attitudes can contribute to delayed recovery and chronicity. If symptoms last for >1yr, they are likely to be permanent.[332]

Other car-crash neck sprains (Seen in ⅓ of car users soon after crashes.) Symptoms may be delayed and persist for years. The best treatment may be to give NSAIDs, a cervical collar, and review in the next clinic, with referral for immediate physiotherapy if symptoms warrant this. Explain to the patient that head restraints *are* helpful—the usual mistake is that they are adjusted too low.

Bony injuries to the face

The face forms a shock absorber which protects the brain from injury. The most common fractures to the facial bones lie along 2 hoops, from ear to ear. One is formed by the zygomatic arch, body, infraorbital rim and nose. The other is formed by the mandible (**fig 1**). Major blunt trauma can cause a fracture to the entire middle third of the face, which has been classified by Le Fort, but since the advent of seat belts these are less common.[333]

Zygoma fractures *The arch:* Before swelling arrives, there is a depression in front of the ear, and lateral jaw excursions or jaw opening may be limited and painful. A suitable radiograph is the submentovertex view (SMV). *The complex:* The zygoma's body has 4 extensions: **1** frontozygomatic; **2** arch; **3** maxillary buttress (in mouth); **4** infraorbital rim. Fractures may be palpated at these points, or disproportionately severe pain elicited on palpation. Occipitomental views are most suitable. *Orbital floor injuries* Blunt trauma around the eye can cause fracture to the orbital floor. Imaging: CT is best, but OM views may show trap door sign in the maxillary sinus.

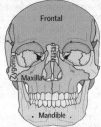
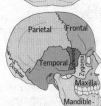

Fig 1. Skull **a** AP **b** lateral.

Clinical exam for periorbital trauma:
- Is there CSF rhinorrhoea, p560? (yes in ≤25%).[334]
- Check zygomatic arch by assessing range of mandibular lateral excursions and opening. Also palpate over the arch (just under the skin) and compare with the unaffected side.
- Patient sitting, doctor standing above and behind, place index fingers on the cheeks and look down from above for asymmetry.
- Check the orbit floor for: diplopia on upward gaze (≈trapped orbital contents); enophthalmos; numbness in the distribution of the infraorbital nerve (suggests fracture).

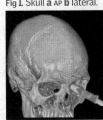

Fig 2. 3D CT of a nasty injury to the eye. ►►On no account remove the knife.

Courtesy of Prof Peter Scally.

- Small risk of retrobulbar haemorrhage: catastrophic if missed: severe pain at back of eye; proptosis; loss of visual acuity. ►Prompt exam is essential.

NB: if the eye is very swollen, application of a rubber glove filled with ice is invaluable, especially if you ask a specialist to travel to check patient; they can no more open a swollen eye than you. *Treatment:* Unless vision↓, or there is significant risk of infection, admission on presentation is not mandatory: seeing at the next fracture clinic is adequate. If in doubt, consult the relevant specialist. Explain about not blowing the nose in fractures in continuity with the maxillary sinus (risks periorbital emphysema and infection).

►**Medicolegal issues** Facial injuries commonly result from assault. Your notes may be used in criminal injuries claims or as evidence in court. Often the individual is drunk and abusive, it is late, and you are busy, but you must make accurate notes (use a ruler) with diagrams. Other people will definitely take time to study and criticize what you have written. Don't forget photographs if assault is particularly serious or children are involved. Document that the patient has given, or refused, permission for statements to be made to the police or legal professionals (the medical notes are confidential).

Neurapraxia implies temporary loss of nerve conduction often via ischaemia following pressure (eg to the lateral popliteal nerve as it crosses the neck of the fibula, see below). In mixed nerves, the motor modality is the more vulnerable component. *Axonotmesis* entails damage to the nerve fibre but the epineural tube is intact, providing guidance to the regrowing nerve. Good recovery is the rule. Growth rate is 1–3mm/day. *Neurotmesis* means division of the whole nerve. As there is no guidance from the endoneural tube, regrowing fibrils cause a traumatic neuroma if they are unable to bridge the gap. The current surgical standard is epineural repair with nylon sutures. To span gaps that primary repair cannot bridge without excess tension, nerve-cable interfascicular autografts are used. Results of nerve repair are fair (at best), with ~50% of regaining useful function. There is much current research regarding drugs, immune system modulators, enhancing factors, and entubulation chambers.[335] *Management* depends on type of injury; refer all complete injuries from laceration or penetration to a specialist for surgical exploration and repair.

Median nerve (C5–T1) The nerve of *grasp.* Injury above the antecubital fossa causes: •Inability to flex index finger interphalangeal joints on clasping the hands (Ochner's test) •Inability to flex the terminal phalanx of the thumb (flexor pollicis longus) •Loss of sensation over the thenar half of the palm.

If the lesion is at the wrist, the only muscle reliably affected is abductor pollicis brevis. Test it by holding the hand palm up. Can the patient raise the thumb out of the plane of the hand? The area of sensory loss is smaller than that for more proximal lesions. See box, 'Median nerve anatomy'.

Ulnar nerve (C8–T1) This is the nerve of finger abduction and adduction (among other roles). One subtle sign of an ulnar nerve lesion is inability to cross the fingers in the 'good luck' sign. Injury level determines severity of the claw deformity. In a distal lesion of the ulnar nerve, there will be more clawing of the 4th and 5th fingers compared with a proximal, more complete lesion at the elbow. This is the *ulnar paradox*, and comes about because higher lesions paralyse flexors too (eg flexor digitorum profundus, FDP).[336] *Froment's paper sign:* On holding a piece of paper between thumb and finger (both hands), there is flexion of the thumb's distal phalanx on trying to pull apart (flexor pollicis longus, is recruited to overcome adductor pollicis weakness). Sensory loss is over the little finger and a variable area of the ring finger (palmar & dorsal).

Radial nerve (C5–T1) This is the nerve of extension of the elbow, wrist, and fingers. It opens the fist. Injury will produce wrist-drop. Test for this with the elbow flexed and the forearm pronated. Sensory loss is variable, but always includes the dorsal aspect of the root of the thumb.

Sciatic nerve (L4–S2) Complete lesions will affect all muscles below the knee, and sensation below the knee laterally.

Lateral popliteal (common peroneal) nerve (L4–S2) The commonest lower limb nerve injury. Lesions lead to equinovarus with inability to dorsiflex the foot and toes. Sensory loss is over the dorsum of the foot.[337]

Tibial nerve (S1–3) Loss causes calcaneovalgus and inability to stand on tiptoe or invert the foot. Sensory loss is over the sole.

Injuries to arteries Bleeding is usually controllable by pressure and elevation of the part. After any injury in which an artery may have been damaged, examine distal pulses carefully. If they are not felt, do not assume that this is due to spasm, but request expert help. Exploration with end-to-end suture, or reversed vein grafts may be needed. The prognosis is not so bad if there are good collaterals (eg to the femoral artery, compared with the popliteal artery).

Complications: Gangrene, contractures, false aneurysm, and arteriovenous fistulae. ▶See *OHCM* p658 for acute limb ischaemia.

Sensory relearning after median nerve repair: the Lundborg–Rosén metaphor

Tactile gnosis This is tested by 2-point discrimination and tactile recognition of objects. Restoration of tactile gnosis in the hand is the main challenge of median nerve repair. It is easy to point out that touch is a major way we interact with our world.

More subtle is how the brain performs *cross-modal interpretation* of our world—ie integrating touch, sound, and vision, and producing meaning out of this integration. Loss of one modality is not a simple case of subtraction, but gives rise to complex compensatory mechanisms. Interpretation of textures, for example, is not usually regained after major injury to a nerve trunk in adults, but there is more plasticity in children: here, cortical remodelling allows meaningful interpretation from misconnected regrown axons.

Best results of repair are seen before the age of 10yrs. By 18yrs, there has been a rapid decline in relearning ability. There is an unexplained temporary increase in learning ability in the late twenties. This pattern, intriguingly, follows that of our ability to learn a new language. So the notion that the problem after nerve injury/repair is that 'the hand is speaking a new language to the brain' is more than an metaphor; accepting this metaphor leads to the idea that education and training are vital to successful nerve repair.[338]

Median nerve anatomy

The median nerve arises from C5, C6, C7, C8, & T1 as a condensation of lateral & medial cords of brachial plexus (p765). It crosses medial to the brachial artery in antecubital fossa. It has no branches above the elbow. ~5cm distal to elbow it gives off its anterior interosseous branch (motor to flexor policis longus (FPL), flexor digitorum profundus (FDP,) index finger & pronator quadratus). The palmar cutaneous branch (sensory to thenar skin) arises ~5cm proximal to wrist and overlies the flexor retinaculum. The recurrent motor branch to the thenar muscles arises at the distal end of carpal tunnel. The median nerve is motor to PT (pronator teres), FCR (flexor carpi radialis), PL (palmaris longus), FDS (flexor digitorum superficialis), LOAF (radial 2 lumbricals, opponens pollicis, abductor pollicis, flexor pollicis brevis). Sensation: radial 3-and-a-half digits. See fig 1, p669 for a cross-sectional diagram of the carpal tunnel.

Orthopaedics and trauma

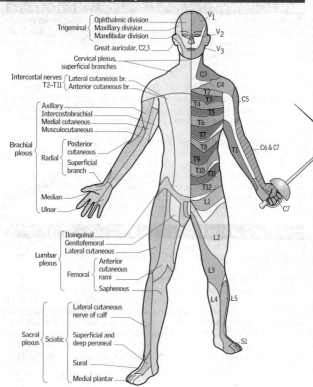

Fig 1. These images reflect the 2011 evidence-based dermatomes, which have revealed much more individual variation than originally thought, so much so that some areas have been left blank (white) because no single best option can be given.

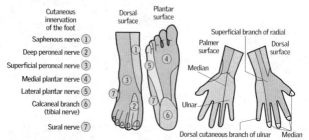

Cutaneous innervation of the foot

Saphenous nerve ①
Deep peroneal nerve ②
Superficial peroneal nerve ③
Medial plantar nerve ④
Lateral plantar nerve ⑤
Calcaneal branch ⑥ (tibial nerve)
Sural nerve ⑦

Fig 3. Feet and hands

See p716 for testing peripheral motor nerves.

Figs 1 and 2 adapted from Lee MWL, McPhee, RW, Stringer MD (2008) 'An evidence-based approach to human dermatomes', *Clinical Anatomy* 21: 363–373, with permission from John Wiley & Sons.

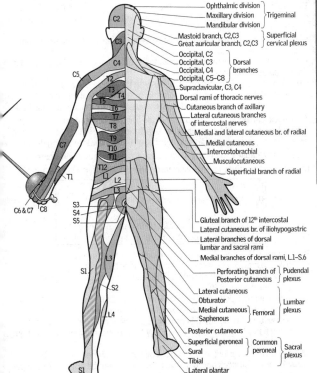

Fig 2. Posterior view

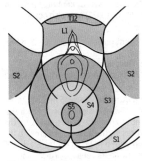

Fig 4. Perineal dermatomes.

Aim to keep a few key dermatomes up your sleeve.

C3–4	Clavicles
C6–7	Lateral arm/forearm
T1	Medial side of arm
C6	Thumb
C7	Middle finger
C8	Little finger
T4	Nipples
T10	Umbilicus
L2–L3	Anterior & inner leg
L5	Medial side of big toe
L5, S1–2	Posterior & outer leg
S1	Lateral margin of foot and little toe
S2–4	Perineum

The above is a rough approximation

The brachial plexus extends from the intervertebral foramina to the axilla spanning a distance of ~15cm. Useful landmarks on its route from cord to arm worth remembering are:

- The roots leave the vertebral column between the scalenus medius and anterior muscles (see fig 2).
- The creation of divisions from trunks takes place under the clavicle, **medial** to the coracoid process.
- The plexus has an intimate relationship with the subclavian and then axillary arteries, with the median nerve forming from the medial and lateral cords anterior to the latter. Look for the characteristic 'M' formation: see figs 1 & 3.

Traumatic causes *Direct* eg shoulder girdle fracture, penetrating or iatrogenic. *Indirect* eg avulsion/traction injuries, due to excessive lateral flexion of the neck—as may occur in motorcycle injuries, or to the newborn during delivery.

Atraumatic causes Tumours (eg Pancoast, from lung), radiation, neuropathy.

Classifying the injury can be done according to the Leffert classification:[339]

I	Open
II	Closed (IIa supraclavicular, IIb infraclavicular)
III	Radiation
IV	Obstetric; (IVa upper root (Erb's palsy), IVb lower root (Klumpke's palsy), IVc mixed)

Root injuries There are 4 types: high, middle, low or complete.

- *High lesions: Erb's palsy* (c5, c6) Damage affects the suprascapular, musculocutaneous and axillary nerves. This leads to paralysis of supraspinatus (abduction), infraspinatus (external rotation), biceps (supination), brachialis (flexion of elbow), deltoid (abduction) and teres minor (external rotation). As a result the arm is held internally rotated, pronated, extended and adducted in the 'waiter's tip' position. Sensation is impaired over deltoid, lateral forearm, and hand. Difficult deliveries (or any trauma in a downwards direction) can produce this sign in neonates.
- *Middle (Brunelli) lesions:* (c7) Produced by anteroposterior trauma (11%).[340]
- *Low lesions: Klumpke's paralysis* (c8, T1) Occurs when the arm is pulled superiorly (forced abduction)—for example trying to break a fall from height by grabbing onto something. Damage to the c8, T1 roots leads to a combination of median and ulnar nerve injury which may produce 'claw hand' (extension at mcp joints, with flexion at dip/pip joints) due to loss of lumbrical function. The arm is held in adduction. Horner's syndrome (p424) may also occur.

Injury to the cords (in green in fig 1)

- *Injury to the lateral cord of the plexus*: Absent power in the biceps and brachioradialis (flexes the forearm at the elbow).
- *Posterior cord injury:* Teres major & deltoid inaction; radial nerve palsy.
- *Medial cord injury:* Affects the ulnar and median nerves. Sensation is absent over the medial arm and hand.

Recovery With incomplete trunk lesions recovery may take >5 months. Prognosis is poor in lesions proximal to the dorsal root ganglion (DRG). For intradermal histamine (1%, into the affected limb) to produce an arterial flare, the route to the DRG must be intact, so if this is present the lesion is proximal to the DRG. MRI gives the best images. Early liaison with a regional centre is advised as early exploration improves the outcome of nerve repair. Surgical options include nerve grafting of viable roots, nerve transfer (from intercostal nerves,) free functioning muscle transfers and tendon transfers.[341]

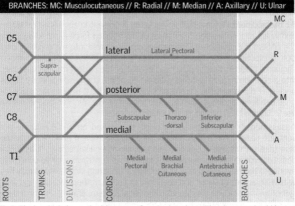

BRANCHES: MC: Musculocutaneous // R: Radial // M: Median // A: Axillary // U: Ulnar

Fig 1. The brachial plexus, the *bête noire* of medical students. This diagram should be just memorizable the night before an exam.   Image courtesy of Luke Famery.

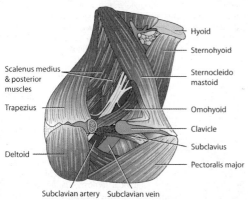

Fig 2. The proximal brachial plexus. The purpose of this figure and **fig 3**, is to show where the brachial plexus is, and not what the brachial plexus is.

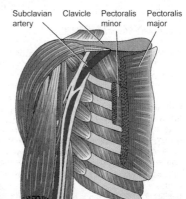

Fig 3. The distal brachial plexus: note the relationship with the axillary artery.

At the accident Assume that spinal injury is present in any serious accident, and in all accidents when the nature of the injuring force is not known, and the patient is unconscious. The patient can be moved into the recovery position (protection of the airway is always the first priority)—but all movement should be planned. Keeping the neck in neutral, the patient may be 'log-rolled' into a semi-prone position (not lateral, see p799). If any spinal injury is suspected at the scene, the paramedics will apply a hard neck collar, place the head between sandbags, and strap the patient onto a spinal board—some will use inflatable bean bag boards to reduce pressure.[342]

Assessment[343] Inital assessment must be focused on ABCs. Intubate and ventilate patients with high tetraplegia early on. Prevent and treat hypotension (aim for SBP >90). Look for, and exclude other injuries before assigning cause of hypotension to neurogenic shock. Restore intravascular volume (don't overload) then consider use of vasopressors. Checking lactate levels may help with assessment of shock and need for fluid resuscitation. Monitor and treat symptomatic bradycardia. Monitor and regulate temperature. Perform serial neurological examinations to assess for deterioration.

Imaging Don't rely on mobile equipment; if possible, take to the radiology department, supervising all movements closely. If there is a clear spinal cord injury, and the patient is stable, CT is the first line of imaging. Image the whole spine as there may be more than one injury.[343] MRI shows fractures, subluxations, disc disruption and protrusion, and cord contusion—and helps establish prognosis. ▶NB: it is hard to arrange in emergency settings, and takes a lot longer than CT (eg 20min vs 20s).

Consequences of injury *Respiratory insufficiency:* Check vital capacity repeatedly. If <500–600mL, intubation and ventilation will be needed. Monitor arterial blood gases. Intubation may produce vagal bradycardia, so give **atropine** 0.3–0.6mg IV before intubation and suction. If abdominal distension is causing respiratory embarrassment, pass an NGT. *Fluid balance:* There is likely to be hypotension below the lesion (sympathetic interruption and resultant neurogenic shock—↓BP and pulse rate). This is not due to hypovolaemia, and it is dangerous to give large volumes of fluid. Use IV not oral fluids for 48h and while ileus persists. *The skin:* Turn every 2h between supine and right and left lateral positions. The Stoke Mandeville bed does this electronically. Use pillows to separate the legs and maintain a lumbar lordosis. *The bladder:* Pass a 12-gauge silicone 5mL balloon catheter before the bladder volume exceeds 500mL (overstretching of detrusor can delay the return of automatic bladder function). See p772.

Treatment *Steroids:* ✦▶**Methylprednisolone** use is controversial. It is recommended in a Cochrane review in 2002[344] (updated in 2009) but the data is contested and other guidelines/systematic reviews suggest it should not be used.[343,345,346] Use within UK centres varies considerably.[347] Seek specialist advice prior to use. *Early surgical decompression:* ✦ Get expert advice on removing damaging bone & disc fragments. (Late internal fusions may also be tried.) There may be no difference in neurologic or functional improvement with early vs late surgery.[348] *Traction:* Skeletal traction will be needed for cervical injuries. Spring-loaded Gardner–Wells skull tongs are preferable to Crutchfield calipers, which need incisions. *Anticoagulation:* Acute cord injury patients are at very high risk of developing VTE, with asymptomatic DVT demonstrable in 60–100% of patients. LMWH (eg enoxaparin 40mg/24h sc) is currently recommended over unfractionated heparin regimens by the American College of Chest Physician guidelines for prevention of VTE. Start warfarin later, and continue prophylaxis for at least 3 months or until completion of inpatient rehabilitation.[349,350] ▶Arrange early and expert transfer to a spinal injuries unit.

Orthopaedics and trauma

Does this patient have a spinal cord injury?[351]

In any unexplained trauma, suspect cord injury if:
• Responds to pain only above clavicle.
• Dermatomal pattern of sensory loss.
• Breathing—diaphragmatic without use of accessory respiratory muscles.
• Muscles—hypotonic, including reduced anal tone (do a PR).
• Reflexes—hyporeflexic.
• Absence of movement in both legs.
• Slow pulse and ↓BP, but in the presence of normovolaemia.
• Priapism[1] or urinary retention.
• Unexplained ileus.
• Clonus in an unconscious trauma patient without decerebrate rigidity.
• Poikilothermia (poor temperature regulation).

The ASIA scale can be used to describe the completeness of the injury:

[ASIA=American Spinal Injury Association]

A	Complete; no sensory or motor function in sacral segments S4–S5
B	Injury incomplete; sensory but not motor function preserved below the neurological level, and extending through sacral segments S4–S5
C	Incomplete; motor function preserved below the level; most key muscles weaker than grade 3 (ie no movement against gravity)
D	Incomplete; motor function preserved below the level; most key muscles are stronger than grade 3, ie active movement against gravity
E	Normal motor and sensory function

▶NB: in the paediatric population SCIWORA (p658) is more common, and so careful clinical examination must be undertaken. Good knowledge of anatomical and developmental variation is also required when assessing plain radiographs—eg pseudosubluxation of C2 on C3 mimicking injury.

What are the mechanisms of injury?

Primary injury (immediate) is easy to understand: within seconds, the cord expands to occupy the entire diameter of the spinal canal. Glutamate floods out of neurons, overexciting their neighbours. Calcium floods in, leading to the formation of toxic free radicals.

Secondary injury (delayed, eg unfolding over weeks) is a response to release of neurotoxins and apoptosis (cell death) which may spread up to 4 segments away from the trauma site.[352]

How long can immobilization go on?

Neck collars and spine immobilization protocol can remain on an unconscious patient for as long as 48h after presentation, usually because it has not been possible to safely clear the spine from injury in the presence of more immediately life-threatening problems. However, immobilization is given such an initial priority because it can be done immediately and does not hinder progress of treatment. It would be a tragedy for a patient to survive life-threatening trauma, only to be paraplegic on account of inattention.

▶▶NB: Remember that a spinal cord injury causing anaesthesia may be masking serious injury below the lesion (eg compartment syndrome, acute abdomen).

---

1 **Priapism** is when pathologic stimuli (eg cervical cord lesions) cause prolonged erection (>4h), or when normal stimuli occurring under pathologic circumstances—eg stasis from sickle-cell disease or leukaemia with leucostasis (wcc↑↑) cause prolonged erections. As it can cause permanent damage, get help. Bilateral shunting between the corpus cavernosum and corpus spongiosum may be needed.

Priapism is named after Priapus, the son of Aphrodite (the goddess of love). He, though, is ugly in most depictions—with a penis so large that he is generally relegated to the position of a scarecrow in the fields. From this position he is happy to be the god of gardens, bees, goats, sheep—and fertility.

Orthopaedics and trauma

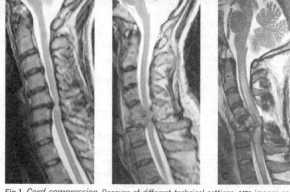

Fig 1. *Cord compression*. Because of different technical settings, MRI images can be called T1 or T2 weighted. These images can be recognized as T2 weighted because the CSF is white (see *OHCM* p749). Compression of the cord has occurred as a result of: a disc protrusion, b metastatic deposit, and c trauma.

Images © Prof Peter Scally.

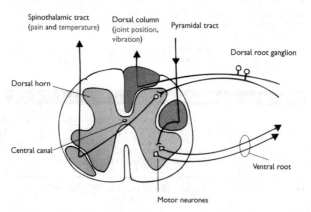

Fig 2. *Cross-section of the spinal cord*. The only neurons to decussate at (or near) their spinal cord level are those in the spinothalamic tract. Pyramidal tract fibres decussate in the medulla and the dorsal column fibres decussate after the gracile and cuneate nuclei of the medulla. Incomplete spinal cord injuries (see figs **3–5**) and younger patients have a better prognosis.[353]

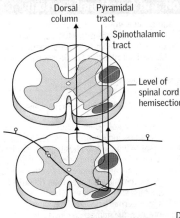

Fig 3. *Brown–Séquard syndrome* (*OHCM*, p710). In this rare injury pattern, there is hemisection of the spinal cord (more often seen after penetrating rather than blunt trauma), causing ipsilateral loss of dorsal column sensation and motor function below the lesion and contralateral loss of spinothalamic sensation from a few levels below the lesion.

NB: spinothalamic tract fibres ascend for a few levels on the same side as cord entry before they decussate.

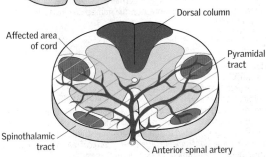

Fig 4. *Anterior cord syndrome*. There is infarction of the spinal cord in the distribution of the anterior spinal artery, causing complete loss of motor function and pain and temperature sensation below the lesion. Vibration and joint position sense are retained. This injury pattern has the worst prognosis of the incomplete injuries.

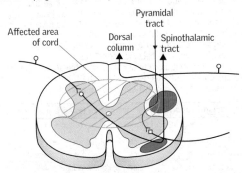

Fig 5. *Central cord syndrome*. Usually seen after a hyperextension injury in someone with pre-existing spinal canal stenosis (most often in the cervical region). There is greater loss of motor power in the upper extremities compared to the lower extremities combined with varying patterns of sensory loss and sphincter dysfunction.

Figs 2-5 adapted from
Donaghy, M. *Oxford Core Texts: Neurology* with permission from OUP

The 'tightest fit' between cord and canal is in the thoracic spine; this region also has the poorest blood supply. These facts explain why thoracic lesions are more likely to be complete than cervical or lumbar lesions. Ischaemic injury often spreads below the level of the mechanical injury. For the segment of the cord involved with injury at a specific vertebra, see below.

Cord compression For causes, see MINIBOX. Root pain (p674) and lower motor neurone signs occur at the level of the lesion with upper motor neurone signs and sensory changes below the lesion (spastic weakness, brisk reflexes, upgoing plantars, loss of co-ordination, joint position sense, vibration sense, temperature and pain).

Causes:
• Bone displacement
• Disc prolapse
• Local tumour
• Abscess
• Haematoma

Cord anatomy (p768) is such that dorsal column sensibilities (light touch, joint position sense, vibration sense) are affected on the same side as the insult, but spinothalamic tract interruption affects pain and temperature sensation for the opposite side of the body 2–3 dermatome levels lower than the affected sensory level. As the cord ends at L1, compression at this vertebral level affects information in the cord relating to lower dermatomes. To determine the cord level affected behind a given vertebra, add the number in blue to that of the vertebra concerned, thus:

• C2–7: **+1**
• T1–6: **+2**
• T7–9: **+3**
• T10 has L1 and L2 levels behind it
• T11 has L3 and 4
• L1 has sacral and coccygeal segments.

It can be difficult to determine the level: MRI will help clarify this.

Lower lumbar problems can cause cauda equina compression (▶▶p675) characterized by muscular pain, dermatomal sensory changes (if the lowest sacral dermatomes are affected the genitals are anaesthetic), and retention of urine ± faeces. ▶*These signs indicate urgent neurosurgical referral with imaging eg to confirm or exclude a tumour or extradural abscess.*

Spinal shock There is anaesthesia and flaccid paralysis of all segments, and muscles innervated below the level (hence areflexia) and there is retention of urine. A 'stage of reorganization' then occurs (reflex emptying of bladder and rectum; sweating). Later, flexion at hip and knee may be induced by stimuli (notably cold), often with emptying of the bladder and rectum (Head and Riddoch's mass reflexes). The legs may become permanently

Spinal or neurogenic?
▶NB: don't confuse *spinal shock* with *neurogenic shock*: the latter is BP↓ without tachycardia, caused by impairment of the descending spinal sympathetic pathways.

fixed in a drawn up position, with dorsiflexion of the ankles (spastic paraplegia in flexion). Over months, tendon reflexes return, and proprioceptive stimuli give rise to 'mass extension'. Exact duration is not predictable.

Paraplegia/quadriplegia levels (See also p716 for testing motor nerves)				
Levels fluctuate (as does interpretation), so examine often:				
Raises elbow to horizontal: *deltoid*	**C5**	Flexes hip: *iliopsoas*		**L2**
Flexes forearm: *biceps*	**C6**	Extends knee: *quadriceps*		**L3**
Extends forearm: *triceps*	**C7**	Dorsiflexes ankle: *tibialis anterior*		**L4**
Flexes wrist and fingers	**C8**	Extends great toe: *Extensor hallucis longus*		**L5**
Spreads fingers	**T1**	Plantarflexes ankle: *gastrocnemius*		**S1**

Orthopaedics and trauma

Restoring lost function: is it possible?

The following is not a list of well-tried treatment options: the field is too new. Here we present a way of thinking about cord injury, and preparing our minds for discussions with experts. Most patients prioritize their wishes for restoration of functions in this order: bowel and bladder control; sexual function; hand function; breathing. Options might be:

- Glutamate receptor blockers to limit secondary injury (p767).
- Anti-apoptotic agents, eg NT-3 (neurotrophin-3), BDNF (brain-derived neurotrophic factor), and ICE-protease (interleukin-1β-converting enzyme) inhibitors.
- Chemical prevention of action potential dissipation from demyelinated areas ± agents to remyelinate axons.
- Blocking natural inhibitors of regeneration, eg IN-1 (inhibitor neutralizing antibody).
- Promotion of axonal regeneration—eg BDNF & NT-3, (see above). Note that guidance of axons must be arranged, eg via guidance molecules such as netrins, cell adhesion molecules, and specific matrix proteins.
- Replacement of lost cells (cloned embryonic stem cells are one option; use of endogenous progenitor cells is another option).

Often these options seem a long way off, but note that only 10% of damaged neurones need to be replaced to enable useful locomotion.[354,355]

Segment injury—a guide to possible subsequent function:

C4	Can use electric chairs with chin control; type with mouthstick; use a 'Possum' environmental control system to turn on lights & open doors.
C5	With special devices, he can feed, wash face, comb hair, and help with dressing the upper body. He may be able to push a wheelchair along the flat, if pushing gloves are worn, and there are capstan rims on the wheels. The NHS will supply an electric wheelchair (indoor use only). Unable to transfer from wheelchair to toilet.
C6	Still needs a strap to aid feeding and washing. Dresses top half of body; helps dress lower half. Can drive with hand controls.
C7	Can transfer, dress, feed himself.
C8	Independent wheelchair life.

Orthopaedics and trauma

One major problem is urinary incontinence and reflex detrusor activity (after acontractility in the period of spinal shock) and the presence of residual urine. This predisposes to infection and ureteric reflux. These are major causes of renal failure, morbidity, and mortality.

Methods of bladder drainage Management in the first few days typically requires an indwelling urethral catheter. This should be secured with a waist band to prevent urethral traction. By the first weeks after cord injury use suprapubic or clean intermittent urethral catheterization[356] (OHCM fig 3, p777) with a 12 or 14 FG Nelaton® catheter. Culture the urine every week, and aim to eradicate infection (particularly important with *Proteus* which induces stones in infected alkaline urine). In some patients it may be possible to induce voiding by tapping the suprapubic area for ~20sec. Initially, catheterization is still necessary to drain the residual urine, but when this is <80mL (on 3 consecutive occasions), discontinue the catheter. If this does not occur, and particularly if the detrusor is non-contractile (conus medullaris or cauda equina injury), intermittent self-catheterization (eg with a silver catheter in women) may be used, as soon as the patient can sit. If reflex voiding occurs, **propantheline** 15–30mg/8–12h PO 1h AC may reduce detrusor activity and obviate the need for wearing drainage devices continuously. It may also help reduce hyperhidrosis.[357] The elderly may require an indwelling silicone catheter, with 6-weekly changes. Weekly washouts (eg Suby-G®) may prevent stones. Aim for an output of >3L/day. Use clamps to achieve volumes of 300mL. Artificial sphincters are available for acontractile bladders.

Complications Genitourinary complications are among the commonest causes for rehospitalization in spinal cord injury patients, so effective management, involvement and education are vital.[358]

Urinary infection: Historically used to be a serious cause of mortality (along with infected skin ulceration).[359] It may be prevented by a high fluid intake, ensuring effective bladder emptying, and acidification of the urine (eg **ascorbic acid** 1g/6h PO).

Detrusor-sphincter dyssynergia: The external urethral sphincter fails to relax or actively contracts during detrusor contraction. There is poor bladder emptying and vesicoureteric reflux, predisposing to pyelonephritis, hydronephrosis, and renal failure. It is wise to do U&E, creatinine, and IVU as early baseline tests. *Treatment:* Endoscopic external sphincterotomy.

Autonomic dysreflexia: In those with lesions above the sympathetic outflow (ie above T6) bladder distension (eg with a blocked catheter) may result in sympathetic overactivity below the level of the lesion. There is vasoconstriction and hypertension (may cause strokes/seizures/intra-cranial haemorrhage and death). The patient may have a headache, a feeling of anxiety, sweaty/blotchy skin above the lesion with pale, dry skin below the levely of lesion. The carotid baroreceptors are stimulated causing reflex vagal bradycardia, but the signals which would normally produce relieving vasodilatation are unable to pass down the cord. Other stimuli which may produce this effect include UTI, calculi, constipation, labour, ejaculation, and bladder or colonic irrigation.[360] *Treatment:* [361] Remove the cause; put in an upright position and loosen tight clothing. Give **nifedipine** (10mg—bite the capsule) with **glyceryl trinitrate** 0.5mg (not if patient has used sildenafil in the prior 24h). Captopril may also be useful in the acute management. Prazosin may be useful in its prevention.

On-demand urination There have been encouraging trials in those with ASIA-A lesions (p767) of the Brindley–Finetech Vocare implantable bladder system which activates anterior sacral nerve roots to regulate bladder and large bowel and urethral/anal contraction. This leads to cost savings (fewer catheters), fewer UTIs, and a better life.[355]

►*Sexual counselling is an integral part of rehabilitation.* It is important in itself, but we should recognize that sexuality interacts with important determinants of our patient's quality of life, eg levels of dependency, aggression, self-esteem, and autonomy.[362]

We should enlist expert help, but we can all counter myths that disabled men cannot sexually satisfy able-bodied women; and that the cord-injured cannot have intercourse. Don't be shy and don't be shocked: for help with discussing sexual issues, see p328. ►Given a knowing and patient partner, most persons with spinal injury can enjoy a satisfying sex life.[363,364]

Be aware that sexuality encompasses more than physical attractiveness and penile–vaginal intercourse. With spinal cord injury, use of sexual imagery and concentration on body areas that retain sensation have especial importance, as does a certain inventiveness and readiness to experiment.[365]

When helping these patients it is important to distinguish sexual drive and sexual satisfaction from fertility and parenting needs. Both need addressing in a systematic way within the broader contexts of psychosocial, emotional, and relationship aspects—and also in terms of cognitive-genital dissociation, perceived sexual disenfranchisement, and sexual rediscovery. Cognitive-genital dissociation may take various forms, eg indicating that for some, sexual activity is more like watching a graphic movie than engaging in a physical experience.[366] It is equally important to assess the partner's needs and responses to the injury. This takes time.[367]

Do not concentrate on physical aspects alone: nevertheless it may be helpful to familiarize yourself with some statistics, and to emphasize that individuals vary. In some studies, locomotor impairment and dysreflexia were more frequently given as causes of reduced sexual pleasure than specific sexual dysfunctions.[365]

In women, only 17% with complete lower motor neuron dysfunction affecting the s2–s5 spinal segments can achieve orgasm, compared with 59% of women with other levels and degrees of injury.

In men with lesions between T6 and L5, 75% can expect improvement in erections with use of **sildenafil**.[368,369]

Fertility issues in men centre around performance and sperm quality, which may be reduced by scrotal hyperthermia, retrograde ejaculation, prostatic fluid stasis, and testicular denervation. Electro-ejaculation and intracytoplasmic sperm injection have a useful role (p293).

In women, pregnancy rates vary from ~10% to 60%.[370] Autonomic dysreflexia is serious risk, especially in lesions at or above the level of T6. Pregnancy and childbirth can be successful and rewarding for all involved when careful planning and communication take place—eg incorporating child care issues into the rehabilitation process.[371]

Orthopaedics and trauma

The **occupational therapist** (ot) is a key person in maximizing the levels of achievement outlined above. She is also in a position to arrange a home visit with a member of the spinal injuries team, and a community liaison nurse or social worker. The aim is to construct a plan with local social services and the local domiciliary ot, so that the patient's (and his family's) hopes can be realized to the fullest extent. She can arrange the necessary home modifications, and give invaluable advice about the level of independence which is realistic to strive for. As ever, the aims of the ot extend into augmenting self-esteem, and helping the patient come to terms with loss of role, and loss of confidence, and to mitigate the effects of disability by arranging for as much purposeful activity as possible, in the realms of both work and leisure. She will also be able to make plans for acquiring of social skills to assist the patient in his new way of life.

Nursing & physiotherapy • *The chest:* Regular physio with coughing and breathing exercises prevents sputum retention and pneumonia which are likely to follow diaphragmatic partial paralysis (eg c3–4 dislocation). If the lesion is above t10 segmental level, there is no effective coughing.

• *The straight lift:* (for transferring patients) One attendant supports the head with both hands under the neck so that the head lies on the arms. 3 lifters standing on the same side insert their arms under the patient, one at a time, starting at the top. After the lift, withdraw in the reverse order.

• *The log-roll:* (learn from observation; see fig 1, p799) 3 lifters stand on the same side of the patient. The one near the head has both arms under the patient's trunk and over the patient's further arm; the 2nd has one arm under the legs and the other arm holds the patient's iliac crest. The 3rd lifter supports the calves. A 4th person controls the head and neck, and gives the command to turn. The patient is then gently rolled laterally, with pillows to support the lumbar curve and to keep the position stable.

• *Posture:* Place joints in a full range of positions. Avoid hyperextensions. Keep the feet flexed at 90° with a pillow between soles and bed-end.

• *Bowels:* From the second day of injury gentle manual evacuation using plenty of lubricant is needed. A flatus tube may be helpful in relieving distension once the ileus of spinal shock has passed. Irrigation may improve quality of life.[372]

• *Wheelchairs:* The patient should be kept sitting erect; adjust the footplates so that the thighs are supported on the wheelchair cushion and there is no undue pressure on the sacrum. ►Regular relief of pressure on sacral and ischial areas is vital. Independence in transferring to bed or toilet will be a suitable aim for some patients with paraplegia. Expert skill is needed in assigning the correct wheelchair for any particular patient.

• *Standing and walking:* Using a 'tilt table', or the Oswestry standing frame with trunk support straps, the tetraplegic patient can become upright. If the injury level is at l2–4, below-knee calipers and crutches enable walking to take place. If the lesion is at t1–8, 'swing to gait' may be possible. The crutches are placed a short distance in front of the feet. By leaning on them and pushing down with the shoulders, both legs can be lifted and moved forwards together. The goal is to promote re-establishment of functional connections in neuronal networks and shaping the motor patterns that they generate.[373]

• *Sport:* Consider archery, darts, snooker, table tennis, and swimming for those with paraplegia. Many other sports may also be suitable. There are interesting and important factors to consider such as the optimal heart rate (eg with lesions above t4 there is severely diminished cardiac acceleration, and a maximal rate of ~130bpm) and the reduction in bone density below the lesion.[374]

Personal qualities in therapists are almost as important as exact anatomic lesion. There may be big mood swings from euphoria to despair as the patient accustoms himself to his loss and his new body image.

"I seemed to have been asleep nearly all of my life."
"...But when did you wake up?"
"I don't know that I ever did, or ever have." *Sons & Lovers*, 274

'Persistent vegetative state' aims to describe the behaviour of severely brain damaged people who show sleep–awake behaviour, but in whom there is absent cognition and awareness.

Causes:
• Trauma
• Anoxia
• Vascular causes
• Encephalitis

Making the diagnosis Persistent vegetative states are rare, and liable to misdiagnosis by non-specialist neurologists and neurosurgeons—it requires careful repeated assessment and taking into account observations made by family and carers. ▸*The harder you look, the more likely you are to find signs of active cognition, so negating the diagnosis of a vegetative state.* The patient in a vegetative state (vs) "appears at times to be wakeful, with cycles of eye closure and eye opening resembling those of sleep and waking". But they lack signs of awareness—there is no evidence they can perceive the environment or their own body.[375] Persistent vegetative state refers to a vs which has continued from more than 4 weeks. Permanent vegetative state refers to a vs that has lasted 12 months following a traumatic brain injury, or 6 months following other causes of brain injury. Patients that show awareness are said to be in a minimally conscious state rather than a vegetative state.

Investigations In addition to history and neurological examination, there are a number of methods that can be used to aid the decision as to whether there is cognitive brain function present: eg somatosensory evoked potentials (SSEPs) and electroencephalography (EEG). However, the problem is that these tests not only have to be 100% specific (an impossibility) but they also need to be able to predict *return* of cognitive function, and not just its presence. To make matters even more complicated, pharmacological and metabolic changes can also interfere with the accuracy of such tests.[376] One review has quoted that with the absence of somatosensory evoked potentials in patients with hypoxic ischaemic encephalopathy, the chances of waking are less than 1%.[377]

Another method of showing awareness and cognition is by demonstrating communication, eg by following a simple request to press a buzzer or to look at a named object. These switches are particularly suited to those who can only manage a tiny amount of voluntary movement. Other ways of communicating include listener scanning: the therapist goes through A–z slowly, and the patient buzzes when the required letter is reached. It may take weeks or months to establish that the patient can communicate. Rancho scale assessment establishes the level of cognition—from confused-and-inappropriate (level 5) to purposeful-and-appropriate (level 8).

fMRI has shown that some patients with the diagnosis of a vegetative state can have patterns of brain activity detectable which are suggestive of higher mental activity thus indicating a degree of consciousness of self and environment.[378] Whether this makes an ethically significant difference in the management of such patients is unresolved.[379]

Management Seek expert rehabilitative help. While waiting for any recovery, aim to provide vigorous nursing care to maintain nutrition, and to prevent pressure sores, and tracheostomy and muscle contracture complications. No drugs are known to help, although there is anecdotal evidence that bromocriptine may do so. Randomized trials indicate that multimodal stimulation (arousal programmes) help. These programmes involve stimulation of all senses every 15min for up to 11h per day.

Once it is agreed that there will be no recovery (the difficult issue), discussions on withdrawing active treatment and nutrition raise big ethical questions—which are only partly mitigated if the patient has an advance directive (an unlikely event). Ethicists, medical specialists, nurses, physiotherapists, judges, and the family must all be allowed to have their say. None is infallible.

NB: also see **Death: diagnosis and management**, *OHCM*, p6.

Orthopaedics and trauma

Muddled over death, brain death and persistent vegetative states?

When the Buddha was ailing, he was at first mispronounced dead by Ananda, his attendant for 25 years. Ananda was then 'corrected' by a top monk who stated that the Buddha had entered a deep yogic trance in which no vital signs could be discerned (as might occur in hypothermia).[380] How do you tell? First, recognize that death is a *process*, and in some instances (such as hypothermia) all processes are suspended—so not even death can unfold (or it may unfold slowly). Next, accept that absent brainstem reflexes is a only a useful short-hand for death of the brainstem—which itself is only a shorthand for brain death (functions remain, such as thermoregulation and production of CNS hormones, etc). And death of the brain is just a useful shorthand for death itself. According to ancient Buddhist authorities, death occurs when the body is bereft of *vitality* (ayu), *heat* (usma), and *sentiency* (viññana). In many ways the senior monk was right. First know your patient, and take into account past history[1] and the current medical and moral context in which the diagnosis of brain death or persistent vegetative states is being made. Then ask a colleague, and keep an open mind—especially when organ donation is contemplated.[2]

---

1 Contexts such as barbiturate poisoning and Bickerstaff's brainstem encephalitis can give a brain-death picture—*but are reversible* (worryingly so—more for ethicists than the patient).
2 Patients who have 'confirmed' brain death and who are suitable for organ donation would be heart-beating donors. However, organ retrieval is never straightforward, and so the Maastricht criteria exist for the categorization of non-heart-beating organ donors: 1 Dead on arrival at hospital; 2 Unsuccessful resuscitation; 3 Awaiting cardiac arrest (eg after withdrawal of treatment); 4 Cardiac arrest after confirmation of brainstem death.[381]

Does he need a radiograph?

The aim is to provide information that will alter management, without exposing patients to unnecessary radiation. The following is based on the advice of the UK Royal College of Radiologists, and other bodies.

Twisting injury of foot or ankle An ankle radiograph is indicated if patients cannot bear weight; or if there is tenderness on the posterior edge of either the lateral or medial malleolus. A foot radiograph is required if there is pain in the midfoot, tenderness at the base of the 5th metatarsal or over the navicular.—but all rules have exceptions, and, on occasion, we've all seen patients walk on a fractured ankle.[1]

Injury to the cervical spine: The consequences of a missed cervical spine injury are disastrous, and so c-spine radiography is always performed for major trauma. But in patients who have been subjected to less violent trauma, what can be used as a guide to requesting imaging? Until you become more experienced in these situations, liaison with a senior colleague is wise. Nonetheless, in the presence of NSAID:

- Neurological exam reveals a focal deficit.
- Spine exam reveals tenderness (posterior midline).
- Alteration in consciousness.
- Intoxication.
- Distracting injury—i.e. long bone fracture, clavicle fracture, chest trauma etc.

...request imaging.[382] Based on the NEXUS criteria for imaging of c-spine blunt injury, all these factors are important, though may have the drawback of a low sensitivity if applied as the sole criteria for imaging.[383,384] The Canadian C-spine rules are more specific but more complicated. High risk factors (dangerous mechanism, age >65, focal neurology) mandate a radiograph. Absence of these allows consideration of low risk factors (simple rear end RTA, sitting up in A&E, ambulatory at any time, delayed onset of pain, absence of midline C-spine tenderness)—the presence of any one allows clinical examination of the neck: if the patient can rotate their neck 45° left and right they do not need a radiograph.[385]

'Possible' neck injury in minor head injury A radiograph is not indicated if fully conscious and there are no symptoms or signs related to the neck.

Nose injury Imaging in A&E is not indicated in simple nasal injury.

Rib injury Only a posteroanterior CXR is indicated if you suspect a pneumothorax; rib views are not needed in uncomplicated blunt injury.

Lumbar spine pain Avoid early radiographs (in 1st 6 weeks) if there are no factors suggesting serious disease, eg trauma, focal neurology, fever, weight↓, anaemia, ESR↑ (so do blood tests first). Each examination=2.2mSv=40 CXRs. The Sievert (Sv) is the SI unit of radiation absorbed by biological tissues—see OHCM p733. This dose may be expected to cause 16 malignancies/yr in the UK at current rates of exposure. It is impossible to protect the ovaries.

Abdominal pain Plain films are rarely needed; request only an erect chest film in suspected gastrointestinal perforation. Erect abdominal films are generally not indicated in most patients with abdominal pain.

Foreign bodies Always do radiography if the presence of glass is possible (glass is usually radiopaque). Ultrasound can also be used in foreign body detection and to guide removal, especially for those that are not radio-opaque (eg splinters).

NB: lumbar spine radiographs deliver a significant dose of radiation to the gonads—similarly for skull and facial radiographs to the eyes (lens cataracts are the risk). These guidelines yield substantial savings in costs and in patients' waiting times, without compromising patient care.

1 Ottawa rules: www.bmj.com/cgi/content/full/326/7386/417. If the rule says 'don't x-ray' it will be right in 98.6% of cases assuming a # prevalence of 15%. Specificity ('do x-ray' and # is present) is worse.[386]

Does he need a CT?

Quick, accurate, and available: good reasons to think of CT as 1st-line imaging for trauma patients. But there are caveats, as any radiologist who has seen images arriving at their workstation monitor, only to have to comment that the patient's heart has stopped, will tell you. The appropriateness of scanning in an acute trauma must be decided on the balance of risk and benefit to the patient. It is not that radiologists don't want sick patients in their department; radiology departments just aren't the best place to be if you are very sick. ►*Ensure that the patient is haemodynamically stable before moving them to the relatively resource-poor radiology department.* Some centres have tried to overcome this problem by bringing CT to the emergency department, imaging patients as they come through the door, and while CT may well become the new stethoscope, this approach will also have its faults. Remember that: *Radiation can do harm:* It cannot be used limitlessly (OHCM p733). *Imaging is just a snapshot:* A 'normal' scan mustn't allow for complacency in patient observation. ►*Always be on the lookout for clinical deterioration requiring prompt intervention.* Imaging takes time: Transfers and interpretation take the longest: CT itself may only take 20s. This is time that the patient is at risk and also time delaying definitive management. For this reason, you may be paradoxically encouraged to request *more* imaging (eg including c-spine), given that having to come back to the department for a second scan doubles the risk.

The Canadian CT head rule CT is only required for minor head injury if one of the following is present:[387]
• Glasgow coma scale <15 at 2h post-injury.
• Suspected open or depressed skull fracture.
• Signs of basal skull fracture: haematotympanum (blood in middle ear/tympanic cavity) raccoon eyes, CSF otorrhoea/rhinorrhoea, Battle's sign, p728).
• Age >65
• Vomiting >2 times
• Amnesia before impact of >30min.
• Dangerous mechanism (pedestrian struck by car; car occupant ejected, fall from a height of >1m, or downstairs).

The NICE guidelines on head injury adds post-traumatic seizure, coagulopathy and focal neurological deficit as indications for a CT head.[388]

CT of the cervical spine CT assessment of the cervical spine is quick and effective. Meta-analysis suggests that CT be used as the first line investigation in those with a depressed mental status, though not as a matter of course for less severe injury, in which plain radiography should still be used.[389] It also has cost-benefit implications.[217] It is indicated if an injury is seen on the plain film series and if there is inadequate visualization (C7/T1 can be difficult to image in full with plain x-ray.) A similar approach applies for other spinal injuries, but remember that MRI will be needed to assess the vital soft tissue structures.

CT of the chest Evidence of traumatic injury on CXR that warrants further imaging: • Haemothorax • Pneumothorax • Widened mediastinum (all difficult to spot on a supine film) • Pneumomediastinum • Posterior rib fractures • Fractures of ribs 1 or 2 • Pulmonary contusion.

CT of the abdomen and pelvis Usually done together. Indications may include: • Free fluid noted on FAST scan (p727), but beware US algorithms for assessment in blunt abdominal trauma)[223] • Suspicion of retroperitoneal haemorrhage (shock but not cause found) • Renal trauma (macroscopic haematuria, microscopic haematuria + shock).

CT of the appendicular skeleton Part of pre-operative planning for complex injury patterns.

►*Remember to think of patterns of injury:* eg rib fractures with bilateral pulmonary contusions have a high coincidence of intra-abdominal injury

Appropriate use of Emergency Departments

From our point of view, the ideal scenario is to have a pristine, ever-ready but empty trauma department with the doctors and nurses educating themselves (etcetera) in the coffee room, occasionally being called out by paramedics to save a few lives in a brief display of energy and technical brilliance. This is not how the public sees our role. If in shock, having just run over a hedge-hog, some people feel they need attention *now*. All Emergency Departments are abused—because it is always doctors who define what abuse is. Thus up to 70% of users have been deemed inappropriate in some studies. This figure dwindles towards nothingness if abuse is defined as those consultations where all 3 parties to the visit, on reflection, concur that it was inappropriate: the doctor, the patient ± family, and the patient's GP (who may have sent them).

Overcrowding and 'exit-block'[390] This is a major problem in Emergency Departments the world over—partly reflecting centrally determined reductions in acute bed provision and availability, and partly reflecting access problems for populations seeking prompt help with immediate (and, sometimes, chronic) problems. If the inpatient side of a hospital is full, patients will stack up in Emergency Departments, awaiting admission. If overcrowding is cumulative, ambulances may be redirected to other hospitals (adding to delay and danger) and patients with genuine needs may, catastrophically, decide they cannot wait any more hours for help.

How to cope with inappropriate attendance

- *Triage* by a trained nurse is one way to reduce inappropriate attendance. (In the UK, triage is mandatory.) Is this condition *life-threatening, urgent, or semi-urgent* or is *delay acceptable*? These are the chief categories. If the most urgent patients are seen first, patients who do not really need to be in the department can wait for ages, and many will begin to drift away. Note that if long waits become essential because of dealing with life-threatening conditions, this should be explained to patients (under the terms of the UK health charter—and as a matter of common courtesy).
- Another way to reduce unnecessary spending is to have primary care facilities within the Emergency Department, or, more radically, to have GPs as the casualty officers—because they use resources more sparingly and are used to dealing with mismatches between patient's expectations and reality. Is this expectation borne out in practice? In one careful randomized study of patient-contacts with the Emergency Department in Dublin ($N=4684$), GPs treating people with semi-urgent problems investigated less (by 20%), referred to other hospital services less (by 39%), admitted fewer patients (45%) and prescribed more often (43%): there were no differences in measures of outcome.[391] It is not clear whether the more economical style of the GPs was to do with being a GP, or because these doctors were older and more experienced than their emergency department counterparts.[1]

Risk management strategy when overwhelmed by the work to be done:
- Prioritize the waiting tasks and then concentrate on the task in hand.
- At times you may feel you are working at a pace that is faster than is comfortable. This is part of 'continuous learning', and as you get better this unease will abate. Look on it as practice for emergency situations where quick decisions are vital. Working faster need not mean making more errors.
- Have good techniques of clinical decision-making, which you continue to refine. Start with something like the system on p532.
- Keep the goal in mind: *What to do for the best for this patient.*

1 UK GPs are an established part of the team at the front line seeing patients in Emergency Departments: they join the growing team of *emergency nurse practitioners*, *junior doctors*, and *consultants* (eg in a 'meet & greet' capacity) to tackle the turnover of patients with more minor injuries and ailments. Medical specialists (eg dedicated *emergency paediatricians*) are also increasingly involved.

Another busy shift?

In the middle of any horrendous Emergency Department shift, you may be forgiven for wondering what on earth is happening outside to prompt such a heave in the number of attendances. Rumours circulate that sunshine means that children are out in force at the local playgrounds, or rain means that old ladies will be slipping up on the kerb. Perhaps late on a Friday night you despair at the number of alcohol-related incidents? Similarly, you hear that because the Grand National is on, the shift is going to be a quiet one...until the race finishes and people are out spending their winnings (or drowning their losses).

Factors that have been suggested to be correlated with an increase in the number of Emergency Department attendances include:

• Warm, dry and sunny weather conditions.[392]
• Season, especially winter for the over-65s and the under 1s.[393,394]
• Local music festivals (despite on-site facilities).[395]
• An at-home winning national sports side (sadly, for assault).[396]
• Major natural disasters (eg a hurricane, though with an understandable reduction on the day of the disaster).[397]
• And yes...Mondays.[394]

Other studies have suggested that attendances may be reduced by major televised sporting events.[398,399]

It is a complicated mix which depends on where in the world you are working and it is not always clear whether these factors are delaying, precipitating, or causative (though logic may point the finger of causality).[1]

Ultimately, the aim of such epidemiological studies is to help in emergency department staffing and logistics, and taken with a pinch of salt, one message is clear: ▸*Don't despair, as all of these factors are well beyond your control!*

---

1 Why not have a look at your own departmental data...

Bites, stings and foreign bodies

Mammal bites All animal bites are contaminated, especially those of human animals: *everything that comes out of the human mouth is poison.* John Steinbeck Cannery Row. Clean well with soap and water, debriding if needed. See p746. ▶Avoid suturing unless cosmetically essential. Give antibiotics covering anaerobes unless very trivial and not high-risk (risk↑ if: ♀, >50yrs, immunosuppressed, wound is to the hand, face or foot, delayed presentation, penetration of underlying structures, crush wound), eg co-amoxiclav 500/125 tab/8h PO (clindamycin 300mg/6h PO if allergic to penicillin—but beware pseudomembranous colitis).[231,400] Bites from monkeys (specifically macaques) require treatment with valaciclovir to prevent transmission of *Cercopithecine herpesvirus 1* which in humans leads to a fatal encephalitis. NB: dog bites may lead to crush injuries, so x-ray to check no underlying fracture or foreign body, bites from cats may not be as trivial as they look: they carry *Pasteurella multocida*, streps, and fusibacteria. Is tetanus prophylaxis needed (p730)? Consider rabies if bitten outside UK. (Post-exposure rabies prophylaxis: phone the UK Central Public Health Lab/Health Protection Agency, 020 8200 6868; after hours, 020 8200 4400.)[401]

Snake bites Britain's only poisonous snake, the adder, is very rarely lethal. There are about 100 bites per year in the UK.[402] Australia has ~3000 bites per year, with 1–2 fatalities. The WHO considers envenomation to be a neglected tropical disease, with >10000 envenomations occurring in India alone. Bites are usually on the hand or foot.[403] R: Wrap the entire affected limb in a crepe bandage and immobilize it. Identify the species if possible and move the patient to hospital. Treat ABCs—respiratory paralysis, hypotension, cardiac arrest and seizures can occur. Check clotting time (many venoms are anticoagulant), renal function, CK, d-dimer, FBC, urine for myoglobinuria. Venom detection kits exist—use if there are clinical signs (nausea, ↓LOC, ptosis, weakness, coagulopathy, muscle pain) or abnormal biochemistry. (Indications for antivenom treatment include abnormal biochemical/clinical signs.) In the UK, give European viper venom antiserum (see *BNF*) 1 vial IV over 15min. Use the same dose for children. It may be repeated after 1h, if there is no improvement. Have adrenaline to hand (p237). If the bite is from a foreign snake or spider, the relevant antivenom may be held at pharmacies in London or Liverpool[UK]—they are available via the National Poisons Information Service and via www.toxbase.org. ▶Avoid tourniquets, incisions, and sucking the wound (but a limb bandage may help confine venom).

Lesser weever fish stings (*Echiicthys vipera*)—eg in barefoot UK bathers. It is not serious, and may be relieved by immersion of the leg for 5–20min in water which is as hot as can be tolerated (eg <45°C).

Scorpion venom Signs: BP ↓ or ↑, renal failure, LVF. R: Lidocaine sc at the site relieves pain. Antidotes prepared from animal antisera are effective against some species of scorpion.[404] Prazosin & L-carnitine 660mg/8h PO *may* help.[405,406]

Airgun pellets These are common, and can be hard to remove. Deaths have occurred, eg when a pellet enters brain through the eye. Get 2 radiographic views to position the foreign body. Ultrasound guidance may also help localize the pellet, but be aware that only shadow or reverberation artefact may be visible, and not the pellet itself. If it has just penetrated the skin, inject local anaesthetic carefully so you can still palpate it: if you cannot remove it easily, leave it *in situ* rather than risk extensive tissue destruction trying to find it; give antibiotics. Pellets tracking subcutaneously, or which have penetrated deeply, must be sought. ▶

Other foreign bodies ▶*Always do radiography if there may be glass/metal/stone in a wound.* Tiny shards may be left *in situ*. Even large shards can be hard to find, needing exploration under GA to remove. Ultrasound may be useful. ▶Always do orbit radiography for a high-velocity metallic foreign body that cannot be seen (eg grinding/hammering injury).

Ingestion of a metallic object[407]

Pathways for metallic foreign body (FB) ingestion management may differ from hospital to hospital, so check your local guidelines. In general:

• *Do CXR* to tell you whether the object has progressed to below the diaphragm, beyond which it is most likely to be safe. There are very rare reports of objects lodging at the pylorus, resulting in gastric erosion.[408]

• *If displaying neck/upper airway symptoms:* Do a lateral neck radiograph: with a CXR, this should enable you to differentiate GI and respiratory tract location. Foreign bodies can occasionally sit asymptomatically at the *valleculae* (= 'little ditches', which are the recesses between mucosal folds at the base of the epiglottis), or in the piriform fossae (which are recesses in the upper oesophagus, either side of the laryngeal inlet).

• *AXR:* Recommended in children—many will have a second FB elsewhere.

• *If in upper ⅓ of oesophagus:* There is risk of perforation, and the object needs endoscopic removal. Ensure there are no more foreign bodies before removing the scope. If lower down, repeat radiography after 12–24h. If the coin is still in the oesophagus, remove endoscopically under GA. ►Button batteries lodged anyway in the oesophagus need urgent removal.

• *If below diaphragm:* Let it pass. The stool can be screened for passage of the object, eg manually, with x-rays or with a metal detector.

The same principles hold for button/tube battery ingestion—reports of heavy metal poisoning are very rare.[409] Surgical removal is warranted for the rare cases of GI obstruction and maybe for persistence of failure to pass.

Fish bones are the chief foreign body to stick in the upper airway/GI tract. Radio-opacity may be species dependent.[410] Lateral neck radiographs are insensitive: CT may be needed, followed by endoscopic removal.[411]

►**Heimlich manoeuvre and back blows** See p795.

Bee stings

Scrape them out gently with a knife or credit card *quickly*.[412] This technique is better at removing a sting than pinching it out, because bee stingers are barbed (fig 1), whereas wasp stingers are smooth. As a consequence, the stinger is left in the skin, still attached to the poison sac and tip of the abdomen, meaning that her first sting will likely be her last.[1]

Pheromones released from the expiring bee attract more bees, but you may be able to outrun them if you see them coming. NB: although always fatal to the bee, a single sting almost never kills you (risk <1 in 1,000,000; ~4 deaths/yr in UK). Fatalities are more likely if you get >200 stings (but >1000 is survivable). Ice ±calamine lotion help itch. Give antihistamines for severe swelling/itch. ►►Anaphylaxis, p237.[413]

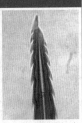
Fig 1. Bee stinger (×40).
Courtesy of Jeff Beck

Killer bee stings (Africanized honeybees: *Apis mellifera scutellata*) Despite treatment on ITU (antihistamines, corticosteroids, bronchodilators, vasodilators, bicarbonate, mannitol, and ventilation), deaths occur ~1–3 days after the attacks (>100 stings), from ARDS, BP↑↑, hepatic and subendocardial necrosis, haemolysis, rhabdomyolysis, acute tubular necrosis, and DIC.[414]

---

1 Bees that sting are ♀. The stinger is a vestigial ovipositor that has subsequently become a stinging organ, evolved for defence purposes (against both other bees and larger, thicker-skinned interferers).

Orthopaedics and trauma

...t, ask the trauma nurse: she will have seen it all before.

...nered my finger, doctor" This usually causes a subungual haema-
...elieved by expressing the blood through a hole trephined in the nail,
...a 19G needle. No force is needed. Simply twiddle the needle vertically on
...nail: the cutting edge will make a suitable hole (p747).

"I've swallowed a fish bone and it's stuck" Always examine the throat and
tonsils carefully. Often the bone has only grazed the mucosa. Use a good light,
and grip the tongue with gauze to move it out of the way before removing any
visible bones with forceps. If you fail, refer to ENT (see p567).

"My fish hook has barbed my finger" Infiltrate with plain lidocaine and
push the hook on through the finger, provided no important structures are in
its way. Once the barb is through, cut it off. Remove the hook where it entered.

"My tooth has been knocked out" Try to replace permanent teeth. Send
deciduous teeth to the tooth fairy. If the former, after the patient sucks it
clean (do not use water) transport in milk—or reinsert it, stabilizing with finger pressure (or biting). Go to a dentist for splinting.

Plaster 'backslabs' (for undisplaced forearm fractures).
- Remove anything which impairs finger circulation (eg rings).
- Protect yourself and your patient with a plastic apron.
- Measure the length for the back slab—from knuckles to just below elbow, so
  that the fingers and elbow will remain mobile.
- Cut a piece of plaster-impregnated bandage 5 times longer than the desired
  length. Fold it into 5-ply. Then see fig 1, ①, OPPOSITE.
- Cut off one corner so that it does not impinge on the thumb.
- Cut a wedge off the other end with the wedge's thick end on the same side as
  the thumb. This aids elbow movement. ②
- Roll stockinette over the forearm, to well above the elbow.
- Wind a roll of wool padding over the stockingette (turns must overlap by
  50%, so protecting flesh from the hard plaster). ③
- Immerse the plaster bandage in tepid water and apply it to the dorsum of
  the arm—without pitting it with your finger tips. ④
- Reflect the stockinette down from the elbow and up from the wrist making
  comfortable top and bottom ends to the plaster. ⑤
- Place a bandage right around the forearm to keep everything in place, securing its end with a strip of wet plaster. ⑥
- Setting takes place over 4min: sooner if warm water is used.
- Put the arm in a sling for 1 day—after which encourage movement of shoulder, elbow, and fingers to prevent stiffness. ▸*Cautions for the patient:* 1 Return immediately to A&E if the fingers go blue, swell, or you cannot move
  them. 2 Do not get the plaster wet. 3 Do not lift heavy weights with the
  hand. Give the patient a plaster care information card.

Removing a tight ring from a swollen finger Pass a No.4 silk suture through
the ring from distal to proximal. Wind the distal end around the finger in a
distal direction. Then unwind from the proximal end distally (should pull the
ring over the coil). Lubrication + compression + traction may also make for
success and a relieved patient. If not, try using a ring cutter (though not for
brass or steel).

"I've caught my penis in my zip" Failing copious lubrication with mineral
oil, the most elegant method is to cut out the bridge from the slider of the zip
with strong wire-cutters as shown in fig 2. The zip then falls apart and all that
is needed is a new zip. (Beware the bridge flying off at speed: hold gauze by
it.) What if the trousers are of immense value? Try the Savile Row technique:
infiltrate the skin with 1% lidocaine (no adrenaline!); carefully manipulate the
prepuce along the side of the slider by an unzipping movement.[415]

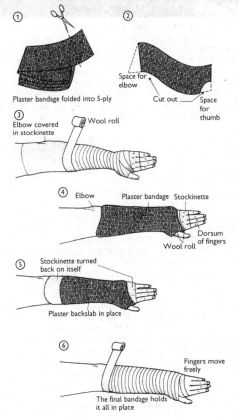

Fig 1. Plaster backslab.

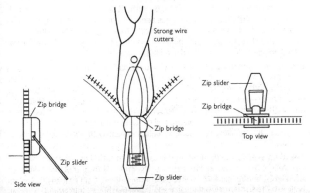

Fig 2. Solution to the zipped penis problem.

Worldwide, around 400,000 drowning deaths occur yearly: most are children.[416] Drowning is the 3rd leading cause of unintentional injury death worldwide. In general children under 5 are at greatest risk, New Zealand and Canada are exceptional in that adult males in these countries drown at higher rates than children. Many drownings in adults are associated with alcohol. Most drownings in children occur in those who are poorly supervised near water. It is quite common for a toddler to bath with a slightly older sibling 'in charge'—the mother thinking that as the child can sit up, he can also save himself from drowning should he topple over. Males are at greater risk of drowning than females.

In communities wealthy enough to have many private swimming pools there are summertime spates of drownings. An adult is temporarily distracted and leaves the garden, and, on return, finds a corpse in the pool. When such a child is brought to A&E the chief concerns are: 1 Cardiac arrest 2 Hypothermia, *OHCM* p860 3 Acidaemia 4 Pulmonary oedema.

Management focuses on ABCDE (p725)

- Immobilize the cervical spine as you open the airway—there may have been trauma here through cause or effect. Clear vomit from mouth.
- Give 100% O_2 to prevent hypoxia—water in alveoli will dilute surfactant and increase atelectasis. CPAP or PEEP may be required.
- Expect BP to drop after leaving the water. Transport with a minimum of rough handling and in the horizontal position (although not always possible in extreme environments). This helps reduce cardiovascular instability.[417]
- If pulseless, start cardiopulmonary resuscitation.
- Monitor ECG. Defibrillate if VF (APLS, p239). For the first shock, give ~2J/kg body weight (~20J at 12 months, 40J at 4yrs, 60J at 8yrs, and 80J at 12yrs). Defibrillation often fails until core T° >30°C. Heroic measures have been tried without clearly affecting outcome[418]—eg rapid core rewarming (warm-water immersion, warm IV fluids at 40°C, breathing heated humidified gas,[419] peritoneal dialysis, thoracotomy for heart irrigation, or heart bypass).
- Do Glasgow Coma Scale, p720; if <6 the prognosis is poor.
- Monitor core T°. Remove wet clothing and examine for signs of other injury.
- If T° <35°C, monitor rectal T° often and rewarm using high ambient T°. Circulatory support may be needed to counter rewarming vasodilatation. Measuring left atrial pressure helps guide IV fluid: too much will ↑ICP.
- Pass a nasogastric tube to relieve gastric dilatation.
- Check U&E, blood gases, and Hb. Get expert advice on the problem of acidosis.
- In the case of continuing resuscitation without success, it is vital not to halt proceedings until full rewarming has been achieved and asystole is noted on ECG. Children and adults have been reported to make a full recovery.[420]
- Remember to consider that drowning may not have been the only life-threatening insult.[421] The coroner will need to be informed of deaths.

Effects of asphyxia and fresh water overload The child usually swallows large amounts of water before final aspiration. This leads to gastric dilatation, vomiting, and further aspiration.[416] ARDS can occur, leading to the major villain, hypoxaemia—hence cerebral oedema and ↑ICP. To combat these, steroids and antibiotics are sometimes given, but without proof of efficacy. As the raised intracranial pressure (ICP) is due to cell death (cytotoxic oedema), steroids do not lower ICP (unlike the vasogenic oedema seen with space-occupying lesions).

The diving reflex Children retain this useful adaptation to our earlier aquatic way of life. As cold water hits the face, the pulse slows and blood is diverted from limbs and muscles to vital areas (brain, kidney). Cold reduces the metabolic rate. This is the physiological explanation for remarkable stories of recovery from prolonged (eg 20min) total immersion.

Preventing death by drowning

In richer parts of the world, drownings in garden ponds are getting commoner, while those in natural freshwater sites are declining. Toddlers have the highest drowning rates—so prevention must target toddlers:

- Constant supervision of infants in baths by adults. Even brief moments away, eg to answer the doorbell, can be disastrous.
- Isolation fencing that *surrounds* the pool, separating it from the home.[422]
- Not swimming alone or in remote, unguarded sites.

Training of the public in basic life support. If given promptly, neurological outcomes are better.[423]

t exhaustion/heat injury

y occurs when core body tempera- eg to >39°C. Basal metabolic rate 100kcal/h; radiation from the sun can contribute 300kcal/h, and strenuous muscular activity 900kcal/h (enough to raise the core temperature by 1°C every 5min). Cooling is achieved mainly by evaporation. Above environmental temperatures of 35°C, 75% of heat loss is by sweating. Convection usually accounts for 15% of heat loss (more if conditions are windy), but if the environment is very hot it can contribute heat gain. Acclimatization to a hot environment (metabolic and cardiovascular changes reduce body core temperature and reduce the threshold for sweating), is mainly completed by 7–12 days.

Risk factors
• Elderly (↓reserves)
• Obese (↓reserves)
• Children (↓sweating)
• Exercising in the heat
• military personnel[424]
• athletes[425]
• Acute febrile illness
• Chronic illness
• Drugs[426]
• cocaine
• ecstasy
• lysergic acid diethylamide
• tricyclic antidepressants
• amphetamines
• phenothiazines
• Dehydration

Forms in the spectrum of heat illness

- *Oedema:* There is swelling of hands, feet, and ankles in the first days of exposure (worse after long-haul flights). It settles spontaneously over 28 days. Avoid diuretics.
- *Heat cramps:* Painful large muscle cramps after a lot of sweating. Treat with oral rehydration (half teaspoonful salt to each litre of water). Painful rhabdomyolysis (*OHCM*, p307) can also contribute.
- *Heat tetany:* Hyperventilation induced by rapid change in temperature. Treat as for usual hyperventilation.
- *Heat exhaustion/syncope:* Weakness, fatigue, light-headedness, nausea, vomiting, cramps, pilo-erection. Core temperature is <40°C. Treat with copious fluids eg 1L/h PO; and cooling with moist spray and increased convection (fan). Rarely, IV fluids are needed. The exact aetiology is unclear.[427]
- *Heat stroke:* Acute neurological impairment with core temperature ≥40°C. Typically associated with organ dysfunction. There are two types—'classic' or non-exertional, and exertional heat stroke. 'Classic' type—is seen when those who have poor cardiovascular reserve, such as infants or the elderly are subjected to environmental heat stress.[428] This form of heat stroke can be the most severe. Tachycardia, tachypnoea, hypotension, irritability, confusion, seizures (± hyponatraemia), and coma may occur. Skin may be hot and dry. Mortality: ~10%. Complications include persistent neurological damage, congestive cardiac failure, centrilobular liver necrosis (which can lead to liver failure), acute renal failure (especially in those in whom exercise contributes) due to rhabdomyolysis. Haematuria and proteinuria feature early, DIC can occur at 12–36h. Exertional heat stroke is seen in athletes/healthy individuals involved in vigorous activity who may not be acclimatized to their environment. Treatment is through rapid cooling (aim for <38.9° within 30mins of initiating treatment). Evaporative cooling is the safest method—wet the patient with tepid water and fan the skin. Ice packs can be used in axillae and groin. Cooling blankets may be used as can immersion in an ice bath. More invasive methods of cooling have no clear benefit. IV fluids and electrolyte replacement may be necessary.[429]

Prevention of heat illness[430]

1. Avoid exercise in extreme heat. For those voluntarily undertaking exercise in extreme conditions, acclimatization is vital.
2. Wear loose-fitting clothing only.
3. Keep well hydrated—especially if exercising; eg 500mL PO prior to exercising and 200mL/15min whilst exercising. As much as 2L/h oral fluid can be required in desert conditions.

▶▶Electric shock injuries

This accounts for 1000 deaths per year in the USA. Lightning strikes kill 150–300 people per year and seriously injuries 1000–1500. Utility workers and those working with electricity lines are the most commonly affected. Injuries within the home are usually due to using improperly earthed appliances or using electrical appliances near water.

Factors that increase the severity of injury [431]

1 *Type of current:* Alternating current (AC) is more dangerous than direct current (DC) of the same magnitude, causing muscle spasm that may make it impossible for the victim to let go of the source. DC usually produces a single large muscular contraction.

2 *Energy delivered:* This is a product of the applied voltage and subsequent current. Extreme heating of tissues may occur, causing internal and external burns and coagulation necrosis.

3 *Current pathway:* The route that the current takes through the body is also an important factor. If it passes through the head or chest (eg entry in one arm and exit from the other), fatal injury is more likely.

4 *Resistance encountered:* Fluid and electrolyte-rich tissues conduct electricity well. Bone is the most resistant tissue, whereas skin thickness (∴ resistance) is important in limiting the amount of current that passes through the body. Tissues designed to conduct electricity—heart and nerves—do badly, and they may sustain preferential damage when other tissues remain intact. ▶Check carefully for nerve damage, even if the surface appearances are mild. DC usually causes asystole, and AC causes VF.

5 *Contact duration:* The briefer the electrocution episode, the better!

Treatment of electric shock

• Ensure the source of current is turned off before attempting rescue.
• Use paradoxical triage: resuscitate the apparently 'dead' before attending to the living. Using standard resuscitation techniques, resuscitate long and aggressively—remarkable recoveries have been reported.
• Assume blunt trauma (stabilize the spine).
• If there are burns (p732), more fluid replacement is required than for normal thermal burns as electrical burns may penetrate deeper(start at 7mL/kg/% rather than the standard 4mL/kg/% and adjust to a target urine output of 1-2mL/kg/hr). ▶Check for rhabdomyolysis.
• Treat arrhythmias conventionally.
• Occult internal damage can lead to compartment syndrome, most frequently in the legs. See p738.

TASER injuries[432]

• The TASER is a conducted electricity device used by law enforcement in the US, UK and Australasia.
• The TASER was invented by Jack Cover, and is an acronym for 'Thomas A Swift's Electric Rifle'—named after a fictional character who developed an electric rifle.
• TASERS fire barbed copper wires which attach to a subject's skin or clothing, and discharge upto 50,000 volts of electricity.
• TASER injuries may be related to barb injuries, electrical injuries or secondary injuries from falling.
• Barbs should be removed, unless embedded in the orbits or genitalia (pinch the metal part of the barb and pull directly backwards whilst stabilizing the tissue with the other hand).
• Patients who have been tasered require an ECG to check for arrhythmia (not shown to persist beyond time of being tasered).
• Examination for secondary injuries due to muscle contraction should be carried out.

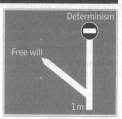

Fig 1. If we take a **deterministic** world view, accidents are inevitable. But proponents of **free will** counter that accidents are preventable (see BOX). If we allow ourselves to be carried along a road that we feel is laid out for us, then do we relinquish authority to prevent these accidents? There is a paradox here: it seems both views co-exist and contradict, so which is the **real world** view?[1]

In German we note that accidents don't just happen: they are built (*einen Umfall bauen*).

Image created by Dr Tom Turmezei.

Relevant pages in other chapters Glasgow Coma Scale (p720); ABCDE – immediate approach to trauma life support (p725); Child Coma Scale (p201); adult basic life support algorithm (p721); cardiorespiratory arrest (p238-9 & OHCM endpapers); drowning (p786); burns & smoke inhalation (p732); spinal injury (p766); heat exhaustion (p788); electrocution (p789); pneumothorax (OHCM p182); asthma (p164).

Sources The best text we have found is *Pre-hospital Medicine* by I Greaves & K Porter, Arnold. For a more concise companion, the same authors have also published the *Oxford Handbook of Pre-Hospital Care*, OUP. *EBM and pre-hospital care:* See F Bunn *et al* Report of WHO Pre-hospital Care Steering Committee.

Definition Pre-hospital *Immediate Care* is the provision of skilled medical help at the scene of an accident or medical emergency, or while in transit to hospital. The Diploma in Immediate Medical Care (DIMC) is a benchmark for professional standards in this area (nurses, doctors, and paramedics may apply).[1]

History Baron Dominique Larrey, Napoleon's Surgeon Marshall, may have provided the first skilled help at the scene with his *ambulances volantes* ('flying ambulances'), and was the first to apply the principle of triage—to sort the injured into priorities for treatment (p796-7).

Note The aim of this chapter is not to provide a full account of the care of *any* patient prior to hospitalization—this is by and large the province of the general practitioner. Rather, our aim here is to highlight those circumstances when doctor and paramedic can work together effectively to save life.

'Accidents' are in fact predictable and preventable

Road crashes affect 1 in 4 people in their lifetime. Each day ~3400 people die and >50,000 people are injured on the world's roads. 90% of fatalities are in low- and middle-income countries, even though they contain <50% of the world's vehicles. Crashes are a chief cause of death in those <45yrs; most deaths in the 15–19 age group are preventable.

Proven life-savers[3]
- Booster seats
- Fencing around water areas
- Flame-resistant clothes
- Smoke detectors

India has the worst record (14 fatalities/10,000 vehicles /yr ≈ 106,000 deaths/ yr).[2] In the UK, road deaths have fallen since 1966 despite a >50% ↑ in numbers of vehicles. There were 2,222 deaths and ~27,000 serious injuries in Britain in 2009.[4] Car users accounted for almost half of all deaths, cyclists for ~5%, motorcyclists for ~22% and pedestrians for ~26%.

Data analysis shows little impact on the rate of decline in fatal accidents in the UK from the seat-belt law (1983). One reason may be *risk compensation*, ie safety improvements are transferred by drivers into increased speed or recklessness, showing that public health experts must recognize our complex emotional and cognitive reactions to safety issues.[5]

Air bags also give a complex picture. They reduce fatalities, but front seat children without a seat belt and infants in passenger-side rear-facing car seats are at risk of fatal injury. Burns, high-frequency hearing loss, corneal and retinal injuries also occur.[6] Age factors: babies are rarely killed as their *risk exposure* is less. Deaths fall in middle age, rising again before falling in old age. In children, death rates are higher in lower social classes and more deprived socioeconomic areas.[7]

Alcohol is involved in 17% of fatal crashes. 24% of drivers and 33% of pedestrians killed have blood alcohol levels > the legal limit of 80mg/100mL (17.4mmol/L). This rises to ~50% of drivers and 75% of pedestrians killed between 10PM & 4AM.[4] There is evidence that older drivers compensate for alcohol-impaired performance by driving carefully; young drivers can compensate in this way, but may choose not to do so (peer group pressure or a delight in risk-taking). Chronic *marijuana* use is also associated with an ↑ risk of car crash—interestingly, the same study showed that after controlling for other risk factors, acute use was not.[8]

Benzodiazepines, antidepressants, antihistamines, and mobile phone use (the latter illegal in UK since 2003) also contribute to road crashes, and it is important that patients are advised not to drive while on these.[9]

▶*If a patient has epilepsy or diabetes with hypoglycaemic attacks (or is otherwise unfit to drive, p526) it is his duty to inform the licensing authorities, and the doctor's duty to request him to do so.*

Prevention A vital cognitive shift occurs if the word *accident* is replaced by *preventable occurrence*, implying that accidents are predictable—often resulting from laziness, haste, ignorance, bad design, false economy, and failure to apply existing knowledge. *Safety education can* change behaviour.[10]

Schemes can help drivers who abuse alcohol, eg the *Driver Improvement System* for traffic violators, and re-education by driving instructors. Psychotherapy helps more than lectures. Health education posters picturing tragic consequences to a girl- or boyfriend are successful.

Laws can save lives—car roadworthiness, drink-driving, seat-belt laws, speed restrictions, and speed cameras[11][12] (especially if infringement leads to re-education/speed awareness courses rather than licence endorsements).[13]

Another effective way of reducing alcohol-related road crashes is to provide good lighting at difficult bends or junctions. Injury in homes may be prevented by such simple measures as child-proof containers, putting holes in polythene bags, using toughened glass throughout the home, and using cooking pans with handles turned in away from toddlers.

Injuries continue to rank as one of the biggest global causes of morbidity and mortality. However, there is a wide variation in the profile of accident statistics throughout the world according to factors such as geography and relative level of average income. The World Health Organization (WHO) publishes statistics on global injury rates.[14] Here we discuss Great Britain, where injury is the commonest cause of death in the first four decades of life.

UK deaths and other injuries[15–17]	
On the roads	
Deaths	2,222
Serious injuries	24,690
Less serious injuries	195,234
Children's deaths	81
Children seriously injured	2590
Deaths in those >65yrs old	609
Home-based accidents	
Deaths	4000
Injuries leading to A&E presentation	2,700,000
Work-based accidents	
Deaths at work	152
Injuries at work	233,000
(of which are serious)	(26,061)

Accidents in the home Old people are particularly at risk. Over half the males and three-quarters of females who die from accidents in their homes are 65 years old or older. About 30% of those falling and fracturing their hip will be dead in 1 year (p752). The commonest cause of accidental death in children is fires; in the 15–44 age group it is poisoning, and in the over-45s the chief cause is falls.

Hospital attendances for accidents 6 million people/year in the UK attend an accident and emergency department following an 'accident'. 2 million of these involve children. This costs ~£146million. Half these accidents occur in the home. *Many more receive treatment from their general practitioner.*

Accidents in children
- ~10,000 children are permanently disabled by accidents each year.
- Accidents cause 1 child in 5 to attend the A&E department each year.
- Accidents are the commonest cause of death among children aged 1-14yrs, and they cause half of all deaths in those aged 10-14yrs.
- Road traffic accidents are the most common fatal accidents in children—around half occur with children as pedestrian victims
- School age children (4-14yrs) in road crashes restrained with a seat belt are 2–10 times as safe as unbelted children, and are at least as well protected as adults wearing seat belts.[2]

Useful contacts and addresses:
- British Safety Council, 70 Chancellors Road, London W6 9RS (UK).[18]
- Royal Society for the Prevention of Accidents (ROSPA), RoSPA House 28 Calthorpe Road, Edgbaston, Birmingham B15 1RP (tel. UK 0121 248 2000)[1].[19]
- Construction Health and Safety Group, St Ann's Road, Chertsey, Surrey KT16 9AT (UK); tel. 020 8741 1231.[20]
- Scottish Chamber of Safety, www.scos.org.uk[21]

Synonyms Artificial respiration; cardiopulmonary resuscitation (CPR).

Definition BLS is the provision of life support—expired air (your own) ventilation + external chest compression, without any equipment. The guidelines here are in line with the recommendations from the Resuscitation Council (UK).[23]

SAFE approach
• As you approach the patient shout for help (pointing to an individual if possible, to activate him or her).
• Approach him with care—are there any hazards to yourself (p800)?
• Free the patient from immediate danger.
• Evaluate the patient's 'ABC' (see below)[1].

> **The SAFE approach**
> Shout for help
> Approach with care
> Free from danger
> Evaluate ABC (Airway, Breathing, Circulation)

Establish unresponsiveness Shake gently by the shoulder while stabilizing the forehead with the other hand. Ask "Are you all right?". If he responds, leave him in that position and further evaluate him—if not, *call for help* and then check airway and breathing.

Airway & Breathing Open the airway using a chin lift. If breathing, put in the recovery position; if not, go to get help *now*. Once help has been summoned, give 30 chest compressions, open the airway and give 2 rescue breaths (slow inflations, just enough to make the chest rise—and achieve a tidal volume of ~400-500mL) and then perform another 30 chest compressions.

> **Nose-to-mouth breaths**
> Nose-to-mouth rescue breaths may be used if:
> • A good seal cannot be made with mouth-to-mouth
> • There is mouth trauma
> • Underwater

Circulation The latest BLS guidelines do not involve assessment of the circulation (for lay rescuers). Chest compressions and rescue breaths continue at a ratio of 30:2 until the victim breaths, or the rescuer becomes exhausted. Compressions should be at a rate of 100-120 min^{-1}, and to a depth of 5-6cm (adults). Compression only CPR may be as effective as combined compression/ventilation resuscitation in the first few minutes (in adults).[24]

Infants (<1yr) and children (1-8yrs) are now rescued with the same algorithm involving 5 immediate rescue breaths if not breathing normally, followed by chest compressions and rescue breaths at a ratio of 15:2. For compressions use one hand one finger breadth above xiphisternum (rate 100/min). Avoid blind finger sweep—may impact foreign body in conical upper airway; do look into the airway for easily removable foreign body. See p238.

▶See p238 for the paediatric algorithm of the European guidelines for basic and advanced life support.

▶See p721 for the adult basic life support algorithm.

▶Both adult **basic** and **advanced** life support algorithms are inside the back cover of *OHCM*.

---

1 BLS by soldiers is deemed inappropriate on the battlefield if the victim has no vital signs.[25]

Choking

Respiratory obstruction by choking on a foreign body is not an infrequent cause of death—which may be prevented by performing the Heimlich manoeuvre. If the person who is choking is conscious and standing, first ask him to bend forward and cough. If this fails, get behind him, and with your arms encircle his abdomen, mid-way between umbilicus and xiphoid process. One hand makes a fist, positioned thumb-to-abdomen. The other hand grasps this fist, and with a sharp movement presses it up and into the abdomen, to dislodge the foreign body. If the victim is already comatose, this manoeuvre can be accomplished with him lying on his back—using the heel of the hand to press with, rather than a fist. Repeated thrusts may be needed. In adults, sweep the mouth with a finger to remove the foreign body.

▶Do not perform this manoeuvre on children <1 year, instead use back blows (below) and chest thrusts (similar to cardiac compressions).

Complications (Rare) If applied incorrectly, direct trauma to abdominal viscera may result ± thrombosis of an abdominal aortic aneurysm or dislodgement of thrombus causing bilateral acute leg ischaemia.[26]

Back blows These are no better, and no worse, than the Heimlich manoeuvre in relieving foreign body obstruction. Neither should be taught or practised to the exclusion of the other. Alternate 5 back blows with 5 abdominal/chest thrusts. Use the heel of the hand to strike forcefully between the scapulae, with the patient leaning forwards.

Use of automatic external defibrillators (AED)

Each year in the UK, 30,000 people undergo an out-of-hospital cardiac arrest. The chances of successful defibrillation decrease by 10% with each minute of delay prior to first shock. The Resuscitation Council of the UK recommends that although layperson training in the use of AEDs is to be encouraged, it is not necessary for their use by members of the public.

▶▶Place one pad to the right of the sternum, below the clavicle, and the other in the left mid-axillary line approximately over the position of the V6 ECG electrode. Whilst most pads are labelled left and right (or have a picture indicating position) it does not matter if their positions are switched. Laypeople should then follow the AED voice/visual prompts, ensuring that if a shock is indicated nobody is touching the victim.

If you are the first on the scene, the following page (which assumes a highly organized response) will seem impossible on a dark night, alone. So the first priority is to get help. You may be surprised in how short a time it all becomes organized to give the picture described below. Requesting the fire service when dialling emergency services may be the quickest way to get a dozen trained first-aiders to the scene with unrivalled skill in extrication.

The distribution of trauma deaths is trimodal—*immediate* (aortic deceleration injury; head injury), *early* (hypoxia and hypovolaemia), and *delayed* (sepsis; multiple organ failure). Prevention (speed restriction; road lighting; seat-belt laws; no drunken-driving; air bags) is better than cure—and medical intervention is too late for the immediate deaths (but did given to victims in the first 'golden hour' can be lifesaving, p723). Use the following for prioritization at the scene (and see MINIBOX).

Command Once in attendance the doctor is responsible for providing all medical care. She will work
closely with the ambulance service, but will have additional skills (eg giving potent IV analgesia).

Priorities at scene
• Command
• Safety
• Communications
• Assessment
• Triage
• Treatment
• Evacuation

Safety *Yourself:* First ensure your own safety; do not approach fire or chemical hazards (p800) until the fire service have made the area safe. Always consider the possibility of a **CBRN** risk (chemical, biological, radiological, nuclear).²⁷ Wear high-visibility clothing, and carry gloves/eye protection/ear defenders. *The scene:* If first to arrive, park obliquely behind the incident ('fend off') and leave hazard lights/ green beacon on. *The casualties:* Remove from any immediate danger; protect from further injury during extrication (eg cover with blanket when windows broken). ▶Check for a hidden victim, eg under a car or over a wall.

Communications Liaise with police (they are in overall command), fire service (for any hazards; they can remove the casualty quickly if he is about to die, or in a very controlled manner, eg if an isolated spinal injury), and paramedics (identify if they have extended skills; use appropriately). Speak to the receiving hospital by radio or telephone (p804, radio procedure), and relay the number and severity of casualties.

Assessment Relate vehicle damage to potential injuries in the casualty ('reading the wreckage'). Is the casualty trapped—relative (cannot move a broken arm to open the door), or absolute (eg feet caught in pedals)?

Triage From the French *trier*, to sift or sort (coffee beans), this process sorts casualties into priorities for treatment. Divide into **IMMEDIATE** (colour-code RED, will die in a few minutes if no treatment, eg obstructed airway, tension pneumo-thorax); **URGENT** (YELLOW, may die in 1-2h if no treatment, eg hypovolaemia); and **DELAYED** (GREEN, can wait eg >4h, eg minor fractures). Those who will certainly die are labelled **EXPECTANT**—to treat them may delay you helping the salvageable, who then die unnecessarily (BLUE, but not all triage labels have this colour—use GREEN). Do not forget to label the dead (WHITE or BLACK), otherwise emergency personnel may repeatedly take a doctor to the same victim, so wasting time and resources. Note that alcohol or drug abuse (eg cannabis²⁸,²⁹) which may have caused the accident in the first place may make assessing casualties much harder. ▶*Note that triage is dynamic.* It starts with a brief-look assessment (see OPPO-SITE), but later may involve a detailed examination. Priorities (and label colour) will change while awaiting, and after treatment. Triage in children is even more specialist, and depends on factors such as height, age, or weight.

---

1 RTA (road traffic accident) is a misnomer: most result from speed and carelessness, and are all too predict-able, rather than being truly accidental.³⁰

How to triage[31]

This is a simple system: its main virtue is *speed*. All casualties should be re-assessed when time and resources allow. Go through the following sequence until you arrive at a triage priority (in coloured CAPITALS and in the table below)—assign its colour label to the casualty and move immediately to the next.
►► *DO NOT STOP TO TREAT*, or you will surrender control of the incident.

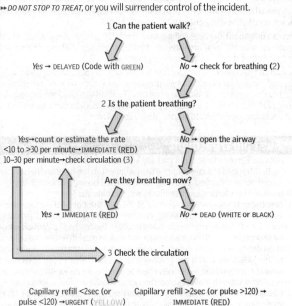

1 Can the patient walk?

Yes → DELAYED (Code with GREEN)   *No* → check for breathing (2)

2 Is the patient breathing?

Yes→count or estimate the rate   *No* → open the airway
<10 to >30 per minute→IMMEDIATE (RED)
10–30 per minute→check circulation (3)

Are they breathing now?

Yes → IMMEDIATE (RED)   *No* → DEAD (WHITE or BLACK)

3 Check the circulation

Capillary refill <2sec (or   Capillary refill >2sec (or pulse >120) →
pulse <120) →URGENT (YELLOW)   IMMEDIATE (RED)

Triage categories		
Colour code	**Category**	**Expectancy**
■	Immediate	Few minutes
	Urgent	1-2h
■	Delayed	>4h
■ or ■	Expectant	Moments
□ or ■	Dead	N/A

Pre-hospital immediate care

In your car boot carry the following minimum equipment:

Oropharyngeal airway(s)	Dressings	Bandages
IV cannulae (14G & 16G)	IV fluid (eg Gelofusine®)	Giving set
Sticky tape	Scissors + Torch	Fire extinguisher

You should give a high priority to making yourself safe and visible, eg: reflective jacket, hard hat, wellington boots.

Extra equipment Cervical collars; Mini-Trach II® (cricothyrotomy kit); chest drain set; sutures; local anaesthetic; analgesia; splints; stethoscope (more a badge of office than a useful tool owing to noise).

Personal transport Remember also to take care of your own transport vehicle, making regular checks of tyre pressures and treads, oil level, windscreen washer fluid and wipers, and spare fuel can. The Road Vehicle Licensing Regulations 1984 also allow for emergency medical responders to carry green lights, but check the regulations to ensure you are compliant.

▶▶First aid treatment
see also p725

A: *Airway:* Remove false teeth and any vomit. Lie in the lateral position (see fig 1). If trapped in a car, continue to manually stabilize head and neck when a rigid collar is applied. Extricate on to a spinal board, and immobilize the head and neck with foam headblocks and securing straps.

B: *Breathing:* If spontaneous, give O₂ at 15L/min via tight-fitting face mask with reservoir. If not breathing, ventilate mouth-to-mouth.[32] If available give 100% O₂ via bag-valve-mask and intubate the trachea.[1] If *tension pneumothorax* suspected (cyanosis, engorged neck veins, shifted trachea), pierce chest with a large IV cannula in 2nd intercostal space in the midclavicular line, on the side from which the trachea is deviated. If there is an *open chest wound*, cover with an Asherman chest seal (adhesive disc with central rubber flutter valve that allows blood and air to escape without re-entering).[33]

C: *Circulation:* Is there a pulse? If not, start external cardiac massage. (Survival from traumatic cardiac arrest with no vital signs at the accident scene approaches 0%.) If there is bleeding, this will almost always be stopped by pressure and elevation of the part. Avoid tourniquets: these are often forgotten and left on too long. Insert 2 large IV cannulae (eg antecubital fossae 14G or 16G; secure these well and splint the arm, eg Armlok®) and start fluid resuscitation (eg Gelofusine®). A policeman or fireman makes a willing dripstand. Ensure that the cannula is not pulled out when the patient is moved. Suspected internal bleeding and fractures of long bones indicate that IV fluid is needed, as blood loss may be considerable (fractured pelvis 2L, femur 1L, tibia, ankle and fractures of several ribs ~½L each). Splinting (eg one leg to the other) helps reduce blood loss as well as relieving pain. NB: the ATLS® target is definitive haemorrhage control, rather than plasma volume normalization.

D: *Disability:* Assess responsiveness rapidly with AVPU:

A = Alert
V = responds to Vocal stimuli
P = responds to Pain
U = Unresponsive

E: *Exposure* = head-to-toe exam (secondary survey), but is often not practical outside hospital. Reassess ABC; quantify coma level (adult Glasgow Coma Scale, p720; child, p201). Remember to give analgesia (p802).

Transport: Keep the injured warm. Procedures (eg IV cannulation) can be performed in moving ambulances if the patient can be extricated quickly.

---

1 Rapid sequence intubation (RSI, p626) is as do-able in the field as in hospital.[34]

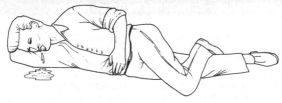

Fig 1. How to vomit. The above is one way of positioning the comatose so vomit is not inhaled and the cervical spine is supported in the midline—minimizing risk of cord injury. It helps if there are 2-3 people to 'log-roll' the casualty into this position, so that the neck is never out of alignment with the body. There have been reports of neurovascular risk to the arm supporting the head, so other positions are being tried, but none has been formally validated.

'Scoop and run'—or 'stay and play'?

'Scoop and run' refers to rapid evacuation of casualties to trauma centres (or A&E unit) usually with only basic life support measures (maintenance of spinal precautions / fracture splinting, bag-mask ventilation etc.); 'stay and play' entails detailed resuscitation at the scene of trauma (intubation, IV access, fluid resuscitation). In deciding which is better, take the following into account.

- There is no single answer for all circumstances. Local geography and the speed and efficiency of the response service play a part, as does the fitness of the casualty. Only experience can tell which option is most appropriate—and luck may well play its part too.
- 'Scoop and run' and 'stay and play' are two ends of a spectrum of activity. Often a minimal amount of resuscitation can be done without causing too much delay, ie get the best of both worlds.[35] For example, to place vascular access during transport rather than before it.[36]
- Penetrating chest injuries have been studied in a pseudo-randomized trial (N=289; full randomization was impossible but 'scoop and run' operated for one day, and 'stay and play' for the next). This showed that the balance of benefit probably lies in 'scoop and run' for this type of injury. Fluid resuscitation aiming for normotension without an operating theatre to hand may be dangerous, as clot may be displaced by the rising BP—with subsequent fatal haemorrhage, which could only have been prevented by major surgery. In this study, 70% in the delayed-resuscitation group survived, compared with 62% who received immediate fluid resuscitation. Duration of hospital stay was shorter for survivors in the delayed-resuscitation group. But note that the results only achieved significance when pre-op and post-op deaths were pooled, and that rates of complications were similar in the two groups (eg respiratory distress syndrome, coagulopathy, wound infection, and pneumonia).[37,38] n=598
- An American review concluded there was insufficient data to suggest blunt or penetrating trauma patients benefit from prehospital fluid resuscitation, but in patients with penetrating injuries and short transport times (<30mins) fluids should be witheld if a palpable radial pulse if present and the patient coherent.[35] If fluids are necessary they should be given in 250mL boluses. During active bleeding titration of fluids to a systolic blood pressure (SBP) >70 is no worse in terms of mortality than a titration to a SBP >100.[39]
- Patients with traumatic brain injury require fluids to be titrated to a SBP >90mmHg.[40]

Hazards

Fire: <5% of road traffic crashes result in fire, and <1:500 result in significant burns. The world's worst ever pile-up was in the Salang Tunnel, Afghanistan, in November 1982, which involved a petrol tanker explosion with an estimated 1100–2700 killed.

Electricity: Power shorts are common, eg from bird strike, and power may be restored after 20min without investigation—you must phone the power company to ensure the source is turned off. High tension cables can be lethal even when standing several metres away.

Rail: An electrified rail can be short circuited by a bar carried by the fire service, or the operating rail authority. Remember that cutting power does not stop diesel locomotives that may also operate on the same line: trains may be stopped by signal lights, red flags, or a series of charges placed on the rail—the noise warns the driver.

Underground/Tube/Metro: In addition to the rail hazards above, this scenario may pose additional quandaries—eg lack of lighting and ventilation, cramped conditions, difficult access to and exit from from accident site.

Chemical: Lorries carrying hazardous loads must display an orange 'HAZCHEM' board (see OPPOSITE). This contains information on how to fight a fire, what protective equipment to wear, if the chemical can be safely washed down the storm drains, and whether to evacuate the area (TOP LEFT); a United Nations (UN) product identification number of four digits (MIDDLE LEFT)—eg 1270 = petrol; a pictorial hazard diamond warning (TOP RIGHT); and an emergency contact number (BOTTOM LEFT). A white plate means the load is non-toxic. The European 'Kemler' plate contains only the UN product number (BOTTOM) and a numerical hazard code (TOP—note repeated number means intensified hazard).

As a concession to freight carriers, mixed loads of <500kg need only be identified by a plain orange square at the front and rear.

To obtain information about the chemical at the scene of an accident look at the transport emergency card (TREM card) carried in the driver's cab; the fire service will be linked with CHEMDATA—a computer database at the National Chemical Information Centre at Harwell; alternatively phone the National Poisons Information Service (eg 0844 892 0111), or use Toxbase® (www.toxbase.org).

▶*Do not approach a chemical incident until declared safe by the fire service.*

Principles of extrication

- Stabilize the vehicle where it lies—movement may exacerbate injury.
- Make the vehicle safe—switch off ignition; immobilize the battery; swill away any petrol.
- Identify the time-critical patient—some will die unless rapidly removed from the vehicle, at whatever cost.
- Read the wreckage—relate the damage of the vehicle to potential injuries: steering wheel deformed = chest injury; dashboard intrusion = patella/femur fracture ± posterior dislocation of the hip. Bodies are softer than metal: major bodywork distortion = major injury.
- The easiest way to enter a car is through the door—try this before removing the windscreen or the roof!
- Remove the wreckage from the casualty, not the casualty from the wreckage; don't try to manoeuvre the casualty through too small a hole.
- Don't move from one entrapment situation straight into another—if necessary spend a short time stabilizing the patient before moving into the back of the ambulance.

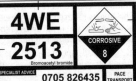

Hazchem advice for the control of the chemical

Substance identification number and name

Hazard symbol and description in a diamond on white square background (rest of label is black lettering on an orange background)

Specialist advice and telephone number

Supplier's name (optional)

Danger labels

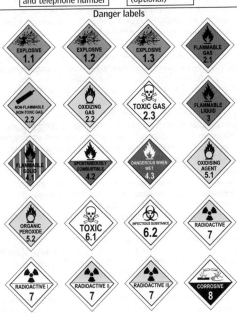

NFPA (National Fire Protection Association)

The US NFPA uses a 'fire diamond' for immediate risk identification for emergency personnel. A number from 0 to 4 (4 being most dangerous) is placed in each coloured sub-diamond: BLUE for 'health', RED for 'flammability', YELLOW for 'reactivity'. The WHITE diamond contains further 'special' information, eg COR for corrosive, ALK for alkaline. NFPA 704 has codes for a large number of dangerous chemicals, eg benzene (3 4 0), hydrogen peroxide (2 0 1 COR).[41]

Why should I give pain relief? There are more than humanitarian reasons for giving analgesia. Catecholamines released with pain may further reduce peripheral perfusion and oxygen delivery in hypovolaemic shock, and increase myocardial oxygen demand following myocardial infarction.

When do I give pain relief? Unless all hope of life and rescue has been abandoned, the priorities of securing an airway and stabilizing the cervical spine, maintaining ventilation, and optimizing the circulation always come before analgesia. The effects of any drugs must be weighed against their potential side-effects (respiratory depression; sedation).

How do I relieve pain? *Psychological:* Beecher noted in 1944 at Anzio[1] that soldiers were indifferent to serious injury. This is unlikely in road crashes; a soldier is released from war horrors by his injuries, but a crash victim is just beginning his nightmare. Reassurance that "the doctor is here" is important.

Splintage: Simple splints can be improvised from clothing; an uninjured leg can splint the injured one. Inflatable air splints are not very robust, although are light and easy to apply. Box splints (fold around the limb) are popular but poorly accommodate a deformed limb, when a vacuum splint (full of tiny beads) is better. Traction splints should be used for a fractured femur: they also reduce blood loss, morbidity, and mortality (the Thomas splint reduced mortality of open fractured femur from 80% to 20% in World War I).

Gaseous: **Nitrous oxide** provides comparable analgesia to 10mg morphine. It is mixed with 50% O_2 as Entonox® or Nitronox® in blue cylinders with a white top. It separates at -6°C (O_2 on top). ►*Do not* use in decompression sickness, p813, pneumothorax (may tension), acute head injury or bowel obstruction.

Opioids: **Morphine** is the gold standard. Give 0.1mg/kg (5–10mg) as starting dose, if fit/healthy person with significant pain, otherwise in small aliquots (1–2mg) IV. **Naloxone** must be available at all times. Dose example: 0.1–0.2mg IV eg repeated at 2min if needed. Fentanyl is at least as effective as morphine and may be easier to titrate given faster onset of action. A typical adult dose starts at 25–50micrograms.[42]

NSAIDs: IM NSAIDs (**diclofenac** 75mg IM, repeated once only, at 30min if needed, or **ketorolac** 10mg IM stat then 10–30mg/4–6h as needed, max 90mg/day, ↓ to 60mg/day in elderly or if <50kg) has a role in musculoskeletal pain—and it doesn't entail monitoring for sedative effects; not recommended for children.[43] Ketorolac can be given IV over ≥15sec; avoid in: hypovolaemia; labour; asthma.

Ketamine: This is a potent, short-acting analgesic at 0.1–0.5mg/kg IV.[44] At higher doses it can be used as sole anaesthetic agent (2mg/kg IV will produce 5–10min of surgical anaesthesia); 'emergence delirium' is common unless a benzodiazepine (**midazolam** ~2mg IV) is also given.[45]

Sedation: An anxious or aggressive patient is often in pain or hypoxic. Reassurance, a clear airway with supplemental oxygen and analgesia is better than sedation, although this is needed rarely: give small aliquots of **midazolam** (p630, up to 1.5mg in elderly—have **flumazenil** to hand).

Local anaesthesia: (p632) Peripheral nerve blocks aid release of a trapped limb. Femoral nerve block is most used and provides complete analgesia (anaesthesia) for femoral fractures (less effective for low shaft fracture). Locate the artery in the groin and put 10–20mL 1% plain **lidocaine** in a fan shape lateral to the artery. Aspirate frequently to avoid intravascular injection. Maximum dose <3mg/kg or 0.28mL/kg of 1% (p731).

---

1 Anzio, 33 miles south of Rome, was a crucial Allied beachhead in the recapturing the 'Eternal City' (5/6/44).

Keeping records

In the controlled bustle of activity at a pre-hospital emergency scene, the same focus that is applied to care provision also needs to be applied to recording of the care given. Recording procedures and drugs is

Essence of keeping records
• Good practice = safe practice
• Treat first, then make records
• Use well-known formats

vital for safe, and therefore good, practice (see MINIBOX). On arrival at hospital, a full dose of morphine given on top of an unknown administration in the field can be enough to lead to overdose.

Care provision will inevitably have to come first, but then it is vital to create accurate records (and dare we say, 'undoctored' in retrospect). Importantly, if using a pre-prepared sheet, use those that are widespread and not your own customised layout that may cause confusion from delay in interpretation. Good record keeping is also vital for trauma scoring (p810).

Treading along the 'thin blue line' (UK)

Very few would think that in passing through a red traffic light with your green emergency lights flashing (p798) to get to an accident scene, or that in smashing a front door to get to a trapped victim you would be open to legal action: ▶just remember that you could be.

In most circumstances, however, provided that you observe the correct codes (eg a red light means 'give way' and is not a simply thoroughfare in your favour) legal action is unlikely.

Ultimately a life-saving decision may fall into your hands, so in preparing to make the *right* the decision, you will get it *right*. Don't be put off from these challenges, as they are part of the essence of the specialty. Consider the following scenarios:

- *Breaking and entering:* Doctors and paramedics cannot legally force entry to a private address, but you would be unlikely to face repercussions if doing so in an attempt to save a life.
- *Driving:* For example, as long as appropriate sirens/lights are used, you: **can** exceed the statutory speed limit by 20mph; **can** use bus lane; **can** stop and park on clearways; **can** treat red light as 'give way'; **cannot** ignore one-way signs; **cannot** cross double white lines; **cannot** ignore stop signs.
- *Consent:* This is too large a topic to cover here completely. Consider that if there is a situation where obtaining informed consent may be an issue (eg unconscious, mental health issues, <16yrs old in absence of parent or guardian) life-saving treatment can probably be administered without fear of repercussion. Further non-life-saving treatment beyond this may raise problems. See also *OHCM* p570.
- *Restraint:* Unless restraining an aggressive or violent individual for safety reasons, medical practitioners have no right to restrain an individual: to do so would constitute assault.
- *Confidentiality:* Be aware that the open environment of a pre-hospital setting is more vulnerable to breaches in confidentiality in the form of both verbal and written communication.

▶Check that you have the appropriate *clinical indemnity* to cover your practice.

The radio net A radio user is identified by a 'call sign'. Messages are usually passed through a central controller (call sign 'control', or 'zero') without being able to hear other users—'two-frequency simplex'; but on some nets all users can hear and talk directly to each other—'single-frequency simplex'.

Acquiring a 'radio voice' This takes practice: *rhythm* should be steady; *speed* is slower than normal speech; *volume*—do not shout or whisper; *pitch* should be raised if the voice is gruff. Remember: '**RSVP**'.

Using a radio Switch on and check battery light (switch off to change battery). Listen (single-frequency) or look (two-frequency) at the 'channel busy' light—you do not want to interrupt any message. Wait 1–2sec after pressing the transmit button before speaking, or the important first few words are lost. Release the transmit button after speaking, or you will prevent others from transmitting. VHF radios have a longer range than UHF.

Messaging To *initiate* say the receiver's call sign then your own. Say "over" to indicate when the receiver should reply. To *continue* a message always start with your own call sign when you speak. To *end* a transmission say "out".

> *Example:* "Zero from Mike One, message over."
> "Zero, go ahead over."
> "Mike One, moving now to new location out."

Remember that anyone can be listening: don't be a comic ("Send the rover over, over"); don't swear; address by appointment rather than name.

Key words Spell long or difficult words using the NATO phonetic alphabet (see OPPOSITE)—you do not want an "empty box" when you asked for "Entonox". Long numbers (drug dose; grid reference) are given whole, then digit by digit (eg 1000 = "one thousand, figures one-zero-zero-zero"). "Roger" or "OK" means you have understood: they are pro-words (see BOX 2); "say again" means repeat the message. ("Repeat" is the order for artillery to fire again and is avoided, at least on military networks!) ETA/ETD are common abbreviations for estimated time of arrival/departure. Avoid radio gibberish ("roger dodger/ten four/over and out"; "negative" and "positive" for "yes" and "no").

Telephone Mobile telephones are useful for pre-hospital communication. However, in major incidents all cells are rapidly utilized (often by the press). In the UK, on application to the Cabinet Office the telephone may be registered to operate on a number of restricted cells in cases where the system is overloaded—this is ACCess OverLoad Control (ACCOLC).

Some UK emergency service ranks			
Epaulette	**Police**	**Fire**	**Ambulance**
2 pips	Inspector	Station Officer	Officer band 1
3 pips	Chief Inspector	Asst. Divisional Officer	Officer band 2
Crown	Superintendent		
Laurel 'U'		Asst. Senior Officer	
Laurel 'U' around pip	Divisional Officer		

UK fire service helmets		
Colour	**Black bands**	**Rank**
Yellow	Nil	Firefighter
Yellow	1 thin	Leading fireman
Yellow	2 thin	Sub-officer
White	1 thin	Station Officer
White	1 thick	Assistant Divisional Officer
White	1 thick (18mm), 1 thin (12mm)	Divisional Officer

NATO phonetic alphabet & number pronunciation for radio use

A ALPHA	B BRAVO	C CHARLIE	D DELTA ("DELL TAH")	E ECHO
F FOXTROT	G GOLF	H HOTEL	I INDIA ("IN DEE AH")	J JULIET
K KILO	L LIMA	M MIKE	N NOVEMBER ("NO VEM BER")	O OSCAR
P PAPA	Q QUEBEC	R ROMEO	S SIERRA ("SEE AIR RAH")	T TANGO
U UNIFORM	V VICTOR	W WHISKEY	X XRAY ("ECKS RAY")	Y YANKEE Z ZULU
1 WUN	2 TOO	3 THUREE	4 FOWER	5 FIYIV
6 SIX	7 SEVEN	8 ATE	9 NINER	0 ZERO . DECIMAL

Pro-word examples (in blue) in a dialogue between OHCS9 and FY1

OHCS9: "Foxtrot Yankee Wun, Foxtrot Yankee Wun, this is Oscar Hotel Charlie Sierra Niner. Request rendezvous Too Decimal Fiyiv centimetres south-east of McBurney's point. **Read back for check**. Over."

FY1: "Oscar Hotel Charlie Sierra Niner, this is Foxtrot Yankee Wun. I **read back**: Too decimal fiyiv centimetres south-east of McBurney's point. **Over**."

OHCS9: "Foxtrot Yankee Wun, Foxtrot Yankee Wun, this is Oscar Hotel Charlie Sierra Niner. **Correct**. **Out**.

Go ahead means "I have got your initial call; pass the rest of your message".

Roger (or **Romeo**) means "ok".

Over means "this is the end of my transmission and I await reply".

Out terminates a dialogue. NB: "over and out" is contradictory.

Wilco means "I will comply" and implies Roger (so "Roger wilco" contains redundancy—don't use). It is wise to precede 'wilco' with the instruction you are going to comply with—in case you are have misheard it.

Station calling is used when addressing an unidentified station which has just hailed the receiver, eg if OHCS9 has received a transmission from an unidentified station we will reply:

"**Station calling** OHCS9—**this is** OHCS9. **Over**." 'This is...' means this transmission is from the station whose designator immediately follows. **Say again** means "I have not understood your message, please repeat" (**all after** x means those words after x **all before** means all words before x).

Emergency radio messages (using an example at sea)

- **Mayday** is the international distress call for when death is at hand (from the French phrase M'aidez; help me!). ➤➤Ensure the radio is on (hi-power). Use channel 16 (the default). Press the microphone button. MIPDANIO tells you how to order your call: say "Mayday, mayday, mayday"→Identify yourself: "**this is**..." (type of vehicle; its name)→Position→Distress type (eg "fire")→Assistance needed→Number of people at risk→Information (eg "abandoning ship; no life-raft")→Over. Release microphone button. Wait 2min. Resend if no response.
- **Pan-pan** ×3 (said as 'pon pon') means urgency short of imminent demise.
- **Securite** ×3 (said as 'say-cure-ee-tay') means "I have important safety information to transmit." Follow 'pan-pan' and 'securite' by saying "all stations, all stations, all stations: this is...(ID→Position)" to alert all listeners. Explain the danger (eg "I am adrift without power in shipping lane...").

Pre-hospital immediate care

Planning For a hospital to be prepared to cope with multiple casualties there must be planning. Each hospital will produce a detailed *Major Incident Plan*, but additionally the tasks of key personnel can be distributed on individual *Action Cards*.

At the scene A medical incident officer (MIO) will be requested from the nearest hospital or BASICS scheme (eg GP or paramedic volunteers from the British Association for Immediate Care www.basics.org.uk). Mobile medical teams (eg A&E senior doctor/surgeon + anaesthetist + 2-4 nurses) should come from hospitals not accepting the main casualties. BASICS doctors should be requested to the scene by radio via the ambulance station). Further BASICS doctors make valuable treatment officers, as they arrive.

Safety: Is paramount—your own and others. Be visible (luminous monogrammed jacket) and wear protective clothing where appropriate (safety helmet; waterproofs; boots; respirator in chemical environment).

Triage: See p796-7.

Communications: Are essential—and frequently an area where improvements are needed.[46] The police are in overall control of the scene. Each emergency service will dispatch a control vehicle and will have a designated incident officer for liaison. Support medical staff from hospital report to the medical commander (SILVER rank medical incident officer, OPPOSITE): his job is to assess then communicate to the receiving hospital the number and severity of casualties, to assess need for further medical teams, to oversee triage (p797) and treatment (with the Ambulance Incident Officer). He must resist temptation to treat casualties as this compromises his role.

Equipment: Must be portable (in small cases/backpacks) and include: triage labels, intubation and cricothyrotomy equipment; intravenous fluids (colloid); bandages and dressings; chest drain (plus flutter valve); amputation kit (when required ideally two doctors should concur); drugs—*analgesic:* morphine; *anaesthetic:* ketamine (p802); *specific antidote* if a chemical threat; cardiac resuscitation drugs; drugs to cover common medical emergencies; eg GTN spray, salbutamol inhaler; limb splints; defibrillator/monitor; ± pulse oximeter; 'comfort bag' for staff and others (£1 coins, sweets, toilet paper, etc).

Evacuation: Remember: with immediate treatment on scene, the priority for evacuation may be reduced (eg a tension pneumothorax—RED—relieved can wait for evacuation—becomes YELLOW, but those who may suffer by delay at the scene must go first (eg unconscious closed head injury; myocardial infarct). Send any severed limbs to the same hospital as the patient, if possible keeping them on ice (not *in* ice as freezing harms tissues).

At the hospital a 'major incident' is declared (eg if >10 serious injuries). A control room is established and the medical coordinator ensures staff have been summoned, nominates a triage officer and supervises the best use of inpatient beds, intensive care, and theatre resources. When the incident is declared clear of casualties, the major incident may still continue for some time at the hospital.[46]

When do major incidents become complex emergencies?

- If the context involves administrative, political, or economic anarchy.
- If the incident sparks a self-perpetuating chain of violence.
- If the incident is not a random event, but focused on one ethnic group.
- If competition for wholly inadequate resources compounds their inadequacy.
- If the incident leads to displacement of children.
- If the incident promotes a state of war.

At the scene of a major incident

The following structure has been developed in the UK for the command and control of a major incident:

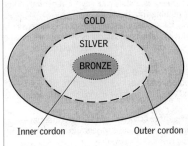

Inner cordon   Outer cordon

The actual incident site is surrounded by the inner cordon in the BRONZE area. The outer cordon surrounds the SILVER area, within which is the entire incident site, including the various incident stations and the SILVER commands. The GOLD area is the regional area within which the incident has occurred.

Each area has a command for each branch of the services: police, fire, ambulance & medical. Concentrating on the medical service, the BRONZE command (*forward medical officer*) will be responsible for supervising doctors in the BRONZE area (eg immediate treatment and primary triage) as well as directing medical equipment in and out and (most importantly) communicating with the *medical commander*. The *medical commander* is also the medical SILVER command. His role is to communicate with the other SILVER command officers (police, fire & ambulance), delegating tasks to available staff, overseeing secondary triage, and continuing an overall medical assessment of the scene. GOLD command is sited away from the main site eg at a regional headquarters. Their responsibility is to liaise with neighbouring area services and independent agencies (eg Environment Agency) for support as needed. This is a simplification of the overall more complex picture; see the *Oxford Handbook of Pre-hospital Care* for an in-depth description.

Command tabards

Recognize the command officers from their tabards:

- Police
- Fire
- Ambulance
- ~ Medical (text only 'medical commander')

IMAGE ADAPTED FROM OXFORD HANDBOOK OF PRE-HOSPITAL CARE, GREAVES ET AL OUP, WITH PERMISSION.

Joining forces

In a major incident the police, fire service, ambulance service, emergency medical service and the armed forces may all be present. Structures for management have been greatly enhanced over recent years, with clear communication across these services vital for effective planning and execution. We learn more from each major incident as it passes, but importantly co-operation between these services during theoretical and practice sessions away from the real emergencies has brought together the experiences from each individual force with great effect.

Pre-hospital immediate care

▶It is often better to spend 30min transporting serious injuries to a well-resourced trauma centre with consultants standing by, than to spend 10min transporting such a person to a small hospital where the most skilled help is not *immediately* available (see MINIBOX). If the small hospital has to transfer the casualty to a trauma centre, no significant savings may be made compared with immediate

Indications for air ambulance transfer
• Difficult scene access
• Weather conditions adverse to ground but not air travel
• Difficult road terrain
• >15 miles from nearest land base

helicopter transfer to the centre.[48] Identifying appropriateness for transport is also important to reduce helicopter overuse, as there is a still tendency for most helicopter transfers to be made in cases of non-life-threatening injury.[49]

The importance of helicopters for casualty rescue/transport is increasingly recognized—but be aware of the limitations and dangers. Helicopters may be used for transporting casualties to hospital, or for interhospital transfer.

Advantages:
• Speed over long distances; access to remote areas
• Delivery of highly trained doctors and special equipment to the scene—eg ready to intubate, paralyse and ventilate, and give mannitol IVI if head injury.[50]

Disadvantages:
• Mid-air crashes in air ambulances have occurred, and are hard to survive.
• Noise and general stress, leading to anxiety and disorientation, and hampering communication—reassure and provide with a headset.
• Vibration exacerbating bleeding and pain from fracture sites.
• Cold—beware in those hypothermic rescues from sea or mountain.
• Problems related to altitude; aircraft limitations, eg weather, landing site, limited carriage space (especially if additional medical personnel).
• Police craft don't allow ECG monitor/oximeter due to magnetic radiation.
• Many published reports of the advantages of air ambulances lack rigour.

The gains of helicopter transfer depend on how many severe injuries occur. One UK study concluded that only ~13 lives would be saved per year in London if it was reserved for the severest cases (injury severity score, ISS, >15, p810); in lesser trauma, there is evidence that outcome is *less* good.[51]

Helicopter safety
• Always approach from the front of the aircraft, in full view of the pilot.
• Secure loose items, eg headgear.
• Do not enter/leave the rotor disc area without permission (thumbs up signal from pilot). Lower your head in the rotor disc area.
• Do not touch the winch strop/cable until the earthing lead has contacted the ground. Also, be sure to avoid the tail rotor.
• Make sure no one is smoking within 50m of the aircraft.

Specific problems
• Decompression sickness (p813): if air is breathed under pressure (divers), nitrogen dissolves in blood and tissues. On rapid ascent after a dive the nitrogen will come out of solution as bubbles, producing joint pains ('the bends') ± rashes, CNS defects and paraesthesia. ▶Do not fly within 12h of a single dive <30m, or within 24h following multiple dives, dives to >30m or any dive requiring a decompression stop.
• Ischaemic chest pain or infarction is not a contraindication to flying.
• Psychiatric illness (eg mania) may preclude safe air transport.
• Burns >20% need preflight nasogastric tube insertion (prevents gas expansion of an ileus) ± in-flight pressure-controlled ventilation.[52]

First steps to improving care after major injury

The National Audit Office finds that 450–600 lives would be saved/yr in England if these points were acted on: tinyurl.com/ybt7w9g

1 Don't simply take the casualty to the nearest hospital. Assess complexity of the injuries and take to a hospital with the necessary skills. Helicopter transport may be the most efficient way to do this.

2 A trauma team with fully-trained neurosurgical and orthopaedic staff (with immediate CT available) should meet the patient at the door. In the NHS, 60% of the time the casualty waits to see the most junior doctor and if the nature of the injuries is recognized, he is passed in stages up the line, perhaps only reaching the definitive specialist when it is too late.

3 More regional trauma networks must be set up. Remember that trauma is the chief cause of death in those <40yrs, and numbers are growing (now about 20,000 major trauma cases/yr in England).

All this happens in other countries such as the USA: ►survival is 20% better.

Problems of altitude   (see high-altitude medicine, p814)

• Hypoxia is unlikely unless there is cardiac or lung disease, anaemia, shock, or chest trauma, as helicopters rarely fly high enough to cause P_aO_2 to fall.

• Reduction in atmospheric pressure results in an expansion of enclosed gases on ascent. This produces pain in blocked sinuses, expansion of a pneumothorax, abdominal wound dehiscence (avoid flying for 10 days post-surgery if possible), and renewed bleeding from a peptic ulcer.

• Drips may also slow down.

• On descent, beware of endotracheal tube cuffs and military antishock trousers (MAST*) deflating significantly (particularly if applied at altitude eg on hillside). Rapid descent may induce barotrauma.

*MAST (=medical anti-shock trousers)

Invented during the Vietnam War, MAST were intended to reduce blood flow to the lower limbs, thereby increasing perfusion to vital thoracic organs and the brain. Their use has decreased since the 80s and 90s due to concerns about their benefit. MAST inflation may impair breathing & ventricular function.[53] They can do damage in those with moderate hypotension (systolic BP 50–90mmHg) who face only a short ride to a hospital, especially those with thoracic injuries. MAST's role in severe shock or long pre-hospital transport times remains unclear. However, a Cochrane review suggested that there was no evidence that they reduced mortality, hospital or ICU stay, and some evidence they worsened outcomes.[54]

Essence Trauma scoring can be used at the roadside to predict the probability of survival (*Ps*),◆ and thus the severity of injury, which may influence where to take the patient (nearby district general hospital, regional hospital, or Trauma Centre?); however experts generally consider it purely an audit and research tool. Retrospectively, physiological data may be combined with an anatomical injury score to compare performance (expected *vs* actual survivors) between hospitals. NB: trauma scoring in children is problematic. See expert literature.[56]

Trauma Score (TS) The original score introduced in 1981 in USA to allow paramedics to make an objective decision on whether patient needed Trauma Centre facilities. Measures respiratory rate + effort; systolic BP; capillary refill; Glasgow Coma Scale (GCS). Maximum score 16. Score ≤13 means mortality ≥10%—USA take to Level 1 Trauma Centre; UK take to large hospital and alert trauma team en route.

Revised Trauma Score (RTS) Measures respiratory rate (RR), systolic BP (sBP), and GCS only: other parameters were found to be poorly reproducible on analysis of a large North American database. Each parameter has values coded to give score of 0-4 (see table, OPPOSITE). These scores are multiplied by a weighting coefficient, then added together to produce the RTS—it is not a suitable roadside tool. RTS has a more reliable correlation with *Ps* than does TS.

Triage Revised Trauma Score (TRTS) This uses the same coded values of respiratory rate, systolic BP, and GCS from the RTS, but a fall by one point in any parameter is taken as significant (thus TRTS ≤11 is significant). This is the most useful pre-hospital trauma triage tool.

Limitations: These scoring systems are not validated for the very young or elderly; up to 20% may have severity underestimated on their initial assessment (if attended rapidly, before physiological decompensation).

Injury Severity Score (ISS) TS, RTS, and TRTS use *physiological* variables to predict *Ps*; these have the advantage of changing with the patient's condition. *Anatomical injury* (data from operation or *post mortem* notes, which does not generally change throughout an episode) can also be used—injuries are scored from 1 (minor) to 6 (fatal) using tables from the Abbreviated Injury Scale (AIS). The body is divided into 6 regions and the 3 highest scores from different regions are squared and added. Maximum score is 75 (5 squared × 3) since AIS 6 in any body region is fatal—and therefore awarded a score of 75. ISS correlates closely with *Ps*. ISS ≥16 implies mortality ≥10% and is termed 'major trauma'.

Limitations: Injuries can be difficult to code; isolated head injury with AIS of 3 has high mortality, but is excluded from 'major trauma' outcome analysis.

TRISS methodology Trauma audit programmes are established in USA and UK—*Major Trauma Outcome Study* (MTOS).[57] TRISS is a complex formula combining RTS, ISS, age, and whether blunt or penetrating trauma. It is poor at predicting individual outcome, but allows comparison of overall performance between hospitals, or the same hospital following, say, introduction of trauma teams. ASCOT (*a severity characterization of trauma*) is newer but not necessarily better.[58] Similarly, TRISS has been combined with physiological categorizations (SAPS-II)[1] to improve reliability.

Z & M statistics compare outcome in different populations. *Z* measures the difference between the actual and predicted number of deaths. *M* (the 'injury severity match') compares the range of injury severity with the main database—if *M* <0.88, *Z* is invalid.[59]

---

1 SAPS = Simplified Acute Physiology Score.[60]

Revised Trauma Score (RTS)[61]

For each of GCS, SBP (systolic BP) and RR determine the attributed value:

GCS	SBP (mmHg)	RR (bpm)	Value
13–15	>89	10–29	4
9–12	76–89	>29	3
6–8	50–75	6–9	2
4–5	1–49	1–5	1
3	0	0	0

Then put into the equation:
(0.9368 × GCS value) + (0.7326 × systolic BP value) + (0.2908 × RR value) = RTS

Blast injury may be encountered in domestic (eg gas explosion) or industrial (eg mining) accidents, or as the result of a terrorist bomb. Terrorism worldwide is responsible for at least 15,000 injured or killed in the last 20 years and most casualties are from bombs. Death may occur without any obvious external injury, often due to air emboli, the correct cause first being recognized by Pierre Jars in 1758 as a *'dilatation d'air'* (ie blast wave). Blast injury is split into 4 phases:
• *Primary:* injury from the blast wave itself.
• *Secondary:* injury from missiles & projectile debris striking the victim.
• *Tertiary:* the victim is thrown by the blast wind, striking surrounding objects.
• *Quaternary:* other injuries caused by explosions—eg burns, asphyxia, crush injuries and toxic inhalations.

Explosions cause injury in seven ways:

1 **Blast wave** A transient (milliseconds) wave of overpressure expands rapidly away from the point of explosion, its intensity inversely proportional to the distance cubed. It produces: (a) cellular disruption at air-tissue interface ('spalling'), ie perforated ear-drum at 100kPa (deafness should prompt thoughts of significant blast injury), 'blast lung' at 175kPa; (b) shearing forces along tissue planes: submucosal/subserosal haemorrhage; (c) re-expansion of compressed trapped gas: bowel perforation, fatal air embolism (coronary artery or cerebral).

2 **Blast lung** may be delayed (up to 48h). Suspect it if there is a perforated drum, but this is *not* a prerequisite (as position of drum in relation to blast wave is critical). Intra-alveolar haemorrhage causes acute respiratory distress syndrome (*OHCM* p178). Most patients who survive lung blast injury regain good lung function within a year.[62][n=11]

3 **Blast wind** Air displaced by the explosion will totally disrupt a body in the immediate vicinity. Others may suffer avulsive amputations. Bodies can be carried by the wind with deceleration injuries on landing (tertiary injury, as above). Glass, wood, stones, and other objects are also carried and act as secondary missiles.[63]

4 **Missiles** Penetration or laceration from missiles are by far the commonest injuries. Missiles can arise from the bomb fragmentation: *primary* if from the casing or *secondary* if from preformed fragments (eg nails, nuts, bolts, ball-bearings) or from the environmental fabric (eg glass and wood particularly).

5 **Flash burns** These are usually superficial and occur on exposed skin (hands/face) in those close to explosion. Flame burns arise through ignition of materials in the environment.

6 **Crush injuries** Can be the result of eg falling masonry or tertiary injury.

7 **Psychological** Acute fear and panic is the aim of the terrorist. Later, chronic intrusive thoughts, anxiety, and poor concentration may form the basis of a post-traumatic stress disorder (p347). This may be augmented by repeated watchings of the event on TV/Video.[64]

Treatment

▶*Do not approach the scene until the possibility of a secondary device has been excluded and it has been declared safe to approach.*

▶*Also remember that you are at a forensic scene, so do not disturb the environs (or any dead bodies) unless necessary to treat a patient.*

Approach the same as any major trauma with priority to airway and cervical spine, breathing, and circulation with haemorrhage control. Rest and observe any suspected of exposure to significant blast, but without other injury. Sudden death or renal failure may follow release of a limb after prolonged crush injury (hyperkalaemia and myoglobinuria): ensure continuous ECG and good hydration. Facial burns may compromise airway, which should be secured by intubation or surgical airway. Psychological support will be needed.

Diving accidents

Thousands go diving every year for recreation. Because of speedy world travel, complications of diving may present to doctors miles from diving centres: for this reason we all need to be familiar with the contraindications and complications of diving, *whatever* our specialty. Do not underestimate the stress of diving: a depth change of 7 metres produces changes in ambient pressure equal to a trip from sea level to the top of Everest.[1]

Contraindications to diving
- Migraine + vomiting attacks
- Otitis (media or externa)
- Hypoglycaemia risk (eg DM)
- Patent foramen ovale[1]

- Lung diseases
- Epilepsy
- Ménière's disease
- Pregnancy

- Pneumothorax history
- Angina; arrhythmias
- Perforated ear drum
- Bleeding disorders.

Complications of diving
- Drowning (p786)
- Marine bites or stings (p782)
- Surface accidents (boating)

- Barotrauma
- Air embolism
- Hypothermia

- Decompression illness
- Pulmonary oedema
- Nitrogen narcosis.

Acute decompression illness Nitrogen is more soluble in lipid than in water, so as N₂ tension increases, it accumulates in CNS, marrow, and fat. On ascent, N₂ bubbles form in these tissues and in venous blood (arterial blood is pressure-equilibrated having just passed through the lungs). Symptoms appear from 1 to 36h after surfacing. *Risk factors:* Multiple dives, ignoring proper decompression stops, rapid ascent, obesity, increasing age, previous decompression sickness, alcohol ingestion, subsequent ascent to high altitude (p808).

Presentation:
- Vomiting
- Throbbing muscle/joint pains
- Migrating skin mottling/rashes
- Pruritus; paraesthesiae

- Mood changes
- Cough; chest pain
- Cyanosis; shock
- Osteonecrosis

- Deafness/nystagmus
- Fits; CNS signs
- Cognitive changes
- Headache.

Management: Speed of response is vital. If recompression starts ≤30min after the onset of symptoms, 80% will respond; if 6h delay, only 50% respond. If air embolism is suspected, place on the left side and give 100% O₂ (15L/min through tight-fitting facemask with reservoir). Seek expert help. Transfer to a hyperbaric facility.[2] If airlift needed, maximally pressurize the cabin, if the route does not allow flying at sea-level. Transport the breathing apparatus and his diving partner (will give the history, but may himself also be at risk). If there is hypothermia, expect BP to drop after leaving the water, and be sure to transport in the horizontal position, and keep cardiovascular instability to a minimum.

Preventing diving accidents
- Augment swimming fitness.
- Avoid dehydration (no alcohol or caffeine for >24h before the dive).
- Do the deepest part of the dive first. Time your ascent.
- Plan 'no-stop' dive profiles (ie avoid decompression stops).
- Make a safety stop at 5m. Avoid remaining under water for longer than is recommended by decompression tables or dive computers.
- Rest before the dive, and keep warm during the dive.
- After the dive avoid sitting still for long periods (decreases regional blood flow and nitrogen removal). Avoid boarding aircraft for about 24h.
- No diving if pregnant: there is (uncertain) risk to the fetus as right-to-left shunting diverts blood from the lungs—which are the best filters of micro-bubbles. (The role of the placenta in this task is unknown.)[65]

---

1 A careful MRI study in 160 asymptomatic scuba divers found many CNS lesions (?akin to multi-infarct dementia) associated with a patent foramen ovale (or other shunt, eg in the lung) allowing paradoxical embolism of venous nitrogen bubbles (venous bubbles occur after ascent from as little as 3m (these bubbles are normally filtered by the lungs).[66]
2 Telephone numbers: UK: Hyperbaric Medicine Unit, Aberdeen Royal Infirmary 0845 4086008; Royal Navy: 07831 151523; Diving Diseases Research Centre: 01752 209999; USA: Diver's Alert Network (919 684 8111) or US Navy (904 234 4351) or Air Force (512 538 3281 or 512 536 3278)

WHO estimates that 140 million people live at altitudes >2500m and 40 million lowland dwellers travel to high altitude each year to ski, trek (fig 1) or work.[67] High-altitude illness refers to conditions afflicting individuals ascending to altitudes faster than their bodies can acclimatize. It chiefly[1] comprises: 1 Acute mountain sickness (AMS) 2 High-altitude cerebral oedema (HACE) and 3 High-altitude pulmonary oedema (HAPE). The latter 2 may be rapidly fatal if untreated.

Acclimatizing to high altitudes During ascent, partial pressure of O_2 in blood falls as barometric pressure drops. Carotid body and medullary chemo-receptors respond to this hypobaric hypoxia by ↑ rate and depth of ventilation. The kidneys respond to the ensuing respiratory alkalosis over a period of days by excreting bicarbonate and reabsorbing hydrogen ions. A true ↑ in the red cell count (RCC) resulting from renal erythropoietin secretion takes weeks to develop. Acclimatization does not return the body to its sea level state.[68]

There is considerable individual variation in the rate and extent of altitude acclimatization. Above 3000m, each night's sleeping altitude should be no higher than 300m above the previous night, with a rest day every 2–3 days or 1000m ascended. High-altitude mental and physical deterioration occurs during prolonged stays at extreme altitude (>5500m).

Acute mountain sickness (AMS) Mild AMS is common at altitudes of >2500m. It may result from ↑ cerebral blood flow and mild cerebral oedema with an input from oxidative stress mediated by oxygen free radicals. Mild AMS is managed conservatively with rest, hydration, analgesia and antiemetics. For management of severe AMS (inability to walk, care for oneself, disturbed consciousness) see OPPOSITE.

Risk factors for AMS:
• Rate of ascent
• Absolute altitude
• Blunted ventilatory response to hypoxia (unreliable sign)[69]
• Level of exertion (NB: physical fitness does not protect)
• Permanent home at <900m
• Previous AMS
• Concurrent URTI
• Neck irradiation or surgery

High-altitude cerebral oedema (HACE) HACE is a potentially rapidly fatal encephalopathy with a change in mental status ± ataxia which is usually preceded by AMS. It may co-exist with HAPE. The exact incidence varies between studies but may be as much as 0.5–1%. It arises from vasogenic cerebral oedema caused by disruption of the blood–brain barrier ± cytotoxic oedema. HACE requires a greater degree of descent than HAPE and recovery takes longer.

High-altitude pulmonary oedema (HAPE) HAPE is more common than HACE and may accompany AMS, typically 2–4 days after ascent to altitudes of >3000m.
Symptoms: Cough, dyspnoea at rest, haemoptysis, extreme lethargy.
Signs: Tachycardia, tachypnoea, cyanosis ± crackles (often right middle lobe; listen in the axilla). HAPE arises from patchy pulmonary vasoconstriction leading to stress failure of pulmonary capillaries and pulmonary oedema. People with a strong hypoxic pulmonary vasoconstrictor response, concurrent respiratory infection or congenital absence of a pulmonary artery are most susceptible.

Using acetazolamide Acetazolamide is a carbonic anhydrase inhibitor that causes ↑bicarbonate excretion by the kidneys, thus accelerating acclimatization.
• It does *NOT* hide symptoms of AMS.
• It may be used as prophylaxis at a dose of 250mg/12h PO (until one day after the maximum altitude is reached) in those with past severe AMS, or those making a forced rapid ascent.
• It can also aid sleep by ↓periodic breathing (dose: 125mg PO 1h before bed).
• Contraindication: sulfa allergy. Give a test dose prior to travel.
• Side effects: paraesthesiae, carbonated beverages taste flat.

---

1 Other high-altitude illnesses: retinal haemorrhage (common; rarely problematic); chronic mountain sickness (polycythaemia, headache, somnolence, depression); subacute mountain sickness. NB: harmless swelling of extremities, more common in females, does not predict AMS.

Golden rules at high altitude

- 'Climb high, sleep low' to promote acclimatization.
- Avoid undue exertion at high altitude.
- Avoid alcohol, sedating antihistamines or sedative-hypnotics.
- Feeling unwell at altitude=altitude illness until proved otherwise.
- Never ascend with AMS symptoms
- Never leave someone with AMS alone.
- If you are worsening, or developing HACE or HAPE...▶descend immediately.

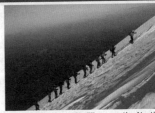

Fig 1. Trekking on Mt. Elbrus on the North Iranian Plateau, where it unites Russia and Europe. At 5642m (18,442 ft) it is the highest peak in both land masses. Of the 7 continental summits it is closest in height to Kilimanjaro (5895m).

Lake Louise consensus criteria for the diagnosis of AMS

AMS is defined as the presence of headache plus at least one of the following symptoms occurring several hours after reaching a higher altitude:
- Gastrointestinal upset
- Fatigue or weakness
- Dizziness or light-headedness
- Difficulty sleeping.

▶▶Emergency management of severe high-altitude illness

Severe AMS (acute mountain sickness)			
DESCENT	Acetazolamide 250mg/8h po	Dexamethasone 4mg/6h PO	Trekkers should *NOT* ascend on dexamethasone

HACE (high-altitude cerebral oedema)			
DESCENT	Acetazolamide 250mg/8h PO	Dexamethasone 8mg IM then 4mg/6h PO	Portable hyperbaric chamber (fig 2) Consider O₂ 4L/min

HAPE (high-altitude pulmonary oedema)			Role unclear
DESCENT	Portable hyperbaric chamber Consider O₂ at 4L/min	Nifedipine SR 20mg/12h PO	Acetazolamide 250mg/8h PO / Dexamethasone 8mg IM then 4mg/6h PO / Inhaled salmeterol / Sildenafil by mouth

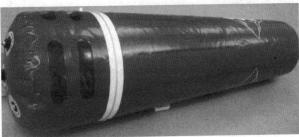

Fig 2. Portable hyperbaric chamber.⁶⁶

We thank Dr Gerard Flaherty for supplying both images and compiling this page for us.

Cracks in the teacup, and chinks of darkness

With our plummy accents and polite manners we have now served you 815 cups of tea in the fine porcelain provided by OUP's typography. And would you like another cup? And do you take sugar? And can we tempt you with a morsel from our plateful of platitudes? Everything here seems clean, sweetly ordered, and well-mannered. But life at the bedside is rarely like this, and we now report that there is a crack in our teacup which OUP cannot mend. Somehow, we knew all the time it was there—and it is through our narrow right-hand vertical columns that we can see chinks of darkness cast their shadow on the aOHCSbsurdly sunny glades in our fool's paradise where no real patient ever trod or bled.

So what is this vertical text, where are these right hand columns, and what do they mean—p99, for example. Here the voice in the narrow right-hand column can subvert, be politically incorrect, swear, and hint at other worlds. It is where a less-polished world intrudes with its scepticism, its cynicism, and its habit of subverting our best-laid plans. Do not fall into the trap of asking which world is true? Right or left? Yin or yang? Nor be fooled by the neat answer that each column represent two ends of a spectrum, and the truth lies somewhere in between. The truth *is* the spectrum, and we cannot see it all.

The helix, the spiral, and a penultimate point

Spirals and helices, beautiful (p534) and deadly (p99), are weaving their way through this book—to what central point? Unlike the circle, the spiral never returns us to our starting place, and recognizes that the person who set out reading this book is not the same as the person who, now exhausted and probably filled-to-bursting, has reached this penultimate point. So reflect on your spiritual journey, and guess its direction—in towards the centre, concentrating on ever finer, but vital detail—or away from the centre, towards infinity?

The last word

It is a pleasure to end this work with a chapter which is really a new beginning: the patient on his way to hospital. So far we have concentrated on what we can bring to the patient. Now let us turn to what the patient brings to us. All too often, time and circumstance lead us to the view that patients are tireless devourers of our energies, and that for all practical purposes, we must go on giving until we die, or give up the unequal struggle with Nature and her diseases. This is to negate the view of patients as food: not just in the sense of giving us our daily bread and butter, but also in the sense of nourishing our personalities. They do this by telling us about ourselves. You may think that you are kind and wise, or clumsy and inadequate, and it takes our patients to disabuse us of these illusions, and to show us that some days we are good, and some days we are bad. Thanks to our patients, we never stay the same. After practising medicine for a few decades, our minds become populated by the ghosts of former patients, beckoning us, warning us, reminding us of the things we cannot control—and the ideals to which we aspire.

We are lucky to work in a profession in which experience counts for more than knowledge, and it is to augment this thirst for experience that we urge our readers to turn away from learning by rote: let us read novels, cultivate our friends, travel far—and try to keep forever curious, for then, if we are lucky, we stand to gain that priceless therapeutic asset: a rich and compassionate personality, and we will be all the more inclined to reformulate this tiresome and inconvenient patient who now confronts us into a lovable series of imperfections, which match and reflect, and reveal our own foibles.

Index

Abbreviations: i refers to an image; t refers to a table; syn.=syndrome; dis.=disease.

U

We thank Bernard Ho, Ayoma Ratnappuli, Mark Cassar, Shahzad Arain, Manish Verma, Mathuranayagham Niroshan, and James Sewell for their help with the index.

Ishihara colour deficiency test
selected plates

Reproduced with permission from the Isshinkai Foundation.
NB: These plates should *not* be used for diagnostic purposes.

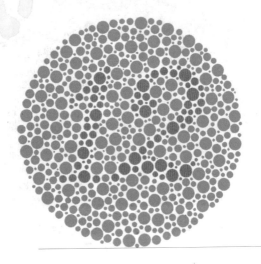

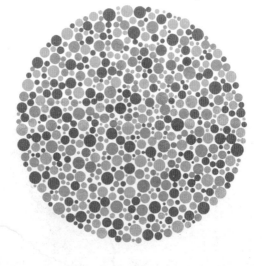

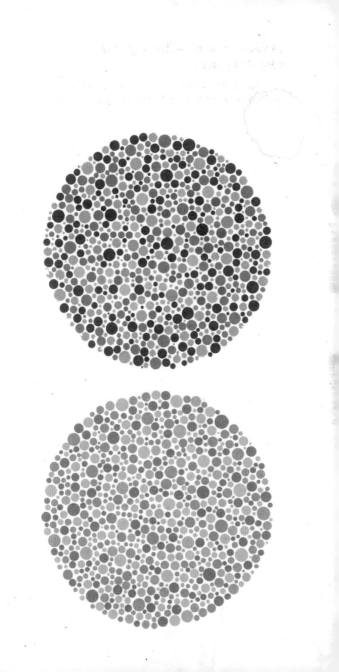

Reference intervals—biochemistry

See p220 for children and p15 for obstetric reference intervals

►All laboratory discourse is probabilistic. ►Drugs may interfere with any chemical method; as these effects may be method-dependent, it is difficult for us to be aware of all possibilities. If in doubt, discuss with the lab.

Substance	Specimen	Normal value	Your hospital
Adrenocorticotrophic hormone	P	<80ng/L	
Alanine aminotransferase (ALT)	P	5–35IU/L	
Albumin	P¶	35–50g/L	
Aldosterone	P**	100–500pmoL/L	
Alkaline phosphatase	P¶	30–300IU/L (adults)	
α-fetoprotein	S	<10ku/L	
α-amylase	P	0–180 Somogyi u/dL	
Angiotensin II	P**	5–35pmol/L	
Antidiuretic hormone (ADH)	P	0.9–4.6pmol/L	
Aspartate transaminase	P	5–35IU/L	
Bicarbonate	P¶	24–30mmol/L	
Bilirubin	P	3–17μmol/L (0.25–1.5mg/100/mL)	
Calcitonin	P	<0.1μg/L	
Calcium (ionized)	P	1.0–1.25mmol/L	
Calcium (total)	P¶	2.12–2.65mmol/L	
Chloride	P	95–105mmol/L	
*Cholesterol (see p654)	P	3.9–7.8mmol/L	
VLDL (see p654)	P	0.128–0.645mmol/L	
LDL	P	1.55–4.4mmol/L	
HDL	P	0.9–1.93mmol/L	
Cortisol	P	a.m. 450–700nmol/L midnight 80–280nmol/L	
Creatine kinase (CK)	P	♂ 25–195IU/L; ♀ 25–170	
Creatinine (*related to lean body mass*)	P¶	70–≤150μmol/L	
Ferritin	P	12–200μg/L	
Folate	S	2.1μg/L	
Follicle-stimulating hormone (FSH)	P/S	2–8u/L (luteal): ovulatory peak 8–15 follicular phase, & ♂: 0.5–5 postmenopausal: >30	
Gamma-glutamyl transpeptidase	P	♂ 11–51; ♀ 7–33IU/L	
Glucose (fasting)	P	3.5–5.5mmol/L	
Glycated (glycosylated) haemoglobin	B	5–8%	
Growth hormone	P	<20mu/L	
Iron	S	♂ 14–31μmol/L; ♀ 11–30	
Lactate dehydrogenase (LDH)	P	70–250IU/L	
Lead	B	<1.8mmol/L	
Luteinizing hormone (LH)	P/S	premenopausal: 3–13u/L follicular: 3–12 ovulatory peak: 20–80 luteal: 3–16 postmenopausal: >30	
Magnesium	P	0.75–1.05mmol/L	
Osmolality	P	278–305mosmol/kg	
Parathyroid hormone (PTH)	P	<0.8–8.5pmol/L	
Phosphate (inorganic)	P	0.8–1.45mmol/L	
Potassium	P	3.5–5.0mmol/L	
Prolactin	P	♂ <450u/L; ♀ <600u/L	
Prostate specific antigen	P	0–4 nanograms/mL	
Protein (total)	P	60–80g/L	
Red cell folate	B	0.36–1.44μmol/L (160–640μg/L)	
Renin (erect/recumbent)	P**	2.8–4.5/1.1–2.7pmol/mL/h	